CONGRATULATIONS

You now have access to Mosby's "Get Smart" Bonus Package!

Here's what's included to help you "Get Smart"

sign on at:

http://www.mosby.com/MERLIN/Wilson/assessment/

A website just for you as you learn health assessment with the new 2nd edition of **Health Assessment for Nursing Practice**

what you will receive:

Whether you're a student, an instructor, or a clinician, you'll find information just for you. Things like:

- Teaching Tips
- Study Questions
- Author Information... and more
- Frequently Asked Questions
- Links to Related Products

plus:

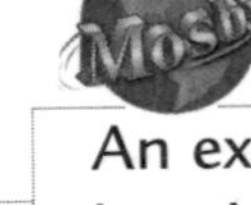

WebLinks

An exciting new program that allows you to directly access hundreds of active websites keyed specifically to the content of this book. The WebLinks are continually updated, with new ones added as they develop. **Peel the top layer only from the sticker on this page and register with the listed passcode.**

n
to
nc.

If passcode sticker is removed, this textbook cannot be returned to Mosby, Inc.

Free CD-ROM

with every copy of **Health Assessment for Nursing Practice,** 2nd Edition

This Valuable Electronic Workbook on CD-ROM Features:

A variety of interactive student activities including multiple-choice questions, matching, crossword puzzles, a hangman game, risk factor exercises, anatomy activities, symptom analysis, and a "Day in the Clinic" exercise.

Health Assessment Laboratory Guides that can be printed off and used in lab settings.

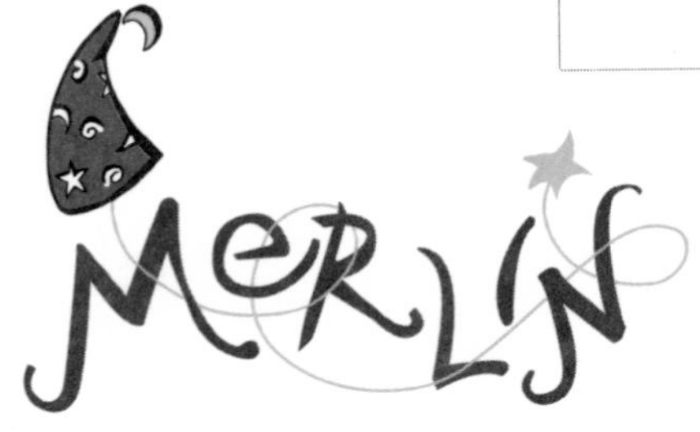

Mosby's Electronic Resource Links & Information Network

Mosby
A Harcourt Health Sciences Company

HEALTH ASSESSMENT for NURSING PRACTICE

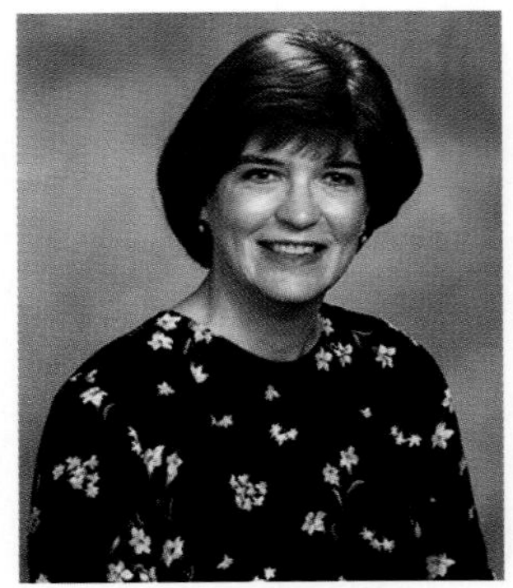

Susan Wilson, a family nurse practitioner, has 28 years of teaching experience, including 20 years teaching health assessment. She has cared for adult clients in a variety of settings from critical care to rehabilitation. Dr. Wilson has taught undergraduate and graduate students in the care of clients in hospital and clinic settings. This text is a synthesis of all that she has learned about health assessment and about teaching health assessment, as well as how to handle the difficulties that she knows students experience in learning health assessment.

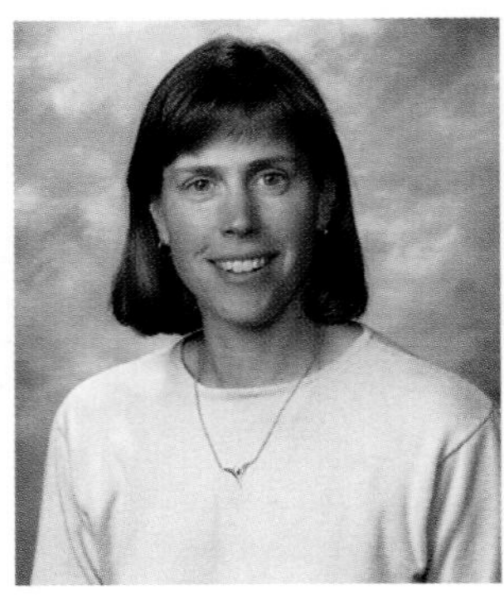

Jean Giddens has been involved in nursing education since 1984. She has taught in several nursing programs including University of New Mexico, University of Texas at El Paso, and most recently at Mesa State College in Colorado. Her content areas in nursing education include health assessment, nursing process, nursing fundamentals, medical-surgical nursing, and nursing pharmacology. Ms. Giddens earned a Bachelor of Science in Nursing at the University of Kansas, and a Master of Science in Nursing at the University of Texas at El Paso. Currently, she is pursuing a Ph.D. in Educational Leadership at Colorado State University. Ms. Giddens is a Certified Clinical Specialist in medical-surgical nursing. In addition to teaching, she works part-time as an emergency department nurse.

HEALTH ASSESSMENT for NURSING PRACTICE

Susan F. **Wilson**
RN, PhD, CS, FNP

Associate Professor
Texas Christian University
College of Health and Human Sciences
Harris School of Nursing
Fort Worth, Texas

Jean Foret **Giddens**
MSN, RN, CS

Assistant Professor
Mesa State College
Department of Nursing and Radiologic Sciences
Grand Junction, Colorado

with 936 illustrations

second edition

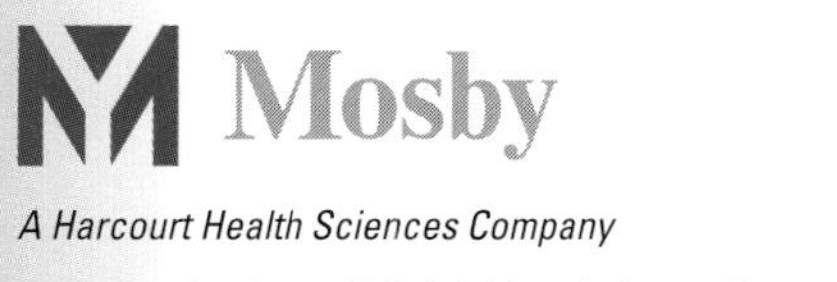

A Harcourt Health Sciences Company

St. Louis London Philadelphia Sydney Toronto

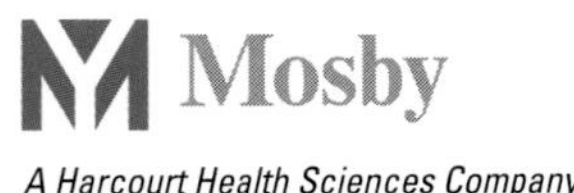

Vice-President, Nursing Editorial Director: Sally Schrefer
Executive Editors: June Thompson, Robin Carter
Developmental Editors: Billi Carcheri Sharp, Kristin Geen
Project Manager: John Rogers
Project Specialist: Kathleen L. Teal
Designer: Amy Buxton

Printed in the United States of America

Mosby, Inc.
A Harcourt Health Sciences Company
11830 Westline Industrial Drive
St. Louis, Missouri 63146

ISBN 0-323-00876-3

00 01 02 03 04 CL/KPT 9 8 7 6 5 4 3 2 1

To my mother, Sara Borden, and my daughter, Megan, for their continued love, patience, and support;
to June Thompson for giving me the opportunity to publish;
to Dr. Ken Katzen for giving me the opportunity to practice in the real world;
and to the faculty, colleagues, and students who have taught me through the years.

SFW

To Jay, Chris, and John for their unconditional support and minimal
complaints of the time I spent on this project;
and to my students past, present, and future.

JFG

REVIEWERS

Joanne Bartram, RN, MS
Instructor, College of Nursing
University of New Mexico
Albuquerque, New Mexico

Elaine J. Beaupre, RN, MEd, MSN
Nursing Instructor
Quincy College
Quincy, Massachusetts

Betty G. Davis, RN, MS
Associate Professor
Mary Black School of Nursing
University of South Carolina–Spartanburg
Spartanburg, South Carolina

Susan Falck, BSN, PA-C
Altru Health Institute
Grand Forks, North Dakota

Michelle Grodner, EdD, CHES
Professor and Chairperson
Department of Community Health
William Paterson University
Wayne, New Jersey

Carl A. Kirton, RN, MA, ACRN, ANP-CS
Clinical Assistant Professor of Nursing
Adult Nurse Practitioner
New York University
New York, New York

Lori Klabunde, FNP, PA-C
The Bone and Joint Center
Bismark, North Dakota

Mary Ann Lambert, MSN, RN
Assistant Professor
Orvis School of Nursing
University of Nevada–Reno
Reno, Nevada

Roberta Prazak, BSN, RN
Registered Nurse I
Memorial Hermann Health Care System
Houston, Texas

Sylvia M. Root, EdD, CFNP
Associate Professor
College of Nursing
Arizona State University
Phoenix, Arizona

■ SPECIAL CONSULTANT

Sue K. Goebel, RNC, MS, WHNP
Assistant Professor of Nursing
Mesa State College
Grand Junction, Colorado

PREFACE

If a teacher is indeed wise, he does not bid you enter the house of his wisdom, but rather leads you to the threshold of your own mind.

Kahlil Gibran
The Prophet

Following this teaching we have revised this text of *Health Assessment for Nursing Practice* to retain the strong features and add others. The underlying principles of the first edition are steadfast. Like the first edition, the *second edition* is based on the assumption that every client from neonate to older person is an interactive complex being who is more than a collection of his or her parts. Each client's health status depends on the interactions of physiologic, psychologic, sociocultural, and spiritual factors. These interactions occur within their physical environments (what they eat, drink, and breathe); what kind of activity and work they participate in and where they live; their social environments and health beliefs (friends, family, and support systems and when and how they seek health care); and their internal environments (what they eat and drink, how they sleep, and how often they exercise).

As faculty, we are challenged with several responsibilities. First, we are challenged to demonstrate caring and compassion when we interact with clients to act as role models for students. Second, we are challenged to help students become knowledgeable and skilled in history taking and physical assessment. Third, we are challenged to model for students as well as teach them how to be objective and nonjudgmental. Finally, we are challenged to assist students to mobilize their resources to apply health assessment knowledge and skills to clients of all ages and from a multitude of cultures and ethnic groups. We know that this content will be needed for the remainder of their professional lives. This textbook is a toolbox of information and techniques. As a wise teacher you lead students to the threshold.

■ ORGANIZATION

Chapters 1 to 10 provide a solid foundation for students, covering such issues as *Developmental Assessment Through the Life Span, Ethnic and Cultural Considerations, Interviewing to Obtain a Health History,* and *Equipment and Techniques for Physical Assessment.* Also included are three new chapters on *Mental Health Assessment, Comfort and Pain Assessment,* and *Sleep and Rest Assessment.* Retained from the first edition are descriptions of how to assess clients with special needs, how to lead clients to improve their health and reduce their risks of illness or injury, and how to synthesize data in order to select nursing diagnoses.

Chapters 10 to 25 are organized by body system, and Chapter 26 discusses *Assessment of the Pregnant Client.* These chapters contain health history questions with rationales in a two-column format that is easy to follow. Likewise the examination techniques with expected findings are described next to abnormal findings in a two-column format for each body system.

Each chapter begins with a review of **Anatomy and Physiology.** This content begins the chapter because physical assessment techniques allow the student to answer the question "How does this client's anatomy and physiology compare with that expected for his or her age and ethnic group?" The **Health History** section that follows instructs the student on history data to collect by providing sample questions to ask the clients along with the reasons for asking those questions. The second column of the Health History section describes the variances that the student may find. **Health Promotion** content in the first edition has been moved to follow the Health History section so that data are collected at the time of history taking. From data collected, the student can identify teaching needed to help the client maintain health. Included in the Health History section are new headings for **Present Health Status, Past Medical History,** and **Problem-Based History.**

The **Examination** section begins with a list of equipment and why it is needed. This section sequentially guides the student in the techniques of performing a physical assessment of an adult, telling what to do, how to do it, and what to expect. Photographs are provided to enhance learning. The left column, **Procedures and Techniques With Normal Findings,** details the techniques of the assessment and the normal findings, while the right column describes **Abnormal Findings.** Following the Examination section is a section on **Age-Related Variations** describing how to individualize the examination for clients of different ages. This section covers infants, children, adolescents, and older adults, and includes subheadings for Anatomy and Physiology, Health History, and Examination. The next section is **Clients With Situational Variations,** which may include examinations of clients who are hearing-impaired or paralyzed. Included here, where appropriate, is a special subheading for **Ethnic & Cultural Variations.** Following is a section on **Examination Summary** providing a review of procedures, a new **Summary of Findings** table, and the **Health**

Promotion section. The **Common Problems and Conditions** section at the end of each chapter has been updated with many new photographs added. **Clinical Application and Critical Thinking,** a new section at the end of the chapter, contains **Sample Documentation** of a client assessment of that body system as well as new **Critical Thinking Questions** and **Case Studies.** Answers for these questions are included in the back of the book to facilitate self-study.

Special **Risk Factors** boxes for disorders in each body system, along with the Health Promotion sections, remind students to discuss these behaviors with clients to help them maintain health and reduce risk of disease. Also included throughout body system chapters are special **Ethnic & Cultural Variations** and **Cultural Note** boxes that contain racial and cultural variations the nurse should consider when assessing clients.

Chapter 27 provides guidelines for putting all of the body system assessments together into one comprehensive examination.

A **Glossary** at the end of the book provides definitions to enhance student comprehension of key concepts and terms.

■ NEW TO THE SECOND EDITION

A new author, Jean Giddens, has added her expertise and creativity to the strength of the content from the first edition.

The textbook has been expanded to 27 chapters. Consider each chapter a different type of tool from the toolbox. Collectively they provide all that students will need to perform a comprehensive health assessment.

New Chapters

- Chapter 7: *Mental Health Assessment* describes the data collection about the client's mental and emotional health.
- Chapter 8: *Comfort and Pain Assessment* describes how to collect data about the physiologic, psychologic, and cultural factors that influence a client's response to pain.
- Chapter 9: *Sleep and Rest Assessment* describes how to obtain data about adequacy of client's sleep and rest cycles.
- Chapter 10: *Nutritional Assessment* was updated and reorganized into the same format used in the body system chapters.
- Chapter 26: *Assessment of the Pregnant Client* compiles all the assessment data related to the pregnant client into one chapter.

The remaining chapters were updated and revised based on the feedback from users, both faculty and students.

New Format and Features

- The Health History section in each body system chapter has been reorganized using the subheadings of **Present Health Status, Past Medical History,** and **Problem-Based History.**
- Special **Risk Factors boxes** highlight information specific to various body systems and disorders.
- **Summary of Findings** tables in each body system chapter contrast Normal Findings, Typical Variations, and Findings Associated With Disorders for that system. These include specific findings for adults, infants and children, adolescents, and older adults.
- **Advanced Practice Skills** are distinguished from basic skills and identified with a special icon ❖. This new feature has been added to bridge the gap between undergraduate and advanced practice education. Advanced content is denoted with a symbol to highlight this material for advanced practice students without being obtrusive for undergraduate students.
- **Functional Health Patterns Involved** and **Collaborative Problems** have been added to the Sample Documentation exercises at the end of body system chapters.
- At the end of each chapter is a section on **Clinical Application and Critical Thinking.** Included is the Sample Documentation exercise and two new learning activities: **Critical Thinking Questions** and a **Case Study** followed by questions. Answers to these activities are located in the back of the text to help students evaluate their learning.

■ TEACHING AND LEARNING AIDS

- An **Electronic Workbook on CD-ROM** packaged free with each text offers a variety of student activities designed to provide a mechanism for application of concepts. Activities include multiple-choice questions, matching, crossword puzzles, a hangman game, risk factor exercises, anatomy activities, symptom analysis, and a "Day in the Clinic" activity. Also included are **Health Assessment Laboratory Guides** that can be printed off by the student and brought to class as assigned for use in the laboratory setting. A special **CD icon** in the text indicates where related study questions or exercises can be found on the CD-ROM.
- The comprehensive **Instructor's Resource Manual with Test Bank** includes Chapter Objectives, Lecture Outlines, and Teaching and Evaluation Strategies for use with classroom lectures. Also included are **Laboratory Checklists** organized by body system. The Physical Assessment Performance Checklists can be used to

assess student performance of various skills, and other useful checklists can be used by students to record subjective and objective data during the examination. The **Test Bank** has been thoroughly revised and includes approximately 1,000 test questions. Also available is a **Computerized Test Bank.**

- The new **MERLIN Website** for this book contains **WebLinks** for each chapter, **Teaching Tips,** and **Frequently Asked Questions** for students and instructors. It can be accessed at http://www.mosby.com/MERLIN/Wilson/assessment/. This dynamic educational component allows students, faculty, and clinicians to access the most current information and resources for further study and research. MERLIN
- **Electronic Image Collection on CD-ROM** to accompany *Mosby's Guide to Physical Examination* contains hundreds of full-color images that can be used to make transparencies or imported into PowerPoint for use in classroom lectures. A chart in the *Instructor's Resource Manual* cross-references these images to related illustrations and content in this text.

The authors and Mosby thank you for choosing this text and sincerely wish you the best. We welcome any comments and suggestions from faculty and students.

CONTENTS

HEALTH ASSESSMENT for NURSING PRACTICE

REMEMBER to check out your **companion CD-ROM**

1 Why Learn Health Assessment?

www.mosby.com/MERLIN/wilson/assessment/

You are sitting at the clinic desk, and a woman with mussed hair and a distressed look on her face tells you that she needs to see someone. You ask her how you can help, and she starts to cry softly. She quickly goes on to tell you that she has a headache that won't go away, that she can't keep going on like this, that she can't eat or sleep, and that she hurts all over. As you take a careful look at her, you note that she has bruises on the side of her face and that her lower lip is swollen and split open. You sit back in your chair, and the wheels of your mind turn. What do you think? What should you do?*

Every time you interact with a client, a family, or the parents of a young child, you initiate the nursing process. The nursing process as endorsed by the American Nurses Association (ANA) (1991) has six steps: (1) to systematically collect objective and subjective information about the client (assessment), (2) to make a clinical judgment about the actual or potential health condition or needs of the client (diagnosis), (3) to identify the desired outcomes with goals to meet the client's needs or improve the client's health condition (outcome identification), (4) to create a comprehensive plan of care to attain the desired outcomes (planning), (5) to carry out the plan of action (implementation), and finally (6) to determine if the desired outcomes were achieved by the interventions (evaluation) (Box 1-1). The first and foundational step is assessment. Without the ability to systematically collect and synthesize information, the entire nursing process is weakened. So whether you are dealing with a client like the one described, caring for a client in the intensive care unit (ICU) who has a sudden onset of shortness of breath and pink frothy sputum, or performing a "well" evaluation or "checkup" of a 50-year-old American Indian man, your interaction always begins with assessment.

Assessment is defined by the ANA as "a systematic, dynamic process by which the nurse, through interaction with the client, significant others, and health care providers, collects and analyzes data about the client." Note that there are two steps in the assessment process. The first involves the collection of data (Box 1-2), and the second involves the interpretation or analysis of the data. These two components of assessment are used differently by nurses in different settings and with different levels of expertise and experience.

*Thanks to Vicki Flynn, from Madison, Connecticut, who as a student nurse in 1995 suggested the idea of this case presentation. She believes that every nurse should be alert to the signs and symptoms of domestic violence. We couldn't agree more and think this example shows the subtle way that a client may present with a significant problem. Thanks, Vicki.

Now consider the case presented above. What do you do with the information the client tells you (symptoms) and your physical observations (signs) (Box 1-3)?

- If you are new to the profession and have not had much experience, you may collect initial data and seek assistance for the client from someone with more experience.
- More experienced nurses may interact with the client and collect more information about each of the client's signs and symptoms and may then determine what clinic and what type of health care provider may best assist the client to ensure quality care that is timely and cost effective.
- The very experienced nurse may reach into his or her past experience, question the client further about the possibility of domestic abuse, determine appropriate referrals, and ensure that the client receives appropriate immediate care and appropriate follow-up and community referrals.
- If the nurse is a nurse practitioner or clinical nurse specialist responsible for case management, he or she may perform both in-depth subjective (the history) and objective (the physical examination) data collection, determine appropriate interventions, actually manage the client's total care during both this and future clinic visits, and make and possibly coordinate the appropriate community referrals.

Although all the nurses listed performed some type of assessment based on the same initial signs and symptoms, each collected and analyzed the data slightly differently because of his or her knowledge and experience.

WHAT HEALTH ASSESSMENT TELLS US

Health assessment provides a systematic method of collecting all types of data that identify the client's strengths, weaknesses, physiologic status, knowledge, motivation, support systems, and coping ability that may influence the client's health either positively or negatively. The nurse collects information and compares the client's state of health to the ideal state of health for the individual, taking into account the client's age, gender, culture, and physical, psychologic, and socioeconomic status. The weaknesses, problems, or deficits found should guide the plan for assisting the client to maximize his or her health potential. For example, if a 42-year-old Hispanic man is admitted to the hospital for pneumonia and the nurse notices his cholesterol level is 260 mg/dl, the nurse should follow the therapeutic medical plan for the pneumonia in addition to developing a nursing plan based on a comprehensive assessment of the client's disease state and his response to the medical treatment. When the time is appropriate and the client is receptive, the nurse

Box 1-1 The Nursing Process

ASSESSMENT

A systematic, dynamic process by which the nurse, through interaction with the client, significant others, and health care providers, collects and analyzes data about the client.

DIAGNOSIS*

A clinical judgment about the client's response to actual or potential health conditions or needs based on an analysis of the data collected.

OUTCOME IDENTIFICATION

Accomplished by establishing measurable, expected, client-focused goals to meet the client's needs or improve his or her health condition.

PLANNING

Creating a plan of care that is a comprehensive outline of care to be delivered to attain the outcomes.

IMPLEMENTATION

May include activities or interventions needed to attain the outcome. The client, significant other, or health care provider may be designated to implement the intervention within the plan of care.

EVALUATION

The process of determining both the client's progress toward the attainment of expected outcomes and the effectiveness of nursing care.

Reprinted with permission from American Nurses Association: *Standards of clinical nursing practice,* ed 2, Washington DC, 1998, American Nurses Foundation/American Nurses.

*Diagnosis includes identification of either a nursing diagnosis or a collaborative problem. A collaborative problem is also referred to as a potential complication (PC).

Box 1-2 Types of Health Assessment Data

SUBJECTIVE DATA

Those things told to the nurse by clients when asked to describe their current state of health, their previous illnesses and surgeries, and their family history. If the subjective data are acquired from a family member instead of from the client himself or herself, it is referred to as a secondary source of data. Subjective data may also be referred to as the *history.*

OBJECTIVE DATA

Data collected from a variety of data sources. During a physical examination, data are obtained using the techniques of inspection, palpation, percussion, and auscultation. Additional data include measurements of the client's height, weight, pulse, blood pressure, temperature, and respiratory rate. Other sources of objective data include urine, blood, other body excretions, x-ray examination, and imaging.

Box 1-3 Signs and Symptoms

SYMPTOMS

Data that the client or family tells the nurse. They include subjective information about the problem or situation. Examples are pain and itching.

SIGNS

Data that are observed, felt, heard, or measured by the nurse. They include the objective information or findings collected by the examiner about a problem or situation. Examples of signs are fever, rash, enlarged lymph nodes, and muscle weakness.

teaches the importance of lowering the cholesterol level and ways to accomplish this through diet and exercise.

WHAT HEALTH ASSESSMENT IS PERFORMED WHERE?

Let's be realistic about where and to what extent health assessment is performed. Many times the student is led to believe that every client in every situation needs a full and complete health assessment performed, but this is unrealistic. The setting or the reason the client seeks health care determines the type of assessment performed by the nurse. There are different types of health assessments performed, such as a screening assessment or a comprehensive assessment. These will be discussed further in Chapter 4, which presents the full spectrum of history questions that may be asked. It is not intended that you ask every client you care for every question on every page. What is important is that you learn all of these questions so that when the situation is appropriate you will know what to ask, how to ask it, and what the client's response means. Certainly clinical judgment is needed to ensure that the complete complement of questions is asked for any given situation. For example, if you are performing a complete health assessment with a client for the first time in a well-client setting, you will want to collect comprehensive subjective and objective information. On the other hand, if you are working in an episodic care clinic or emergency department and the client presents with burns on her hand and chest, that is not the time to conduct a comprehensive assessment. It is important, however, to conduct a focused assessment ensuring comprehensive data collection about all subjective and objective elements that may have direct or indirect impact on the management of the client's burn and potential risk for future injury. For example, it would be important to inquire about the client's last tetanus injection, chronic medical conditions, and current medications. In addition, if you assess the client to be at risk or in need of further health evaluation, it is very important that the client be referred to a more appropriate site at a later date so that a comprehensive assessment may be made.

The expertise of the nurse performing the examination is another factor determining the type of assessment to be conducted. Certainly a clinical nurse specialist, a nurse practitioner, or a nurse who is very experienced in a given area will be capable of conducting more thorough examinations than a nurse with less experience. For example, a nurse working in an adult intensive care unit will have expertise assessing a client with hemodynamic instability; and a family nurse practitioner working in a women's clinic will have expertise in performing routine pelvic examinations.

This textbook covers assessment techniques from basic to advanced. It is not realistic for the beginning student to learn every assessment technique presented. Although advanced assessment techniques are quite obvious to the experienced nurse, they may not be obvious to the beginning student. Throughout this textbook advanced assessment techniques will be indicated with the following symbol: ❖

DOCUMENTATION OF DATA

Data collected from health assessment must be documented so that other health care providers can use the information. Complete, accurate, and descriptive documentation of health assessment improves the effectiveness of the entire health care team. Documenting these data also prevents the client from having to provide the same information to another health care provider. The written record serves as a legal document and permanent record of the client's health status at the time of the nurse-client interaction. Thus it serves as a baseline for evaluation or subsequent changes and decisions related to care. Using an outline of data to collect and taking brief notes during the encounter will facilitate the documentation and increase its accuracy. The nurse must record data concisely, without bias or opinion. Health assessment documentation is discussed further in Chapter 27.

WHAT DO YOU DO WITH ALL THESE DATA?

The outcome of a health assessment is a portrait of the client's physical status, strengths and weaknesses, abilities, support systems, health beliefs, and activities to maintain health, as well as his or her health problems and lack of resources for maintaining health. The nurse must analyze the subjective and objective data collected from the client to identify problems and to initiate a nursing plan of care (Fig. 1-1). Data analysis involves clustering data so that the problems may present themselves more clearly. Assessment forms historically have been organized under a body system format (e.g., cardiovascular, musculoskeletal, auditory, visual). Although organization of data in such a format is useful to nurses, it is incomplete because it does not include data from other important areas such as sleep, activity, or health promotion activities. Functional health patterns, proposed by Gordon (1994), is a framework for organizing data by areas of health status or function rather than body systems (Table 1-1). Data organized in a functional health pattern format help the nurse and client identify areas of wellness (or positive function), as well as problems and nursing diagnoses. In addition, the North American Nursing Diagnosis Association (NANDA) has proposed a new taxonomy that incorporates concepts similar to functional health patterns (NANDA, 1999). A list of the current NANDA nursing diagnoses is presented in Appendix B of this text (NANDA, 1999).

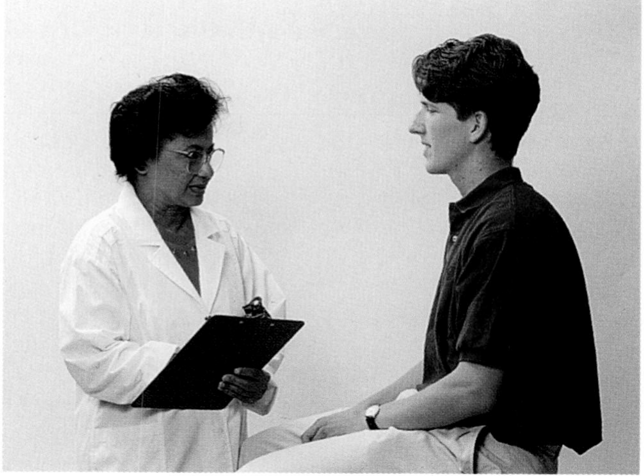

Fig. 1-1 The written record serves as a legal document and permanent record of the client's health status at the time of the nurse-client interaction.

Now consider the woman who came to the clinic desk in the beginning of this chapter. This woman—let's call her Stacy—has more than mussed hair, a distressed face, headache, facial bruises, a split lip, and general body aching. Stacy is a woman with a physical, psychologic, emotional, spiritual, and socioeconomic history. Data analysis can begin only after some health care professional takes the time to systematically collect comprehensive health assessment information about all aspects of Stacy's presenting situation and her motivation for seeking care.

You are now challenged to diligently study this health assessment text to learn how and when to collect and use both subjective and objective data so that you can be the best nurse possible. Someday you may be the nurse behind the clinic desk with whom a client shares a very difficult problem. You need to be prepared to collect accurate and comprehensive health assessment data about the client, to make accurate clinical judgments about the client's situation, and to develop an intervention to assist the client or to provide care that will improve the client's actual or potential health status. If you are able to do this, then the client will have been well served. An accurate and comprehensive health assessment is indeed one of the important cornerstones of the art and science of professional nursing.

Table 1-1 Functional Health Pattern Organization

FUNCTIONAL HEALTH PATTERN	DESCRIPTION
Health perception–health management	Client's perceived level of health, practices for maintaining health, and adherence to medical or nursing prescriptions
Nutrition–metabolism	Pattern of foods and fluids consumed relative to the metabolic need, appetite and food preferences, weight loss/weight gain; also focuses on metabolic activity and tissue integrity
Elimination	Patterns of bowel and urinary elimination, problems with control, and use of assistive devices; also explores skin excretion
Activity–exercise	Client's level of activity, including leisure activities, exercise, level of energy with expenditure, ability to complete activities of daily living
Sleep–rest	Client's routines and function related to sleep, resting, and relaxing
Cognitive–perceptual	Client's comprehension and sensory abilities, such as vision, hearing and touch, pain, and decision-making abilities
Self-perception–self-concept	Attitudes towards self, including body image, self-identity, and sense of self-worth and self-esteem
Role–relationship	Patterns of relationships, satisfaction of relationships and role responsibilities
Sexuality–reproduction	Menstrual and reproductive history, sexual activity and function, and satisfaction with sexual activity
Coping–stress tolerance	Client's perception of stress, response to stresses, and coping strategies
Value–belief	Values and beliefs or goals held by the client and family and perceived conflicts with value system

Data from Gordon MJ: *Nursing diagnosis: process and application,* ed 3, St. Louis, 1994, Mosby.

CLINICAL APPLICATION and CRITICAL THINKING

CRITICAL THINKING QUESTIONS

For each of the following scenarios, describe what type of health assessment (comprehensive or focused) would be conducted on the child and mother. Defend your answers.

1. A mother runs into the emergency department with her 6-year-old son, stating that he fell 15 feet from a tree. You observe a child who is screaming and who has an open fracture to the left forearm.
2. A mother brings her 6-year-old son to the asthma clinic, stating that her physician suggested routine visits to monitor the child's progress and to learn to manage his illness.

CASE STUDY 1

Sharon is a 42-year-old woman admitted to the hospital with a diagnosis of acute cholecystitis. She tells the nurse she has pain in her right abdomen that feels like a knife—and that it goes all the way to her shoulder. Sharon is also very nauseated. She tells the nurse that she is exhausted and has not slept for three nights because the pain keeps her awake. The nurse observes dark circles under Sharon's eyes. Her vital signs are as follows:

Blood pressure (BP): ***132/90 mm Hg***
Pulse: ***104 beats/min***
Respirations: ***22 per minute***
Temperature: ***101.8° F (38.8° C)***

A complete blood count (CBC) reveals that Sharon has an elevated white blood cell (WBC) count. She lies in her bed in a fetal position and tells the nurse that it hurts too much to get up and move.

1. List the subjective data described in Case Study 1.
2. List the objective data described in Case Study 1.
3. List the functional health patterns in which the client may have negative function.
4. List some of the NANDA-approved nursing diagnoses that may be applicable to Sharon's care, based on what you now know.

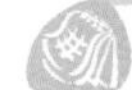

CASE STUDY 2

Linda is a client on the orthopedic unit. Listed below are data collected by the nurse during an interview and assessment.

Interview Data

Linda states, "I fell off my horse while riding. The horse stepped on my leg and crushed the bone in my upper leg."

She complains of pain in her right leg. The pain medication helps only a little. She wants to move but can't because of the traction. Linda says, "My butt hurts because I can't move around." She tells the nurse, "I have not had a bowel movement for 3 days now, and the last time the stool looked like hard, dry rabbit turds. Normally at home I go every day." Linda has not been hungry either. She says that "the food is horrible." Linda also complains that she is so bored she can't stand it. "I am used to being active," she says, "so being stuck in bed is driving me crazy. TV shows are not worth watching."

Examination Data

- 41-year-old woman; occupation: schoolteacher.
- **Vital signs:** BP, 108/72 mm Hg; pulse, 88 beats/min; respirations, 16 per minute; temperature, 98.1° F (36.7° C); height, 5′5″ (165 cm); weight, 135 lb (61 kg).
- **Medication:** Percocet 1 or 2 by mouth (PO) every 4 to 6 hours as needed for pain. She has taken these every 6 hours.
- **Diet:** Regular diet. Has eaten, on average, 30% of meals. Fluid intake has averaged 1000 ml/day.
- **Activity:** Client is on complete bed rest.
- **Respiratory:** Breathing even/unlabored. Lungs are clear to auscultation bilaterally.
- **Cardiovascular:** Pulses palpable. Heart rate and rhythm regular. No peripheral edema.
- **Abdomen:** Slightly distended. Bowel sounds auscultated throughout abdomen.
- **Musculoskeletal:** Right leg in skeletal traction. Normal sensation to foot/toes, rapid capillary refill. Other extremities: Full range of motion. No pain over joints and muscles.
- **Integumentary:** Skin warm and dry. Pin sites for traction without redness or drainage. Two-inch-diameter redness over sacrum. Skin intact.

Listed below are four functional health patterns in which the nurse has identified negative functioning with a nursing diagnosis for each. Using data from the case study above, cluster data under each problem. The data should be consistent with the functional health pattern and support the diagnosis. Some data may be placed under more than one problem.

1. Functional health pattern: cognitive–perceptual
   Nursing diagnosis: *pain* related to right leg injury
   a. Subjective data
   b. Objective data
2. Functional health pattern: elimination
   Nursing diagnosis: *colonic constipation* related to inactivity and analgesics
   a. Subjective data
   b. Objective data
3. Functional health pattern: nutrition–metabolic
   Nursing diagnosis: *risk for impaired skin integrity* related to immobility
   a. Subjective data
   b. Objective data
4. Functional health pattern: activity–exercise
   Nursing diagnosis: *diversional activity deficit* related to complete bed rest
   a. Subjective data
   b. Objective data

2 Developmental Assessment Through the Life Span

REMEMBER to check out your **companion CD-ROM**

www.mosby.com/MERLIN/wilson/assessment/

A comprehensive approach to nursing practice includes the assessment of physical, behavioral, and cognitive aspects of development. Since all of these aspects influence health, they must be considered when the nurse interacts with clients.

This chapter is organized by chronologic age divisions that correlate with developmental periods. Each division discusses all three aspects of assessment and describes some assessment tools applicable to that age group. Behavioral and psychosocial development for each age division are summarized using Duvall's and Miller's developmental tasks. During the first 6 years, however, physical growth and development are so dramatic that additional data are used to describe motor development, social-adaptive behaviors, and language development.

- *Motor development* has two components: gross and fine motor behavior. Gross motor behavior refers to postural reactions such as head balance, sitting, standing, creeping, and walking. Fine motor behavior refers to the use of hands and fingers in the prehensile approach to grasping and manipulating an object.
- *Social-adaptive behavior* refers to the interactions of the infant or child with other persons and the ability to organize stimuli, to perceive relationships between objects, to dissect a whole into its component parts, to reintegrate these parts in a meaningful fashion, and to solve practical problems. Examples are smiling at other persons and learning to feed self crackers.
- *Language behavior* is used broadly to include visible and audible forms of communication, whether facial expression, gesture, postural movements, or vocalizations (words, phrases, or sentences). Language also includes the comprehension of communication by others.

THEORIES OF DEVELOPMENT

By using theories of development nurses can describe and predict growth and development through the life span. Two widely used theories of behavioral and cognitive development are described briefly. These theories were developed by Erik Erikson and Jean Piaget.

Personality Development: Erikson's Theory

Erik Erikson (1902-1994) believed that the ego was the primary seat of personality functioning (Erikson, 1963). He viewed social and cultural influences as the driving forces that create inner conflicts accompanying psychosocial maturation and growth. His psychodynamic theory of development defines eight specific developmental stages, by chronologic age, in which the resolution of polar conflicts leads to personality development (Table 2-1). The successful outcome of each stage results in specific lasting effects. For example, in the first stage, during infancy, the conflict is trust versus mistrust. When the infant develops trusting relationships with others, usually the mother, then the lasting outcome tends to be ambition, enthusiasm, and motivation. By contrast, when trust is not developed, that person tends to develop apathy and indifference. Accomplishing each successive task provides the foundation for a healthy self-identity. Each stage depends on the previous stage and must be accomplished for the person to successfully complete the next one. Other people and environmental factors influence a person's accomplishment of these tasks; however, the motivation to achieve a healthy identity arises from within each person. Although each conflict is described at a particular developmental stage, all the conflicts exist in each person to some extent throughout life. Even though the conflict may be resolved at one time in a person's life, it may recur in similar circumstances (Erikson, 1963).

Cognitive Development: Piaget's Theory

Jean Piaget (1896-1980) described stages of cognitive development from birth to about 15 years of age. Cognition is defined as how a person perceives and processes information about the world. Piaget believed the child's main goal was to master the environment to establish equilibrium between self and environment.

Piaget believed the child's view of the world developed from simple reflex behavior to complex logical and abstract thought. To fully develop cognition, the child needs a functioning neurologic system and sufficient environmental stimuli. There are four distinct, sequential levels of cognitive development (Table 2-2). Each stage represents a qualitative change of thinking and behaving. All children move through the stages in sequential order but not necessarily at the same age (Piaget and Inhelder, 1969).

Adult Intelligence

Though Piaget's work represents the most complete work in cognitive development, it does not progress through adulthood. Theorists of adult intelligence propose the assessment of "practical" intelligence. They believe intelligence develops through an interaction of biologic and environmental factors. Intellectual abilities of adults can be sustained or improved until late adulthood. Two types of adult intelligence

Table 2-1 Erikson's Eight Stages of Human Development

STAGE (APPROXIMATE)	PSYCHOSOCIAL STAGE	LASTING OUTCOMES
Infancy	Basic trust versus basic mistrust	Drive and hope
Toddlerhood	Autonomy versus shame and doubt	Self-control and will power
Preschool	Initiative versus guilt	Direction and purpose
Middle childhood (school age)	Industry versus inferiority	Method and competence
Adolescence	Identity versus role confusion	Devotion and fidelity
Young adulthood	Intimacy versus isolation	Affiliation and love
Middle adulthood	Generativity versus stagnation	Production and care
Older adulthood	Ego integrity versus despair	Renunciation and wisdom

Modified from Erikson EH: *Childhood and society,* ed 2, New York, 1963, Norton.

Table 2-2 Piaget's Levels of Cognitive Development

STAGE	AGE	CHARACTERISTICS
Sensorimotor	0-2 years	Thought dominated by physical manipulation of objects and events.
Preoperational	2-7 years	Functions symbolically using language as major tool.
Concrete operations	7-11 years	Mental reasoning processes assume logical approaches to solving concrete problems.
Formal operations	11-15 years	True logical thought and manipulation of abstract concepts emerge.

Modified from Schuster C, Ashburn S: *The process of human development: a holistic life-span approach,* Boston, 1992, Lippincott.

have been described: fluid and crystallized. Fluid intelligence represents the ability to perceive complex situations and engage in short-term memory, concept formation, reasoning, and abstraction. This type of intelligence is dependent on central nervous system function and declines with age and physiologic change. Crystallized intelligence is associated with those skills and knowledge learned as a part of growing up in a given culture, such as verbal comprehension, vocabulary, and ability to evaluate life experiences. It is dependent on life experiences and education and remains stable or increases with maturity (Shaie, 1990). In addition to innate ability, other factors such as social class, illness, personality, and motivation affect adult intelligence. For example, adults of average intelligence who have the opportunities for education and are sufficiently motivated reveal greater increases in intelligence throughout adulthood. Fluid intelligence begins to decline at about age 35 to 40, but crystallized intelligence is maintained longer (Merriam and Caffarella, 1999).

Several theorists believe that the academic type of testing used to assess intelligence in children is not appropriate for adults. A great deal of intelligence in adults is gained from "real world" experiences that are difficult to measure by standardized tests. Sternberg is a theorist who proposed a three-pronged theory of intelligence. The first was the componential subtheory, which described the internal analytic mental mechanisms. The experiential subtheory focused on how a person's learning through life experiences, combined with insight and creativity, affects the person's thinking. The third was the contextual subtheory, which focused on the role of the external environment in determining what constitutes intelligence in a particular situation (Sternberg, 1986). Factors contributing to the presumption of intellectual decline in older adults are their diminished vision and slower response time.

INFANTS

Infancy refers to the first year of life. The rapid growth and development that occur during these first 12 months are evident from the data given in Table 2-3, which lists changes in the infant by month, whereas subsequent tables document changes by intervals of 6 months to 1 year. During this time extensive neurologic and physical development occur in addition to the acquisition of psychosocial skills.

Physical Growth Height, weight, and head circumference are measured to assess infant growth. Growth proceeds from head to toe (cephalocaudal) as evidenced by the infant's development of head control before sitting and mastery of sitting before standing. Healthy newborns weigh between 5 lb 8 oz and 8 lb 13 oz (between 2500 and 4000 g). The newborn period is the first 28 days of life. Commonly newborns lose 10% of their birth weight in the first week but regain it in 10 to 14 days. In general they double their birth weight by 4 to 5 months of age and triple it by 12 months of age. The infant grows 1 inch (2.5 cm) monthly for the first 6 months, followed by ½ inch (1.3 cm) a month

Table 2-3 Expected Development of Infants

AGE	FINE MOTOR	GROSS MOTOR	SOCIAL-ADAPTIVE	LANGUAGE
1 month	Follows with eyes to midline Hands predominantly closed Strong grasp reflex	Turns head to side Keeps knees tucked under abdomen When pulled to sitting position, has gross head lag and rounded, swayed back	Regards face	Responds to bell Cries in response to displeasure Makes sounds during feeding
2 months	Follows objects well; may not follow past midline Hands frequently open	Holds head in same plane as rest of body Can raise head and maintain position; looks downward	Smiles responsively	Vocalizes (not crying) Cries become differentiated Coos
3 months	Follows past midline When in supine position puts hands together; will hold hands in front of face Pulls at blanket and clothes	Raises head to 45° angle Maintains posture Looks around with head May turn from prone to side position When pulled into sitting position, shows only slight head lag	Shows interest in surroundings	Laughs Coos, babbles, chuckles
4 months	Grasps rattle Plays with hands together Inspects hands Carries objects to mouth	Actively lifts head up and looks around (Fig. 2-1) Will roll from prone to supine position When pulled to sitting position, no longer has head lag When held in standing position, attempts to maintain some weight support	Becomes bored when left alone Begins to show memory	Squeals Vocalizations change with mood
5 months	Can reach and pick up object May play with toes	Able to push up from prone position and maintain weight on forearms Rolls from prone to supine and back to prone Maintains straight back when in sitting position	Smiles spontaneously Playful, with rapid mood changes Distinguishes family	Uses vowel-like cooing sounds with consonantal sounds (e.g., *ah-goo*)
6 months	Will hold spoon or rattle Will drop object and reach for second offered object Holds bottle	Begins to raise abdomen off table Sits, but posture still shaky May sit with legs apart; holds arms straight as prop between legs Supports almost full weight when pulled to standing position	Recognizes parents Holds out arms to be picked up	Begins to imitate sounds Uses one-syllable sounds (e.g., *ma, mu, da, di*)

Table 2-3 Expected Development of Infants—cont'd

AGE	FINE MOTOR	GROSS MOTOR	SOCIAL-ADAPTIVE	LANGUAGE
7 months	Can transfer object from one hand to other Grasps objects in each hand Bangs cube on table	Sits alone; still uses hands for support When held in standing position, bounces Puts feet to mouth	Fearful of strangers Plays peekaboo Keeps lips closed when dislikes food	Says four distinct vowel sounds "Talks" when others are talking
8 months	Beginning thumb-finger grasping Releases object at will Grasps for toys out of reach	Sits securely without support Bears weight on legs when supported May stand holding on	Responds to word *no* Dislikes diaper changes	Makes consonant sounds *t, d, w* Uses two syllables such as *da-da,* but does not ascribe meaning to them
9 months	Continued development of thumb-finger grasp May bang objects together Use of dominant hand evident	Steady sitting; can lean forward and still maintain position Begins creeping (abdomen off floor) Can stand holding onto established object when placed in that position	Seems interested in pleasing parent Show fears of going to bed and being left alone	Responds to simple commands Comprehends *no-no*
10 months	Practices picking up small objects Points with one finger Will offer toys to people but unable to let go of objects	Can pull self into sitting position; unable to let self down again Stands while holding on to furniture	Inhibits behavior in response to command *no-no* Repeats actions that attract attention Plays interactive games such as pat-a-cake Cries when scolded	Says *da-da, ma-ma* with meaning Comprehends *bye-bye*
11 months	Holds crayon to mark on paper Drops object deliberately for it to be picked up	Moves about room holding onto objects Preparing to walk independently; wide-base stance Stands securely holding on with one hand	Experiences satisfaction when task is accomplished Reacts to restrictions with frustration Rolls a ball to another upon request	Imitates speech sounds
12 months (1 year)	May hold cup and spoon and feed self fairly well with practice Can offer toys and release them Releases cube in cup	Able to twist and turn and maintain posture Able to sit from standing position May stand alone, at least momentarily	Shows emotions of jealousy, affection, anger, fear May develop habit of "security blanket" or favorite toy	*Da-da* or *ma-ma* specific Recognizes objects by name Imitates animal sounds Understands simple verbal commands (e.g., "Give it to me")

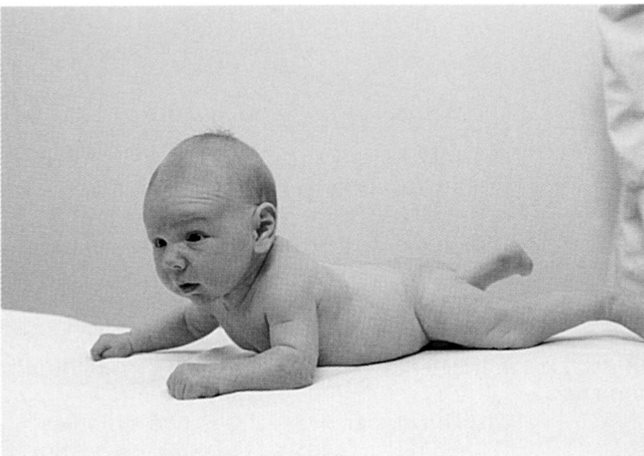

Fig. 2-1 At 4 months infant actively lifts head and looks about.

from age 6 months to 12 months. Expected head circumference for term newborns averages from 13 to 14 inches (33 to 36 cm) and increases ½ inch (1.3 cm) monthly for the first 6 months. By 6 months teeth begin to erupt, with a total of 6 to 8 teeth by the end of the first year.

Behavioral and Cognitive Development A summary of the expected developmental milestones is found in Table 2-3. The psychosocial crisis at this age is called trust versus mistrust. Infants develop trust relationships with the mother or primary caregiver. The important criterion is the quality and consistency of the mother-child relationship. Infants who receive consistent, loving care learn that they can depend on people around them to meet their needs. By contrast, care that is inconsistent, abusive, or undependable may result in mistrust of people.

Piaget identifies sensorimotor development as the primary task of infancy. Infants utilize their sensorimotor abilities to master motor milestones and to launch relationships with others. Not only can infants advance from crawling to walking and eating some foods, but they also have the ability to win the hearts and attention of others with an intentional smile and showing preference for familiar caregivers. Bonding takes place with caregivers; at about 1 month different cries can be identified as being related to different needs, expressive language progresses to the first word, and receptive language is developed enough to understand and briefly respond to simple disciplinary commands. Learning at the sensorimotor level of cognitive development occurs through the five senses as infants interact with the environment. Infants learn object permanence, which means that objects and people still exist when they are out of sight.

The developmental tasks of infancy according to Duvall and Miller (1985) are listed in Box 2-1.

Assessment tools for the infant focus on physical growth and psychosocial development, as well as determining the mother's and father's interactions with the infant. Selected tools are listed in Table 2-4.

Box 2-1 Developmental Tasks of Infants

- Achieving physiologic equilibrium following birth
  - Learning to take food satisfactorily
- Learning to adjust to other person
  - Reacting positively to both familiar and strange persons
- Learning to love and be loved
  - Responding affectionately to others through cuddling, smiling, and loving
  - Beginning to give self spontaneously and trustingly to others
- Developing system of communication
  - Learning patterns of recognition and responses
  - Establishing nonverbal, preverbal, and verbal communication
- Learning to express and to control feelings
  - Developing a sense of trust and confidence with the world
- Laying a foundation for self-awareness
  - Seeing oneself as a separate entity
  - Finding personal fulfillment with and without others

Data from Duvall EM, Miller BC: *Marriage and family development,* ed 6, New York, 1985, Harper & Row.

CHILDREN

Toddlers

Toddlerhood is the period of growth and development from 12 to 36 months. During this period the child's locomotion is increasing, and the child becomes more independent in moving about. Toddlers have a strong quest for exploration and mastery of the surrounding world and environment. Parents seeking to foster their children's exploratory and inquiring spirit, along with the mastery of motor skills, often feel extremely overwhelmed and exhausted at the end of the day. This exhaustion, coupled with the toddler's low tolerance for frustration, has led to this stage being labeled the "terrible twos."

Physical Growth A slower but steady growth in height and weight occurs during toddlerhood. By 24 months, chest circumference exceeds head circumference. Children are half their adult height by age 2. By 30 months the birth weight is quadrupled. The usual appearance of a toddler includes a potbelly, swayback, and short legs. The toddler may be ready for daytime control of bowel and bladder function by age 24 months. Teeth continue to erupt, with 20 teeth expected by 30 months.

Behavioral and Cognitive Development Autonomy versus shame and doubt describes the psychosocial crisis for toddlers. The terms "holding on" and "letting go" are used to describe this stage. Now that they are walking and talking, they yearn for independence; however, they lack judgment to maintain their safety. They learn when it is safe to hold on to furniture and when to let go. The

Table 2-4 Summary of Assessment Instruments

NAME	AGE	ASSESSMENT FOCUS	COMMENTS
*NBAS: Neonatal Behavioral Assessment Scale (Brazelton & Nugent, 1995)	Newborn	Neurologic deficits	The most widely used neonatal behavioral assessment scale. Used with all cultural groups. Special training required to administer test. Data from the test may be used to enhance parenting skills and sensitivity to infant behaviors.
National Child Assessment Form (Kaufman and McMurrian, 1992)	0-3 years	Social-emotional, language, cognitive, gross and fine motor	Developmental progression is noted through visual representation. Behavior is considered either consistently present, occasionally present, or not present. *Format:* checklist.
Assessment Tool for Measuring Maternal Attachment Behaviors (Cropley, Lester, and Pennington, 1976)	Infancy	Maternal attachment	Used to monitor progression of maternal attachment, evaluate interventions for stimulating and fostering maternal attachment, and identify at-risk situations. *Format:* checklist.
BSID-II: Bayley Scale of Infant Development (Bayley, 1993)	1-42 months	Mental, psychomotor behavior	Used with children at risk for or suspected risk of developmental delay.
BINS: Bayley Infant Neurodevelopmental Screener (Bayley, 1993)	3-24 months	Mental, psychomotor	Abbreviated form of the BSID II.
Portage Guide to Early Education (*Portage project,* 1994)	Birth-6 years	Cognitive, motor, self-help, social, communication	A home-teaching program assesses child's development, serves as an educational guide to enhance family functioning, and supports parent in child's development. Translated into 35 languages. *Format:* checklist.
Lollipop Test (Chew, 1992)	5 years	School readiness—visual perception, numeric ability, color recognition and visual discrimination, spatial recognition	Diagnostic screening tool.
Fathering Assessment Tool (Murphy, 1979)	Not age-specific Infancy-young child	Father-child interactions	Measures father-infant interactions, role gratification, growth potential, and family support. *Format:* Likert scale.
*Denver II (1994)	0-6 years	Personal—social, fine motor–adaptive, language, and gross motor (direct observation)	Used worldwide. Screens for early detection of developmental delays.
Prescreening Developmental Questionnaire (PDQ, RPDQ) (Denver, 1994)	3 months-6 years	Personal—social, fine motor–adaptive, language, and gross motor (completed by parent or during interview)	Abbreviated form of Denver II. Collects data about child from parents. *Format:* questionnaire.

*Requires training to use

Continued

Table 2-4 Summary of Assessment Instruments—cont'd

NAME	AGE	ASSESSMENT FOCUS	COMMENTS
CABS: Children's Adaptive Behavior Scale Revised (Kicklighter and Richmond, 1983)	5 years to 10 years, 11 months	Language and psychosocial	Describes language development, independent functioning, family role performance, economic-vocational activity, and socialization. Used to develop educational plans for handicapped.
Washington Guide to Promoting Development in the Young Child (Powell, 1981)	0-5 years	Feeding, sleep, play, motor, language, toilet training, discipline, dressing	Focuses on social development, requires direct observation; no score calculated; offers objective identification of developmental levels.
Goodenough-Harris Drawing Test (Goodenough, 1926; Harris, 1983)	3-15 years	Mental age, intelligence quotient	Test is composed of two scales: man and woman. Each drawing is scored on 75 specific characteristics.
Social Readjustment Rating Scale (Holmes and Rahe, 1967)	Adult	Stress	Measures the amount of change an individual has experienced within the last year. Based on the belief that change is stressful.
Change in Life Events Scale for Children (Coddington, 1972)	Preschool-senior high	Stress	Same as Social Readjustment Rating Scale.
Overload Index Pace of Life Index (Kemper, Giuffre, and Drabinski, 1986)	Adolescent-adult	Stress from lack of time management and pacing life	Ten- and 15-question indexes to help recognize sources of daily stress and teach health promotion strategies.
VII: Vocational Interest Inventory (Lunneborg, 1981)	Adult	Career interest	
CAI: Career Assessment Inventory (Johansson and Johansson, 1978)	Adult	Career interest	
Personal Assessment of Intimacy Relationships (Schaefer and Olson, 1981)	Adult	Perception of intimacy and goals for the relationship	Five types of intimacy assessed: emotional, social, sexual, intellectual, and recreational.
*Myers-Briggs Type Indicator (Myers and Briggs-Myers, 1980)	Adult	Personality	Used by pastors, counselors, educators. Used in premarital counseling and coworker-manager interactions. Describes the continuum of complementary vs. opposing personality types in terms of sensing/intuitive, thinking/feeling, perceptive/judging, introvert/extrovert.
Job Descriptive Index (Smith, Kendall, and Hulin, 1969)	Adult	Job satisfaction (tasks)	Determines satisfaction with tasks performed in vocation.
Social Rewards Satisfaction Scale (Goldstein and Hersen, 1984)	Adult	Job social rewards	Determines satisfaction with workplace social environment.

*Requires training to use

Table 2-4 Summary of Assessment Instruments—cont'd

NAME	AGE	ASSESSMENT FOCUS	COMMENTS
Intrinsic and Extrinsic Rewards Satisfaction Scale (Goldstein and Hersen, 1984)	Adult	Job satisfaction	Determines satisfaction of internal and external rewards of vocation.
Need Satisfaction Questionnaire (Porter, 1961)	Adult	Personal needs in job	Determines how well vocation meets personal needs.
CRICHT: Chrichton Geriatric Rating Scale (Robinson, 1964)	65+	Behavior and functioning	Rates behavior and ability to perform activities of daily living.
SGSS: Stokes/Gordon Stress Scale (1986)	65+	Stress	Similar to Social Readjustment Rating Scale, using belief that change is stressful.
Modes of Adaptation Patterns Scale (Kane and Kane, 1984)	Older adult	Coping skills	Results in four adaptive styles: high activity plus high morale (conformist), high activity plus low morale (ritualist), low activity plus high morale (passive-contented), low activity plus low morale (retreatist).
Sandoz Clinical Assessment—Geriatric (SCAG) (Shader, Harmatz, and Salzman, 1974)	Older adult	Behavior and functioning	Assesses behavior and ability to perform activities of daily living.
Calgary Family Assessment (Wright and Leahey, 1984)	Families	Structure, development, function	Developed for use by nurses. Tool is easily modified to fit family being assessed.
FES: Family Environment Scale (Moos and Moos, 1976)	Families	Social environment	Compares real and ideal family social environments. Ten subscales measure relationships, personal growth, system maintenance. Results used as guide for family therapy and education.
Evaluation of Family Functioning Scale (Reidy and Thibaudeau, 1984)	Families	Functioning regarding health	Developed for use by community health nurses. Dimensions evaluated include health/illness, problem-solving and coping abilities.
Parenting Satisfaction Scale	Adult	Parent-child relationship	Self-report. *Format:* Likert scale.
FACES: Family Adaptability and Cohesion Evaluation Scales I, II, III (Olson, 1986)	Adult	Family functioning	Families are defined as enmeshed vs. disengaged and structurally rigid vs. chaotically formed.
FILE: Family Inventory of Life Events and Changes (McCubbin and Patterson, 1987)	Family	Stress	FILE and A-FILE are similar to Social Readjustment Rating Scale for life stressors. *Format:* questionnaire.
A-FILE: Adolescent-Family Inventory of Life Events and Changes (McCubbin and Patterson, 1987)	Adolescent/family	Stress	FILE and A-FILE are similar to Social Readjustment Rating Scale for life stressors. Format: questionnaire.

Box 2-2 Developmental Tasks of Toddlers

- Achieving physiologic equilibrium following birth
  - Learning the know-how and the where-when of elimination
  - Learning to manage one's body effectively
- Learning to adjust to other persons
  - Responding to others' expectations
  - Recognizing parental authority and controls
  - Learning the do's and don'ts of the immediate world
- Learning to love and be loved
  - Meeting emotional needs through widening spheres and variety of contacts
- Developing system of communication
  - Acquiring basic concepts such as yes/no
  - Mastering basic language fundamentals
- Learning to express and to control feelings
  - Healthy management of feelings of fear and anxiety
  - Handling feelings of frustration, disappointment, and anger appropriately for age
  - Moderating demanding attitudes
- Laying a foundation for self-awareness
  - Exploring the rights and privileges of being an individual

Data from Duvall EM, Miller BC: *Marriage and family development*, ed 6, New York, 1985, Harper & Row.

parents or caregivers try to balance their control between allowing toddlers to be independent enough to explore the environment and learn and keeping them safe from injury. The "holding on" and "letting go" also apply to bowel control established at this time. In their attempts to be independent, toddlers may fail to achieve their goals. Repeated failures may lead to feelings of shame and doubt in their abilities.

Cognitive development of the toddler remains in the sensorimotor level. At about 2 years Piaget's preoperational stage begins when toddlers learn by trial and error and by exploration. Using their motor skills, they move around the environment and pick up objects, and, using their senses, they see, feel, smell, taste, and hear what they find.

Developmental tasks of toddlers are listed in Box 2-2. A summary of the expected development milestones, including fine and gross motor, social-adaptive, and language behaviors, are found in Table 2-5 (Fig. 2-2).

The tool used most frequently by nurses to assess development is the Denver II, used for children age 1 month to 6 years. This tool replaced the original Denver Developmental Screening Test (DDST) and the revised DDST in 1994. The Denver II differs from the DDST by having an increased number of language items, two articulation items, a new age scale, a new category of item interpretation to identify milder delays, a behavior rating scale, and new training materials. The Denver II form is shown in Fig. 2-3, pp. 16-17.

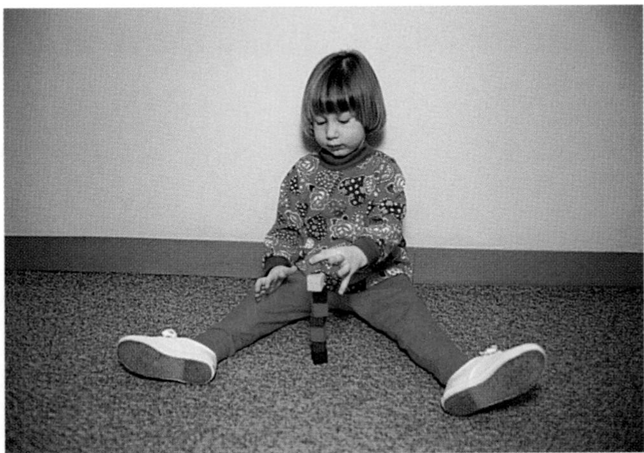

Fig. 2-2 Child building block tower demonstrates fine motor skills.

Preschoolers

The preschooler ranges in age from 3 to 5 years. As children's locomotion and language mature, they move away from the protective yet confining care of parental figures. Children begin to understand concepts and meanings in a more "real" sense and begin increased forms of independent play and decision making.

Physical Growth Typical preschoolers grow 2 to 2¾ inches (5 to 7 cm) a year. By age 4, birth length has doubled, and weight increases by 3 to 5 pounds (1.4 to 2.3 kg) a year. Appearance changes as the long bones grow more than the trunk, and preschoolers lose their baby fat and their potbellies. By age 5, children begin to lose deciduous teeth, and first permanent teeth erupt.

Behavioral and Cognitive Development During the preschool years children become more autonomous, communicate easily, become toilet trained, have an active imagination, demonstrate basic social skills, can delay gratification, use more acceptable outlets to express frustration, and expand their environment beyond home. The psychosocial crisis described by Erikson is initiative versus guilt. Preschoolers continue to explore their environments with greater skills and a new enthusiasm and motivation. When family members praise children for their activities, they learn that they are meeting parental expectations and become independent and self-sufficient. At this stage their conscience develops, that inner voice that provides a sense of right and wrong. When family members persistently ridicule children, the children may develop guilt about their behavior.

Cognitive development continues at the preoperational level. Children begin the symbolic function, in which they develop concepts and classifications to associate one event, object, or person with a similar one. Children demonstrate this when they act out an event they have seen or experienced, but they emphasize only one aspect of the event. At this level children become egocentric, when they are self-centered and unable to understand others' viewpoint.

Table 2-5 Expected Development of Toddlers

AGE	FINE MOTOR	GROSS MOTOR	SOCIAL-ADAPTIVE	LANGUAGE
15 months	Can put raisins into bottle Will take off shoes and pull toys Builds tower of two cubes Scribbles spontaneously Uses cup well, but rotates spoon	Walks alone well Able to seat self in chair Creeps up stairs Cannot throw ball without falling	Tolerates some separation from parents Begins to imitate parents' activities (e.g., sweeping, mowing lawn)	Says 10 or more words "Asks" for objects by pointing Uses *no* even when agreeing with request
18 months	Builds tower of three to four cubes Turns pages in book two or three at a time Manages spoon without rotating	May walk up and down stairs holding hand May show running ability	Imitates housework Temper tantrums may be more evident Has beginning awareness of ownership (e.g., *my toy*)	Says 10 or more words Points to two or three body parts
24 months (2 years)	Able to turn doorknob Able to take off shoes and socks Able to build seven- to eight-block tower (Fig. 2-2) Dumps raisins from bottle following demonstration Turns pages in book one at a time	May walk up stairs by self, two feet on each step Able to walk backward Able to kick ball	Parallel play demonstrated Pulls people to show them something Increased independence from mother	Has vocabulary of 300 words Uses two- or three-word phrases Uses pronouns *I, you* Uses first name Refers to self by name
30 months (2½ years)	Able to build eight-block tower Scribbling techniques continue Feeding self with increased neatness Dumps raisins from bottle spontaneously	Able to jump from object Walking becomes more stable; wide-base gait decreases Throws ball overhanded	Separates easily from mother In play, helps put things away In toileting, only needs help to wipe Begins to notice sex differences	Gives first and last name Uses plurals Refers to self by appropriate pronoun Names one color

The developmental tasks for preschoolers as described by Duvall and Miller are listed in Box 2-3 on p. 18. A summary of the expected development including fine and gross motor, social-adaptive, and language behaviors of preschoolers is found in Table 2-6 on p. 18.

Assessment tools focus on readiness for school and social assessment (see Table 2-4).

School-Age Children

The beginning of school is a developmental landmark for children. Entering school brings a new influential environment into children's lives. Information about concepts, life, and interpersonal relationships expands beyond the confines of the family home. Teacher and peer influences may be noticed in school-age children's reactions and behavior. The school-age period lasts from approximately 6 to 12 years of age.

Physical Growth The growth continues at a slow pace, with about a 5-pound weight gain and 2-inch height increase per year. Growth rates for boys and girls are similar until the growth spurt starts between the ages of 10 and 12 years. By age 8 or 9 there is increased smoothness and speed in motor control, making the child more agile and graceful. Bone replaces cartilage and continues to ossify. Bones of the face and jaw grow at a faster rate than they have in previous years. The school-age child is slimmer, with less body fat and a lower center of gravity. Eyes and hands are well coordinated, and muscles are stronger and more developed. These changes in growth facilitate fine motor activities such as drawing, needlework, and playing musical instruments,

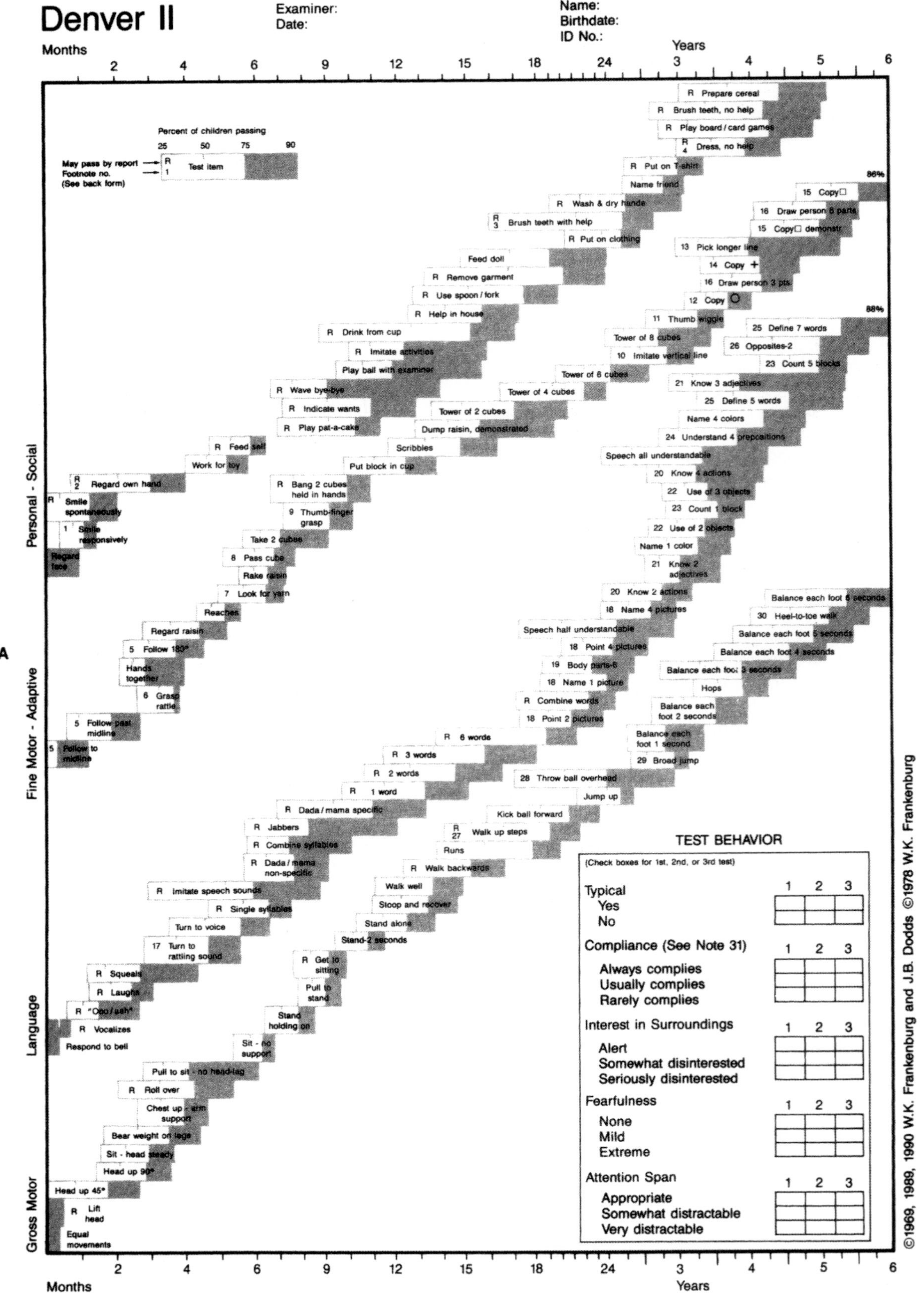

Fig. 2-3 Denver II. (From Frankenburg et al, 1992.)

DIRECTIONS FOR ADMINISTRATION

1. Try to get child to smile by smiling, talking or waving. Do not touch him/her.
2. Child must stare at hand several seconds.
3. Parent may help guide toothbrush and put toothpaste on brush.
4. Child does not have to be able to tie shoes or button/zip in the back.
5. Move yarn slowly in an arc from one side to the other, about 8" above child's face.
6. Pass if child grasps rattle when it is touched to the backs or tips of fingers.
7. Pass if child tries to see where yarn went. Yarn should be dropped quickly from sight from tester's hand without arm movement.
8. Child must transfer cube from hand to hand without help of body, mouth, or table.
9. Pass if child picks up raisin with any part of thumb and finger.
10. Line can vary only 30 degrees or less from tester's line.
11. Make a fist with thumb pointing upward and wiggle only the thumb. Pass if child imitates and does not move any fingers other than the thumb.

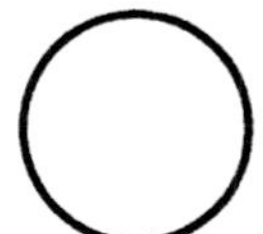

12. Pass any enclosed form. Fail continuous round motions.

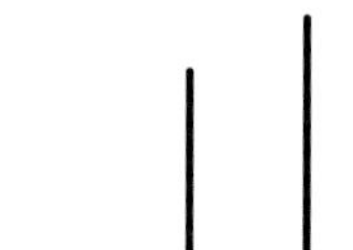

13. Which line is longer? (Not bigger.) Turn paper upside down and repeat. (pass 3 of 3 or 5 of 6)

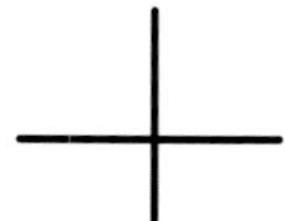

14. Pass any lines crossing near midpoint.

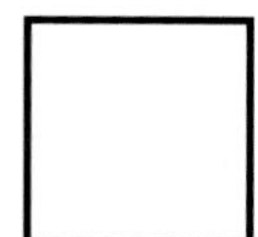

15. Have child copy first. If failed, demonstrate.

When giving items 12, 14, and 15, do not name the forms. Do not demonstrate 12 and 14.

16. When scoring, each pair (2 arms, 2 legs, etc.) counts as one part.
17. Place one cube in cup and shake gently near child's ear, but out of sight. Repeat for other ear.

B

18. Point to picture and have child name it. (No credit is given for sounds only.)
    If less than 4 pictures are named correctly, have child point to picture as each is named by tester.

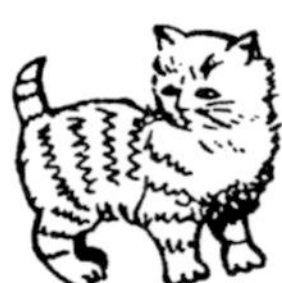
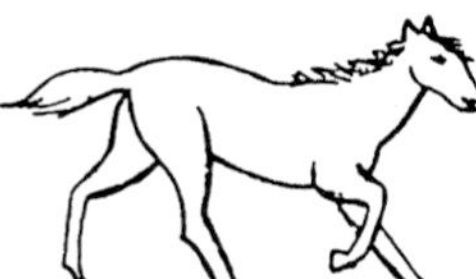
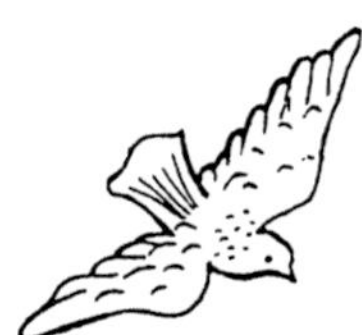
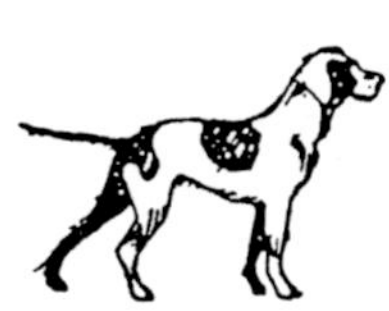
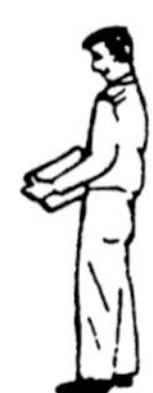

19. Using doll, tell child: Show me the nose, eyes, ears, mouth, hands, feet, tummy, hair. Pass 6 of 8.
20. Using pictures, ask child: Which one flies?... says meow?... talks?... barks?... gallops? Pass 2 of 5, 4 of 5.
21. Ask child: What do you do when you are cold?... tired?... hungry? Pass 2 of 3, 3 of 3.
22. Ask child: What do you do with a cup? What is a chair used for? What is a pencil used for? Action words must be included in answers.
23. Pass if child correctly places and says how many blocks are on paper. (1, 5).
24. Tell child: Put block **on** table; **under** table; **in front of** me, **behind** me. Pass 4 of 4. (Do not help child by pointing, moving head or eyes.)
25. Ask child: What is a ball?... lake?... desk?... house?... banana?... curtain?... fence?... ceiling? Pass if defined in terms of use, shape, what it is made of, or general category (such as banana is fruit, not just yellow). Pass 5 of 8, 7 of 8.
26. Ask child: If a horse is big, a mouse is __? If fire is hot, ice is __? If the sun shines during the day, the moon shines during the __? Pass 2 of 3.
27. Child may use wall or rail only, not person. May not crawl.
28. Child must throw ball overhand 3 feet to within arm's reach of tester.
29. Child must perform standing broad jump over width of test sheet (8 1/2 inches).
30. Tell child to walk forward, → heel within 1 inch of toe. Tester may demonstrate. Child must walk 4 consecutive steps.
31. In the second year, half of normal children are non-compliant.

OBSERVATIONS:

Fig. 2-3, cont'd Denver II.

Box 2-3 Developmental Tasks of Preschoolers

- Settling into healthy daily routines
  - Enjoying a variety of active play
  - Being more flexible and capable of accepting change
  - Mastering good eating habits
  - Mastering the basics of toilet training
  - Developing physical skills
- Becoming a participating member of the family
  - Assuming responsibility within the family
  - Giving and receiving affection and gifts freely
  - Identifying with the parent of the same sex
  - Developing an ability to share parents with others
  - Recognizing the family's unique ways
- Beginning to master impulses and to conform to expectations of others
  - Outgrowing impulsivity
  - Learning to share, take turns, enjoy companionship
  - Developing sympathy and cooperation
  - Adopting situationally appropriate behavior
- Developing healthy emotional expressions
  - Acting out feelings during play
  - Delaying gratification
  - Expressing hostility/making up
  - Discriminating between a variety of emotions, feelings
- Learning to communicate effectively with others
  - Developing a vocabulary and speech ability
  - Learning to listen, follow directions, increase attention span
  - Acquiring social skills that allow more comfortable interactions with others
- Developing ability to handle potentially dangerous situations
  - Respecting potential hazards
  - Effectively using caution and safety practices
  - Being able to accept assistance when needed
- Learning to be autonomous with initiative and a conscience of his or her own
  - Becoming increasingly responsible
  - Taking initiative to be involved in situations
  - Internalizing expectations, demands of family and culture
  - Being self-sufficient for stage of development
- Laying foundation for understanding the meaning of life
  - Developing gender awareness
  - Trying to understand the nature of the physical world
  - Accepting religious faith of parents, learning about spirituality

Data from Duvall EM, Miller BC: *Marriage and family development,* ed 6, New York, 1985, Harper & Row.

Table 2-6 Expected Development of Preschoolers

AGE	FINE MOTOR	GROSS MOTOR	SOCIAL-ADAPTIVE	LANGUAGE
36 months (3 years)	Can unbutton front buttons (Fig. 2-4) Copies vertical lines within 30° Copies zero Begins to use fork	Walks up stairs, alternating feet on steps Walks down stairs, two feet on each step Pedals tricycle Jumps in place Able to perform broad jump	Dresses self with help with back buttons Pulls on shoes Parallel play Able to share toys	Vocabulary of 900 words Uses complete sentences Constantly asks questions
48 months (4 years)	Able to copy plus sign (+) Picks longer line three out of three times Uses scissors Can lace shoes	Walks down stairs, alternating feet on steps Able to button large front buttons Able to balance on one foot for approximately 5 seconds Catches ball	Play is associative Imaginary friend is common Boasts and tattles Selfish, impatient, rebellious	Gives first and last name Has 1500-word vocabulary Uses words without knowing meaning Questioning is at a peak
60 months (5 years)	Able to dress self with minimal assistance Able to draw three-part human figure Draws square (■) following demonstration Colors within lines	Hops on one foot Catches ball bounced to him or her two out of three times Able to demonstrate heel-toe walking Jumps rope	Eager to follow rules Less rebellious Relies on outside authority to control the world	Has 2100-word vocabulary Recognizes three colors Asks meanings of words Uses sentences of six to eight words

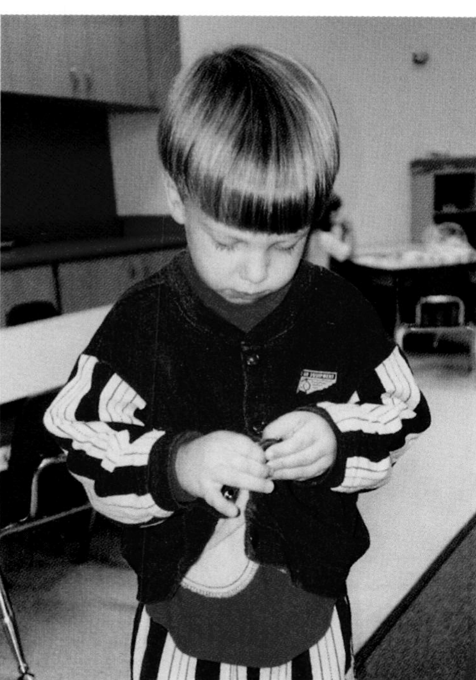

Fig. 2-4 Preschooler develops the ability to help dress self.

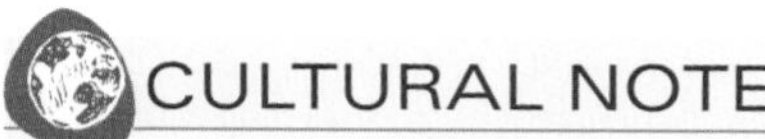

CULTURAL NOTE

There are height variations among children of different races. Asian children are the shortest with Hispanic children being the next taller group. African Americans and whites are the tallest group with Native Americans being as tall or a little shorter.

African-American children achieve their growth earlier than whites. White boys match with their African-American counterparts by age 9 or 10 years, whereas white girls match by age 14 or 15 years.

Within the same racial group, obese children tend to be taller than slim children. Children from lower socioeconomic status tend to be shorter than children from high socioeconomic status (Dewey et al, 1986; Hamill, Johnston, Lemeshow, 1973; Lin, 1992; Malina, Zavaleta, Little, 1987. In Seidel et al, 1999.)

CULTURAL NOTE

Mexican-American children tend to have higher weight-for-height ratio than the average American child. By contrast Chinese and Southeast Asian children often are in the tenth percentile on the National Center for Health Statistics (NCHS) growth curves.

Body weight variations may be due to differences in bone density and musculature of the race rather than body fat. Asian and African-American children usually are the lightest, followed by white children, Native American children, and then Mexican-American children (Ryan et al, 1990; Strauss, 1993. In Seidel et al, 1999.)

Box 2-4 Developmental Tasks of School-Age Children

- Learning the basic skills required for school (Fig. 2-5)
  - Mastering reading and writing
  - Developing reflective thinking
  - Mastering physical skills
- Mastering money management
  - Obtaining money through socially acceptable ways
  - Buying wisely
  - Saving
  - Delaying gratification
  - Understanding role of money and place in life
- Becoming an active and cooperative member of the family
  - Participating in family discussions
  - Joining in family decision making
  - Being responsible for household chores
  - Participating in reciprocal gift giving
- Extending abilities to relate to others
  - Asserting rights
  - Developing leadership skills
  - Following social mores and customs
  - Cooperating in group situations
  - Maintaining close friendships
- Managing feelings and impulses
  - Coping with frustrations
  - Managing anger appropriately
  - Expressing feelings in the right time, place, and manner and to the right person
- Identifying the sex and gender role
  - Differentiating expectations based on gender
  - Understanding reproduction and gender-specific physical development
  - Managing physical growth spurts
  - Conceptualizing life as a mature man or woman
- Identifying self as worthy individual
  - Gaining status and respect
  - Growing in self-esteem and self-confidence
  - Establishing unique identity
- Developing conscience and morality
  - Determining right from wrong
  - Developing moral-guided control over behavior
  - Learning to live according to identified values

Data from Duvall EM, Miller BC: *Marriage and family development*, ed 6, New York, 1985, Harper & Row.

and gross motor activities such as jumping, biking, and swimming. By age 12 the rest of the teeth (except the wisdom teeth) erupt.

Behavioral and Cognitive Development

The psychosocial crisis for this age is industry versus inferiority. Interactions with children and teachers at school broaden children's social contacts. Industry influences a desire to achieve. They learn how to compete and how to cooperate with others. School relationships provide social sup-

Box 2-5 Preventive Services Recommended From Birth to 10 Years of Age*

SCREENING

Periodic height and weight measurements
Hemoglobinopathy screen at birth
Phenylalanine level at birth
T_4 (thyroxine) and/or thyroid-stimulating hormone (TSH) level at birth
Blood pressure with a cuff from age 3 years
Vision screen by age 3 years

COUNSELING

Injury Prevention

Child safety seats for children less than 5 years of age
Lap-shoulder belts at 5 years and older
Bicycle helmet; avoid bicycling near traffic
Smoke detector, flame-retardant sleepwear
Hot water heater temperature less than 120° to 130° F (49° to 54° C)
Window and stair guards, pool fences
Safe storage of drugs, toxic substances, firearms, and matches
Syrup of ipecac, poison control numbers
Cardiopulmonary resuscitation (CPR) training for parents and caretakers

Diet and Exercise

Breast-feeding, iron-enriched formula and foods (infants and toddlers)
Limit fat and cholesterol; maintain caloric balance; emphasize grain, fruits, vegetables (ages 2 to 10)

Substance Use

Effects of passive smoke
Antitobacco message

DENTAL HEALTH

Regular visits to dental care provider
Floss, brush with fluoride toothpaste daily
Advice about baby-bottle tooth decay

IMMUNIZATIONS (See Table 2-7)

CHEMOPROPHYLAXIS

Ocular antibiotic prophylaxis at birth

Data from Report of the U.S. Preventive Services Task Force: *Guide to clinical preventive services,* ed 2, Baltimore, Maryland, 1996, Williams & Wilkins.
*The U.S. Preventive Services Task Force recommended interventions—screening tests, counseling interventions, immunizations, and chemoprophylactic regimens—for the prevention of more than 80 target conditions. The clients who receive these services are asymptomatic individuals of all age groups and risk categories. The recommendations are based on a standardized review of current scientific evidence.

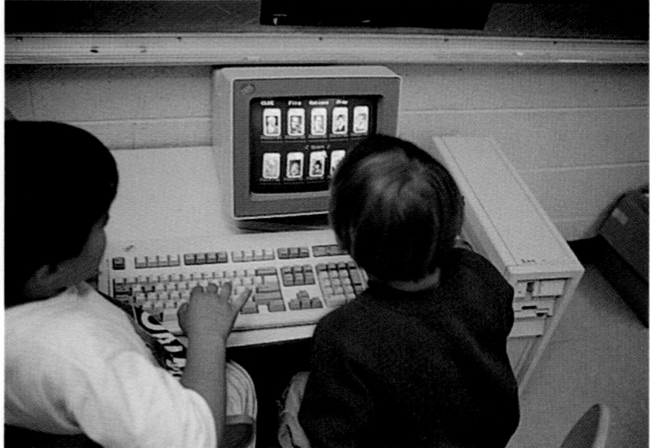

Fig. 2-5 School-age children learn the basic skills required for school.

port outside the home environment, and peer approval becomes important. Inferiority develops when children sense failure in meeting expectations set by self and others. Concrete operations is the level of cognitive development described by Piaget when children learn inductive reasoning and logical operations. In school they learn to use numbers, to read, and to classify. By the time children enter school, their development of fine and gross motor, social-adaptive, and language skills changes more gradually. The focus of assessment changes to identifying the accomplishment of developmental tasks. Tasks for the school-age child are listed in Box 2-4. Preventive services recommended for individuals from birth to 10 years of age are listed in Box 2-5.

Assessment tools for school-age children focus on mental abilities and social and emotional behaviors. Table 2-4 lists selected tools to use with this age group.

ADOLESCENTS

The hallmark of adolescence is puberty, which marks the end of childhood and the onset of adulthood. Adolescence occurs from approximately 12 to 13 years of age to 17 to 18 years of age.

Physical Growth The growth spurt that occurs during puberty is highly variable and accounts for 20% to 25% of the final adult height. Growth frequently occurs during spring and summer months. The normal girl grows from 2 to 4½ inches (5.1 to 11.4 cm), and the normal boy grows from 2 to 5 inches (5.1 to 12.7 cm). This height is accompanied by an increase in weight. The normal girl will increase in weight by 10 to 23 lb (4.5 kg to 10.4 kg), whereas the weight of the normal boy will increase from 12½ to 29 lb (5.7 to 13.2 kg). The growth in girls occurs 18 to 24 months before that in boys, but the average weight gain for boys is 4½ lb (2 kg) per year more than for girls (Neinstein, 1991).

Table 2-7 Recommended Immunization Schedule Through the Life Span[a]

RECOMMENDED AGE[b]	IMMUNIZATIONS[c]	COMMENTS
INFANTS		
Birth	HBV[d]	
1-2 months	HBV[d]	
2 months	DTaP, Hib, IPV	DTaP and IPV can be initiated as early as 4 weeks after birth in areas of high endemicity or during outbreaks. DTaP is the preferred vaccine for all doses of the vaccination series, including completion of the series in children who have received one or more doses of whole-cell DTP.
4 months	DTaP, Hib, IPV	Interval of 2 months (minimum of 6 weeks) is recommended for IPV.
6 months	DTaP, Hib[g]	
6-18 months	HBV,[d] IPV	
TODDLERS		
12-15 months	Hib, MMR	MMR should be given at 12 months of age in high-risk areas; if indicated, Mantoux skin test for tuberculosis may be done at the same visit.
12-18 months	DTaP, Var[f]	The fourth dose (DTaP or DPT) may be administered as early as 12 months of age, provided 6 months have elapsed since the third dose and the child is unlikely to return at age 15 to 18 months.
PRESCHOOLERS		
4-6 years	DTaP, IPV, MMR	MMR is recommended at this age but may be given at any visit provided that at least 1 month has elapsed since the receipt of the first dose and that both doses are given beginning at or after 12 months of age.
SCHOOL-AGE CHILDREN		
11-12 years	MMR, Var	MMR is given if child did not receive between ages 4 and 6 years. Varicella is given if child is susceptible to chickenpox.
ADOLESCENTS		
14-16 years	Td	Repeat every 10 years.
EARLY ADULTHOOD		
20-25 years	Td, PPV	Repeat Td every 10 years. PPV recommended for Alaskan natives and certain Native Americans in adulthood.
MIDDLE ADULTHOOD		
35-65 years	Td	Repeat every 10 years.
OLDER ADULT		
65 years and older	Td, PPV, influenza	Repeat Td booster every 10 years. Clients previously immunized with PPV should receive a dose when they turn 65 if 5 years or more have passed since the first dose. Influenza should be given annually.

Data from www.aap.org/family/parents/immunize.htm (aap *American Academy Pediatrics*), 1999; and Zanca J: Adult vaccines: who should get what, and when? *Newsletter of the Office of Minority Health, U.S. Department of Health and Human Services: closing the gap,* p13, November 1998.

[a]Table is not completely consistent with all package inserts. For products used, also consult manufacturer's package insert for instruction on storage, handling, dosage, and administration. Biologics prepared by different manufacturers vary, and package inserts of the same manufacturer may change from time to time. Therefore the practitioner should be aware of the content of the current package insert.

[b]These recommended ages should not be construed as absolute. For example, 2 months can be 6 to 10 weeks. However, MMR usually should not be given to children younger than 12 months. If measles vaccination is indicated, monovalent measles vaccine is recommended and the MMR should be given subsequently at 12 to 15 months.

[c]Vaccine abbreviations: HBV, hepatitis B virus vaccine; DTaP, diphtheria and tetanus toxoids and acellular pertussis vaccine; Hib, *Haemophilus influenzae* type b conjugate vaccine; IPV, inactivated poliovirus vaccine; MMR, measles, mumps, and rubella virus vaccine live; Td, adult tetanus toxoid (full dose) and diphtheria toxoid (reduced dose) for children older than 7 years and adults; PPV, pneumococcal pneumonia vaccine.

[d]An acceptable alternative to minimize the number of visits for immunizing infants of hepatitis B surface antigen (HBsAg)-negative mothers is to administer dose 1 at birth to 2 months, dose 2 at 4 months, and dose 3 at 6 to 18 months.

[e]Dose 3 of Hib is not indicated if the product for doses 1 and 2 was PedvaxHIB (PRP-OMP).

[f]Susceptible children may receive varicella vaccine (Var) at any visit after the first birthday, and those who lack a reliable history of chickenpox should be immunized during the 11-to-12-year-old visit. Susceptible children 13 years of age or older should receive two doses at least 1 month apart.

Table 2-7 Children Not Immunized in the First Year of Life in the United States—cont'd

RECOMMENDED TIME OR AGE	IMMUNIZATION(S)[g,h]	COMMENTS
YOUNGER THAN 7 YEARS		
First visit	DTaP, Hib, HBV, MMR, IPV	If indicated, Mantoux skin test for tuberculosis may be done at same visit. If child is 5 years of age or older, Hib is not indicated.
Interval After First Visit		
1 month	DTaP, HBV	IPV may be given if accelerated poliomyelitis vaccination is necessary, such as for travelers to areas where polio is endemic.
2 months	DTaP, Hib, IPV	Second dose of Hib is indicated only in children whose first dose was received when younger than 15 months.
≧8 months	DTaP, HBV	IPV is not given if the third dose was given earlier.
4-6 years (at or before school entry)	DTaP or IPV	DTaP is not necessary if the fourth dose was given after fourth birthday; IPV is not necessary if the third dose was given after the fourth birthday.
11-12 years	MMR	Give at entry to middle or junior high school.
10 years later	Td	Repeat every 10 years throughout life.
7 YEARS AND OLDER		
First visit	HBV,[i] IPV,[j] MMR,[k] Td	
Interval After First Visit		
2 months	HBV, IPV, Td	IPV may also be given 1 month after the first visit if accelerated poliomyelitis vaccination is necessary.
8-14 months	HBV, IPV, Td	OPV or IPV is not given if the third dose was given earlier.
11-12 years	MMR	Give at entry to middle or junior high school.
10 years later	Td	Repeat every 10 years throughout life.

Data from Wong DL et al: *Whaley and Wong's Nursing care of infants and children,* ed 6, St Louis, 1999, Mosby www.aap.org/family/parents/immunize.htm.

[g]If all needed vaccines cannot be administered simultaneously, priority should be given to protecting the child against those diseases that pose the greatest immediate risk. In the United States these diseases for children younger than 2 years usually are measles and *H. influenzae* type b infection; for children older than 7 years, they are measles, mumps, and rubella (MMR).

[h]DTaP, HBV, Hib, MMR, and IPV can be given simultaneously at separate sites if the client's return for future immunizations is a concern.

[i]Priority should be given to hepatitis B immunization for adolescents.

[j]If person is 18 years or older, routine poliovirus vaccination (IPV) is not indicated in the United States.

[k]Minimum interval between doses of MMR is 1 month.

Behavioral and Cognitive Development

The psychosocial crisis at this age is described as identity versus role confusion. The adolescent reviews the learning, experiences, and values accepted in earlier stages and modifies them into a unique and personalized identity. During this identity clarification process, the adolescent may decide that previously accepted ideas and beliefs need to be changed. Adolescents may behave in new and different ways, much to the chagrin of their parents, as they "try on" differing roles and values. The adolescent begins testing and evaluating previously accepted notions about life, living, spirituality, relating, and being, some of which come from influence of peers (Fig. 2-6). The early values of the child often are the accepted values from the parental authority in the family. Role confusion develops for adolescents who are unsuccessful in developing their own identity. They may develop low self-esteem, poor to no direction in their lives, and have difficulty making career choices.

Formal operations is the term Piaget gave to the adolescent years. Adolescents are able to perform abstract reasoning and form logical conclusions. They are able to form hypotheses and devise ways to test them. Their analytic skills are used in making judgments about their actions and future lives. Advanced intellectual skills allow them to reexamine accepted ideas, which can be a strain within the family but leads to a stronger sense of self and independence. Developmental tasks for the teen years include those listed in Box 2-6.

Assessment tools for this age group focus on social and emotional behaviors, in addition to identifying and reducing stress. A list of selected tools is found in Table 2-4.

Box 2-6 Developmental Tasks of Adolescents

- Accepting physical changes
  - Coming to terms with physical maturation
  - Accepting one's own body
- Achieving a satisfying and socially accepted role
  - Learning masculine/feminine role
  - Realistic understanding of gender role
  - Adopting acceptable practices
- Developing more mature peer relationships
  - Being accepted by peer group (Fig. 2-6)
  - Making and keeping friends of both sexes
  - Dating
  - Loving and being loved
  - Adapting to variety of peer associations
  - Developing skills in managing and evaluating peer relationships
- Achieving emotional independence
  - Outgrowing childish parental dependence
  - Developing mature affection for parents
  - Being autonomous
  - Developing mature interdependence
- Getting an education
  - Acquiring basic knowledge and skills
  - Clarifying sex-role attitudes toward work and family roles
- Preparing for marriage and family life
  - Formulating sex-role attitudes
  - Enjoying responsibilities
  - Developing responsible attitudes
  - Distinguishing between infatuation and mature love
  - Developing mutually satisfying personal relationships
- Developing knowledge and skills for civic competence
  - Communicating as a citizen
  - Becoming involved in causes outside oneself
  - Acquiring problem-solving skills
  - Developing social concepts
- Establishing one's identity as a socially responsible person
  - Developing philosophy of life
  - Implementing worthy ideals and standards
  - Assuming social obligations
  - Adopting mature sense of values and ethics
  - Dealing effectively with emotional responses

Data from Duvall EM, Miller BC: *Marriage and family development,* ed 6, New York, 1985, Harper & Row.

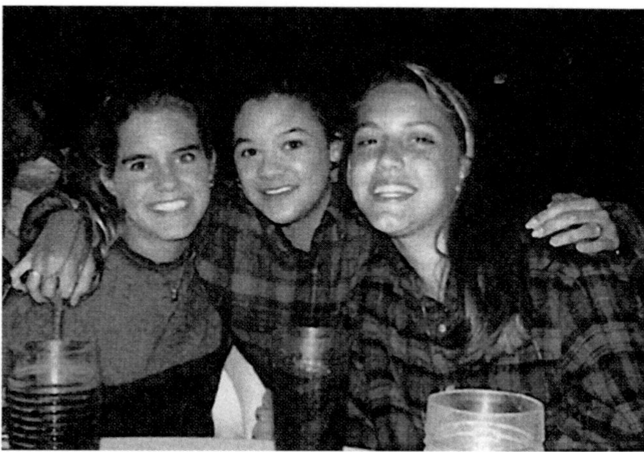

Fig. 2-6 The peer group is a major influence in adolescent development. (From Wong et al, 1999.)

ADULTS

Early Adulthood

Young adults (approximately 20 to 35 years of age) are at the height of physical and cognitive capabilities. The psychologic crisis at this time is intimacy versus isolation. These individuals begin to express their identity through work, recreation, and interpersonal relationships. Adults move away from the dependent role in the family of origin to establishing their own lifestyle. Productivity, self-sufficiency, and intimacy in love relationships are driving tasks for adults, even though adults may shift back and forth in career choices, commitment, and goals as they continually define and redefine a definition of self. The young adult is ready to enter the adult world and assume a position as a responsible citizen. Achievements are the result of self-direction, with goals changing as a result of reevaluation. Mature relationships with others are important in both the work and home environments. Many young adults choose to marry and start a family. Role confusion may develop when young adults have difficulty moving from adolescence and their dependence on parents or family to developing their own identity and adult role responsibilities. The developmental tasks listed in Box 2-7 are those usually accomplished during this stage. Preventive services recommended for individuals from 11 to 24 years are listed in Box 2-8.

The focus of assessment for young adults is on career choice and mate selection.

Career Choice Many assessment tool inventories have been developed for the young adult contemplating career choices. In these inventories, basic interest areas are compared with occupational themes. The inventory responses will cluster similar interest areas and relate them to an occupation or vocational choice. Stability in interest areas is important to the predictive power of the inventory. If an individual has many, varied interests, then the inventory scores may be less reliable and less valid. Career assessment inventories are commonly used by college-bound students, placement and selection agencies, and individuals uncertain of a career choice or those planning a career change (see Table 2-4).

Mate Selection Along with career choice, mate selection is a primary interest area for many individuals in early adulthood. The field of premarital and couple counseling has rapidly expanded since the 1940s, along with the increasing divorce rate in America. Various tools have been used to try to give couples a prediction of potential areas of conflict and mismatching in their relationship. Tools range from diagnostic ratings, inventories, and checklists to personal or couple interviews, questionnaires, and even games (see Table 2-4).

Box 2-7 Developmental Tasks of Young Adults

- Establishing one's autonomy as an individual
- Planning a direction for one's life
- Getting an appropriate education
- Working toward a vocation
- Appraising love and sexual feelings
- Becoming involved in love relationships
- Selecting a mate
- Getting engaged
- Being married

Data from Duvall EM, Miller BC: *Marriage and family development,* ed 6, New York, 1985, Harper & Row.

Middle Adulthood

Entry into the middle years, between ages 35 and 65, may be met with the feeling that one's best years have passed, especially in light of today's emphasis on youth.

Physical Growth There are obvious physical signs of aging, such as wrinkling of the skin, graying or loss of hair, and changes in muscle tone and mass. Changes in vision and hearing may affect social relationships and learning unless corrective actions are taken.

Behavioral and Cognitive Development During this time many decisions have been made concerning career, partner, children, lifestyle, and living arrangements. The psychosocial crisis at this time is generativity versus stagnation. For persons who have successfully met the developmental tasks of earlier stages, this can be a period of stability, self-understanding, and self-actualization. For others this is the time of the midlife crisis, when they feel life is stagnant or incomplete. Frustration drives them to search for new directions and goals in life. During middle age one reaps the benefits of career success, support of family and friends, and experiences of earlier years. With intro-

Box 2-8 Preventive Services Recommended for Individuals From 11 to 24 Years of Age

SCREENING

Height and weight
Blood pressure
Papanicolaou (Pap) test
Chlamydia screen
Rubella serologic tests or vaccination
Assessment for problem drinking

COUNSELING

Injury Prevention

Lap-shoulder belts
Bicycle, motorcycle, all-terrain vehicle (ATV) helmets
Smoke detector
Safe storage or removal of firearms

Substance Abuse

Avoid tobacco use
Avoid underage drinking and illicit drug use
Avoid alcohol and drug use while driving, swimming, boating, etc.

Sexual Behavior

Sexually transmitted disease prevention: abstinence; avoid high-risk behavior; use condoms and/or female barrier with spermicide
Unintended pregnancy: contraception

Diet and Exercise

Limit fat and cholesterol; maintain caloric balance; emphasize grains, fruits, vegetables
Adequate calcium intake (females)
Regular physical activity

Dental Health

Regular visits to dental care provider
Floss, brush with fluoride toothpaste daily

IMMUNIZATIONS (See Table 2-7)

CHEMOPROPHYLAXIS

Multivitamin with folic acid (females planning or capable of pregnancy)

Data from Report of the U.S. Preventive Services Task Force: *Guide to clinical preventive services,* ed 2, Baltimore, Maryland, 1996, Williams & Wilkins.

spection common to this period, wisdom is nurtured. There is an appreciation that there is more to life than the goals set in one's youth and a desire to be an integral part of one's society. New levels of development emerge as one gains a deeper level of self-understanding and self-comfort.

Box 2-9 Developmental Tasks of Middle Adults

- Providing a comfortable and healthful home
- Allocating resources to provide security in later years
- Division of household responsibilities
- Encouragement of both husband and wife roles within and beyond the family
- Maintaining emotional and sexual intimacy
- Incorporating all family members into family circle as family enlarges, and caring for extended family
- Participating in activities outside the home
- Developing competencies that maintain family functioning during crises and encourage achievement

Data from Duvall EM, Miller BC: *Marriage and family development,* ed 6, New York, 1985, Harper & Row.

Most middle-age adults are an integral part of a family. Changes for adults affect not only themselves but also members of their family. Although many adults experience personal struggles as they progress through this stage, most adults meet normal developmental challenges without a crisis.

Despite conflicting research on intellectual changes, the middle years are productive years, with energy directed at maintaining a home, relationships, and work.

Developmental tasks for this stage include those listed in Box 2-9.

Preventive services recommended for individuals from 25 to 64 years of age are listed in Box 2-10.

As the middle-age adult is concerned with life achievements, many of the assessment tools used in this age group focus on career, home, and personal satisfaction with life (see Table 2-4).

Older Adulthood

The later years, beginning with age 65, are for most adults productive years met with a sense of pleasure and enjoyment. Older adults represent the fastest growing population in the United States, and probably the least understood. They are a very diverse group.

Physical Growth Though there are many physical changes that accompany aging, most older adults are active

Box 2-10 Preventive Services Recommended For Individuals From 25 to 64 Years of Age

SCREENING

Blood pressure
Height and weight
Total blood cholesterol level (men age 35 to 64, women age 45 to 64)
Papanicolaou (Pap) test
Fecal occult blood test and/or sigmoidoscopy (men and women over 50)
Mammogram and clinical breast examination (women 50 to 69)
Rubella serologic tests or vaccination history (women of childbearing age)

COUNSELING

Substance Use

Tobacco cessation
Avoid alcohol or drug use while driving, swimming, boating, etc.

Diet and Exercise

Limit fat and cholesterol; maintain caloric balance; emphasize grains, fruits, vegetables
Adequate calcium intake (women)
Regular physical exercise

Injury Prevention

Lap-shoulder belts
Motorcycle, bicycle, all-terrain vehicle (ATV) helmets
Smoke detector
Safe storage or removal of firearms

Sexual Behavior

Sexually transmitted disease prevention: avoid high-risk behavior; use condoms and/or female barrier with spermicide
Unintended pregnancy: contraception

Dental Health

Regular visits to dental care provider
Floss, brush with fluoride toothpaste daily

IMMUNIZATIONS (See Table 2-7)

CHEMOPROPHYLAXIS

Multivitamin with folic acid (women planning or capable of pregnancy)
Discuss hormone prophylaxis (perimenopausal and postmenopausal women)

Data from Report of the U.S. Preventive Services Task Force: *Guide to clinical preventive services,* ed 2, Baltimore, Maryland, 1996, Williams & Wilkins.

Box 2-11 Developmental Tasks of Older Adults

- Making satisfying living arrangements
- Adjusting to retirement
- Establishing comfortable routines
- Maintaining physical and mental health
- Maintaining love, sex, and marital relations
- Remaining in touch with other family members
- Keeping active
- Finding the meaning in life

Data from Duvall EM, Miller BC: *Marriage and family development,* ed 6, New York, 1985, Harper & Row.

members of society and have independent lifestyles. Chronic health problems are common but usually can be managed.

Behavioral and Cognitive Development

The psychosocial crisis at this time is ego integrity versus despair. Despair may develop with the loss of one's spouse or the adjustment related to retirement. Society is becoming more aware of the presence of ageism and stereotyping against a person due to age. The growing number of older Americans has in itself encouraged society to better understand the needs and concerns of this stage of development. In addition, older adults are encouraging positive attitudes about aging and making society aware of the developmental tasks they experience and the barriers to leading a healthy, happy life in a society that values youth. Ego integrity develops as older adults give back to society and as they interact with grandchildren.

Cognitive development in the old-old adult has been studied. In a longitudinal study of subjects ranging from 73 to 99 years of age, researchers found that although many subjects reported some decline in abilities, more than half displayed no decline. A study of 18 people ages 100 to 106 found that these centenarians reported rich late-life learning experiences, the majority of which occurred through social interaction (Merriam and Caffarella, 1999).

Developmental tasks for the aging adult have been summarized in Box 2-11.

The lengthy time span for this age group is divided in several ways. Lueckenotte (2000) describes young-old from ages 65 to 74, middle-old from ages 75 to 84, and old-old as 85 years and older. Separate tasks with different age groupings are identified (Box 2-12). Preventive services recommended for individuals 65 years of age and older are listed in Box 2-13.

As with earlier adult stages, previously discussed tools may be used to assess the adult of later years. However, in the past 10 years there has been an increased focus on geriatric assessment and issues more specific to the later years of life (see Table 2-4). Community resources for the older adult warrant assessment, exploration, and evaluation.

Box 2-12 Developmental Tasks of Young-Old and Old-Old Adults

YOUNG-OLD (APPROXIMATELY 65 TO 85 YEARS)

- Preparing for and adjusting to retirement
- Adjusting to lower and fixed income of retirement
- Establishing physical living arrangements
- Adjusting to new relationships with adult children and their offspring
- Managing leisure time
- Adjusting to slower physical and intellectual responses
- Dealing with death of parents, spouse, and friends

OLD-OLD (APPROXIMATELY OVER 85 YEARS)

- Learning to combine new dependency needs with continued need for independence
- Adapting to living alone
- Accepting and adjusting to possible institutional living
- Establishing affiliation with age group
- Adjusting to increased vulnerability to physical and emotional stress
- Adjusting to loss of physical strength, illness, and approach of one's own death
- Adjusting to losses of spouse, home, and friends

Data from Brown M: *Readings in gerontology,* St. Louis, 1984, Mosby.

FAMILY DEVELOPMENT AND ASSESSMENT

Most individuals in America grow up within the social unit of a family. However, the definition and composition of family structures have changed dramatically over the past several years. Families are no longer traditionally two married heterosexual parents with children who live under one roof. Blended families are composed of stepchildren and children from the current unit. Homosexual couples join as family units, some of which include children. There are single-parent families: some from divorce, some never married, and some formed because of adoption or artificial fertilization. There are also intergenerational families in which multiple generations live together under one roof or in which grandparents or even great-grandparents raise and care for their grandchildren. Thus defining and understanding the contemporary family is a complex challenge. For our purposes, a family shall be defined as two or more individuals who share bonds of commitment, loyalty, and affection. The family unit typically shares some degree of time, financial and physical resources, and responsibilities for the unit maintenance.

Duvall and Miller (1985) define the functions and task of the family unit through stages for the traditional family of the past, that is, the two-parent, married, heterosexual couple with children, in Table 2-8.

Box 2-13 Preventive Services Recommended For Individuals Age 65 and Older

SCREENING

Blood pressure
Height and weight
Fecal occult blood test and/or sigmoidoscopy
Mammogram and clinical breast examination (women under 69)
Papanicolaou (Pap) test (women)
Vision screening
Assessment for hearing impairment
Assessment for problem drinking

COUNSELING

Substance Use

Tobacco cessation
Avoid alcohol or drug use while driving, swimming, boating, etc.

Diet and Exercise

Limit fat and cholesterol; maintain caloric balance; emphasize grains, fruits, vegetables
Adequate calcium intake (women)
Regular physical activity

Injury Prevention

Lap-shoulder belts
Motorcycle and bicycle ATV helmets
Fall prevention
Safe storage or removal of firearms
Smoke detector
Set hot water heater to less than 120° to 130° F (49° to 54° C)
Cardiopulmonary resuscitation (CPR) training for household members

Dental Health

Regular visits to dental care provider
Floss, brush with fluoride toothpaste daily

Sexual Behavior

Sexually transmitted disease prevention: avoid high-risk sexual behavior; use condoms

IMMUNIZATIONS (See Table 2-7)

CHEMOPROPHYLAXIS

Discuss hormone prophylaxis (perimenopausal and postmenopausal women)

Data from Report of the U.S. Preventive Services Task Force: *Guide to clinical preventive services,* ed 2, Baltimore, Maryland, 1996, Williams & Wilkins.

Nonnuclear or nontraditional families within American culture form a growing population that has been studied by Visher and Visher (1979). They note that in adoptive families the children sustained a primary relationship loss with both biologic parents, but usually the household was composed of an adult heterosexual couple. In foster families, the children also sustained a primary relationship loss with a biologic parent, and the household usually had an adult couple serving as head of household. However, in foster families there may be children who are members of more than one household, and the adults in the family may have minimal or even no legal relationship with the foster children.

In stepfamilies, a biologic parent lives elsewhere, and the children commonly move between the homes of two biologic families. Virtually all members of a stepfamily sustain primary relationship loss. The parent and stepparents must repeatedly deal with a part-time relationship with the stepchild if the stepchild is involved with the other biologic parent. The relationship between the adult parents outside of the stepfamily predates the new marriage and the relationship with the stepparent. This can create conflicts and loyalty divisions in parenting strategies and with the child. Children within a stepfamily struggle with being members of more than one household, while stepparents cope with parenting a child to whom they are not related.

Single-parent families are rising in number because of the increasing divorce rate in America and the decreasing social stigma related to unwed mothers. In single-parent families the child lives with one biologic parent. Both the child and the single parent sustain a loss from the absent biologic parent of the child. There is great variation in the involvement of the absent parent of the child; some are actively involved with the child, whereas others have minimal to no involvement. Other children may be added to the single-parent family from the same or different biologic parentage. Financial difficulties are the most noted stressor for single-parent families as only one adult is present to care for the children, care for the home, and provide for the family.

Assessment tools for families focus on structure and function, social environment, interrelationships among members, and identifying and reducing family stress. Selected tools are listed in Table 2-4.

SUMMARY

The growth and development of an individual throughout the life cycle is unique. Despite that uniqueness, commonalities form the basis of understanding psychosocial stages of development throughout life. From that knowledge, tools have been designed to assess both individuals and the family structures in which they are nurtured. Objective assessment can be used to determine whether an individual is progressing within an acceptable range of development, is atrisk for developmental delays, or is experiencing developmental delays. The family can be assessed for style of func-

Table 2-8 Developmental Tasks of the Family

STAGES	THEMES
Married couple	Without children; establishing satisfying marriage; adjusting to pregnancy; fitting into kin network
Childbearing	Oldest child birth to 30 months; nurturing infants; establishing home
Family with preschoolers	Oldest child 2½ to 6; adapting to needs of children; decreased energy and privacy as parents
Family with school-age children	Oldest child 6 to 13; being part of community of school-age families; encouraging educational achievement of children
Family with teenagers	Oldest child 13 to 20; balancing freedom and responsibility; establishing postparental interests
Family launching young adults	First child gone until last child's leaving home; maintaining supportive home base
Middle-age parents	Empty nest to retirement; refocusing on marriage; maintaining kin ties
Aging family members	Retirement to death of both spouses; coping with bereavement; adapting home for aging; adjusting to retirement; living alone

Data from Duvall EM, Miller BC: *Marriage and family development,* ed 6, New York, 1985, Harper & Row.

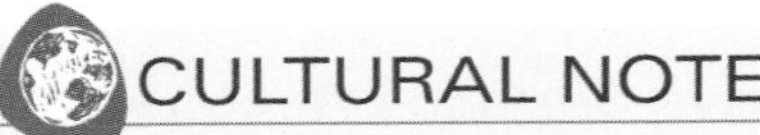

CULTURAL NOTE

Family size and structure vary by racial group. For example, 46% of African-American families are headed by a female. Asian Americans tend to have large families (e.g., Cambodians, Laotians, and Vietnamese average five people per family). Japanese are exceptions with an average of three people per family.

Chinese emphasize loyalty to family and devotion to tradition. A hierarchical structure is common in which older children have authority over young ones. For the Eskimo the family is important for survival in the harsh Arctic environment. The family size is traditionally four people. The foundation of the Mexican family is the nuclear family, and it is the most significant social organization. Marriage and family are the foundation of Navajo life. In the Navajo society women are expected not to achieve more than their husbands (Giger and Davidhizar, 1995).

ioning and success in meeting family tasks. A wide range of assessment instruments is available, with new instruments being developed yearly. Table 2-4 gives a brief summary of the assessment tools discussed in this chapter. The challenge is to identify an appropriate tool for the situation, to determine the level of expertise needed for administration and data interpretation, to use data to most effectively promote psychosocial development, and to be knowledgeable about community resources for both professional assessment and implementation of intervention strategies. Results of assessment can be used to maintain family or individual development or to plan active interventions. Early intervention, at its best, can promote optimal development of healthy individuals and families.

CLINICAL APPLICATION and CRITICAL THINKING

CRITICAL THINKING QUESTIONS

Developmental tasks of the family, as described by Duvall and Miller, are based on the "traditional family" (two-parent married heterosexual couple with children). However, many families do not fall into this description. Consider and answer the following two questions for each type of family: (a) How do these families differ from the "traditional" family? (b) Do the Duvall and Miller developmental tasks of the family apply?

1. Blended families
2. Single-parent families
3. Intergenerational families
4. Foster families

CASE STUDY 3

Mrs. Mildred Cobb is a 78-year-old woman who is brought to the geriatric clinic by her son and daughter-in-law. Mrs. Cobb's son tells the examiner that his father died 5 months ago, and ever since then his mother has "gone downhill." Mr. Cobb indicates that his mother is no longer keeping her house clean or cooking appropriate meals. Also, her personal

hygiene habits have dramatically changed. She has lost interest in getting her hair done, and she no longer likes to get dressed for the day. Mr. Cobb tells the examiner, "When I suggest a retirement home, she becomes very angry and tells me to mind my own business. I am just worried about Mom, and I want to make sure she is well cared for." During this conversation Mrs. Cobb sits quietly. She interjects only to say, "I have taken care of you, your brother, and your father. Now all of a sudden you think I am helpless and want to lock me away." Mrs. Cobb appears clean, although her hair is matted and her clothes are badly wrinkled and do not match. Her speech is clear, but her overall affect is very dull. She does not make eye contact with her son or the examiner. A physical examination demonstrates normal bodily functioning consistent with her age group.

1. List the interview data described in the case study.
2. List the examination data described in the case study.
3. Which of Erikson's developmental stages is Mrs. Cobb experiencing?
4. Based on what is known from the interview, which developmental tasks of older adults may Mrs. Cobb be struggling with?
5. What additional assessment or focus of assessment is needed?
6. What developmental assessment tools should be considered?

REMEMBER to check out your companion CD-ROM

3 Ethnic and Cultural Considerations

www.mosby.com/MERLIN/wilson/assessment/

The world is becoming one global village. Ethnic and cultural heritage binds groups together through shared values, beliefs, and practices. However, different ethnic and cultural heritages also separate groups and can make them enemies based on these differences (Geissler, 1998). We are indeed a land of many colors, many heritages, and many histories. With this diversity come many challenges. As a health care professional, you are challenged with the responsibility to work with and care for individuals who may not have the same skin color, language, health practices, beliefs, and values as your own. When this occurs, the goal is not to force the client and his or her family to comply with your beliefs, values, and health practices but instead to meet the client where he or she is and to work with his or her belief and value system. The challenge occurs not when the client is of the same heritage and speaks the same language as the nurse, but when the cultures and languages are different. Consider the following scenario:

> You are caring for a 72-year-old Hispanic woman, Rosa Martinez, who speaks Spanish as her primary language. Conversing in broken English, she tells you that she has injured her lower back and now has continuing aches and stiffness. She does not want to be at the clinic but is here because her daughter forced her to come. She says that she hasn't seen a physician in years because Maria, her *cuerandera,* takes good care of her. When you inquire whether she has seen Maria for her back, she replies yes and then goes on to tell you that Maria had given her an herbal formula to take internally and had made herbal poultices to use at home. The client tells you that she believes that these remedies are working and she is not sure why her daughter made her come to the clinic.

The nurse caring for Mrs. Martinez is potentially challenged by three issues: (1) the language barrier; (2) an alternative health care provider, Maria the *cuerandera,* in whom Mrs. Martinez has much confidence; and (3) the use of alternative folk remedies—the herbal formulas and poultices. How the nurse interacts with this client and her family will depend partly on the nurse's own heritage and culture and partly on her knowledge of and attitude toward other cultures and other cultural health beliefs and practices.

As health care professionals we are each challenged to be as knowledgeable as possible about the health beliefs, practices, and values of cultural and racial groups other than our own. An individual may be from one of the major racial and cultural groups, such as American Indian, African American, Asian, white American, or Hispanic, or one of the often unrecognized cultural groups, such as the homeless, migrant workers, gay men, or lesbians. Each group has special needs, special values, and possibly different beliefs that may affect the type of health care that is sought, needed, and, most important, understood as affecting the client's health. Because the racial and cultural diversity among us is so great, we cannot know the health beliefs, practices, and cultural values of all groups. "It isn't a realistic expectation that we should know all the customs and courtesies of all cultures" (Rosemary Prentice in Lester, 1998). To improve cultural awareness and sensitivity, however, we can ask the questions to gather information about the unique beliefs and value systems of people of other cultures and backgrounds. Improving cultural awareness requires several steps. First, develop a sensitivity to the differences between your own culture and the client's; second, don't stereotype; third, learn the facts; and fourth, develop a template that may be used for cultural assessment of the client and the family.

BECOME CULTURALLY COMPETENT

Culturally competent care is defined as care that is sensitive to issues related to culture, race, gender, and sexual orientation (American Academy of Nursing Expert Panel Report, 1992). One model of cultural competence has four components that are listed here separately but that occur simultaneously. The first is the affective component of cultural awareness that is developed by appreciating and being sensitive to the values, beliefs, life ways, and problem-solving practices of a client's culture. The second is the cognitive component, when you read and interview others about world views, beliefs, practices, lifestyles, and problem-solving strategies. The third is a psychomotor component called cultural skill, when you use systematic cultural assessment tools to collect data about your clients. The final component is cultural encounter, when you engage in cross-cultural interactions with clients of diverse backgrounds (Campinha-Bacote, Yahle, and Langenkamp, 1996).

To begin to become culturally competent you must do the following*:

1. Recognize that cultural diversity exists.
2. Recognize the uniqueness of and demonstrate respect for individuals and families of cultures other than your own (Fig. 3-1).
3. Respect the unfamiliar.
4. Identify and explore your own cultural beliefs.
5. Recognize that some cultural groups have definitions of health and illness that may differ from your own.

*Modified from Seidel et al, 1999.

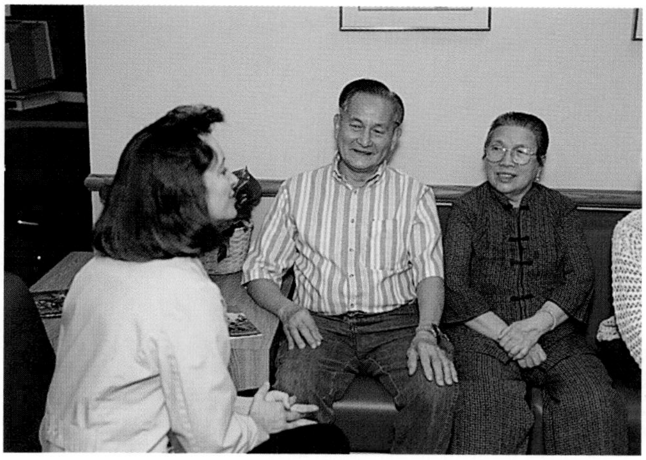

Fig. 3-1 It is important to develop a sensitivity to the differences between your own culture and that of clients from another culture.

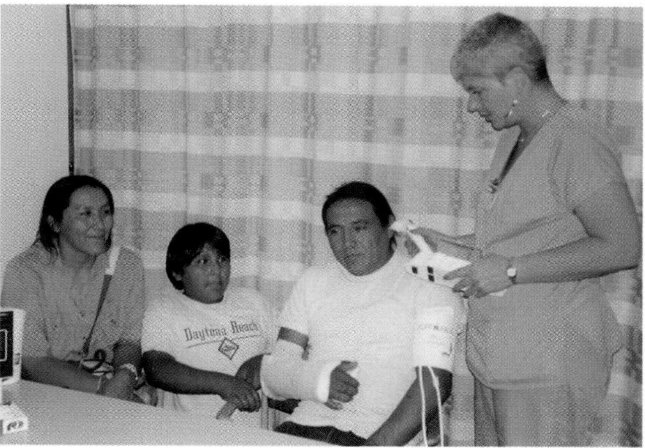

Fig. 3-2 Recognize that some cultural groups maintain health and healing practices that may be different from your own.

6. Recognize that some cultural groups maintain health and healing practices that may be different from your own (Fig. 3-2).
7. Be willing to modify health care delivery to be more congruent with the client's cultural background.
8. Recognize the cultural diversity and uniqueness of individuals within a recognized cultural group.
9. Recognize and appreciate that each person's cultural values are ingrained and therefore very difficult to change.

DON'T STEREOTYPE

Every individual on this earth is unique. Regardless of a person's skin color, physical features, cultural heritage, or social group, realize that individual's uniqueness. Cultural heritage plays an important part in helping to identify the individual's "roots" and perhaps helps to explain attitudes, beliefs, and health practices, but each major cultural group is made up of unique individuals and families who may have values and attitudes that differ from the cultural norm. Don't assume that because individuals or families are Asian or Pacific Islander that they all share culturally similar beliefs. For example, within the Asian or Pacific Islander people are Chinese, Filipino, Japanese, Asian Indian, Korean, Vietnamese, Cambodian, Thai, Bangladeshi, Burmese, Indonesian, Malayan, Laotian, Kampuchean, Pakistani, Sri Lankan, Hawaiian, Samoan, Tongon, Tahitian, Palauan, Fijian, and Northern Mariana Islanders, and each of these groups has a unique heritage and set of beliefs.

Personal beliefs and knowledge about other cultures in the United States have been influenced by stereotyped images and misinformation presented through the media, educational and political institutions, and family beliefs. Some common misbeliefs and stereotyped images include the following:

- All African Americans have large families.
- All African Americans and Hispanics are on welfare.
- All welfare recipients are minorities.
- The color black connotes evil; the color white connotes goodness and purity.
- All Asians excel in math and science.
- All American Indians are alcoholics.
- All American Indians are supported by the government.
- All Hispanics speak Spanish.

If you learn nothing else from this text, learn that we are all unique individuals deserving of a unique and personalized assessment of our beliefs, our values, and our culture.

LEARN THE FACTS

In addition to the just-mentioned thesis that every individual is unique and should be respected accordingly, facts about five major cultural groups provide background information from which the nurse can work (Table 3-1). Religious beliefs concerning health care are presented in Table 3-2 on pp. 42-43. Box 3-1 on p. 44 lists the treatments for "hot" and "cold" conditions used to reestablish harmony and balance. Although these tables provide information about major cultural groups and religions, remember that there are numerous other groups who share different beliefs and practices. A cultural assessment should be completed for all clients (Campinha-Bacote et al, 1996). By performing cultural assessments, nurses and other health care providers learn about clients' unique cultures and the cultures' influences on them.

DEVELOP A TEMPLATE FOR ASSESSMENT

When assessing the client and family, it is important to include a direct assessment of the client's health beliefs and practices that may reflect his or her cultural heritage. Knowing the risks of stereotyping, perform a focused interview that will provide information about the client's personal beliefs, values, and attitudes.

Introductory Questions

Where were you born?
With what particular cultural group do you identify?

Text continued on p. 44

Table 3-1 Facts About Major Cultural Groups

	AFRICAN AMERICAN	HISPANIC/MEXICAN	ASIAN/PACIFIC ISLANDER	AMERICAN INDIAN/ ALASKAN NATIVE	WHITE AMERICAN
DEMOGRAPHIC TRENDS	In 1998 African Americans made up 12.8% of the U.S. population, and are the single largest minority group in the country. There were 34,598,000 African Americans in the United States in 1996. As a group they are young (over 41% are under age 29), urban (80%), and female (53%). Over 45% of the families are headed by females with no spouse present, compared with 12.7% for all races. The proportion of African Americans below the poverty level was 23.6% in 1996, compared with 13.7% for all races In 1997 the median family income for this group was $28,602 compared with $42,300 for all races.	Hispanics, including Mexicans, Puerto Ricans, Cubans, and persons from Central and South America, make up 11% of the U.S. population, which makes them the second largest minority. There were 29,703,000 Hispanics in this country in 1997. The Hispanic population is young, with 40% under the age of 19 years. The percentage of families below the poverty level was 29.4% in 1997. Most Hispanics live in urban areas. The five states in which Hispanics are more than 10% of the total state population are New Mexico, Texas, California, Arizona, and Colorado. The median family income for Hispanics in 1996 was $26,178.	Asians and Pacific Islanders make up 3.7% of the U.S. population and are the fastest-growing minority in this country. In 1997 there were 10,071,000 Asians and Pacific Islanders. There are over 20 categories for Asians and Pacific Islanders. About 30% are under the age of 19 years. In 1997, 9.9% of the families were headed by females with no spouse present. In 1996, 14.5% of Asians/Pacific Islanders lived below the poverty level. According to 1997 data, 95% of Asian Americans lived in metropolitan areas, compared with 75% of the general population. The majority of the Asian Americans in the United States live in California. The median family income for Asian Americans in 1997 was $49,105.	American Indians and Alaskan natives are a diverse group of people from varied cultural backgrounds. More than 500 tribal groups are recognized by the federal government. In 1990 the number of American Indians/Alaskan natives was 1,931,391, or 0.78% of the entire U.S. population. The American Indian and Alaskan native population served by the Indian Health Service is young (30% below the age of 15), and is growing at a rate of almost 3% per year. Almost 26% of all American Indian and Alaskan native households are headed by women. The number of Indians living below the poverty level in 1990 was 31% with higher levels among the Navajo, 49%, and Sioux, 44%. In 1990 the median family income was $21,619. Before 1940, 90% of Indians lived on reservations, but by 1980 more than 50% lived in urban areas.	In 1997, there were 191,791,000 white Americans, who made up 71.8% of the U.S. population. One third of the white population was under the age of 24 years. In 1997 8.9% of families were headed by females with no spouse present. The percentage of whites living below the poverty level was 6.3% in 1997. According to 1998 data, 79% of whites live in metropolitan areas. The mean household income for whites in 1997 was $47,023.

				The average family has between four and five members, which makes it the largest family size of any minority or nonminority group.	
EDUCATION AND EMPLOYMENT	The percentage of African Americans completing high school is 87% and college is 15%. Unemployment rate for African Americans in 1996 was 13.1% compared with 5.9% for all races.	The percentage of Hispanics completing high school is 54.7% and college is 10.3%. The unemployment rate for Hispanic males was 9.2% in 1996.	The percentage of Asian Americans completing high school is 84.9% and college is 42.2%. The unemployment rate for Asian Americans in 1997 was 5.1%.	The proportion of American Indians and Alaskan natives finishing college is less than half that of all races in the United States, and the unemployment rate is twice as high as all other combined races. The unemployment rate for Indian males was 16.2% in 1990.	The percentage of whites completing high school is 88% and college is 22%. The unemployment rate for whites in 1997 was 4.5%.
HEALTH CARE UTILIZATION	In 1994 about 52% of African Americans under the age of 65 had private health insurance, 24.5% had Medicaid, and 21.5% had no health insurance. For those over 65 years, 42.4% had Medicare and private health insurance, 15% had Medicare and Medicaid, and 34.5% had Medicaid only. A greater percentage of African Americans use hospital clinics and emergency departments as their usual source of care than any other single racial group.	In 1994 about 49% of Hispanics under the age of 65 had private health insurance, 17.4% had Medicaid, and 33.5% had no health insurance. For those over 65 years, 49% had Medicare and private health insurance, 19.5% had Medicare and Medicaid, and 23% had Medicaid only. Hispanics who had no health insurance often used public clinics and emergency departments for care.	Asian/Pacific Islanders make visits to physicians less frequently than other ethnic groups. Those Asian Americans over 65 years of age visit the physician half as often as their white counterparts. Asian/Pacific Islanders are more likely to visit pediatricians and obstetricians and less likely to visit surgeons and psychiatrists than other ethnic groups.	Since 1955, the U.S. Public Health Service through its Indian Health Service (IHS) has been responsible for providing comprehensive health service to American Indians and Alaskan natives. In 1995 it is estimated that the IHS provided care for 1.37 million American Indians and Alaskans, or 70% of all Indians. The remainder usually seek care by other private and public health service providers. Care provided by the IHS is given at no cost to the individual clients.	In 1992, 72.3% of whites had private health insurance, 5.0% had Medicaid, and 17% had no health insurance. For those over 65 years, 78.8% had Medicare and private health insurance, 4.4% had Medicare and private health insurance, 4.4% had Medicare and Medicaid, and 13% had Medicaid only.

Demographic data from www.census.gov/population; health statistics from U.S. Department of Health and Human Services: *Health—United States 1995,* DHHS Pub No (PHS) 96-1232, Hyattsville, Md, 1996, ________; additional data from Seidel HM et al: *Mosby's guide to physical examination,* ed 4, St. Louis, 1999, Mosby; www.IHS.gov, 1999; Wong DL et al: *Whaley and Wong's nursing care of infants and children,* ed 6, St. Louis, 1999. Mosby.

Table 3-1 Facts About Major Cultural Groups—cont'd

	AFRICAN AMERICAN	HISPANIC/MEXICAN	ASIAN/PACIFIC ISLANDER	AMERICAN INDIAN/ ALASKAN NATIVE	WHITE AMERICAN
HEALTH CARE UTILIZATION—cont'd				Although medical care is available at no cost via the IHS hospitals and clinics, many Indians live in remote areas where the availability of physicians is half the national average.	
GENERAL HEALTH STATUS	The life expectancy for African-American males is 64.4 years and females is 73.7 years.	Good data about Hispanics are lacking because the national reporting systems often do not list Hispanics as an ethnic group separate from other whites.	The health status of Asian Americans as a group is good. They have a longer life expectancy than whites.	Life expectancy for American Indians and Alaskan natives is 73.2 years, compared to the U.S. expectancy of 75.4 years for all races.	Life expectancy for white men is 73.1 years and for women, 79.5 years.
Illness Patterns	The top 10 causes of death among African Americans, in descending order, are as follows: • Heart disease (#1 men, #1 women) • Malignant neoplasms (#2 men, #2 women) The three most common cancers of African-American males are prostate, lung and bronchus, and colorectal; and for women the most common cancers are breast, colorectal, and lung and bronchus.	Hispanic women are less likely to use any contraceptive than any other minority groups. This puts them at higher risk for pregnancy and sexually transmitted diseases, including HIV. The top 10 causes of death among Hispanics and Mexican Americans, in descending order, are as follows: • Heart disease (#1 men, #1 women) • Malignant neoplasms (#2 men, #2 women)	The top 10 causes of death among Asians and Pacific Islanders, in descending order, are as follows: • Heart diseases (#1 men, #2 women) • Malignant neoplasms (#2 men, #1 women) • Cerebrovascular disease (#3 men, #3 women) • Unintentional injuries (#4 men, #4 women) • Pneumonia and influenza (#5 men, #5 women)	The top 10 causes of death among Native Americans, in descending order, are as follows: • Heart diseases (#1 men, #1 women) • Unintentional injuries (#2 men, #3 women) • Malignant neoplasms (#3 men, #2 women) • Chronic liver disease and cirrhosis (#4 men, #6 women) • Suicide (#5 men, #10 women) • Pneumonia and influenza (#6 men, #7 women)	The top 10 causes of death among white Americans, in descending order, are as follows: • Heart diseases (#1 men, #1 women) • Malignant neoplasms (#2 men, #2 women) • Cerebrovascular disease (#3 men, #3 women) • Chronic obstructive pulmonary disease (#4 men, #4 women) • Unintentional injuries (#5 men, #6 women)

	• Homicide and legal intervention (#3 men, #10 women) African-American males between the ages of 15 and 44 are the highest risk group to be victims of homicide. The lifetime risk of becoming a homicide victim is 1 in 21 for them. • Human immunodeficiency virus (HIV) infection (#4 men, #7 women) • Unintentional injury (#5 men, #5 women) • Cerebrovascular disease (#6 men, #3 women) • Pneumonia and influenza (#7 men, #6 women) • Chronic obstructive pulmonary disease (#8 men, #9 women) • Diabetes mellitus (#9 men, #4 women) African-American women have the highest mortality associated with diabetes at 72.2/100,000. • Conditions in the perinatal period (#10 men, #7 women)	• Unintentional injuries (#3 men, #5 women) • HIV infection (#4 men, #9 women) • Homicide and legal intervention (#5 men) • Cerebrovascular disease (#6 men, #3 women) • Chronic liver disease and cirrhosis (#7 men) • Suicide (#8 men) • Diabetes mellitus (#9 men, #4 women) • Pneumonia and influenza (#10 men, #6 women) • Chronic obstructive pulmonary disease (#7 women) • Conditions originating in the perinatal period (#8 women) • Congenital anomalies (#10 women)	• Chronic obstructive pulmonary disease (#6 men, #7 women) • Homicide and legal intervention (#7 men, #10 women) • Suicide (#8 men, #8 women) • Diabetes mellitus (#9 men, #6 women) • HIV infection (#10 men) • Congenital anomalies (#9 women) Southeast Asian refugees have a higher incidence of intestinal parasites, positive tuberculin test, and presence of hepatitis B antigens and have anemia more often than other Asian Americans and whites in general.	• Cerebrovascular disease (#7 men, #5 women) • Diabetes (#8 men, #4 women) • Homicide and legal interventions (#9 men) • Chronic obstructive pulmonary disease (#10 men, #8 women) • Nephritis, nephrotic syndrome, and nephrosis (#9 women) The more full-blooded the American Indian or Alaskan native, the more likely it is that the individual will manifest type 2 diabetes, with the same manifestations and vascular complications as in non-Indians.	• Pneumonia and influenza (#6 men, #5 women) • Suicide (#7 men) • HIV infection (#8 men) • Diabetes mellitus (#9 men, #7 women) • Conditions originating in the perinatal period (#10 men, #8 women) • Atherosclerosis (#8 women) • Nephritis, nephrotic syndrome, and nephrosis (#9 women) • Septicemia (#10 women)

Demographic data from www.census.gov/population; health statistics from U.S. Department of Health and Human Services: *Health—United States 1995,* DHHS Pub No (PHS) 96-1232, Hyattsville, Md, 1996, ________; additional data from Seidel HM et al: *Mosby's guide to physical examination,* ed 4, St. Louis, 1999, Mosby; www.IHS.gov, 1999; Wong DL: *Whaley and Wong's nursing care of infants and children,* ed 6, St. Louis, 1999, Mosby.

Table 3-1 Facts About Major Cultural Groups—cont'd

	AFRICAN AMERICAN	HISPANIC/MEXICAN	ASIAN/PACIFIC ISLANDER	AMERICAN INDIAN/ ALASKAN NATIVE	WHITE AMERICAN
Births	The birth rate for African-American females under the age 18 was 10.8% in 1993. The rate of low infant birth weights for African-American females is 16.4% compared with 8.6% for all races The rate of African-American women who smoked while pregnant is 12.7%. The infant mortality rate is 16.6 per 1000 live births, and the maternal mortality rate is 20 per 1000 deliveries.	The birth rate for Hispanic females under the age 18 is 7.2%. The rate of low infant birth weight for Mexican-American females is 5.8%. Infant mortality rate was 71 per 1000 live births in 1991.	The percent of live births to Asians or Pacific Islanders under age 18 is 2.1%. The percentage of low infant birth weights is 6.4%. The rate of women from this group who smoked while pregnant is 4.3%. The infant mortality rate in 1991 was 5.8 per 1000 live births.	The rate of low infant births was 7.6% in 1993. The infant mortality rate in 1991 was 13.3 per 1,000 live births. Maternal mortality among Indians is 12% higher than in the population in general.	The birth rate for whites under age 18 is 4.0%. The rate of low infant birth weights for whites was 7.1% in 1993. The rate of whites who smoked while pregnant is 16.8%. The infant mortality rate of whites is 7.1 per 1000 live births.
Lifestyle	The rate of African Americans over age 18 who smoke is 33.2% for men and 19.8% for women. The rate of obesity for African-American men is 32.9% and for women, 49.6%. The rate of high serum cholesterol level (200 mg/dl) for African-American men is 16.1% and for women, 19.7%. The rate of hypertension for African-American men is 37.4% and for women, 31%.	The rate of obesity for Mexican-American males is 35.4% and for females, 47.3%. The rate of high serum cholesterol for Mexican-American males is 16.9% and for females, 15.7%. The rate of hypertension for Mexican-American males is 18.6% and for females, 14.7%.			The rate of whites over age 18 who smoke is 27% for males and 23.7% for women. The rate of obesity for white men is 32.3% and for women, 32.6%. The rate of high cholesterol level (>200 mg/dl) for white men is 19.1% and for women, 20.2%. The rate of hypertension for white men is 25.1% and for women, 18.3%.

HEALTH BELIEFS	Illness may be classified as *natural* (forces of nature) or *unnatural* (evil influences such as witchcraft, voodoo or hex). Some African Americans may believe that serious illness has been sent by God as punishment. Because of this, they may resist health care.	Health beliefs often have a strong religious association. Body balance is a major cause of illness, especially imbalances between *caliente* (hot) and *frio* (cold). Some Hispanics and Mexican Americans believe that good health is the result of "good luck," which is the reward for good behavior. Illness may be seen as punishment from God for wrongdoing, or from forces of nature and the supernatural. Illness may be prevented by eating the proper foods, working the proper amount of time, wearing religious medals or amulets, and sleeping with relics at home.	*Chinese* believe that a healthy body is a gift from the parents and should be cared for. Health is a result of the forces that rule the world: yin (cold) and yang (hot). Illness results when there is an imbalance. *Chi* is innate energy, and the lack of *chi* results in fatigue, poor constitution, and long illness. *Vietnamese* also believe in *yin* and *yang*. Health results from harmony and balance with existing universal order, harmony attained by pleasing good spirits and avoiding evil ones. There are many rituals to prevent illness and to prevent the wrath of evil spirits. *Japanese* have the religious influence of Shinto, which is that humans are inherently good and that evil is caused by outside spirits. Illness is caused by contact with polluting agents, such as bad blood, corpses, or skin diseases. *Filipinos* believe that God's will and supernatural forces govern	Health is a state of harmony with nature and the universe. Illness indicates that there is disharmony, which may be because of a supernatural force. Violation of a restriction or prohibition is thought to cause illness. Many American Indians and Alaskan natives fear witchcraft and may carry objects to protect themselves from witchcraft. Theology and medicine are strongly interwoven.	White Americans believe illness has a cause-and-effect relationship. Illness can be caused by an unhealthy lifestyle, microorganisms, or injury; it is a consequence of an unhealthy lifestyle. Thus, health can be maintained if they eat a healthy diet, exercise, drink alcohol in moderation if at all, and reduce stress when needed. Some religions believe illness is punishment for sins committed.

Demographic data from www.census.gov/population; health statistics from U.S. Department of Health and Human Services: *Health—United States 1995,* DHHS Pub No (PHS) 96-1232, Hyattsville, Md, 1996, ________; additional data from Seidel HM et al: *Mosby's guide to physical examination,* ed 4, St. Louis, 1999, Mosby; www.IHS.gov, 1999; Wong DL: *Whaley and Wong's nursing care of infants and children,* ed 6, St. Louis, 1999, Mosby.

Table 3-1 Facts About Major Cultural Groups—cont'd

	AFRICAN AMERICAN	HISPANIC/MEXICAN	ASIAN/PACIFIC ISLANDER	AMERICAN INDIAN/ ALASKAN NATIVE	WHITE AMERICAN
HEALTH BELIEFS—cont'd			the universe. Illness, injuries, and other misfortunes are God's punishment for violations of His will. Yin and yang balances and imbalances cause health and illness.		
Health Practices	Self-care and folk remedies are quite prevalent. Many folk therapies may have a religious origin. Because of inadequate health insurance and lack of a regular health care provider, it is common for some African Americans to attempt home remedies first and not seek help until the illness is serious. It is more likely that the individual will seek care from the "old lady" (a woman in the community with knowledge of herbs or other remedies), a "spiritualist" (one who received the gift for healing from God), the "priest" (a most powerful voodoo priest or priestess), or the "root doctor" (a healer who uses herbs, oils, candles, and ointments).	To deal with severe illness, Hispanics may often make promises, visit shrines, offer medals and candles, and offer prayers.	*Chinese* believe that the goal of health care is to restore yin and yang. Treatments may include acupuncture, acupressure, tai chi, moxibustion (the application of heat to the skin), or medicinal herbs, They are likely to go to a wide variety of folk healers from herbalists, spiritual healers, or temple healers to fortune healers. *Vietnamese* will use all possible means before seeking care from outside agencies or health providers. Fortune-tellers determine the event that caused the illness. They may pray at the temple to obtain divine instruction about what to do during an illness. They may use special diets to prevent illness and promote health.	Many American Indians and Alaskan natives seek medical care from a medicine person, an altruistic person who must use his or her powers in conjunction with herbs and rituals in a purely positive way to heal the individual. The medicine healer may use negative force powers to act against the sick person's enemies. One type of medicine healer is the diviner-diagnostician, who may diagnose the problem but who does not have the powers or skills to implement medical treatment. Some medicine healers use herbs and curative but nonsacred medical procedures. Others cure by the power of song and the laying on of hands, with powers obtained from supernatural beings.	Health care is believed to be a right, rather than a privilege. When whites have a minor illness, they attempt to treat it with over-the-counter remedies or alternative medicines such as herbs. When these remedies fail or the illness is more serious and they have access to health care, they make an appointment with their health care provider, who may be a doctor, nurse practitioner, physician assistant, or chiropractor. Those who do not have health insurance use the emergency departments or public clinics for health care.

			Japanese remove evil and illness by purification. Treatments may include acupuncture, acupressure, massage, and moxibustion along affected meridians. Most Japanese use a combination of Asian and Western healing methods, including *Kampō* medicine, which is the use of natural herbs. The family is viewed as the party responsible for caring for the ill and disabled. *Filipinos* may use amulets as a shield from witchcraft or as a good-luck charm. Religious medals may also be used.		
Family Relationships	There is often a strong kinship that bonds family members. The family will come together at a time of crisis. They are less likely to view illness as a burden than other groups. When necessary, there is sex-role sharing among parents.	Family is very important. The family has a strong kinship and may include *compadres* (godparents), who are established by ritual kinship. Older family members and parents are respected. If elders become ill, they are usually cared for at home. Children are highly valued, very desired, and seen as a gift from	*Chinese* have strong extended families and have loyalty to the young and the old. Respect for elders is taught at an early age. The behavior of children is a reflection on the family. Males are valued more highly than females; women are submissive to men in the family. *Japanese* believe that the family provides the	The family is an extended family, which includes relatives from both sides. Elder members assume the leadership.	The two-parent nuclear family is declining among whites. High mobility of families locates adults away from their parents and the grandparents of their children. The high divorce rate has created many single-parent families and blended families in which two adults marry for a second time and merge their children

Demographic data from www.census.gov/population; health statistics from U.S. Department of Health and Human Services: *Health—United States 1995,* DHHS Pub No (PHS) 96-1232, Hyattsville, Md, 1996, ________; additional data from Seidel HM et al: *Mosby's guide to physical examination,* ed 4, St. Louis, 1999, Mosby; www.IHS.gov, 1999; Wong DL: *Whaley and Wong's nursing care of infants and children,* ed 6, St. Louis, 1999, Mosby.

Table 3-1 Facts About Major Cultural Groups—cont'd

	AFRICAN AMERICAN	HISPANIC/MEXICAN	ASIAN/PACIFIC ISLANDER	AMERICAN INDIAN/ ALASKAN NATIVE	WHITE AMERICAN
Family Relationships—cont'd		God. They are usually taken everywhere with the family. Children are taught to obey and to respect the parents. The home often has a shrine area, which contains statues and pictures of saints. The family is usually large and home centered, which is the core of their existence. The father is the decision maker and the provider. The wife and children are subordinate.	anchor. They tend to keep problems within the family. They value self-control and self-sufficiency. The concept of *haji* (shame) imposes strong control. The behavior of the children reflects on the family. *Vietnamese* also believe that the family is the central anchor. Many families are multigenerational, with the elders receiving great respect. Men are the decision makers, and women are taught to be submissive. Individual needs and interests are subordinate to those of the family. Although children are highly valued, they are expected to respect their parents.		into a new family. With the increase in working parents, children spend time in day care where others care for them. In other families children spend time at home after school unsupervised when parents are working.
Communication	African Americans are alert to any evidence of discrimination. Often importance is placed on nonverbal behavior. Because of distrust, there may be "testing" behaviors to assess health care providers before seeking care. The best approach by health care providers is to be simple and direct, but caring.	Many Hispanics are bilingual, speaking both English and Spanish. In some areas of the country, the language may be primarily Spanish. Many Hispanics have a strong preference to speak their native tongue and may show no eagerness to learn or speak English.	*Chinese* believe that the open expression of emotions is unacceptable. *Japanese* may also suppress their emotions. When they do not know what to do or what is wanted of them, they may wait silently for direction. *Vietnamese* may avoid direct eye contact as a sign of respect. They	Most American Indians and Alaskan natives are bilingual, speaking both English and their native tongue. Nonverbal communication and respect are very important. Making eye contact may be considered invasive during a conversation.	English is the primary language of whites and they expect everyone to speak it. Few whites are bilingual. Whites make eye contact when talking and use body language and facial expressions as a part of their communication. Some people show their emotions and others work hard to hide them.

			may hesitate to ask questions because asking questions may be considered impolite. *Haitians* may prefer family/friends to act as translators and confidants. They may smile and nod in agreement when they do not understand. Their quiet and gentle communication style and lack of assertiveness may lead the health care provider to falsely believe that they comprehend even when they do not.		
Other Comments	There may be a high level of caution and distrust of majority groups. A history of humiliation, oppression, and loss of dignity may cause some African Americans to express or demonstrate feelings of social anxiety. If the African American's values are compromised, he or she will most likely retain dignity rather than seek care or follow the advice of a health care provider. The African-American minister is a strong influence in the African-American community and a valued resource to the ill individual. About 9% of nursing students are African American.	Hispanics show a high degree of modesty, which is often a deterrent to seeking medical care. They have a relaxed concept of time and consider being slightly late for an appointment as acceptable. The hospital is often considered as the place to go to die. For many, religion is very important. The percentage of nursing students who are Hispanic is 3%.	*Chinese* respect their bodies and believe that it is best to die with their bodies intact. They may therefore refuse surgery. Older members may believe that the hospital is a place to go to die. Many believe in reincarnation. *Japanese* highly value cleanliness. Time is also valuable and should be used wisely. They may be stoic and not openly show evidence of pain or discomfort. *Vietnamese* value status more than money. There is a high value placed on social harmony. There are 3.3% of nursing students who are Asian.	Because the hospital is often considered as the place to die, the client may resist hospitalization. Great respect is shown to the elders of both the family and the tribe. There are 0.7% of nursing students who are Native Americans.	There are 84.4% of nursing students who are white Americans

Demographic data from www.census.gov/population; health statistics from U.S. Department of Health and Human Services: *Health—United States 1995,* DHHS Pub No (PHS) 96-1232, Hyattsville, Md, 1996, ________; additional data from Seidel HM et al: *Mosby's guide to physical examination,* ed 4, St. Louis, 1999, Mosby; www.IHS.gov, 1999; Wong DL: *Whaley and Wong's nursing care of infants and children,* ed 6, St. Louis, 1999, Mosby.

Table 3-2 Religious Beliefs Concerning Medical Care

RELIGION	BELIEFS REGARDING MEDICAL CARE
Adventist (Seventh Day Adventist; Church of God)	May believe in divine healing and practice anointing with oil and use of prayer May desire communion or baptism when ill Believe in man's choice and God's sovereignty May oppose hyponosis as therapy Sabbath: Saturday for many Accept Bible literally
Baptist (27 groups)	"Laying on of hands" (some) May resist some therapies, such as abortion Believe God functions through physician May believe in predestination; may respond passively to care Fundamentalist and conservative groups accept Bible as inspired word of God
Black Muslim	Faith healing unacceptable Always maintain personal habits of cleanliness General adherence to Moslem tenets overlaid, in many instances, by antagonism to whites, especially Christians and Jews
Buddhist Churches of America	Illness believed to be a trial to aid development of soul; illness due to karmic causes May be reluctant to have surgery or certain treatments on holy days Cleanliness believed to be of great importance Family may request Buddhist priest for counseling Optimistic outlook; teach ways to overcome fears, anxieties, apprehension
Church of Christ Scientist (Christian Science)	Deny the existence of health crisis; see sickness and sin as errors of mind that can be altered by prayer Oppose human intervention with drugs or other therapies; however, accept legally required immunizations May adhere to belief that disease is a human mental concept that can be dispelled by "spiritual truth" to extent of refusing all medical treatment May desire services of practitioner or reader; will sometimes refuse even emergency treatment until they have consulted a reader Unlikely to donate organs for transplant
Church of Jesus Christ of Latter Day Saints (Mormons)	Devout adherents believe in divine healing through anointment with oil and "laying on of hands" by church officials (elders) Medical therapy not prohibited Married adults wear special undergarments May request Sacrament on Sunday while in hospital Financial support for sick available through well-funded welfare system Discourage cremation Discourage use of tobacco
Eastern Orthodox (Turkey, Egypt, Syria, Rumania, Bulgaria, Cyprus, Albania, etc.)	Anointment of the sick No conflict with medical science Discourage cremation
Episcopal (Anglican)	May believe in spiritual healing Rite for anointing sick available but not mandatory Religious icons very important Communion four times yearly: Christmas, Easter, June 20, and August 15; may be mandatory for some
Friends (Quakers)	Believe in plain speech and dress Pacifists
Greek Orthodox	Each health crisis handled by ordained priest; deacon may also serve in some cases Holy Communion administered in hospital Some may desire Sacrament of the Holy Unction performed by priest Oppose euthanasia Believe every reasonable effort should be made to preserve life until termination by God Discourage autopsies that may cause dismemberment Prefer burial by cremation

Nursing Diagnosis: Application to clinical practice, ed 4, Philadelphia, 1992, JB Lippincott, Conley L: Childbearing and childbearing practices in Mormonism, *Neonatal Network* 9(3):41-48, 1990; Kozier B, Erb G: *Fundamentals of nursing,* ed 5, Menlo Park, CA, 1995, Addison-Wesley; McQuay JE: Cross cultural customs and beliefs related to health crisis, death, and organ donation/transplantation, *Crit Care Nurs Clin North Am* 7(3):581-594, 1995; Spector RE: *Cultural diversity in health and illness,* ed 4, Stamford, CT, 1996, Appleton & Lange; Wong DL et al: *Whaley and Wong's nursing care of infants and children,* ed 6, St. Louis, 1999, Mosby.

Table 3-2 Religious Beliefs Concerning Medical Care—cont'd

RELIGION	BELIEFS REGARDING MEDICAL CARE
Hindu	Illness or injury believed to represent sins committed in previous life Accept most modern medical practices Cremation preferred
Islam (Muslim/Moslem)	Faith healing not acceptable unless psychologic condition of patient is deteriorating; performed for morale Ritual washing after prayer; prayer takes place five times daily (upon rising, midday, afternoon, early evening, and before bed); during prayer, face Mecca and kneel on prayer rug Older Muslims often have a fatalistic view that may interfere with compliance with therapy May oppose autopsy
Jehovah's Witness	Adherents generally absolutely opposed to blood transfusions, including banking of own blood; individuals can sometimes be persuaded in emergencies May be opposed to use of albumin, globulin, factor replacement (hemophilia), vaccines Often possible to obtain a court order appointing a hospital official as temporary guardian to consent to a child's transfusion when parents refuse consent Autopsy approved only as required by law
Judaism (Orthodox and Conservative)	May resist surgical procedures during Sabbath, which extends from sundown Friday until sundown Saturday Seriously ill and pregnant women exempt from fasting Illness is grounds for violating dietary laws (e.g., client with congestive heart failure not required to use kosher meats, which are high in sodium) Oppose all forms of mutilation, including autopsy; body parts not donated or removed; amputated limbs, organs, or surgically removed tissues should be made available to the family for burial Donation or transplantation of organs requires rabbinical consent May oppose prolongation of life after irreversible brain damage
Lutheran	If grave prognosis, family may request anointing and blessing of sick or visit by church official Accept scientific developments
Mennonite	No illness rituals Deep concern for dignity and self-determination of individual that would conflict with shock treatment or medical treatment affecting personality or will
Methodist	May request communion before surgery or similar crisis Encourage donation of body or body parts to medical science
Nazarene	Church official administers communion and laying on of hands Believe in divine healing but not exclusive of medical treatment Cremation permitted
Pentocostal (Assembly of God, Foursquare)	No restrictions regarding medical care Deliverance from sickness provided for in atonement; may pray for divine intervention in health matters and seek God in prayer for themselves and others when ill May insist illness is divine punishment; most consider it an intrusion of Satan Practice glossolalia (speaking in tongues)
Orthodox Presbyterian	Communion administered when appropriate and convenient Blood transfusion accepted when advisable Pastor or elder should be called for ill person Believe science should be used for relief of suffering Full forgiveness granted for any illness connected with a sin
Roman Catholic	Encourage anointing of sick, although this may be interpreted by older members of church as equivalent to the old terminology "extreme unction" or "last rites"; they may require careful explanation if reluctance associated with fear of imminent death Traditional church teaching does not approve of contraceptives or abortion; however, some clergy advocate more liberal views on these issues Family may request that major amputated limb be buried in consecrated ground Transplant accepted as long as loss of organ does not deprive donor of life or functional integrity of body Autopsy acceptable Religious articles important
Russian Orthodox	Cross necklace is important and should be removed only when necessary and replaced as soon as possible Adherents believe in divine healing, but not exclusive of medical treatment Opposed to autopsy, embalming, or cremation
Unitarian Universalist	Most believe in the general goodness of their fellow humans and appreciate the expression of that goodness by visits from their clergy and follow parishioners during times of illness Cremation preferred to burial

Box 3-1 The Balance of Life: The Hot and the Cold

A naturalistic or holistic approach often assumes that there are external factors, some good, some bad, that must be kept in balance if we are to remain well. The balance of hot and cold is a part of the belief system in many cultural groups, such as the Arab, Chinese, Filipino, and Hispanic. To restore a disturbed balance, that is, to treat, requires the use of opposites, for example, a hot remedy for a cold problem. Different cultures may define hot and cold differently. It is not a matter of temperature, and the words used might vary. For example, the Chinese have named the forces yin (cold) and yang (hot). Western medicine cannot ignore the naturalistic view if many of its patients are to have appropriate treatment for illness as well as disease.

HOT AND COLD CONDITIONS AND THEIR CORRESPONDING TREATMENTS

Hot Conditions	Cold Foods	Cold Medicines and Herbs	Cold Conditions	Hot Foods	Hot Medicines and Herbs
Fever	Fresh vegetables	Orange flower water	Cancer	Chocolate	Penicillin
Infection	Tropical fruits	Linden	Pneumonia	Cheese	Tobacco
Diarrhea	Dairy products	Sage	Malaria	Temperate Zone fruits	Gingerroot
Kidney problem	Meats such as goat, fish, chicken	Milk of magnesia	Joint pain	Eggs	Garlic
Rash	Honey	Bicarbonate of soda	Menstrual period	Peas	Cinnamon
Skin ailment	Cod		Teething	Onions	Anise
Sore throat	Raisins		Earache	Aromatic beverages	Vitamins
Liver problem	Bottled milk		Rheumatism	Hard liquor	Iron preparations
Ulcer	Barley water		Tuberculosis	Oils	Cod-liver oil
Constipation			Cold	Meats such as beef, waterfowl, mutton	Castor oil
			Headache	Goat's milk	Aspirin
			Paralysis	Cereal grains	
			Stomach cramps	Chili peppers	

Modified from Wilson HS, Kneisl CR: *Psychiatric nursing,* ed 3, Menlo Park, Calif, 1988.

What is the Client's Primary Language and Method of Communication?

- What is the language that is usually spoken in your home?
- How well do you speak, read, and write English?
- In what language do you think?
- Do you have to translate in your mind when communicating?
- Are there special rituals of communication in your family? (For example, is there someone special to whom questions should be directed?)
- Are there unique customs in your culture that influence nonverbal or verbal communication?
- Are there signs of indicating respect for others?
- Are there culturally appropriate ways to enter and leave situations?

What are the Client's Personal Beliefs About Health and Illness?

- How do you define health and illness?
- Do you believe that you have control over your health?
- Are there particular practices or rituals that you believe will improve your health?
- Do you or have you used any of the alternative healing methods, such as acupuncture, acupressure, *ayurveda,* healing touch, or herbal products? If so, how effective was the treatment?
- Whom do you consult when you are ill?
- Are there particular practices or rituals that you believe should be used to treat your health problem?
- What are your attitudes toward mental illness? pain? handicapping conditions? chronic disease? death? dying?
- Who makes the health decisions in your family?
- What health topics do you feel uncomfortable talking about or are taboo to discuss?
- What examination procedures do you feel modest about?

What are Religious Influences and Special Rituals That Affect the Client?

- Is there a particular religion that you practice?
- Whom do you look to for guidance and support?
- Are there any special religious practices or beliefs that are likely to feel supportive when you are ill?
- What events, rituals, and ceremonies are considered important within your life cycle, such as birth, baptism, puberty, marriage, and death?

What are the Roles of Individual People in the Family?

- Who makes the decisions in your family?
- What is the composition of your family? How many generations or family members live in your household?
- When the marriage custom is practiced, what is the attitude about separation and divorce?
- What is the role of and attitude toward children in the family?
- When the children are punished, how is it done, and who does it?
- What are the major important events in your family? How are they celebrated?
- Do you or the members of your family have special beliefs and practices surrounding conception, pregnancy, childbirth, lactation, and childrearing?

Does the Client Have Special Dietary Practices?

- What is the main type of diet eaten in your home?
- Are there special types of foods that are forbidden by your culture or foods that are a cultural requirement in observance of a rite or ceremony?
- Who in your family is responsible for food preparation?
- Is the food in your culture prepared in any special way?
- Are there specific beliefs or preferences concerning food, such as those believed to cause or cure illness?

REMEMBER . . .

The most important behaviors in cultural assessment are to be sensitive, to ask questions, to gather information specific to the individual client, to not stereotype, and to not assume that just because you took care of a similar client last week that you know exactly how this client feels and what he or she believes.

Regardless of the client's race or cultural heritage, each individual is unique. Before you become involved in the detailed task of a physical assessment, take the time to first get to know the client and his or her family.

CLINICAL APPLICATION and CRITICAL THINKING

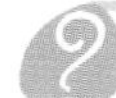

CRITICAL THINKING QUESTIONS

1. A young American Indian child is brought to the emergency department by his mother and grandmother with severe abdominal pain and fever. Upon assessment, the nurse notes a foul-smelling cloth wrapped around the child's abdomen. The cloth will interfere with the examination. What should the nurse do?
2. You are working in a hospital that has a visiting policy of two visitors per client at one time. One client on the medical floor is an elderly Hispanic man who has had multiple visitors throughout the day. When you go into his room, you count 11 visitors (who all claim to be relatives) in the room. How should you handle this situation?
3. You have a minority client who has a chronic illness requiring dietary teaching and education about medications. Listed below are areas for cultural assessment. For each area, list at least one question that might be asked as part of a cultural assessment to better prepare for this client's care.

   Health beliefs and practices:

   Religious and ritual influences:

   Dietary practices:

   Family relationships:

REMEMBER to check out your companion CD-ROM

4 Interviewing to Obtain a Health History

www.mosby.com/MERLIN/wilson/assessment/

The nurse initiates therapeutic relationships by gathering information about clients—finding out about their current state of health and how it can be maintained or improved. To accomplish this, the nurse interviews clients to learn about them and the social, economic, and cultural factors that influence their health and their responses to illness.

PURPOSE OF THE HEALTH HISTORY

The purpose of the health history is to obtain subjective data from clients. Together the nurse and the clients use this database to create a plan to promote health, prevent disease, resolve acute health problems, and minimize limitations related to chronic health problems. Accomplishing this purpose involves meeting both the clients' expectations for health and the nurse's expectations for the health of those clients. Information to be gathered about clients includes how they define health, whether they believe they can attain and maintain health, whether they believe they are responsible for their health, and what health behaviors they practice now and what unhealthy behaviors they are willing to change. The clients' expectations for health are based on their life experiences, the experiences of their families and friends, and the culture in which they live. The nurse has a broader view of health and compares a client's current state of health to a standard needed to attain or maintain optimal health and then determines how far away the client is from the desired standard.

The American Nurses Association (ANA) standards of practice (1991) direct nurses to establish a comprehensive database. Outcome criteria for this standard include (1) obtaining pertinent data using appropriate assessment techniques; (2) involving the client, significant others, and health care providers in data collection, when appropriate; (3) collecting data in a systematic manner; and (4) documenting relevant data in a retrievable form (ANA, 1991, p. 9).

The nursing process is initiated as the nurse begins data collection about the client's history. A variety of factors will have an impact on the outcome of the interviews. These factors include the nurse's personality and behavior, the personality and behavior of the client, how the client is feeling at the time of the interview, the nature of the information being discussed or problem being confronted, and the physical setting. The nurse's approach must be orderly without being rigid. Random approaches often result in an incomplete database and incomplete diagnoses and solutions, which reduce the potential of successful outcomes.

PROVIDING A RELAXED SETTING

Introduce yourself to the clients, offer a handshake, and tell them your role in their care (Fig. 4-1). Be sure you know their names and pronounce them correctly. Address clients by their title (for example, Mr., Mrs., Miss, or Ms.) and their surname. Avoid using the first name with clients unless they request it, except when the client is a child. Also avoid substituting the client's role for his or her name, such as referring to the client as "mom" or "grandpa."

When possible, allow clients to remain in street clothes during the interview to obtain the history and then have them change into a gown for the physical examination. You and the client should sit at a distance from each other that provides a comfortable flow of conversation and allows you to establish eye contact. The client's comfort level is related to personal space, that is, the area that surrounds the person's body. How much space clients want from you will vary and is influenced by their cultures and previous experiences in similar situations. Be attentive to how comfortable a client appears and, if you are not sure, ask "Is this a comfortable seating arrangement for you?" When you are learning the interview process, you may want to use an outline to prompt questions and take brief notes during the interview. Both practices are acceptable as long as they do not interfere with your eye contact with the client or with the flow of information.

DECIDING HOW MUCH DATA TO COLLECT

How much data do you collect at one time? Assessment interviews may be comprehensive or focused. The comprehensive health assessment provides a complete health history, family history, review of all body systems, psychosocial assessment, and physical examination. This type of assessment may be part of an admission to a hospital or the first office or home visit, or it may be used when the client's reason for seeking care is for relief of generalized symptoms such as weight loss or fatigue. This type of assessment requires more time than routine visits because a comprehensive database is being established. Often clients are given questionnaires to complete about their histories before the interview to reduce the time spent in data collection. However, the information gained from questionnaires should be reviewed with the client during the interview for clarification.

The focused health assessment concentrates on episodic health care needs. These needs may be well-child or well-adult visits, screening, or changes in health states that have occurred since the comprehensive health assessment. Well

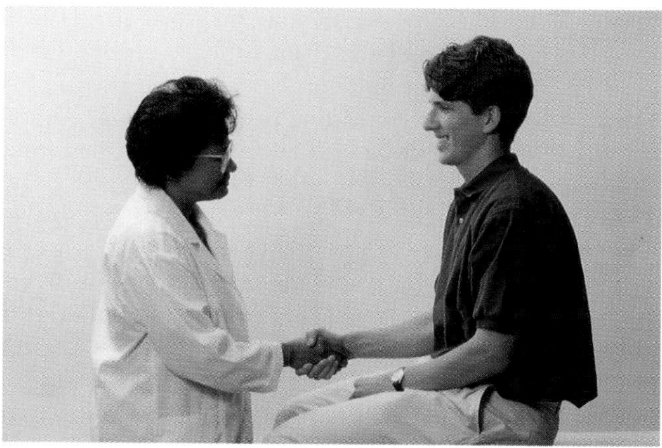

Fig. 4-1 Offer the client a handshake and introduce yourself.

visits include changes in the history since the last visit, a limited physical examination, and education about normal growth and development and health promotion. Screening allows identification of specific risk factors. For example, blood pressure screening provides data on the risk for hypertension. A tuberculin skin test is given to identify those exposed to tuberculosis. A focused interview is also used when the client seeks help to address an urgent problem such as relief from asthma attacks or chest pain. Further data may be collected once the client is stabilized, particularly if the client will require ongoing care.

The admission process for many hospitals includes obtaining a comprehensive database, particularly if the client is expected to have a hospital stay exceeding a couple of days. The condition of the client, however, must be considered. A critically ill client, for instance, is unable to participate in a comprehensive interview, and thus it is inappropriate to pursue. Family members may be of assistance in providing important information to the nurse while the client is seriously ill. Once the client is no longer critically ill, a comprehensive interview should be conducted.

Regardless of the type of history taken, the nurse should determine whether to ask or defer certain questions on a health history because situations exist when certain data are irrelevant to some individuals. In addition, during an interview the nurse may uncover important data requiring further investigation. When this occurs, the nurse must be able to determine what additional questions will help clarify the data.

COMMUNICATING WITH THE CLIENT

From the start there are several points to keep in mind. A stiff, formal demeanor may inhibit the client's ability to communicate, yet being too casual or having a laid-back attitude may fail to instill confidence. Because the client may search for meaning in everything you say, avoid being careless with words. What may seem an innocent comment to you may be vital to the client. Similarly, your face need not be a mask, but avoid the extremes of reaction—startle, surprise, laughter, grimacing—as the client provides information. Your nonverbal demeanor is as important as your words.

The first impression you make starts with the way you appear to the client. The way you are dressed and groomed is important in establishing a positive first impression. Modest dress, clean fingernails, and neat hair are imperative. Avoid extremes in dress and manner so that appearance does not become an obstacle or distraction to the client's response.

Interviewing the client with others in the room may present a challenge. Be careful not to assume relationships among the people in the room. For example, when a woman accompanies a child, do not assume the adult is the child's mother; ask "Are you the mother?" Also, when a man and a woman are together, do not assume what their relationship is; ask. Sometimes the relationship will be explained during introductions but, if not, clarify by asking "What is your relationship?" Trying to interview a mother when her active children are in the room may be disruptive. If the children are too young to wait in the waiting room, find a developmentally appropriate activity for them to do until you complete the interview. When the client speaks a different language, a translator is needed. An objective observer who is the same gender as the client will be a better translator than a family member who may alter the meaning of what is said. The client should respond to the questions if possible. Sometimes the spouse, parent, or another person will answer for the client unless otherwise directed. When this occurs, you must validate with the client that the information is correct. If others persist in answering for the client, you may have to ask the others to allow the client to answer or ask them to wait in another room until the end of the interview.

The Art of Asking Questions

The art of obtaining information from clients and listening carefully to their responses is an essential competency of nurses. Questions you ask must be clearly spoken and understood by the client. Define words the client may not understand, but do not use so many technical terms that the definitions become confusing. Use the client's terms if possible. Slang words may be used if necessary to describe certain conditions. Comply with the client's level of knowledge and understanding.

Encourage the client to be as specific as possible. For example, if you ask how many glasses of water the client drinks each day and he or she says, "Oh, a few," clarify what the client means by asking "How many is a few? Three? Four? Five?" This approach yields a more specific answer and provides the client's interpretation of "a few."

Ask one question at a time and wait for the reply before asking the next question. If you ask several questions at a time, the client may get confused about which question to answer and you may be uncertain about which question the client is answering. For example, you ask "Have you had immunizations for tetanus, hepatitis B, and influenza?" If the client answers yes, you are not sure if he or she means yes to all three or to one.

If you become confused by something a client says, ask for clarification. The explanation may clear up the confusion, or it may indicate that the client has misinformation or some underlying emotional or thought-processing difficulty that impairs understanding.

Be attentive to the feelings that accompany the client's responses to some questions. These responses may signify additional data you need to collect during this interview or a problem that needs to be addressed in the future. For example, if the client reports that her mother died of breast cancer and she begins to cry, this may indicate a future need for discussing coping or adjustment methods with the client.

Clients may ask you questions during the interview. Answer specific questions using terms that they understand. Avoid overburdening them with an in-depth answer that, while correct, is far more information than necessary to satisfy them. If a client asks a question you do not feel prepared to answer at the moment or one that is very broad, you can get additional information by asking "Why do you ask?" This will give you direction in answering the client's specific question. If you do not know the answer to the question, perhaps you can refer the client to the appropriate resource.

Types of Questions to Ask

Begin the interview with *open-ended questions,* such as "How have you been feeling?" This broadly stated question encourages a free-flowing, open response (Northouse and Northouse, 1992). The aim of an open-ended question is to elicit a response that is more than one or two words. Clients will respond to this type of question by describing the onset of signs or symptoms in their own words at their own pace. The open-ended question should, however, focus on the client's health. A question that is too broad, such as "Tell me a little about yourself" may be too general to get any useful information. The risk of asking open-ended questions is that clients may be unable to focus on the topic being asked about or may take excessive time to tell their story. In these cases, you will need to focus the interview. Flexibility is needed when using this type of question, however, because the client's associations may be important, and you must allow clients freedom to pursue them. You may note topics the client mentions that you want to follow up on later in the interview.

To gain more precise details, you must ask more direct, specific, *closed-ended questions* that require one or two words. For example, you might ask "Do you become short of breath?" or "Do you frequently get bruises?" Another reason for using this type of question is to give clients options when answering questions, such as "Is the pain in your stomach sharp, dull, or aching?" This type of question is valuable in collecting data, but it must be used in combination with open-ended questions because failure to allow clients to describe their health in their own words may lead to inaccurate conclusions (Northouse and Northouse, 1992). Directive questions lead the client to focus on one set of thoughts. This type of question is most often used in reviewing systems or in evaluating functional status. An example would be "Describe the drainage you have had from your nose."

Asking questions about sensitive issues can be accomplished by explaining that you have personal or sensitive questions to ask or by describing clients you have interviewed in the past. An example of this type of question is "I need to know about the drugs you have used that are not prescription or over-the-counter; have you ever used illegal drugs?" An alternative is to say "Some clients have experimented with illegal drugs; have you ever used illegal drugs?" This method of questioning has been called permission giving because the nurse gives clients permission to report information about a sensitive topic.

Techniques That Enhance Data Collection

The question-answer format is the essential tool used in obtaining a client history. Data collection can be facilitated by using the following techniques.

Active Listening Active listening is performed by concentrating on what the client is saying and the subtleties of the message being conveyed. Two behaviors that interfere with active listening are formulating your next question while the client is talking and predicting how clients will answer questions. If you are concentrating on how you are going to word your next question, your attention will be shifted away from the information that client is providing you. When you make assumptions about how the client will respond to questions and plan your next question based on your assumptions, your question may be illogical if your assumption is wrong.

Facilitation Facilitation is attained by using phrases to encourage the client to continue talking. These include verbal responses such as "Go on," "Uh-huh," and "Then?" and nonverbal responses such as head nodding and shifting forward in your seat with increased attention.

Clarification Clarification is used to obtain more information about conflicting, vague, or ambiguous statements. Examples might be "What do you mean by 'you almost lost it'?" or "What do you think kept you from returning to work?"

Restatement Restatement involves repeating what clients say using different words; it confirms your interpretation of what they said. For example, "Let me make sure I understand what you said. The pain in your stomach occurs before you eat and is relieved by eating. Is that correct?"

Reflection Reflection is repeating a phrase or sentence the client just said. This encourages elaboration and indicates you are interested in more information.

Client: "I got out of bed and I just didn't feel right."
Nurse: "You didn't feel right?"
Client: "Uh huh, I was dizzy and had to sit back on the bed before I fell over."

Confrontation Confrontation is used when you notice inconsistencies between what the client reports and your observations or other data about the client. For example, "I'm confused here. You say you are staying on your diet and exercising 3 times a week, yet your weight has increased since your last visit? Can you help me to understand this?" Your tone of voice is important when using confrontation; use a tone that communicates confusion or misunderstanding, rather than one that is accusatory and angry.

Interpretation Interpretation is used when you want to share with clients a conclusion you have drawn from data they have given. After hearing your interpretation, clients can confirm, deny, or revise your interpretation. For example, "Let me share my thoughts about what you just told me. The week you were out of the office you exercised, felt no muscle tension, and had a normal blood pressure. I wonder if your work environment is contributing to your high blood pressure?"

Summary A summary condenses and orders data obtained during the interview to help clarify a sequence of events. This is useful when interviewing a client who rambles or does not provide sequential data. Also, summary is useful at the end of the interview to emphasize data that have implications for health promotion, disease prevention, or resolving the client's health problems.

Techniques That Diminish Data Collection

The following communication techniques have been found to interrupt the free flow of the interview, interfere with data collection, and possibly impair the client-nurse relationship. These techniques can be avoided by considering the interview from the client's perspective, such as how you would prefer the flow of the conversation to go and how you would want things explained to you.

Using Professional Terminology You are using professional terminology when you use medical terms or abbreviations not commonly known to clients. Some examples include saying "hypertension" instead of "high blood pressure," "dysphagia" rather than "difficulty in swallowing," "CVA" rather than "stroke," or "CA" rather than "cancer." Using these words may be condescending; furthermore, they inhibit the exchange of information and may create a barrier between you and the client (Sieh and Brentin, 1997).

Expressing Value Judgments Including value judgments in your questions is always a hindrance. For example, you should ask "What kind of protection do you use during intercourse?" rather than saying "You do use protection during intercourse, don't you?" The latter question forces clients to respond in a way that is consistent with your values or causes them to feel guilty or defensive when they must answer to the contrary.

Talking Too Much Interviews are about the clients and how to meet their needs. When you monopolize the conversation by talking, you cannot collect sufficient data about the clients' needs.

Interrupting the Client Allow clients to finish sentences; do not become impatient and finish their sentences for them. The ending you add to a sentence may not be the ending that the client would have used. Associated with interrupting is changing the subject before a client has finished giving information about the last topic discussed. You may feel pressured for time and eager to move on to other topics, but allow clients an opportunity to complete their thoughts.

Being Authoritarian or Paternalistic When you use the approach of "I know what is best for you, and you should do what I say," you risk alienating the client. Despite what you believe is best for clients, you must always remember that their health is their responsibility. They may choose to follow or ignore your advice and teaching.

Using "Why" Questions Using "why" questions may put clients on the defensive. When clients are asked why they did something, the implication is they must defend their choices. Instead of asking "Why didn't you take all the antibiotic?" you might say "I noticed you stopped taking the antibiotics before all the pills were gone" and then wait to see if the client offers an explanation. If no explanation is forthcoming, you can follow up with "I am curious about the reason for not taking all the antibiotic."

Managing Awkward Moments

Answering Personal Questions Clients may ask questions about you from time to time. They are curious about you and your life. Often a brief, direct answer will suffice to satisfy the client's curiosity. You may feel comfortable sharing certain experiences that may support clients, such as parenting issues or how you handle stress. Sharing these mutual experiences may enhance the relationship with clients and increase your credibility.

Dealing With Silence Silence can be awkward. You may have the urge to break the silence with a comment or question. Remember, however, that clients may need the silence as time to reflect or to gather courage. Some issues can be so painful to discuss that silence is necessary and should be accepted. Silence may provide feedback for you that the client may not be ready to discuss this topic now or that your approach needs to be evaluated. Become comfortable with silence; it can be useful.

Cultural Competence Nurses work with clients from many cultural backgrounds. It is essential that the nurse develop cultural competence to identify cultural factors that may influence how a client behaves when ill (Lester, 1998). Culturally sensitive nursing care refers to the variability in nursing approaches needed to provide culturally appropriate and competent care. To deliver culturally sensitive care, nurses must interact with each individual as a unique person who is a product of past experiences, beliefs, and values that have been learned and passed down from one generation to the next (Fig. 4-2). Remember, however, that all individuals within a specific cultural group will not think and behave in a similar manner. Avoid stereotyping clients just because of their culture. There may be as much diversity within a cultural group as there is across

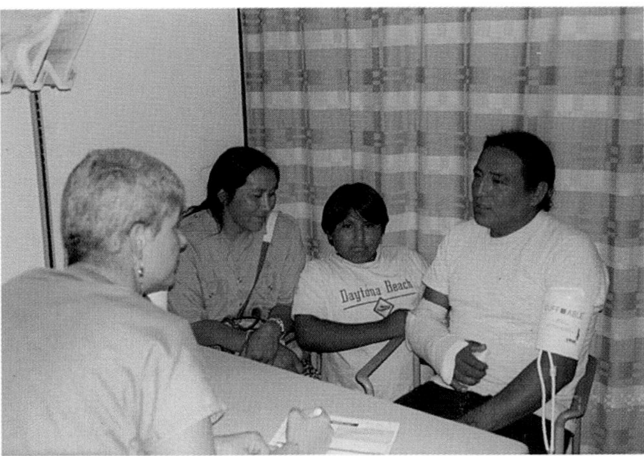

Fig. 4-2 Interact with the client as a unique person and be sensitive to cultural diversities.

cultural groups. Ask clients about experiences that illustrate what has been of value to them and that characterize their culture. This will increase your knowledge about other cultures and endear you to clients for your interest in them as individuals (see Chapter 3).

Displays of Emotion Crying is a natural emotion and should be permitted when it occurs. Saying "Don't cry" is not a therapeutic response. A more appropriate approach is to provide tissues and let the client know it is all right to cry by giving a response such as "Take all the time you need to express your feelings." Postpone further questioning until the client is ready. The crying may indicate a client need that can be addressed at a later time. Compassionate response to a crying client demonstrates caring and may enhance the therapeutic relationship.

Anger of clients may be uncomfortable. The most therapeutic approach is to deal with it directly by first identifying the source of the anger. You may say "You seem angry; can you tell me the reason for your feelings?" If clients choose to discuss the anger, they hopefully will identify whether the anger is directed at someone else or at you. If clients are angry at someone else, you can discuss with them an approach for talking with that person about the reason for the angry feelings. When clients are angry with you, encourage them to discuss their feelings. Acknowledge the angry feelings and, if appropriate, apologize. You may be able to continue working with these clients after the angry feelings are discussed, but if clients would prefer to interact with another nurse, then you should honor their request. Regardless of the outcome, you have modeled for the clients a healthy, appropriate approach to managing anger.

SCOPE OF THE HEALTH HISTORY

The health history format described in this chapter provides a comprehensive format that may take over an hour to complete. The scope of the history includes the following areas:

- Biographic data
- Reason for seeking care
- Present health status
- Past health history
- Family history
- Review of systems
- Psychosocial status
- Environmental health

Box 4-1 Biographic Data

Name
Gender
Address and telephone number
Birth date
Birthplace (important when born in foreign country)
Race—physical features such as skin color, bone structure, or blood group that are genetically determined
Culture—pattern of behavioral responses shaped by values, beliefs, norms, and practices
Religion
Marital status
Family or significant others living in the home
Social security number
Occupation
Contact person
Advance directive (decisions about end-of-life care)
Durable power of attorney for health care
Source of referral
Usual source of health care
Type of health insurance

BIOGRAPHIC DATA

The biographic data are collected at the first visit and then updated as changes occur. These data begin to form a picture of the client as a unique individual. Box 4-1 lists the data to be obtained.

REASON FOR SEEKING CARE

The reason for seeking care, also called the chief complaint (CC), is a brief statement of the client's purpose for requesting the services of a health care provider. The client's reason for seeking care is recorded in direct quotes. When clients have multiple reasons, list them all and ask clients to indicate the priority of the complaints. Some clients may initially be uncomfortable giving you the actual reason for seeking care. In this case, it is possible they may not divulge the true reason they came until the end of the visit, after they begin to feel more comfortable.

The client's condition dictates how the examiner will proceed. Urgency dictates expediency. Clients with severe pain, dyspnea, or injury should not be subjected to a prolonged history. Biographic data may be delayed to pursue the health concern. This approach enables the examiner to hypothesize quickly and identify the cause of the health concern and plan how to alleviate the signs or symptoms. However, clients with depression may need to be given more time to freely divulge feelings and surrounding circumstances.

Box 4-2 Symptom Analysis

LOCATION—Where are the symptoms?
- Is the location in a specific area? vague and generalized? Does symptom radiate?

QUALITY—Describe the characteristics of the symptom
- Describe the sensation: stabbing, dull, aching, throbbing, nagging, sharp, squeezing, itching.
- Describe the drainage: color, texture, composition, appearance, and odor.
- Was the onset slow? abrupt? noticeable to others?
- Was the symptom intermittent or continuous?
- How has symptom interrupted your life (e.g., sleeping, eating, working, activities at home or school)?

QUANTITY—Describe the severity of the symptom
- Describe the size, extent, number, or amount (e.g., of lesion, rash, blister, discharge).
- Was the symptom so severe that it interrupted your activities?
- On a scale of 1 to 10, with 10 being most severe, how would you rate your symptom?

CHRONOLOGY—When did the symptom start?
- Ask specific date, time, day of the week.
- How many times a day, week, month did symptom occur?
- How did client feel in between episodes of the symptom?

SETTING—Where are you when the symptom occurs?
- Does anyone else with whom you have been in contact have a similar symptom?
- Are there psychologic or physical factors in the environment that may be causing the symptom (e.g., stress or smoke or chemicals)?

ASSOCIATED MANIFESTATIONS—Do other symptoms occur at the same time?
- What effect does the symptom have on body function? activities? appetite?

ALLEVIATING FACTORS
- What home remedies have you tried?
- What medications have you tried (over-the-counter and prescription)?
- Are there certain body positions that relieve symptom?

AGGRAVATING FACTORS
- Is symptom aggravated by an activity (e.g., walking, climbing stairs, eating, a body position)?

PRESENT HEALTH STATUS

The present health/illness status gives clients an opportunity to expand on the reason for seeking care. When the reason is to improve current health status, rather than to relieve illness, the data collected include what clients are doing currently to maintain their health and what they think may be hindering the accomplishment of their health goals. Data included here are as follows:

- Current health promotion activities: diet, exercise, stress management, meditation, yoga, spiritual or religious groups
- Client's perceived level of health
- Current medications
  Herbal preparations
  Type of drug (prescription, over-the-counter, vitamins, illegal)
  Prescribed by whom
  When first prescribed
  Reason for prescription
  Dose of medication and frequency per day
  Client's perception of the effectiveness of medication

In contrast, when clients seek relief from illness, then a symptom analysis is completed. A symptom analysis is a systematic way to collect data about the history and status of symptoms and focuses on eight variables: location, quality, quantity, chronology, setting, associated manifestations, alleviating factors, and aggravating factors (Box 4-2).

PAST HEALTH HISTORY

Past health history is important, since past illnesses may have some effect on the client's current health needs and problems. The following categories of data are included:

- *Allergies:* food, drug, environmental factors, and contact substances. Be sure to specifically ask about substances to which the client could be exposed in the health care setting, such as latex and iodine. When asking about allergies, be sure the client knows what is meant by the term *allergies.* Many people do not know the difference between a side effect (such as nausea) and a true allergic reaction. When the client indicates he or she has an allergy to a medication or substance, it is a good idea to ask the client to describe what happens with exposure.
- *Childhood illnesses:* measles, mumps, rubella, chickenpox, pertussis, *Haemophilus influenzae* infection, streptococcal throat infection, otitis media. (Ask if there were complications in later years, such as rheumatic fever or glomerulonephritis that can occur after streptococcal throat infection.)
- *Surgeries:* type, date, outcome
- *Hospitalizations:* illnesses, dates, outcome

- *Accidents or injuries:* fractures, lacerations, loss of consciousness, burns, penetrating wounds
- *Chronic illnesses:* for example, diabetes, hypertension, heart disease, sickle cell anemia, cancer, seizures, chronic obstructive pulmonary disease, arthritis, and mental illness such as depression, anxiety disorders, substance abuse, and schizophrenia. Ask how much the illness interferes with daily activities.
- *Immunizations:* tetanus, diphtheria, pertussis; mumps; rubella; poliomyelitis; hepatitis B; influenza, pneumococcal pneumonia, varicella, and, for foreign-born clients, Bacille Calmette-Gurin (BCG)
- *Last examinations:* physical, dental, vision, hearing, electrocardiogram (ECG), chest radiograph, skin test for tuberculosis; for women: Papanicolaou (Pap) smear, mammogram
- *Obstetric history:* number of pregnancies (gravidity), number of births (parity), and number of abortions/miscarriages. (For each birth document the course of pregnancy, labor, type of delivery [vaginal or cesarean section], weight of neonate, and postpartum course.)

FAMILY HISTORY

Family history of the client's blood relatives, spouse, and children is obtained to identify any illnesses of a genetic, familial, or environmental nature that might affect the client's current or future health. Trace back at least two generations to maternal and paternal parents and grandparents. Also include siblings, uncles, and aunts. Sometimes health information about significant others, sexual partners, and roommates is relevant to the client's health. Questions about the health of family members should include the following:

- Alzheimer's disease
- Cancer (all types)
- Diabetes mellitus
- Heart disease
- Hypertension
- Seizures
- Emotional problems
- Alcoholism/drug abuse
- Mental illness
- Developmental delay
- Endocrine diseases (specify)
- Sickle cell anemia
- Kidney disease
- Cerebrovascular accident

Document the absence of the diseases by writing "No history of (disease name)" so that others who read this history will know that you asked the client about the family

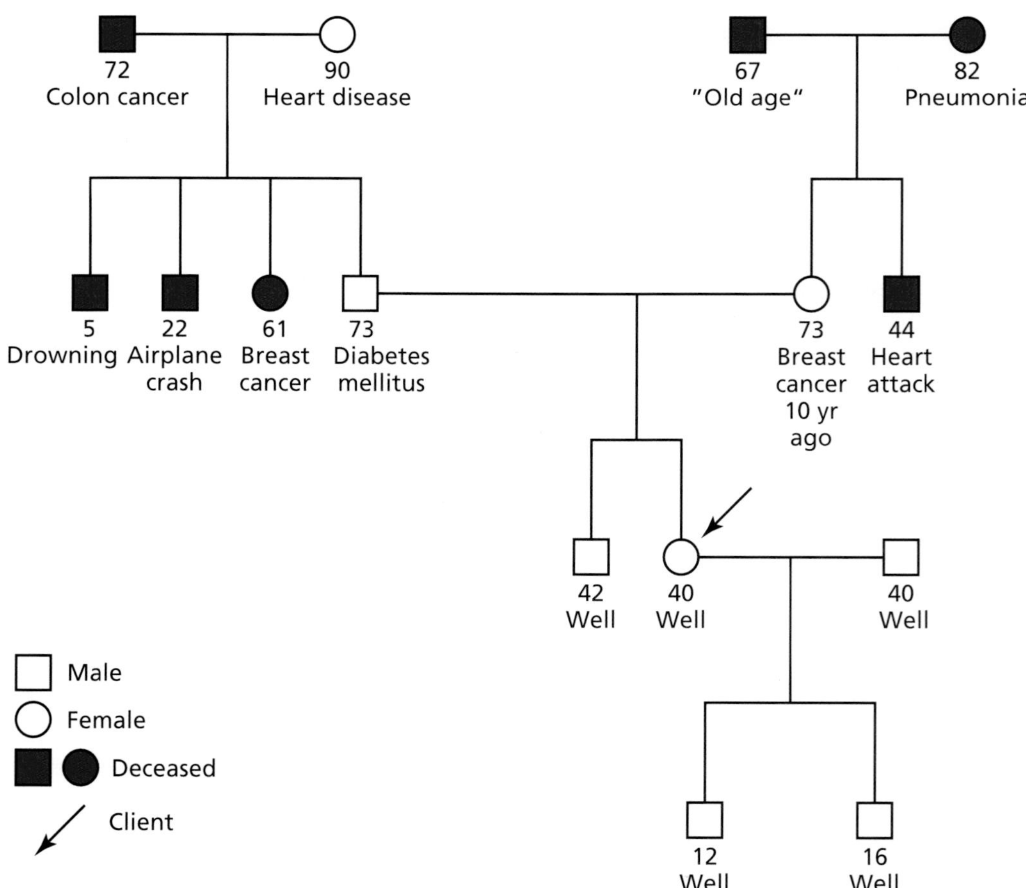

Fig. 4-3 Sample genogram identifying grandparents, parents, aunts and uncles, siblings, spouse, and children.

history of the specific disease. Document the presence of these diseases in a family tree or genogram. Also include the current ages of those who are alive and well and the cause and age at death of those who are deceased (Fig. 4-3).

REVIEW OF SYSTEMS

Review of systems (ROS) is conducted to inquire about the past and present health of each of the client's body systems and to ensure that no significant data were omitted in the present health status section. In the review of the physical systems, when clients respond positively to a symptom, then a symptom analysis is completed. If the data collection from the present health status section has already provided sufficient data on a body system, you do not need to repeat those questions in this section. For example, if you completed a symptom analysis on "cough" when completing the present health status, you need not repeat questions about cough in the review of systems.

Symptoms are listed in this chapter using medical terms, but a brief definition is included as needed to facilitate your interpretation of the term to the client. For example, if you want to know if the client has dyspnea, you ask "Do you become short of breath?" If the client says no, you would document "denies dyspnea" or "no dyspnea," but if the client says yes, you would use questions from the symptom analysis and document your findings. Therefore you will need to know the medical terms for documentation and communication with other health care providers, but only terms understood by the client are used during the interview. While some health promotion (HP) data are included in the previous sections on present health status and past health history, additional information is collected during the review of systems.

Below is an outline, organized by body region or body system, of the symptoms you ask the client about. In a comprehensive health assessment, you ask most of the questions; but in a focused health assessment, you ask about only those systems related to the reason for seeking care.

General Health Status
- Fatigue, weakness
- Sleep patterns
- Weight, unexplained loss or gain
- Self-rating of overall health status

Integumentary System
- *Skin*
  - Skin disease, problems, lesions (wounds, sores, ulcers)
  - Skin growths, tumors, masses
  - Excessive dryness, sweating, odors
  - Pigmentation changes or discolorations
  - Rashes
  - Pruritus (itching)
  - Frequent bruising
  - Texture or temperature change
  - Scalp itching
  - HP: Measures taken to limit sun exposure; use of sunscreen; skin self-examination
- *Hair* (refers to all body hair, not just head and pubic area)
  - Changes in amount, texture, character, distribution
  - Alopecia (loss of hair)
- *Nails*
  - Changes in texture, color, shape
  - HP: Type and frequency of nail care

Head
- Headache
- Past significant trauma
- Vertigo (dizziness)
- Syncope (brief lapse of consciousness)
- HP: Use of protective headgear

Eyes
- Discharge
- Pruritus
- Lacrimation (excessive tearing)
- Pain in eyeball
- Visual disturbances such as blind spots (floaters), halos around lights, or flashing lights
- Swelling around eyes
- Redness
- Unusual sensations or twitching
- Vision changes (generalized or vision field)
- Use of corrective or prosthetic devices
- Diplopia (double vision)
- Blurring vision
- Photophobia (increased sensitivity to light)
- Difficulty reading
- Interference with activities of daily living
- HP: Use of protective eyewear

Ears
- Pain
- Cerumen (wax)
- Infection, earache
- Discharge
- Hearing changes
- Use of prosthetic devices
- Increased sensitivity to environmental noises
- Change in balance
- Tinnitus (ringing or cracking)
- Interference with activities of daily living
- HP: Ear protection from excessively loud noise

Nose, Nasopharynx, and Paranasal Sinuses
- Discharge
- Epistaxis (nosebleed)
- Sneezing
- Obstruction
- Sinus pain
- Postnasal drip
- Change in ability to smell
- Snoring
- Pain over sinuses

Mouth and Oropharynx
- Sore throat
- Tongue or mouth lesion (abscess, sore, ulcer)
- Bleeding gums

Voice changes or hoarseness
Use of prosthetic devices (dentures, bridges)
Altered taste
Dysphagia (difficulty swallowing)
Difficulty chewing
HP: Self-care habits, frequency and kind of dental hygiene

Neck
Lymph node enlargement
Swelling or masses
Pain/tenderness
Limitation of movement
Stiffness

Breasts
Pain/tenderness
Swelling
Nipple discharge
Changes in nipples
Lumps, masses, dimples
HP: Breast self-examination (frequency, method)

Cardiovascular System
Heart
Palpitations
Chest pain
Dyspnea (shortness of breath)
Orthopnea (person must sit to breathe)
Paroxysmal nocturnal dyspnea (periodic dyspnea during sleep)
HP: Monitor fat in diet, exercise regularly

Peripheral vasculature
Coldness, numbness
Discoloration
Peripheral edema
Varicose veins
Intermittent claudication (leg pain with exercise that ceases with rest)
Paresthesia (abnormal sensations)
Leg color changes
HP: Use of support hose if work involves standing
Avoid crossing legs at the knees
Exercise patterns

Respiratory System
Colds
Cough, nonproductive or productive
Hemoptysis (coughing up blood)
Dyspnea (short of breath)
Night sweats
Wheezing
Stridor (abnormal, high-pitched, musical sound)
Pain on inspiration or expiration
Smoking history, exposure to smoke

Gastrointestinal System
Change in taste
Thirst
Indigestion or pain associated with eating
Pyrosis (burning sensation in esophagus and stomach with sour eructation [belching])
Dyspepsia (heartburn or bloating)
Nausea/vomiting
Hematemesis (vomiting blood)
Appetite changes
Food intolerance
Abdominal pain
Jaundice (yellowish color to skin and sclera)
Ascites (abnormal intraperitoneal fluid accumulation)
Bowel habits
Flatus
Constipation
Diarrhea
Changes in stools (color, consistency)
Hemorrhoids (pain, rectal bleeding)
Use of digestive or evacuation aids
HP: Type of diet, compare diet to food pyramid

Urinary System
Characteristics of urine (color, contents)
Hesitancy
Urinary frequency (in 24-hour period)
Urgency
Change in urinary stream
Nocturia (excessive urination at night)
Dysuria (painful urination)
Flank pain (posterior portion of body between ribs and iliac crest)
Hematuria (blood in the urine)
Suprapubic pain
Dribbling or incontinence
Polyuria (excessive excretion of urine)
Oliguria (decreased urination)
Pyuria (white blood cells or pus in urine)
HP: Amount of daily water intake
Females—measures to prevent urinary tract infections

Genitalia
General
Lesions
Discharges
Odors
Pain, burning, pruritus
Painful intercourse
Infertility
HP: Methods of protection from unwanted pregnancy and sexually transmitted diseases

Men
Impotence
Testicular masses/pain
Prostate problems
Change in sex drive
HP: Penis and scrotum self-examination practices

Women
Menstrual history (date of onset, last menstrual period [LMP], length of cycle)

Amenorrhea (absent menstruation)
Menorrhagia (excessive menstruation)
Dysmenorrhea (painful menstruation)
Metrorrhagia (irregular menstruation)
Dyspareunia (pain during intercourse)
Postcoital bleeding (bleeding after intercourse)
Pelvic pain
HP: Genitalia self-examination

Musculoskeletal System

Muscles

Twitching, cramping, pain
Weakness

Bones and joints

Joint swelling, pain, redness, stiffness
Joint deformity
Crepitus (noise with joint movement)
Limitations in joint range of motion
Interference with activities of daily living

Back

Back pain
Limitations in joint range of motion
Interference with activities of daily living
HP: Amount and kind of exercise per week

Central Nervous System

History of central nervous system disease (specify with examples)
Fainting episodes or loss of consciousness
Seizures (characteristics, how treated)
Dysphasia (impairment in speech)
Dysarthria (poorly articulated speech)
Cognitive changes
Inability to remember (recent versus dated)
Disorientation to time, place, person
Hallucinations

Motor-gait

Loss of coordinated movements
Ataxia (balance problems)
Paralysis (partial versus complete)
Paresis
Tic, tremor, spasm
Interference with activities of daily living

Sensory

Paresthesia (abnormal sensations, e.g., "pins and needles," tingling, numbness)
Anesthesia (absent sensation, location)
Pain (describe)

Endocrine System

Changes in skin pigmentation or texture
Changes in or abnormal hair distribution
Sudden or unexplained changes in height or weight
Intolerance of heat or cold
Presence of secondary sex characteristics
Polydipsia (excessive thirst)
Polyphagia (excessive hunger)
Polyuria (excessive urine output)
Anorexia (decreased appetite)
Weakness

PSYCHOSOCIAL STATUS

Psychologic and sociologic data are important aspects of a health history. The following is an outline of information to be obtained:

General statement of client's feelings about self
Degree of satisfaction in interpersonal relationships
Client's position in home relationships
Most significant relationship
Community activities
Work or school relationships
Family cohesiveness
Activities
General description of work, leisure, and rest distribution
Hobbies and methods of relaxation
Family demands
Ability to accomplish all that is desired during period (day, week)
Cultural or religious practices
Occupational history
Jobs held in past
Current employer
Education preparation
Satisfaction with present and past employment
Recent changes or stresses in client's life (e.g., divorce, moving, new job, family illness, new baby, financial stress)
Coping strategies for stressful situations
Changes in personality, behavior, mood
Feelings of anxiety or nervousness
Feelings of depression (e.g., insomnia, crying, fearfulness, marked irritability or anger)
Use of medications or other techniques during times of anxiety, stress, or depression
Habits
Alcohol/drugs
Type of alcohol/drugs
Frequency per week
Pattern over past 5 years; 1 year
Alcohol/drug consumption variances when anxious, stressed, or depressed
Driving or other dangerous activities while under the influence
High-risk groups: Sharing/using unsterilized needles and syringes
Smoking
Kind (cigarette, cigar, pipe)
Amount per day
Pattern over 5 years; 1 year
Smoking variances when anxious or stressed
Desire to quit smoking
Exposure to secondhand smoke
Coffee and tea
Amount per day

Pattern over 5 years; 1 year
Consumption variances when anxious or stressed
Physiologic effects
Other
Overeating, sporadic eating, or fasting
Nail biting
Financial status
Sources of income
Adequacy of income
Recent changes in resources or expenditures

ENVIRONMENTAL HEALTH

An outline of data to be obtained for the environmental health portion of the history includes the following:

General statement of client's assessment of environmental safety and comfort
Hazards of employment (inhalants, noise, heavy lifting, machinery, psychologic stress)
Hazards in the home (concern about fire, smoke detector, stairs to climb, inadequate heat, open gas heaters, pest control, violent behaviors, loud sound systems including earphones)
Hazards in the neighborhood or community (noise, water and air pollution, heavy traffic on surrounding streets, overcrowding, violence, firearms, sale/use of street drugs)
Hazards of travel (use of seat belts, motorcycle or bicycle helmets)
Travel outside the United States (when and which countries visited, length of stay)

HEALTH HISTORY FORMAT BASED ON FUNCTIONAL HEALTH PATTERNS

Not all health histories are organized in a body systems format as previously described. One common interview format used by nurses in many areas is based on functional health patterns. For example, in many hospitals, functional health patterns is the format used for the nursing admission history. As you might recall, the use of functional health patterns as a nursing database was briefly discussed in Chapter 1. In addition to biographic data and the reason for seeking care, a nursing history based on functional health patterns collects and organizes data in each of the following 11 areas (Gordon, 1994):

- Health perception–health management
- Nutrition–metabolism, nutrition–metabolic
- Elimination
- Activity–exercise
- Cognitive–perception
- Sleep-rest
- Self-perception–self-concept
- Role–relationship
- Sexuality–reproduction
- Coping–stress tolerance
- Values–belief

An example of a health history based on functional health patterns is presented in Appendix C.

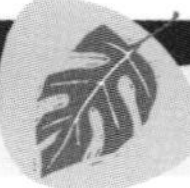

AGE-RELATED VARIATIONS IN THE HEALTH HISTORY

NEWBORN

The terms *newborn* and *neonate* are used interchangeably and refer to the first 27 days of life. Infant is used to describe a baby from 1 to 12 months of age. The gestational age and well-being of the neonate will influence the information needed for the database; therefore newborns who are at risk should receive additional assessment by neonatal experts.

The purpose of this assessment is to determine the newborn's physical condition and transition from intrauterine to extrauterine life. Maternal history is an important aspect of the total health database of the newborn, since the mother's behaviors and experiences during pregnancy also may affect the neonate.

Biographic Data Biographic data should include the following:

- *Name:* mother's name and neonate's name and sex; multiple births may be listed as newborn A, B, etc., until names are given.
- *Age:* gestational age, date and time of birth
- *Birth weight*: in pounds and ounces or in grams
- *Parent's culture:* (pattern of behavioral responses shaped by values, beliefs, norms, and practices)
- *Socioeconomic factors of family:* (e.g., parent's employment, on Medicaid)
- Address and telephone number of parents or family
- Siblings and family in home
- Parent's means of transportation for follow-up examinations of newborn
- Description of parent's home and size and type of community

Reason for Seeking Care The reason for seeking care is reported by the adult bringing the neonate for care. The visit may be a well-baby or a sick-baby visit. Review with the parent or caregiver the schedule for immunizations and well-baby examinations.

Present Health Status Ask the adult accompanying the neonate to elaborate on the reason for seeking care. For a sick-baby visit, complete a symptom analysis (see Box 4-2). For a well-baby visit, the data collected are the same as those listed under the review of systems. Also discuss the physical care of the neonate, including cord care, care after circumcision, use of bulb syringe for suctioning nasal secretions, and proper positioning of the neonate for sleep.

Past Health History The past health history of the neonate begins with the mother's health status during the pregnancy. This should include the following data:

- Extent of prenatal care
- Complications of pregnancy: bleeding, falls, edema of hands and feet, hypertension, proteinuria, unusual weight gain, infections
- Use of tobacco during pregnancy (type, amount)
- Medications taken, including street drugs (include dose, duration, and month of gestation when taken)
- Radiographs taken
- Emotional state of mother during pregnancy: crying or depression states
- Planned pregnancy
- Mother's attitude toward neonate
- Father's attitude toward neonate
- Pregnancy history (parity, gravidity, abortions, miscarriages, time between pregnancies)

Problems that arise during the labor and delivery process also can affect the neonate. The following data should be collected:

Labor and delivery process

- Where delivery occurred (hospital, birth center, home)
- Number of weeks of gestation
- Labor: spontaneous or induced, duration, complications
- Type of delivery: vaginal or cesarean section (planned or emergency cesarean section)
- Type of anesthesia used in delivery
- Presentation of neonate (e.g., vertex, breech)
- Special equipment or procedures required (e.g., forceps)
- Gestational assessment data and neurologic assessment data (Apgar score)
- Medications: vitamin K, hepatitis B immunization initiated, standard eye care, other medications ordered
- Tests performed (e.g., bilirubin, ABO isoimmunization, phenylketonuria)
- Baby's condition in hospital: oxygen requirements, color, feeding, vigor, cry; duration of baby's stay in hospital and whether infant discharged with mother; prescriptions such as bilirubin phototherapy or antibiotics

Family History Family history for the neonate is the same as for the adult, with the addition of congenital anomalies or hereditary disorders in the family.

Review of Systems Review of systems for the neonate is the same as for the adult with the following additions:

General Health Status

Nutrition

Breast- or bottle-fed, reasons for changes, if any; type of formula used, amount offered and consumed, frequency of feeding and weight gain

Sleep

Hours of sleep

HP: Position neonate on side for sleep

Integumentary System

Changes in color of skin or nails

Rashes, petechiae (tiny red spots)

Birthmarks

Healing of cord

HP: Cord care

Eyes

Follows object with eyes

Drainage

Ears

Discharge

Turns toward sounds

Nose, Nasopharynx, and Paranasal Sinuses

Difficulty breathing

Discharge

HP: Use of bulb syringe to suction nose

Mouth and Oropharynx

Strong suck

Respiratory System

Difficulty breathing

Cough, productive or nonproductive

Gastrointestinal System

Frequency and consistency of stools

Urinary System

Number of diapers used per day

Genitalia

Healing of circumcision

Discharge from vagina

HP: Care after circumcision

Musculoskeletal System

Moving extremities symmetrically

Central Nervous System

Describe cry

Is adult able to console neonate?

Response to touch, noise

Sleep cycle, amount

Psychosocial Status Discuss the following with the parent or guardian of the neonate:

- Sibling rivalry, how to deal with it
- Parenting skills
- Stresses of newborn in family, arrangements for infant care, mother's and/or father's plans for return to work

Environmental Health Discussion of the neonate's environmental health should include the following:

- Safety: infant seat and seat belts
- Protection from falls
- Appropriate clothing
- Avoiding drafts
- Supporting infant's head
- Absence of smoking in infant's environment

■ INFANTS

Infancy is the period of life from 1 to 12 months. History for the infant is the same as that for the child.

■ CHILDREN

Health history for the child is similar to that for the adult, with the additions of prenatal care, growth and development, and behavioral and school status histories. Most data are obtained from the adult accompanying the child but include the child as much as appropriate for his or her age (Fig. 4-4). Also observe the interaction between the adult and the child during the examination. Depending on the age of the child, it might be helpful to set a time to collect data from the parent without the child's presence. Collecting a complete history during a well-child visit is more desirable than when the child is sick. The following format parallels the adult history but includes the significant pediatric data.

Biographic Data Biographic data to be gathered for the child include the following:

- Informant: person giving the history (relationship to client)
- Name of child
- Names of children and family members living in the home
- Means of transportation to health care facility, if pertinent
- Description of home, size and type of community

Reason for Seeking Care The reason for seeking care portion of the health assessment is the same as for the adult. Data are usually taken from the adult accompanying the child brought for care.

Present Health Status The same present health status information is recorded for the child as for the adult. If illness is present, record a symptom analysis. If it is a well-child visit, proceed with the data collection about the child's health, growth, and development. (Chapter 2 describes the expected growth and development of children.) Also include information on the following:

- Current medications
  Type (e.g., prescription, over-the-counter, vitamins)
  Prescribed by whom
  Effect of medications
- Allergies (food, drug, environmental factors, contact substances)
- Last examinations (physical, dental, vision, hearing, developmental screening)
- Immunizations: dates administered (see immunization schedule in Chapter 2)

Past Health History Health history of mother during pregnancy is the same as for the newborn.

- Birth order
- Neonatal period is the same as described for the newborn
- Illnesses: injuries, hospitalizations, communicable diseases (e.g., colds, earaches, common childhood diseases such as measles, rubella [German measles], chickenpox, mumps, pertussis [whooping cough], diphtheria, scarlet fever, streptococcal infections, tonsillitis, allergic manifestations)

Family History Family history should include a maternal gestational history, listing all pregnancies and the health status of living children. For deceased children indicate age, cause of death, and duration of pregnancy if miscarriage. Other questions about the health of family members are the same as for the adult.

Review of Systems The review of systems includes the following additions and variations:

General Health Status
Fatigue patterns
Energetic or overactive patterns
Growth: changes in height and weight appropriate for age

Nutrition
Breast- or bottle-fed, reasons for changes, if any; type of formula used, amount offered and consumed, frequency of feeding and weight gain
Present diet and appetite, age of introduction of solids, age when child achieved three meals a day; present feeding patterns; age weaned from bottle or breast; type of milk and daily intake; food preferences
Recent weight gain or loss (describe)
Twenty-four hour recall, including types and amount of food eaten (formula, breast milk, meat, fruits, vegetables, cereals, juices, eggs, milk, sweets, snacks) and frequency
Does child feed self?
Where does child eat?
Who eats with child?
Parent's perception of child's nutritional status
Use of vitamin supplements

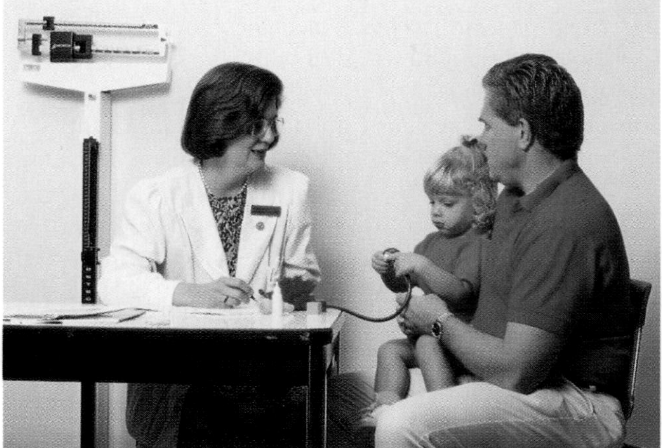

Fig. 4-4 Most data are obtained from the adult accompanying the child.

Integumentary System
Skin
Chronic rashes
Easy bruising, bleeding, or petechiae
Hair
Infections, lice
Nails
Nail biting
Hygiene
Eyes
Crossed eyes
Complaint of vision changes
Reading difficulty
Sits too close to television or video games
Ears
Multiple infections or earaches
Myringotomy tubes in ears
Discharge (describe)
Parent's perception of child's hearing
Mouth and oropharynx
Dentition: age of first teeth, loss of deciduous teeth, eruption of first permanent teeth
Sore throat (frequency, describe)
Tonsils present
Mouth sores
Toothaches, caries
Mouth breathing
HP: toothbrushing and flossing pattern
Breasts
Development of breasts and nipples

Cardiovascular System
Cyanosis (what precipitates it)
Dyspnea (shortness of breath) on exertion
Limitation of activities
Frequent complaints of extremity coldness
Excessive bleeding or easy bruising
Fatigue
Lead exposures

Respiratory System
Snoring

Urinary System
Status of toilet training; plans for; problems
Bed-wetting (associated with emotional upset; family history of bed-wetting)
Use of bubble bath

Genitalia
General
Birth defects
Rashes, irritation
Areas of concern
Girl: If menstruating, refer to adult database for appropriate questions; development of pubic hair
Boy: Development of facial and pubic hair, voice changes, emissions, penile/scrotal enlargement

Musculoskeletal System
Gait ability
Curvature of the spine (age when noted)
Generalized aching

Central Nervous System
Birth injury
Speech
Stuttering
Speech misarticulation
Language delay
Cognitive changes
Passing-out episodes
Staring spells
Learning difficulties
Motor-gait
Developmental clumsiness

Endocrine System
Precocious or delayed puberty

Psychosocial Status The following is an outline of the data collected regarding the child's psychosocial status:

General Status
General statement of child's feelings about self
Parent's observations of child's feelings about self

Development (Following commonly used developmental milestones. Refer to Chapter 2 for comprehensive descriptions.)
Age when able to do the following:
Hold head erect while in sitting position
Roll over from front to back and back to front
Sit alone unsupported
Stand with support and alone
Walk with support and alone
Use words
Talk in sentences
Dress self
Age when toilet trained: approaches to and attitudes regarding toilet training
How sexuality education is handled in the home

Caretakers and Family
Who lives in child's home?
Primary care provider for child
Relationships among members of the household

Friends
Child's relationships with friends, classmates, siblings
Age of playmates
Ability to make friends easily
Imaginary friends or animals

Habits
Behavior patterns: nail biting, thumb sucking, pica (habitual ingestion of nonfood substance), rituals ("security" blanket or toy), and unusual movements (head banging, rocking, overt masturbation, walking on toes)
General description of typical day
Sleep patterns and naps; sound sleeper or fretful; number of hours of sleep per 24 hours; nightmares, night terrors, parent's response

Kinds of play: amount of active and quiet play per 24 hours, television time per 24 hours
Hobbies and methods of relaxation (for older child)

Family

Activities of family as unit
Methods of discipline within family
Effects of discipline
Who disciplines child?
Child's reaction to discipline
Parents or providers: type of employment, type of child care provided if both parents work
Availability of emotional support for parents in care of child and opportunity to be away from child

School

Present grade in school or level of nursery care
School performance
Behavior problems
Learning problems; special classes required, if any
Attitude about school
Rate of absenteeism

Ability to Cope with Stress

Child's ability to adapt to new situations
Recent changes or stresses in child's life, (e.g., new baby, financial stress, divorce/separation, move to new home/neighborhood/school)
Behavior patterns child uses to cope with stress
Change in personality, behavior, mood
History of psychiatric care or counseling

Environmental Health General statement of parent's assessment of environmental safety and comfort.

Hazards in the home, to include survey of the following:
Toys appropriate for age
Storage of firearms, drugs, toxic chemicals, matches
Stairway protection (e.g., use of gates for toddlers or handrails for older children)
Type of bed (protection device to prevent falls)
Pest control
Open space heaters
Peeling of lead paint in older homes

Injury prevention
Safety belts
Smoke detector in the home
Burn prevention
Medication safety
Hot water heater temperature

Hazards in the neighborhood
Unsafe play area
Stranger safety
Heavily traveled streets
No sidewalks
Water or air pollution
Excessive noise
Isolation or overcrowding from neighbors
Bicycle safety

Other primary prevention measures
Effects of passive smoke
Skin protection from ultraviolet light

ADOLESCENTS

History for an adolescent is similar to that for a child. There are several options to consider when assessing the adolescent. The first is choosing which database to use, pediatric or adult. Some nurses prefer to use the pediatric database until the client is 12 to 14 years old and then begin using the adult one, whereas others modify the pediatric tool and use it throughout adolescence. A second option is whether to assess the adolescent with the parent present. Frequently the history is taken with both present, and then the parent is asked to leave so that the adolescent can have time alone with the examiner to discuss health issues privately. Observe the interaction between the adolescent and the parent, as well as that with other children in the family who might attend the assessment. A sense of confidentiality should be established so the teenager feels comfortable with the examiner and trusts him or her enough to discuss delicate subjects. In sensitive areas, the nurse should try to approach the teen with a direct but empathetic and nonjudgmental manner. Time should be left at the end of the assessment to summarize the examination and allow time for the adolescent to ask questions. Often adolescents do not reveal what is actually on their minds until the end of the session, when the time devoted for the examination is almost gone and they have developed the courage to express concerns. There should be an opportunity at the end of the examination for discussing any risk-taking behaviors such as use of drugs or alcohol, drinking and driving, and sexual practices.

The biographic data, reason for seeking care, present health status, past medical history, and family history for an adolescent are the same as for an adult.

Review of Systems Review of systems for the adolescent is the same as that for the adult with the addition of the following:

Gastrointestinal
Satisfaction with diet and weight
Frequency of binge eating, inducing vomiting, abuse of laxatives, excessive exercise, or prolonged fasting

Genitourinary
Males: age of first night ejaculation
Concern about size of penis
Females: age of onset of menses

Psychosocial Status The psychosocial history for adolescents includes those factors listed previously for the adult in addition to specific concerns of this age group. The history is obtained primarily from the adolescent, with or without the parent present. Table 4-1 lists suggested questions to ask the adolescent. The psychosocial history can be summarized using the acronym HEADSS (Home, Education, Activities [including peers], Drugs, Sexuality, Suicide) (Goldenring and Cohen, 1988).

- *Home:* present family members, intactness of family, relationships between adolescent and other family members or extended family

Table 4-1 Questions to Ask Adolescents in Obtaining a Psychosocial History

TOPIC	QUESTION
Home	Where do you live, and who lives there with you?
Education	What are you good at in school? What is hard for you? What grades do you get?
Activities	What do you do for fun? What things do you do with friends? What do you do with your free time?
Drugs	Many teenagers experiment with drugs, alcohol, and cigarettes. Have you or your friends ever tried them? What have you tried? Do any of your family members use drugs, alcohol, or cigarettes?
Sexuality	Have you ever had a sexual relationship with anyone? Most young people become interested in sexual relationships at your age. Have you had any with boys, girls, or both? Tell me about your sex life.
Suicide	How long does it take you to fall asleep at night? How often do you wake up during the night? Has there been a change in your appetite or eating pattern? How satisfied are you with your eating patterns? How do you handle your feelings such as anger, sadness, worry, anxiety?

- *Education:* grade average, school enjoyment and adjustment, preferred subjects, vocational plans
- *Activities:* relationships with the same and opposite sex, interests, hobbies, and free-time activities
- *Drugs:* use of drugs (including alcohol and tobacco) by adolescent, peers, or family members
- *Sexuality:* knowledge of expected bodily changes during adolescence, dating patterns, sexual activity
- *Suicide:* feelings of sadness, loneliness, depression, or suicidal thoughts

Environmental Health The environmental health history for the adolescent is the same as for the adult.

■ OLDER ADULTS

There are a variety of definitions, connotations, and meanings for words such as *aging, aged, old,* and *elderly.* The age range from 65 to 74 years has been termed young-old, 75 to 84 years middle-old, and over 85 years, old-old (Lueckenotte, 2000). Another differentiation is made between healthy elderly and frail elderly. Often older adults are described by their functional status, which defines old by evaluating the functional performance of clients against standard adult performance (Matteson, McConnell, and Linton, 1997). Box 4-3 provides a functional assessment of activities of daily living (ADLs).

Older adult clients are not different from other adult clients. There is no specific age at which concerns related to the aging process warrant additional screening questions to complete an accurate database. The older person may have different concerns and needs due to disability, chronic disease, and changes normal with aging. The older adult client with multiple symptoms, a long history of illness and hospitalizations, and numerous problems at home requires more time for you to adequately analyze the status of each symptom and its interaction with other illnesses. Clients whose speech is impaired from a stroke may need more time to describe their reasons for seeking care.

Reason for Seeking Care Some older adults have chronic diseases to which they have adapted. Determine if the reason for the visit is related to one of the chronic conditions or is an unrelated problem. Certain problems are not easily identified, but, with skilled questioning, they may emerge as the assessment progresses (for instance, depression, weakness, or difficulty caring for self at home).

Clients may attribute new health problems to "getting old" and therefore not report them as significant.

Patience may be required in identifying priorities of the client's concern, which may be different from the priorities of the nurse.

Present Health Status Present health status of the older adult should include the following data about current medications:

Type of drug, reason for taking (over-the-counter and prescribed medications)
Prescribed by whom
When first prescribed
Amount of medication per day (compare prescribed with actual doses per day; include over-the-counter drugs also)
How medication is taken
Effectiveness of medication
Side effects of medications
Is there sharing of medications with others?
Do visual difficulties affect taking medications?
Ability to afford needed medications
Is transportation available to get prescriptions filled?

Past Health History The past health history for an older adult is the same as for the adult. The time span included in the history of course is longer, and the client's memory may not be too accurate. Several visits may be required to obtain a comprehensive past health history from an older person.

Box 4-3 Activities of Daily Living Assessment

A. Self-care
1. Dressing, undressing, clothing
   a. Keeping clothes in good repair (mending)
   b. Accessing clothes
   c. Getting into and out of underwear (bra, girdle, underpants, pantyhose, stockings, garter belt)
   d. Putting on and removing pants
   e. Getting arms in sleeves
   f. Managing zippers, buttons, snaps (especially in back), ties
   g. Putting on socks, shoes, tying laces
   h. Applying prostheses (e.g., glasses, hearing aids)
2. Grooming and hygiene
   a. Washing, drying, brushing hair
   b. Brushing teeth
   c. Cleaning and putting in dentures
   d. Shaving
   e. Caring for nails (feet and hands)
   f. Applying makeup
   g. Preparing bathwater and testing temperature
   h. Getting into and out of tub, shower
   i. Reaching and cleaning all body parts
3. Elimination
   a. Position altered for urination or sitting on toilet
   b. Ability to wipe self
   c. Lowering onto and rising from toilet

B. Mobility
1. Difficulty climbing or descending stairs (Is bedroom or bathroom on upper level? How many stairs or flights to apartment or house?)
2. Sitting up and rising from bed
3. Lowering to or rising from chair
4. Walking (short and long distances); describe necessity for walking
5. Opening doors
6. Reaching items in cupboards
7. Necessity for lifting (and any difficulty)

C. Communication
1. Dialing telephone
2. Reading numbers
3. Hearing over telephone
4. Answering door
5. Immediate access to neighbors, help

D. Eating
1. Access to market
2. Preparing food (opening cans and packages, using stove, reaching dishes, pots, utensils)
3. Handling knife, fork, spoon (cutting meat)
4. Getting food to mouth
5. Chewing, swallowing

E. Housekeeping, laundry, house upkeep
1. Making bed
2. Sweeping, mopping floors
3. Dusting
4. Washing dishes
5. Cleaning tub, bathroom
6. Picking up clutter (to client's satisfaction)
7. Taking out trash, garbage
8. Use of basement (stairs, cleaning)
9. Laundry facilities (in home or near residence, washtub, clothesline)
10. Yard care (garden, bushes, grass)
11. Other home-maintenance concerns (e.g., access to fuse box, storm windows, furnace filters, painting)

F. Medications
1. Large number of prescriptions (may be many)
2. Ability to remember
3. Ability to see labels or directions
4. Medications kept in one area

G. Access to community
1. Bus line
2. Walking
3. Driving (self or service from others)
4. Church, dry cleaning, drugstore, bank, health care facility, dentist, other community agencies

H. Other
1. Caring for spouse, relative, or companion
2. Financial management (able to write checks, make payments, cash checks)
3. Care of pet(s)

Family History Obtaining a family history for an older adult is of questionable value in predicting which diseases the client is at risk for, depending on the age of the client. It does, however, provide data about illnesses and causes of death of relatives.

Review of Systems The ROS is the same as for the adult.

Psychosocial Status Obtain data on the following:

- General statement of client's feelings about self
- Relatives and friends in home or nearby (to meet sexual, affection, support needs)
- If client lives alone, to what extent is living alone tolerated?
- Does client have sufficient and satisfactory access to family and friends? Does client have a pet?

If client lives with family, are relationships satisfactory?
Does client participate in family activities and in family decisions? Is there conflict with family members?
Activities of daily living
Can client independently perform the following: dressing, grooming, bathing, preparing meals, grocery shopping, climbing stairs?
General description of work, leisure, and rest distribution
Hobbies and methods of relaxation
Family demands
Ability to accomplish all that is desired during period (day/week)
Transportation
Automobile: Does client consider self a safe driver? Is maintaining vehicle a financial burden?
Bus: Easy access? Able to step aboard? Does client feel safe when riding bus?
Driving services from others: availability, convenience
Walking: problems with distance, carrying packages, fear of traffic
Occupational/volunteer history
Jobs held in past
Current employment
Volunteer and community activities
Satisfaction with present activities
Work/retirement concerns
Reduced/fixed income
Moving/selling home
Role change/time adjustment
Problems in relationship with spouse because of retirement
Recent changes or stresses in client's life (e.g., moving, retirement, illness of self or family member, financial stress, death of friend or family member, new responsibilities)
General statement about client's ability to cope with situation of stress (may also want to get input from spouse, adult child, or close friend)
History of psychiatric care or counseling
Feelings of fear, anxiety, or nervousness
Feelings of depression (e.g., insomnia, crying, fearfulness, marked irritability or anger)
Changes in personality, behavior, mood
Use of medications or other techniques during times of anxiety, stress, or depression

Environmental Health Data to be obtained should include the following:
General statement of client's assessment of environmental safety and comfort
Hazards of employment (if appropriate): inhalants, noise, heavy lifting, machinery, psychologic stress
Hazards in the home: concern about fire, stairs to climb, inadequate heat, open gas heaters, pest control, fear of falling
Safety at home for client who has difficulty with activities of daily living
Gait or balance problems:
Slippery or irregular surfaces (e.g., icy sidewalks, small rugs, risers on stair not fastened down)
Obstructions or clutter on stairs, extension cords
Steep, dark stairs (e.g., cellar)
Stairs without handrails
Inadequate space for maneuvering walker, wheelchair
Slippery bathtub
Decreased vision requires adequate lighting in dark hallway and on stairs, use of a night-light
Decreased sensitivity to pain and heat requires caution when using heating pads or hot water bottles, and with hot bathwater
Hazards in the neighborhood: noise, water, and air pollution; heavy traffic on surrounding streets; overcrowding; isolation from neighbors; violence; firearms
Community hazards: unavailability of grocery stores, laundry facilities, drugstore, bus line access
Hazard of maintaining a driver's license: Traffic accidents may occur because of slow reaction time, decreased vision, difficulty turning torso, walking too slowly for traffic signals

SUMMARY

Collecting a thorough history accomplishes several goals. It establishes a therapeutic relationship with the client. It also provides a picture of the client and identifies problems mentioned by the client that you can confirm or refute during the physical examination.

Once data are collected they must be organized, synthesized, and documented. When you collect health history data in an organized manner, the documentation becomes easier. See the following example of a health history documentation for an adult.

SAMPLE ADULT HEALTH HISTORY DOCUMENTATION

Biographic Data

Name: Megan S. Brockles
Gender: Female
Address: 5410 Cypress Hill, Irving, Texas 75062

Megan S. Brockles is a 46-year-old, white woman in no acute distress.

Telephone numbers: (214)999-9999, home; (214)444-4444, work
Birth date: 10-13-54
Birthplace: Houston, Texas
Race: White
Culture: American female
Religion: Methodist
Marital status: Married, 25 years
Family: Lives with spouse, two sons, and mother in a four-bedroom home in a suburban area

Social security number: 123-45-6789
Occupation: Counselor in a high school
Contact person: Kristopher Brockles, spouse
Advance directive: Yes, spouse has power of attorney
Source of referral: Colleague at work
Type of insurance: Network Health

Reason for Seeking Care

CC: "need Pap smear and something for these allergies"

Present Health Status

Health has been good during last 5 years; during past year has had sneezing, watery eyes, nasal congestion with clear nasal drainage. (Symptom analysis) Symptoms worse in the spring months, slow onset. Nasal congestion interferes with sleep and sometimes eating. Sneezing "fits" interfere with activity at the time; may sneeze 10 to 15 times in succession. Sneezing "fits" occur every 2 to 3 days at unpredictable times, at home rather than at work. Tearing of eyes occurs with sneezing. Takes over-the-counter allergy-relief medicine, which gives temporary relief. Working in the yard makes symptoms worse.

Current health promotion activities include walking 1.5 miles 2 to 3 times per week; performs breast self-examination each month.

Diet

Usual breakfast: Muffin, 1% milk, fruit juice, coffee
Usual lunch: Eats at school; meat, 1 vegetable, salad, tea
Usual dinner: Meat (turkey, chicken, pork, rarely beef); fruit or tossed salad; 1 green or yellow vegetable; potato, pasta, or rice; dessert; 1% milk
Snacks: Crackers with salsa or peanut butter
Current medications: Multiple vitamin plus vitamin C 1000 mg; zinc 50 mg; vitamin E 400 units; aspirin 325 mg; over-the-counter allergy medications

Past Health History

Allergies: Seasonal allergies, does not know what she is allergic to. Denies allergies to drugs or food
Childhood diseases: 1956-1966 measles, mumps, rubella, chickenpox, streptococcal throat, otitis media. Denies complications
Surgeries: 1958 brachial cleft cyst removed, Houston, Texas, Dr. Skylar; 1979 appendectomy, Irving, Texas, Dr. Reed
Hospitalizations: See obstetric below
Accidents/injuries: Denies
Immunizations: Childhood immunizations for school, denies tetanus immunization since high school
Last examinations
Physical, Pap smear: March 2000
Dentist: June 1999
Vision: September 1999
Hearing: High school
ECG: Denies
Mantoux test: September 1998
Mammogram: Denies
Obstetric history: Gravida 2, para 2, abortions 0
1978 vaginal delivery, 6 lb 14 oz healthy boy, no complications
1982 vaginal delivery, 7 lb healthy boy, no complications
1985 tubal ligation, no complications
Family history: Diabetes mellitus, maternal grandmother

Review of Systems

General: Client considers herself in "good health" except for allergies. Denies fatigue. Feels rested after sleep periods.
Nutritional: Reported height = 5 ft 9 in (175 cm), reported weight = 140 lb (63 kg). Weight consistent

Integumentary System

Skin: Denies lesions, masses, discolorations, rashes. Some pruritus during winter months, clears with lotion
HP: Uses sunscreen when outside 1 hour
Hair: Denies texture changes or loss, uses hair color monthly to cover gray; no scalp irritation reported from hair coloring
Nails: Denies changes in texture, color, shape. Manicures nails weekly
Head: Denies scalp itching, headache, trauma, vertigo, syncope
Eyes: Wears glasses/contacts for nearsighted vision. Eyes water during "allergy attacks." Denies discharge, pruritus, pain, visual disturbances
Ears: Has pierced ears—1970. Cleans ears with cotton-tipped applicator after shower. Denies pain, discharge, tinnitus
Nose, nasopharynx, paranasal sinuses: Clear nasal discharge, sneezing, nasal congestion during "allergy attacks." Denies epistaxis, olfactory deficit, snoring
Mouth and oropharynx: Denies sore throat, lesions, gum irritation, chewing or swallowing difficulties, hoarseness, voice changes
HP: Brushes teeth twice daily followed by flossing
Neck: Denies tenderness or range-of-motion difficulties
Breasts: Tenderness before menstrual periods, takes vitamin E to prevent fibrocystic breast disease; denies discharge, lumps, masses
Cardiovascular system: Denies chest pain, shortness of breath, and palpitations; feet frequently feel cold; denies discoloration and peripheral edema
Respiratory system: Denies breathing difficulties, chronic cough, and shortness of breath
Gastrointestinal system: Denies eating and digestion problems; denies hematemesis, jaundice, ascites; daily bowel movement is formed, brown; denies hemorrhoids
Urinary system: Describes urine as yellow and clear; voiding frequency 4 to 5 times daily; denies voiding difficulties, dysuria, urgency, and flank pain. Denies polyuria and oliguria, and nocturia
Genitalia: LMP July 1999; up until a few years ago, menses was every 28 to 30 days, regular intervals, light to medium flow. Since that time menses became sporadic

with light flow; no menses since July 1999; denies genital lesions, discharge, sexually transmitted disease (STD) history; sexually active, satisfied with sexual activity

Musculoskeletal system: Denies muscular weakness, twitching and pain, gait difficulties and extremity deformities, joint swelling, pain, stiffness and crepitus

Central nervous system: Denies changes in cognitive function, coordination, and sensory deficits

Endocrine system: Denies changes in skin pigment, change in weight, polyuria, polydipsia, polyphagia, anorexia, weakness

Psychosocial Status

Client states she feels good about herself most of the time. She experiences episodes of frustration integrating her mother into the life of her family. She considers her husband her best friend but also speaks of two other very close female friends. She counts on her friends to help her "talk through" stress periods. Considers family very close; communication channels are open most of the time. Her oldest teenage son resists sharing what is going on in his life but has been told that his parents are available if he needs them.

Client's activities include maintaining a home, raising two teenage boys, working full time. Her mother helps to maintain the home and prepare meals. Client is active in a community organization and church activities. A current family demand is disagreements she has with her mother about how to discipline her sons. She would like more time for herself.

She has a master's degree in counseling. She enjoys her job as a high school counselor, which she has held for 16 years. She gets frustrated with the lack of parenting skills of some of her students' parents.

Recent change in her life is a new principal who has just joined the school. She is not sure how well they will interact.

Client denies previous psychiatric counseling or feelings of anxiety or nervousness that she could not cope with. Methods of coping with stress are exercise and talking with her friends. To relax client enjoys drawing, playing piano, and gardening. Client and her spouse have had marriage counseling on two different occasions, which she feels was beneficial.

Drugs/alcohol: Denies drug use; 1 to 2 glasses of wine per week

Smoking: Denies

Coffee/tea: 2 cups coffee and 1 glass tea daily

Financial status: Feels there is adequate money for their activities and saving for college and retirement

Environmental Health

Client believes her home and neighborhood environment are safe and without hazards.

Subjective Problem List

1. Requests Pap smear
2. Seasonal allergies: wants more effective medication treatment
3. Due for tetanus immunization
4. Concerned about fibrocystic disease for which she takes vitamin E
5. Conflict with her mother about discipline of sons
6. Concerned about relation with new principal at work

(Final problem list is developed and priorities are established after physical examination.)

CLINICAL APPLICATION and CRITICAL THINKING

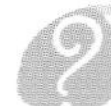

CRITICAL THINKING QUESTIONS

1. A mother brings her 6-week-old baby to the clinic for a well-baby visit. In conducting a comprehensive interview for health history, what information should the nurse explore with the mother regarding past health for a 6-week-old infant?
2. Consider the elements involved in taking the health histories of an infant, a child, and an adolescent. Compare the focus of psychosocial status for each age group.

   Newborn/infant

   Child

   Adolescent
3. How does a health history organized by functional health patterns differ from one organized by body systems? Which one is better?

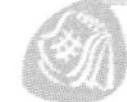

CASE STUDY

Jean is a 37-year-old woman who has been interviewed for a health history, which includes the following family history. Jean is married. Her husband is 43. The couple have a 12-year-old-son, an 11-year-old daughter, and a 10-year-old son, all in good health. Jean has a 42-year-old brother and three sisters who are 32, 36, and 40 years old. All of her siblings are in good health. Both of Jean's parents are alive. Her 70-year-old father has mild emphysema and is an only child. Her mother is 66 and has hypertension. Jean's mother has three siblings. The

oldest brother (Jean's uncle) is 74 and suffers from glaucoma. Another brother is 72 and is in good health. A sister is 69 and has osteoarthritis. All of Jean's grandparents are deceased. Her paternal grandfather died at the age of 89 of prostate cancer. Her paternal grandmother died of congestive heart failure at the age of 91. Jean's maternal grandfather died at the age of 86 of prostate cancer; her maternal grandmother died of "old age" at the age of 96.

1. Draw a genogram for Jean's family history with the information provided.

REMEMBER to check out your **companion CD-ROM**

5 Equipment for Physical Assessment

www.mosby.com/MERLIN/wilson/assessment/

Many of the techniques of physical assessment require the use of instruments to objectively measure or evaluate clinical signs or health status. This chapter describes the equipment most frequently used for physical assessment and the personal protective clothing that may be required during the examination. Use of these instruments is found either in Chapter 6, "Techniques of Physical Assessment," or in the chapters that describe the examination of specific body systems.

THERMOMETERS (TEMPERATURE MEASUREMENT)

Purpose: To assess the functional status of the body's tissues and cells.

Four types of thermometers are commonly in use to evaluate body temperature: mercury-in-glass, electronic, tympanic, and disposable. The most inexpensive, the mercury thermometer (Fig. 5-1, *A*), consists of a glass tube sealed at one end with a mercury-filled bulb at the other. Exposure of the bulb to heat causes the mercury to expand and rise in the enclosed tube. These thermometers may be calibrated in either Fahrenheit or Celsius and may be used to measure oral, axillary, or rectal temperature.

There are safety issues regarding use of mercury-in-glass thermometers. When a glass thermometer breaks, the risk for injury may occur not only because of the broken glass, but also because the mercury released poses a hazard to individuals and to the environment. The mercury must be disposed of appropriately according to institutional guidelines. Another safety risk with use of the glass thermometer is infection. Ineffective disinfection of glass thermometers has been linked to outbreaks of nosocomial infection (Cutter, 1994). In most settings, a disposable plastic sheath is used to cover the thermometer.

The electronic thermometer (Fig. 5-1, *B*) consists of a battery-powered display unit, a thin wire cord, and a temperature-sensitive probe. The probe must be covered with a disposable sheath before use. The probes are color coded (blue or white for oral and red for rectal) for proper use. The advantage of the electronic thermometer over the mercury thermometer is speed (O'Toole, 1997). The electronic thermometer calculates and displays the temperature on a digital screen within 15 to 30 seconds. Many electronic thermometers have a switch on the unit to permit the measurement of temperature in either Fahrenheit or Celsius.

The tympanic thermometer (Fig. 5-1, *C*) is very popular in all clinical settings. Taking the client's temperature with this device requires less than 5 seconds and is very easy. The device works when the temperature-sensitive probe, covered with a disposable sheath, is inserted into the client's ear; the probe measures the temperature of the blood flowing near the tympanic membrane. This provides an accurate measurement of core body temperature. Like the electronic thermometer, tympanic thermometers may be programmed to measure temperature in either Fahrenheit or Celsius.

Disposable, single-use thermometer strips (Fig. 5-1, *D*) are thin strips of plastic with chemically impregnated paper. They are frequently used for temperature evaluation in children. Chemical dots on the strip change color, representing the highest temperature. The strips are configured so that the examiner can identify the highest colored dot and correlate that with the temperature reading.

STETHOSCOPE

Purpose: To hear sounds within the body that are not easily heard with the naked ear.

There are several types of stethoscopes: the acoustic stethoscope, the magnetic stethoscope, the electronic stethoscope, and the stereophonic stethoscope. For routine health assessment, the acoustic stethoscope is most commonly used (Fig. 5-2, *A*).

The acoustic stethoscope is a closed cylinder that transmits sound waves from the source through the tube to the examiner's ears. It does not magnify sound, but, by blocking out extraneous room noise, it permits difficult-to-hear sounds to be more easily heard. The stethoscope consists of three components: the ear pieces, the tubing, and the end piece. The ear pieces, which may be hard or soft, should fit snugly and completely fill the ear canal. **When the ear pieces are correctly placed in the ears, they should point toward the nose.** This alignment fits the contour of the ear canal. The tubing of the stethoscope should be made of thick, firm rubber that is no longer than 12 to 18 inches (30 to 46 cm). If the tubing is longer than 18 inches, the sounds may become distorted. The head of the stethoscope consists of two components: the diaphragm and the bell. The head of the stethoscope should be heavy enough to lie firmly on the body surface without being held. This piece is configured by a closure valve so that only the diaphragm or the bell may be activated at any one time. The diaphragm consists of a flat surface with a rubber or plastic ring edge. It is used to hear high-pitched sounds such as breath sounds, bowel sounds, and normal heart sounds. Its structure screens out low-pitched sounds. The bell of the stethoscope is constructed in a concave shape. It should be used to hear soft,

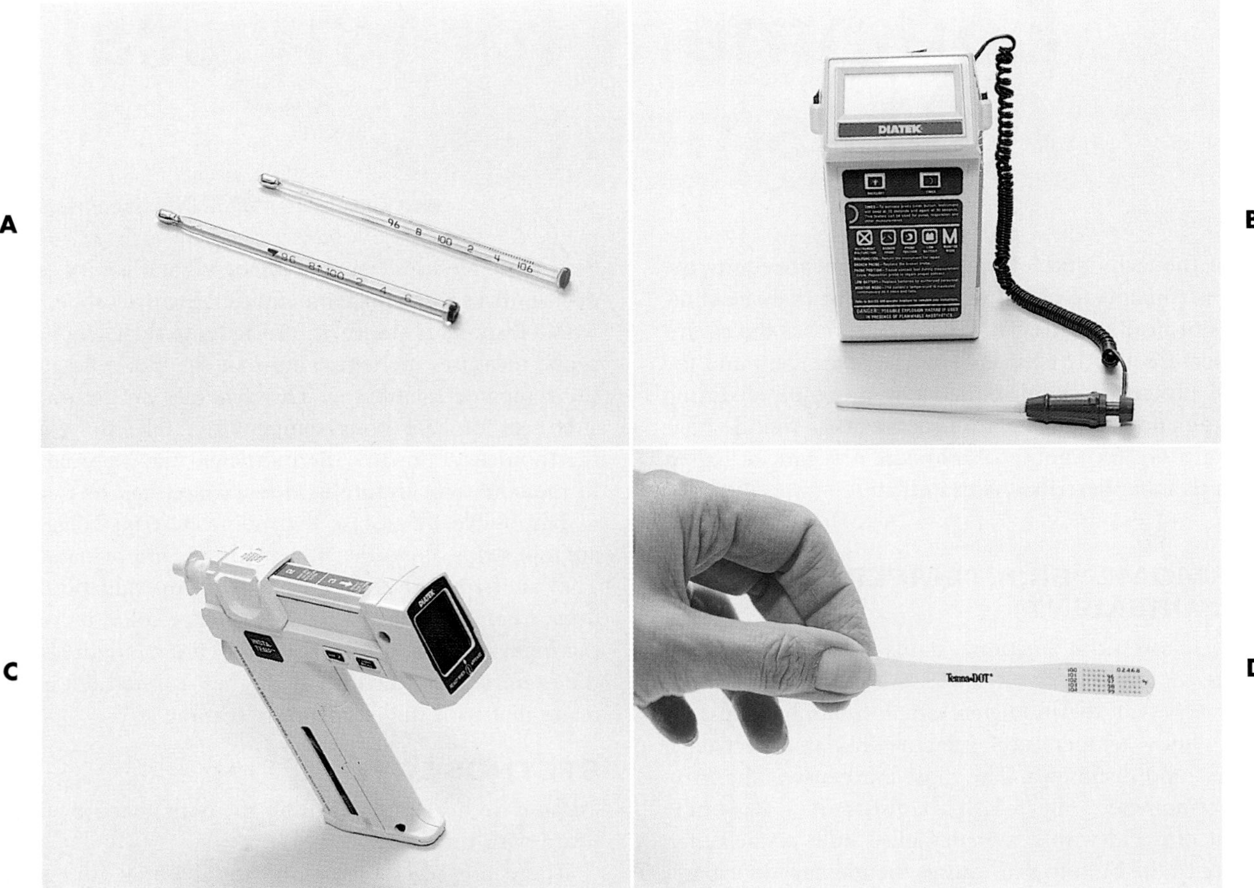

Fig. 5-1 **A,** Mercury thermometer (*rectal,* red tip; *oral,* blue tip). **B,** Electronic thermometer. **C,** Tympanic thermometer. **D,** Disposable, single-use thermometer strips.

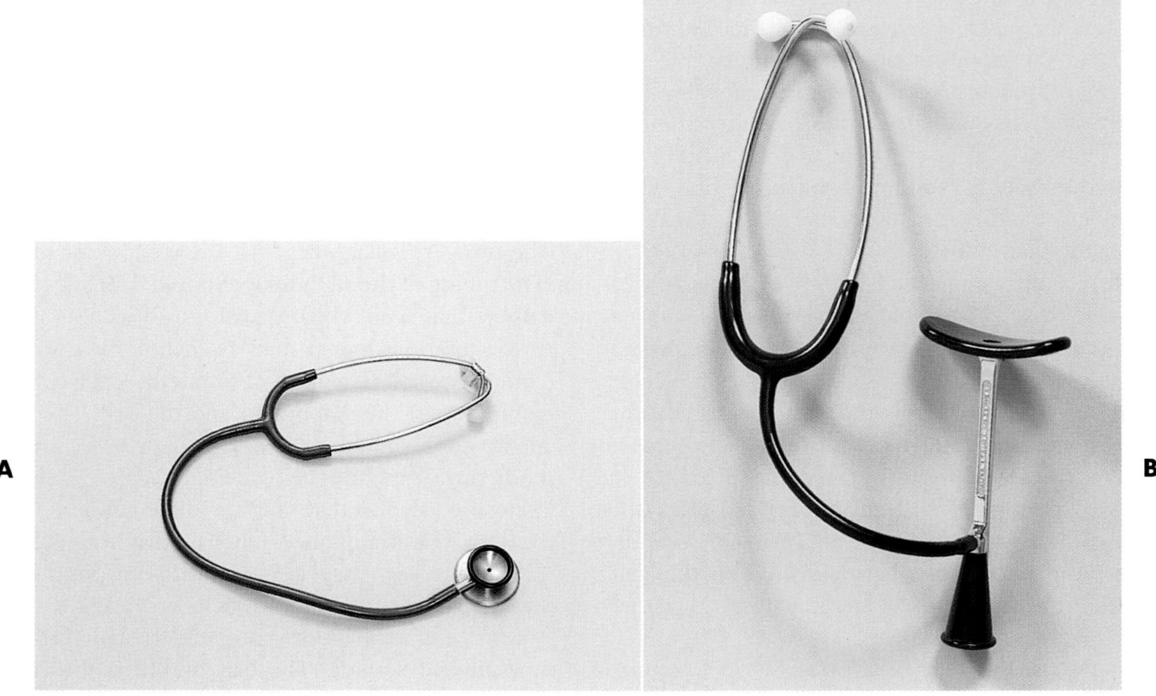

Fig. 5-2 **A,** Acoustic stethoscope. **B,** Fetoscope. (From Seidel et al, 1999.)

low-pitched sounds such as extra heart sounds or vascular sounds (bruit). When using the bell, the examiner should hold it lightly in place to ensure that a complete seal exists around the bell. If the bell is firmly placed on the skin and the concave surface is filled with skin, the bell will convert and function as a diaphragm.

Some stethoscopes have varying sizes of end pieces, which are interchangeable. When examining an infant or young child, the diaphragm and bell should be sized accordingly. Ideally the diaphragm and the bell should span one intercostal space.

A special type of stethoscope known as a fetoscope (Fig. 5-2, *B*) is used to auscultate the fetal heart. The fetoscope has a metal attachment that rests against the head of the examiner. This metal piece aids in the conduction of sound so that heart tones are heard more easily.

BLOOD PRESSURE MEASUREMENT EQUIPMENT

Purpose: To measure the arterial blood pressure.

Blood pressure measurement requires three pieces of equipment: the sphygmomanometer, the cuff, and the stethoscope. Together they may be used to measure blood pressure.

There are three types of sphygmomanometers. Two types, aneroid and mercury, attach to a blood pressure cuff bladder and require manual cuff inflation. A stethoscope must be used in conjunction with these devices to actually assess the blood pressure. The third type is electronic and assesses the blood pressure without the use of a stethoscope.

1. An aneroid sphygmomanometer is a glass-enclosed circular gauge containing a needle that registers in

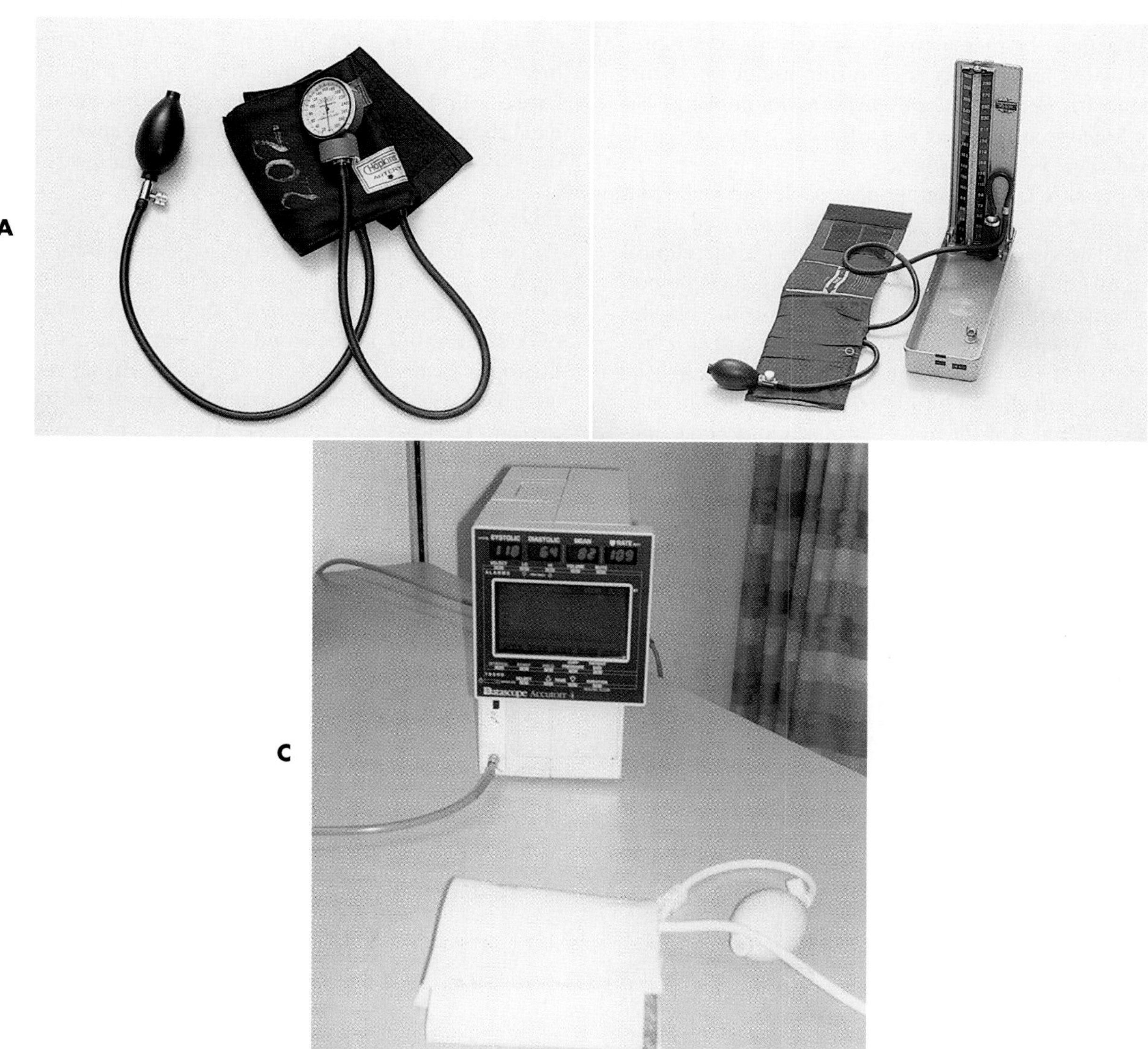

Fig. 5-3 **A,** Aneroid sphygmomanometer. **B,** Mercury manometer tube. **C,** Electronic blood pressure measurement.

millimeter calibrations. The gauge is attached to the blood pressure cuff bladder (Fig. 5-3, *A*). This gauge needs periodic calibration to ensure accurate measurement.

2. A mercury sphygmomanometer is an upright manometer tube containing mercury. The pressure created in the bladder of the cuff moves the column of mercury up against the force of gravity. Millimeter calibrations mark the height of the mercury column (Fig. 5-3, *B*).
3. An electronic sphygmomanometer operates by sensing circulating blood flow vibrations and converting these vibrations into electric impulses. These impulses in turn are translated to a digital readout. The readout generally consists of blood pressure, mean arterial pressure, and pulse rate. The device is not capable of determining quality of the pulse, such as rhythm or intensity. The device may be programmed to repeat the measurements on a scheduled periodic basis and to alarm if the measurements are outside of the precalculated limits. This is especially useful for clients requiring frequent blood pressure monitoring. No stethoscope is required when the electronic device is used (Fig. 5-3, *C*).

Blood pressure cuffs are either disposable and made of a latex substance or reusable and made of a textured fabric (Fig. 5-4). The type of cuff used depends on the clinical situation. All cuffs have a bladder that inflates during blood pressure measurement and a cuff that secures the bladder on the arm. When selecting a blood pressure cuff it is important to select the correct size for the client. Ideally the bladder of the cuff should be 40%, or one third to one half, of the circumference of the limb. On most cuffs, range lines are indicated to assess proper size. When a correctly sized cuff is applied, the cuff edge should lie between the range lines (see Fig. 5-4). Adult cuffs come in two widths. The standard cuff (4 2/3 to 5 1/6 inches) is adequate for most adults. If the adult is large or obese, an oversized cuff (6 to 6 1/3 inches) may be used. If the adult has an extremely obese arm, a thigh cuff can be used. For children, there are many different sizes of cuffs. The width of the cuff should cover two thirds of the child's or infant's upper arm. For both children and adults, if the cuff is too wide, it will underestimate the blood pressure; if it is too narrow, it will overestimate the blood pressure.

DOPPLER

Purpose: To amplify sounds that are difficult to hear with an acoustic stethoscope.

The Doppler uses ultrasonic waves to detect difficult-to-hear vascular sounds, such as fetal heart tones or peripheral pulses (Fig. 5-5). To use the device, coupling gel is applied to the probe; then the transducer is slid over the skin surface until the blood flow source is heard in the examiner's earpieces. As blood in the vessels ebbs and flows, the probe on the distal end of the Doppler picks up and amplifies the subtle changes in pitch. The resulting sound that the examiner hears is a swishing, pulsating sound. Most Dopplers have a sound volume control to amplify the sound. In prenatal clinics the Doppler often is attached to speakers so that the expectant parents may also hear the fetal heart sounds.

PULSE OXIMETRY

Purpose: To estimate the arterial oxygen saturation in the blood.

Pulse oximetry is a noninvasive measurement of arterial oxygen saturation in the blood (Fig. 5-6). This device uses a fiberoptic beam that reflects off the circulating red blood cells. This reflection is used to calculate an estimation of the percentage of oxygen saturation in arterial blood, as well as a pulse rate. The oximeter consists of a cutaneous sensor probe that may be taped or clipped to the client's ear, finger,toe, foot, or wrist. Pulse oximetry is considered highly accurate in the measurement of oxygen saturation over the

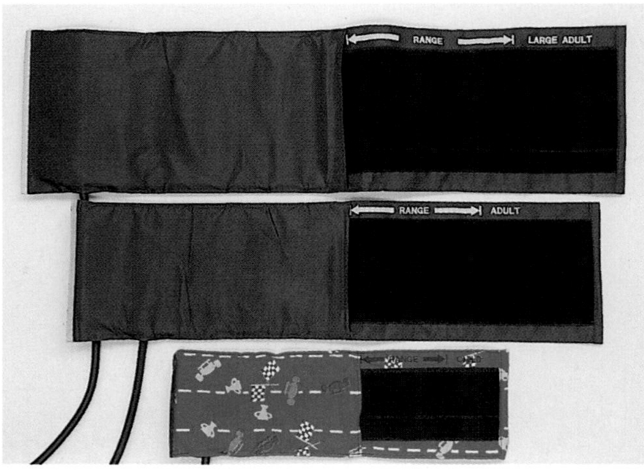

Fig. 5-4 Blood pressure cuffs.

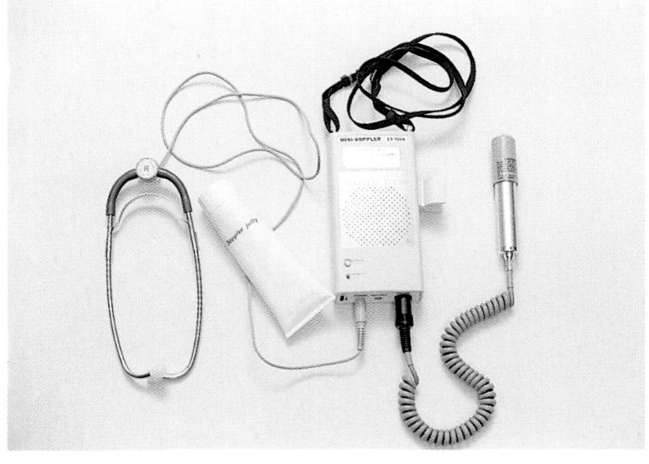

Fig. 5-5 Doppler.

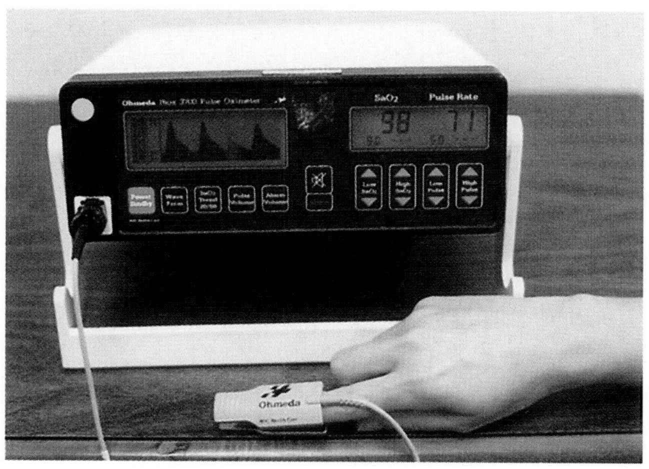

Fig. 5-6 Pulse oximeter.

range of 70% to100%. In many settings, it is sometimes referred to as "the fifth vital sign." As many as 86% of nurses and physicians routinely use pulse oximetry to assess client status (Grap, 1998; Tierney, Whooley, and Saint, 1997).

SNELLEN'S VISUAL ACUITY CHART

Purpose: Used as a screening examination for far, or distant, vision and color perception.

Snellen's chart is a large wall chart hung at a distance of 20 feet from the client (Fig. 5-7, *A*). The chart consists of 11 lines of letters of decreasing size. The letter size indicates the degree of visual acuity when read from a distance of 20 feet. The client should be tested one eye at a time. Beside each line of letters is the corresponding acuity rating that should be recorded (e.g., 20/40, 20/100). The top number of the re-

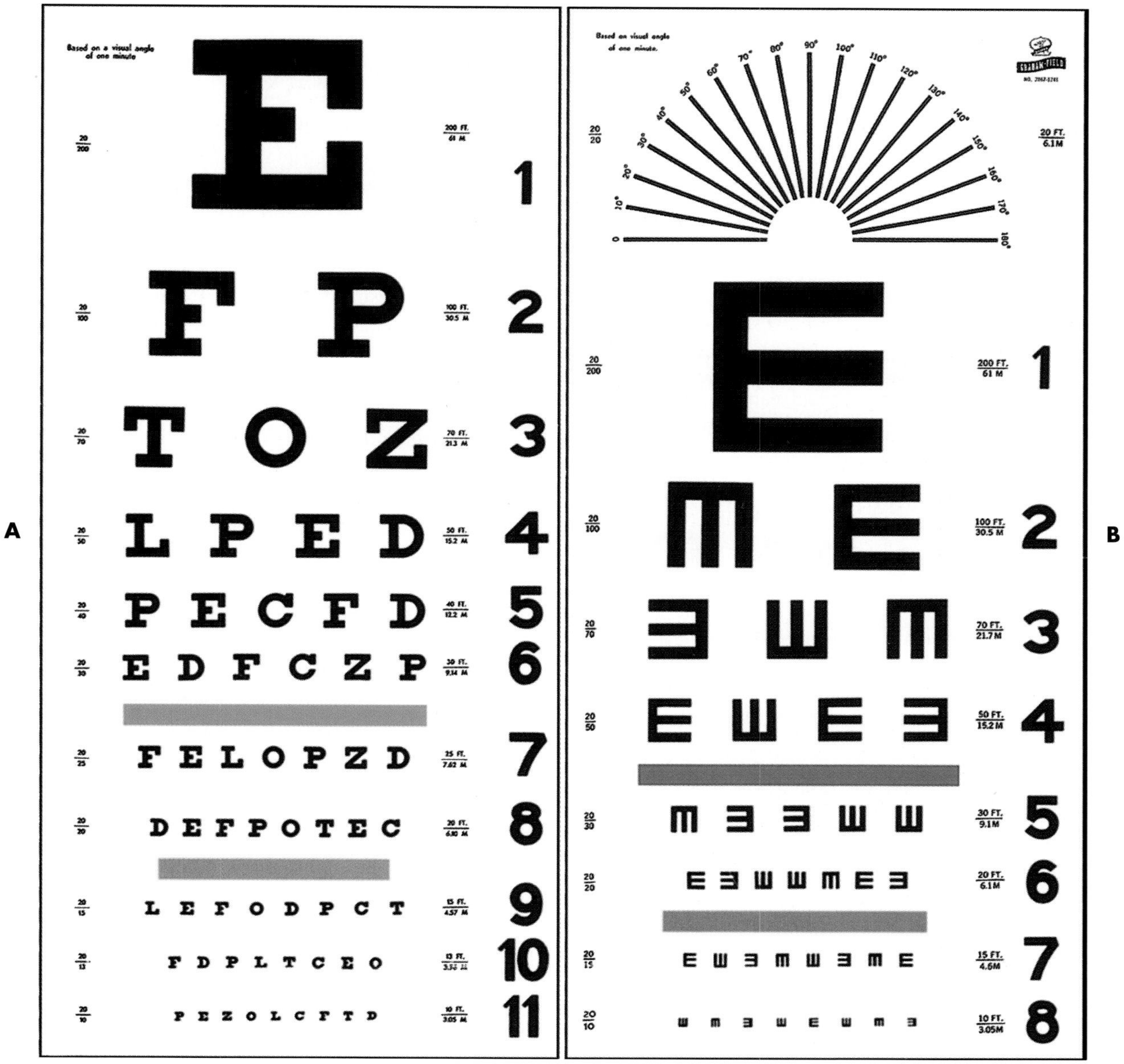

Fig. 5-7 **A,** Snellen's visual acuity chart. **B,** "E" chart. (From Seidel et al, 1999.)

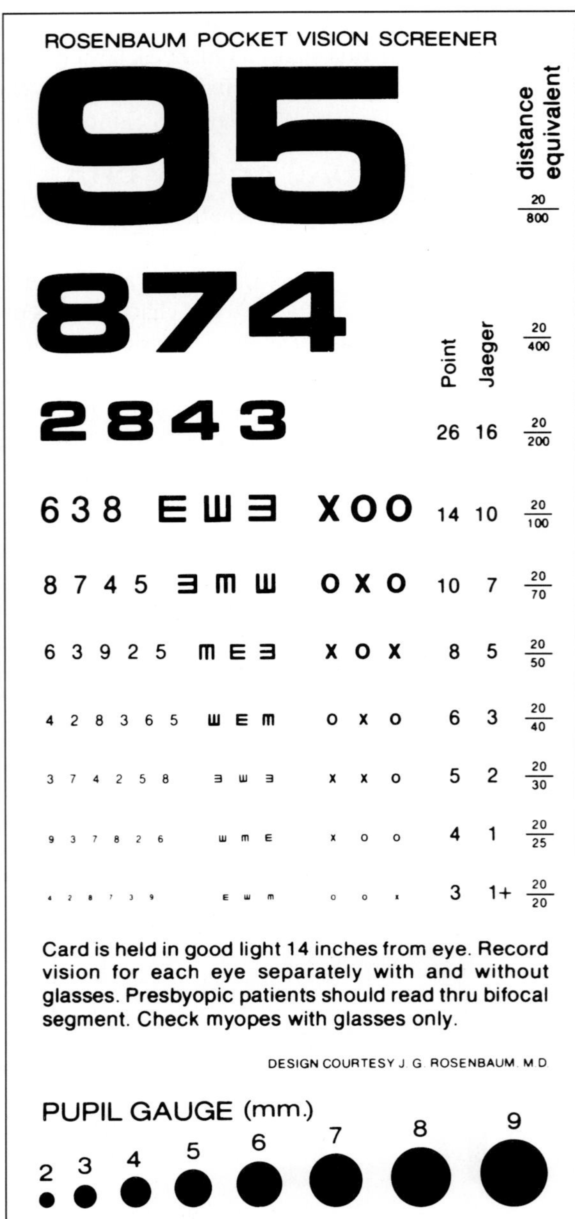

Fig. 5-8 Rosenbaum near-vision chart. (From Seidel et al, 1999.)

cording indicates the distance between the client and the chart and the bottom number indicates the distance at which a person with normal vision should be able to read that line of the chart. Ask the client to name the colors of the horizontal lines as a brief test of color perception. The top line is green, and the bottom line is red. Also, ask the client which line is longer as a brief field perception measurement. The green line is longer.

For young children or non-English-speaking individuals, the "E" chart may be used (Fig. 5-7, *B*). The examiner describes the "E" as a table with legs and asks the client to point in the direction that the legs of the table point. The scoring of the "E" chart is the same as that of Snellen's chart. See Chapter 16 for further information regarding assessment of visual acuity.

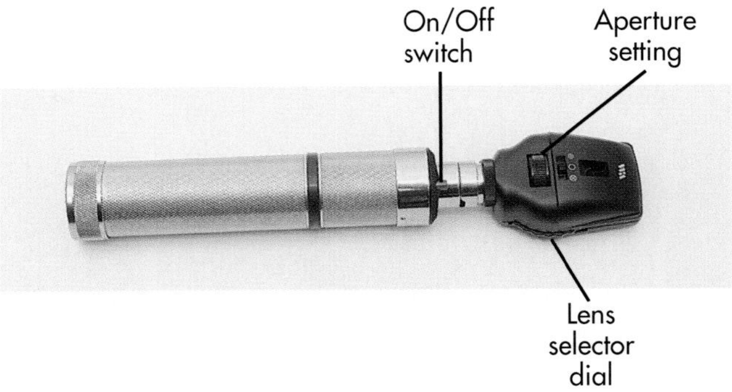

Fig. 5-9 Ophthalmoscope.

NEAR-VISION CHART

Purpose: To assess the client's near, or close-up, vision.

Two charts, the Jaeger and the Rosenbaum, are commonly used to evaluate near vision. The Rosenbaum chart consists of a series of numbers, *E*'s, *X*'s, and *O*'s in graduated sizes (Fig. 5-8). The client should hold the chart 14 inches from the face. Each eye should be individually evaluated for visual acuity. Visual acuity is measured in the same distance equivalents as the far-vision acuity charts, such as 20/20. The Jaeger equivalent is also shown on the Rosenbaum card. The Jaeger equivalent for 20/20 is Jaeger 2.

If a Rosenbaum card is not available, near vision may be approximated by holding a newspaper at a distance of 14 inches from the client's face. The client should be able to read the newsprint without difficulty.

OPHTHALMOSCOPE

Purpose: To examine the internal structures of the eye.

The ophthalmoscope is a system that consists of a series of lenses, mirrors, and light apertures that, when focused correctly, permits the examiner to inspect the detailed internal structures of the eye (Fig. 5-9). The instrument itself consists of the ophthalmoscope head and the handle, which either contains batteries or connects to a wall-mounted electrical source. The head and power source fit together by a turn-and-lock system.

The head of the ophthalmoscope consists of two movable parts: the lens selector dial and the aperture setting. The lenses (diopters) of the ophthalmoscope have varying magnification ranging from -20 to +40. The positive numbers on the lens are shown in black, and the negative numbers are shown in red. When the lens selector dial is turned clockwise, the positive or black-number-sphere lenses are brought into place. Likewise, when the lens selector disk is turned counterclockwise, the negative or red-number-sphere lenses are brought into place. The plus and minus lenses compensate for myopia or hyperopia in either the examiner's or client's eyes and also permit focusing at different places within the client's eye.

The aperture setting has several settings that permit light variations during the examination. If the client's pupils have been dilated, the large light may be used for the internal eye examination. The small light may be used if the client's pupils are very small or if the pupils have not been dilated. The red-free filter actually shines a green beam of light. The filter facilitates the identification of pallor of the disc and permits the recognition of retinal hemorrhages by making the blood appear black. The slit light permits easy examination of the anterior of the eye and determination of elevation or depression of a lesion. The grid light permits the examiner to estimate the size, location, or pattern of a fundal lesion. Eye examination using an ophthalmoscope is discussed further in Chapter 16.

OTOSCOPE

Purpose: To provide illumination and magnification for the examination of the external auditory canal and tympanic membrane.

The otoscope consists of two and sometimes three components: the head, the handle, and sometimes the pneumatic attachment (Fig. 5-10). The head of the otoscope consists of a magnification lens, a light source, and a speculum that is inserted into the auditory canal. Specula come in various sizes. Choose the largest size speculum that will fit into the client's ear canal. The handle of the otoscope either contains batteries or connects to a wall-mounted electrical source. The pneumatic attachment for the otoscope is used to evaluate the fluctuation of the tympanic membrane in children. The attachment consists of a small rubber tube that is attached to the head of the otoscope and a bulb that is attached to the other end of the tubing. When the bulb is squeezed, it produces small puffs of air against the tympanic membrane, causing the membrane to move. No fluctuation of the membrane may indicate pressure behind the membrane. See Chapter 15 for further discussion regarding use of the otoscope.

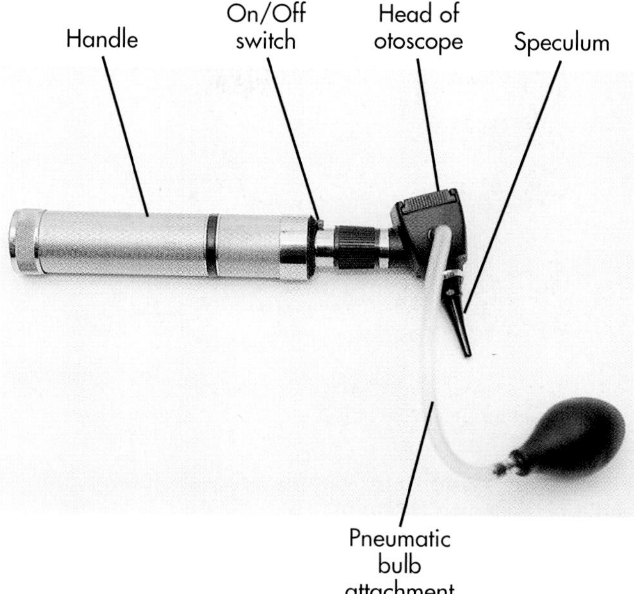

Fig. 5-10 Otoscope with pneumatic bulb.

NASAL SPECULUM

Purpose: To spread the opening of the nares so the internal surfaces of the nose may be examined.

Two instruments may be used as a nasal speculum. The simple nasal speculum is used in conjunction with a penlight to visualize the lower and middle turbinates of the nose (Fig. 5-11). The instrument is used by gently squeezing the handle of the speculum, causing the blades of the speculum to open and spread the nares, which permits internal inspection of the nose. The second type of nasal speculum is a broad-tipped, cone-shaped device that is placed on the end of an otoscope. The nasal cavity may be inspected by using the light source and viewing lens of the otoscope.

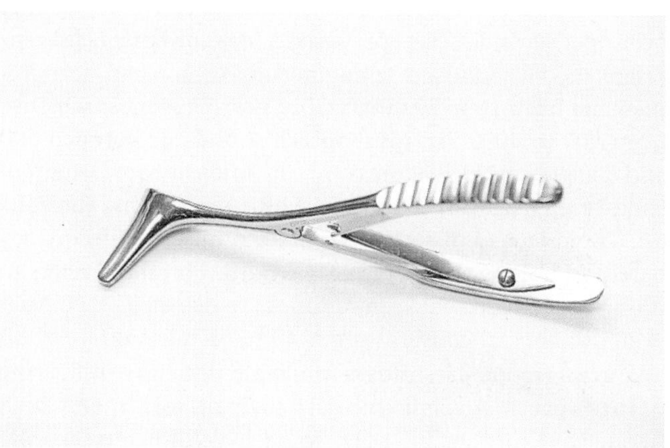

Fig. 5-11 Nasal speculum.

TUNING FORK

Purpose: The tuning fork has two purposes in physical assessment: (1) auditory screening and (2) assessment of vibratory sensation during the neurologic examination.

The tuning fork is used during the physical examination for both sound and vibratory sensation evaluation (Fig. 5-12). For auditory evaluation, a high-pitched tuning fork with a frequency of 500 to 1000 Hz should be used. This frequency fork can estimate hearing loss in the range of normal speech (300 to 3000 Hz). If a lower-frequency fork were used, overestimation of hearing ability could result. For neurologic vibratory evaluation a tuning fork with a pitch between 100 and 400 Hz should be used. To engage, sharply strike the tuning fork on the heel of the hand. See Chapters 15 and 25 for further information on this assessment technique.

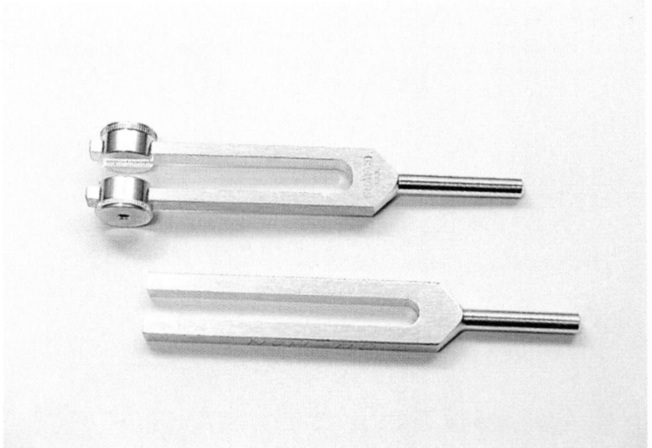

Fig. 5-12 Tuning forks for vibratory sensation (*top*) and auditory screening (*bottom*).

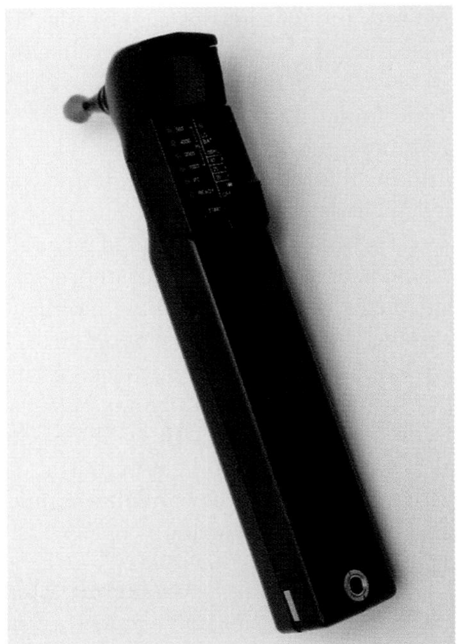

Fig. 5-13 Audiometer.

AUDIOMETER

Purpose: To perform basic screening for hearing acuity.

The audiometer produces pure tones of simple sound waves. Sound is described by the number of vibrations that occur per second. Cycles per second (cps) or hertz (Hz) represent the vibrations. A young healthy person can hear frequencies from 16 to 20,000 Hz, but hearing is most sensitive from 500 to 4000 Hz; most speech sounds lie between 500 and 3000 Hz. A decibel measures the intensity or strength of sound ranging from 0 dB to 140 dB, with 0 being the softest. The intensity of sound required to make any frequency barely audible to the average ear is 0 dB. Threshold refers to the signal level at which pure tones are detected. A whisper is 20 dB; normal conversation is 40 to 65 dB. A 40 to 46 dB loss in all frequencies causes moderate difficulty in hearing normal speech. A client with a 15 to 20 dB loss in only high frequencies such as 4000 Hz would have difficulty hearing high-pitched consonants (Lewis et al, 2000).

The hand-held, battery-operated audiometer (Fig. 5-13) provides a fast, simple test to detect hearing problems. Remove the audiometer from the charging unit. Select the ear speculum that best fits the client's ear canal; a snug fit is desired to screen out surrounding noise. Attach the ear speculum to the audiometer with a clockwise turn. Instruct clients to respond when they hear the tone. Often the client is asked to respond by raising an index finger to indicate hearing a tone. Set the audiometer to 20 dB, and push the start button. The audiometer systematically and automatically creates tones at the different frequencies: 1000, 2000, 4000, and 5000 Hz. A light appears on the audiometer when the specific tone at a given frequency is sounded. The client's raised index finger, indicating perception of a tone, should correspond to the light seen by the examiner on the audiometer. The client should hear the four tones in each ear. If any of the tones is not heard, increase the dB to 25 and repeat the test procedure at the different frequencies. If any of these tones is not heard, use 40 dB. When these tones are not heard at 40 dB, refer the client for further evaluation.

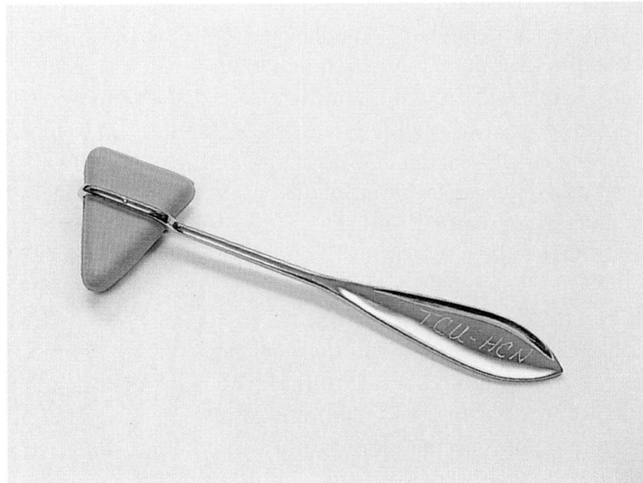

Fig. 5-14 Percussion hammer.

PERCUSSION, OR REFLEX, HAMMER

Purpose: To test deep tendon reflexes.

The percussion, or reflex, hammer consists of a triangular rubber component on the end of a metal handle (Fig. 5-14). The hammer is configured so that either flat or pointed surfaces may be used to elicit the reflex response. The flat surface is most commonly used when striking the tendon directly. The pointed surface may be used either to strike the tendon directly or to strike the examiner's finger,

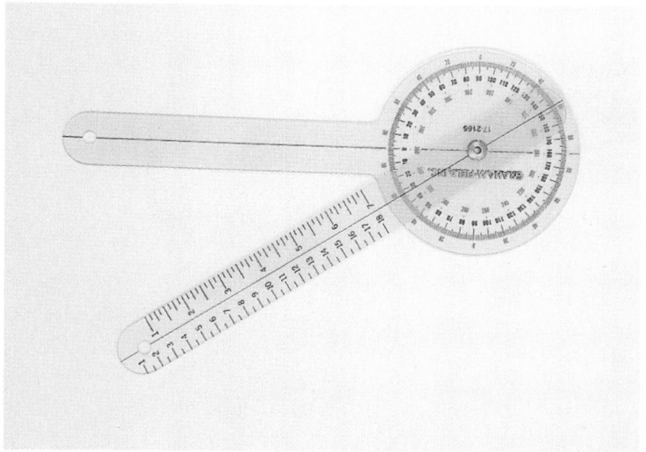

Fig. 5-15 Goniometer.

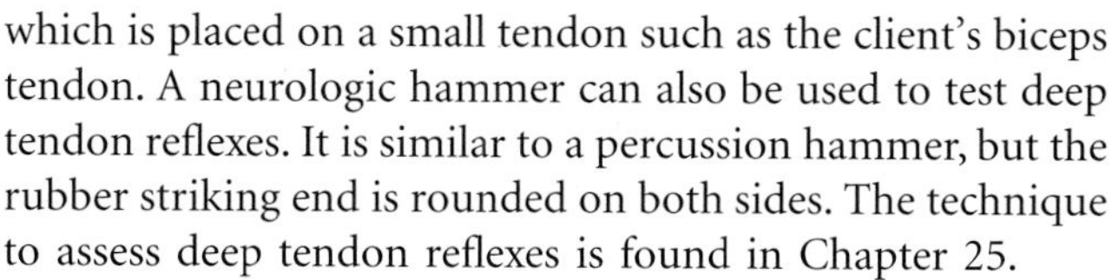

which is placed on a small tendon such as the client's biceps tendon. A neurologic hammer can also be used to test deep tendon reflexes. It is similar to a percussion hammer, but the rubber striking end is rounded on both sides. The technique to assess deep tendon reflexes is found in Chapter 25.

GONIOMETER

Purpose: To determine the degree of flexion or extension of a joint.

The goniometer is a two-piece ruler that is jointed in the middle with a protractor type of measuring device (Fig. 5-15). The goniometer is placed over a joint, and, as the individual extends or flexes the joint, the degrees of flexion and extension are measured on the protractor. This is further discussed in Chapter 24.

PENLIGHT

Purpose: To provide a focused light source during the assessment at any point at which the examiner desires one.

The penlight has many uses during a physical assessment (Fig. 5-16). It may be used to illuminate the inside of the mouth or nose, highlight a lesion, or evaluate pupillary constriction. It is most important that the penlight have a bright light source. If the examiner does not have a penlight, the light transmitted from the otoscope may be substituted as a focused light source.

RULER

Purpose: To measure lesions or other marks on the skin.

A small metric ruler that has both millimeter and centimeter markings is useful for measuring lesions or other marks on the skin (Fig. 5-17). It is helpful if the ruler is transparent.

TAPE MEASURE

Purpose: To measure circumference and length.

A tape measure is convenient in various situations such as measuring the length of an infant or the circumference of a client's head or chest. A tape measure that has inches on one side and centimeters on the reverse side is ideal. To ensure accuracy of measurement, it is imperative that the tape measure be nonstretchable.

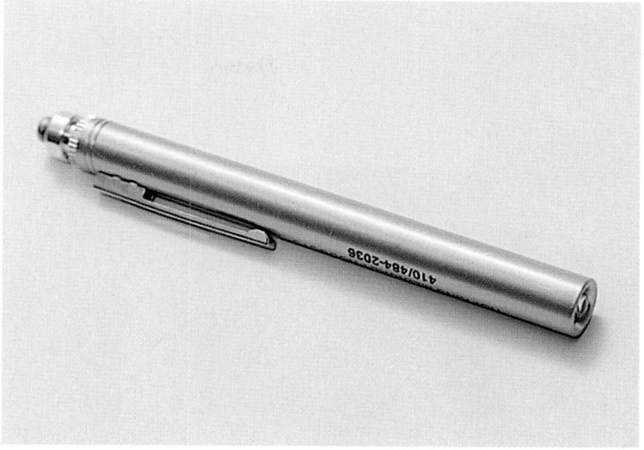

Fig. 5-16 Penlight.

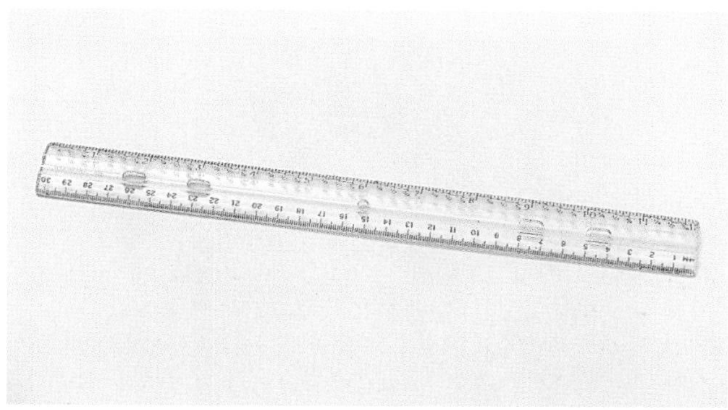

Fig. 5-17 Centimeter ruler.

CALIPERS FOR SKINFOLD THICKNESS

Purpose: To measure the thickness of subcutaneous tissue to estimate the amount of body fat.

Different models of calipers (e.g., Lang or Herpendem) may be used to measure the thickness of subcutaneous tissue at different points on the body (Fig. 5-18). The most frequent location for thickness evaluation is the posterior aspect of the triceps. Use of calipers to measure skinfold thickness is further discussed in Chapter 10.

TRANSILLUMINATOR

Purpose: To differentiate the characteristics of tissue, fluid, and air within a specific body cavity.

A transilluminator consists of a strong light source with a narrow beam at the distal section of the light (Fig. 5-19). When the examination room is darkened and the light is placed directly against the skin over a body cavity such as a sinus area or the scrotum, the transilluminator disseminates

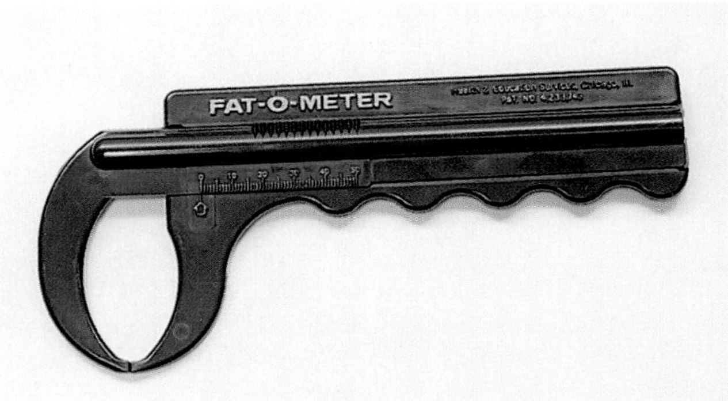

Fig. 5-18 Skinfold calipers.

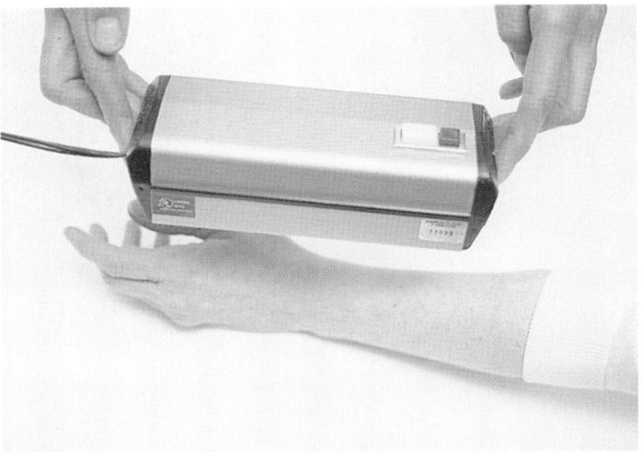

Fig. 5-20 Wood's lamp. The purple color on the skin indicates no fungal infection is present.

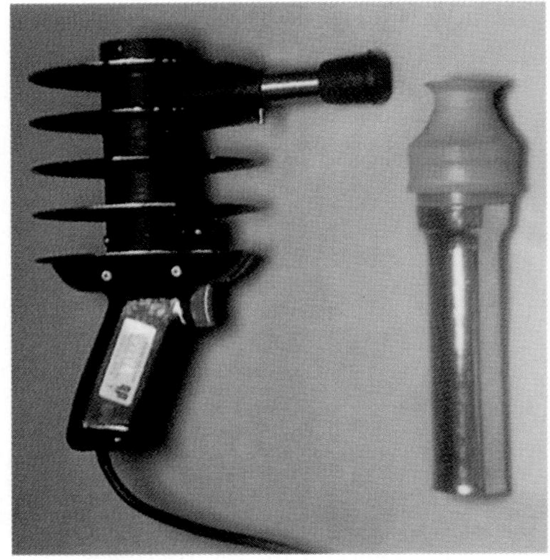

Fig. 5-19 Transilluminator. (From Seidel et al, 1999.)

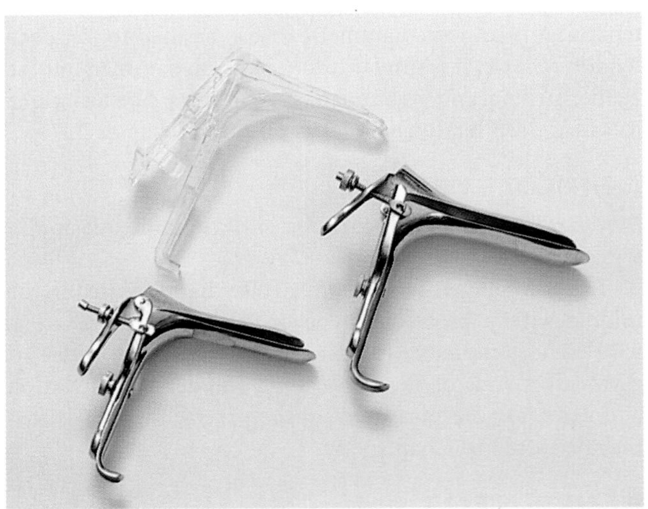

Fig. 5-21 Vaginal specula.

its light source under the surface of the skin. Depending on whether the area under the skin surface is air, fluid, or tissue, the light is transmitted differentially and provides different glowing red tones of light.

WOOD'S LAMP

Purpose: To detect fungal infections of the skin or, used with fluorescein dye, to detect corneal abrasions.

The Wood's lamp produces a black-light effect. It is used to assess for the presence of a fungal infection. Skin lesions caused by a fungal infection will take on a fluorescent yellow-green or blue-green color when examined with a Wood's lamp (Fig. 5-20). The examination room should be darkened to enhance the clinical interpretation of the lesion color.

VAGINAL SPECULUM

Purpose: To spread the walls of the vaginal canal so the examiner can visualize the vaginal tissue and the cervix.

There are three types of vaginal specula: the Graves' speculum, the Pederson speculum, and the pediatric or virginal speculum. All of the specula are composed of two blades and a handle and may be available as either reusable metal or disposable plastic models (Fig. 5-21). The Graves' speculum is available in a variety of sizes, with blades ranging from 3.5 to 5.0 inches in length and 0.75 to 1.25 inches in width. The bottom blade is approximately 0.25 inches longer than the top blade. This conforms to the longer posterior vaginal wall and aids with visualization.

The Pederson speculum has blades that are as long as the Graves' speculum but are much narrower and flatter.

The pediatric or virginal speculum is smaller in all dimensions of width and length.

Plastic and metal specula differ slightly in ease of use and positioning. The metal speculum has two positioning devices. The top blade is hinged and has a thumb lever attached. When the thumb lever is pressed down, the distal end of the top blade rises, thus opening the speculum. The

Box 5-1 Standard Precaution Guidelines

The Centers for Disease Control and Prevention (CDC) Hospital Infection Control Practice Advisory Committee has issued recommendations for isolation precautions in hospitals (Garner, 1996). Many of the recommendations are applicable in all health care settings. Although health assessment is a relatively safe client care activity, the potential for infection transmission exists; thus these guidelines are an important component.

It is recommended that the nurse follow standard precautions during health assessment. Standard precautions are taken to prevent infection transmission not only from the client to the health care worker, but also from the health care worker to the client or from client to client via the hands of the health care provider. Standard precautions will reduce the risk of infection transmission from both recognized and unrecognized sources of infection.

Standard precautions include the following concepts:

1. *Hand washing:* The nurse should always scrupulously wash hands with a germicidal soap both before and after direct contact with the client. This is considered the single most important measure to reduce transmission of infection.
2. *Gloves:* Gloves should be worn when contact with a client's blood and/or body fluid is possible. Specifically, this applies to contact with blood, body fluids (urine, feces, sputum, wound drainage, etc.), nonintact skin, and mucous membranes. Gloves should also be worn if handling equipment contaminated with blood or body fluids. Gloves are worn for three primary reasons:
   - To protect the health care worker from exposure to blood-borne pathogens carried by the client
   - To protect the client from microorganisms on the hands of the health care worker
   - To reduce the potential of infection transmission from one client to another client via the hands of the health care worker

   The use of gloves does not reduce the frequency or importance of hand washing. Hands must be washed before performing a procedure even when gloves are worn, and then again immediately after removal of gloves. Gloves should be changed between procedures on the same client if the gloves have become contaminated. If a glove breaks during a procedure, it should be removed promptly and replaced with a new glove. Health care workers who have open draining lesions or weeping dermatitis should refrain from all direct client care and from handling client care equipment until the condition resolves.
3. *Masks, eye protection, face shields:* The nurse should wear a mask with eye protection or a face shield during procedures that may result in splashes or sprays of the client's blood, body fluids, secretions, or excretions. Such equipment protects the mucous membranes of the eyes, nose, and mouth from contact, thus reducing the likelihood of pathogen transmission. Although not routinely needed for health assessment, situations may occur in which this equipment becomes necessary.
4. *Gown:* A gown should be worn to prevent contamination of skin and clothing during procedures that may result in splashes or sprays of the client's blood or body fluids. A gown may also be indicated when in contact with a client who has a known, epidemiologically important infection in which specific isolation measures are being taken.
5. *Patient care equipment:* The nurse should avoid touching equipment contaminated with blood or body fluids unless gloves are worn. Multiuse patient equipment that has been soiled with blood or body fluids (a vaginal speculum, for instance) should not be reused until it has been adequately cleaned and reprocessed. Single-use items must be properly disposed of after client use. The nurse must take caution when handling contaminated sharp equipment. (Gloves will not provide protection from a sharp injury such as a needle stick.) Appropriate handling of sharps involves the following principles:
   - Never recap a needle after client use.
   - Never attempt to remove a needle from a disposable syringe by hand.
   - After client use, place disposable syringes and needles directly into a "sharps container"—a puncture-resistant container designated for contaminated sharp items.

blade may be locked open at that point by tightening the screw on the thumb lever. The proximal end of the speculum may also be opened wider if necessary by loosening and then tightening another thumbscrew on the handle.

The disposable plastic speculum differs from the metal type in that the bottom blade is fixed to a posterior handle and the upper blade is fixed to the anterior lever handle. When the lever is pressed, the distal end of the top blade opens and, at the same time, the base of the speculum widens. As the speculum opens it goes through a series of clicking sounds until it actually snaps into the desired position. The client should be forewarned about the clicking and snapping sounds. In addition, some of the plastic models have a port where a light source may be inserted directly into the speculum. See Chapter 21 for further discussion on use of the speculum.

PERSONAL PROTECTIVE EQUIPMENT

Standard precautions apply to all clients in all health care settings. Gloves, masks, eye protection, and gowns may be indicated for certain parts of an examination. It is important that all health care professionals are aware of and follow standard precaution guidelines. These guidelines are presented in Box 5-1. It is important to note that the incidence of latex allergy has increased significantly in recent years. Latex is found in gloves and many types of equipment and supplies. Health care professionals are at risk for developing latex allergy because of their frequent exposure to latex. The National Institute for Occupational Safety and Health (NIOSH) has issued recommendations to prevent latex allergy for health care workers, which are summarized in Box 5-2 (NIOSH, 1997). Clients may also have a latex allergy; particularly at risk are children with spina bifida and people who have had multiple medical procedures and surgeries, especially genitourinary surgery (Gritter, 1998). Health care professionals should routinely ask clients about latex allergy.

Box 5-2 Preventing Latex Allergy

- If latex gloves are to be used, use a powder-free, low-allergen glove, if possible.
- Do not use oil-based hand lotions when wearing latex gloves.
- Immediately after removing latex gloves, wash hands with mild soap and dry thoroughly.
- If you develop latex allergy symptoms, avoid direct contact with latex products and see a health care provider knowledgeable about latex allergy. Early symptoms of latex allergy are similar to contact dermatitis (dry itching, irritated areas on the hands or skin in contact with latex). A more severe symptom is a delayed hypersensitivity dermatitis. Lesions resembling poison ivy may appear 1 to 2 days after contact. The lesions can progress to oozing blisters.

CLINICAL APPLICATION and CRITICAL THINKING

CRITICAL THINKING QUESTIONS

1. A 3-week-old baby is brought to the clinic by her mother for a well-baby visit. You are preparing to check the baby's temperature. Considering the different types of thermometers and routes, what would be appropriate?
2. You are preparing to do a comprehensive examination on an adult woman who has no history of infectious disease. What infection control measures should be taken for a routine examination?
3. A pregnant woman comes to the clinic for a routine prenatal visit. During the visit you want to document fetal heart tones. What type of equipment might be used to assess this, and how do the types of equipment differ?
4. You are admitting a woman to the hospital. While conducting the nursing admission history, you learn she has a latex allergy. What measures should be taken to protect her from latex exposure?

REMEMBER to check out your **companion CD-ROM**

6 Techniques of Physical Assessment

www.mosby.com/MERLIN/wilson/assessment/

Data for physical assessment are collected using the techniques of inspection, palpation, percussion, auscultation, and positioning. These techniques are described in this chapter together with assessment of vital signs—pulse, respiration, blood pressure, and temperature—and general assessment techniques of weight and height. Use of selected equipment described in Chapter 5 also is described in this chapter.

TECHNIQUES

Inspection

The definition of inspection is "to look at; to examine critically." This includes all data obtained by looking at the client. (Data obtained by smell are included as a part of inspection, even though smell falls outside the definition.) Inspection begins the moment the examiner meets the client, and it requires attention to detail. For example, data about the neuromuscular system are obtained by observing the client's gait and ease of movement from standing to sitting. Data about emotional and mental status are collected by noting facial expressions, tone of voice, and affect. Does the client maintain eye contact during the history taking? Are the facial expressions and body language appropriate for the conversation? Is the clothing appropriate for the weather? The skin assessment begins by noticing the color of the client's skin. Are any odors detected? When unpleasant odors are detected, examiners must try to suppress reactions that may be communicated through facial expressions. These preliminary observations can be important clues to data needed during the remainder of the examination.

Inspection is a part of assessment in every body system and is hindered by any preconceived assumptions examiners may have about clients. Observe the client thoroughly with a critical eye, comparing the right and left sides to find and explain variations noted during the examination. By concentrating on the client without being distracted, the examiner will not overlook potentially important data about the client.

During inspection, the client is draped appropriately to maintain modesty but provide sufficient exposure. Adequate lighting is essential and should be direct enough to allow examiners to see color, texture, and mobility without distortions or shadows. Shadows can be useful, however, for observing contour and variations in body surface. Shadows are created with tangential lighting by directing the light from a penlight or adjustable lamp at right angles to the area being inspected (Fig. 6-1). At times instruments, such as an otoscope, ophthalmoscope, or vaginal speculum, are used to enhance inspection. Use of these instruments is described in subsequent chapters on assessment of specific body systems. Although inspection at first may seem like an easy assessment technique to master, examiners must practice to develop this skill, as with any other.

Palpation

Palpation is the use of sensation of the examiner's hands to feel texture, size, shape, consistency, and location of certain parts of the client's body and also to identify areas the client reports as being tender or painful. This assessment technique requires the examiner to move into the client's personal space. It is important that the touch is gentle, hands are warm, and nails are short to prevent discomfort or injury to the client. Touch has cultural significance and symbolism. Each culture has its own understanding about the uses and meanings of touch. As a result, it is of utmost importance that examiners tell clients the purpose of their touch (e.g., "I'm feeling for lymph nodes now") and manner and location of touch (e.g., "I'm going to press deeply on your abdomen to feel the organs"). Gloves are worn when palpating mucous membranes or any other area where contact with body fluids is likely.

The palmar surface of fingers and finger pads are more sensitive than fingertips and are used to determine position, texture, size, consistency, masses, fluid, and crepitus. The ulnar surface of the hand extending to the fifth finger is the most sensitive to vibration, whereas the dorsal surface of the hand is best for assessing temperature.

Uses of palpation for specific body systems are discussed in subsequent chapters. Palpation using the palmar surfaces of the fingers may be light or deep and is controlled by the amount of pressure applied with hands or fingers. For example, the following technique is used to assess the abdomen. Light palpation is accomplished by pressing to a depth of 1 cm (0.4 inches) and is used to assess skin, pulsations, and tenderness. Deep palpation is done by using one or both hands to press in about 4 cm (1.6 inches) and is used to determine organ size and contour. Light palpation should always precede deep palpation because palpation may cause tenderness or disrupt fluid, which would interfere with collecting data by light palpation.

One of the purposes of palpation is to determine the size of tissue such as lymph nodes or nodules. To accomplish this purpose, examiners need to know the width of their fingers to use them as approximate measures as needed.

A bimanual technique of palpation uses both hands, one anterior and one posterior, to entrap an organ or mass be-

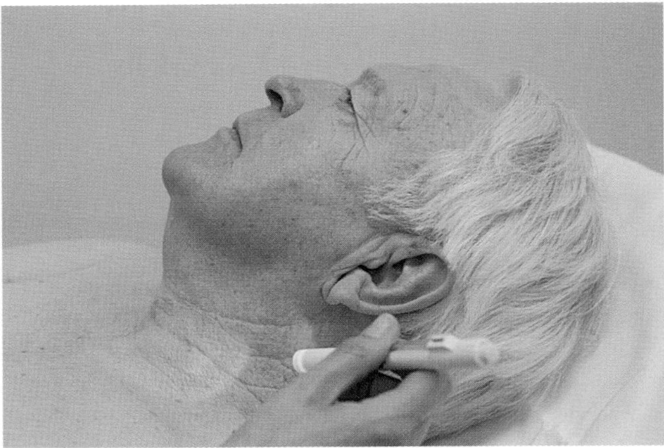

Fig. 6-1 Tangential light used to inspect jugular vein pulsation.

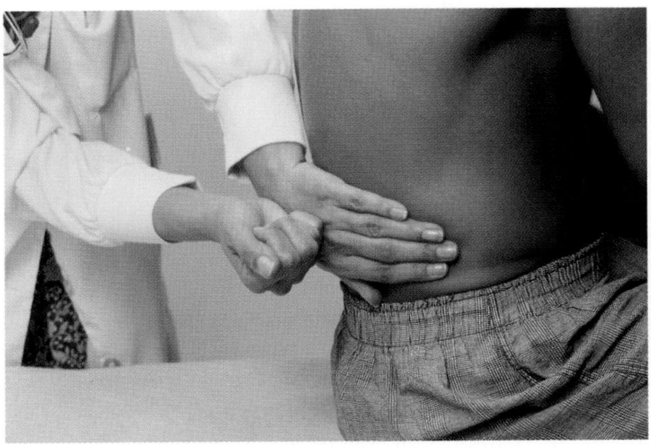

Fig. 6-3 Hand position for indirect fist percussion of kidney.

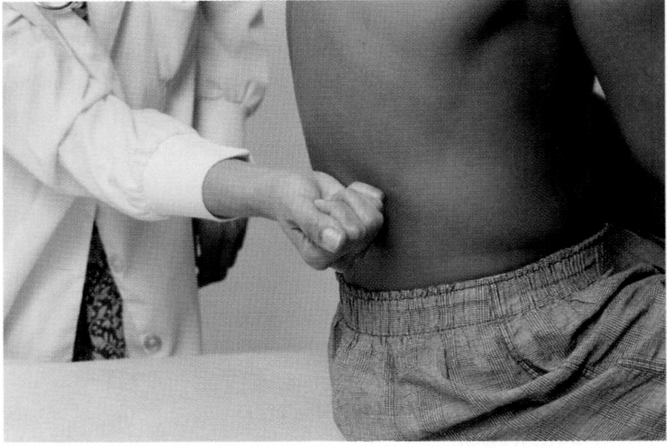

Fig. 6-2 Hand position for direct fist percussion of kidney.

tween the fingertips to assess size and shape. This technique is used to assess the kidneys and uterus.

Percussion

Percussion is performed to evaluate the size, borders, and consistency of some internal organs, to detect tenderness, and to determine the extent of fluid in a body cavity. There are two percussion techniques, direct and indirect.

Direct percussion involves striking a finger or hand directly against the client's body. The examiner may use direct percussion technique to evaluate the sinus of an adult client (by use of a finger) or to elicit tenderness over the kidney by striking the costovertebral angle (CVA) directly with a fist (Fig. 6-2).

Indirect percussion requires both hands and is done by different methods depending on which body system is being assessed. Indirect fist percussion of the kidney is performed by placing the nondominant hand palm down, fingers together over the CVA, and gently striking the fingers with the lateral aspect of the fist of the dominant hand (Fig. 6-3).

Indirect percussion of the thorax or abdomen is performed by placing the distal phalanx of the middle finger of the nondominant hand against the skin over the organ being percussed. This finger is sometimes referred to as the pleximeter. The other fingers of that hand are spread apart and slightly elevated off the client's skin so that they do not dampen the vibration. With the tip of the middle finger of the dominant hand (plexor), the examiner strikes the distal interphalangeal joint, or just distal to the joint, that lies against the client's skin. The tip of the striking finger hits the middle finger, which is against the skin, between the cuticle and first joint. Some examiners use both the index and the middle fingers as plexors. The force of the downward snap of the striking finger(s) comes from rapid flexion of the wrist. The wrist must be relaxed and loose while the forearm remains stationary (Fig. 6-4). The nail of the plexor must be trimmed to avoid piercing the client with long fingernails. Rebound the plexor finger as soon as it strikes the pleximeter so that the vibration is not muffled. Listen for the vibrations created by one finger striking another. The tapping produces a vibration 1 1/2 to 2 inches (4 to 5 cm) deep in body tissue and subsequent sound waves. Percuss two or three times in one location before moving to another. Stronger percussion will be needed for obese or very muscular clients, since thickness of tissue can impair the vibrations. The denser the tissue, the quieter the percussion tones. The percussion tone over air is loud, over fluid is less loud, and over solid areas is soft. Five percussion tones are described in Table 6-1. Tympany is a loud, high-pitched sound heard over the abdomen. Resonance is heard over normal lung tissue, whereas hyperresonance is heard in overinflated lungs (as in emphysema). Dullness is heard over the liver, and flatness is heard over bones and muscle. Detecting sound changes is easier when moving from resonance to dullness (e.g., from the lung to the liver). Indirect percussion is an awkward technique at first but can be mastered with practice.

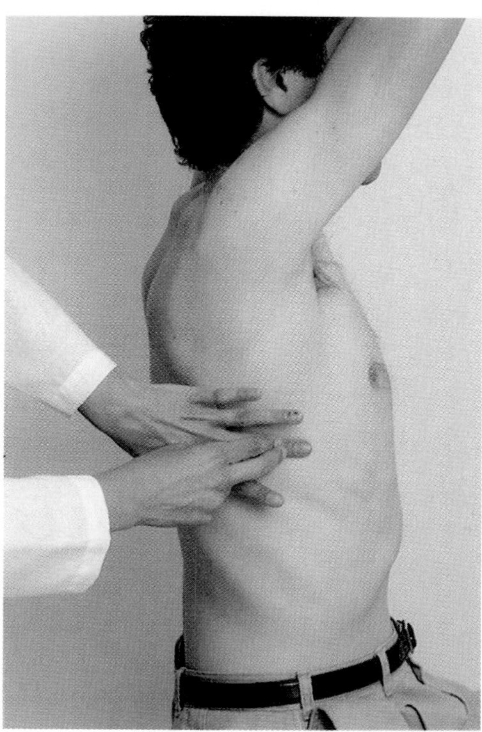

Fig. 6-4 Indirect percussion of lateral chest wall.

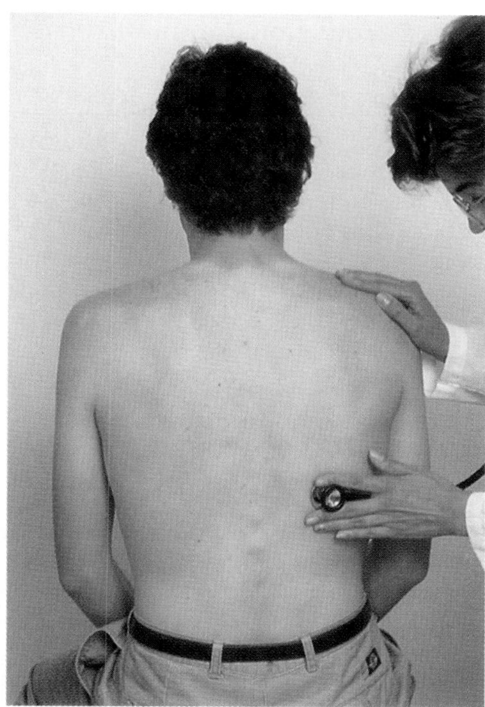

Fig. 6-5 The diaphragm of the stethoscope is stabilized between the index and middle fingers.

Auscultation

Auscultation is the act of listening for sounds. The examiner uses auscultation without any assistive devices when evaluating sounds such as coughing, speech, and percussion tones. A stethoscope is an assistive device used in auscultation to block out extraneous sounds when evaluating the condition of the heart, blood vessels, lungs, pleura, and intestines. As described in the previous chapter, the head of the stethoscope consists of two components: the bell and the diaphragm. The bell of the stethoscope is used to hear soft, low-pitched (low-frequency) sounds such as vascular sounds and extra heart sounds, whereas the diaphragm is used to hear high-pitched (high-frequency) sounds such as breath and bowel sounds. Frequently the examiner will use both the bell and diaphragm during an examination.

Examiners should warm the stethoscope before placing it on clients. If clients become cold and shiver, the involuntary muscle contractions could interfere with normal sounds. The bell or diaphragm of the stethoscope is placed directly against the skin, since clothes obscure or alter sounds. Auscultating a hairy chest can seem to produce an abnormal lung sound (crackles) when actually the sound is the friction of the chest hair against the diaphragm. When this occurs, examiners should moisten the hair before auscultating.

The diaphragm is held firmly against the client's skin, stabilizing it between the index and middle fingers (Fig. 6-5). When the bell is used, avoid pressing too firmly against the skin, because this will stretch the skin so that it acts like the diaphragm of the stethoscope and thus inhibits vibrations. The examiner listens for the sound and also its characteristics: intensity, pitch, duration, and quality (Box 6-1). Examiners concentrate as they listen because sounds may be transitory or subtle. Closing the eyes may improve listening because it reduces distracting visual stimuli. Examiners try to isolate the specific sounds, such as sounds of air during inspiration or a single heart sound, sometimes referred to as selective listening.

POSITIONING

The sitting and supine positions are the most common for the client during the physical examination. These plus other positions used in an examination are shown in Table 6-2. The inability of a client to assume a position not only may require use of an alternate examination position, but also may be a significant finding about the client's physical status. For example, a client who is short of breath may not be able to lie supine. To assess the abdomen of this client, the examiner may need to use an examining table that has an elevated headrest or defer the abdominal examination (if it is not an urgent problem) until the respiratory condition is treated. The client is draped appropriately in the various positions to provide for modesty, while allowing exposure needed for the examination.

VITAL SIGNS

The temperature, pulse, respiration, and blood pressure are often referred to as vital signs because they are baseline indicators of a client's health status. They are measured

Table 6-1 Percussion Tones

AREA PERCUSSED	TONE	INTENSITY	PITCH	DURATION	QUALITY
Lungs	Resonant	Loud	Low	Long	Hollow
Bone and muscle	Flat	Soft	High	Short	Extremely dull
Viscera and liver borders	Dull	Medium	Medium high	Medium	Thudlike
Stomach and gas bubbles in intestines	Tympanic	Loud	High	Medium	Drumlike
Air trapped in lung (emphysema)	Hyperresonant	Very loud	Very low	Longer	Booming

Box 6-1 Characteristics of Sounds Heard by Auscultation

- *Intensity* is the loudness of the sound, described as soft, medium, or loud.
- *Pitch* is the frequency or number of sound waves generated per second. High-pitched sounds have high frequencies. Expected high-pitched sounds are breath sounds, whereas cardiac sounds are low pitched.
- *Duration* of sound vibrations is short, medium, or long. Layers of soft tissue dampen the duration of sound from deep organs.
- *Quality* refers to the description of the sounds (e.g., hollow, dull, crackle).

early in the physical examination or integrated into the examination.

Temperature

Body temperature is maintained by a thermostat located in the hypothalamus. Heat is gained through the processes of metabolism and exercise and lost through radiation, convection, conduction, and evaporation. The expected temperature ranges from 96.4° F to 99.1° F (35.8° C to 37.3° C) with an average of 98.6° F (37° C). This is the stable core temperature at which cellular metabolism is most efficient.

Temperature changes occur due to normal variations and activities. Diurnal variations of 1° F to 1.5° F (.6° C to .9° C) occur with the lowest temperature early in the morning and the highest in the late afternoon and early evening. During menstrual cycles a woman's temperature increases .5° F to 1.0° F (.3° C to .6° C) at ovulation and remains elevated until menses ceases. This elevation is due to progesterone secretion. Moderate to vigorous exercise increases temperature.

Temperature can be measured by several routes: oral, tympanic, axillary, and rectal. Devices measure body temperature in Fahrenheit or Celsius; some devices measure in both. Conversion between the two measurements is easily done by simple math (Box 6-2).

Box 6-2 Conversion of Fahrenheit to Celsius

Degrees C = 5/9 (degrees F) − 32
Degrees F = 9/5 (degrees C) + 32

Oral Temperature Temperature measurement by the oral route is safe and accurate. However, delay taking the oral temperature for 15 minutes if the client has smoked or ingested hot or cold liquids or food (Cole, 1993). To take a temperature with a mercury-in-glass thermometer, shake the thermometer to move the mercury down below 95° F (35° C). Place plastic sheath on thermometer, if available. Place the thermometer under the client's tongue in the right or left posterior sublingual pocket, which receives its blood supply from the carotid artery, which reflects inner core temperature. Ask the client to keep the mouth closed while temperature is being measured. Leave the thermometer in place for 3 minutes, then remove and read the temperature at the mercury level on the scale (Potter and Perry, 1997). The examiner must be aware of the potential risk of injury when a glass thermometer is used with young children or confused adults.

When using an electronic thermometer, cover the blue or white probe with a disposable sheath. Place the probe under the client's tongue as just described. Ask the client to keep the mouth closed while temperature is being measured. An electronic oral thermometer remains in place for 15 to 30 seconds until the audible signal occurs and the temperature registers on the display screen. Assessment of oral temperature with this type of thermometer is safe for use with children or confused adults since the plastic sheath will not break.

Tympanic Membrane Temperature Electronic thermometers that measure temperature from the tympanic surface are convenient. The probe is covered with a protective sheath and placed inside the external ear canal with firm but gentle pressure. The probe must come in contact with all sides of the ear canal. (The probe does not extend all the way to the tympanic membrane.) The thermometer is removed after the audible signal occurs (about 2 to 3 seconds) and the temperature reading is displayed.

Axillary Temperature Measurement of axillary temperature has long been considered safe and accurate. Results from research, however, raise questions regarding the accuracy in measurement, especially in the febrile client. Compared with other temperature measurement devices, axillary temperatures have a low sensitivity in their ability to

Table 6-2 Positions for Examination

POSITION	AREAS ASSESSED	RATIONALE	LIMITATIONS
Sitting	Head and neck, back, posterior thorax and lungs, anterior thorax and lungs, breasts, axillae, heart, vital signs, and upper extremities	Sitting upright provides full expansion of lungs and provides better visualization of symmetry of upper body parts.	Physically weakened client may be unable to sit. Examiner should use supine position with head of bed elevated instead.
Supine	Head and neck, anterior thorax and lungs, breasts, axillae, heart, abdomen, extremities, pulses	This is the most normally relaxed position. It provides easy access to pulse sites.	If client becomes short of breath easily, examiner may need to raise head of bed.
Dorsal recumbent	Head and neck, anterior thorax and lungs, breasts, axillae, heart, abdomen	This position is used for abdominal assessment because it promotes relaxation of abdominal muscles.	Clients with painful disorders are more comfortable with knees flexed.
Lithotomy*	Female genitalia and genital tract	This position provides maximal exposure of genitalia and facilitates insertion of vaginal speculum.	Lithotomy position is embarrassing and uncomfortable, so examiner minimizes time that client spends in it. Client is kept well draped.
Sims'	Rectum and vagina	Flexion of hip and knee improves exposure of rectal area.	Joint deformities may hinder client's ability to bend hip and knee.
Prone	Musculoskeletal system	This position is used only to assess extension of hip joint.	This position is poorly tolerated in clients with respiratory difficulties.
Lateral recumbent	Heart	This position aids in detecting murmurs.	This position is poorly tolerated in clients with respiratory difficulties.
Knee-chest*	Rectum	This position provides maximal exposure of rectal area.	This position is embarrassing and uncomfortable.

*Clients with arthritis or other joint deformities may be unable to assume this position.
From Potter PA, Perry AG: *Basic nursing: a critical thinking approach,* ed 4, St Louis, 1999, Mosby.

detect fever in a febrile group (Haddock et al, 1996; Schmitz et al, 1995). Axillary temperature can be measured with a glass thermometer or an electronic thermometer. When using a glass thermometer, begin by shaking down the mercury as described previously. Place the thermometer in the axilla, and hold the arm against the body for 5 to 10 minutes. Withdraw the thermometer, and read the level of mercury on the scale.

When using an electronic thermometer, the probe is held in the middle of the axilla, with the arm held against the

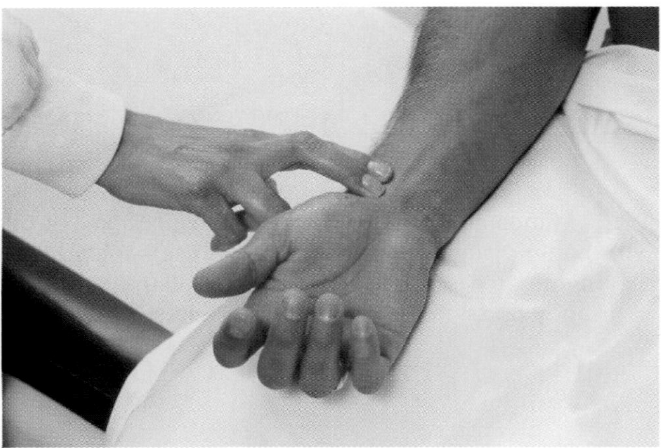

Fig. 6-6 Radial pulse.

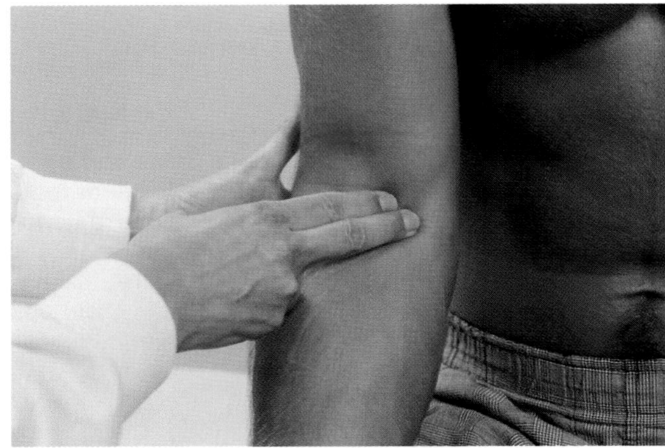

Fig. 6-7 Brachial pulse.

body, until the audible signal occurs and the temperature appears on the screen.

Rectal Temperature Rectal temperatures are taken less frequently with the advent of methods such as the tympanic thermometer. Rectal temperatures may be used when other routes are not possible. The rectal route is not recommended in infants, particularly those under the age of 3 months because of the risk of rectal perforation (Wong and Perry, 1998). The client is frequently placed in a Sims' position with the upper leg flexed. Appropriate privacy should be provided. When using a rectal mercury-in-glass thermometer, prepare it by shaking down the mercury as described above. Place the thermometer in a plastic sleeve, and apply a water-soluble lubricant. Insert the thermometer into the rectum 1 to 1.5 inches (2.5 to 3.8 cm), and hold in place 2 minutes. A rectal electronic thermometer is used by covering the red probe with a disposable sheath, inserting it into the rectum 1.5 inches (3.8 cm), and holding it in place until the audible signal occurs and the temperature is displayed on the screen.

Pulse

Palpation of arterial pulses provides valuable information about the cardiovascular system. When assessing vital signs, the pulse is taken to determine heart rate and rhythm. The rate is the number of times in a minute the pulsation is felt. The rhythm is the regularity of the pulsations, that is, the time between each beat. Pulses are palpated using the finger pads of the index and middle fingers. Firm pressure is applied over the pulse, but not so hard that the pulsation is occluded. If pulses are difficult to locate, then the amount of pressure is varied and the area around the pulse is palpated.

Although a pulse can be taken in many areas, the radial artery is most frequently used to measure heart rate because it is accessible and easily palpated. The radial pulse is found at the radial, or thumb, side of the forearm at the wrist (Fig. 6-6). The brachial and carotid arteries are common alternative sites for pulse assessment. The brachial pulse is located in the groove between the biceps and triceps muscle just medial to the biceps tendon at the antecubital fossa (in the bend of the elbow) (Fig. 6-7). The carotid pulse is found by palpating along the medial edge of the sternocleidomastoid muscle in the lower third of the neck (Fig. 6-8). Heart rate is also assessed by counting the apical pulse, but this requires auscultation with a stethoscope.

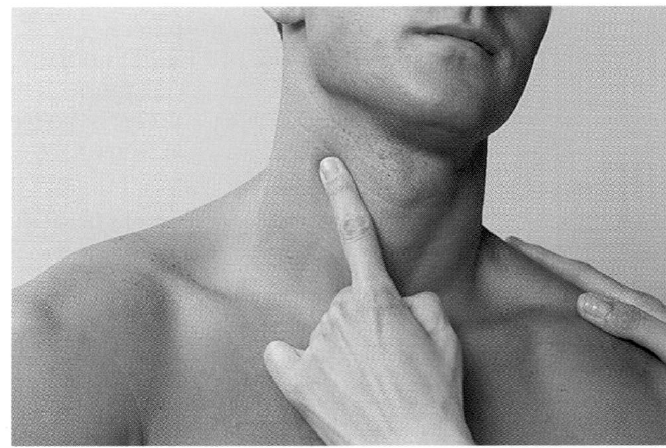

Fig. 6-8 Carotid pulse.

To take a pulse, place your fingers over the artery and feel for the pulsations and the rhythm. If the rhythm is regular (time between each beat is consistent), count the number of pulsations palpated for 30 seconds and multiply by 2 or count for 15 seconds and multiply by 4. If the pulse rhythm feels irregular (time between each beat varies), count the number of pulsations for a full minute. Expected heart rates are listed in Table 6-3.

The palpation of pulses also provides important information regarding the strength of the pulse and perfusion of blood to various parts of the body. This will be discussed further in Chapter 18.

Respiration

After assessing pulses, examiners often leave their fingers on the pulse (e.g., radial pulse) while they assess the client's

Table 6-3 Normal Heart Rates

AGE	HEART RATE (BEATS/MIN)
Infants	120-160
Toddlers	90-140
Preschoolers	80-110
School-agers	75-100
Adolescents	60-90
Adults	60-100

Data from Hazinski MF, editor: *Nursing care of the critically ill child,* St Louis, 1984, Mosby; and Kinney MR et al: *AACN's clinical reference for critical care nursing,* ed 3, St Louis, 1993, Mosby. In Potter PA, Perry AG: *Basic nursing: a critical thinking approach,* ed 4, St Louis, 1999, Mosby.

Table 6-4 Ranges of Expected Respiratory Rates by Age

AGE	RESPIRATORY RATE PER MINUTE
Newborn	30-50
1 year	20-40
3 years	20-30
6 years	18-26
10 years	16-22
16 years	14-20
18 years and over	12-20

breathing for respiratory rate, rhythm, and depth. Using inspection, they count the number of breaths per minute without the client's knowledge of their assessment. This will prevent the client from becoming self-conscious because of the assessment and perhaps changing the rate or depth of breathing.

The respiratory rate is the number of times the client completes one ventilatory cycle (inhalation and exhalation) each minute. Respiration rates vary with age (Table 6-4). Other factors that increase respiratory rate are fever, anxiety, exercise, and increased altitude. Rhythm is the regularity of breathing; the expected finding when the client is sitting or lying quietly is equal spacing between breaths. Rhythm is described as regular or irregular. Depth is assessed by observing the excursion or movement of the chest wall. Depth is described as deep (full lung expansion with full exhalation), normal, or shallow (small amount of air moves in and out of lungs and may be difficult to observe). Men usually breathe diaphragmatically, which increases the movement of the abdomen, whereas women breathe thoracically with movement of the thoracic cage.

Blood Pressure

Blood pressure is the force of blood against the arterial walls. It reflects the relationship between cardiac output and peripheral resistance. The cardiac output is the volume of blood ejected from the heart each minute. Peripheral resistance is the force that opposes the flow of blood through vessels. For example, when the arteries are narrow, the peripheral resistance to blood flow is high, which is reflected in an elevated blood pressure. Blood pressure is dependent on the velocity of the blood, intravascular blood volume, and elasticity of the vessel walls.

Table 6-5 Normal Blood Pressures

AGE	SYSTOLIC	DIASTOLIC
Infants	60-96 mm Hg	30-62 mm Hg
Age 2	78-112 mm Hg	48-78 mm Hg
Age 8	85-114 mm Hg	52-85 mm Hg
Age 12	95-135 mm Hg	58-88 mm Hg
Adult	100-140 mm Hg	60-90 mm Hg

Systolic pressure in the thigh can be higher by 10 to 40 mm Hg as compared with brachial artery pressure. Diastolic pressure remains the same.
From Canobbio MM: *Cardiovascular disorders,* St. Louis, 1990, Mosby.

Blood pressure is measured in millimeters of mercury (mm Hg). The measurement indicates the height to which the blood pressure can raise a column of mercury. Systolic blood pressure is the maximum pressure exerted on arteries when the ventricles eject blood from the heart. When the ventricles relax, the blood remaining in arteries exerting a minimum pressure is called the diastolic blood pressure. Blood pressure is recorded with the systolic pressure written on top of the diastolic pressure (e.g., 130/76), but it is not a fraction. The difference between the systolic and diastolic pressures is called the pulse pressure, which normally ranges from 30 to 40 mm Hg. Expected blood pressure ranges are shown in Table 6-5.

Systemic blood pressure can be measured directly or indirectly. Direct measurement is accomplished by inserting a small catheter into an artery that provides continuous blood pressure measurements and arterial waveforms. This direct measurement is done in the critical care setting when close monitoring is required. Blood pressure is more commonly assessed indirectly by an auscultation method using a sphygmomanometer and a stethoscope. Two types of sphygmomanometers are used: mercury and aneroid (see Chapter 5). The mercury sphygmomanometer is considered the more accurate and reliable indirect measure of systemic blood pressure. The procedure for assessing blood pressure is described in Box 6-3.

Mechanism of Blood Pressure Measurement Blood flows freely through the artery until the inflated cuff occludes the artery enough to interrupt blood flow. As the cuff pressure is slowly released, the examiner listens for the sound of the blood pulsating through the artery again. This sound indicates the return of blood flow and the systolic blood pressure. This sound is called the first Korotkoff sound, named for the Russian physician who first

Box 6-3 Procedure for Measuring Blood Pressure

- With the client sitting or lying down, position the client's upper arm at heart level with the palm turned up. Palpate either branchial pulse (in the antecubital space), and apply the blood pressure cuff 1 inch (2.5 cm) above the site of brachial pulsation.
- Center the bladder of the cuff over the artery (Fig. 6-9). Wrap the deflated cuff evenly and snugly around the upper arm.
- Position the manometer at eye level no more than 1 yard (1 m) away. Close the valve on the pressure bulb clockwise until it is tight but easily releasable with one hand.
- Palpate the brachial or radial pulse with fingertips of one hand while inflating the cuff rapidly to 30 mm Hg above the point where the pulse disappears. Release the valve slowly to deflate the cuff and note the point when the pulse reappears; this is the palpated systolic pressure.
- Deflate the cuff and wait 30 seconds. Place the stethoscope over the brachial pulse (Fig. 6-10).
- Close the valve on the pressure bulb again and inflate the cuff to 30 mm Hg above the palpated systolic pressure. Slowly release the valve and allow the mercury to fall at a rate of 2 to 3 mm Hg per second.
- Note the mamometer pressure reading when the first clear sound (first Korotkoff sound) is heard; this is the systolic pressure.
- Continue to deflate the cuff, noting the point at which the sound disappears; this is the diastolic pressure.
- Deflate the cuff and remove from client's arm.
- If this is the first blood pressure assessment, repeat the procedure on the other arm. Also, the blood pressure often is taken while clients are lying, sitting, and standing so that comparisons can be made.
- Tell the client the blood pressure measurement, record the data, and compare it with previous readings.

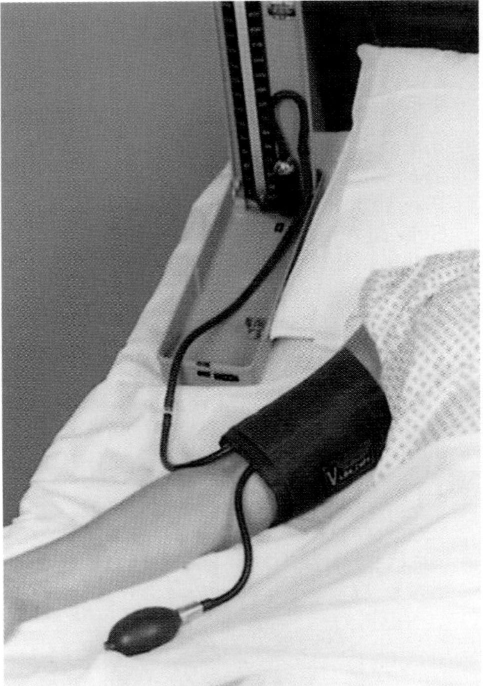

Fig. 6-9 Center the bladder of the blood pressure cuff over artery. (From Potter and Perry, 1999.)

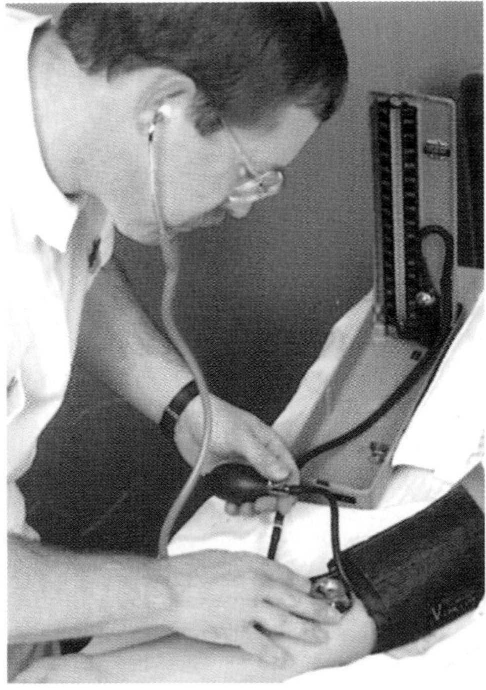

Fig. 6-10 Listening for Korotkoff sounds to assess blood pressure. (From Potter and Perry, 1999.)

described it. The first Korotkoff sound is a clear, rhythmic thumping corresponding to the pulse rate that gradually increases in intensity (Fig. 6-11). The pressure reading at which this sound is heard is noted and indicates the systolic pressure. The swishing sound heard as the cuff continues to deflate is the second Korotkoff sound. The third Korotkoff sound is a softer thump than phase one. The fourth Korotkoff sound becomes muffled and low pitched as the cuff is further deflated. The fifth Korotkoff sound occurs at the pressure at which there is no sound, indicating the artery is completely open. In adolescents and adults the manometer pressure noted at the fifth Korotkoff sound is the diastolic pressure. It takes a great deal of practice to differentiate all five sounds. Differentiation of the five sounds is ordinarily not necessary. In most cases only two numbers are recorded: the first (systolic) and last (diastolic) Korotkoff sounds.

Systolic blood pressure can be measured in the leg when the arms cannot be used. With the client in the prone posi-

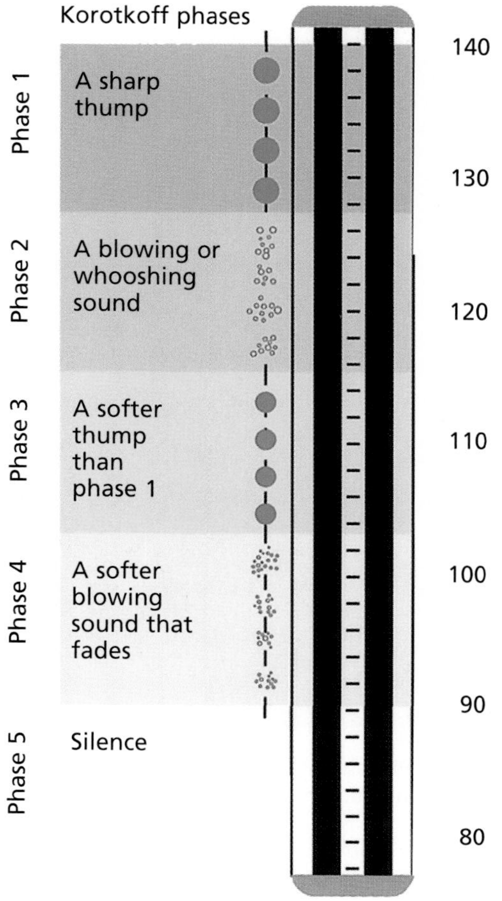

Fig. 6-11 Sounds auscultated during blood pressure measurement can be differentiated into five Korotkoff phases. In this example the blood pressure is 140/90. (From Potter and Perry, 1999.)

tion, wrap a large cuff 7 to 7.9 inches (18 to 20 cm) around the lower third of the thigh, centering the bladder of the cuff over the popliteal artery. Follow the same procedure for taking a blood pressure measurement in the arm. Normally the systolic blood pressure is 10 to 40 mm Hg higher in the leg than in the arm. The diastolic pressures of arms and legs are similar.

Factors That Affect Blood Pressure Measurements

1. Characteristics of clients that may alter blood pressure:
   - *Age:* From childhood to adulthood there is a gradual rise.
   - *Gender:* After puberty, females usually have a lower blood pressure than males; however, after menopause, women's blood pressure is often higher than men's.
   - *Race:* The incidence of hypertension is twice as high in African Americans as in whites.
   - *Diurnal variations:* Blood pressure is lower in the early morning and peaks in later afternoon or early evening.
   - *Emotions:* Feeling anxious, angry, or stressed may stimulate the sympathetic nervous system to increase the blood pressure.
   - *Pain:* Experiencing pain can increase blood pressure.
   - *Personal habits:* Ingesting caffeine or smoking a cigarette within 30 minutes before measurement may increase blood pressure.
   - *Weight:* Obese clients tend to have higher blood pressures than nonobese clients.
2. Examiner error causing falsely high blood pressures:
   - Positioning client's arm above the level of the heart
   - Examiner's eyes not level with the manometer—looking up at the meniscus
   - Using a cuff that is too narrow
   - Wrapping the cuff too loosely or unevenly
   - Deflating the cuff too slowly
3. Examiner error causing falsely low blood pressures:
   - Positioning client's arm below the level of the heart
   - Examiner's eyes not level with the manometer—looking down at the meniscus
   - Positioning the manometer higher than the client's heart
   - Using a cuff that is too wide
   - Not inflating the cuff enough
   - Deflating the cuff too rapidly
   - Pressing the diaphragm too firmly on the brachial artery
   - Reinflating the cuff without completely deflating the cuff

GENERAL ASSESSMENT

Weight

The amount of one's body weight or mass is determined by genetics, dietary intake, exercise, and fluid volume. Genetics influence height and body size, including bone structure, muscle mass, and gender. A diet high in fat may increase body weight, particularly when clients do not exercise regularly. Fat distribution varies by gender and age. In men total body fat is evenly distributed, whereas in women additional fat is distributed over the shoulders, breasts, buttocks, and lateral aspects of thighs and pubic symphysis, which can dramatically alter body shape. Why females deposit fat in specific locations is unknown, but the fat in breasts protects the mammary glands and provides energy for future gestation and lactation needs (Rofles and DeBruyne, 1990).

An unintentional change in weight can be a significant finding. For example, an increase in weight may be the first sign of fluid retention. For every liter of fluid retained (1000 ml or about 1 quart), weight increases 2.2 lb (1 kg). Also, unexplained weight loss may be one indication of suspected malignancy or disease process.

Measure weight using a balance scale by asking the client to stand in the middle of the scale platform while the large and small weights are balanced. The scale uses a counterbalance system of adding or subtracting weights in increments as small as 1/4 lb (0.1 kg) to achieve a level horizontal balance beam on the scale. Move the larger weight to the 50-lb (22.7-kg) increment less than the client's weight. Adjust the smaller weight to balance the scale. Read the weight to the nearest 1/4 lb (0.1 kg).

Electronic scales are available in many clinical settings. These provide a digital reading of the client's weight seconds after the client steps on the scale. There are also electronic scales available for clients unable to stand.

Height

One's height is determined by genetics and dietary intake. Genetics influence height and body size, bone structure, muscle mass, and gender. Dietary factors influence bone and muscle growth. Height is measured on a platform scale with a height attachment. The height attachment is pulled up and the horizontal headpiece extended before the client steps on the scale to avoid poking the client as the headpiece is extended. The attachment then is lowered until the horizontal headpiece touches the client's crown. The vertical measuring scale can be in inches or centimeters. Height peaks during the adolescent growth spurt, which is highly variable from adolescent to adolescent. Adult height is attained between ages 18 and 20 (Neinstein, 1991). Height for an adult usually is measured as a baseline only.

Skinfold Thickness

Skinfold calipers are used to measure skinfold or fat-fold thickness of fat in the subcutaneous tissue to estimate the extent of overnutrition or undernutrition. (See Fig. 5-18 in Chapter 5.) Measures of body fat are useful in determining nutritional status. About half the body fat is directly beneath the skin, and its thickness reflects total body fat.

Three measurements are taken, and the two closest measurements are averaged. The most common site for measuring fat folds is the triceps, using a vertical fold on the back of the arm between the shoulder and the elbow. The examiner uses the thumb and index finger to grasp and lift a fold of skin and fat about 1/2 inch (1.27 cm) on the posterior aspect of the client's arm halfway between the olecranon process (tip of the elbow) and acromial process on the lateral aspect of the scapula. Opened caliper jaws are placed horizontally to the raised skinfold; then the examiner releases the lever of the calipers to make the measurement to the nearest millimeter (Fig. 6-12).

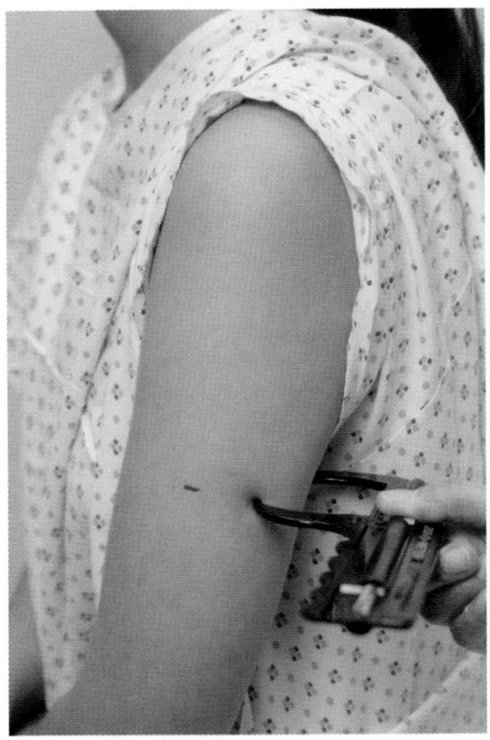

Fig. 6-12 Placement of calipers for triceps skinfold thickness measurement.

Another skinfold site is the thigh (a vertical fold on the anterior thigh midway between the iliac crest and patella). Additional sites for men are the chest (diagonal fold midway between the shoulder crease and nipple) and abdomen (vertical fold just to the side of the umbilicus). Another site for women is just above the iliac crest at the midaxillary line. Expected skinfold measurements for men and women are shown in Table 10-4. Repeated fat-fold measurements over time document the increase or decrease in fat stores in the body (Rolfes and DeBruyne, 1990). Body fat percentage can be more precisely determined by water displacement analysis.

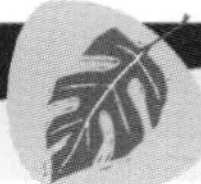

AGE-RELATED VARIATIONS

NEWBORNS AND INFANTS

In addition to measuring weight and height (recumbent length) of an infant, measurements of head circumference and, when necessary, chest circumference are taken to assess growth and development. Monitoring growth of infants is important and can easily be accomplished by plotting the height and weight by age on growth charts at each visit. Recumbent length, weight, and head circumference are plotted on the growth chart to assess patterns of growth and to evaluate growth compared to infants of the same age and gender. The percentile in which the infant's length and weight falls is identified and shared with the caregiver. The most frequently used growth charts in the United States are from the National Center for Health Statistics (NCHS). These are found in Appendix F.

Weight The platform scale is used for weighing newborns, infants, and small children (Fig. 6-13). The scale has curved sides to prevent the infant from rolling. A paper is

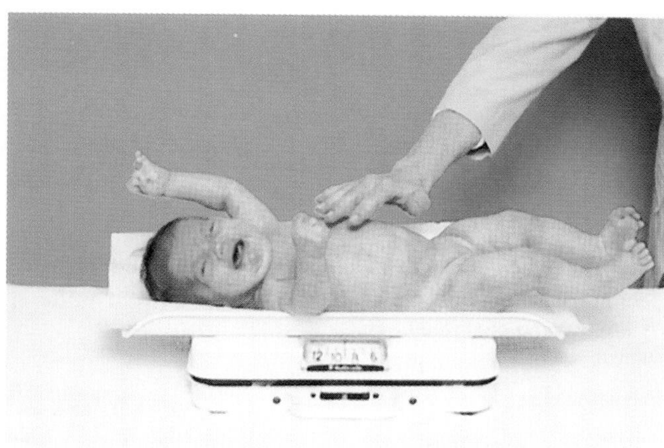

Fig. 6-13 Weighing an infant. (From Wong et al, 1999.)

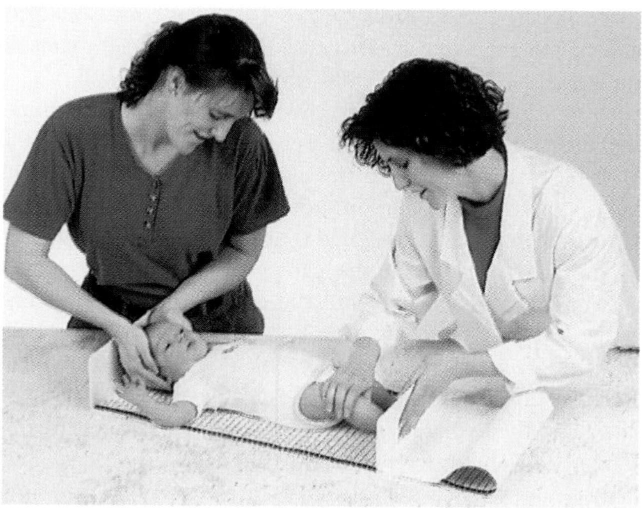

Fig. 6-14 Measurement of recumbent length. (Courtesy Seca Corporation.)

placed on the scale, and the unclothed newborn is laid on the paper. The newborn is weighed by balancing the scale just as for the adult. The weight is recorded to the nearest 1/2 oz or 14 g.

Healthy newborns weigh between 5 lb 8 oz and 8 lb 13 oz (2500 and 4000 g). Newborns commonly lose 10% of their birth weight in the first week but regain it in 10 to 14 days. In general, they double their birth weight by 4 to 5 months of age and triple their birth weight by 12 months of age.

Recumbent Length Recumbent length of newborns and infants can be measured by using an infant measuring mat, consisting of a soft rubber graduated mat attached to a plastic footboard (Fig. 6-14). The infant lies on the mat with the head against the headboard. The infant's knees are held together and pressed gently against the mat with one hand, while the footboard is moved against the heels. The height can be recorded in inches or centimeters.

Another device for measuring height of infants has a rigid headboard and movable footboard. The measuring board can be placed horizontally on a table. The barefoot infant lies supine on the measuring board until the infant's head touches the headboard. The footboard is then moved until it touches the bottom of the infant's feet.

When height-measuring devices are not available, the examiner improvises. Using a safety pin at one end of the blanket, the examiner lays the infant's head at the pin, extends the infant's body as just described, and marks the location of the foot on the blanket with another pin. The distance between pins is measured to determine the infant's height. Also, the examiner can place the infant on a piece of paper and mark at the head and feet with a pen.

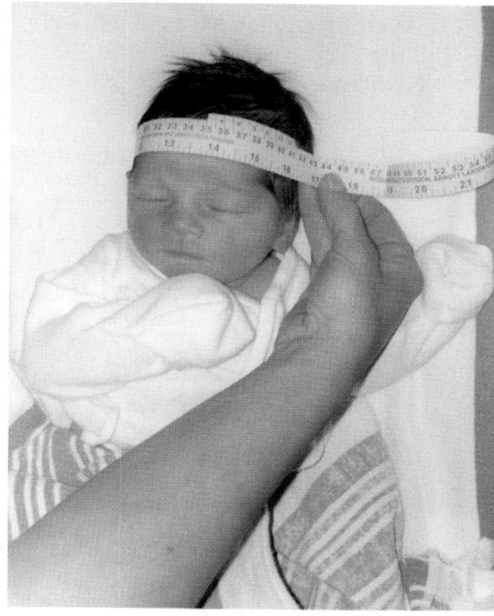

Fig. 6-15 Measuring head circumference of a neonate.

Head Circumference Head circumference should be measured at every well-child visit up to the age of 2 years, then yearly until age 6. The measuring tape is wrapped snugly around the infant's head at the largest circumference, usually just above the eyebrows, the pinna of the ears, and the occipital prominence at the back of the skull (Fig. 6-15). The tape measure is read to the nearest 1/8 inch (0.5 cm). Head circumference is measured at least twice to check for accuracy.

Expected head circumference for term newborns averages from 13 to 14 inches (33 to 36 cm). The head circumference is plotted on a growth curve appropriate for age and gender and compared with the population standard (Table 6-6). Head circumference should be about 1 inch (2 to 3 cm) larger than chest circumference. A head circumference that is rapidly increasing suggests increased intracranial pressure. A head circumference below the fifth percentile suggests microcephaly.

Table 6-6 Average Chest and Head Circumference of U.S. Children

AGE	CHEST CIRCUMFERENCE (cm)	HEAD CIRCUMFERENCE (cm) MALES	FEMALES
Birth	35	35.3	34.7
3 months	40	40.9	40.0
6 months	44	43.9	42.8
12 months	47	47.3	45.8
18 months	48	48.7	47.1
2 years	50	49.7	48.1
3 years	52	50.4	49.3

Data from Lowrey GH: *Growth and development of children,* ed 8, Chicago, 1986, Mosby; and Waring WW, Jeansonne LO: *Practical manual of pediatrics,* ed 2, St Louis, 1982, Mosby. In Seidel HM et al: *Mosby's guide to physical examination,* ed 4, St Louis, 1999, Mosby.

Chest Circumference Chest circumference is usually not assessed unless an abnormal head or chest size is suspected. The chest circumference is measured at the nipples, pulling the tape measure firmly without causing an indentation in the skin. The measurement is noted between inspiration and expiration and recorded to the nearest 1/8 inch (0.5 cm) (Fig. 6-16). At birth the infant's chest circumference may be equal to or slightly less than the head circumference. Between 1 and 2 years of age, the infant's chest circumference should closely approximate the head circumference (see Table 6-6).

Vital Signs

Temperature. Wide variations are found in temperatures of newborns and infants because they have less effective heat-control mechanisms. Temperature can be measured at several sites in the body. The safest ways to measure temperature in newborns are at tympanic or axillary sites. Rectal temperatures are contraindicated in newborns because of the risk of rectal perforation (Wong and Perry, 1998).

Pulse and Respirations. Pulse and respirations are assessed for the same qualities as in the adult, but at a time when the infant is quiet. If the infant is quiet at the beginning of the assessment, the examiner listens to the apical pulse for a full minute and counts the respirations before proceeding to other parts of the assessment. Expected heart rates for infants and children are listed in Table 6-3.

Respiratory rates are counted using the same procedure as for adults; however, infants usually breathe diaphragmatically, which requires observation of the abdominal movement. Respirations are counted for a full minute because an infant's respiratory rate may be irregular as a normal variation.

■ CHILDREN

Height and Weight To measure the height of a child who can stand but is too short for the adult scale, the examiner uses a platform with a movable headboard. The child stands erect on the platform, and the headboard is lowered until it touches the child's head. Height is recorded in inches or centimeters on the growth chart appropriate for the child's age and gender (Fig. 6-17). A tape measure also can be attached to a wall so that the child's height can be measured by having the child stand against the wall.

Monitoring the weight of children is essential. Continuing the graph of height and weight begun in infancy is a valuable screening tool to track the child's growth in comparison with the population standard (see Appendix F). The percentile in which the child's height and weight falls is noted and shared with the caregiver. Height and weight measurements continue until the end of the growth spurt between ages 18 and 20.

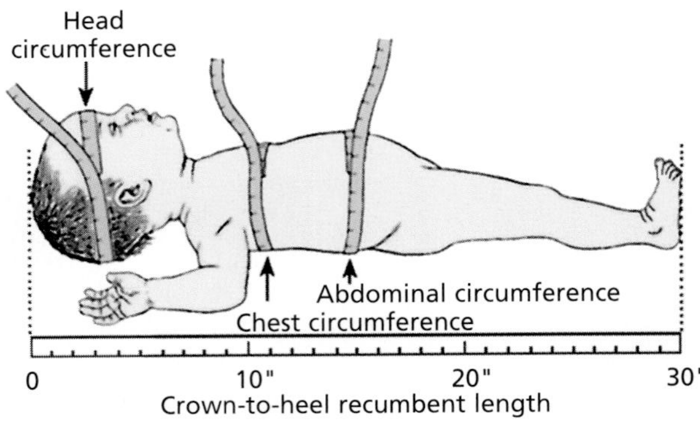

Fig. 6-16 Measurement of head, chest, and abdominal circumference and crown-to-heel (recumbent) length. (From Wong et al, 1999.)

Head and Chest Circumference Head circumference should be measured at every well-child visit until age 2 and then annually until age 6. By 2 years of age the infant's head circumference is two thirds its adult size. The head circumference is measured as described previously and plotted on the growth chart to compare the growth of the child with a population standard.

Between 5 months and 2 years of age, the infant's chest circumference should closely approximate the head circumference. After 2 years of age the chest circumference should exceed the head circumference.

Vital Signs

Temperature. Temperatures can be taken safely in children using electronic thermometers or tympanic membrane sensors. Mercury-in-glass thermometers should not be used until the child is at least 5 years old and can be trusted to keep the thermometer under the tongue with the mouth closed without biting the thermometer. Before this age, taking an axillary temperature using a mercury-in-glass thermometer is safe and accurate.

Rectal temperatures should be taken as a last resort. A convenient position for taking a rectal temperature is with the child side-lying with knees flexed toward the abdomen.

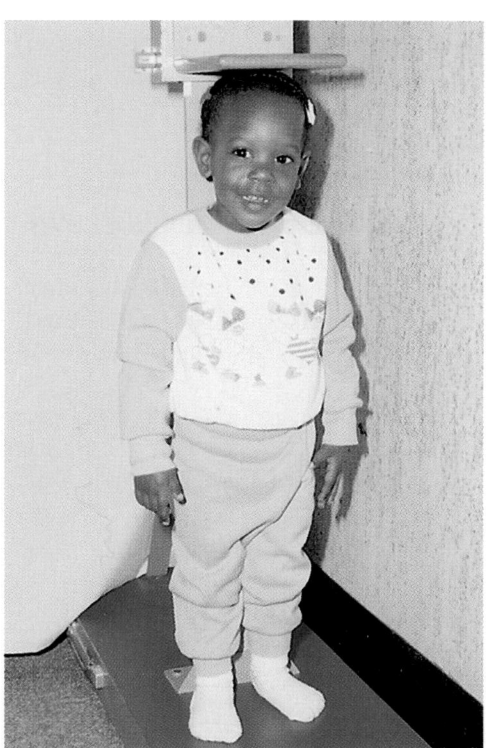

Fig. 6-17 Measuring the height of a child. (From Seidel et al, 1999.)

This position is maintained with one of the examiner's hands while the lubricated thermometer is held in the rectum a maximum of 1 inch (2.5 cm).

Blood pressure. The American Heart Association (AHA) recommends that blood pressure be measured annually in children from age 3 through adolescence. For an accurate reading the appropriate cuff size must be used (see Chapter 5). Show the equipment to be used to the child and explain the procedure before applying the cuff to help enlist the child's cooperation. The AHA recommends using the fourth Korotkoff sound as an indication of the diastolic pressure in children (Report of the Second Task Force, 1987).

■ ADOLESCENTS

Weight and Height These measurements should be obtained at least annually. Before puberty, the differences in male and female body composition are minimal. Sex differences in the skeletal system, lean body mass, and fat stores become apparent during the adolescent growth spurt. Just before the growth spurt, body fat begins to increase.

■ OLDER ADULTS

Weight and Height Older adults tend to weigh less and become shorter. For those in their 80s and beyond, body weight may decrease due to muscle wasting or chronic diseases. Also, total body water declines, which contributes to weight loss. Subcutaneous fat distribution shifts from the face and extremities to the abdomen and hips. This age group also has decreased bone formation, which may result in reduced height due to shortening of the vertebrae and thinning of the vertebral disks. If kyphosis or flexion of knees or hips occurs, arms and legs look longer and out of proportion.

Vital Signs Older adults tend to have lower normal temperatures, with an average of 97.2° F (36.2° C). Those who have arteriosclerosis tend to have higher blood pressures. As the aorta becomes rigid, the systolic blood pressure increases. Those with diabetes mellitus may have reduced compliance of vessels, resulting in high systolic blood pressures.

CLINICAL APPLICATION and CRITICAL THINKING

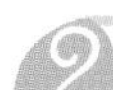

CRITICAL THINKING QUESTIONS

1. You are attempting to auscultate a client's chest with the diaphragm of the stethoscope during an examination. Describe measures you should take to enhance the auscultation process.
2. A father brings his 8-week-old baby to the clinic for a well-baby visit. What measurements are routinely done to evaluate growth and development? How is this information recorded for comparison purposes?
3. Your female client is 5 feet 5 inches tall, weighs 140 lb, and has a medium frame. A skinfold thickness at the triceps was taken at 25 mm. Where does your client fall in percentiles of weight and skinfold thickness? (Refer to Table 10-4.)

REMEMBER to check out your **companion CD-ROM**

7 Mental Health Assessment

www.mosby.com/MERLIN/wilson/assessment/

A comprehensive assessment of an individual includes mental and emotional health as well as physical health. Mental health is an elusive concept because data are based on a description of an individual's behavior by the health professional performing the assessment. Furthermore, the issue of persistence of behavior must be considered. How long must a person engage in a particular behavior or mood before health professionals determine the person has an alteration in mental health? These issues make quantifying mental health assessment a challenge. Changes in clients' lives may affect their mental health, requiring periodic mental health assessment. Factors influencing mental health include self-concept, interpersonal relationships, stress management abilities, spiritual and belief systems, genetic factors, and physiologic functioning of the limbic system and neurotransmitters.

ANATOMY AND PHYSIOLOGY

The limbic system is called the emotional brain because it is believed to regulate emotions and memory. It forms a border of subcortical structures that surround the corpus callosum (Fig. 7-1). There is a lobe of the limbic system in each cerebral hemisphere that provides communication links between and among different structures. For example, when a person sees something that recalls a memory of happy emotions, there is communication among the occipital lobe for vision, prefrontal lobe for memory, and limbic lobe for emotion and memory. The communication function of the limbic system may initiate or inhibit other parts of the brain such as the cerebral cortex, brainstem, or hypothalamus to normalize expressions of emotion, influence their ultimate expression to other than normal, or affect the biologic rhythm, sexual behavior, and motivation of an individual (McKenry and Salerno, 1998).

Several neurotransmitters are associated with mental health. Neurotransmitters are substances that carry messages from neuron to neuron or from neuron to muscle cell. They are synthesized in the neuron, released in the synaptic cleft, and bind to receptor sites on another neuron or effector cell. There are three neurotransmitters that facilitate or initiate activity: norepinephrine, serotonin, and dopamine. Norepinephrine is thought to help regulate mood and maintain arousal. Cocaine and amphetamines increase release and block the reuptake of norepinephrine, causing overstimulation of the postsynaptic neurons. Serotonin pathways are similar to norepinephrine and have similar effects. Levels of serotonin are elevated in schizophrenia, contributing to delusions, hallucination, and withdrawal. Dopamine acts in the midbrain on emotions and memory and in the hypothalamus and pituitary gland, affecting emotional responses and stress reactions. Gamma-aminobutyric acid (GABA) is an inhibitory neurotransmitter that suppresses activity; insufficient GABA may contribute to anxiety.

HEALTH HISTORY

The focus of a mental health history is to determine how the client compares with the characteristics of a healthy personality listed in Box 7-1. Since mental health assessment is based primarily on subjective data, the history for mental health assessment is longer than in other systems.

Data collection begins when the nurse first sees the client. Is the client dressed appropriately for the weather? Does his or her mood seem appropriate? Is the affect (emotional state) appropriate? What is the client's body posture? Is the client slumped over and looking at the ground with a sad facial expression or walking tall with a brisk step and a smiling face? What is the client's tone of voice? Does he or she talk in a monotone or a happy, expressive tone? Does the client's conversation flow in a logical sequence? Table 7-1 lists conversational styles consistent with alterations in thought processes.

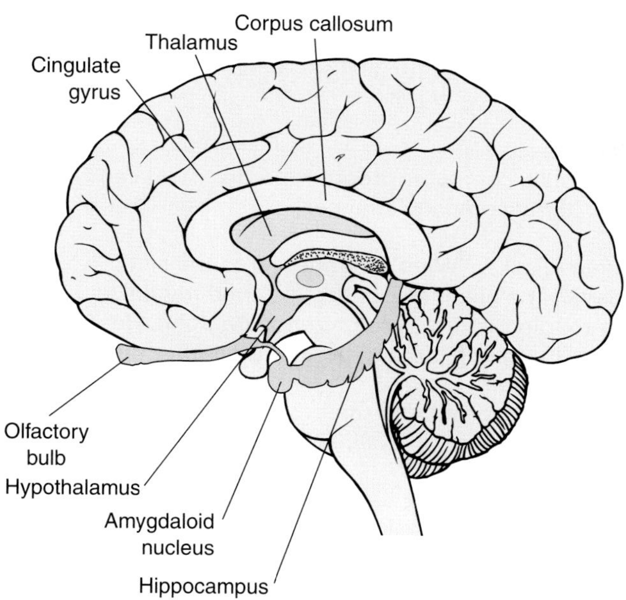

Fig. 7-1 The limbic system. (From McKenry and Salerno, 1998.)

Box 7-1 Characteristics of Mentally Healthy Persons

- They demonstrate high-control behavior, as evidenced by being considerate, farsighted, cautious, punctual, and norm oriented.
- They are socially adaptable, as evidenced by being well adapted, task oriented, and honest with strong superegos.
- They demonstrate high mental health, as evidenced by being self-confident, energetic, active, good problem solvers, calm, well balanced, and autonomous and by demonstrating willpower.
- They are self-actualized, as evidenced by being assertive, dominant, lively, casual, spontaneous, well tempered, and creative.

From Becker P, Korchin SJ, and Minsel B: A cross-cultural view of positive mental health. Two orthogonal main factors replicable in four countries, *Journal of cross-cultural psychology,* 22:157-181, 1991, © Western Washington University. Reprinted by permission of Sage Publications, Inc. In Varcarolis EM: *Foundations of psychiatric mental health nursing,* ed 3, Philadelphia, 1998, Saunders.

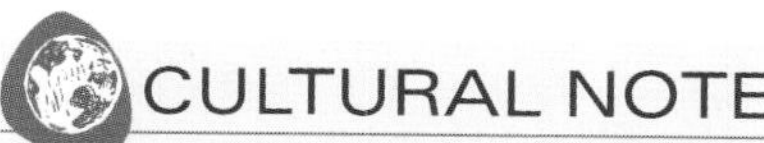

CULTURAL NOTE

CULTURALLY RELEVANT PHENOMENA IN MENTAL HEALTH NURSING

Mental health is the degree to which a person is able to fulfill the cultural expectations of his or her society. Thus mental health and deviance from mental health are derived from cultural expectations (Arnault, 1998).

Phenomena include the following:

- Perception of reality—may be culturally prescribed, spiritually induced in a traditional healing system, or otherwise sanctioned by the cultural group. For example, a Native American client may appear to a white American to have lost touch with reality, but the Native American is practicing his or her spiritual healing ritual that is important to attain or maintain health.
- Needs, feelings, thoughts of others and self—clients need to attend to their needs, feelings, and thoughts of self and others, whether they are internal or external. Events considered as stressors vary from one culture to another. For example, Kenyans are taught not to discuss or show their feelings of sadness or pain. If a Kenyan was seen by an American health care provider for a suspected mental health disorder, he or she would not willingly share feelings, which is a large part of the health history for mental health nursing. This client may be seen as uncooperative, when in fact he or she is complying with the Kenyan culture.
- Decision making—the ability to make decisions may be culturally prescribed so that families and cultures designate decision makers, which may include health care decisions. Inability to make decisions is a clinical manifestation of depression and anxiety. For example, in traditional Vietnamese families, the oldest male makes decisions about health care. As a result, a female client may delay seeking health care until she consults with the oldest male in the family.

Data from Arnault DS: Framework for culturally relevant psychiatric nursing. In Varcarolis EM: *Foundations of psychiatric mental health nursing,* ed 3, Philadelphia, 1998, Saunders.

Table 7-1 Problems of Word Usage Associated With Alterations in Thought Processes

DEFINITION	EXAMPLE
Blocking occurs with thought disorganization when clients have difficulty articulating a response or stop in midsentence as if they were stuck.	"I work as a computer programmer for . . . I can't think of my company's name."
Confabulation is a fabrication of experiences or situations, explained in detailed and plausible ways to cover up gaps in memory. Often used as a defense mechanism by alcoholics and persons with head injuries, dementia, or lead poisoning.	The nurse asks, "What brought you to the clinic today?" The client responds, "I turned my ankle. I was running a new pass pattern with John. He was right on target, a 30-yard pass, but another player got in my way, and I fell."
Neologism is a word or term used with a new meaning known only to the client, who is often delusional, psychotic, or delirious.	"I turned the corner and there was a huge *combaster* headed right for me. Well, you can imagine how I felt."
Circumstantiality is a speech pattern in which a client has difficulty separating relevant from irrelevant information. While describing an event, the client uses so much detail that the original thought becomes lost. Circumstantiality may be a sign of chronic brain syndrome.	The nurse says, "How did you feel when you won the award?" The client responds, "Well, I jumped out of my chair, I wore the black backless gown, but I seriously considered wearing the red sequin gown, with diamond stud earrings and necklace, but the shoes were uncomfortable, you know, with 3-inch heels, I would just fall over getting up to get my award, but then I could have borrowed shoes from Lisa, her apartment is so well decorated with the country look . . . ."
Loosening (loose association) is a disturbance in thinking in which the association of ideas and thought patterns becomes so vague, diffuse, and unfocused as to lack any logical sequence or relationship to any preceding topics of conversation.	"I have three sisters . . . living in the north is so cold . . . but typing is what I do best . . . so when I started the car I heard a funny noise . . . you know."
Flight of ideas is a continuous talking in which the client switches rapidly from one topic to another with each topic being incoherent or unrelated to the previous one or stimulated by some environmental stimuli. Flight of ideas is a frequent symptom of manic states and schizophrenia.	"Hi, I came in today . . . that coffee smells great, but the caffeine . . . chocolate has caffeine, but so much fat . . . need to walk 3 miles every day to keep the weight off . . . I bought a new swim suit, it's a two-piece."
Word salad is a jumble of words and phrases that lacks logical coherence and meaning. Word salad occurs when clients are disoriented or have schizophrenia.	"Dog bark . . . sunshine today . . . fill . . . form . . . reclining chair . . . grass . . . hamburger . . . flowers . . . vacation . . . steamship."
Perseveration is the involuntary and pathologic persistent repetition of words, ideas, and phrases regardless of the stimulus or its duration. This is consistent with clients who have brain damage or organic mental disorders, although it may appear in schizophrenia.	*Nurse:* "Ready to see your family?" *Client:* "Ready set go." *Nurse:* "They are in the snack bar." *Client:* "Ready set go."
Echolalia is the automatic and meaningless repetition of another's words or phrases, seen in clients with schizophrenia	*Nurse:* "Ready to see your family?" *Client:* "See your family, see your family, see your family."
Clanging (clang association) is the mental connection between dissociated ideas made because of similarity in the sounds of the words used to describe ideas. This occurs frequently in the manic phases of bipolar disorder.	"I went to bed . . . head on straight . . . wait . . . full . . . pull the cart . . . heart to heart . . . part . . . should . . . should you . . . no you better not . . . heart . . . cart . . . part my hair . . . hair there."

Data from Varcarolis EM: *Foundations of psychiatric mental health nursing,* ed 3, Philadelphia, 1998, Saunders.

HEALTH HISTORY

Mental Health

QUESTIONS | RATIONALE

PRESENT HEALTH STATUS

➤ How have you been feeling about yourself? Do you consider your present feelings to be a problem in your daily life? If so, do you feel the problem is temporary or curable?

■ This invites the client to discuss feelings and may help to begin to identify problems (e.g., depression, stress, anger).

➤ What medical problems do you have?

■ Some medical problems may cause changes in mood or behavior (e.g., endocrine disorders).

➤ What medications are you taking?

■ Side effects of some medications may cause changes in mood and behavior. Also the nurse needs to know if the client is taking medications for mental health disorders.

Self-Concept

➤ How would you describe yourself to others? What are your best characteristics? What do you like about yourself?

■ This determines how clients perceive themselves. Those with positive self-esteem regard themselves favorably and can name their positive attributes.

Interpersonal Relationships

➤ How satisfied are you with your interpersonal relationships? Do you have friends you socialize with? Are there people to whom you can talk about feelings and problems?

■ Achievement of satisfying interpersonal relationships is needed for mental health. Clients who have few to no interpersonal relationships may be depressed or out of touch with reality. Having sources of social support is important for interpersonal relationships.

➤ Do you prefer to be alone or with other people?

■ Clients who prefer to be alone may be experiencing emotional problems.

Stressors

➤ Have there been any recent changes in your life? Were these changes stressors for you? What are the major stressors in your life now?

How do you deal with stress? What actions do you take to relieve stress? Are those methods of stress relief currently effective for you? (Inquire about stressors such as money, intimate relationships, death or illness of a family member or friend, employment problems.) (Box 7-2 lists some coping strategies frequently used.) One way to inquire further about stress is to administer the Holmes Social Readjustment Rating Scale (Table 7-2).

■ Coping with the stress of daily life is essential to maintain mental health. Answers to these questions help to identify the client's stressors and how well they are being managed.

Anger

➤ Have you been feeling angry? Do you feel angry now? How do you react when you are angry: verbally, physically, or do you keep your anger inside? Can you talk about what has caused this anger?

■ Knowing how clients react to anger can help them find an acceptable way to express their feelings (e.g., hit a pillow instead of a person, verbally express anger in an empty room or elevator). Talking about the cause of the anger can be therapeutic and provides an opportunity for the nurse to make referrals for help.

Box 7-2 Coping Strategies

SINGLE COPING STRATEGIES

- Pray, trust in God
- Take out tension on someone or something else
- Blame someone else for your problem
- Resign yourself to the situation because it looks hopeless
- Do nothing, hoping the problem will resolve itself
- Try to put the problem out of your mind
- Daydream, fantasize
- Drink alcoholic beverages, take drugs
- Meditation, yoga, biofeedback

COPING STRATEGIES THAT ARE OPPOSITES (EMPHASIZES THE INDIVIDUALITY OF EACH PERSON AND EACH STRESSFUL SITUATION)

Worry	Want to be alone, withdraw from the situation
Seek comfort from a friend	Get mad, swear, curse
Laugh it off, believing that things could be worse	Get prepared for the worst
Go to sleep, things will look better in the morning	Physical activity, exercise
Don't worry about it, everything will be fine	

Modified from Jalowiec A, Powers MJ: Stress coping in hypertensive and emergency room patients, *Nurs Res* 30:13, 1981.

Table 7-2 Holmes Social Readjustment Rating Scale

EVENT	EVENT VALUE	EVENT	EVENT VALUE
1. Death of a spouse	100	22. Change in responsibilities at work	29
2. Divorce	73	23. Son or daughter leaving home	29
3. Marital separation	65	24. Trouble with in-laws	29
4. Jail term	63	25. Outstanding personal achievement	28
5. Death of a close family member	63	26. Spouse begins or stops work	26
6. Personal injury or illness	53	27. Begin or end school	26
7. Marriage	50	28. Change in living conditions	25
8. Fired at work	47	29. Revision of personal habits	24
9. Marital reconciliation	45	30. Trouble with boss	23
10. Retirement	45	31. Change in work hours or conditions	20
11. Change in health of family member	44	32. Change in residence	20
12. Pregnancy	40	33. Change in schools	20
13. Sex difficulties	39	34. Change in recreation	19
14. Gain of a new family member	39	35. Change in church activities	19
15. Business readjustment	39	36. Change in social activities	19
16. Change in financial state	38	37. Change in sleeping habits	16
17. Death of a close friend	37	38. Change in number of family get-togethers	15
18. Change to different line of work	36	39. Vacation	13
19. Change in number of arguments	35	40. Christmas	12
20. Mortgage or loan over $10,000	31	41. Minor violations of the law	11
21. Foreclosure of mortgage or loan	30	Total Points	

Directions for completion: Add up the point values for each of the events that you have experienced during the past 12 months.

Scoring

Below 150 points:

The amount of stress you are experiencing as a result of changes in your life is normal and manageable. There is only a 1 in 3 chance that you might develop a serious illness over the next 2 years based on stress alone. Consider practicing a daily relaxation technique to reduce your chance of illness even more.

150 to 300 points:

The amount of stress you are experiencing as a result of changes in your life is moderate. Based on stress alone, you have a 50/50 chance of developing a serious illness over the next 2 years. You can reduce these odds by practicing stress management and relaxation techniques on a daily basis.

Over 300 points:

The amount of stress you are experiencing as a result of changes in your life is high. Based on stress alone, your chances of developing a serious illness during the next 2 years approaches 90%, unless you are already practicing good coping skills and regular relaxation techniques. You can reduce the chance of illness by practicing coping strategies and relaxation techniques daily.

QUESTIONS | **RATIONALE**

Alcohol Abuse

➤ Do you ever drink alcohol, including beer, wine, or liquor?

■ Current guidelines recommend screening every adult and adolescent for problem drinking.

➤ If yes, ask the following questions:
-What is the maximum number of drinks you've had on any given occasion during the last month?
-On a typical day when you drink, how many drinks do you have?
-On average, how many days per week do you drink alcohol?

■ These question help identify the quantity of alcohol drunk.

➤ The four CAGE questions are used as a screening tool. CAGE is an acronym for *C*ut down, *A*nnoyed, *G*uilty, *E*ye opener.

1. Have you ever felt you should *cut down* on your drinking?
2. Have people *annoyed* you by criticizing your drinking?
3. Have you ever felt bad or *guilty* about your drinking?
4. Have you ever had a drink first thing in the morning to steady your nerves, get rid of a hangover (*eye opener*), or get the day started (Smith-Dijulio, 1998)?

■ The CAGE is the most popular screening tool for primary care. It is less sensitive for early problem drinking or heavy drinking (Report of U.S. Preventive Task Force, 1996).

➤ AUDIT (*A*lcohol, *U*se, *D*isorders *I*dentification *T*est), is another screening tool. It is a 10-item scale with a score from 0 to 4 on each item (Table 7-3) (Report of the U.S. Preventive Services Task Force, 1996).

■ These 10 AUDIT questions ask about quantity and frequency of drinking, binging, and drinking consequences.

Drug Abuse

➤ Do you use illegal or street drugs? What drugs do you use? Box 7-3 is a glossary of drug jargon. How often do you use these drugs? The CAGE or AUDIT screening tools may be adapted to ask questions about drug abuse.

■ Use of illegal drugs needs to be documented since it contributes to health problems.

PROBLEM-BASED HISTORY

Depression

➤ Risk factors for depression are listed in the box on p. 100. Are you able to fall *asleep* and stay asleep without difficulty? Have you noticed any marked change in your *eating habits?* Have you recently gained or lost weight without trying to? Have you noticed a change in the amount of energy you have *(fatigue)?* Do you have *crying* spells? Have you recently experienced a loss, such as a job, friend, or spouse? Do you have difficulty *making decisions?* Have you noticed less interest in participating in your usual activities?

■ These questions help to identify *possible symptoms of depression.* Some clients can recognize symptoms but do not realize that the group of symptoms may indicate depression.

➤ Describe your *mood.* Have you noticed an increase in *irritability?* Do you ever feel as though you do not care about anything? Do you spend much time alone? (Estimate the number of waking hours per day per week.)

■ Depressed people feel sad, blue, helpless, and alone.

➤ Do you have friends whom you can trust and who are available when you need them?

■ Friends may be a source of social support to listen to the client's feelings and demonstrate their caring for the client.

Box 7-3 Glossary of Drug Jargon

AMPHETAMINES

Bams
Beans
Benn
Bennies
Black beauties
Black cadillacs
Black dex
Bombido (injectable)
Browns
Cartwheels
Chalk
Co-pilots
Cranks
Cross
Crystal
Dexies
Dice
Doe
Drives
Eyeopeners
Fives (5 mg)
Footballs
Goofballs
Green hearts
Greenies
Greens
Heart(s)
Horse hearts
Jolly babies
Leapers
Lid rollers
Lightning
Meth
Orange hearts
Peaches
Pep pills
Rippers
Roses
Speed
Splash
Thrusters
Truck drivers
Wake-up
White crosses
White dexies
Whites
Yellow bams
Zeeters
Zip

BARBITURATES (GENERAL)

Barbs
Courage pills
Downers
Golf balls
Goofers
Idiot pills
Nimbie
Nimbles
Peanuts
Sleepers

BARBITURATES (SPECIFIC)

Blue birds (amobarbital)
Blue devils (amobarbital)
Blue heaven (amobarbital)
Canary (pentobarbital)
Christmas trees (mixtures)
Downers (amobarbital)
F-40s (secobarbital)
F-66s (amobarbital sodium and secobarbital sodium) (gorilla pills)
Mexican yellows (pentobarbital)
Nemmies (pentobarbital)
Pink ladies (secobarbital)
Pinks (secobarbital)
Rainbow (secobarbital; amobarbital)
Red birds (secobarbital)
Red devils (secobarbital)
Reds (secobarbital)
Seggy, seccy (secobarbital)
Tooies (tuinal)
Yellow jackets (pentobarbital)
Yellows (pentobarbital)

COCAINE

Bernies flake
C
Candy
Cecil
Charlie
Coca-cola
Coke
Cokomo (Kokomo)
Crack
Dust
Flake
Gift of the Sun God
Gold dust
Happy trails
Incentive
Lady snow
Leaf (the)
Movie star drug
Nose
Nose candy
Pimp
Pimp's drug
Rich man's drug
Rock
Schoolboy
Snow
Society high
Star-spangled powder
Stardust
White horse
White stuff

HEROIN

Big Harry
Blanco
Boy
Caballo
Chiva
Deuce (a $2 packet)
Doojee
Dust
H
Harry; hairy
Horse
Joy powder
Scag
Scat
Smack
Stuff
Sugar
Ticata
White lady
White stuff

MORPHINE

Dreamer
Dust
Emma (Miss)
Emsel
Hard stuff
Hocus
M
Monkey
Morf
Morpho
Unkie
White stuff

From Wong DL et al: *Whaley & Wong's nursing care of infants and children,* ed 5, St Louis, 1995, Mosby.

Box 7-3 Glossary of Drug Jargon—cont'd

MARIJUANA

Acapulco gold (potent)
Bush
Butter
Flower
Grass
Griffo
Hemp
Hooch
Hooter
Indian hay
J
Jive
Joint
Kif
Mary Jane
Mohasky
Mooters
Mu
Mutah
Panama red
Pot
Reefer (cigarette)
Rockets
Smoke
Splimi
Stick (cigarette)
Straw
Superjoint
Texas tea
Tie stick (mixed with opium and tied to a popsicle stick)
Weed

LSD (LYSERGIC ACID DIETHYLAMIDE)

Acid
Blotter acid (on paper)
Blue microdot
Cube (the)
D (big)
Heavenly blue
Purple haze
Royal blue
Sugar
Wedding bells
Windowpane

PCP (PHENCYCLIDINE)

Angel dust
Busy bee
DOA
Elephant
Goon
Hog (also chloral hydrate)
Horse tranquilizer
Magic mist
Peace pills
Rocket fuel
Sherman's
White horizon
Wobble

OTHER HALLUCINOGENS

DMT (dimethyltryptamine): businessman's special
DMZ (benactyzine)
DOM (4-methyl-2,5-dimethoxyamphetamine), STP
Hashish: black has; black Russian (potent)
STP (dimethoxymethylamphetamine), DOM (syndicate acid, tranquility)
THC (tetrahydrocannabinol): hallucinogen in marijuana and hashish

MIXED SUBSTANCES

Chicago green (marijuana/opium)
Double trouble (amobarbital/secobarbital)
Fours (actaminophen with 60 mg codeine)
Fuel (marijuana/insecticide)
Hog (phencyclidine/vegetable material [veterinary drug])
In-betweens (barbiturates/amphetamines)
Mickey Finn (chloral hydrate/alcohol)
Speedball (heroin/cocaine; Percodan/methedrine)
Star-spangled powder (heroin/cocaine)

MISCELLANEOUS

Alcohol: mountain dew, alley juice (methyl alcohol) moonshine (ethyl alcohol), sauce, hootch, booze, juice
Amyl nitrite: aimes, snappers
Chloral hydrate: joy juice
Ethchlorvynol (Placidyl): dyls, plastic red, K-H, K-N
Meperidine hydrochloride: Diane
Mescaline: chief, mesc, mescalito, mescal beans
Methadone: dolls, dollies fizzies (tablets)
Methaqualone (Quaalude): 714, ludes, sopors, westcoast, lemons
Opium for smoking: black stuff
Paregoric: licorice, bitter
Peyote: button, cactus, Hikori, Kikuli, Huatari, Wokouri, seni, tops
Tobacco: coffin, deck (pack), fag

Table 7-3 AUDIT Structured Interview[a]

QUESTION	SCORE 0	1	2	3	4
How often do you have a drink containing alcohol?	Never	Monthly or less	2-4 times/mo	2-3 times/wk	4 or more times/wk
How many drinks do you have on a typical day when you are drinking?	None	1 or 2	3 or 4	5 or 6	7-9*
How often do you have 6 or more drinks on one occasion?	Never	Less than monthly	Monthly	Weekly	Daily or almost daily
How often during the last year have you found that you were unable to stop drinking once you had started?	Never	Less than monthly	Monthly	Weekly	Daily or almost daily
How often last year have you failed to do what was normally expected from you because of drinking?	Never	Less than monthly	Monthly	Weekly	Daily or almost daily
How often during the last year have you needed a first drink in the morning to get yourself going after a heavy drinking session?	Never	Less than monthly	Monthly	Weekly	Daily or almost daily
How often during the last year have you had a feeling of guilt or remorse after drinking?	Never	Less than monthly	Monthly	Weekly	Daily or almost daily
How often during the last year have you been unable to remember what happened the night before because you had been drinking?	Never	Less than monthly	Monthly	Weekly	Daily or almost daily
Have you or someone else been injured as a result of your drinking?	Never	Yes, but not in last year (2 points)		Yes, during the last year (4 points)	
Has a relative, doctor, or other health worker been concerned about your drinking or suggested you cut down?	Never	Yes, but not in last year (2 points)		Yes, during the last year (4 points)	

From Report of the U.S. Preventive Services Task Force: *Guide to clinical preventive services,* ed 2, Baltimore, Maryland, 1996, Williams & Wilkins.
[a]Score of greater than 8 (out of 41) suggestive of problem drinking and indicates need for more in-depth assessment. Cut-off of 10 points recommended by some to provide greater specificity.
*5 points if response is 10 or more drinks on a typical day.

Risk Factors

COMMON RISK FACTORS ASSOCIATED WITH Depression

AT-RISK POPULATIONS

Women are at risk for depression 2:1 over men.

Adolescents are at risk for depression and anxiety due to peer pressure and desire to fit in and to be independent of parents.

Children whose mothers abused drugs, including alcohol, during their pregnancy are at risk for a variety of altered mental health states.

RISK FACTORS

Depression—loss of significant other, family member, job, home, or status

Stress—feeling overwhelmed, too much to do, unexpected life changes, usual coping skills have not been effective

Anxiety—threats to biologic safety and basic human need, unmet needs for status and prestige, guilt, discrepancies between self-view and actual behavior, fear of the unknown

QUESTIONS | **RATIONALE**

➤ How long have you had these feelings?

■ Depressed feelings for 2 weeks is one criterion for a diagnosis of depression.

➤ Have you had feelings like this before? What did you do about depressive feelings at that time?

■ Depression may be a recurring disorder. Treatment that was successful in the past may be useful again.

➤ Have you ever thought about hurting yourself or ending your life? (If so, describe past methods and any specific plans for the future.) Depression can be assessed by administering the Beck Depression Inventory (Fig. 7-2).

■ A client who has a specific plan for suicide is at higher risk than one who has no plan.

Anxiety

➤ Have you had *difficulty concentrating or making decisions?* Have you been *preoccupied or forgetful?* How well have you been sleeping? Are you able to fall *asleep* and stay asleep without difficulty? Have you noticed a change in the amount of energy you have *(fatigue)?* Have you been more *irritable* than usual? Do your *muscles seem tense?* Do you feel a *tightening in your throat?*

■ These are *symptoms of anxiety.* See the description of the four levels of anxiety under Common Problems and Conditions on pp. 107-108.

➤ Have you felt nauseated? Does your heart feel as though it is racing? Have you had to urinate more often than usual?

■ Nausea, urinary frequency, and palpitations may be physiologic responses to anxiety.

➤ Have you noticed a change in your feelings?

■ Feelings of anger, guilt, worthlessness, and anguish often accompany anxiety. Clients may report feeling that he or she is going to die or having a sense of impending doom.

➤ You seem anxious or uncomfortable.

■ Giving the client feedback on nonverbal behavior gives him or her an opportunity to confirm or deny the presence of anxiety. An anxious person moves around, paces, repeats the same question or statement, and seems unable to focus on the interview.

❖ ➤ The Mini-Mental State Examination (MMSE) is a standardized screening tool used to estimate cognitive function or document changes in cognitive function (Fig. 7-3). It is a useful screening tool for detecting organic brain disease. It includes assessment of orientation, registration, attention and calculation, recall, and language.

Beck Depression Inventory, Short Form

Instructions: This is a questionnaire. On the questionnaire are groups of statements. Please read the entire group of statements in each category. Then pick out the one statement in that group which best describes the way you feel today, that is, *right now!* Circle the number beside the statement you have chosen. If several statements in the group seem to apply equally well, circle each one.

Be sure to read all the statements in each group before making your choice.

A. (Sadness)
- **3** I am so sad or unhappy that I can't stand it.
- **2** I am blue or sad all the time and I can't snap out of it.
- **1** I feel sad or blue.
- **0** I do not feel sad.

B. (Pessimism)
- **3** I feel that the future is hopeless and that things cannot improve.
- **2** I feel I have nothing to look forward to.
- **1** I feel discouraged about the future.
- **0** I am not particularly pessimistic or discouraged about the future.

C. (Sense of failure)
- **3** I feel I am a complete failure as a person (parent, husband, wife).
- **2** As I look back on my life, all I can see is a lot of failures.
- **1** I feel I have failed more than the average person.
- **0** I do not feel like a failure.

D. (Dissatisfaction)
- **3** I am dissatisfied with everything.
- **2** I don't get satisfaction out of anything anymore.
- **1** I don't enjoy things the way I used to.
- **0** I am not particularly dissatisfied.

E. (Guilt)
- **3** I feel as though I am very bad or worthless.
- **2** I feel quite guilty.
- **1** I feel bad or unworthy a good part of the time.
- **0** I don't feel particularly guilty.

F. (Self-dislike)
- **3** I hate myself.
- **2** I am disgusted with myself.
- **1** I am dissapointed in myself.
- **0** I don't feel disappointed in myself.

G. (Self-harm)
- **3** I would kill myself if I had the chance.
- **2** I have definite plans about committing suicide.
- **1** I feel I would be better off dead.
- **0** I don't have any thoughts about harming myself.

H. (Social withdrawal)
- **3** I have lost all of my interest in other people and don't care about most of them at all.
- **2** I have lost most of my interest in other people and have little feeling for them.
- **1** I am less interested in other people than I used to be.
- **0** I have not lost interest in other people.

I. (Indecisiveness)
- **3** I can't make any decisions at all anymore.
- **2** I have great difficulty in making decisions.
- **1** I try to put off making decisions.
- **0** I make decisions about as well as ever.

J. (Self-image change)
- **3** I feel that I am ugly or repulsive-looking.
- **2** I feel that there are permanent changes in my appearance and they make me look unattractive.
- **1** I am worried that I am looking old or unattractive.
- **0** I don't feel that I look any worse than I used to.

K. (Work difficulty)
- **3** I can't do any work at all.
- **2** I have to push myself very hard to do anything.
- **1** It takes extra effort to get started at doing something.
- **0** I can work about as well as before.

L. (Fatigability)
- **3** I get too tired to do anything.
- **2** I get tired from doing anything.
- **1** I get tired more easily than I used to.
- **0** I don't get any more tired than usual.

M. (Anorexia)
- **3** I have no appetite at all anymore.
- **2** My appetite is much worse now.
- **1** My appetite is not as good as it used to be.
- **0** My appetite is no worse than usual.

Scoring

- **0-4** None or minimal depression
- **5-7** Mild depression
- **8-15** Moderate depression
- **16+** Severe depression

Fig. 7-2 Beck Depression Inventory, Short Form. (From Beck and Beck, 1972.)

Patient..................................
Examiner...............................
Date...................................

"MINI-MENTAL STATE"

Maximum Score	Score	
		ORIENTATION
5	( )	What is the (year) (season) (date) (day) (month)?
5	( )	Where are we: (state) (county) (town) (hospital) (floor).
		REGISTRATION
3	( )	Name 3 objects: 1 second to say each. Then ask the patient all 3 after you have said them. Give 1 point for each correct answer. Then repeat them until he learns all 3. Count trials and record. Trials
		ATTENTION AND CALCULATION
5	( )	Serial 7's. 1 point for each correct. Stop after 5 answers. Alternatively spell "world" backwards.
		RECALL
3	( )	Ask for the 3 objects repeated above. Give 1 point for each correct.
		LANGUAGE
9	( )	Name a pencil, and watch (2 points)
		Repeat the following "No ifs, ands or buts." (1 point)
		Follow a 3-stage command: "Take a paper in your right hand, fold it in half, and put in on the floor" (3 points)
		Read and obey the following: CLOSE YOUR EYES (1 point)
		Write a sentence (1 point)
		Copy design (1 point)
	_______	Total score
		ASSESS level of consciousness along a continuum _______________ Alert Drowsy Stupor Coma

INSTRUCTIONS FOR ADMINISTRATION OF
MINI-MENTAL STATE EXAMINATION

ORIENTATION

(1) Ask for the date. Then ask specifically for parts omitted, e.g., "Can you also tell me what season it is?" One point for each correct.

(2) Ask in turn "Can you tell me the name of this hospital?" (town, county, etc.). One point for each correct.

REGISTRATION

Ask the patient if you may test his memory. Then say the name of 3 unrelated objects, clearly and slowly, about one second for each. After you have said 3, ask him to repeat them. The first repetition determines his score (0-3) but keep saying them until he can repeat all 3, up to 6 trials. If he does not eventually learn all 3, recall cannot be meaningfully tested.

ATTENTION AND CALCULATION

Ask the patient to begin with 100 and count backwards by 7. Stop after 5 subtracations (93,86,79,72,65). Score the total number of correct answers.

If the patient cannot or will not perform this task, ask him to spell the word "world" backwards. The score is the number of letters in correct order. E.g. dlrow = 5, dlorw = 3.

RECALL

Ask the patient if he can recall the 3 words you previously asked him to remember. Score 0-3.

LANGUAGE

Naming: Show the patient a wrist watch and ask him what it is. Repeat for pencil. Score 0-2.

Repetition: Ask the patient to repeat the sentence after you. Allow only one trial. Score 0 or 1.

3-Stage command: Give the patient a piece of plain blank paper and repeat the command. Score 1 point for each part correctly executed.

Reading: On a blank piece of paper print the sentence "Close your eyes", in letters large enough for the patient to see clearly. Ask him to read it and do what it says. Score 1 point only if he actually closes his eyes.

Writing: Give the patient a blank piece of paper and ask him to write a sentence for you. Do not dictate a sentence, it is to be written spontaneously. It must contain a subject and verb to be sensible. Correct grammer and puncuation are not necessary.

Copying: On a clean piece of paper, draw intersecting pentagons, each side about 1 in., and ask him to copy it exactly as it is. All 10 angles must be present and 2 must intersect to score 1 point. Tremor and rotation are ignored.

Estimate the patient's level of sensorium along a continuum, from alert on the left to coma on the right.

Fig. 7-3 Mini-Mental State examination, a standardized screening tool of mental status. The maximum score is 30. Depressed clients without dementia usually score between 24 and 30. A score of 20 or less is found in clients with dementia, delirium, schizophrenia, or an affective disorder. ("Mini-Mental State." A practical guide for grading the cognitive state of patients for the clinician, *Journal of Psychiatric Research,* (12)3:189-198, 1975.)

EXAMINATION

Equipment

- Scale with height measurement
- Stethoscope
- Sphygmomanometer

PROCEDURES AND TECHNIQUES WITH NORMAL FINDINGS	ABNORMAL FINDINGS
➤**MEASURE the height and weight of the client.** Refer to average height/weight table for expected norms, Appendix F.	■ Weight loss or gain can occur with depression.
➤**PALPATE, then AUSCULTATE the brachial artery to evaluate arterial blood pressure.** Blood pressure varies with sex, body weight, and time of day, but the upper limits for adults are 140 mm Hg systolic and 90 mm Hg diastolic.	■ Anxiety, especially severe anxiety or panic, may cause elevated blood pressure due to the sympathetic stimulation.
➤**PALPATE the brachial pulse for rate, rhythm, amplitude, and contour.** (See Chapter 18 for descriptions.) *Rate:* 60 to 100 beats/min *Rhythm:* Regular (equal spacing between beats) *Amplitude:* Easily palpable, smooth upstroke *Contour:* Smooth and rounded, a series of pulse strokes, unvaried, symmetric responses	■ Pulse rates for clients with anxiety may be elevated due to sympathetic stimulation.
➤**OBSERVE and COUNT respirations for rate and breathing pattern.** Note the respiratory rate. Breathing should be smooth and even. In adults breathing should occur at a rate of 12 to 20 breaths per minute. Evaluate the rhythm or pattern of breathing. The chest wall should symmetrically rise and expand then relax. It should appear easy, without effort.	■ Respiratory rate may be increased during anxiety due to sympathetic stimulation. The client may appear to be dyspneic. Respiratory rate may be decreased during depression, and the breathing pattern may include frequent, deep sighs.
➤**OBSERVE for changes in voice tone, rate of speech, perspiration, and muscle tension or tremors.**	■ Other physical signs of anxiety include changes in tone of voice and rate of speech, body tremors, increased muscle tension, perspiration, sweaty palms.

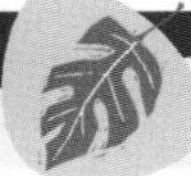

AGE-RELATED VARIATIONS

■ INFANTS

Health History

Questions to ask the parent or guardian when the client is a neonate or infant include the following:

- Did client's mother take illegal or street drugs while she was pregnant? What kind of drugs and how often were they used?
- Did the mother drink alcohol during the pregnancy? How much and how often?

Rationale Alcohol and other drugs cross the placenta and can alter development of the neonate's central nervous system.

Examination

Normal and Aabnormal Findings. Normal findings for the infant would be consistent with expected growth and development described in Chapter 2. Fetal alcohol syndrome (FAS) is found in infants of alcoholic women. Physical and mental deficits include severe growth deficiency, heart defects, malformed facial features, mental retardation, low birth weights, learning problems, and hyperactivity. Although the physical features are evident in the neonate, the behaviors at this age are nonspecific and may go undetected until the infant is older. The defects are irreversible.

Narcotic abstinence syndrome (NAS) describes a set of behaviors exhibited by infants exposed to narcotics in utero, causing a withdrawal effect. Low–molecular weight narcotics cross the placenta into fetal circulation. When a pregnant woman habitually uses narcotics, especially heroine or methadone, the infant becomes passively addicted. The manifestations become most pronounced between 48 and

72 hours after birth and may last 6 to 8 weeks. Clinical manifestations of the autonomic nervous system may last 3 to 4 months and include tremors, restlessness, hyperactive reflexes, increased muscle tone, tachypnea, and a high-pitched shrill cry. Although these neonates suck on their fists and have an exaggerated rooting reflex, they are poor feeders with ineffective sucking and swallowing reflexes. Regurgitation and vomiting are common, as is diarrhea (Wong et al, 1999).

Fetal cocaine exposure occurs when cocaine crosses the placenta. Mothers who use cocaine while pregnant develop hypertension and decreased uterine blood flow. These infants experience cerebral infarcts, renal defects, cardiac anomalies, low birth weight and length, and a decreased head circumference. Infants with prenatal cocaine exposure are at risk for sudden infant death syndrome (SIDS) (Wong et al, 1999).

Adolescents

Health History

The following are questions to ask adolescents:

- Adolescence can be a rough time of life. How do you cope with your stress?
- Do you have a group that you hang out with?
- I know many schools have drug problems. Does your school have such a problem?
- Do most of your friends drink alcohol or do drugs?
- Have you ever been ill because of alcohol or drugs?

Rationale These questions are asked to identify teens who have poor self-esteem or lack social or positive interpersonal relationships, as well as those who turn to drugs to solve their problems. These characteristics put teens at risk for altered mental health status.

Box 7-4 contains a 12-question quiz to help determine if a teenager has a drinking problem.

Questions to ask the parents or guardians of adolescents when there is a concern about drug or alcohol abuse:

- Does your son or daughter spend many hours in his or her bedroom apparently doing nothing?
- Does your son or daughter resist talking to family members or isolate himself or herself from the family?
- Has there been a definite change in your son's or daughter's attitude toward school? with his or her friends?
- Has your son or daughter dropped out of school or community activities?

Box 7-4 How to Tell When Teenage Drinking Is a Problem

The teen years provide young men and women with more independence and freedom. Most teenagers want to try new things: different ways of acting or dressing, perhaps a different hair style or color. Just as teens want to be different from the way they were, they want to be accepted by their peers. Drinking alcohol may be one of the behaviors they try, and they may be encouraged to drink by their peers.

The following quiz will help teens recognize whether they have a drinking problem. If they answer "yes" to *any one* of the 12 questions, they should be encouraged to take a serious look at their drinking habits and what their drinking might be doing to them. Teenagers and parents who would like help or more information can be referred to their local Alcoholics Anonymous office.

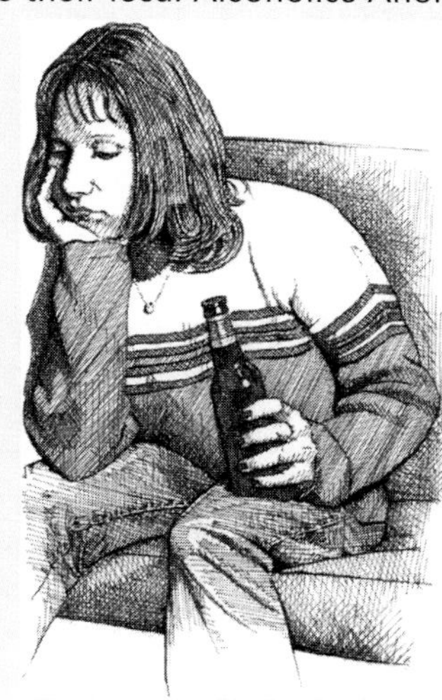

ILLUSTRATION: KATE MCKEON

A SIMPLE 12-QUESTION QUIZ DESIGNED TO HELP YOU DECIDE

1. Do you drink because you have problems? To relax?
2. Do you drink when you get mad at other people, your friends or parents?
3. Do you prefer to drink alone, rather than with others?
4. Are your grades starting to slip? Are you goofing off on your job?
5. Did you ever try to stop drinking or to drink less—and fail?
6. Have you begun to drink in the morning, before school or work?
7. Do you gulp your drinks?
8. Do you ever have loss of memory due to your drinking?
9. Do you lie about your drinking?
10. Do you ever get into trouble when you're drinking?
11. Do you get drunk when you drink, even when you don't mean to?
12. Do you think it's cool to be able to hold your liquor?

From Lucas B: Recognizing and treating patients with drinking problems, *Patient Care Nurse Pract* 1(12):51, 1998.

- Have you noticed swings in mood and increased irritability and angry outbursts?
- Does your son or daughter seem unhappy and less able to cope with frustration then he or she used to?
- Has your son or daughter become more manipulative? Has there been lying to avoid confrontation or to not get caught?

Rationale These questions assess parents' awareness of their teenager's behavior and try to identify those teens at risk for mental health disorders (Schonberg, 1988).

Adolescence is a time of emotional turmoil and may be characterized by mood lability, gloomy introspection, great drama, and heightened sensitivity. It is also a time of rebellion and behavioral experimentation. The diagnosis of depression can be missed in adolescence when the parents and/or health care provider dismiss indications of depression as expected adolescent behavior. The chief complaint may be behavior or conduct problems in school, substance or alcohol abuse, or family turmoil.

Examination

Normal and Abnormal Findings. For normal findings, refer to Box 7-1. The presenting symptoms of depression in adolescents are the same as in adults: sadness, difficulty sleeping, and lack of motivation. The expression of these symptoms may be different; for example, wearing black clothing, writing poetry or stories with morbid themes, or preoccupation with nihilistic themes in song lyrics may indicate sadness. Watching television all night, having difficulty waking up for school, and sleeping during the day may indicate an inability to sleep at night. A decline in grades may indicate lack of sleep, as well as a loss of concentration and slowed thinking, lower energy levels, and lack of motivation. Boredom may be an expression of depression. Lack of appetite may lead to anorexia or bulimia (Blackman, 1995).

■ Older Adults

Anatomy and Physiology

Metabolic activity in the brain decreases with age. Cerebral blood flow is markedly reduced in clients with late-onset depression compared with younger clients with depression. Also there are decreased concentrations of serotonin, dopamine, and norepinephrine in older adults with a reduction in beta-adrenergic receptor binding sites in the frontal lobes. These expected physiologic changes may contribute to depression (Ruggles, 1998).

Depression in the elderly may be overlooked. When they report a decrease in appetite, low energy, or fatigue, it may be explained as the result of a decrease in metabolism or loss of taste buds that occur with aging. When they report problems concentrating or sleeping, it may be interpreted as an expected change in aging. Other illnesses or medication side effects may cause depression. It may also follow the death or illness of significant others. Many older adults think that depression will go away by itself, that they are too old to get help, or that reporting their sadness is a sign of weakness. They must be encouraged to report their feelings to health care providers, who in turn must consider depression as a possibility.

Examination

Normal and Abnormal Findings. For normal findings, refer to Box 7-1. Depression is assessed in older adults in the same way as in other adults. The Yesavage Geriatric Depression Scale, Short Form has been validated for use with this age group (Fig. 7-4).

Yesavage Geriatric Depression Scale, Short Form

Read the following 15 questions. Circle the response (*yes* or *no*) at the end of the question if it applies to you; that is, if it describes how you are feeling. If the answer given at the end of the question does NOT apply to you, then do not write anything for that question.

1. Are you basically satisfied with your life? (no)
2. Have you dropped many of your activities and interests? (yes)
3. Do you feel that your life is empty? (yes)
4. Do you often get bored? (yes)
5. Are you in good spirits most of the time? (no)
6. Are you afraid that something bad is going to happen to you? (yes)
7. Do you feel happy most of the time? (no)
8. Do you often feel helpless? (yes)
9. Do you prefer to stay home at night, rather than go out and do new things? (yes)
10. Do you feel that you have more problems with memory than most? (yes)
11. Do you think it is wonderful to be alive now? (no)
12. Do you feel pretty worthless the way you are now? (yes)
13. Do you feel full of energy? (no)
14. Do you feel that your situation is hopeless? (yes)
15. Do you think that most persons are better off than you are? (yes)

Score 1 point for each response that matches the yes or no answer after the question.

Fig. 7-4 Yesavage Geriatric Depression Scale, Short Form. (Reprinted from *Journal of Psychosomatic Research,* volume 17, Yesavage JA, Brink TL, Development and validation of a geriatric depression screening scale: A preliminary report, pp. 37-49, copyright 1983, with permission from Elsevier Science.)

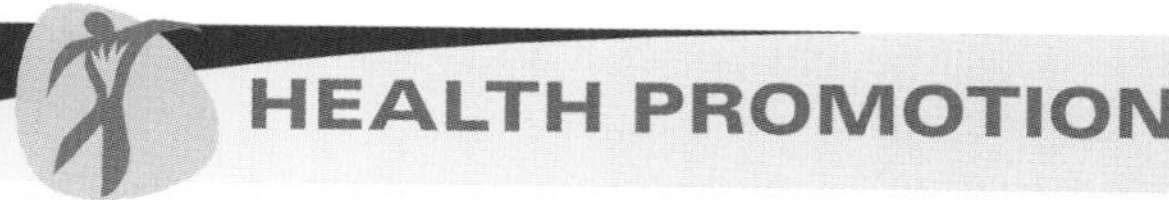

HEALTH PROMOTION

STRESS MANAGEMENT

Using stress management techniques can help reduce anxiety or depression and potential physical illnesses that can result from stress. Researchers have found that it is the *perception* of a life event that determines the person's emotional and psychologic reactions it to. A number of stress reduction techniques can be used, including relaxation, yoga, tai chi, meditation, physical exercise, music therapy, prayer, writing in a journal, and art therapy. Three positive coping styles to stress are figuring out how to deal with the situation (problem solving), using social supports to allow others to help in dealing with the stressful situation, and looking for "the silver lining," or reframing the situation to see the positive as well as the negative side (Varcarolis, 1998). Coping strategies are listed in Box 7-2.

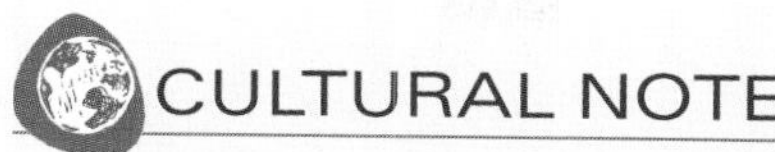

CULTURAL NOTE

Researchers have found that it is the *perception* of a recent life event that determines a person's emotional or psychologic reaction to it. Each culture influences how a stressful event is perceived and how members of that culture are expected to respond. Some cultures allow a verbal or physical response, whereas others refrain from any outward reaction at all. The Western European and North American cultures believe that stress from an emotional state can lead to somatic illness. Since some cultures do not believe that stress contributes to disease, their members would not understand the need for stress management (Varcarolis, 1998).

SCREENING FOR ALCOHOLISM AND DRUG ABUSE

Every comprehensive health history of an adolescent or adult must ask questions about use of alcohol and drugs. Abuse of drugs and alcohol can alter a person's behavior, resulting in damage to interpersonal relationships, loss of employment, and alienation from social support systems. This type of abuse also interferes with sleep and causes a variety of physical illnesses. Questions for screening are in the section on alcohol abuse in the discussion of the health history. The AUDIT (see Table 7-3) is another screening tool to use. Teaching clients the difference between use and abuse is important for health promotion.

COMMON PROBLEMS AND CONDITIONS

Mental Health

ALTERATIONS OF MOOD AND AFFECT

Major Depression

Major depression is an abnormal mood state in which a person characteristically has a sense of sadness, hopelessness, helplessness, worthlessness, and despair resulting from some personal loss or tragedy. A person may experience a single episode or may have recurrent episodes of depression. Feeling depressed is not the same thing as the illness of depression. A person must have been in a depressed mood or have lost interest or pleasure for at least 2 weeks, accompanied by significant distress or impairment and at least four of the classic symptoms before a diagnosis of major depression is made. These symptoms include weight loss or weight gain, insomnia or hypersomnia, psychomotor agitation or retardation, excessive fatigue, intense feelings of worthlessness or guilt, difficulty concentrating and making decisions, and suicidal thoughts. Depression is more common in women than men. While psychosocial factors contribute to depression in women, the fluctuations of estrogen and progesterone during menses, pregnancy, and menopause are associated with affective and mood changes.

Anxiety

Anxiety is a feeling of uneasiness or discomfort experienced in varying degrees, from mild anxiety to panic. Unlike fear, which is a response to an actual object or event, anxiety is a response to no specific source or actual object. The energy that anxiety provides may mobilize a person to take constructive action such as solving a major problem or filling an unmet need. When used destructively, it can immobilize a person. A mildly anxious person has a broad perceptual field because the anxiety heightens awareness to sensory stimuli. The person sees more, hears more, and thinks more logically. Learning occurs during mild anxiety. The moderately anxious person has a more narrow field of perception and uses selective inattention to ignore stimuli in the environment to focus on a specific concern. The severely anxious person has reduced perception of stimuli and develops compulsive mechanisms to avoid the anxiety-provoking object or situation. During severe anxiety the person experiences impaired memory attention and concentration, difficulty solving problems, and is unable to focus on events in the environment. The panic level of anxiety is characterized by complete disruption of the perceptual field. The person experiences intense terror and is unable to think logically or make decisions. Physical manifestations of anxiety represent sympathetic nervous system stimulation. The person experiences muscle tension, tachycardia, dyspnea, hypertension, increased respiration, and profuse perspiration.

ALTERATIONS OF THOUGHT CONTENT

Phobia

Phobia is an anxiety disorder characterized by an obsessive, irrational, and intense fear of a specific object, such as an animal; an activity, such as leaving a familiar place like home; or a physical situation, such as heights. Typical manifestations of phobia are faintness, fatigue, palpitations, perspiration, nausea, tremor, and panic.

Hypochondriasis

Hypochondriasis is a chronic, abnormal preoccupation with one's health. It is characterized by extreme anxiety or depression and unrealistic interpretation of real or imagined physical symptoms as indication of serious illness despite medical evidence to the contrary.

Delusions

Delusions are persistent aberrant (deviant) beliefs or perceptions held by a client despite evidence to the contrary. Examples include delusion of being controlled, in which clients believe that an external force is controlling their feelings, beliefs, thoughts, or actions. Delusion of grandeur is an exaggeration of one's importance, wealth, power, or talents, as seen in paranoid schizophrenia. Delusion of persecution is a morbid belief that one is being mistreated, harassed, or conspired against, as seen in paranoia and paranoid schizophrenia.

SUBSTANCE ABUSE DISORDERS

Alcohol Withdrawal Syndrome

Ethyl alcohol, or ethanol, is a central nervous system depressant found in alcoholic beverages. The blood alcohol level (BAL) is used to measure the amount of alcohol in blood. The legal intoxication level in most states is 100 mg/dl (0.10%), with some states using 0.08%. Alcohol inhibits the inhibitory neurotransmitter GABA, which may cause an initial euphoria, but as the consumption continues, the central nervous system becomes depressed. Early manifestations of alcohol withdrawal include tremors, anorexia, anxiety, restlessness, and insomnia that begin 6 to 8 hours after the last drink. For the next 2 to 3 days the client may experience disorientation, nightmares, abdominal pain, nausea, and diaphoresis. Also temperature, pulse rate, and blood pressure are elevated. Visual and auditory hallucination may occur. Severe withdrawal manifestations are called delirium tremens (DTs), in which the client experiences cardiac dysrhythmias, hypertension, increased respirations, profuse sweating, delusion, and hallucinations.

DRUG INTOXICATION

Table 7-4 presents signs and symptoms of intoxication from drugs commonly abused (cannabis, cocaine, opiates, barbiturates, amphetamines, hallucinogenic agents).

Table 7-4 Signs and Symptoms of Acute Drug Intoxication

DRUG(S) ABUSED	SIGNS AND SYMPTOMS
Cannabis drugs	Tachycardia and postural hypotension, conjunctival vascular congestion, distortions of perception, dryness of mouth and throat, possible panic
Cocaine	Increased stimulation, euphoria, increased blood pressure and heart rate, anorexia, insomnia, agitation; in overdose, increased body temperature, hallucinations, seizures, death
Opiates	Depressed blood pressure and respiration; fixed, pinpoint pupils; depressed sensorium; coma; pulmonary edema
Barbiturates and other general CNS depressants	Depressed blood pressure and respirations; ataxia, slurred speech, confusion, depressed tendon reflexes, coma, shock
Amphetamines	Elevated blood pressure, tachycardia, other cardiac dysrhythmias, hyperactive tendon reflexes, pupils dilated and reactive to light, hyperpyrexia, perspiration, shallow respirations, circulatory collapse, clear or confused sensorium, possible hallucinations, paranoid feelings
Hallucinogenic agents	Elevated blood pressure, hyperactive tendon reflexes, piloerection, perspiration, pupils dilated and reactive to light, anxiety, distortion of body image and perception, delusions, hallucinations

From McKenry LM, Salerno E: *Mosby's pharmacology in nursing,* ed 20, St Louis, 1998, Mosby.

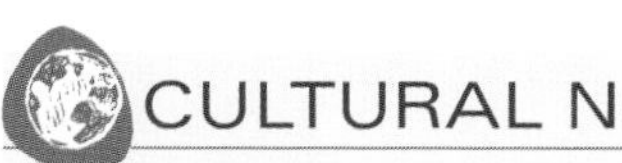

CULTURAL NOTE

Drugs that are considered illegal in one society are considered legal and useful in another. For example, in the United States and parts of Western Europe, caffeine, alcohol, and nicotine are used widely and accepted. In the Middle East cannabis is considered a legal drug, whereas alcohol is forbidden. Some Native American tribes use peyote, a hallucinogen causing visual and auditory hallucination, for religious services (McKenry and Salerno, 1998).

DISORDERS

Delirium

Delirium is defined as a clinical state characterized by attention deficits, disorganized thinking, confusion, disorientation, restlessness, incoherence, anxiety, excitement, and at times illusions. This condition is caused by disturbances in cerebral function due to a variety of metabolic conditions. Symptoms are of a short duration and are reversible with treatment.

Dementia

Dementia is a progressive, organic mental disorder characterized by chronic personality disintegration, confusion, disorientation, stupor, deterioration of intellectual capacity with impairment of memory, judgment, and impulses. Kinds of dementia include Alzheimer's disease, senile dementia, toxic dementia, and paralytic dementia.

Schizophrenia

Schizophrenia is any one of a large group of psychotic disorders characterized by gross distortion of reality, disturbances of language and communication, withdrawal from social interaction, and the disorganization and fragmentation of thought perception and emotion reaction. Clinical manifestations include apathy and confusion; delusions and hallucinations; rambling or stylized patterns of speech, such as echolalia, incoherence, or evasiveness; withdrawn, regressive, and bizarre behavior; and emotional lability. The condition may be mild or require prolonged hospitalization.

Bipolar Disorder

Bipolar disorder is a mood disorder characterized by episodes of mania, depression, or mixed moods. Characteristics of the manic phase are excessive emotional displays, excitement, euphoria, hyperactivity accompanied by elation, boisterousness, impaired ability to concentrate, decreased need for sleep, and limitless energy, often accompanied by delusion of grandeur. In contrast, in the depressive phase there is marked apathy and feelings of profound sadness, loneliness, guilt, and lowered self-esteem.

Obsessive-Compulsive Disorder

Obsessive-compulsive disorder is classified as an anxiety disorder because of the anxiety symptoms that develop when the client tries to resist an obsession or compulsion. An obsession is a persistent thought or impulse that cannot be dismissed from consciousness. These thoughts may be trivial or morbid, but they are always anxiety producing. A compulsion is an uncontrollable, persistent urge to perform certain acts to relieve anxiety and reduce tension. These clients have a need to control themselves, others, and their environment.

CLINICAL APPLICATION AND CRITICAL THINKING

CRITICAL THINKING QUESTIONS

1. What assessment questions distinguish between stress and anxiety?
2. While assessing mental status, the nurse can collect valuable objective data with a brief, general survey. What types of things should the examiner consider?
3. Compare and contrast assessment findings of an infant with fetal alcohol syndrome, an infant with narcotic abstinence syndrome, and one with fetal cocaine exposure.
4. How are delirium and dementia similar, and how are they different?

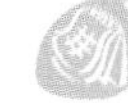

CASE STUDY

Sarah comes to the student health clinic with complaints of fatigue. Below are data collected by the nurse practitioner from interview and examination.

Interview Data

Sarah tells the nurse she has felt constantly tired, and all she wants to do is sleep. Sarah tells the nurse she does not have time to be tired, because final examinations are approaching, and she is very concerned about her grades and begins to cry. "I am so afraid I will not pass my classes. If I don't pass, my parents will not help me with school anymore." When asked to describe herself, Sarah replies, "Friendly, but not very smart." Sarah goes on to tell the nurse that she has a boyfriend but only sees him occasionally since he lives in another state. When asked about other friends, Sarah replies, "I know all of the people in my class."

Examination Data

- **Vital signs:** Blood pressure, 128/84 mm Hg; pulse, 96 beats/min; respiration 18 per minute, temperature, 98.6° F (36.7° C).
- **General survey:** Well nourished, overweight young woman appearing unkept, with slightly swollen red eyes from crying. Makes infrequent eye contact.
- **Height:** 5′ 3″ (160 cm).
- **Weight:** 148 lb. (67 kg).
- **Mental status:** Oriented to person, place, and time. Slow speech pattern with flat affect.
- All body system findings within normal limits.

1. What data deviate from normal findings, suggesting to the nurse that Sarah may have a mental health issue?
2. What additional information should the nurse ask or assess for?
3. In what functional health patterns does data deviate from normal?
4. What nursing diagnosis and/or collaborative problems should be considered for this situation?

8

Comfort and Pain Assessment

REMEMBER to check out your **companion CD-ROM**

www.mosby.com/MERLIN/wilson/assessment/

Just as health is more than the absence of disease, so comfort is more than the absence of pain. Although providing for comfort is a central concept of nursing, it is difficult to assess because clients' perception of comfort depends on their culture and experience (Table 8-1). A person's perception of comfort may pertain to bodily sensations; interpersonal, family, and societal relationships; internal awareness of self, including esteem, sexuality, meaning of life, and one's relationship to a higher power; or to the external background such as light, noise, color, temperature, and natural versus synthetic elements (Kolcaba, 1995). The definitions of comfort include to strengthen, encourage, aid, and support; to refresh, sustain, strengthen, and invigorate; or to relieve a specific cause of discomfort. This last definition frequently is associated with relief from pain.

What distinguishes pain from discomfort is the intensity of the feeling and the pain experiences of the client. A group of 200 clients ranging in age from 16 to 82 years were asked to name experiences that caused pain and those that caused discomfort. Painful experiences reported were slamming a finger in a door, a throbbing headache, a sharp sensation in the chest, an incision the first day after surgery, muscle cramps, and coughing that caused incisional pain. The sensations of discomfort included itching, being in one position too long, being unable to have anything by mouth (NPO), full feeling in the abdomen, nausea, dull headache, shortness of breath, muscular aches, limitation of physical activity, insertion of a tube into the rectum or the stomach, sore throat, waiting for test results and for a procedure to be done (Jacox, 1979).

Pain is difficult to define because of its multidimensional aspects. It is defined as an unpleasant sensory and emotional experience associated with actual or potential tissue damage (McCaffery and Pasero, 1999). Pain is an experience, not an objective finding, so the client's subjective experience is the gold standard of assessing pain severity (Schneider, 1998). The most accurate and reliable evidence of the existence of pain and its intensity is the client's report (Turk and Melzack, 1992).

The literature describes three types of pain: acute, chronic malignant, and chronic non-malignant pain. A clear distinction among these types of pain is often not possible and invariably results in overlap or omission. Acute pain has a sudden onset with limited duration that subsides as healing occurs. As malignancies progress and metastasize, approximately 90% of clients will experience pain. Cancer pain may be caused by infection and inflammation, pressure from a growing tumor on nerve endings, stretching of visceral surfaces, or obstruction of ducts and intestines (McCance and Huether, 1998). Cancer pain is described in three stages: early, intermediate, and late. Early cancer pain occurs after initial surgery for diagnosis or treatment. This pain usually subsides the third day and overlaps with acute pain. Intermediate pain results from postoperative contraction of scars and nerve entrapment or from cancer recurrence or metastasis. This type of pain may be controlled by palliation such as radiation, chemotherapy, neurosurgery, and analgesics. The later stage of cancer pain occurs when therapy no longer controls the disease. This pain overlaps chronic, nonmalignant pain and may slowly increase in intensity and at times may be intractable (Deters, 1999). Chronic, malignant pain is persistent, lasting at least 6 months, and often does not respond to usual therapy.

The pain threshold is the point at which a stimulus is perceived as pain. This threshold does not vary significantly among people or in the same person over time. In contrast, pain tolerance is the time or intensity of pain a person will endure before outwardly responding to it. A person's culture, pain experience, expectations, role behaviors, and physical and emotional health influence pain tolerance.

ANATOMY AND PHYSIOLOGY

The physiology of pain involves a journey from the site of stimulation of peripheral receptors to the spinal cord (transduction), up the spinal cord (transmission) to the cerebral cortex (perception), and back down the spinal cord (modulation).

The first step in the pain process is transduction. It is conversion of mechanical, thermal, chemical, or electrical stimuli that activate somatic and visceral free nerve endings called nociceptors located at the ends of small, thinly myelinated or unmyelinated fibers. Cell damage causes release of

Table 8-1 Response to Pain* in Selected Countries

COUNTRY	PREDOMINANT ETHNIC GROUP	RESPONSE TO PAIN
Algeria	Arab Berber	Pain is expressed only in private or with close relatives or friends; pain during labor and delivery is expressive.
Australia	White	Pain is expressed verbally within limits.
Bahrain	Bahraini	Clients expect immediate pain relief and may request it persistently. Because they believe that energy conservation is needed for recovery, they resist therapies requiring exertion.
Belize	Mestizo, Creole	Expressive pain reactions predominate. Cancer is usually suspected if a reason for the pain cannot be found. It is believed that if pain is denied, it will go away. Home remedies and over-the counter medications are used before seeking medical care.
Brazil	White	Pain is expressed verbally.
Cambodia (Kampuchea)	Khmer (Cambodian)	Pain reactions may be severe before relief is requested.
China	Han Chinese	A display of emotion is considered a weakness of character. Thus, feelings such as anger and pain often are suppressed. Pain relief interventions should be offered more than once, because it is considered impolite to accept something the first time it is offered.
Dominican Republic	Mixed (Hispanic)	Loud expressive reactions are seen along with praying and complaining. Pain is perceived as an inevitable part of illness or injury by many and as a punishment from God by others. Pain medicines may not be available or may be in limited supply in some health care facilities here.
Egypt	Eastern Hamitic	Pain relief is expected to be immediate and may be requested persistently. Pain is expressed privately or in the company of close friends or relatives, except during labor and delivery. Because they believe that energy conservation is needed for recovery, they resist therapies requiring exertion.
Ethiopia	Oromo, Amhara and Tigrean	People are stoic and may refuse pain medications even when they are ordered and available.
Finland	Finnish	People are willing to communicate pain, however they are not expressive.
Germany	German	Strong, stoic behavior is exhibited. Pain is an expected part of the healing process and may be tolerated.
Ghana	Akan	Clients may select inappropriate analgesia for pain relief and take any analgesic they can get in any quantity.
Haiti	Black	A high tolerance for pain and discomfort exists, although some sources indicate a low pain threshold. Loud verbal expressions may be heard during labor.
Iceland	Icelandish	Clients do not complain of pain; therefore, pain is probably severe when medication is given. They also report not wanting to bother the nurse for pain medication.
India	Indo-Aryan	Clients have a quiet acceptance for pain, but will accept some relief measures.
Iran	Persian	Pain usually is expressed, the women may yell throughout labor. The custom is to compensate them for their suffering during childbirth by giving them gifts.
Iraq	Arab	Pain relief is expected to be immediate and may be requested persistently. Because they believe that energy conservation is needed for recovery, they resist therapies requiring exertion. Pain is usually expressed privately or only with close relative and friends. However, during labor and delivery, pain is expressed vehemently.
Ireland	Irish	The Irish are typically inexpressive and stoic; they do not vocalize pain and are less likely to describe pain as intense. They will try to hide pain from family and friends.

Data from Geissler EM: *Pocket guide to cultural assessment,* ed 2, St Louis, 1998, Mosby.

*Remember, these descriptions are for the "typical" client from these countries. To avoid stereotyping you must validate with each client whether he or she has the pain reactions described below. For example, to an Irishman you might say, "I read that people from Ireland do not express their pain even when it is intense. Is that true for you?"

Table 8-1 Response to Pain* in Selected Countries—cont'd

COUNTRY	PREDOMINANT ETHNIC GROUP	RESPONSE TO PAIN
Israel	Jewish	Jewish clients describe their pain in great detail and display overt suffering as a way to get help and sympathy.
Italy	Italian	Expressive, loud reactions communicate distress or call for reassurance, especially with chronic pain. People are likely to blame themselves for pain. They do not describe pain in great detail.
Japan	Japanese	Clients are stoic and withstand discomfort.
Jordan	Arab	Same as that for Iraq. Arabs are the predominant ethnic group in this country.
Kenya	Kikuyu, Luhya, Luo	Pain relief measures are not common. Some believe that pain is necessary for healing. Pain relief is not used during labor and delivery. The woman shows her strength by withstanding this pain.
Korea (South)	Korean	People tend to be stoic. It is proper to display no facial expressions of pain.
Kuwait	Kuwaiti	Same as for Iraq.
Laos	Lao (Lao Lum)	Pain may be severe before relief is requested.
Lebanon	Arab	Same as for Iraq.
Libya	Arab Berber	Same as for Iraq.
Lithuanua	Luthuanian	Pain tolerance is valued. Pain medications are in limited supply. During labor and delivery women are encouraged to keep silent and be stoic.
Madagascar	Malayo-Indonesian	Pain is shown and expressed.
Mexico	Mestizo	Pain relief might be refused as a means of atonement. Emotional self-restraint and stoic inhibition of strong feelings and emotional expression are seen. Expressions of pain may be self-help relief mechanisms.
Morocco	Arab Berber	Same as for Iraq.
Netherlands	Dutch	During labor and delivery, pain relief is expected.
Nigeria	Hausa, Yoruba	Many Muslim Nigerians are stoic, and they may offer their pain to Allah.
Philippines	Christian Malay	Clients may be stoic if they believe that pain is the will of God and that God will give them the strength to bear it.
Poland	Polish	Tolerance to pain is valued. Pain may be expressed by facial expression or by crying out.
Romania	Romanian	During labor and delivery in hospitals, woman receive no analgesia and are expected not to make any sounds.
Russia	Russian	Some are communicative about pain and others are stoic. Injection is the preferred method of delivery for pain medication.
Saudi Arabia	Arab	Pain is expressed verbally and nonverbally with emotion, especially to the family. Immediate pain relief is desired. A great deal of analgesia may be needed for pain relief. Some clients may want to remain sufficiently alert to be able to pray.
Spain	Spanish	In general, pain is not well tolerated and pain relief medications will be requested.
Sweden	Swedish	Pain is expressed verbally and nonverbally. Immediate pain relief is expected.
Syria	Arab	Same as for Iraq.
Tunisia	Arab	Same as for Iraq.
Turkey	Turkish	Pain is considered a part of life and is tolerated. Pain is not commonly expressed.
United Arab Emirates	Arab	Same as Iraq.
Vietnam	Vietnamese	Clients are stoic. Pain may be severe before relief is requested. Clients may remain quiet and even smile while experiencing pain.

A

NOCICEPTION: BASIC PROCESS OF NORMAL PAIN TRANSMISSION

1 **Transduction:** Conversion of one energy from another. This process occurs in the periphery when a noxious stimulus causes tissue damage. The damaged cells release substances that activate or sensitize nociceptors. This activation leads to the generation of an action potential.

A. **Sensitizing substances** released by damaged cells:
- Prostaglandins (PG)
- Bradykinin (BK)
- Serotonin (5HT)
- Substance P (SP)
- Histamine (H)

B. An **action potential** results from:
- Release of the above sensitizing substances (nociceptive pain) + a change in the charge along the neuronal membrane

or
- Abnormal processing of stimuli by the nervous system (neuropathic pain) + a change in the charge along the neuronal membrane

The change in charge occurs when Na^+ moves into the cell and other ion transfers occur.

2 **Transmission:** The action potential continues from the site of damage to the spinal cord and ascends to higher centers. Transmission may be considered in three phases:
- Injury site to spinal cord. Nociceptors terminate in the spinal cord.
- Spinal cord to brain stem and thalamus. Release of substance P and other neurotransmitters continues the impulse across the synaptic cleft between the nociceptors and the dorsal horn neurons. From the dorsal horn of the spinal cord, neurons such as the spinothalamic tract ascend to the thalamus. Other tracts carry the message to different centers in the brain.
- Thalamus to cortex. Thalamus acts as a relay station sending the impulse to central structures for processing.

3 **Perception of pain:** Conscious experience of pain.

4 **Modulation:** Inhibition of nociceptive impulses. Neurons originating in the brain stem descend to the spinal cord and release substances such as endogenous opioids, serotonin (5HT), and norepinephrine (NE) that inhibit the transmission of nociceptive impulses.

Fig. 8-1 **A,** Outlines the four basic processes involved in nociception: *1,* transduction; *2,* transmission; *3,* perception; and *4,* modulation. (From McCaffery and Pasero, 1999.)

several substances that facilitate the movement of the pain impulse from the periphery to the spinal cord as shown in Fig. 8-1. These substances include prostaglandins (PGs), bradykinin (BK), serotonin (5HT), substance P (SP), and histamine (H) (McCaffery and Pasero, 1999). Table 8-2 lists examples of these stimuli, their sources, and the pathophysiologic processes they initiate.

The next step in the journey, transmission, begins with stimulation of one of the four types of nerves by the nociceptors (see Fig. 8-1). These nerve fibers are large myelinated A-alpha fibers, large myelinated A-beta fibers, small myelinated A-delta fibers, and small unmyelinated C fibers. These are afferent (sensory) nerves that carry the impulses from the periphery to the spinal cord. The A-delta fibers are associated with sharp, pricking, acute, well-localized pain of short duration. The C fibers are associated with dull, aching, throbbing, or burning sensation that has a diffuse nature, slow onset, and relatively long duration.

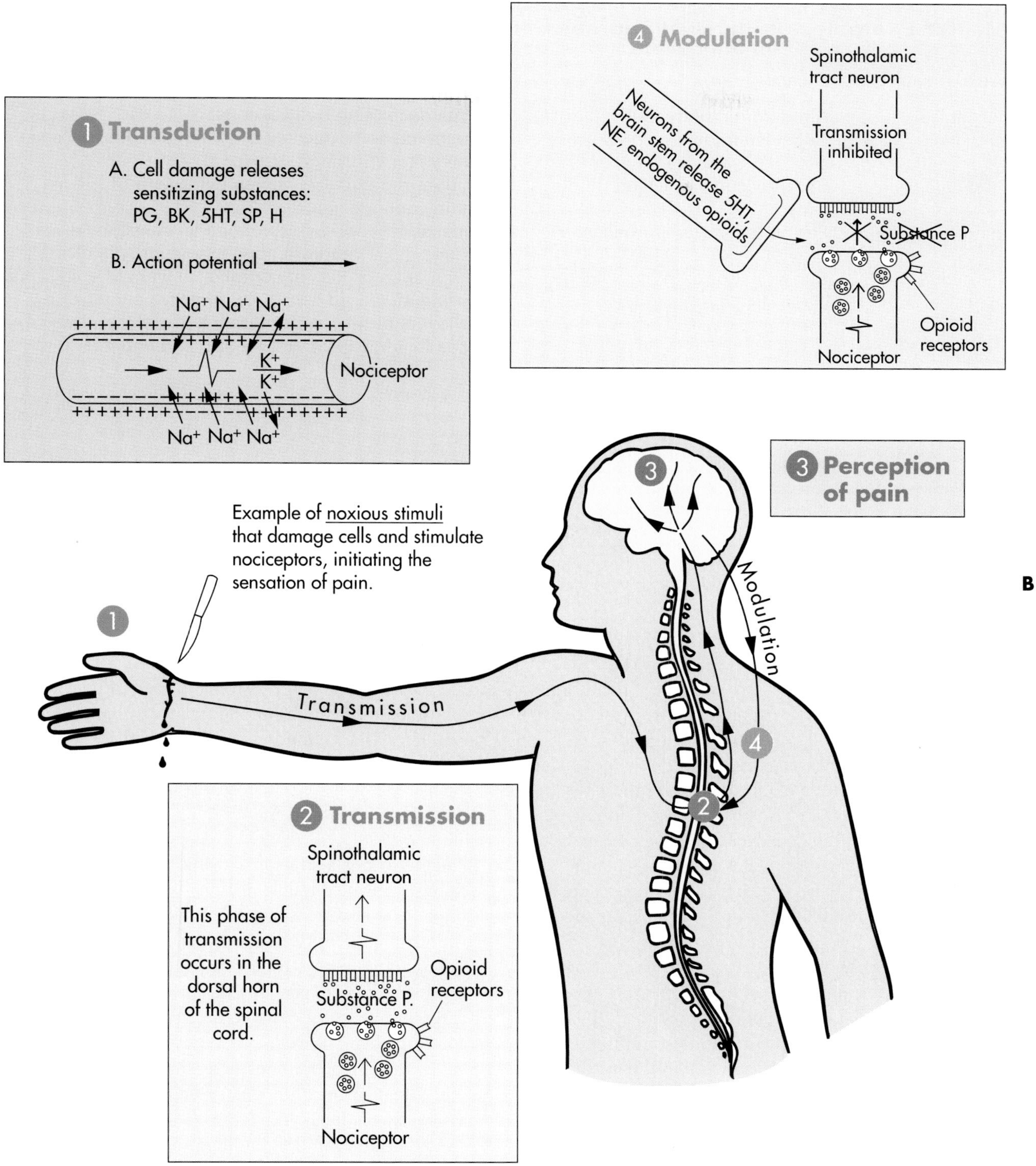

Fig. 8-1, cont'd **B,** Illustrates the four basic processes involved in nociception: *1,* transduction; *2,* transmission; *3,* perception; and *4,* modulation. (From McCaffery and Pasero, 1999.)

The nociceptors carrying impulses from the periphery terminate in the dorsal horn of the spinal cord. The neurotransmitters such as substance P are needed to continue the pain impulse across the synaptic cleft between the nociceptors and the dorsal horn neurons (McCaffery and Pasero, 1999). According to gate theory of pain, when the "gate" is opened, pain impulses enter the spinal cord to ascend to the brain, where pain perception occurs. The gate is the substantia gelatinosa that is located in the dorsal horn of the spinal cord. When the gate is closed, the impulses carried by afferent fibers are prevented from entering the spinal cord. The gate is closed by stimulation from large myelinated

Table 8-2 Examples of Physical Sources of Pain

TYPE OF STIMULUS	SOURCE	PATHOPHYSIOLOGIC PROCESS
Mechanical	Alteration in body fluids	Edema distending body tissues
	Duct distention	Overstretching of duct's narrow lumen (e.g., passage of kidney stone through ureter)
	Space-occupying lesion (tumor)	Irritation of peripheral nerves by growth of lesion within confined space
Chemical	Perforated visceral organ	Chemical irritation by secretions on sensitive nerve endings (e.g., ruptured appendix, duodenal ulcer)
Thermal	Burn (heat or extreme cold)	Inflammation or loss of superficial layers of epidermis, causing increased sensitivity of nerve endings
Electrical	Burn	Skin layers burned with muscle and subcutaneous tissue injury, causing injury to nerve endings

From Potter PA, Perry AG: *Basic nursing: a critical thinking approach,* ed 4, St Louis, 1999, Mosby.

A-alpha and A-beta fibers. Massage and vibration are mechanical stimuli that close the gate by stimulating the A-alpha and A-beta myelinated nerves. The gate is opened by stimulation from small myelinated A-delta fibers and small unmyelinated C fibers. When afferent impulses open the gate, they are carried up the spinal cord to the brain in the spinothalamic and spinoreticular tracts.

The thalamus and parietal lobe of the cerebral cortex are sites of pain perception. Although the journey of the pain stimulus takes a fraction of a second to reach the brain, people do not know they hurt until the parietal lobe is stimulated.

The pain journey ends with modulation, defined as an alteration in the magnitude of electrical current; that is, the body produces substances to reduce pain perception. On the way to the thalamus, afferent nerve fibers travel through the brainstem, where they stimulate efferent (descending) nerves that inhibit nociceptor stimuli. These nerves are descending fibers because they start in the brainstem and descend to the dorsal horn of the spinal cord. These descending efferent nerves release substances such as endogenous opioids (e.g., endorphins and enkephalin), 5HT, norepinephrine (NE), and gamma-aminobutyric acid (GABA) that inhibit the transmission of noxious stimuli and produce analgesia (McCaffery and Pasero, 1999). For example, endorphins and enkephalins act on the opioid receptor sites throughout the brain and spinal cord to decrease the afferent stimulation of pain.

Pain is classified by the location of pathophysiology involved (Fig. 8-2). The first classification, nociceptive pain, is subdivided into somatic and visceral pain. The second classification of pain, neuropathic pain, is subdivided into centrally generated pain and peripherally generated pain.

Referred pain is the term used when clients describe pain felt at a site different from that of an injured or diseased organ. It commonly occurs during visceral pain because many organs have no pain receptors; thus when afferent nerves enter the spinal cord, they stimulate sensory nerves from unaffected organs in the same spinal cord segment as those neurons in areas where injury or disease is located. For example, gallbladder disease causes referred pain to the right shoulder, and myocardial infarction causes referred pain to the left shoulder, arm, or jaw.

Phantom pain is pain that a person feels in an amputated extremity after the stump has healed. It commonly occurs in a person who experienced pain in that limb before amputation. If the nerve pathway from the amputated extremity is stimulated anywhere along the pathway, nerve impulses ascend to the cerebral cortex so that the person perceives pain even though the limb is no longer there. Phantom pain also is influenced by emotions and sympathetic stimulation. This type of pain may be associated with trigger points, which are small hypersentivity areas in muscle or connective tissue located close to the tissues removed (McCance and Huether, 1998).

Acute pain is a stressor that initiates a generalized stress response causing physiologic signs associated with pain. The sympathetic nervous system responds to acute pain of low-to-moderate intensity and superficial pain by causing bronchial dilation, increased heart rate, peripheral vasoconstriction, hypertension, diaphoresis, increased muscle tension, dilated pupils, and decreased gastrointestinal motility. The parasympathetic nervous system responds to severe or deep pain by causing pallor, muscle tension, decreased heart rate; rapid, irregular breathing; nausea and vomiting; and weakness or exhaustion.

In addition to understanding the physiology of pain, the nurse must understand the many other factors that influence the pain experience. The perception of pain varies with the age of the client. This is discussed in the section on age-related variations. Two studies of chronic pain found no differences between genders in the effects of pain. In the first study of 202 men and 226 women with chronic, nonmalignant pain, no differences were reported in pain severity, emotional distress, interference of pain with life, or impact of pain on functional activities. In a second study of 143 clients with chronic malignant pain (91 men and 52 women), no differences were found in demographic variables, dura-

CLASSIFICATION OF PAIN BY INFERRED PATHOLOGY

Two Major Types of Pain

I. Nociceptive Pain	II. Neuropathic Pain
A. Somatic Pain B. Visceral Pain	A. Centrally Generated Pain B. Peripherally Generated Pain

I. Nociceptive Pain: Normal processing of stimuli that damages normal tissues or has the potential to do so if prolonged; usually responsive to nonopioids and/or opioids.

A. Somatic Pain: Arises from bone, joint, muscle, skin, or connective tissue. It is usually aching or throbbing in quality and is well localized.

B. Visceral Pain: Arises from visceral organs, such as the GI tract and pancreas. This may be subdivided:

1. Tumor involvement of the organ capsule that causes aching and fairly well-localized pain.
2. Obstruction of hollow viscus, which causes intermittent cramping and poorly localized pain.

II. Neuropathic Pain: Abnormal processing of sensory input by the peripheral or central nervous system; treatment usually includes adjuvant analgesics.

A. Centrally Generated Pain

1. Deafferentation pain. Injury to either the peripheral or central nervous system. Examples: Phantom pain may reflect injury to the peripheral nervous system; burning pain below the level of a spinal cord lesion reflects injury to the central nervous system.
2. Sympathetically maintained pain. Associated with dysregulation of the autonomic nervous system. Examples: May include some of the pain associated with reflex sympathetic dystrophy/causalgia (complex regional pain syndrome, type I, type II).

B. Peripherally Generated Pain

1. Painful polyneuropathies. Pain is felt along the distribution of many peripheral nerves. Examples: diabetic neuropathy, alcohol-nutritional neuropathy, and those associated with Guillain-Barré syndrome.
2. Painful mononeuropathies. Usually associated with a known peripheral nerve injury, and pain is felt at least partly along the distribution of the damaged nerve. Examples: nerve root compression, nerve entrapment, trigeminal neuralgia.

Fig. 8-2 A method of classifying pain is by the pathophysiology involved. *I,* Nociceptive pain (stimuli from somatic and visceral structures); *II,* Neuropathic pain (stimuli abnormally processed by nervous system). (From McCaffery and Pasero, 1999.)

tion of pain, severity of pain, or functional limitations (Turk and Okifuji, 1998).

Clients associate different meanings with their pain. For example, some perceive the pain as a punishment, threat, or loss, whereas others view pain as a challenge. The more attention clients focus on the pain, the more intense the experience. Thus, using distraction to divert attention away from pain may be a valuable pain-relief intervention. Anxiety and fatigue are known to increase the pain perception. When clients are anxious about their diagnosis, they may report more intense pain than they report after they know the diagnosis. Previous experience with pain may influence the response. If clients have had a similar type of pain experience in the past, they know how to relieve the pain, they are less anxious, and they feel more in control of their pain. In contrast, clients may experience more intense pain if they have not previously experienced intense pain and have no past coping skills to use or if they have a pain experience that is different from the one they had earlier.

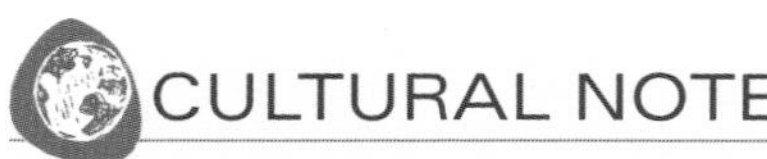

Culture influences how people learn to react to and express pain. Likewise, the culture of nurses influences the degree of pain they infer that patients have. Nurses who report their own experiences as painful tend to infer more patient pain. Nurses from eastern and southern European and African backgrounds tend to infer greater suffering than do nurses of northern European backgrounds. Years of experience, current position, and area of clinical practice are unrelated to nurses' inferences of suffering (Ludwig-Beymer, 1995). Native Americans and Asians tend to be stoic in their pain responses, whereas Italians and Hispanics are more vocal about their pain. Some Mexican Americans rarely acknowledge symptoms of pain because they consider that a lack of stamina and a sign of weakness. Moaning is an acceptable expression of pain and may be used as an attempt to relieve pain. Japanese also tend to be stoic in their pain response. The same is true of Kenyans, who expect to have pain as a part of illness or after surgery and do not expect pain-relieving medication. Remember that these descriptions of pain responses are general tendencies of individuals from these cultures. Nurses must not assume that all persons of a particular culture will respond the same way to pain. Thus the assessment of each client's response to pain is important for individualized care.

HEALTH HISTORY

Comfort and Pain

Because pain is a complex, multidimensional, subjective experience, there are many questions to ask in the health history. The subjective part of pain assessment can be organized by the *ABCD*'s of clients' pain experience. *A* is the affective response, which is clients' emotional response, such as anger, fear, anxiety, or depression. *B* is the behavioral response that is synonymous with the alleviating factors and refers to how clients act when they feel the pain, such as posture they assume for pain relief or action they take to relieve the pain, such as slow deep breathing or distraction techniques. *C* is the cognitive response, which refers to the meaning of the pain for them, their belief about the purpose of the pain, and their attitude about the pain, which is influenced by past experiences with pain (Wilkie and Boss, 1996). *D* is the description that clients provide of their pain, which includes the usual symptom analysis: location, quality, quantity, chronology, setting, associated manifestations, alleviating factors, and aggravating factors. Because clients are frequently eager to describe their pain, those questions usually are asked first.

QUESTIONS	RATIONALE
DESCRIPTION OF PAIN	
Location	
➤ Where is your pain? Can you point to the location(s)?	■ Location may provide information about the cause of pain and its type (e.g., somatic versus visceral) (see Fig. 8-2).
Quality	
➤ Can you describe what the pain feels like? Does it feel as if the pain is internal or external? Box 8-1 provides pain quality descriptors. Fig. 8-3 is the McGill Pain Questionnaire, which helps clients describe their pain.	■ Somatic pain is usually aching or throbbing in quality, while visceral pain is aching and well-localized if from tumor or intermittent, cramping and poorly localized if from obstruction (see Fig. 8-2).

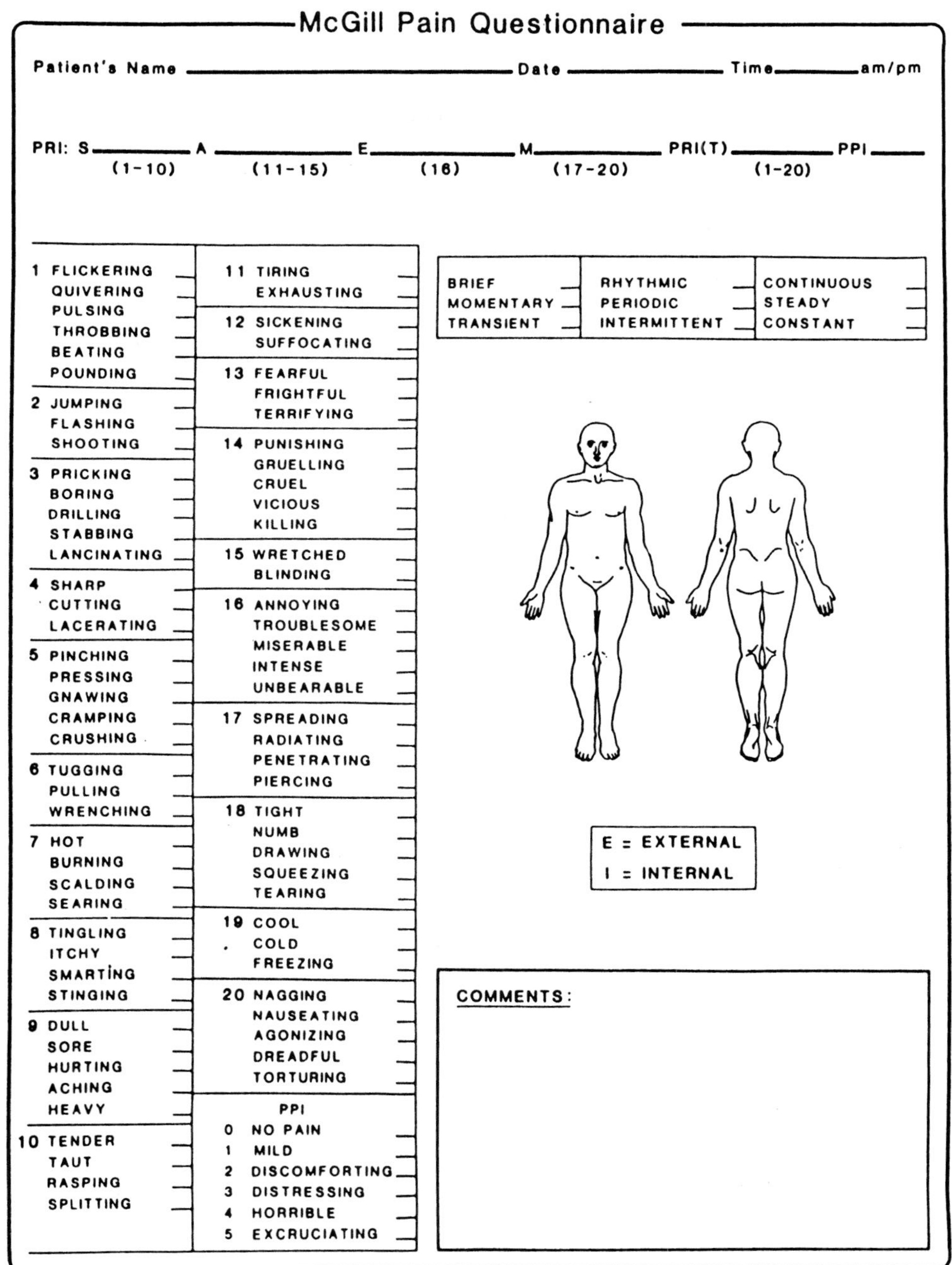

McGill Pain Questionnaire

Patient's Name ______ Date ______ Time ______ am/pm

PRI: S ______ (1-10) A ______ (11-15) E ______ (16) M ______ (17-20) PRI(T) ______ (1-20) PPI ______

1 FLICKERING, QUIVERING, PULSING, THROBBING, BEATING, POUNDING

2 JUMPING, FLASHING, SHOOTING

3 PRICKING, BORING, DRILLING, STABBING, LANCINATING

4 SHARP, CUTTING, LACERATING

5 PINCHING, PRESSING, GNAWING, CRAMPING, CRUSHING

6 TUGGING, PULLING, WRENCHING

7 HOT, BURNING, SCALDING, SEARING

8 TINGLING, ITCHY, SMARTING, STINGING

9 DULL, SORE, HURTING, ACHING, HEAVY

10 TENDER, TAUT, RASPING, SPLITTING

11 TIRING, EXHAUSTING

12 SICKENING, SUFFOCATING

13 FEARFUL, FRIGHTFUL, TERRIFYING

14 PUNISHING, GRUELLING, CRUEL, VICIOUS, KILLING

15 WRETCHED, BLINDING

16 ANNOYING, TROUBLESOME, MISERABLE, INTENSE, UNBEARABLE

17 SPREADING, RADIATING, PENETRATING, PIERCING

18 TIGHT, NUMB, DRAWING, SQUEEZING, TEARING

19 COOL, COLD, FREEZING

20 NAGGING, NAUSEATING, AGONIZING, DREADFUL, TORTURING

PPI

0 NO PAIN
1 MILD
2 DISCOMFORTING
3 DISTRESSING
4 HORRIBLE
5 EXCRUCIATING

BRIEF	RHYTHMIC	CONTINUOUS
MOMENTARY	PERIODIC	STEADY
TRANSIENT	INTERMITTENT	CONSTANT

E = EXTERNAL
I = INTERNAL

COMMENTS:

Fig. 8-3 McGill Pain Questionnaire. The descriptors fall into four major groups: sensory, 1 to 10; affective, 11 to 15; evaluative, 16; and miscellaneous, 17 to 20. The rank value of each descriptor is based on its position in the word set. The sum of the rank values is the pain rating index (PRI). The present pain intensity (PPI) is based on a scale of 0 to 5. (From Melzack and Katz, 1994.)

Box 8-1 Pain Quality Descriptors Most Commonly Used to Describe the Nature of Pain

Some of the words below describe your *present* pain.
Circle *only* those words that best describe it.

1	2
Throbbing	Tiring
Shooting	Exhausting
Stabbing	Sickening
Sharp	Terrifying
Gnawing	Torturing
Burning	3
Aching	Nagging
Tender	Annoying
Heavy	Intense
Tight	Unbearable

From Wilkie DJ et al: Use of the McGill Pain Questionnaire to measure pain: a meta-analysis, *Nurs Res* 39:36, 1990. In Lewis SM, Heitkemper MM, Dirksen SR: *Medical-surgical nursing: assessment and management of clinical problems,* ed 5, St Louis, 2000, Mosby.

QUESTIONS

Quantity

➤ How would you describe the intensity, strength, or severity of the pain on a scale of 1 to 10, with 1 being very mild pain and 10 being the most intense pain possible?

Figs. 8-4, 8-5, 8-6, and 8-7 provide scales and instruments to measure perception of pain intensity and quality.

RATIONALE: ■ This provides further description of how "bad" the pain feels to the client. The client's rating is subjective since pain is a subjective experience, but scales allow the client to communicate how severe the pain feels (pain quantity) and can be used as a subjective measure of pain relief after interventions are implemented.

Chronology

➤ When does the pain occur? During activity? Before or after eating?

■ Physical activity may aggravate pain. Eating may increase peptic ulcer pain.

➤ Does the pain occur suddenly or gradually?

■ Acute pain has a sudden onset. Ischemic pain gradually increases in intensity.

Setting

➤ Where are you when the pain occurs? Does the pain change if you change locations? Are there any factors in the environment that contribute to the pain?

■ These questions are trying to determine if environment contributes to pain, such as chemicals or gases in the air or a hot, dry environment versus a cold and damp one.

Associated Manifestations

➤ What other symptoms do you have during the pain, such as nausea, vomiting, palpitations, shortness of breath, or sweating?

■ Acute pain stimulates the sympathetic nervous system, which can cause physiologic symptoms that may accompany the pain.

Alleviating Factors (See Behavioral Response to Pain)

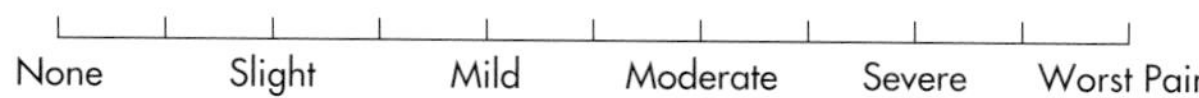

Fig. 8-4 Descriptive Pain Intensity Scale. (From Seidel et al, 1999.)

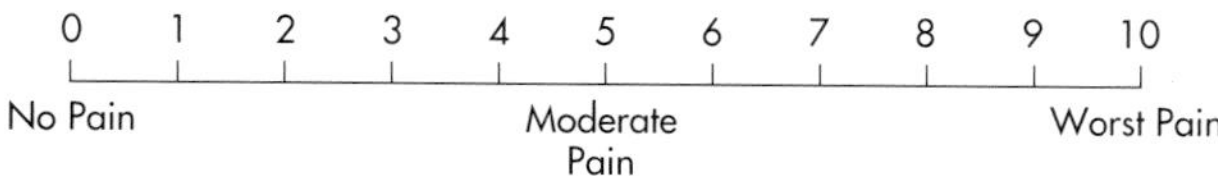

Fig. 8-5 Numeric Pain Intensity Scale. (From Seidel et al, 1999.)

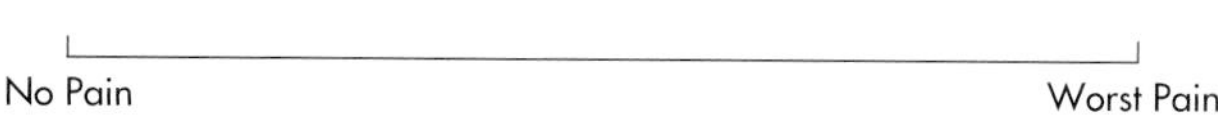

Fig. 8-6 Visual Analogic Scale. (From Seidel et al, 1999.)

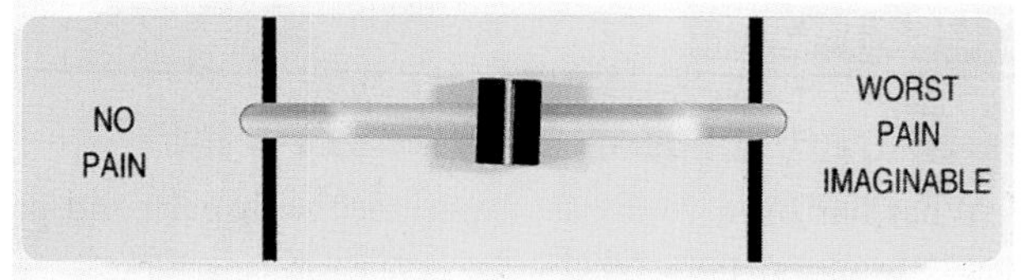

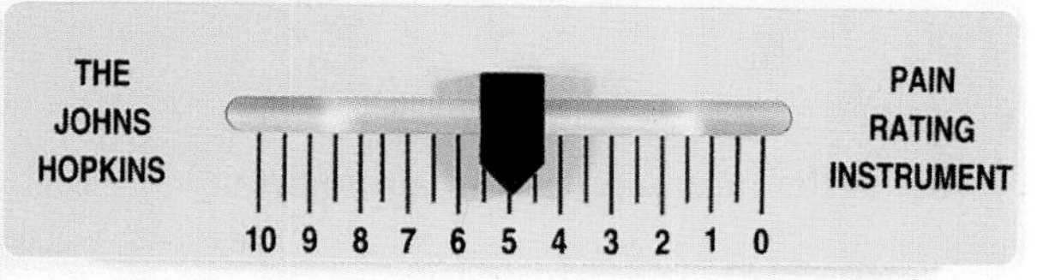

Fig. 8-7 Self-contained, portable, pain-rating instrument that can provide immediate assessment of pain. It is a 5 × 20 cm plastic visual analog scale with a sliding marker that moves within a 10-cm groove. The side facing the client **(A)** resembles a traditional analog scale, whereas the opposite side **(B)** is marked in centimeters to quantify pain intensity. The tool has been shown to be valid to measure pain intensity. (Reprinted from *Journal of Pain and Symptom Management,* volume 7, Grossman SA et al, A comparison of the Hopkins Pain Rating Scales in patients with standard visual analogue and verbal descriptor scales in patients with cancer pain, pp. 196-203, copyright 1992, with permission from Elsevier Science.)

QUESTIONS | **RATIONALE**

Aggravating Factors

➤ What makes the pain worse?

■ The answer may help to determine the cause of the pain.

➤ For clients with chronic pain ask: How has the pain affected your quality of life? How has your life been constricted by the pain?

■ This question helps differentiate between addiction and appropriate dependency on opioid analgesics. One who is addicted often reports that his or her life is constricted, but those who use appropriate opioid therapy report an enhancement of life (Schneider, 1998).

AFFECTIVE RESPONSE TO PAIN

➤ What kinds of emotions do you feel when you are experiencing the pain?

■ This question assesses the affective response to pain. Clients may feel anger, fear, depression, or anxiety.

➤ What is your attitude toward the use of medications for pain relief?

■ Some clients will not ask for pain relief medications for fear of addiction. This misconception can be remedied when it exists.

BEHAVIORAL RESPONSE TO PAIN

➤ How do you react to your pain? How do you express your pain?

■ This determines the behavioral component of pain. Some clients are demonstrative in their responses to pain. Knowing the answer can help nurses to help clients relieve their pain.

➤ What relieves the pain (e.g., medication, certain position, distraction, rest, restricted activity)?

■ The answer may help determine the cause and the treatment.

QUESTIONS	RATIONALE
COGNITIVE RESPONSE TO PAIN	
➤ What has been your past experience with pain and pain relief? What are your expectations for pain relief?	■ These questions address the cognitive response to pain. Clients use their past experiences to respond to pain. When nurses know what those past experiences are, they can be more helpful in helping clients relieve their pain.
➤ What is the meaning of this pain for you?	■ The meaning of pain is unique for each person. For some people the meaning is that they should not have behaved in the way that hurt them (e.g., "I should not have tried to steal home base"). To others the meaning is spiritual or psychologic, that they are being punished, that they have had impure thoughts. Knowing the meaning of the pain helps the nurse understand the client's subjective experience of pain.

EXAMINATION

Objective determination of pain may not be possible for all clients, particularly those who have chronic pain, malignant or nonmalignant. *Although acute pain is associated with observable physical and autonomic changes described below, these changes are not usually observed in clients with chronic pain (Schneider, 1998). "Observation of behavior and vital signs should not be used instead of self-report"* (Acute Pain Management Guideline Panel, 1992, p. 7).

PROCEDURES AND TECHNIQUES WITH NORMAL FINDINGS	ABNORMAL FINDINGS
➤**OBSERVE client for posture and hand movement.** Posture should be erect, and hand movement should not be excessive.	■ Guarding of a painful body part, rubbing or pressing the painful area, distorted posture, or fixed or continuous movement may indicate acute pain. Clients may lie very still to avoid movement or may be restless. Head rocking, pacing, or inability to keep hands still maybe other signs of acute pain.
➤**OBSERVE facial expressions.**	■ Acute pain may be manifested by wrinkled forehead, tightly closed eyes, lackluster eyes, grimace, clenched teeth, or lip biting.
➤**LISTEN for sounds the client makes.** Sounds other than those of conversation are not expected.	■ Moaning, grunting, screaming, crying, or gasping may indicate acute pain.
➤**INSPECT skin for color, temperature, and moisture.** Skin should be expected color for race, warm, and moist with elastic turgor.	■ Pale or diaphoretic skin is due to sympathetic response. Warm, dry skin is due to parasympathetic response.

PROCEDURES AND TECHNIQUES WITH NORMAL FINDINGS	ABNORMAL FINDINGS
➤**MEASURE blood pressure and pulse.** They should be within normal limits for age.	■ Systolic blood pressure and heart rate are increased by the sympathetic stimulation.
➤**COUNT respirations.** They should be within normal limits for age.	■ Respiratory rate increases with sympathetic stimulation and may be variable with parasympathetic stimulation.
➤**OBSERVE pupillary size and reaction to light.** Pupils should be 3 to 5 mm in diameter, equal, and reactive to light.	■ Pupil dilation is due to sympathetic stimulation, and constriction is due to parasympathetic stimulation.

AGE-RELATED VARIATIONS

■ NEONATES AND INFANTS

At one time it was believed that nerve pathways of neonates were not developed enough to transmit painful stimuli. This misconception has been refuted by a number of research studies that indicate that infants, both preterm and full term, perceive and react to pain in much the same way as a child or adult. The physiologic responses of neonates to pain are manifested by a global stress response. This pain response is evidenced by increased heart rate, hypertension, decreased oxygen saturation, pallor, and sweating (Wong et al, 1999).

Like neonates, infants perceive pain. Older infants try to avoid pain by physical resistance.

■ TODDLERS AND PRESCHOOLERS

Young children have difficulty understanding pain and the procedures that cause pain. They have developed a basic ability to describe pain and its intensity and location. They often respond by crying or with anger. Children may perceive the pain as a threat to their security or as punishment, and they hold someone accountable for their pain. Use of a rational explanation for the pain is often unsuccessful. Some young children have little or no experience with pain. The physiology of pain, however, is the same in children as it is in adults. The Wong/Baker FACES Rating Scale (Fig. 8-8) and the Oucher Scale (Figs. 8-9, 8-10, and 8-11) are examples of reliable and valid pain scales useful with children as young as 3 years of age. The child is asked to select the face that fits his or her level of pain. The Oucher Scale has versions with white, African-American, and Hispanic children.

■ SCHOOL-AGE CHILDREN

At this age children are better able to describe pain location and pattern. They try to be brave and are responsive to explanation about the reason for the pain. If pain persists, their behavior may regress.

Children's temperaments affect how they cope. One study found children who were passive and cooperative rated pain of a lumbar puncture as more intense than children who resisted the procedure (Broome et al, 1990).

■ ADOLESCENTS

Voicing feelings of pain may be considered a weakness. In the presence of peers, they want to appear brave.

■ OLDER ADULTS

Although transmission and perception of pain may be slowed in the older person, the pain that is felt is no different from that of any other adult. They have a long lifetime of experience in coping with pain. Pain is not an expected part of aging. Pain in the older person is assessed in the same way as for any adult.

Some older persons may interpret pain as an expected aspect of aging that they must endure. They may deny the pain because they associate the pain with getting older, or they may use distraction to prevent the pain from interfering with their daily activities. Indicators of pain may be fatigue, lethargy, or anorexia. They may fear the expenses of diagnostic tests and treatment or that the medication to relieve the pain or its side effects will make their daily lives more difficult or change their personalities or behavior.

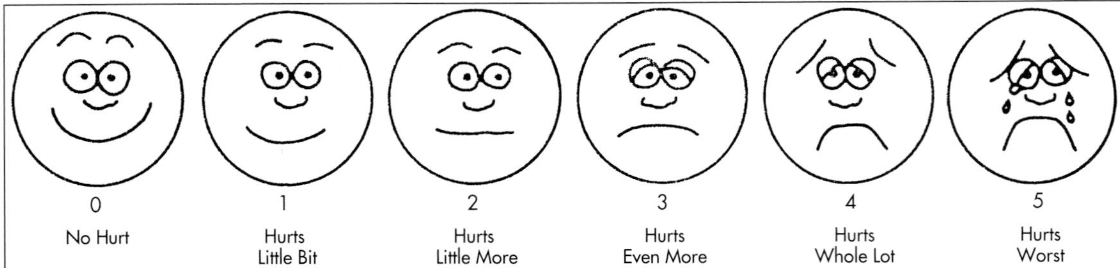

Fig. 8-8 Wong/Baker FACES Rating Scale. Explain to the client that each face is a person who feels happy because he or she has no pain (hurt) or sad because he or she has some or a lot of pain. **Face 0** is very happy because there is no hurt. **Face 1** hurts just a little bit. **Face 2** hurts a little more. **Face 3** hurts even more. **Face 4** hurts a whole lot. **Face 5** hurts as much as you can imagine, although you don't have to be crying to feel this bad. Ask the client to choose the face that best describes how he or she is feeling. Recommended for persons 3 years of age and older. (From Wong DL, Hockenberry-Eaton M, Wilson D, Winkelstein ML, Ahmann E, DiVito-Thomas PA: *Whaley & Wong's Nursing care of infants and children,* ed 6, St Louis, 1999, Mosby, p. 1153. Copyrighted by Mosby. Reprinted by permission.

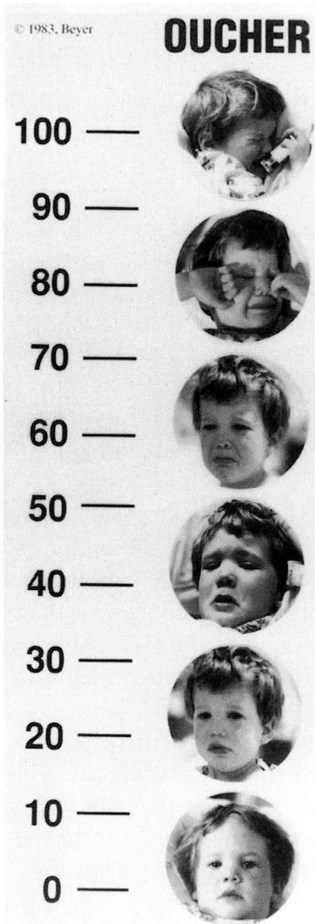

Fig. 8-9 Oucher Scale (Caucasian). (Caucasian Oucher developed and copyrighted by Judith E. Beyer, 1983, currently at the University of Kansas.)

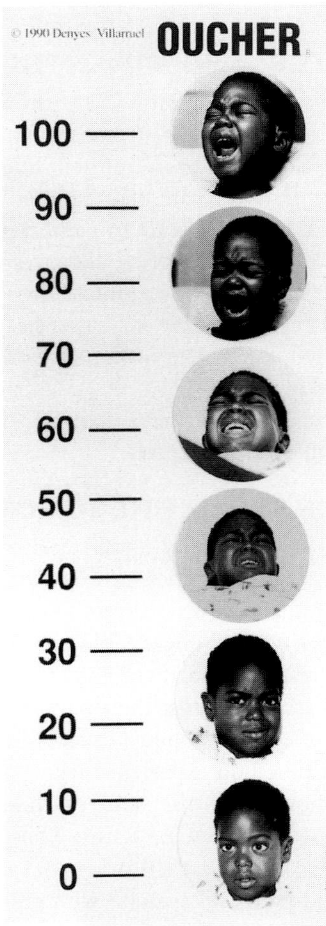

Fig. 8-10 Oucher Scale (African-American). (Courtesy Antonia Villarruel, PhD, FAAN, RN.)

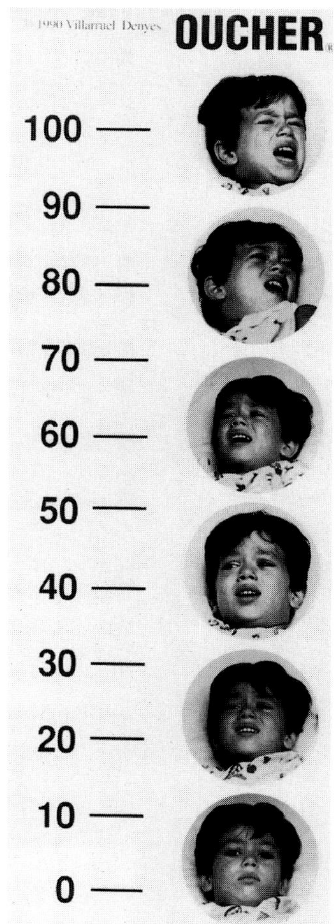

Fig. 8-11 Oucher Scale (Hispanic). (Courtesy Antonia Villarruel, PhD, FAAN, RN.)

EXAMINATION SUMMARY

Comfort and Pain

- Observe for posture and hand movements.
- Observe facial expressions.
- Listen to sounds client makes.
- Inspect skin for:
  - Color
  - Temperature
  - Moisture
- Measure blood pressure, pulse, and respiration.
- Observe pupillary size and reaction to light.

CLINICAL APPLICATION and CRITICAL THINKING

CRITICAL THINKING QUESTIONS

1. You are caring for three clients who have pain. The first client is Janie Baker, a 42-year-old African-American woman who had her gallbladder out this morning and is complaining of pain in the upper right quadrant of her abdomen. The second client is William Sanford, a 65-year-old white man who has terminal cancer and had an intestinal obstruction removed this morning to relieve intraabdominal pressure. The third client is Esther Martinez, a 52-year-old Hispanic woman who had a fusion of her right ankle this morning to treat her chronic rheumatoid arthritis.
   - **a.** How will your assessment of each client be the same?
   - **b.** How will your assessment of each client differ and why?
2. You are caring for the following clients who have pain:
   A man who is an Arab from Iraq
   A woman from Cambodia
   A man from China
   A man from Israel
   A woman from the Philippines

   Based on the clients' ethnic beliefs about pain reaction, how will your approaches to their pain assessment vary and why?

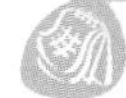

CASE STUDY

Mike Moore is a 46-year-old man who comes to the emergency department with a chief complaint of severe right abdominal and flank pain.

Interview Data

Mr. Moore tells the nurse, "The pain came on rather suddenly about an hour ago; I was doing some work at my desk, and it suddenly started." The pain is described as mainly in the right flank area, but it extends into the right lower abdominal area as well. Mr. Moore describes the pain as "severe" sharp pain. On a scale of 1 to 10, Mr. Moore states, "This is off your pain scale—at least a 12." The pain is described as constant, with intensity being intermittent as it may lighten slightly and intensify again. The other symptom Mr. Moore describes is nausea.

Examination Data

- **Vital signs:** Temperature, 101.8° F (38.8° C); Pulse rate, 108 beats/min; Blood pressure, 128/96 mm Hg; Respirations, 24 breaths per minute.
- **General survey:** Client curled up on stretcher in fetal position; appears uncomfortable, groaning.
- **Skin:** Skin is pale, diaphoretic, and warm to touch.
- **Abdomen:** Flat, no scars observed; bowel sounds active in all four quadrants; soft, nontender to palpation.

1. What data deviate from normal findings, suggesting a need for further investigation?
2. What additional questions could the nurse to ask to clarify symptoms?
3. What additional physical assessment, if any, should the nurse complete?
4. What nursing diagnoses and/or collaborative problems should be considered for this situation?

REMEMBER to check out your companion CD-ROM

9 Sleep and Rest Assessment

www.mosby.com/MERLIN/wilson/assessment/

ANATOMY AND PHYSIOLOGY

Sleep and rest are needed for health and well-being. Sleep is a state of reduced consciousness from which a person can be aroused through the use of sensory stimuli: sounds, touch, bright light, or smells. During this reduced state of consciousness there is diminished skeletal muscle activity and decreased metabolism. Rest is a period of inactivity that provides relief from anything distressing, disturbing, annoying, or tiring and creates peace of mind and mental and emotional calm. The terms rest and sleep are sometimes used synonymously.

Sleep physiology is a complex process involving the activation of several neurotransmitters in various areas of the brain. Structures of the brain believed to be involved with sleep are the reticular activating system (RAS) in the upper brainstem, the bulbar synchronizing region (BSR) in the pons and forebrain, the hypothalamus and thalamus in the diencephalon, and the frontal lobe in the cerebral cortex. The RAS receives sensory input to maintain wakefulness (Fig. 9-1). Norepinephrine, dopamine, acetylcholine, and gamma-aminobutyric acid (GABA) are neurotransmitters that contribute to wakefulness. Release of serotonin from the BSR contributes to sleep.

Sleep is necessary to allow the body time to restore itself and to prepare for the next day. An example of this restorative function is the repair of epithelial and specialized cells that occurs. During sleep the workload of the heart is decreased. The heart rate slows from the usual 70 to 80 beats/min to 60 to 70 beats/min, accompanied by a 5% to 10% reduction in systemic blood pressure.

Sleep patterns may be disrupted by physical or psychologic illnesses, by environmental factors such as noise or room temperature, by maturational factors such as age, and by drugs such as alcohol, hypnotics, antidepressants, and narcotics. When people are deprived of sleep, they have difficulty coping with stress, their immune system becomes impaired, and they feel fatigued, with decreased ability to concentrate. They may demonstrate perceptual difficulties such as confusion, paranoia, and hallucinations with increased anxiety and short-term memory loss. Sleep patterns are identified in laboratories where data are collected while individuals sleep. These data are collected using an electroencephalogram (EEG), which measures electrical activity in the brain, an electrocardiogram (ECG), which measures electrical impulses of the heart, an electromyogram (EMG), which measures muscle tone, and an electrooculogram (EOG), which measures tone of muscles that move the eyeball.

Stages of Sleep

Data from the EEG, ECG, and EOG are used to identify two distinct phases of sleep: non-rapid eye movement (NREM) sleep followed by rapid eye movement (REM) sleep. Characteristics of the four stages of NREM sleep and REM sleep are listed in Box 9-1. Activities that occur during NREM sleep are snoring; slow, regular respiration; low heart rate and blood pressure; absence of body movement; and slow, regular brain activity. The subsequent phase, REM sleep, or active sleep, is characterized by irregular respiration, variable heart rate and blood pressure, absence of snoring, rapid eye movement, and twitching of the face and fingers. Dreaming is closely associated with REM sleep.

A person's sleep patterns are highly individualized and change throughout life as the daily requirement for sleep gradually decreases. Although each person is different, the typical adult falls asleep in 8 to10 minutes and sleeps 7.5 to 8 hours, with about 95% of that time spent sleeping, 30 minutes or more in deep REM sleep and 2 hours dreaming (Wynsberghe, 1995). Sleep for an adult consists of three to five sleep cycles beginning with stage 1 NREM and progressing through to REM sleep and then back to one of the stages of NREM sleep. An average sleep cycle lasts 90 minutes, but each cycle has varying amounts of NREM and REM sleep. Figure 9-2 illustrates the normal adult sleep cycle and stages of sleep. The first cycle usually follows an orderly progression from stage 1 to stage 4 of NREM sleep followed by the REM sleep phase. The subsequent cycles may omit stage 1 and proceed in a different order from stage 4 to stage 2 and then to REM sleep. During the first sleep cycle the NREM phase is longer than the REM phase. But as sleep continues, the time spent in NREM sleep decreases and REM sleep increases.

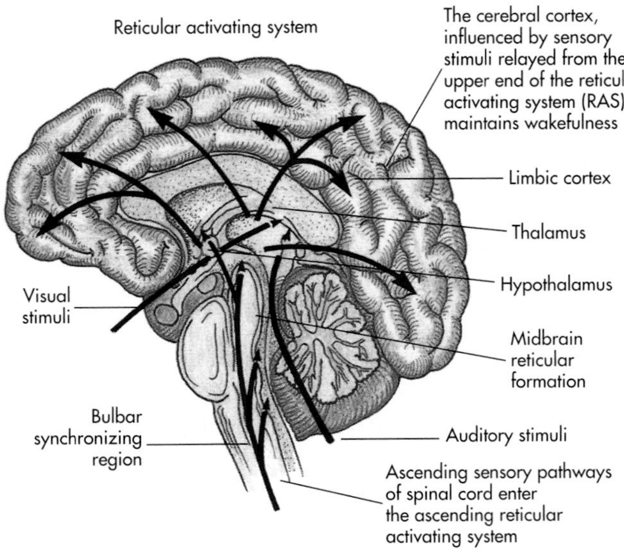

Fig. 9-1 The RAS and BSR control sensory input, intermittently activating and suppressing the brain's higher centers to control sleep and wakefulness. (From Potter and Perry, 1999.)

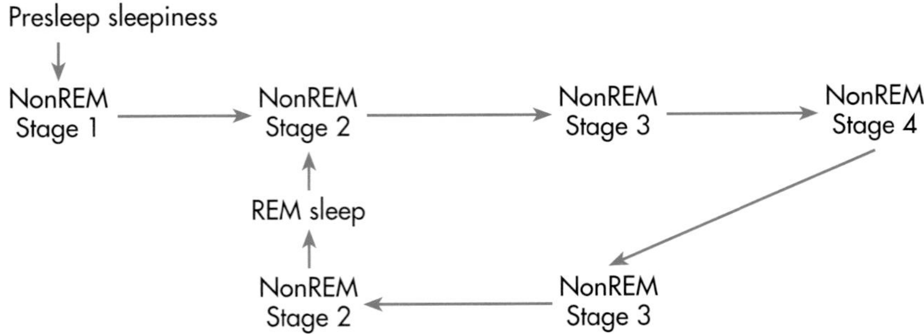

Fig. 9-2 The stages of the adult sleep cycle. (From Potter and Perry, 1999.)

Box 9-1 Stages of Sleep

STAGE 1: NONREM

Lightest level of sleep
Lasts a few minutes
Decreased physiological activity beginning with a gradual fall in vital signs and metabolism
Person easily aroused by sensory stimuli such as noise
If person awakes, feels as though daydreaming has occurred
Reduction in autonomic activities (e.g., heart rate)

STAGE 2: NONREM

Period of sound sleep
Relaxation progresses
Arousal still easy
Lasts 10 to 20 minutes
Body functions still slowing

STAGE 3: NONREM

Initial stages of deep sleep
Sleeper difficult to arouse and rarely moves
Muscles completely relaxed
Vital signs decline but remain regular
Lasts 15 to 30 minutes
Hormonal response includes secretion of growth hormone

STAGE 4: NONREM

Deepest stage of sleep
Very difficult to arouse sleeper
If sleep loss has occurred, sleeper will spend most of night in this stage
Restores and rests the body
Vital signs significantly lower than during waking hours
Lasts approximately 15 to 30 minutes
Possible sleepwalking and enuresis
Hormonal response continues

REM SLEEP

Stage of vivid, full-color dreaming (less vivid dreaming may occur in other stages)
First occurs approximately 90 minutes after sleep has begun, thereafter occurs at end of each NREM cycle
Typified by autonomic response of rapidly moving eyes, fluctuating heart and respiratory rates, and increased or fluctuating blood pressure
Loss of skeletal muscle tone
Responsible for mental restoration
Stage in which sleeper is most difficult to arouse
Duration increasing with each cycle and averaging 20 minutes

From Potter PA, Perry AG: *Basic nursing: a critical thinking approach,* ed 4, St Louis, 1999, Mosby.

HEALTH HISTORY

Sleep and Rest

QUESTIONS	RATIONALE
PRESENT HEALTH STATUS	
➤ How many hours do you usually sleep per day?	■ Data are used to compare usual sleep pattern with the expected norms for the client's age.
➤ During what hours do you usually sleep? Are there variations in the time of day that you sleep?	■ Someone who rotates shifts at work, creating a inconsistent sleep-wake cycle, may develop altered sleep cycles.
➤ Do you feel rested when you wake up from sleep?	■ This is a subjective indication of the quality of sleep time.
➤ How often do you take naps? If so, how long do you typically sleep?	■ Need for napping during day may suggest inadequate length or quality of sleep at night. Long naps (longer than 1 1/2 to 2 hours) may disrupt nighttime sleep.
➤ What is your usual bedtime routine (e.g., brushing teeth, bathing, reading, watching television, listening to music)?	■ Sleep may be disturbed when the usual ritual is changed.
➤ What medication(s) do you take?	■ Side effects of many drugs may interfere with sleep (Box 9-2).
PROBLEM-BASED HISTORY	
➤ Do you have difficulty falling asleep or staying asleep? Do you wake up frequently during sleep?	■ Positive response suggests disorders of initiating and maintaining sleep (DIMS) such as psychologic or persistent insomnia.
➤ How often does it happen? How long does it last? When this happens, how easy is it for you to go back to sleep?	■ Knowing the frequency and duration can help to identify the cause.
➤ What are factors that keep you from sleeping? Examples are work-related issues, personal relationships, financial concerns, family concerns, dealing with stress, or anxiety or depression.	■ Responses help to identify therapy for sleeplessness. Stress may cause tension that makes falling asleep difficult; stress causes release of adrenaline and corticosteroids that cause sleeplessness. ■ As anxiety and depression increase so does lack of sleep, while lack of sleep increases anxiety and depression.
➤ Do you drink alcohol before bedtime?	■ Alcohol speeds onset of sleep, disrupts REM sleep, and causes difficulty in returning to sleep.
➤ Do you eat or drink caffeine before bedtime?	■ Caffeine prevents client from falling asleep and may cause awakening during night.
➤ What factors make sleeping worse?	■ This allows the client to add data to the assessment not previously asked.

Box 9-2 Drugs and Their Effects on Sleep

HYPNOTICS

Interfere with reaching deeper sleep stages
Provide only temporary (1 week) increase in quantity of sleep
Eventually cause "hangover" during day: excess drowsiness, confusion, decreased energy
May worsen sleep apnea in older adults

DIURETICS

Cause nocturia

ANTIDEPRESSANTS AND STIMULANTS

Suppress REM sleep

ALCOHOL

Speeds onset of sleep
Disrupts REM sleep
Awakens person during the night and causes difficulty in returning to sleep

CAFFEINE

Prevents person from falling asleep
May cause person to awaken during night

DIGOXIN

Causes nightmares

BETA BLOCKERS

Cause nightmares
Cause insomnia
Cause awakening from sleep

VALIUM

Decreases stages 2, 4, and REM sleep
Decreases awakenings

NARCOTICS (MORPHINE/DEMEROL)

Suppress REM sleep
If discontinued quickly, can increase risk of cardiac dysrhythmias because of "rebound REM" periods
Cause increased awakenings and drowsiness

From Potter PA, Perry AG: *Basic nursing: a critical thinking approach,* ed 4, St Louis, 1999, Mosby.

EXAMINATION

Equipment

- Sphygmomanometer and stethoscope for measuring blood pressure
- Scale for measuring weight
- Nasal speculum for inspecting nasal septum

PROCEDURES AND TECHNIQUES WITH NORMAL FINDINGS	ABNORMAL FINDINGS
➤**INTERVIEW the client to assess mental status, thought patterns, speech patterns.**	■ Slow or confused thought processes or slow or slurred speech may indicate sleep deprivation.
➤**OBSERVE facial appearance.**	■ Sad expression or flat affect may indicate depression.
➤**OBSERVE gross motor movements and posture.**	■ Slow, exaggerated movements and/or slumped posture may indicate sleep deprivation.
➤**MEASURE blood pressure and body weight.**	■ Hypertension and obesity are risk factors for sleep apnea.
➤**INSPECT nasal septum for patency and deviation.**	■ Deviated septum may obstruct nasal passages, contributing to airway obstruction that may contribute to sleep apnea.
➤**INSPECT neck for size.**	■ Clients with sleep apnea often have short, thick neck.
➤**INSPECT pharynx for tonsillar hypertrophy.**	■ Large tonsils may obstruct airway during sleep.

AGE-RELATED VARIATIONS

■ NEONATES, INFANTS, AND CHILDREN

During the first few weeks of life a neonate may sleep as much as 20 hours daily with half the sleep time in the REM stage. The newborn has five distinct states of sleep: regular sleep, irregular sleep, drowsiness, alert inactivity, and waking and crying (Wynsberghe, 1995). Wrapping newborns snugly in a blanket and rocking them horizontally promotes sleep.

Infants develop a nighttime pattern of sleep by 3 to 4 months of age. They take several naps daily and sleep an average of 8 to 10 hours at night. Their sleep is predominantly REM sleep. Breast-fed infants wake more frequently than bottle-fed infants (Wong et al, 1999).

By age 2 children usually sleep through the night and take daily naps. The total sleep averages 12 hour per day. Naps often cease by age 3 years.

Sleep obtained by school-aged children varies with their level of activity and state of health. The 90-minute adult sleep cycle begins at this age. Naps usually are not needed. Older children may resist sleeping because they don't want to miss any activity or they need to be independent.

Health History

- In what position is the infant placed for sleep?
  Rationale The recommended sleeping position for infants is on their back or side to prevent sudden infant death syndrome (SIDS) (Wong et al, 1999).
- Is the infant breast-fed or bottle-fed?
  Rationale Breast-fed babies wake up more often than bottle-fed babies.
- How many naps is the infant or child taking, and how long do they last?
  Rationale Excessively long naps may interfere with nighttime sleep. Infants take several naps, by age 2 one nap is taken, and by age 3 naps usually cease.
- Where does the child fall asleep—own crib, parent's bed, couch, someone's lap?
  Rationale Child may awaken when moved to bed.
- What is the bedtime ritual (e.g., brushing teeth, bathing, reading, storytelling)?
  Rationale A consistent routine facilitates sleep.
- Does the child awaken during the night frightened? What is the parental response to the child's fear?
  Rationale Nightmares are common during childhood. Consistent parental assurance of safety helps the child return to sleep.
- Does the child resist going to bed because of fears of the dark, strange noises, or intruders?
  Rationale School-age children often have bedtime resistance for which the cause is not always known.

CULTURAL NOTE

Many experts recommend that infants and children sleep in their own crib or bed; however, co-sleeping or the family bed is common and accepted in some cultures, for example, African-American, Hispanic, and Japanese. Other groups adopting this habit are single and working parents (Wong et al, 1999).

■ ADOLESCENTS

Teenagers sleep 8 to 9 hours per day, of which a total of about 2 hours is spent in REM sleep. An adolescent may sleep late in the morning after staying up late at night. Rapid growth and active lifestyle may cause fatigue.

Health History

- Are stresses from the peer group or performance in school interfering with sleep?
  Rationale Pleasing peers, social acceptance, or pressure for academic performance may be stressors for this group that interfere with sleep.

■ OLDER ADULTS

Young-Old Adults

The time in nighttime sleep declines, with shortening of REM sleep and a decrease in stages 3 and 4 of NREM sleep.

Old-Old Adults

The typical 80-year-old adult takes 18 to 20 minutes to fall asleep and sleeps about 6 hours; about 80% of that time is spent sleeping, with a few minutes in deep REM sleep and about 1 hour dreaming (Wynsberghe, 1995). An 80-year-old adult experiences more frequent awakenings and is aroused more easily than a 65-year-old adult (Allen et al, 1991).

Older adults may experience frequent awakening during the night and take more time to fall back asleep. This change in sleep pattern may require a nap during the day.

Health History

- Do you wake up frequently while sleeping? Is there something specific that awakens you, such as shortness of breath, the need to urinate, or pain?
  Rationale Knowing what awakens clients may help solve the problem of sleep disturbance.
- Do you take naps during the day?
  Rationale An increase in the number or length of naps during the day may indicate a sleep problem during the night or may contribute to a sleep problem during the night.

COMMON PROBLEMS AND CONDITIONS

Sleep and Rest

Transient Psychophysiologic Insomnia

Transient psychophysiolgic insomnia is the most common sleep disorder even though clients rarely seek health care for it. Insomnia is defined as difficulty getting to sleep or waking up and being unable to go back to sleep. It is not a disease. Transient psychophysiologic insomnia lasts less than 3 weeks and has an abrupt onset related to an identifiable precipitating stressor. The stressor usually is a domestic or occupational problem, but the cause may be a reduction or cessation of addictive substances such as tobacco, alcohol, antianxiety drugs, or even sleeping medications.*

Persistent Insomnia

Persistent insomnia is defined as insomnia lasting longer then 3 weeks. These clients feel fatigue during the day but function appropriately. Clients who have been diagnosed with anxiety disorders such as obsessive thoughts or phobias may experience this kind of insomnia.

Excessive Somnolence

Excessive somnolence, also called hypersomnia, is defined as excessive daytime sleepiness. Causes include substance abuse, medication side effects, sleep apnea, and narcolepsy. Symptoms may range from tiredness throughout the day and interference with social activities to severe accidents caused by marked sleepiness.*

Transient Hypersomnia

Transient hypersomnia lasting less than 3 weeks is usually due to psychologic response to stress. Onset is abrupt with symptoms of persistent fatigue and loss of energy. Persistent hypersomnia lasting more than 3 weeks may indicate sleep apnea or narcolepsy.*

Sleep Apnea

Sleep apnea is characterized by breathing abnormalities that vary from reduction of airflow (hypopnea) to complete cessation of airflow (apnea). Sleep apnea may be due to central apnea, with cessation of respiratory effort and thus no airflow, or obstructive apnea from occlusion of upper airway with continued respiratory effort. Central sleep apnea occurs in infants and adults over age 65 years. Obstructive sleep apnea frequently occurs in obese men who have presenting symptoms of loud snoring and daytime sleepiness. The apnea ends when they twitch and awaken. Other clinical manifestations may include choking or gasping episodes at night and systemic and pulmonary hypertension. The sleepiness may range from subtle decrease in alertness to falling asleep in the middle of a conversation. Most data are collected from the bed partner since clients are unaware of their breathing pattern.*

Narcolepsy

Narcolepsy is defined as a sudden onset of excessive daytime sleepiness that lasts from 10 to 30 minutes. It is accompanied by one or more of the following conditions: cataplexy, a transient loss of postural muscle tone; sleep paralysis, an awakening with transient inability to speak or move; hypnagogic hallucinations, dreamlike visual hallucinations occurring at the transitions from wakefulness to sleep; and finally, disturbed nocturnal sleep, frequent, brief awakening during a night's sleep.

Sleep Terror Disorder

Sleep terror disorder, also called night terrors, occurs in children between the ages of 1 and 12 years and is characterized as a loud, uncontrollable screaming. It occurs usually during the transition from stage 4 to stage 1 of NREM sleep and occurs approximately 90 to 120 minutes after the onset of sleep. The child does not wake up and has no memory of the event; however, it does disturb the family members' sleep. Adults in their twenties and thirties may have sleep terrors characterized by sudden awakenings in the first third of sleep with a profound sense of dread. Contributing factors are fatigue, stress, or tricyclic antidepressants at bedtime. In both children and adults there are signs of autonomic activity e.g. tachycardia and diaphoresis.*

Sleepwalking (Somnambulism)

Sleepwalking (somnambulism) commonly occurs in boys more often than girls and is seen between the ages of 6 and 12 years. Occasionally it occurs in adults who had a history of sleepwalking in childhood with complete remission until the age of 20 or 30, when it recurs for several years. Sleepwalking occurs during the first third of the sleep period during the transition from stage 4 to stage 1 of NREM sleep. The sleepwalking lasts from a few seconds to several minutes, and the person has partial or no recollection of the activity. Persons who sleepwalk are under stress or fatigued, or they take a sedative or hypnotic at bedtime. Other predisposing factors are seizure disorders, central nervous system infections, and trauma. Arousal from sleepwalking is difficult, and walking is complicated by clumsy gait. Safety for the sleepwalker is a concern.*

Nocturnal Enuresis

Nocturnal enuresis, or bed-wetting, occurs in children at age 5 until puberty. It is seen in boys more frequently than

*Neubauer et al, 1998.

*Neubauer et al, 1998.

girls. Urination occurs prior to entering REM sleep. The child awakens because of the wet clothing. When enuresis persists beyond adolescence, the possibilities are epilepsy, psychologic disturbance, neurogenic bladder, dementia, or sleep apnea.*

■ OTHER SLEEP DISORDERS

Effects of Alcohol and Hypnotic Drugs on Sleep

Alcohol is a depressant, and people use it as a sleeping aide. Alcohol, however, reduces serotonin, causing sleep fragmentation. Alcohol speeds the onset of sleep but decreases REM sleep. The rebound causes the person to awaken during the night and have difficulty returning to sleep. This may lead to subsequent alcohol intake to get back to sleep quickly, but this further disrupts REM sleep.

Hypnotic drugs are taken to fall asleep faster or to sleep longer. Most hypnotic drugs suppress REM sleep. When the drug is discontinued, even after a single dose, there is a rebound in REM sleep with vivid dreams and increasing awakening.

*Neubauer et al, 1998.

CLINICAL APPLICATION and CRITICAL THINKING

CRITICAL THINKING QUESTIONS

1. Why is it necessary to assess client's sleep patterns?
2. What are the consequences of inadequate sleep?
3. Each of the following clients takes a nap daily:
   A 2-year-old girl
   A 3-year-old boy
   A 16-year-old girl
   An 85-year-old man
   a. Is a nap an expected behavior of each client?
   b. What do you think could be the reason for the nap for each one?
   c. What assessment questions would you ask each client/family member to get more information?

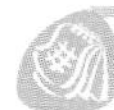

CASE STUDY

Brian is a 32-year-old man who comes to the clinic with a general complaint of feeling tired and not sleeping well. Below are data collected by the nurse from an interview and assessment.

Interview Data

Brian tells the nurse he has not been sleeping well and wants something to help him sleep better. He states that lately he never feels rested. When asked about sleep routine, he tells the nurse, "I go to bed about 11 PM each night and fall asleep quickly, but then I wake up around 2 AM and can't go back to sleep–I just end up tossing and turning." Brian tells the nurse that he does not have any specific routine before sleeping. "I just go to bed." When asked about stress in his life, Brian tells the nurse he is going through a divorce and may have to file bankruptcy. He states, "There has been so much stress lately that I have been having a couple of drinks every night to help me unwind."

Examination Data

- **Vital signs:** Blood pressure, 116/78 mm Hg; Pulse rate, 92 beats/min; Respirations, 20 breaths per minute; Temperature, 98.6° F (37° C).
- **General survey:** Well-nourished adult male, ambulates slowly but smoothly. Hair matted. Slumped posture.
- **Mental status:** Oriented to person, place, and time. Speech slow with flat affect.
- All body system findings within normal limits.

1. What data deviate from normal findings, suggesting to the nurse that Brian has a sleep pattern disturbance?
2. What additional information should the nurse ask or assess for?
3. In what functional health patterns does the data deviate from normal?
4. What nursing diagnosis and/or collaborative problems should be considered for this situation?

REMEMBER to check out your **companion CD-ROM**

10 Nutritional Assessment

www.mosby.com/MERLIN/wilson/assessment/

A nutritional assessment of the client is an integral part of the total health assessment because food and fluid are basic biologic needs of all human beings. Nutritional assessment includes an assessment of current nutritional status, but also identification of risk factors for nutritional problems. Four types of data collected include dietary history, anthropometric measurement, biochemical tests, and clinical evaluation. Although data collection will vary with age group, the general approach is consistent throughout the life cycle.

ANATOMY AND PHYSIOLOGY

Nutrients are necessary to provide the body calories for energy, to build and maintain body tissues, and to regulate body processes. The base energy requirement is called the basal metabolic rate (BMR), which is influenced by several factors. Activity levels, illness, injury, infection, ingestion of food, and starvation can all affect the BMR. When caloric intake meets energy needs, no weight change occurs. When energy needs exceed caloric intake, weight loss occurs; caloric intake exceeding energy needs results in weight gain. Nutrients are classified into one of three groups: macronutrients, micronutrients, and water.

MACRONUTRIENTS

Carbohydrates, proteins, and fats are considered macronutrients, meaning nutrients needed in large amounts.

Carbohydrate is the main source of energy and fiber in the diet. Each gram of carbohydrate produces 4 kcal of energy. Fiber passes through the digestive tract partially undigested, providing bulk that stimulates peristalsis. The two main sources of carbohydrates are plant foods (fruits, vegetables, and grains) and lactose (from milk). Although a small amount of carbohydrate is stored in the liver and muscle (in the form of glycogen) to serve as energy reserves between meals, moderate amounts of carbohydrates must be ingested at regular intervals to meet the energy demands of the body. If more carbohydrate is ingested than needed, the excess is stored as adipose tissue. The recommended carbohydrate intake in the diet is 55% to 60% of total calories (or at least 100 g/day for adults) (Williams, 1999).

Protein plays an essential role in building body tissue that facilitates growth and repair of body tissues. Protein is a source of energy. The simplest form of a protein is an amino acid. There are 20 different amino acids, and these combine in a number of different ways to form proteins. Ten of the amino acids are considered essential in the diet because they are not synthesized by the body (Williams, 1999). A complete-protein food contains all of the essential amino acids; complete proteins are also referred to as high-biologic-value proteins. Foods containing complete proteins include meat, fish, poultry, milk, and eggs. Foods that contain incomplete proteins include cereals, legumes, and some vegetables. Combinations of incomplete-protein foods can provide all the essential amino acids. If more protein is ingested than needed, the extra is used to supply energy or is stored as fat in adipose tissue. Each gram of protein provides 4 kcal of energy. The recommended protein intake in the diet is 15% to 20% of total calories, (about 45 g/day for adults).

Fat is the main source of fatty acids, which are essential for normal growth and development. Other functions of fat include synthesis and regulation of certain hormones, tissue structure, nerve impulse transmission, energy, insulation, and protection of vital organs. There are two essential fatty acids for metabolic processes: linoleic and linolenic acids. Fat is the body's major form of stored energy. If energy needs exceed carbohydrate intake, fat can be converted to glucose by a process known as gluconeogenesis. If more fat is ingested than needed, it is stored in adipose tissues. One gram of fat has 9 kcal of energy. The recommended fat intake in the diet is less than 30% of total calories (about 66 g/day for adults). When fats provide less then 10% of total calories, nutritional deficiencies may occur (Williams, 1999). Fats account for 35% to 45% of the typical diet of Americans.

MICRONUTRIENTS

Micronutrients are those nutrients that are required in small quantities by the body. The two groups of nutrients that make up this category are vitamins and minerals. These nutrients are essential for growth, development, and metabolic processes that occur continuously throughout the body.

Box 10-1 Vitamins

FAT-SOLUBLE VITAMINS

Vitamin A
Vitamin D
Vitamin E
Vitamin K

WATER-SOLUBLE VITAMINS

Vitamin C
B vitamins
- Thiamin
- Riboflavin
- Niacin
- Pyridoxine (B_6)
- Pantothenic acid
- Biotin
- Folate
- Cobalamin (B_{12})

Table 10-1 Minerals

	TRACE MINERALS	
MAJOR MINERALS	ESSENTIAL	UNCLEAR ROLE
Calcium	Iron	Silicon
Phosphorus	Iodine	Vanadium
Magnesium	Zinc	Nickel
Sodium	Copper	Tin
Potassium	Manganese	Cadmium
Chloride	Chromium	Arsenic
Sulfur	Cobalt	Aluminum
	Selenium	Boron
	Molybdenum	
	Fluoride	

Vitamins are classified as water soluble or fat soluble (Box 10-1). Water-soluble vitamins cannot be stored in the body; thus they must be ingested in the diet daily. Fat-soluble vitamins can be stored in the body, and in fact vitamin toxicity can result if they are taken in large quantity. Deficiencies or toxicities in micronutrients result in nutritionally based disease and may be clinically observed with examination.

Minerals are grouped into two categories: major minerals and trace minerals (Table 10-1). Major minerals are present in the body in large amounts with a required intake over 100 mg/day. Trace minerals are present in the body in smaller amounts; 10 of these are considered essential and have a required intake under 100 mg/day. The role of the remaining 8 is unclear.

WATER

Water composes 60% to 70% of total body weight, making it a critical component of the body. Cellular function depends on a well-hydrated environment. Since water is continually lost from the body, water replacement is required on a continual basis as well. Without water, an individual can survive for only a few days. The average adult metabolizes 2 1/2 to 3 L of water every day in the form of both foods and fluids (Williams, 1999). Fluid needs are increased in certain situations, especially fever, infection, gastrointestinal (GI) losses, and respiratory illness.

HEALTH HISTORY

Nutrition

A dietary history includes a collection of data to assess the client's actual or potential nutritional needs. The history must also assess problems the client may have related to nutritional status. Data gained from the history are used to evaluate the adequacy of the diet and to identify areas needed for client education (Fig. 10-1).

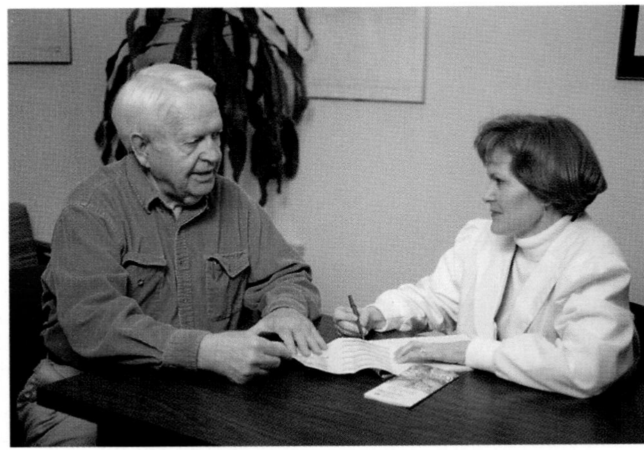

Fig. 10-1 Patient education is vital for improving the nutritional status of a client.

QUESTIONS	RATIONALE
PRESENT HEALTH STATUS	
➤ How would you describe your overall health?	■ Input from an individual regarding his or her health status may provide insight regarding nutritional problems.
➤ Do you have any chronic illnesses? If so, describe.	■ Many chronic illnesses are associated with nutritional problems and/or require special dietary measures and referral to a registered dietitian (examples include diabetes, cystic fibrosis, phenylketonuria, celiac disease, congestive heart failure, renal failure, and cancer).
➤ Do you take any medications? If so, what do you take and how often?	■ Many medications can affect an individual's nutrition. Some medications affect appetite, others may cause gastrointestinal discomfort such as nausea, fullness, constipation, or diarrhea. Some medications are affected by foods ingested; thus food restrictions may be necessary.
➤ How would you describe your appetite?	■ A change in appetite may be a clue to problems with food intake, weight gain, or weight loss.
➤ What are your food preferences? food dislikes?	■ Food preferences and dislikes are perhaps the strongest influence on a diet.

QUESTIONS

➤ Do you have any dietary restrictions or use any dietary supplements?

➤ Describe what you typically eat in a day for breakfast, lunch, dinner, and snacks.

➤ What is your typical fluid intake (type, amounts)?

➤ Have you noticed any changes in your weight in the last 6 months? If so, describe.

➤ Do you have any food intolerance or allergies? If so, describe.

RATIONALE

■ Some individuals are on special diets or use nutritional supplements to manage a disease (such as diabetes or renal disease), for weight loss, for weight gain, or even just to improve their health.

■ A 24-hour recall provides a history of an individual's food intake, allowing an estimation of the adequacy of the diet. Other tools useful for collecting data include a food diary and a food-frequency questionnaire. (See Appendix G for nutrition screening forms.)

■ Fluid intake should be assessed for adequacy of amount and type of intake. Many persons consume large quantities of empty calories through alcoholic beverages and soft drinks. Drinks containing caffeine have diuretic effects and thus may contribute to excessive water loss.

■ Weight should remain fairly stable over time. Significant rapid changes in weight require further evaluation.

■ Many persons have intolerance to foods such as lactose or food allergies such as nuts or shellfish (75% of the world population has lactose intolerance) (Williams, 1999).

CULTURAL NOTE

Lactose intolerance among adults has been reported among most of the populations of the world but affects a larger percentage of some cultural groups than others. This intolerance affects the following percentages of various groups:

Asians	94%
Black Africans	90%
American Indians	79%
Black Americans	75%
Hispanic Americans	50%
White Americans	17%

(Overfield, 1995.)

QUESTIONS

RATIONALE

➤ Do you have any problems obtaining, preparing, or eating foods? If so describe.

■ Obtaining adequate nutrition may be a problem for low-income groups or those with disabilities. Preparation of food must also be considered. Individuals with physical deficits or illness may have difficulty with food procurement and preparation. If this is an issue, assess support systems for someone willing to purchase and prepare food or assess for community resources.

➤ Do you use street drugs or drink alcohol? If so, describe.

■ The use of drugs or alcohol can contribute to nutritional deficiencies. Alcohol is a source of "empty" calories, that is, calories that supply no nutrients, which in turn suppresses the appetite. Alcohol also impairs the absorption of nutrients. Additionally, money spent on drugs and alcohol may replace money available for the purchase of food. Professionals believe alcohol consumption is underreported by 50% in clients with alcoholic histories (Zeman and Ney, 1988).

Past Medical History or Family History

➤ Have you ever had problems with your weight or problems eating in the past? If so, describe.

■ A personal history of excessive weight gain (such as during a pregnancy) or weight loss with an illness is important to note.

➤ Have you or anyone in your family ever had nutritional problems?

■ Obesity in one or both parents makes an individual at higher risk for excessive weight—which is partly genetic and partly from learned patterns of behavior regarding eating.

PROBLEM-BASED HISTORY

The most commonly reported problems related to nutrition include weight loss, weight gain, difficulty chewing and swallowing, and loss of appetite or nausea. As with symptoms in all areas of health assessment, a symptom analysis is completed, which includes the location, quality, quantity, chronology, setting, associated manifestations, alleviating factors, and aggravating factors (see Box 4-2 in Chapter 4).

Weight Loss

➤ When did the weight loss start? What is your "normal weight"? What is your weight now? How many pounds have you lost in the last 6 months?

■ Determine onset of weight loss and extent of weight loss. It is also important to determine if weight loss has been sudden or gradual.

➤ What do you attribute the weight loss to?
- Desired weight loss—change in eating habits, increase in exercise, etc.
- Undesired weight loss—loss of appetite, vomiting, illness, stress, medications, etc.
- Preoccupation with body weight—strict calorie intake, fasting, bulimia, laxative abuse, excessive exercise, etc.

■ It is important to note if weight loss is desired or undesired. If desired, consider if weight loss is acceptable; if not desired, identify contributing factors. Individuals generally will be able to explain what they think is causing the weight loss.

QUESTIONS

RATIONALE

RISK FACTORS

COMMON RISK FACTORS ASSOCIATED WITH Eating Disorders
- Preoccupation with weight
- Perfectionist
- Poor self-esteem
- Self-image disturbances
- Cultural—Peer pressure
- Athlete—Drive to excel in sports
- Compulsive or binge eating

➤ Have you had any symptoms associated with the loss of weight, such as fatigue, headaches, bruising, constipation, hair loss, or cracks in corners of mouth?

■ Excessive weight loss may cause a number of symptoms because of inadequate energy and protein and insufficient vitamins and minerals.

Weight Gain

➤ When did you start gaining weight? What do you consider your normal weight? What is your weight now? How many pounds have you gained in the last 6 months?

■ Establish the total weight gained and the time frame over which it occurred, whether sudden or gradual.

➤ What do you attribute the weight gain to?
-Desired—intentional increase in calories; dietary supplements.
-Undesired—decrease in activity levels, change in eating habits, increased appetite, medications, stopped smoking etc.

■ Determine if the weight gain is desired or undesired and if the weight gain is perceived as a problem to the client.

Difficulty Chewing and/or Swallowing

➤ Do you have problems with chewing food? If so, describe. When did this start?

■ Ask the client what the nature of the problem is. Determine the time frame over which this has occurred.

➤ Do you have problems swallowing food? If so, describe. When did this start?

■ Identify the time frame and determine the nature of the swallowing problem. Choking and coughing are common symptoms associated with impaired swallowing.

➤ What types of foods give you the most problems?

■ Thin liquids and foods requiring forceful chewing (such as meat) may not be tolerated well.

➤ What types of foods are you able to consume without difficulty?

■ Foods that are soft and highly viscous are most easily chewed and swallowed.

➤ Have you had a change of weight since this problem developed?

■ Weight loss, particularly if undesired, may be an indication that food intake is hampered by chewing or swallowing difficulties.

Loss of Appetite or Nausea

➤ Do you have problems with your appetite? Do you have problems with nausea? If so, describe.

■ Appetite may fluctuate from time to time. A reduction in appetite over an extended period of time may result in nutritional deficiencies.

➤ When did this problem start?

■ Establish the onset of the problem—this may provide clues as to the cause and potential nutritional deficiencies.

QUESTIONS	RATIONALE
➤ What do you attribute this problem to? (medications, illness, pregnancy, depression, etc.)	■ Many times the client will have an idea what is causing a change in appetite or nausea. Medications can cause this as well as illnesses, pregnancy, and depression.
➤ What types of foods are the most offensive or do you find most intolerable? What types of foods are you able to consume without difficulty?	■ In some cases, an individual may avoid an entire food group and eat from another. It is important to determine if foods from all groups are eaten.
➤ Have you had a change of weight since this problem developed?	■ A significant change in weight is indicative of a significant problem and may suggest nutritional deficiencies as well.

Once the client's eating habits have been established, the nurse uses these data to evaluate the adequacy of the diet—known as dietary assessment. The most accurate approach to date is to compare the client's intake with the recommended dietary allowances (RDAs); however, a major revision is underway to replace the RDAs. The revised recommendations, called dietary references intakes (DRIs), are a collaboration between Canada and the United States. The DRI is a generic term used to refer to at least three types of reference values: estimated average requirement (EAR), RDA, and tolerable upper intake level (UL). The EAR is the intake value estimated to provide adequate nutrition to 50% (an average) of age- and gender-specific groups; thus the intakes recommended would not meet the needs of the remaining 50%. The RDA is the dietary intake that is sufficient to meet nutrition requirements of nearly all individuals in the group. The UL is the maximum level of daily nutrients that is unlikely to pose health risks for most individuals in the group (Whitney, Cataldo, and Rolfes, 1998). Updates for the DRI will continue through 2003, but the current RDA and DRI recommendations are listed in Table 10-2. Box 10-2 shows how to convert percentages of calories from fats, proteins, and carbohydrates to grams.

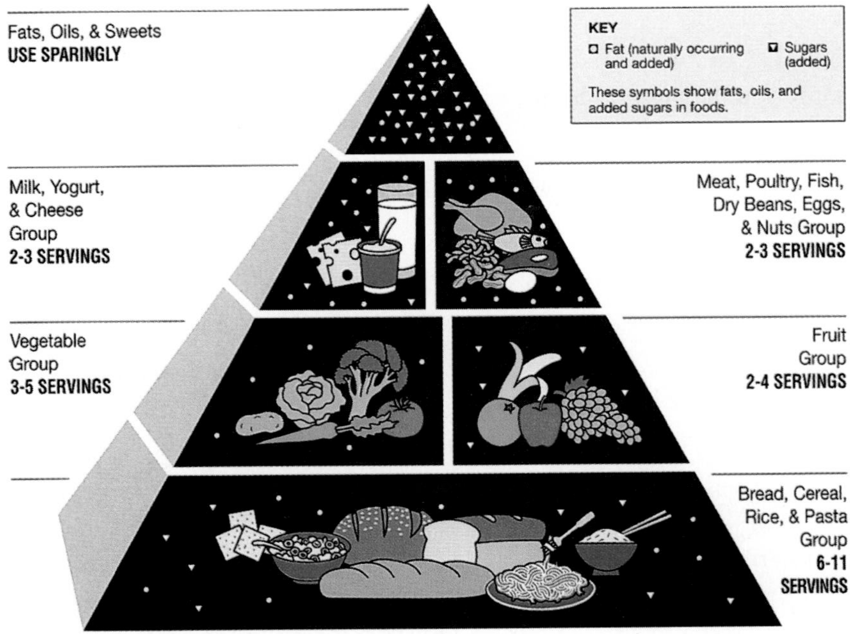

Fig. 10-2 Food guide pyramid.

Comparing diet intake against the food guide pyramid is another approach to dietary assessment. Determine the number of servings per day for each of the six groups, and compare food intake with the recommended number of servings. The original food guide pyramid (Fig. 10-2) gives recommended servings for each of six food groups. The vegetarian food pyramid was developed to meet needs of vegetarian clients, whose food choices do not fit the original pyramid (Fig. 10-3).

Once the diet has been evaluated, interventions may be necessary, which may range from dietary teaching to referral to a registered dietitian. Box 10-3 has some helpful suggestions regarding dietary teaching.

Table 10-2 1997-1998 Dietary Reference Intakes (DRI)

	RECOMMENDED DIETARY ALLOWANCES (RDA)								ADEQUATE INTAKES (AI)					
AGE (yr)	THIAMIN (mg)	RIBOFLAVIN (mg)	NIACIN (mg NE)‡	VITAMIN B_6 (mg)	FOLATE (μg DFE)	VITAMIN B_{12} (μg)	PHOSPHORUS (mg)	MAGNESIUM (mg)	VITAMIN D (μg)	PANTOTHENIC ACID (mg)	BIOTIN (μg)	CHOLINE (mg)	CALCIUM (mg)	FLUORIDE (mg)
INFANTS†														
0.0-0.5	0.2	0.3	2§	0.1	65	0.4	100	30	5	1.7	5	125	210	0.01
0.5-1.0	0.3	0.4	4	0.3	80	0.5	275	75	5	1.8	6	150	270	0.5
CHILDREN														
1-3	0.5	0.5	6	0.5	150	0.9	460	80	5	2.0	8	200	500	0.7
4-8	0.6	0.6	8	0.6	200	1.2	500	130	5	3.0	12	250	800	1.1
MALES														
9-13	0.9	0.9	12	1.0	300	1.8	1250	240	5	4.0	20	375	1300	2.0
14-18	1.2	1.3	16	1.3	400	2.4	1250	410	5	5.0	25	550	1300	3.2
19-30	1.2	1.3	16	1.3	400	2.4	700	400	5	5.0	30	550	1000	3.8
31-50	1.2	1.3	16	1.3	400	2.4	700	420	5	5.0	30	550	1000	3.8
51-70	1.2	1.3	16	1.7	400	2.4	700	420	10	5.0	30	550	1200	3.8
>70	1.2	1.3	16	1.7	400	2.4	700	420	15	5.0	30	550	1200	3.8
FEMALES														
9-13	0.9	0.9	12	1.0	300	1.8	1250	240	5	4.0	20	375	1300	2.0
14-18	1.0	1.0	14	1.2	400	2.4	1250	360	5	5.0	25	400	1300	2.9
19-30	1.1	1.1	14	1.3	400	2.4	700	310	5	5.0	30	425	1000	3.1
31-50	1.1	1.1	14	1.3	400	2.4	700	320	5	5.0	30	425	1000	3.1
51-70	1.1	1.1	14	1.5	400	2.4	700	320	10	5.0	30	425	1200	3.1
>70	1.1	1.1	14	1.5	400	2.4	700	320	15	5.0	30	425	1200	3.1
PREGNANCY	1.4	1.4	18	1.9	600	2.6	*	+40	*	6.0	30	450	*	*
LACTATION	1.5	1.6	17	2.0	500	2.8	*	*	*	7.0	35	550	*	*

Modified with permission from National Academy of Sciences, Food and Nutrition Board, National Research Council: *Recommended dietary allowances,* ed 10, Washington, DC, 1989, National Academy Press; National Academy of Sciences Institute of Medicine: *Dietary reference intakes for thiamin, riboflavin, niacin, vitamin B_6, folate, vitamin B_{12}, pantothenic acid, biotin, and choline,* Washington, DC, 1997-1998, National Academy Press; and National Academy of Sciences, Institute of Medicine: *Dietary reference intakes for calcium, phosphorus, magnesium, vitamin D, and fluoride,* Washington, DC, 1997-1998, National Academy Press. Courtesy of National Academy Press, Washington DC.

*Values for these nutrients do not change with pregnancy or lactation. Use the value listed for women of comparable age.

†For all nutrients, an AI was established instead of an RDA as the goal for infants; for the B vitamins and choline, the age groupings are 0 through 5 months and 6 through 11 months.

‡Abbreviations: *NE,* niacin equivalents; *DFE,* dietary folate equivalents; *RE,* retinol equivalents; *TE,* α-tocopherol equivalents.

§The AI for niacin for this age group only is stated as milligrams of preformed niacin instead of niacin equivalents.

THE VEGETARIAN FOOD PYRAMID
A daily guide to food choices
Vegetable fats and oils, sweets, and salt
Eat sparingly
OIL
HONEY
Low-fat or non-fat, milk, yogurt, fresh cheese, and fortified alternative group
2-3 servings
Eat moderately
MILK
Non-Dairy Soy Drink
Yogurt
Cottage Cheese
Legume, nut, seed, and meat alternative group
2-3 servings
Eat moderately
SOYBEANS
TOFU
Vegetable group
3-5 servings
Eat generously
Fruit group
2-4 servings
Eat generously
RAISINS

Whole grain bread, cereal, pasta, and rice group
6-11 servings
Eat liberally
OAT MEAL
Shredded Wheat
Pasta

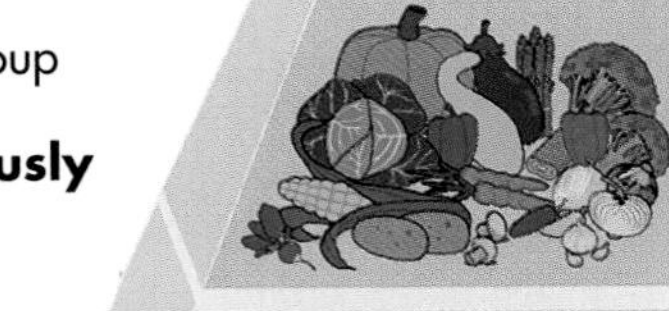

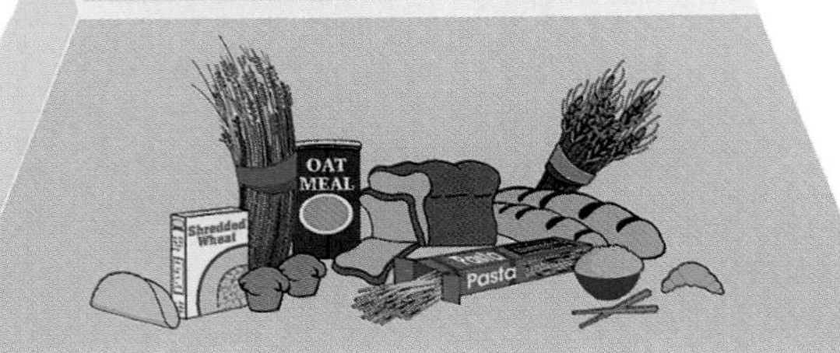

Fig. 10-3 Vegetarian food pyramid. (From The Health Connection, 1994. Illustration by Merle Poirer. The Vegetarian Food Guide Pyramid is available as posters and handouts by calling The Health Connection at 1-800-548-8700 or 301-790-9735.)

Box 10-2 Calculating Percentages of Nutrients

In a well-balanced diet for a healthy person, intake should be as follows:

10% to 20% of kcal should come from protein.
30% or less of kcal should come from fat.
50% to 60% of kcal should come from carbohydrate.

HOW MANY CALORIES IN EACH CATEGORY CAN BE CONSUMED?

Determine the ideal daily caloric goal; then take the percentage of that goal.

Example: 2000-calorie diet:

15% of 2000 kcal is about 300 kcal protein per day
30% of 2000 kcal is about 600 kcal fat per day
55% of 2000 kcal is about 1100 kcal carbohydrates per day

HOW MANY GRAMS IN EACH CATEGORY CAN BE CONSUMED?

Divide the number of calories per gram of each macronutrient by the number of calories allowed.

Protein yields 4 kcal
Fat yields 9 kcal
Carbohydrate yields 4 kcal

300 kcal of protein per day divided by 4 kcal/g = 75 g of protein per day.

600 kcal of fat per day divided by 9 kcal/g = 66.6 g of fat per day.

1100 calories of carbohydrate per day divided by 4 kcal/g = 275 g of carbohydrate per day.

Box 10-3 Guidelines for Dietary Teaching for Healthy Eating

- Assess the literacy of the client, and tailor recommendations to his or her level. Low-literacy clients would benefit from handouts with pictures or video education tools.
- Consider the client's cultural food choices when teaching healthy eating.
- Encourage the client to add fruit and vegetable servings throughout the day (as opposed to only at dinner) to help increase the total number of vegetable servings.
- Use a visual image of meat as a "side dish" and grains and vegetables as the "main course" to enhance the client's understanding of portions.
- Meat, poultry, and fish portions can be described as the size of a deck of cards (3 oz). Healthy eating guidelines recommend only 4 to 6 oz of meat, poultry, and fish per day.

When discussing various types of fat, remember that saturated fat is solid at room temperature, whereas monounsaturated and polyunsaturated fats are liquid at room temperature. Saturated fats should be minimized. In small quantities, monounsaturated and polyunsaturated fats are preferred.

EXAMINATION

Equipment

- Tape measure (to measure midarm circumference)
- Weight scale (to measure body weight)
- Height scale (to measure height)
- Skinfold calipers (to measure triceps skinfold)
- Calculator (to calculate nutrition estimates)

PROCEDURES AND TECHNIQUES WITH NORMAL FINDINGS

ABNORMAL FINDINGS

ANTHROPOMETRIC MEASURMENTS

The common measurements taken in anthropometrics include height, weight, triceps skinfold measurements, and midarm circumference.

➤**MEASURE height and weight for body mass index (BMI).** Body mass index is a weight-to-height ratio used to assess nutritional status. Using the BMI table (Table 10-3), mark the values for height and weight. If you don't have a BMI table, the BMI can be calculated by using the formula in Box 10-4. The normal range for BMI is 20 to 25.

■ Clients increase their risk of developing nutrition-related problems the further their weight varies from the normal range.

BMI <20	Underweight
BMI 25-30	Overweight
BMI >30	Obesity
BMI >40	Severe Obesity

(Williams, 1999).

Table 10-4 presents mean BMI data and the prevalence of overweight people among the United States population.

Box 10-4 Calculation of BMI

CALCULATION USING KILOGRAMS AND METERS

$$\text{BMI} = \frac{\text{Weight (kg)}}{\text{Height (m}^2\text{)}}$$

CALCULATION USING POUNDS AND INCHES

$$\text{BMI} = \frac{\text{Weight (lb)} \times 705}{\text{Height (in)}^2}$$

Example: A woman is 65 inches tall and weighs 156 pounds.

$$\frac{156 \times 705}{65^2} = \frac{109980}{4225} = \text{BMI } 26.03$$

➤**COMPARE client's body weight to the desirable body weight (DBW).** Calculate the client's DBW and compare this to the actual body weight by using the following formula:

Females: 100 lb (45.5 kg) for the first 5 feet + 5 lb (2.27 kg) for each inch greater than 5 feet ± 10%

Males: 106 lb (48 kg) for the first 5 feet + 6 lb (2.7 kg) for each inch greater than 5 feet ± 10%

Express the weight as a percentage of DBW by dividing the current weight by the DBW and multiplying by 100.

$$\frac{\text{Current Weight}}{\text{DBW}} \times 100 = \%\ \text{DBW}$$

Example:

$$\frac{\text{Current weight 150 pounds}}{\text{DBW 160 pounds}} = .9375 \times 100 = 93.8\%\ \text{of DBW}$$

■ Clients increase their risk of developing nutrition-related problems the further their weight varies from 100% DBW.

Severely underweight	70% or less of DBW
Moderately underweight	80% or less of DBW
Mild obesity	20% to 40% above DBW
Moderate obesity	40% to 100% above DBW
Morbid obesity	Over 100% above DBW or over 45 kg higher than DBW.

(Yanovski, 1993).

Table 10-3 Body Mass Index Chart

BMI→	19	20	21	22	23	24	25	26	27	28	29	30	31	32	33	34	35
HEIGHT (inches)	BODY WEIGHT (pounds)																
58	91	96	100	105	110	115	119	124	129	134	138	143	148	153	158	162	167
59	94	99	104	109	114	119	124	128	133	138	143	148	153	158	163	168	173
60	97	102	107	112	118	123	128	133	138	143	148	153	158	163	168	174	179
61	100	106	111	116	122	127	132	137	143	148	153	158	164	169	174	180	185
62	104	109	115	120	126	131	136	142	147	153	158	164	169	175	180	186	191
63	107	113	118	124	130	135	141	146	152	158	163	169	175	180	186	191	197
64	110	116	122	128	134	140	145	151	157	163	169	174	180	186	192	197	204
65	114	120	126	132	138	144	150	156	162	168	174	180	186	192	198	204	210
66	118	124	130	136	142	148	155	161	167	173	179	186	192	198	204	210	216
67	121	127	134	140	146	153	159	166	172	178	185	191	198	204	211	217	223
68	125	131	138	144	151	158	164	171	177	184	190	197	203	210	216	223	230
69	128	135	142	149	155	162	169	176	182	189	196	203	209	216	223	230	236
70	132	139	146	153	160	167	174	181	188	195	202	209	216	222	229	236	243
71	136	143	150	157	165	172	179	186	193	200	208	215	222	229	236	243	250
72	140	147	154	162	169	177	184	191	199	206	213	221	228	235	242	250	258
73	144	151	159	166	174	182	189	197	204	212	219	227	235	242	250	257	265
74	148	155	163	171	179	186	194	202	210	218	225	233	241	249	256	264	272
75	152	160	168	176	184	192	200	208	216	224	232	240	248	256	264	272	279
76	156	164	172	180	189	197	205	213	221	230	238	246	254	263	271	279	287

To use the table, find the appropriate height in the left-hand column. Move across to a given weight. The number at the top of the column is the BMI at that height and weight. Pounds have been rounded off.

From National Institutes of Health/National Heart, Lung, and Blood Institute: *Clinical guidelines on the identification, evaluation, and treatment of overweight and obesity in adults: the evidence report,* June 1998, National Institutes of Health.

Table 10-4 Prevalence of Overweight and Mean Body Mass Index (BMI) of the U.S. Population Ages 20 to 74 Years by Race and Gender

RACE/GENDER	PREVALENCE OF OVERWEIGHT (%)	MEAN BMI
White		
Men	32.0	26.3
Women	32.2	25.9
Black		
Men	31.8	26.5
Women	49.1	28.3
Hispanic-American		
Men	39.8	27.1
Women	48.1	27.8

From Kuczmarski RJ, Flegal KM, Campbell SM, Johnson CL: Increasing prevalence of overweight among U.S. adults: the National Health and Nutrition Surveys, 1960 to 1991, *JAMA* 272:205-211, 1994. (Data collected 1988-1991.)

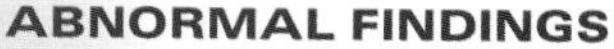

PROCEDURES AND TECHNIQUES WITH NORMAL FINDINGS

ABNORMAL FINDINGS

These calculations allow you to express the current weight as a percentage of the DBW. Ideally, the client will be fall between 90% and 110% of DBW. The calculated weight can be increased or decreased by 10% to account for bone structure and amount of muscle or fat tissue. This information should be considered a component of assessment.

➤COMPARE client's current body weight to the usual body weight (UBW). Documentation of the amount of weight loss over a period of up to 6 months may be helpful in determining the severity of weight loss. To determine the rate of weight loss, one can calculate the percentage change of weight by dividing current body weight by the usual body weight and multiplying by 100.

$$\frac{\text{Current Body Weight}}{\text{Usual Body Weight}} \times 100 = \%\ \text{UBW}$$

■ A weight loss of 5% in1 month, 7.5% over 3 months, or 10% over 6 months is considered significant and should be referred for evaluation and treatment of malnutrition.

❖ **➤ESTIMATE body fat by measuring triceps skinfold.** Skinfold measurements provide a good estimate of total body fat (Fig. 10-4). Triceps skinfold measurements are made with skinfold calipers at the midpoint between the acromial process and the olecranon of the nondominant arm (See Fig. 6-12 in Chapter 6). One limitation of the skinfold test is that the fat may be thicker under the skin in one area than another. To overcome this limitation, three measurements should be taken and the results averaged (Whitney, Cataldo, and Rolfes, 1998). Normal ranges for skinfold fat measurements for men and women are included in Table 10-5. The desired skinfold measurement falls at or near the 50th percentile. Accuracy of this measurement is affected by the skill of the examiner taking the measurements.

■ Values significantly higher than normal can indicate increased fat mass. Values significantly lower than normal can indicate decreased fat mass secondary to either an increase in lean mass or depleted fat stores (Whitney, Cataldo, and Rolfes, 1998).

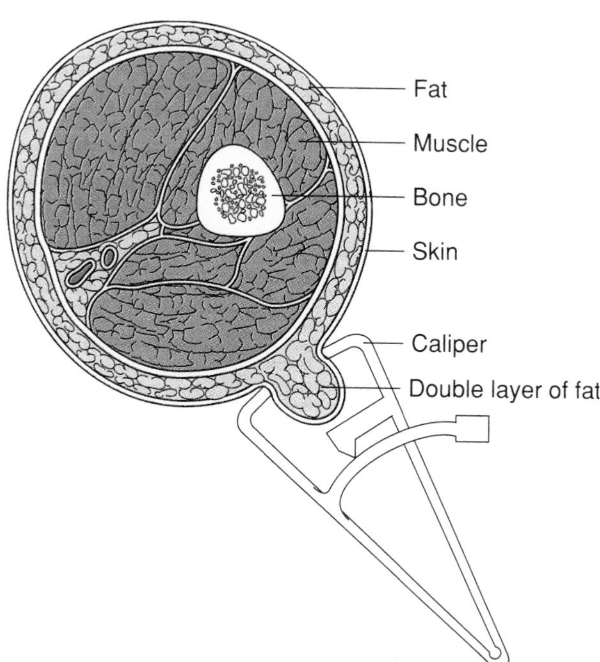

Fig. 10-4 Cross-section of arm with triceps skinfold measurement. (From Barkauskus et al, 1998.)

Table 10-5 Percentiles for Triceps Skinfold Measurements (Adults)

	TRICEPS SKINFOLD		
GENDER	5th	50th	95th
MALES			
18-19	4	9	24
19-25	4	10	22
25-34	5	12	24
35-45	5	12	23
45-54	6	12	25
55-64	5	11	22
65-74	4	11	22
FEMALES			
18-19	10	18	30
19-25	10	18	34
25-34	10	21	37
35-45	12	23	38
45-54	12	25	40
55-64	12	25	38
65-74	12	24	36

Data from Frisancho AR: New norms of upper limb fat and muscle areas for assessment of nutritional status, *Am J Clin Nutr* 34:2540-2545, 1981.

PROCEDURES AND TECHNIQUES WITH NORMAL FINDINGS

❖ ➤**ESTIMATE midarm muscle circumference (MAMC).** Although not routinely measured, these data provide an estimation of skeletal muscle mass and available protein and fat stores. First, measure the midarm circumference (MAC). Use a measuring tape to measure (in centimeters) the circumference of the client's bare arm midway between the tips of the olecranon and the acromial processes (use the same arm and the same location where skinfold thickness was measured) (Fig. 10-5). Use the MAC measurement and the triceps skinfold measurement (TSF) to calculate MAMC using the formula below. Normal ranges for MAC and MAMC are found in Table 10-6.

$$\text{MAC (cm)} - [0.314 \times \text{TSF (mm)}] = \text{MAMC cm}$$

Example: A 53-year-old woman has a midarm circumference of 27 cm and triceps skinfold of 20 mm. MAMC is calculated as follows:

$$27\text{ cm} - (0.314 \times 20) = 27 - 6.28 = 20.72\text{ MAMC cm}$$

ABNORMAL FINDINGS

■ MAMC is decreased in the presence of protein malnutrition (Williams, 1999).

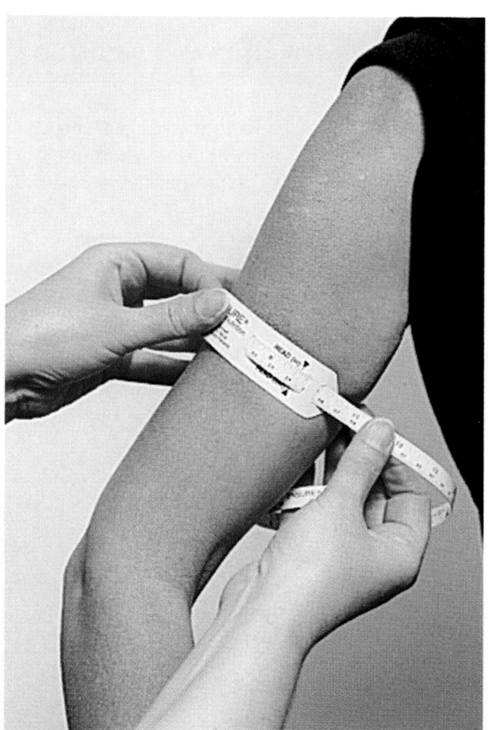

Fig. 10-5 Measurement of mid–upper arm circumference. (From Seidel et al, 1999.)

Table 10-6 Percentiles for Midarm Circumference and Midarm Muscle Circumference (Adults)

	MIDARM CIRCUMFERENCE (cm)			MIDARM MUSCLE CIRCUMFERENCE (cm)		
GENDER	5th	50th	95th	5th	50th	95th
MALES						
18-19	24.5	29.7	37.9	22.6	26.4	32.4
19-25	26.2	30.8	37.2	23.8	27.3	32.1
25-34	27.1	31.9	37.5	24.3	27.9	32.6
35-45	27.8	32.6	37.4	24.7	28.6	32.7
45-54	26.7	32.2	37.6	23.9	28.1	32.6
55-64	25.8	31.7	36.9	32.6	27.8	32.0
65-74	24.8	30.7	35.5	22.3	26.8	30.6
FEMALES						
18-19	22.2	25.8	32.5	17.4	20.2	24.5
19-25	22.1	26.5	34.5	17.9	20.7	24.9
25-34	23.3	27.7	36.8	18.3	21.2	26.4
35-45	24.1	29.0	37.8	18.6	21.8	27.2
45-54	24.2	29.9	38.4	18.7	22.0	27.4
55-64	24.3	30.3	38.5	18.7	22.5	28.0
65-74	24.0	29.9	37.3	18.5	22.5	27.9

Data from Frisancho AR: New norms of upper body limb fat and muscle areas for assessment of nutritional status, *Am J Clin Nutr* 34:2540-2545, 1981.

PROCEDURES AND TECHNIQUES WITH NORMAL FINDINGS

ABNORMAL FINDINGS

❖ ➤**CALCULATE the waist-to-hip ratio.** Waist-to-hip ratio is an indication of the risk of unhealthy fat distribution. To obtain the waist-to-hip ratio, measure the waist at the narrowest point, then measure the hips at the widest point. Calculate the waist-to-hip ratio using the formula below.

$$\frac{\text{Waist (cm)}}{\text{Hip (cm)}}$$

For example, if a man has a 44-inch waist (112 cm) and 40-inch hips (101 cm), the calculation would be:

$$112 \text{ cm}/101 \text{ cm} = 1.1 \text{ waist to hip ratio}$$

The desired waist-to-hip ratio for women is 0.8 or less and for men is 1.0 or less. Women typically collect fat in their hips, giving their bodies a pear (gynecoid) shape. Men, however, build up fat around their waists, giving them an apple (android) shape. People whose fat is concentrated in the abdomen are more likely to develop health problems associated with obesity.

■ A ratio that exceeds the desired ratio is indicative of upper body obesity. This increases the risk of developing health problems related to obesity (e.g., diabetes, hypertension, coronary artery disease, gallbladder disease, osteoarthritis, and sleep apnea) (www.nihhk.nih.gov, 1999).

Box 10-5 Normal Adult Values for Laboratory Tests Used for Nutritional Assessment*

SERUM ALBUMIN

3.5 = 5-5.0 g/dl or 35-50 g/L (SI units)

PREALBUMIN

15-36 mg/dl or 150-360 mg/L (SI units)

HEMOGLOBIN

Male	14-16 g/dl or 8.7-11.2 mmol/L (SI units)
Female	12-16 g/dl or 7.4-9.9 mmol/L
Pregnant female	>11 g/dl

HEMATOCRIT

Male	42%-52% or 0.42-0.52 volume fraction (SI units)
Female	37%-47% or 0.37-0.47 volume fraction
Pregnant female	>33%

BLOOD GLUCOSE

75-110 mg/dl or 4.0-6.0 mmol/L (SI units)

SERUM CHOLESTEROL

<200 mg/dl or 5.20 mmol/L (SI units)

SERUM TRIGLYCERIDE

Male	40-160 mg/dl or 0.45-1.81 mmol/L
Female	35-135 mg/dl or 0.40-1.52 mmol/L

HIGH-DENSITY LIPOPROTEIN (HDL)

Male	>45 mg/dl or >0.75mmol/L
Female	>55 mg/dl or >0.91 mmol/L

LOW-DENSITY LIPOPROTEINS (LDL)

Male and Female 60-180 mg/dl or <3.7 mmol/L

CHOLESTEROL TO HDL

Male	5.0
Female	4.4

Data from Pagana KD, Pagana TJ: *Mosby's manual of diagnostic and laboratory tests,* St. Louis, 1998, Mosby.
*Values for infants and children may vary—refer to laboratory manual for other age groups.

PROCEDURES AND TECHNIQUES WITH NORMAL FINDINGS

ABNORMAL FINDINGS

LABORATORY TESTS

➤**ASSESS nutritional status by reviewing laboratory tests.** Many laboratory tests are helpful in assessment of nutritional status. Not all of these tests are indicated for all situations. Refer to Box 10-5 for normal ranges for adults.

Serum albumin measures circulating protein. Albumin levels can be affected by fluid status, blood loss, liver function, trauma, and surgery. Fluctuation of albumin levels occurs over a 3- to 4-week period.

Prealbumin is a reflection of protein and calorie intake for the previous 2 to 3 days.

Hemoglobin and hematocrit provide information regarding erythrocytes. These are clinically useful to screen for anemia due to dietary deficiency such as iron, folate, and vitamin B_{12}.

Serum glucose reflects carbohydrate metabolism. A fasting glucose level is used to screen for the presence of diabetes mellitus or glucose intolerance.

Lipid profile includes several tests that are indicators of lipid metabolism and are important determinants of risk factors for cardiovascular disease. Total cholesterol and triglyceride levels, high-density lipoprotein (HDL) level, low-density lipoprotein (LDL) level, and cholesterol/high-density lipoprotein ratio are included in a lipid profile. (The cholesterol-to-HDL ratio is calculated by dividing the total cholesterol value by the HDL value.)

■ Abnormal Biochemical Tests

Low albumin levels suggest protein calorie malnutrition. Levels between 2.8 and 3.5 g/dl is consistent with moderate protein deficiency; levels below 2.5 g/dl represent severe protein depletion. Rapid changes in albumin are most likely due to factors other than nutrition.

A deficiency of either calories or protein can cause prealbumin to decline. A malnourished individual undergoing refeeding therapy can produce rises in prealbumin levels.

Low hemoglobin and hematocrit levels suggest anemia. The causes of anemia are numerous, but dietary deficiencies of iron, B_{12}, or folate are a few possible causes. Elevated hemoglobin and hematocrit levels may occur in dehydration, chronic anoxia, and polycythemia.

Hypoglycemia (blood glucose level less than 75 mg/dl) may indicate inadequate caloric intake.

Hyperglycemia (blood glucose level over 126 mg/dl) may be an indication of diabetes mellitus (Committee on the Diagnosis and Classification of Diabetes Mellitus, 1997).

Values equal to or greater than 200 mg/dl for total cholesterol and triglyceride levels indicate the client is at increased risk. A complete lipid profile and cardiovascular risk assessment are recommended for clients with total cholesterol or triglyceride level above 200 mg/dl (Grundy et al, 1993). Elevations of total cholesterol, triglycerides, and LDL increase the risk for developing coronary heart disease; elevated HDL levels reduce the risk.

CLINICAL EXAMINATION

Many nutritional deficiencies become apparent through clinical evaluation. Table 10-7 summarizes common findings with nutritional deficiencies.

➤**ASSESS general appearance and level of orientation.** A well-nourished individual is alert and has a body weight within normal ranges.

■ Poor nutritional status may be recognized from general observation. Excessive obesity, cachexia, or generalized edema are obvious indicators of poor nutritional status. Prominent cheek and clavicle bones or wasted-appearing limbs suggest malnutrition. A client with insufficient caloric intake may be irritable or have a flat affect. Disorientation can be caused by niacin deficiency.

Table 10-7 Clinical Signs and Symptoms of Various Nutrient Deficiencies

AREA OF EXAMINATION	SIGN/SYMPTOM	POTENTIAL NUTRIENT DEFICIENCY
Hair	Alopecia	Zinc, essential fatty acids
	Easy pluckability	Protein, essential fatty acids
	Lackluster	Protein, zinc
	"Corkscrew" hair	Vitamin C, vitamin A
	Decreased pigmentation	Protein, copper
Eyes	Xerosis of conjunctiva	Vitamin A
	Corneal vascularization	Riboflavin
	Keratomalacia	Vitamin A
	Bitot' spots	Vitamin A
GI tract	Nausea, vomiting	Pyridoxine
	Diarrhea	Zinc, niacin
	Stomatitis	Pyridoxine, riboflavin, iron
	Cheilosis	Pyridoxine, iron
	Glossitis	Pyridoxine, zinc, niacin, folate, vitamin B_{12}
	Magenta tongue	Riboflavin
	Swollen, bleeding gums	Vitamin C
	Fissured tongue	Niacin
	Hepatomegaly	Protein
Skin	Dry and scaling	Vitamin A, essential fatty acids, zinc
	Petechiae/ecchymoses	Vitamin C, vitamin K
	Follicular hyperkeratosis	Vitamin A, essential fatty acids
	Nasolabial seborrhea	Niacin, pyridoxine, riboflavin
	Bilateral dermatitis	Niacin, zinc
Extremities	Subcutaneous fat loss	Kcalories
	Muscle wastage	Kcalories, protein
	Edema	Protein
	Osteomalacia, bone pain, rickets	Vitamin D
	Arthralgia	Vitamin C
Neurologic	Disorientation	Niacin, thiamin
	Confabulation	Thiamin
	Neuropathy	Thiamin, pyridoxine, chromium
	Paresthesia	Thiamin, pyridoxine, vitamin B_{12}
Cardiovascular	Congestive heart failure, cardiomegaly, tachycardia	Thiamin
	Cardiomyopathy	Selenium

Data from Ross Products Division, Abbott Laboratories Inc. In Seidel HM et al: *Mosby's guide to physical examination,* ed 4, St Louis, 1999, Mosby.

PROCEDURES AND TECHNIQUES WITH NORMAL FINDINGS

ABNORMAL FINDINGS

➤**INSPECT the skin for surface characteristics, hydration, and lesions.** The skin should be smooth, elastic, and without lesions, cracks, or bruising.

■ Many nutritional deficiencies and fluid imbalance can be recognized by changes to the skin. The presence of edema indicates fluid retention (which may reflect protein depletion), whereas dry skin and decreased skin turgor may reflect dehydration. Multiple bruises are associated with vitamin C and K deficiencies; essential fatty acid deficiencies lead to dry flaking skin and eczema. Cracks or lesions on the skin may be the result of niacin deficiency. Follicular hyperkeratosis is associated with vitamin A deficiency (Fig. 10-6).

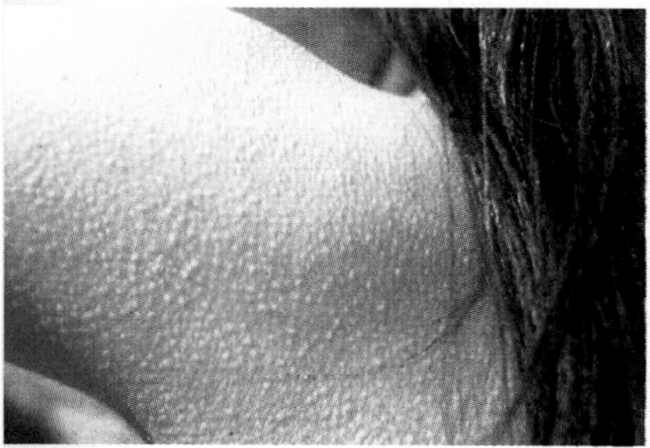

Fig. 10-6 Follicular hyperkeratosis. (From McLaren, 1992.)

➤**INSPECT the hair and nails for appearance and texture.** In well-nourished individuals, hair appears shiny, smooth, and firm. Nails should be pink, smooth, intact, and firm.

■ Hair that is dull and falls out easily or observable hair loss is indicative of protein and fatty acid deficiencies. Spoon-shaped nails may be associated with iron deficiency.

➤**INSPECT the eyes for surface characteristics.** Mucous membranes (conjunctivae) around the eyes should be pink and free of lesions or drainage. The corneas should be clear and

■ Conjunctiva that is pale may be a sign of anemia. Excessively red conjunctiva may indicate riboflavin deficiency. Foamy-looking areas on the eyes (known as Bitot's spots) or excessively dry eyes are caused by vitamin A deficiency. With end-stage deficiency the cornea becomes dry and hard, a condition known as xerophthalmia (Fig. 10-7). shiny.

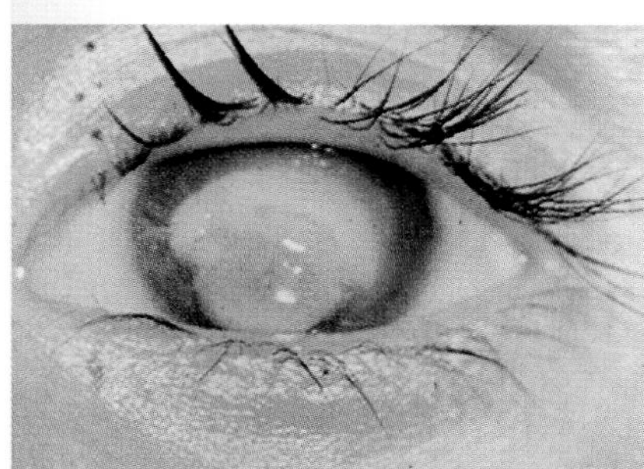

Fig. 10-7 Xerophthalmia. (From McLaren, 1992.)

PROCEDURES AND TECHNIQUES WITH NORMAL FINDINGS

➤INSPECT the oral cavity for dentition and intact mucous membranes. The teeth should be present, clean, and intact; dentures, if present, should be assessed for fit. The mucous membranes and gums should be moist, pink, and free of lesions. The tongue and lips should be pinkish red, smooth, and without lesions.

➤INSPECT and PALPATE the extremities for shape, size, coordinated movement, and sensation. Well-developed muscles should be observed, and these should be bilaterally equal. The client should have muscle strength and coordinated muscle movement. The client should have full sensation to extremities.

ABNORMAL FINDINGS

■ Poor dentition and painful oral lesions can negatively affect food intake. Dry mucous membranes may be indicative of dehydration. Bleeding gums may be a sign of vitamin C deficiency; vitamin B complex deficiency can cause cracks in the corners of the mouth or on the lips or an excessively red tongue. A purplish tongue can be caused by riboflavin deficiency.

■ Muscle weakness and wasting is a sign of inadequate protein intake or excessive protein wasting. Uncoordinated muscle movements may interfere with the ability to feed self. Vitamin D deficiency can cause skeletal malformation (Fig. 10-8). Thiamin deficiency can cause peripheral neuropathy and paraesthesia.

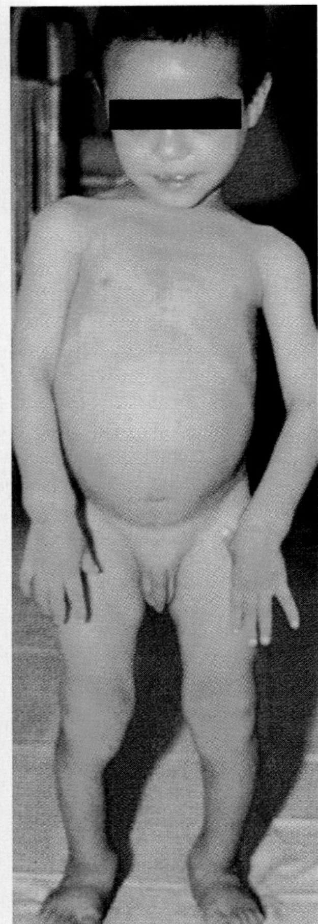

Fig. 10-8 Rickets. (From McLaren, 1992.)

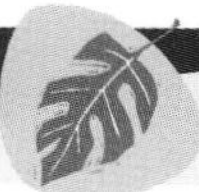

AGE-RELATED VARIATIONS

■ NEONATES AND INFANTS

Anatomy and Physiology

The first year of life is associated with rapid growth; thus adequate nutrition is essential. Breast-feeding is recommended for the first year of life because the composition of breast milk promotes normal infant growth and offers natural immunity. Infants typically double their birth weight within the first 4 months and triple their weight by the end of the first year.

Health History

During the first year of life, a comprehensive diet history of the infant's feeding habits, types and tolerance to foods and formula, and an estimate of amounts consumed will give valuable information to the examiner.

- How are you feeding your infant (breast-feeding or formula)?

  Rationale Establish feeding method.

- If breast-feeding: How often and how long does your baby feed? Do you think your baby is getting enough to eat?

  Rationale Assess the adequacy of feedings. Mother should have baby feed from both breasts.

- If formula-fed: What type of formula do you give the baby? How do you prepare it? How much does the baby take at each feeding? Has your baby experienced problems with constipation, diarrhea, vomiting, or skin rashes?

  Rationale Assess the adequacy of feedings. Assess for adequate preparation of formula, particularly if it is mixed. Symptoms listed above are commonly associated with formula intolerance.

- Do you give your infant water? If so, how much? How often?

  Rationale During the first month of life, the ability of neonates to excrete excess water is still not fully developed; thus routine water supplementation can result in oral water intoxication (Scariati et al, 1997). Older infants, however, should be offered water on a regular basis.

- Have you started to introduce solid foods to your infant? If so, what foods have been offered and at what age? Has your infant developed any rashes, vomiting, or diarrhea?

  Rationale Solid foods should be introduced between 4 and 6 months. Food should be introduced gradually and one at a time. Symptoms may be caused by food intolerance or allergies.

Examination

Procedures and Techniques Anthropometric measurements for the infant include body weight, height (length), and circumference of head (see Chapter 6). The measurements obtained not only provide baseline parameters of the newborn's nutritional status at birth, but also reflect overall intrauterine growth and development. Skinfold measurements and biochemical tests are not recommended for the well newborn or during the first year of life. The nurse should review biochemical tests if an abnormality is suspected. Also observe the newborn infant for rooting reflex and effective suck effort and swallowing.

Normal and Abnormal Findings The newborn infant should have a strong rooting reflex. Suck effort should be strong without evidence of swallowing difficulties. Neonates having birth measurements that fall between the 5th and 95th percentile of the intrauterine growth chart may be considered as having appropriate growth for gestational age (AGA). Large for gestational age (LGA) are infants with growth parameters greater than the 95th percentile. These neonates should be closely monitored during the first 24 hours for hypoglycemia (Wong et al, 1999). Small for gestational age (SGA) refers to those neonates born weighing less than the 5th percentile on the intrauterine growth charts (Metcoff, 1994).

■ CHILDREN

Anatomy and Physiology

The rapid growth that occurs during the first year typically slows down during the toddler and school-age years. School-aged children should gain approximately 4 ½ to 8 ½ lb (2 to 4 kg) per year until adolescence.

Health History

The history should be conducted as previously discussed for the adult. The DRIs/RDAs (see Table 10-2) provide a guideline for estimating nutrient needs for healthy children. National Cholesterol Education Program (NCEP) guidelines for children over the age of 2 years are the same as for the general population (Grundy and Bilheimer, 1993). Children on vegetarian diets may be at risk for many nutritional deficiencies, including iron, calcium, zinc, vitamin D, and vitamin B_{12} (Sinatra and Sinatra, 1996). Unhealthy nutrition habits early in life may contribute to such chronic disease as obesity, abnormal glucose tolerance, hypertension, and elevated cholesterol and triglyceride levels.

Examination

Procedures and Techniques The examination is the same as described for the adult. Weight-for-height is the most reliable indicator for growth for this age group. Plot data on growth charts with each visit. The BMI may be an important indicator after the first year but is not routinely calculated. Triceps skinfold and biochemical tests are not routinely evaluated in the well child. These may be clinically indicated if the child is malnourished or obese. Finally, inspect the child's teeth for presence and general appearance.

Normal and Abnormal Findings Height and weight falling between the fifth and 95th percentiles is an expected finding. Children who fall below the fifth percentile or above the ninety-fifth percentile should be further evaluated. The identification of the malnourished or failure-to-thrive (FTT) is a high priority during toddlerhood. This may occur as a result of inadequate availability of nutrients and from parents underfeeding the child to prevent obesity. Teeth should be present and in good condition without presence of decay. Tooth decay of primary teeth, caused by intake of carbohydrate-containing beverages such as milk or juice before a nap or bedtime, is a common abnormal finding with this age group. Several terms are used to describe this, including baby bottle tooth decay, nursing bottle caries, and nursing bottle syndrome.

■ ADOLESCENTS

Anatomy and Physiology

Adolescence is a time for rapid growth. If the growth is outside the expected parameters, close follow-up may be necessary. Obesity and eating disorders are problems that may be identified in this age group.

Health History

The nutritional history should be the same as previously described for the adult. Questions should specifically address obesity and eating disorders since these are common problems in this age group. Establishment of eating patterns may reveal poor eating habits associated with multiple school or athletic activities. Girls who have reached sexual maturity should be questioned about menstruation, as iron deficiency anemia could occur. If the adolescent is pregnant, referral for intensive nutritional counseling is necessary.

Examination

Procedures and Techniques Examination of the adolescent proceeds as described for the adult. Weight-for-height continues to be plotted on growth charts. The BMI may be calculated with this age group, particularly if weight-for-height is outside normal parameters. Skinfold measurements and biochemical tests are not necessary for healthy adolescents, although lipid screening may be indicated for obese adolescents.

Normal and Abnormal Findings An adolescent with a BMI greater than 30 or less than 20 should be referred for medical treatment (Himes and Dietz, 1994).

■ OLDER ADULTS

Anatomy and Physiology

Older adults require fewer calories, have decreased taste sensation, and decreased absorption from the GI tract. Dehydration is the most common fluid and electrolyte disorder among older adults and is responsible for a large number of hospitalizations in this population. Chewing and swallowing difficulties are most prevalent in this age group.

Health History

The nutritional history should be the same as previously described for the adult with some additional considerations, including medications and assessing social interactions, living arrangements, and functional ability.

- What medications do you currently take?

  Rationale Older adults take more prescription medications than do any other age group (Valassi and Clark, 1992). Potential food and drug interactions must be evaluated because some medications have negative effects on nutritional status by decreasing appetite or absorption of nutrients. Table 10-8 lists common drugs taken by older adults and possible nutritional deficiencies that may occur.

- Whom do you live with? If lives alone: What is your routine for purchasing and preparing food? What kind of social activities do you participate in? How often?

  Rationale Many older adults live alone and have limited access to food (Valassi and Clark, 1992). Social isolation, loneliness, and living alone are significant risk factors for inadequate nutritional intake. Among older

Table 10-8 Nutritional Deficiences Caused by Common Drugs Taken by the Elderly

DRUG AND DRUG GROUP	DEFICIENCY
CARDIAC GLYCOSIDES	
Digitalis	Anorexia→ protein energy malnutrition Zinc and magnesium deficiency
DIURETICS	
Thiazides→ Furosemide Ethacrynic acid	Potassium, zinc, and magnesium depletion
Triamterene→	Folic acid deficiency
ANTIINFLAMMATORY DRUGS	
Aspirin Indomethacin→	GI blood loss→ iron deficiency
Colchicine→	Malabsorption of fat-soluble and water-soluble vitamins
ANTACIDS (ANTACID ABUSE)	Phosphate depletion; osteomalacia
LAXATIVES (LAXATIVE ABUSE)	
Mineral oil→	Deficiency of vitamins A, D, and K Potassium deficiency Multiple nutrient deficiencies due to malabsorption Folic acid and vitamin D deficiency

From Roe DA: *Geriatric nutrition,* ed 2. Copyright © 1987 by Allyn & Bacon. Reprinted/adapted by permission.

adults who live alone, men have a greater tendency to consume poor-quality diets than do women. One study found that older adult participants in congregate meal programs were less likely to skip meals than older adult clients with meals delivered to their homes (Frongilli et al, 1992).

- What activities are you capable of doing for yourself? What sorts of activities do you need assistance with?
  Rationale The level of activities of daily living has an impact on nutritional status of older adults.

Examination

Procedures and Techniques Evaluation of the older client is similar to that previously described for adults. The BMI is a reliable indicator of obesity in this age group. The TSF and MAC measurements may not be as accurate as with a younger person because of changes in fat distribution, declining muscle mass, and sagging skin. Routine screening of serum glucose, hemoglobin, and hematocrit levels is recommended in the older adult population. Total cholesterol level may have a decreased significance in older adults. Elevated serum cholesterol in clients over 70 years of age with no other risk factors for cardiovascular disease does not increase the risk for cardiovascular events (Krumholz et al, 1994). Observing the client while he or she eats is important to determining if the client is able to carry food to his or her mouth, has muscle strength for chewing, and has the ability to swallow.

EXAMINATION SUMMARY

Nutrition

PROCEDURE

Anthropometric Measurements

- Measure height and weight for body mass index (BMI).
- Compare client's body weight to the desirable body weight (DBW).
- Compare client's current body weight to usual body weight (UBW).
- ❖ Estimate body fat by taking triceps skinfold measurements.
- ❖ Estimate mid–arm muscle circumference (MAMC).
- ❖ Calculate hip-to-waist ratio.

Biochemical Measurements

- Assess nutritional status by reviewing laboratory tests.

Clinical Evaluation

- Assess general appearance and level of orientation.
- Inspect the skin for surface characteristics, hydration, and lesions.
- Inspect the hair and nails for appearance and texture.
- Inspect the eyes for surface characteristics.
- Inspect the oral cavity for dentition and intact mucous membranes.
- Inspect and palpate the extremities for shape, muscle size, tone, and sensation.

SUMMARY OF FINDINGS

Age Group	Normal Findings	Findings Associated With Nutritional Disorders
Infants	*Length-for-weight:* Within 5th and 95th percentiles; consistent weight gain.	*Length-for-weight:* <5th or >95th percentile; poor weight gain pattern.
	Head circumference: Within 5th and 95th percentiles.	*Head circumference:* <5th or >95th percentile.
	General appearance: Alert, active.	*General appearance:* Lethargic; irritable.
	Feeding patterns: Strong suck reflex; consistent with age.	*Feeding patterns:* Food intolerance; poor or weak suck reflex; problems swallowing.

Age Group	Normal Findings	Findings Associated With Nutritional Disorders
Children	*Height for weight:* Within 5th and 95th percentiles.	*Height for weight:* $<5^{th}$ or $>95^{th}$ percentile.
	Oral cavity: Presence of teeth, clean without decay.	*Oral cavity:* Tooth decay.
Adolescent	Same as adult.	Same as adult.
Adults	*BMI:* 20-25	*BMI* : <20—underweight >30—obesity
	Current weight: Within 10% to 15% of DBW.	*Current weight:* 20% more or less than DBW.
	Triceps skinfold: Near 50th percentile.	*Triceps skinfold:* $\leq 5^{th}$ or $\geq 95^{th}$ percentile.
	MAC, MAMC: Near 50th percentile.	*MAC, MAMC:* $\leq 5^{th}$ or $\geq 95^{th}$ percentile.
	Hip-to-waist ratio: Men $\leq$1.0 Women $\leq$0.8	*Hip-to-waist ratio:* Men >1.0 Women >0.8
	General appearance: Alert, appears to be well-nourished.	*General appearance:* Flat affect; irritability or disorientation; obvious obesity or cachexia.
	Skin/nails: Smooth, normal skin tone for ethnicity; free of lesions or cracks, well hydrated, elastic. Nails smooth, intact, rounded.	*Skin/nails:* Skin color pale, texture rough, with flaking skin, cracks, or lesions; decreased skin turgor; bruises; nails may appear spoon shaped or be brittle.
	Hair: Shiny, smooth.	*Hair:* Coarse, dull, brittle, falls out easily.
	Eyes: Cornea clear, shiny; conjunctiva pink without lesions or drainage.	*Eyes:* Pale or very red conjunctiva; drainage, lesions.
	Oral cavity: Teeth intact, good repair, mucous membranes moist, no lesions, no cracks; tongue pink and smooth.	*Oral cavity:* Teeth missing or in poor condition or poorly fitting dentures; dry mucous membranes; lesions, cracks, pale or bleeding gums; tongue red or purple.
	Extremities: Well-developed muscles with coordinated movement; full sensation; no lesions; reflexes within normal limits; full sensation to extremities.	*Extremities:* Muscle wasting, muscle weakness, decreased reflexes, paresthesia, or peripheral neuropathy.
Older Adult	Same as adult.	Same as adult.

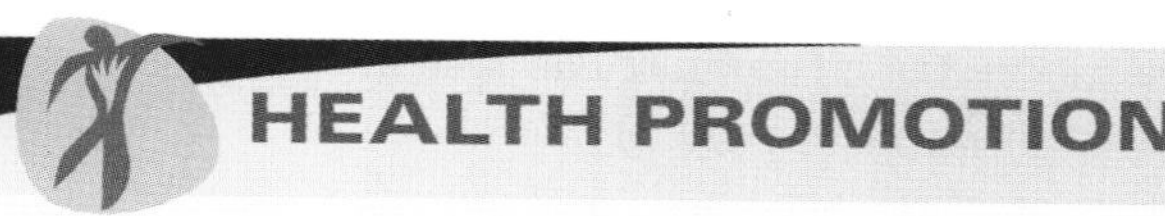

HEALTH PROMOTION

HEALTHY EATING HABITS

Eating in a manner consistent with the food guide pyramid provides adequate nutrients and energy to promote health, prepare tissue, and in some cases prevent disease. Adults need to be positive role models for children and adolescents in providing healthy food and snacks. This does not prevent the periodic hot fudge sundae or pizza as long as that kind of high fat intake does not become the norm. Dietary recommendations for health are as follows:

- Limit total fat intake to 30% or less of calories. Reduce saturated fat intake to less than 10% of calories and the intake of cholesterol to less than 300 mg daily.*

CALORIES BY AGE GROUP*

Age	Kcal/day
1 year	1,000
3 years	1,300
10 years	2,000
Adolescent	2,000 to 4,000 depending on activity
Adult	1,500 to 2,400+ depending on activity
Older adult (>65 years)	Decrease calories by 5% per decade

- Increase intake of starches and other complex carbohydrates (55% of calories).* Maintain protein intake at moderate levels (15% of calories).*
- Balance food intake and physical activity to maintain appropriate body weight.
- For those who drink alcoholic beverages, limit consumption to the equivalent of less than 1 oz of pure alcohol daily. Pregnant women should avoid alcoholic beverages. A drink is any alcoholic beverage that delivers ½ ounce of pure ethanol. For example, 1 1/4 ounces of hard liquor (e.g., 80-proof whiskey, gin, rum, vodka) is equal to 4 to 5 oz of wine, 10 oz of wine cooler, or 12 oz of beer.*
- Limit total daily intake of salt to 6 g or less.
- Maintain adequate calcium intake (refer to DRI tables for various age groups and conditions).
- Maintain an optimal intake of fluoride, particularly during the years of primary and secondary tooth formation and growth (6 months to 3 years, 0.25 mg/day; 3 to 6 years, 0.50 mg/day; 6 to 16 years, 1.0 mg/day†; women, 3.1 mg/day; men, 3.8 mg/day.*

These recommendations can be accomplished by eating 6 to 11 servings of bread, cereal, rice, and pasta; 2 to 4 servings of fruit; 3 to 5 servings of vegetables; 2 to 3 servings of milk, yogurt, and cheese; and 2 to 3 servings of meat, poultry, fish, dry beans, eggs, and nuts. A serving is ½ cup or 4 oz.

WEIGHT REDUCTION AND GAIN

Remember that just as weight goes on over time, it comes off over time. A realistic goal is loss of 1 lb/week. One pound equals 3,500 calories. If 3,500 kcal is divided by 7 days a week, you must decrease your caloric intake by 500 calories a day to meet this goal. The weight loss is more rapid if the calorie reduction is combined with physical exercise for at least 30 minutes 3 times a week.

If weight gain is the goal, exercise is still important for general health. Increasing calories by 500 a day while still selecting foods from the food pyramid will facilitate weight gain.

*Whitney, Cataldo, and Rolfes, 1998.

*Whitney, Cataldo, and Rolfes, 1998.
†U.S. Preventive Services Task Force, 1996.

COMMON PROBLEMS AND CONDITIONS

Nutrition

OBESITY

Obesity is defined as a body mass index greater than 30 and occurs when there is an imbalance between energy intake and energy expenditure. Causes of obesity include fat cell development, genetics, overeating, and inactivity. When more energy is consumed than is used, it is stored in fat cells. The amount of fat in a person's body reflects the number and size of fat cells. The number of fat cells increases during growth periods in childhood and puberty. The number of fat cells increases more rapidly in obese children than lean children. When fat cells reach their maximum size, they divide.

Genetics play an important part in determining a person's body weight and height. When both parents are obese, the chance that the children will be obese is high (80%). Overeating increases energy intake, whereas inactivity inhibits energy expenditure.

Obesity may contribute to four of the leading causes of death: heart disease, cancer, stroke, and diabetes mellitus. Other disorders that are associated with obesity are hypertension, sleep apnea, gout, low back pain, gallbladder disease, respiratory problems, and complications from surgery (Whitney, Cataldo, and Rolfes, 1998).

UNDERWEIGHT

Underweight is defined as a body mass index of less than 20. Although not as common a problem as obesity in the United States, this affects about 10% of the American population (Williams, 1999). People who are underweight may not consume enough nutrients for tissue healing and effective immune function. This increases the risk of infection and decreases the effectiveness of the physiologic response to stress. Underweight women become infertile because a certain percentage of body fat is necessary for proper reproductive functioning. Those who do conceive have a higher rate of giving birth to an underweight or unhealthy neonate. Self-esteem may be affected due to the underweight condition.

BULIMIA

Bulimia is a psychologic disorder manifested as an eating disorder. It is characterized by repeated episodes of binge eating followed by purging through self-induced vomiting, misuse of laxatives or diuretics, or excessive exercise. It is estimated that as many as 20% of college women engage in bulemic behavior (Williams, 1999). During the binge period (usually within a 2-hour period), the person feels he or she cannot stop eating; there is a lack of control over eating. The purging then is a compensatory behavior to prevent becoming overweight. The vomiting and diarrhea can cause deficits of sodium, potassium, and magnesium. The hydrochloric acid from vomiting causes irritation and infection of the pharynx, esophagus, and salivary glands; erosion of teeth; and dental caries (Whitney, Cataldo, and Rolfes, 1998).

ANOREXIA NERVOSA

Anorexia nervosa is a psychologic disorder related to body image and an abnormal fear of becoming obese. This disorder is commonly seen during adolescence and young adulthood, primarily among girls. It is characterized by prolonged reduction of food intake, resulting in emaciation, and is often associated with emotional stress or conflict. The starvation that results contributes to anemia, amenorrhea, irregular heart rate, slowed gastrointestinal tract motility, and impaired immune function. Other effects of starvation include low serum albumin; dry, thin skin; abnormal nerve functioning; reduced body temperature; and hypotension. (Whitney, Cataldo, and Rolfes, 1998).

VITAMIN D DEFICIENCY

A deficiency in vitamin D is called rickets in children and adult rickets or osteomalacia in adults. Normally vitamin D facilitates the production of a protein that binds calcium. Inadequate vitamin D in the diet along with inadequate exposure to sunlight results in rickets. With the lack of vitamin D there is inadequate calcium-binding protein to absorb calcium from the gut. In children the signs are faulty calcification, resulting in bowed legs, slow bone growth, deformed ribs, prolonged closing of fontanels, slow eruption of teeth, and malformed, decay-prone teeth (see Fig. 10-8). The effect on the neuromuscular system is lax smooth muscles, causing protrusion of the abdomen and muscle spasms.

Adults who develop osteomalacia are more often women who have repeated pregnancies and periods of lactation, low calcium intake, and little exposure to the sun. Signs of osteomalacia are demineralization of bones, causing deformities and fractures of limbs, spine, and thorax and pain in the pelvis, lower back, and legs (Whitney, Cataldo, and Rolfes, 1998).

THIAMIN DEFICIENCY

Thiamin (vitamin B_1) deficiencies are commonly diagnosed in individuals with chronic alcohol ingestion and in the homeless due to poor dietary intake. The medical term for thiamin deficiency is beriberi, but this term is rarely used. Sources of thiamin are pork, ham, bacon, whole grains or enriched breads and cereals, legumes, and nuts. Thiamin is needed for energy metabolism and nerve function. Signs of thiamin deficiency include cardiovascular system changes such as edema, enlarged heart, abnormal heart rhythms, and heart failure. Nervous and muscular systems signs are muscle degeneration, weakness, painful calf muscles, low morale, difficulty walking, loss of ankle and knee jerk reflexes, and mental confusion (Whitney, Cataldo, and Rolfes, 1998) (Fig. 10-9).

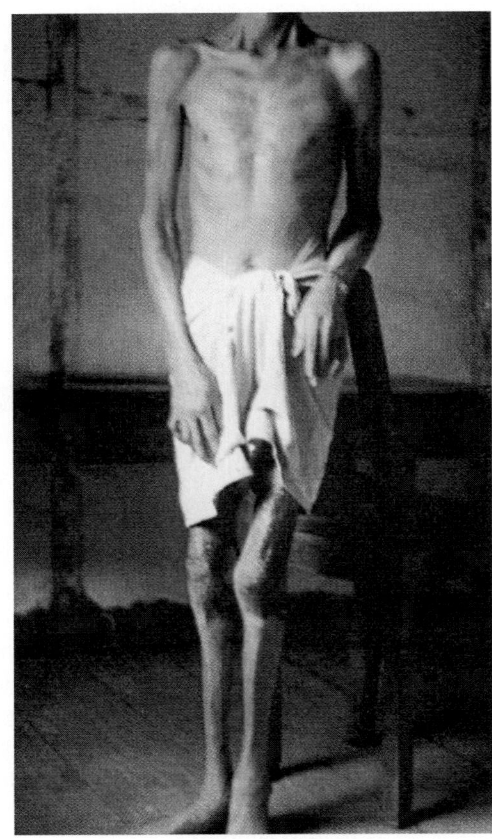

Fig. 10-9 Severe thiamin deficiency. (From McLaren, 1992.)

CLINICAL APPLICATION and CRITICAL THINKING

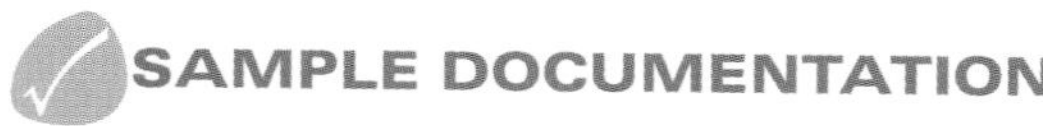

SAMPLE DOCUMENTATION

CASE 1

L.D. is a 73-year-old woman who comes as a new patient to the clinic.

Subjective Data

A 73-year-old woman, new to the community; is seeking health care professional for management of hypertension. States in good health; current medication: diuretic (furosemide 40 mg daily) for blood pressure control. No chronic illness other than hypertension, admits to always having a weight problem, but has had no weight changes for several years. Appetite described as "good," eats three meals per day; has a preference for fried foods. Verbalizes no food dislikes or intolerances. Has been told to eat a low-salt diet in the past, admits does not know what that means. Drinks 5 to 6 glasses of water per day. Believes she is at risk for "heart problems" and would like assistance reducing her risk.

Objective Data

Vital signs: Temperature, 98.3° F (36.8° C); Pulse rate, 82 beats/min; Respirations, 18; Blood pressure, 142/100 mm Hg. Height, 5′3″ (160 cm); weight, 155 lb (70 kg); BMI, 27.5; DBW, 115 lb; 35% over DBW.
Serum cholesterol, 220 mg/dl; HDL, 55 mg/dl; LDL, 258 mg/dl.
General survey: Moderate obesity; walks without difficulty.
Skin: Without dryness, lesions, or edema; pink skin tone.
Hair: Gray; thick, full.
Mucous membranes: Pink, moist without lesions or cracks.
Eyes: Wears glasses; conjunctiva pink, no lesions or discharge.

Functional Health Patterns Involved

- Health perception–health management
- Nutrition–metabolic

Medical Diagnosis

Hypertension, overweight

Nursing Diagnosis and Collaborative Problems

- *Altered nutrition: more than body requirements* related to food intake/energy expenditure imbalance as manifested by: BMI-27.5.
- *Health-seeking behaviors:* desire for reducing risk factor for cardiovascular disease.

PC: Coronary artery disease related to risk factors.
PC: Hypokalemia related to diuretic therapy.

CASE 2

B.A is 43-year-old man who seeks a preemployment examination.

Subjective Data

A 43-year-old man; employment examination for general laborer with construction company. States health is excellent. No medical problems; no medications; denies drug use; drinks 1 to 2 beers each PM. Appetite described as "huge," eats everything in sight. Eats three meals a day, plus snacks between meals. Has always had problems keeping weight up. Works construction; very physically demanding job. No special dietary needs; no supplementation. Drinks coffee in AM.; several glasses of milk and water daily; becomes easily dehydrated on days he works.

Objective Data

Vital signs: Temperature, 98.8° F (37° C); Pulse rate, 72 beats/min; Respirations, 14; Blood pressure, 110/68 mm Hg. Height, 6′2″ (109 cm); Weight, 155 lb (70 kg); BMI, 20.3; DBW, 177 lb; 12% below DBW.
General survey: Tall, slender; muscles well developed; well defined.
Skin: Smooth, dry, without lesions.
Mucous membranes: Moist, pink, without cracks or lesions.
Hair: Dark brown with some graying; thin, balding.

Functional Health Patterns Involved

- Nutrition–metabolic

Medical Diagnosis

None.

Nursing Diagnosis and Collaborative Problems

- *Altered nutrition: less than body requirements* related to energy exceeding nutritional intake as manifested by: Current body weight 12% below DBW.
- *Risk for fluid volume deficit* related to insufficient fluid intake for exercise.

CRITICAL THINKING QUESTIONS

1. An 85-year-old man is admitted to the hospital with dehydration and generalized weakness. He currently is 5′9″ (175 cm) tall and weighs 150 lb (68 kg). He suffered a mild cerebrovascular accident (CVA) 3 months ago. His wife states that since that time he has lost weight. What should specifically be addressed as his nutritional status is evaluated?

2. A mother brings her 1-week-old baby to the nurse practitioner's office for a well-baby visit. How is nutritional status assessed?
3. Two men are seen in a clinic. The first man is 5′ 3″ (160 cm) and weighs 160 lb (72.7 kg). The second man is 6′4″ (187 cm) and weighs 220 lb (100 kg). Both men have a BMI of about 26. How is it possible they have the same BMI?
4. A 52-year-old man comes to the clinic complaining of decreased appetite and weight loss over the last 6 months. He is 5′10″ (178 cm) tall and currently weighs 145 lb. He tells you that his usual weight is 170 lb (77 kg). Calculate his BMI, the DBW, and the percentage of DBW. Also calculate his percentage of weight loss based on his UBW. Based on these values, what conclusions can you make?

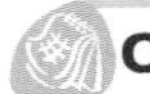

CASE STUDY

Marian is a 45-year-old woman who is brought to the hospital after an episode of fainting.

Interview Data

Marian states she has been very tired lately and gets short of breath and fatigued very easily. She also complains of cracks in the corners of her mouth that won't heal. When asked about her diet, she tells the nurse she is a "new vegetarian." She states she started a vegetarian diet about 4 months ago "to prevent diseases and because animals are unclean." She acknowledges weight loss since starting the diet but states, "I am healthy because of what I eat and because I am thin." She refuses foods that contain meat or animal products. Her diet is described as "healthy," typically eating beans, rice, breads, and salad. She is not specific about portions, stating, "I eat the amount I am hungry for." Her fluid intake consists of coffee, tea, and water. She does not use drugs or alcohol. She also tells the nurse that her financial resources are very limited.

Examination Data

- **Vital signs:** Blood pressure, 118/76 mm Hg; Pulse rate, 92 beats/min; Respirations, 20; Temperature, 98.2° F (36.8° C); Height, 5′4″ (162 cm); Weight, 110 lb (50 kg).
- **General observation:** Very thin, protruding bony prominence to cheeks and clavicles.
- **Skin:** Warm, very dry with scaling—especially on arms/legs.
- **Hair:** Thin, dull, easily plucked.
- **Oral cavity:** Pink, moist mucous membranes without lesions. Teeth present, in good repair. Cracks noted in corners of mouth.
- **Eyes:** Conjunctiva pale; no drainage.

1. What data deviate from normal findings, suggesting a need for further investigation?
2. What additional information should the nurse ask or assess for?
3. In what functional health patterns does data deviate from normal?
4. What nursing diagnosis and/or collaborative problems should be considered for this situation?

REMEMBER to check out your companion CD-ROM

11 Skin, Hair, and Nails

www.mosby.com/MERLIN/wilson/assessment/

ANATOMY AND PHYSIOLOGY

The skin is an elastic, self-regenerating, protective cover for the entire body, protecting against microbial and foreign-substance invasion and minor physical trauma while keeping vital body fluids and components safely contained. Protection is its most important function, but it is not the only one. The skin and its appendages provide the body with its primary contact with the outside world, providing sensory input about the environment. Its sensitive surface detects and reports—via nerve endings and specialized receptors—comfort factors such as temperature and surface textures, enabling the body to adapt through either temperature regulation or position changes. This regulation of body temperature is accomplished continuously through radiation, conduction, convection, and evaporation. Other functions of the skin include production of vitamin D; excretion of sweat, urea, and lactic acid; expression of emotion (e.g., blushing); and even repair of its own surface wounds by exaggerating the normal process of cell replacement.

The skin is composed of three layers that are functionally related: the epidermis, the dermis, and the hypodermis. The main components of each of these layers and their functional and spatial relationships are shown in Fig. 11-1.

EPIDERMIS

The outermost layer, the epidermis, has an exposed, cornified layer that serves as a protective barrier and regulates water loss. The underlying epidermal layers fold into the dermis and contain hair roots, apocrine sweat glands, eccrine sweat glands, and sebaceous glands. Hair and nails arise from these underlying layers and are composed primarily of keratin (produced by keratin cells, which are generated in the epidermis) (Habif, 1996). Melanocytes, located in the base epidermal layer, secrete melanin, which provides pigment for the skin and hair and serves as a shield against ultraviolet radiation. The epidermis is avascular and is shed and replaced with new cells about every 14 to 30 days (Lewis et al, 2000).

DERMIS

The dermis is made up of highly vascular connective tissue. The blood vessels dilate and constrict in response to external heat and cold and to internal stimuli such as anxiety or hemorrhage, resulting in the regulation of body temperature and blood pressure. The dermal blood nourishes the epidermis, and the dermal connective tissue provides support for the outer layer. The dermis also contains sensory fibers that react to touch, pain, and temperature. The arrangement of connective tissue enables the dermis to stretch and contract with body movement. Dermal thickness varies from 1 to 4 mm in different parts of the body.

HYPODERMIS

The hypodermis is composed primarily of loose connective tissue interspersed with subcutaneous fat. These fatty cells help to retain heat and to provide a protective cushion and storage for calories.

APPENDAGES

At junctions between the epidermis and the dermis, the hair, nails, and several glands are formed; the skin glands include the eccrine sweat glands, the apocrine sweat glands, and the sebaceous glands.

Hair

Hair is formed by epidermal cells in the dermis. Each hair consists of a root, a shaft, and a follicle (the root and its covering). At the base of the follicle, the papilla—a loop of capillaries—supplies nourishment for growth. Melanocytes in the shaft provide color.

Nails

Nails are really epidermal cells converted to hard plates of keratin. The site of nail growth occurs at the white crescent-shaped area extending beyond the proximal end of the nail (Fig. 11-2).

Eccrine Sweat Glands

These glands regulate body temperature by water secretion through the skin's surface. They are distributed almost everywhere throughout the skin's surface.

Apocrine Sweat Glands

These structures are much larger, deeper, and not nearly as widely spread as the eccrine glands; they are found only in the axillae, nipples, areolae, anogenital area, eyelids, and external ears. In response to emotional stimuli, the glands se-

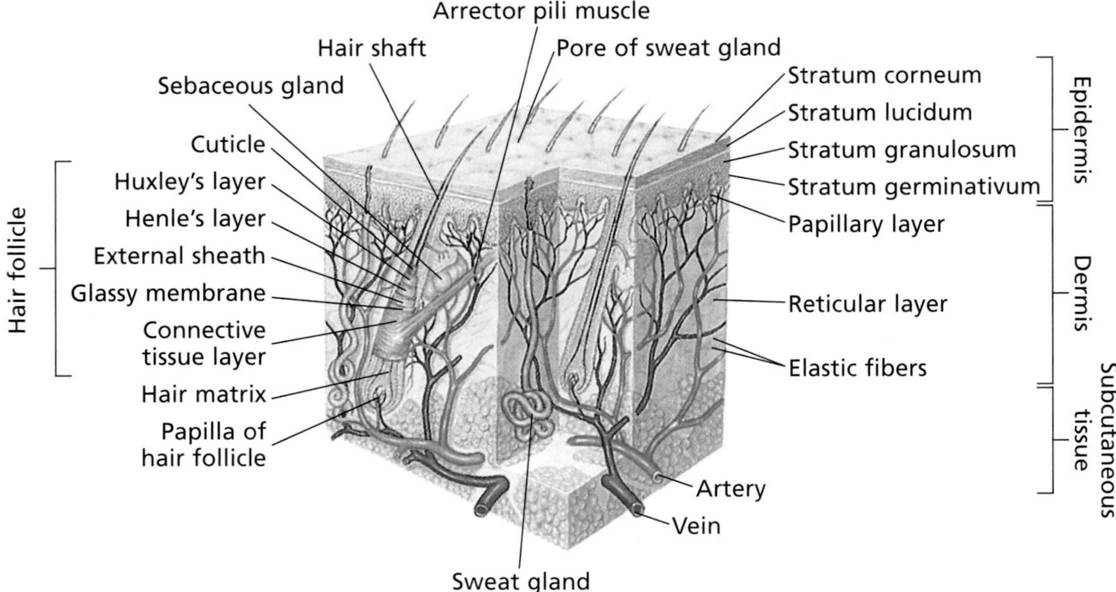

Fig. 11-1 Anatomic structures of the skin. (From Seidel et al, 1999.)

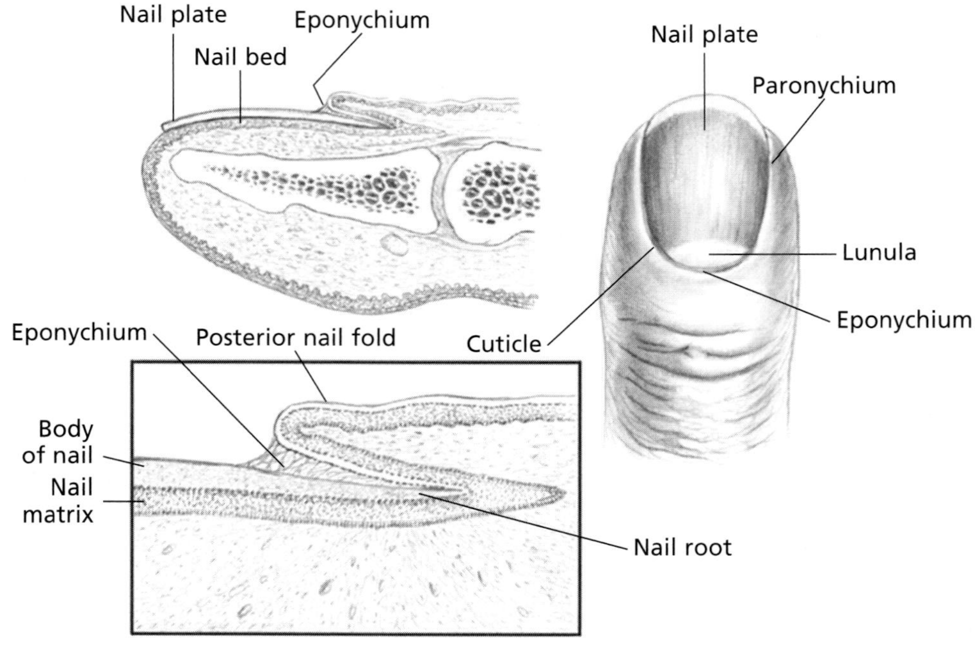

Fig. 11-2 Structures of the nail. (From Thompson et al, 1997.)

crete an odorless fluid containing protein, carbohydrates, and other substances. Decomposition of apocrine sweat produces what we associate with body odor.

Sebaceous Glands

These glands secrete a lipid-rich substance, sebum, which keeps the skin and hair from drying out. The secretion, which is stimulated by sex hormone activity, varies throughout the life span, according to hormone levels at different stages of the life span.

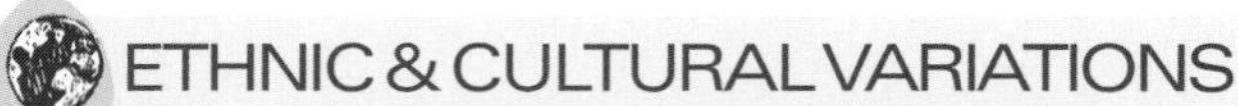

American Indians, Alaskan natives, Pacific Islanders, and Asian Americans have fewer apocrine glands than whites. They sweat less and produce a milder body odor. In Alaskan natives, most eccrine sweat glands are located in the face. Chloride concentrations in sweat decrease as skin color darkens. (Matsunaga, 1962; Petrakis, 1971.)

HEALTH HISTORY

Skin, Hair, and Nails

QUESTIONS	RATIONALE
PRESENT HEALTH STATUS	
➤ How would you describe your overall health?	■ Determine what the client's perception of his or her overall health is. This may give clues as to diagnosed or undiagnosed chronic conditions.
➤ Do you have any chronic illnesses? If so, describe.	■ Some chronic illnesses cause changes to the skin such as pruritus, excessive dryness, and skin lesions.
➤ Do you take any medications? If so, what do you take and how often?	■ Both prescription and over-the-counter medications should be noted. Assess if the client is taking medications as prescribed. Medications can cause a number of side effects to the skin, including allergic reactions in the form of hives or rashes, lesions associated with photosensitivity, or other systemic effects such as acne breakouts, thinning of the skin, and stretch marks (Nicol, 1997).
➤ How would you describe the condition of your skin and your hair?	■ Determine what the client's perception of his or her skin and hair is.
➤ What do you do to keep your skin healthy? (hygiene measures, use of lotions, protection)	■ Health care practices may be clues for underlying skin problems. Specifically determine frequency and products used.
➤ Do you routinely do anything to limit or avoid sun exposure to your skin? Do you use sunscreen protection?	■ Sun exposure/protection practices are important data to identify clients with risk factors for skin cancers.
➤ Have you noticed any changes in the way your skin and hair looks or feels? Any changes in the sensation of your skin? If so, where? Describe.	■ Ask the client if he or she has noticed changes as opposed to asking them if they have any problems. A client may have a pathologic skin condition yet may not be aware of it or may not consider it a problem. This information helps identify clients at risk for injury to their skin or development of skin ulcers.
➤ Do you often have wounds? When you have a wound, describe how it heals.	■ Wounds should heal quickly. Those that do not may indicate metabolic problems or problems with circulation, or they may be associated with a neoplastic disease.
➤ Does the ingestion of certain foods cause itching, burning, or eruption of rashes? If so, which ones? Do you have skin irritation when in contact with certain types of clothing, metals, chemicals, or plants?	■ Many clients have known food or drug allergies that result in skin rash or lesions. Keep in mind that not all skin allergies are caused by food or medication; they can also be caused by contact with a substance including wool, metal, plants, etc.

QUESTIONS | RATIONALE

Past Medical History or Family History

➤ Have you had problems with your skin in the past? If so, describe.

■ Past skin problems are important to document. These may be clues to current skin lesions.

➤ Has anyone in your family ever had skin problems? Cancer of the skin?

■ A family history helps to determine predisposition to certain skin disorders. Some skin disorders have familial or genetic links, others may be associated with lifestyle or living environment.

PROBLEM-BASED HISTORY

The most commonly reported problems related to the skin include rashes, discomfort, pruritus, and lesions. As with symptoms in all areas of health assessment, a symptom analysis is completed, which includes the location, quality, quantity, chronology, setting, associated manifestations, alleviating factors, and aggravating factors (see Box 4-2 in Chapter 4).

Skin

Rash

➤ When did the rash start? Where did you first notice the rash? Describe what the rash looked like initially: flat? raised? How long has the rash persisted?

■ Determine onset, location, and duration of the rash.

➤ Does the rash itch or burn? What makes it better? Worse? (Does exposure to the sun make it worse?) What have you done to treat it? Have you noticed any other symptoms associated with this rash such as joint pains, fatigue, or fever?

■ Document accompanying symptoms, aggravating and relieving factors, and self-treatment factors.

➤ Do you have any known allergies to pets, foods, drugs, plants, soaps, deodorants, etc? Are you currently taking any medications, either prescription or over-the-counter? If so, what? Does anyone else in your family have a similar rash? Have you been exposed to others with a similar rash? If so, have they been seen or treated for their problem?

■ A rash is not generally a disease in itself, but rather a symptom of an allergic response, skin disorder, or systemic illness. Some of these questions help to differentiate the cause of the rash.

➤ Do you have or have you recently had any fleabites or been exposed to any environmental irritants?

■ If the client has fleabites, he or she should be evaluated for plague. Prevalence of the disease is highest in the western states of Arizona, New Mexico, Colorado, and California.

Pain/Discomfort to Skin

➤ Have you had or do you currently have pain or discomfort associated with your skin? If so, when did the pain start? Describe the location of the pain. Does the pain or discomfort extend from where it started? Does it spread anywhere? Does the pain stay on the skin surface, or does it go deep inside?

■ Document onset and location of the pain.

➤ Describe the pain or discomfort—sharp, dull, achy, burning, itching, etc. How bad is your pain on a scale of 1 to 10? Is the pain constant, or does it come and go? If constant, does the pain vary? If pain comes and goes, how long does the pain last?

■ Document characteristics of the pain or discomfort.

➤ What triggers the pain? Are there things that make the pain worse? Better? (Box 11-1.)

■ Document aggravating and relieving factors for the discomfort.

Itching (Pruritus) and Hives

➤ When did the itching or the hives first start? Where did it start? Has it spread?

■ Document onset and location of the itching or hives.

➤ Does anything make the itching worse? Is there anything that relieves it? What have you done to treat yourself?

■ Document characteristics and aggravating and relieving factors of the itching or hives.

QUESTIONS

RATIONALE

Box 11-1 Focus on Pain: Skin, Hair, and Nails

When a client complains of pain and/or discomfort associated with the skin, hair, and nails, the nurse should conduct a focused symptom analysis, including onset, location, pattern, intensity, and description of the pain; aggravating and alleviating factors; and treatment modalities. Pain and discomfort are associated with a number of skin and nail disorders ranging from mild discomfort (such as pruritus associated with dry skin) to intense, severe pain (such as pain associated with a large abscess or herpes zoster). The degree of pain one experiences is highly individualized and may vary by the severity or stage of the disorder. Additionally, the effect of a lesion on body image can have a tremendous impact on the pain perceived by an individual.

➤ What were the circumstances when you first noticed the itching? Taking medications? Contact with possible allergens such as animals, foods, drugs, plants?

■ Pruritus may be caused by an allergic response or may occur secondary to an infestation of scabies, lice, or insect bites. Systemic diseases such as biliary cirrhosis and some types of cancer such as lymphoma may also cause pruritus.

➤ Do you have dry or sensitive skin?

■ Dry or sensitive skin may make an individual more prone to itching or hives.

Change in Skin Color or Change in Moles

➤ Has there been any generalized change in your skin color, such as a yellowish tone or paleness?

■ Changes in overall skin color may have a number of causes, including medications, anemia, or an internal systemic disease such as liver disease causing jaundice.

➤ Have there been any localized changes in your skin color, such as discoloration of one or both feet, bluish tone to the fingernails, or areas of bruises or patches?

■ Localized changes may be associated with changes in tissue perfusion, causing a discoloration to the affected area, cyanosis, bruising (may be a sign of a hematologic condition, abuse, frequent falls, etc.) or vitiligo—a loss of pigmentation in the skin.

➤ Have you noticed any change in a mole, or are you getting more moles? If so, describe. (Changes in moles may include color, shape, texture, tenderness, bleeding, or itching.)

■ A changing or irregular mole may be a sign suggesting a malignant neoplasm or melanoma.

Skin Texture

➤ Has the texture of your skin changed, such as skin thinning, or has it become fragile?

■ Changes in the skin texture may be a normal change associated with aging or indicate a metabolic or nutritional problem.

➤ Do you have excessively dry (xerosis) or oily (seborrhea) skin? If so, is it seasonal, intermittent, or continuous? What do you do to treat it?

■ A history of dry skin may provide information about an existing system disease (e.g., thyroid disease), or it may be related to an environmental condition such as low humidity or hard water. Dry skin may also be associated with poor skin lubrication.

QUESTIONS	RATIONALE
Wounds	
➤ Do you have any wounds? If so, for how long?	■ The location of a wound and how long it has been there are important to document.
➤ What have you done to treat the wound?	■ Self-treatment of a wound may provide insight to the appearance of a wound, particularly if client reports problems associated with wound healing.
➤ Do you have problems with wound healing?	■ A history of problems associated with wound healing can point to nutritional or metabolic problems or infection or indicate poor circulation.
Hair	
➤ Has the condition or quality of your hair changed in the past 6 to 12 months? If so, describe. When did you notice the change? Did the change occur suddenly?	■ Establish onset and nature of the changes with the hair.
➤ Was the change related to stress? Fever? Other illness? Itching? What kinds of hair products have been used on your hair recently?	■ Reports of changes in the hair such as excessive dryness or brittle hair may indicate stress or systemic disease. Exposure to hair care products may account for changes in texture or condition of hair.
➤ Has there been a change in your diet in the last few months?	■ Changes in hair texture can be affected by one's diet.
➤ Have you noticed any changes in the distribution of hair growth on your arms or legs?	■ A decrease in hair growth on an extremity, particularly the lower extremity, may indicate problems with circulation. Increases in hair growth may be caused by an ovarian or adrenal tumor.
Nails	
➤ Do you have any problems with your nails? If so, when did you first notice the changes, and what are those changes?	■ The health and consistency of the fingernails and toenails may be an important sign about the client's general health. Establish onset of the changes or problem.
➤ Have you been exposed to or do you handle any chemicals at home or work?	■ Exposure to chemicals can cause the nails to change in appearance or consistency.
➤ Are your nails brittle? Have you noticed a pitting type of pattern to your nail?	■ Pitting, brittle nails, crumbling, and changes in color can be caused by nutritional deficiencies, systemic diseases, or localized fungal infections.
➤ Do you chew your nails? Do you have now or have you ever had an infection of the nail or around the nail bed? If so, describe.	■ Clients who have a habit of nail biting may use the biting as an unconscious way to handle stress. The nails may show signs of local infection such as fungal infection.
➤ Do you have difficulty keeping your nails clean? Do your nails appear dirty?	■ Hyperthyroidism may cause the nail to separate from the nail bed and make the nail appear "dirty."

RISK FACTORS

COMMON RISK FACTORS FOR PROBLEMS ASSOCIATED WITH Skin, Hair, and Nails

- Systemic disease (liver, kidney, collagen, endocrine)
- Previous trauma or surgery
- Infection—viral, bacterial, or fungal
- Immobility
- Frequent sun exposure (especially unprotected)
- Exposure to chemicals
- Exposures to allergens
- Taking medications associated with photosensitive response

EXAMINATION

Equipment

- Magnifying lens to visualize lesions or skin texture as needed
- Centimeter ruler (clear, see-through plastic if possible) to measure size of lesions
- Light source (gooseneck lamp, penlight, flashlight, etc) to aid in inspection of lesions
- Wood's lamp (optional) to identify fungal lesions
- Gloves to palpate lesions (if the client has open lesions)

PROCEDURES AND TECHNIQUES WITH NORMAL FINDINGS | **ABNORMAL FINDINGS**

SKIN

Start with a general survey noting the color of the skin, general pigmentation, vascularity or bruising, and lesions or discoloration. Note any unusual odors. Next, examine the skin more closely, moving systematically from the head and neck to the trunk, arms, and legs. Then move behind the client and carefully examine the back. If the client is lying down, the buttocks should also be examined at this time. In a head-to-toe assessment the skin can be examined in conjunction with other body systems. Before you begin, be sure to have adequate lighting. Subtle changes to the skin may be missed without adequate lighting (Butler, 1997).

➤**INSPECT the skin for general color.** Inspect the skin for general color and uniformity of color. The skin color should be consistent over the body surface, with the exception of vascular areas such as the cheeks, upper chest, and genitalia, which may appear pink or have a reddish purple tone. The normal range of skin color varies from whitish pink to olive tones to deep brown. Table 11-1 describes special considerations for examining clients with dark skin. Sun-exposed areas may show evidence of a slightly darker pigmentation or freckles.

■ By carefully inspecting the skin, you may find evidence of local or systemic disease. Signs of particular importance include the following:

- *Cyanosis:* In light skin it will appear as a blue tinge, especially of the palpebral conjunctiva, nail beds, lips, oral membranes, palms, and soles of feet; in dark skin cyanosis will appear as an ashen or gray color of the lips and under the tongue and loss of the normal "shine" or "glow" of well-oxygenated skin.

Table 11-1 Special Considerations for Examining Dark-Skinned Clients

CLINICAL SIGN	LIGHT SKIN	DARK SKIN
Cyanosis	Grayish blue tone, especially in nail beds, earlobes, lips, mucous membranes, palms, and soles of feet	Ashen-gray color most easily seen in the conjunctiva of the eye, oral mucous membranes, and nail beds.
Ecchymosis (bruise)	Dark red, purple, yellow, or green color, depending on age of bruise	Deeper bluish or black tone, difficult to see unless it occurs in an area of light pigmentation.
Erythema	Reddish tone with evidence of increased skin temperature secondary to inflammation	Deeper brown or purple skin tone with evidence of increased skin temperature secondary to inflammation.
Jaundice	Yellowish color of skin, sclera of eyes, fingernails, palms of hands, and oral mucosa	Yellowish green color most obviously seen in sclera of eye (don't confuse with yellow eye pigmentation, which may be evident in dark-skinned clients), palms of hands, and soles of feet.
Pallor	Pale skin color that may appear white	Skin tone will appear lighter than normal. Light-skinned African Americans may have yellowish brown skin; dark-skinned African Americans may appear ashen. Specifically evident is a loss of the underlying healthy red tones of the skin.
Petechiae	Lesions appear as small, reddish purple pinpoints	Difficult to see; may be evident in the buccal mucosa of the mouth or sclera of the eye.
Rash	May be visualized as well as felt with light palpation	Not easily visualized but may be felt with light palpation.
Scar	Generally heals, showing narrow scar line	Frequently has keloid development, resulting in a thickened, raised scar.

PROCEDURES AND TECHNIQUES WITH NORMAL FINDINGS

ABNORMAL FINDINGS

- *Pallor:* In light skin it will appear as a loss of "rosy glow" in skin, appearing pale instead; in dark skin pallor will appear as an ashen or gray appearance of black skin, more yellowish brown in brown skin, with loss of the underlying red tones. Pallor is easiest to see in the mucous membranes, lips, nail beds, and the palpebral conjunctiva.
- *Jaundice:* Light-skinned clients will have a yellowish color, seen most clearly in the sclera of the eyes, oral mucosa, palms of hands, and soles of feet; dark-skinned clients will also have a yellowing of the sclera of the eyes, oral mucosa, palms of hands, and soles of feet.

PROCEDURES AND TECHNIQUES WITH NORMAL FINDINGS

➤INSPECT the skin for areas of variation in skin color. Almost all healthy individuals have variations in skin color. Some variations are normal for individuals of darker skin pigmentation. Also note intentional changes in skin color to certain areas including coining and tattoos. If a tattoo is present, its location and the characteristics of the surrounding areas should be examined and documented. Normal variations of the skin include such findings as the following:

- *Striae:* Silver or pink "stretch marks" secondary to weight gain or pregnancy (Fig. 11-3).

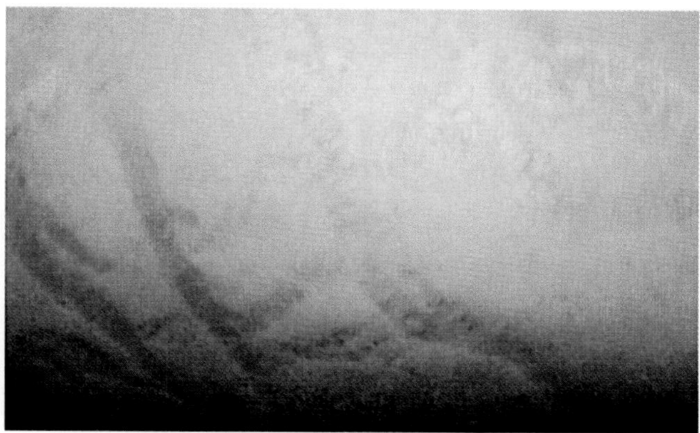

Fig. 11-3 Striae. (From Seidel et al, 1999; courtesy Antoinette Hood, MD, Department of Dermatology, University of Indiana School of Medicine, Indianapolis.)

- *Vitiligo:* An area of unpigmented skin secondary to a lack of melanin. Vitiligo may appear in all races but is more prevalent in dark-skinned races (see Table 11-2 on pp. 170-173).
- *Moles (pigmented nevi):* May be tan to dark brown in color and may be raised or flat (see Table 11-2).
- *Freckles:* Small, flat macules that may appear anywhere on the body. The most common locations are on the face, arms, and back.
- *Birthmarks:* May be tan, reddish, or brown and are generally flat. Types of birthmarks include port-wine stains (nevus flammeus), strawberry mark (immature hemangioma), cavernous hemangioma, and mongolian spots (see section on infant age-related variations).
- *Calluses:* Callused areas most commonly appear on hands, feet, elbows, and knees and may appear yellowish.

CULTURAL NOTE

- "Coining" is a treatment practiced by Cambodians and Vietnamese. The body is rubbed vigorously with a coin while exerting pressure until red marks appear over the bony prominence of the rib cage on the back and chest. Marks created by this treatment frequently have been mistaken as signs of abuse or mistreatment.
- "Cupping" is a treatment for arthritis, stomachaches, bruises, and paralysis. A cup is heated and placed on the skin. As a result of the heat, the cup adheres to the skin and may leave a reddened area or mark. This is practiced by Latin American and Russian cultures. (Monteleone, 1996)

ABNORMAL FINDINGS

■ Marked hyperpigmentation is an abnormal finding. A new tattoo should be examined for presence of infection.

Table 11-2 Primary Skin Lesions

SKIN LESIONS	EXAMPLES		
MACULE A flat, circumscribed area that is a change in the color of the skin; less than 1 cm in diameter	Freckles, flat moles (nevi), petechiae, measles, scarlet fever	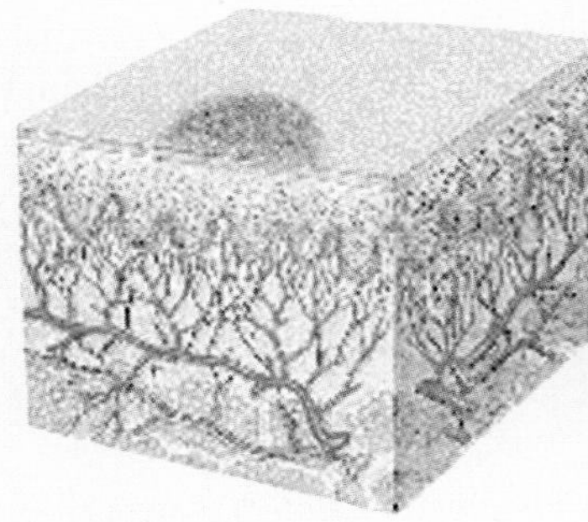	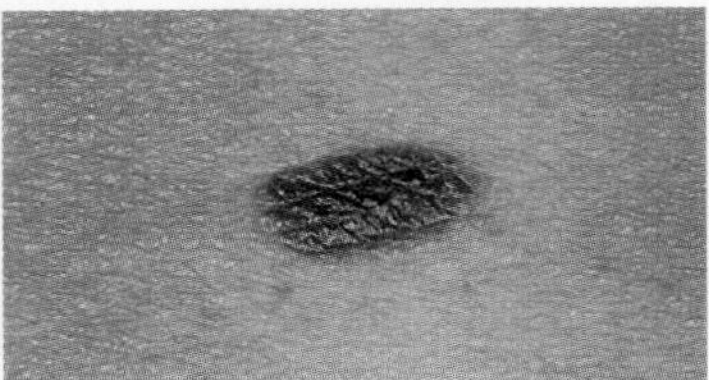 Flat nevi. (From Habif, 1990.)
PAPULE An elevated, firm, circumscribed area less than 1 cm in diameter	Wart (verruca), elevated moles, lichen planus, cherry angioma, skin tag	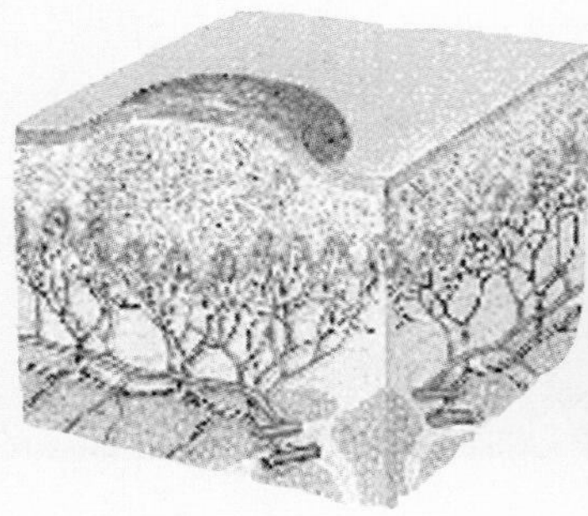	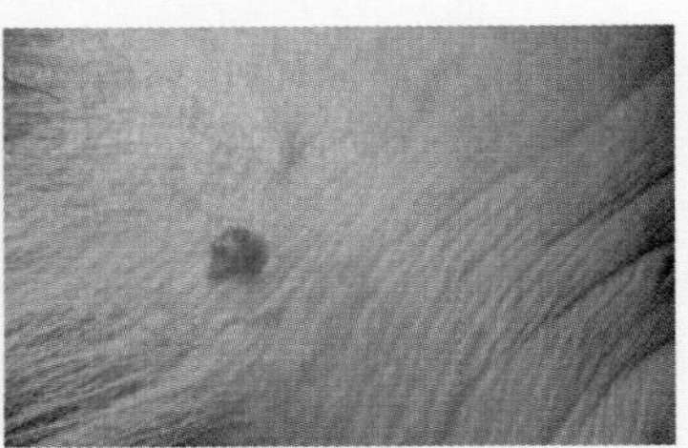 Cherry angioma. (From Baran et al, 1991.)
PATCH A flat, nonpalpable, irregular-shaped macule more than 1 cm in diameter	Vitiligo, port-wine stains, mongolian spots, café au lait spots	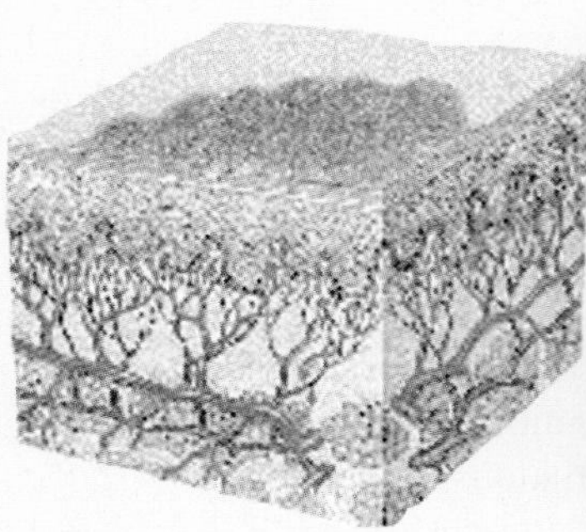	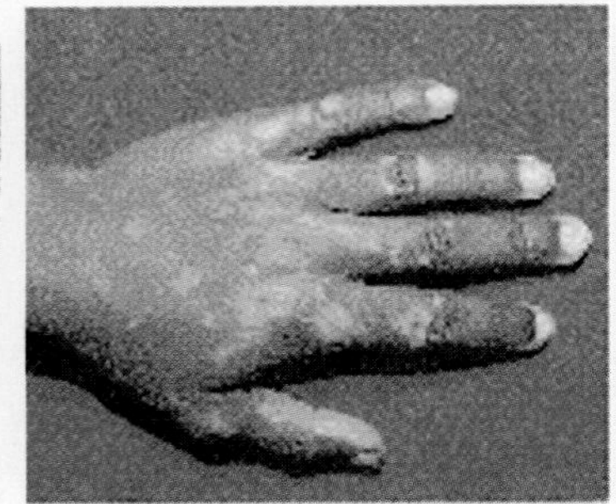 Vitiligo. (From Weston and Lane, 1991.)
PLAQUE Elevated, firm, and rough lesion with flat top surface greater than 1 cm in diameter	Psoriasis, seborrheic and actinic keratoses, eczema	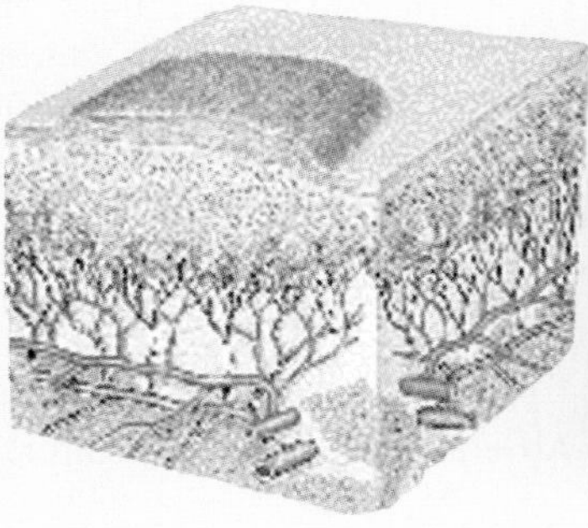	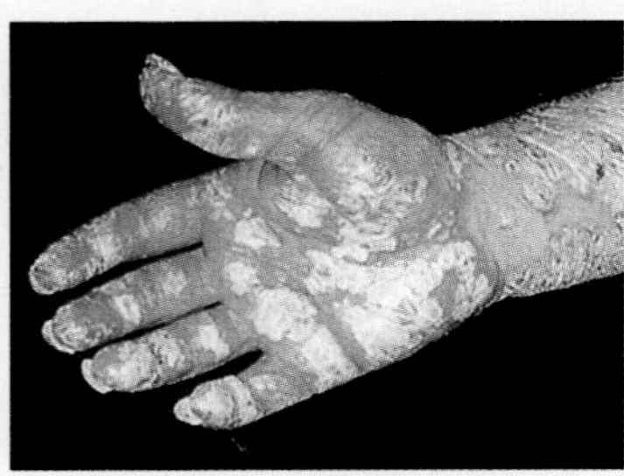 Plaque type of psorias. (From Goldstein and Goldstein, 1997.)

Table 11-2 Primary Skin Lesions—cont'd

SKIN LESIONS	EXAMPLES
WHEAL Elevated irregular-shaped area of cutaneous edema; solid, transient; variable diameter	Insect bites, urticaria, allergic reaction, lupus
NODULE Elevated, firm, circumscribed lesion; deeper in dermis than a papule; 1 to 2 cm in diameter	Dermatofibroma erythema nodosum, lipomas, melanoma, hemangioma, neurofibroma
TUMOR Elevated and solid lesion; may or may not be clearly demarcated; deeper in dermis; greater than 2 cm in diameter	Neoplasms, lipoma, hemangioma
VESICLE Elevated, circumscribed, superficial, not into dermis; filled with serous fluid; less than 1 cm in diameter	Varicella (chickenpox), herpes zoster (shingles), impetigo, acute eczema

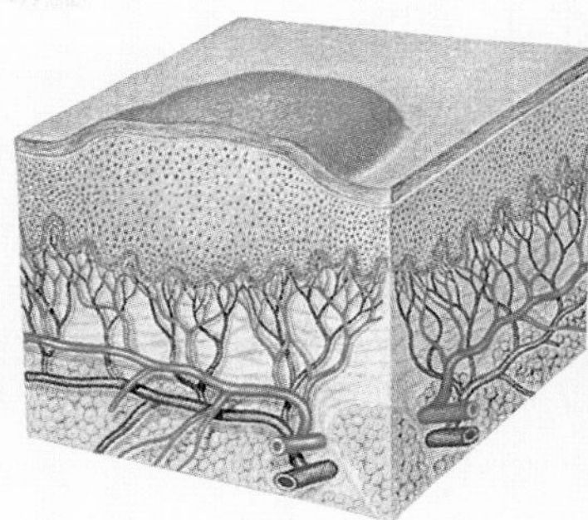
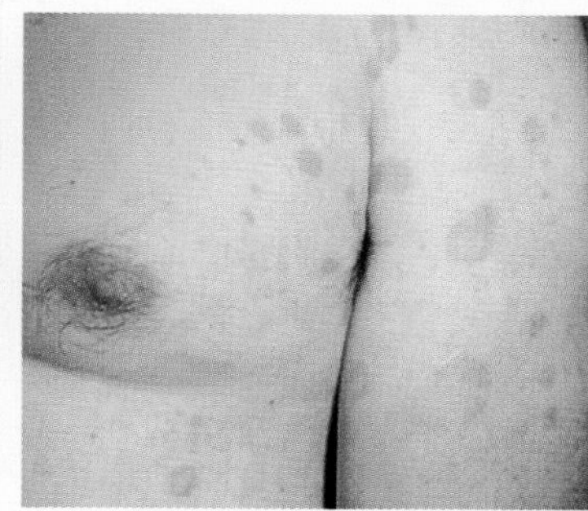

Wheals of urticaria.
(From Goldstein and Goldstein, 1997.)

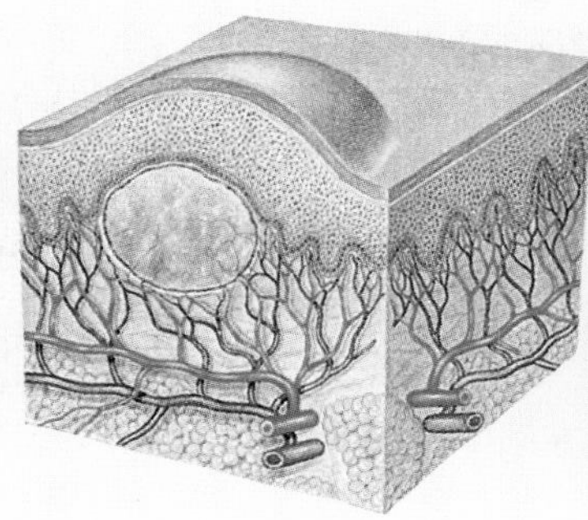
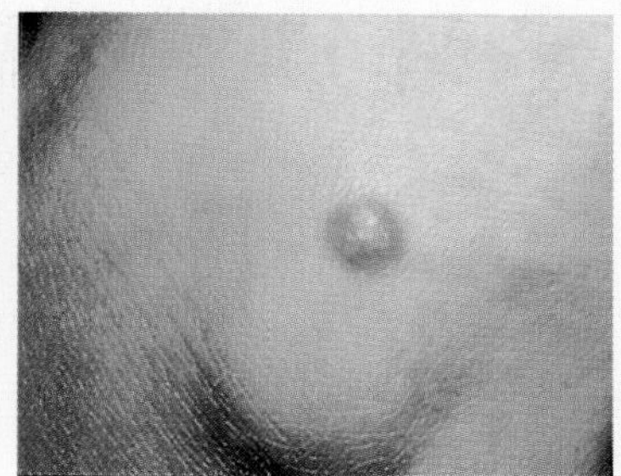

Dermatofibroma.
(From Goldstein and Goldstein, 1997.)

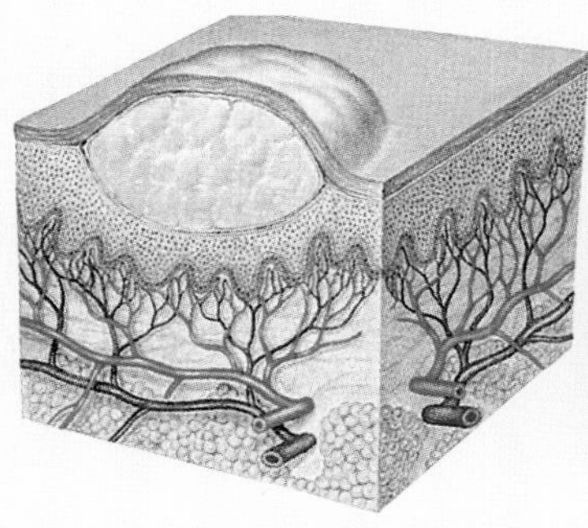
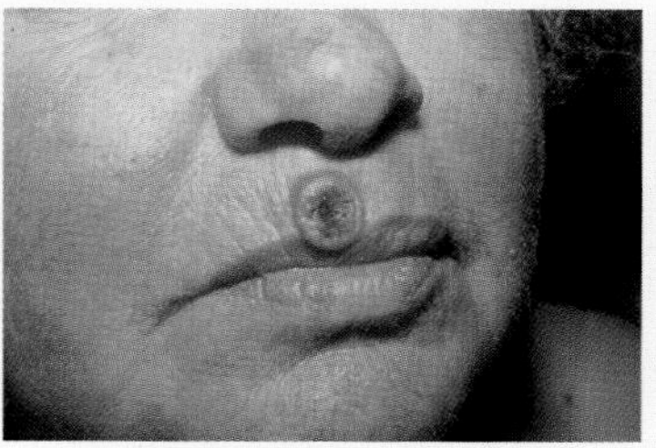

Tumor of upper lip.
(From Goldstein and Goldstein, 1997.)

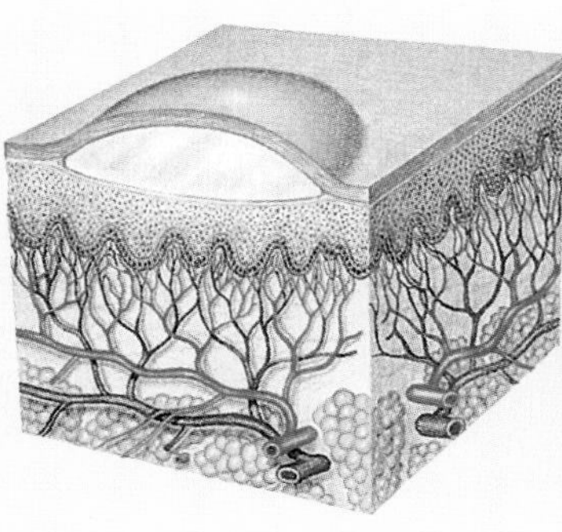
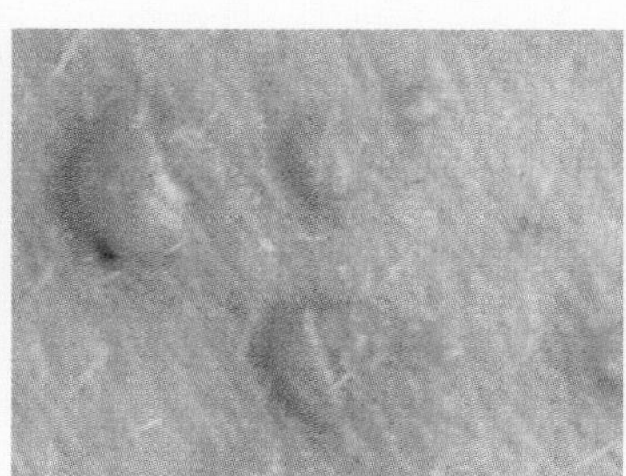

Vesicles. (From Farrar et al, 1992.)

Continued

Table 11-2 Primary Skin Lesions—cont'd

SKIN LESIONS	EXAMPLES
BULLA Vesicle greater than 1 cm in diameter	Blister, pemphigus vulgaris, lupus, impetigo, drug reaction
PUSTULE Elevated, superficial lesion; similar to a vesicle but filled with purulent fluid	Impetigo, acne, folliculitis, herpes simplex
CYST Elevated, circumscribed, encapsulated lesion; in dermis or subcutaneous layer; filled with liquid or semisolid material	Sebaceous cyst, cystic acne
TELANGIECTASIA Fine, irregular red lines produced by capillary dilation	Telangiectasia in rosacea, vascular spider, lupus erythematosus

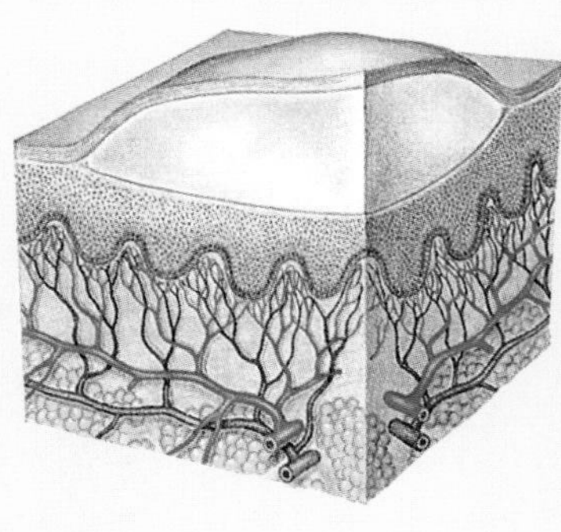

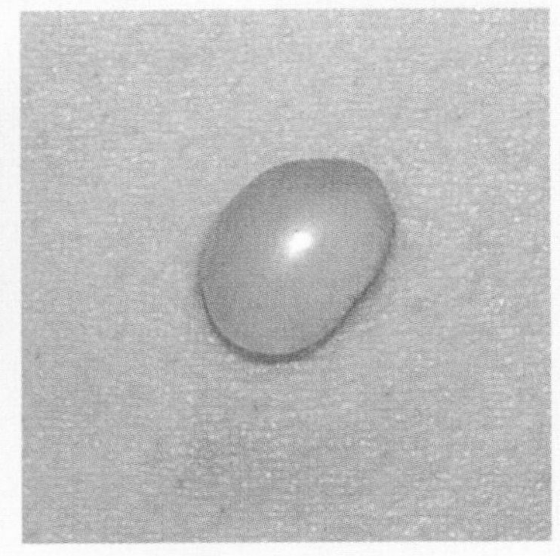

Blister. (From White, 1994.)

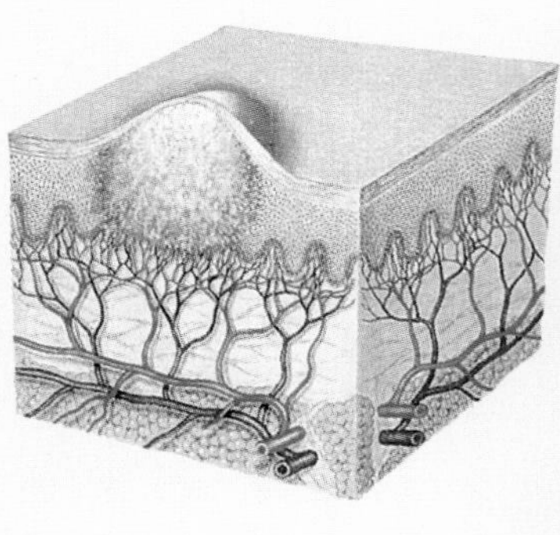

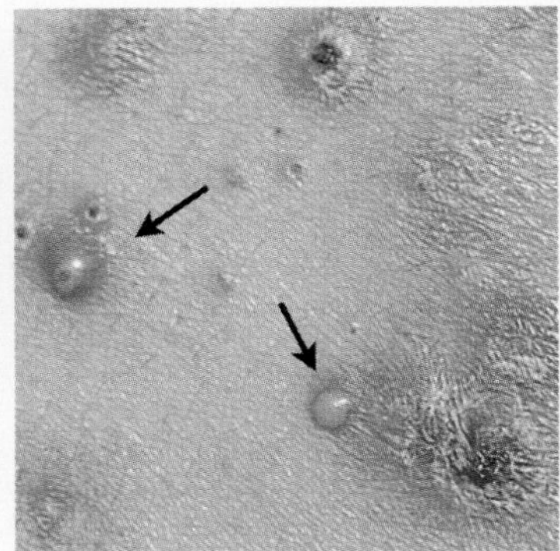

Acne.
(From Weston, Lane, and Morelli,1996.)

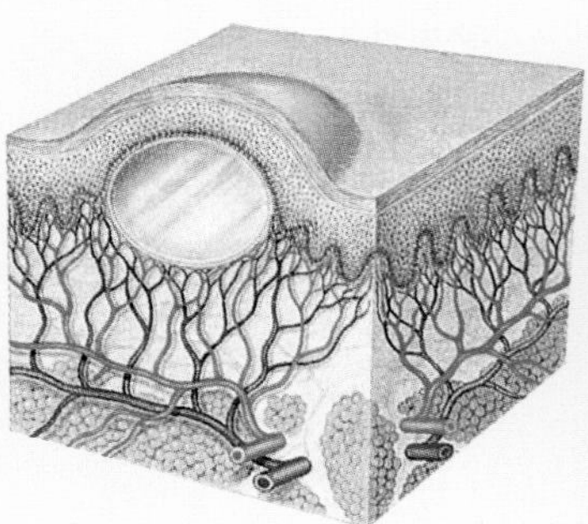

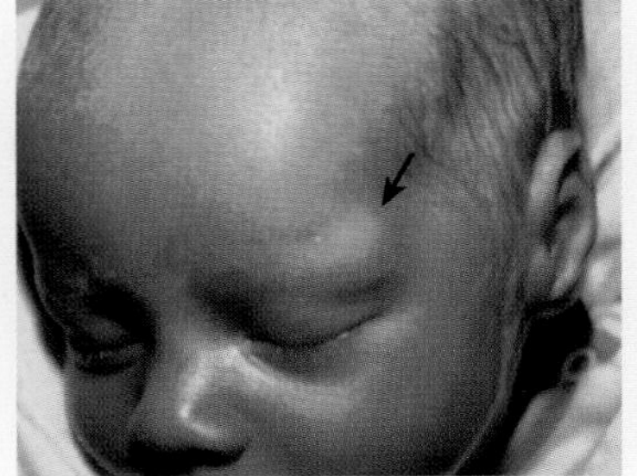

Sebaceous cyst.
(From Weston, Lane, and Morelli, 1996.)

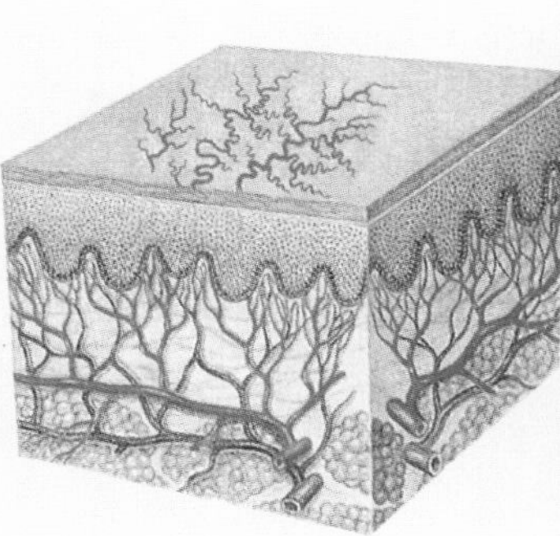

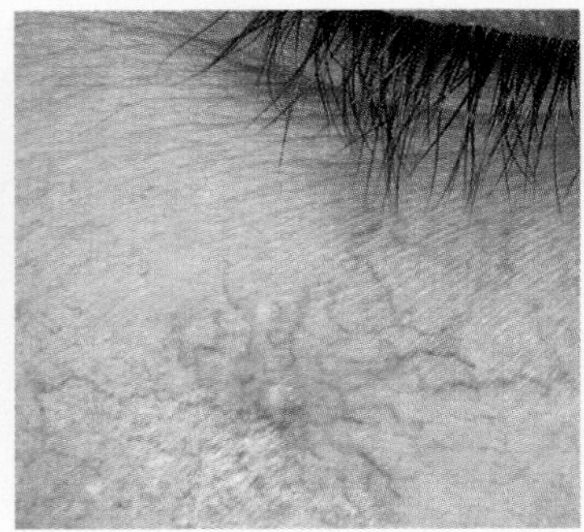

Vascular spider. (From Habif, 1996.)

PROCEDURES AND TECHNIQUES WITH NORMAL FINDINGS

➤**INSPECT and PALPATE the skin for lesions.** The term *lesion* is used to describe any observable change from normal skin structure. When a lesion is identified, the examiner should observe and palpate the lesion to determine its characteristics. The lesion is documented based on its characteristics, including location, distribution, color, pattern, edges, flat or raised, and size. (Box 11-2 and Fig. 11-4.) Use a centimeter ruler to measure the size of lesions. A strong light source is helpful to determine the exact color, elevation, and borders. Lesions are divided into two categories: primary lesions (see Table 11-2) and secondary lesions (see Table 11-3 on pp. 175-177) (Goldstein and Goldstein, 1997). It is important to note that many different pathologic conditions can cause similar types of lesions, and lesions caused by some conditions (chickenpox, for example) can overlap categories. The value of learning the categories is to help the examiner describe the type of lesion seen, not necessarily what is causing it.

❖ Use a Wood's lamp to identify fluorescing lesions, indicating fungal infection. Darken the room and shine the light on the area to be examined. If there is no fungal infection, the light tone on the skin will appear soft violet.

Box 11-2 Lesion Characteristics to be Noted During Examination

- Note the **location and distribution** of the lesion. Is the lesion generalized over the entire body or section of the body, or is it localized to a specific area such as around the waist, under a piece of jewelry, or just in the hair?
- Describe the **color** of the lesion and describe how this lesion may be different in color from other lesions noted on the body (e.g., a mole or freckle). Has the patient noticed a change in the color of the lesion?
- What is the **pattern** of the lesion? Are the lesions clustered? Are they in a line? How does the patient describe the development of the pattern of the lesion? (See Fig. 11-4.)
- What are the **edges** of the lesion like? Is the edge of the lesion regular or irregular? Has the patient noticed a change in the shape of the lesion?
- Is the lesion **flat, raised, or sunken?**
- What is the current **size** of the lesion? Measure using a centimeter ruler. Has the patient noticed a change in the size of the lesion?
- What are the **characteristics** of the lesion? Is it hard, soft, or fluid filled? If there is an exudate, what is the color of the drainage fluid? Does the exudate have an odor? Note both the color and odor if present. Has the patient noticed a change in either the characteristics or drainage of the lesion? If so, how and when?

ABNORMAL FINDINGS

■ The common characteristics of primary and secondary lesions are described in Tables 11-2 and 11-3. Scarring caused by needle-track marks are generally indicative of intravenous drug use.

❖A yellow-green or blue-green fluorescence indicates the presence of fungal infection.

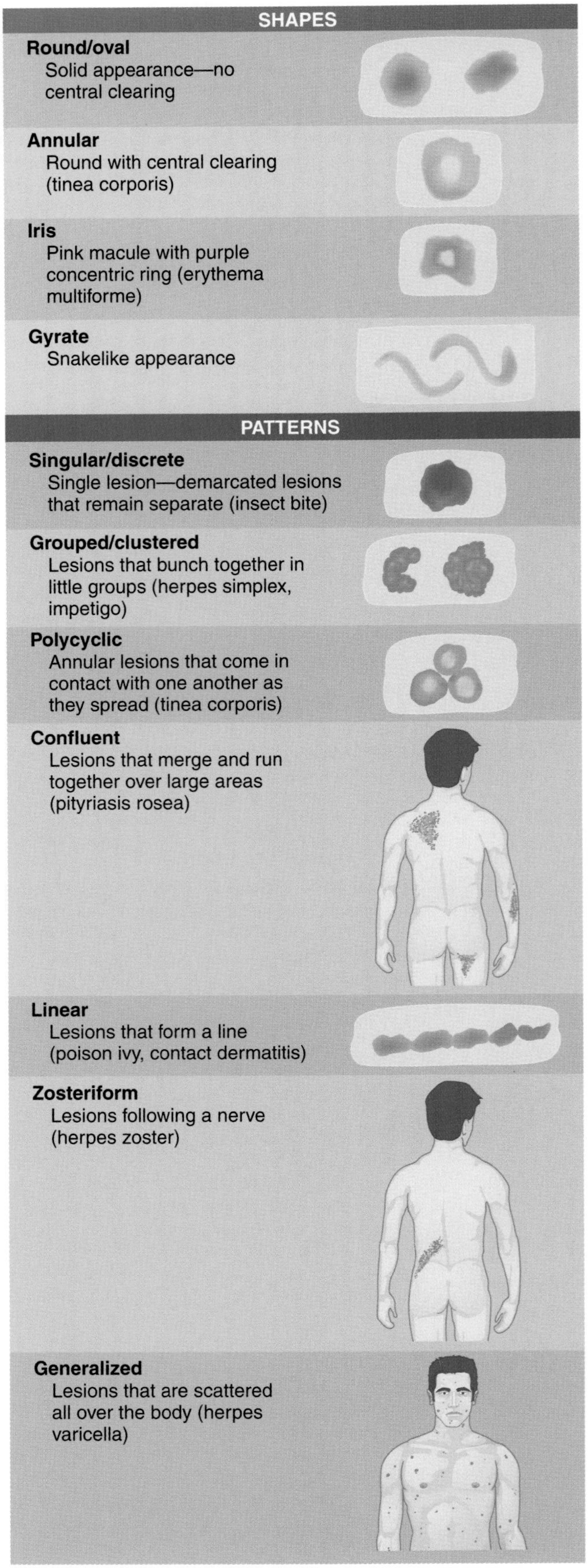

SHAPES

Round/oval
Solid appearance—no central clearing

Annular
Round with central clearing (tinea corporis)

Iris
Pink macule with purple concentric ring (erythema multiforme)

Gyrate
Snakelike appearance

PATTERNS

Singular/discrete
Single lesion—demarcated lesions that remain separate (insect bite)

Grouped/clustered
Lesions that bunch together in little groups (herpes simplex, impetigo)

Polycyclic
Annular lesions that come in contact with one another as they spread (tinea corporis)

Confluent
Lesions that merge and run together over large areas (pityriasis rosea)

Linear
Lesions that form a line (poison ivy, contact dermatitis)

Zosteriform
Lesions following a nerve (herpes zoster)

Generalized
Lesions that are scattered all over the body (herpes varicella)

Fig. 11-4 Shapes and patterns of lesions.

Table 11-3 Secondary Skin Lesions

SKIN LESIONS	EXAMPLES		
SCALE Heaped-up keratinized cells; flaky skin; irregular; thick or thin; dry or oily; variation in size	Flaking of skin with seborrheic dermatitis following scarlet fever, or flaking of skin following a drug reaction; dry skin, pityriasis rosea, eczema, xerosis	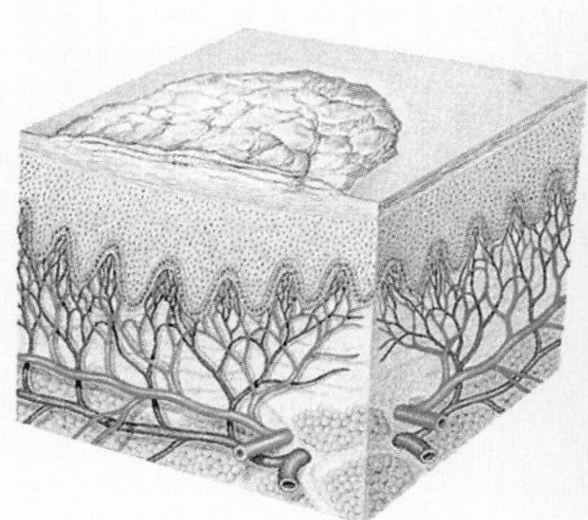	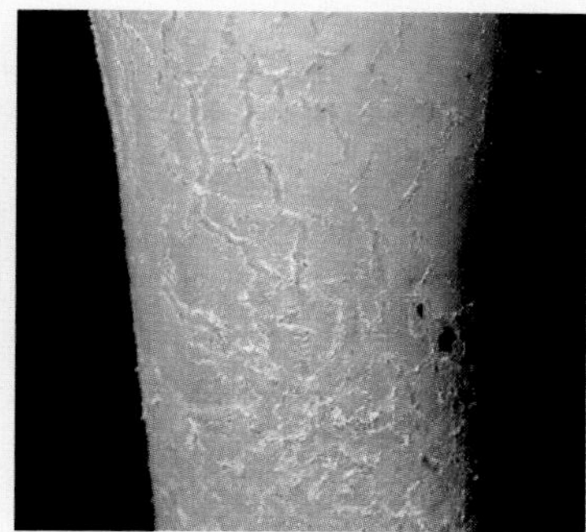 Scaling. (From Habif, 1996.)
LICHENIFICATION Rough, thickened epidermis secondary to persistent rubbing, itching, or skin irritation; often involves flexor surface of extremity	Chronic dermatitis	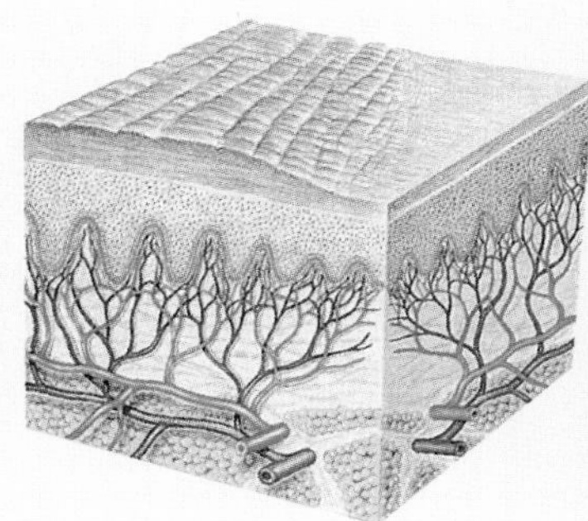	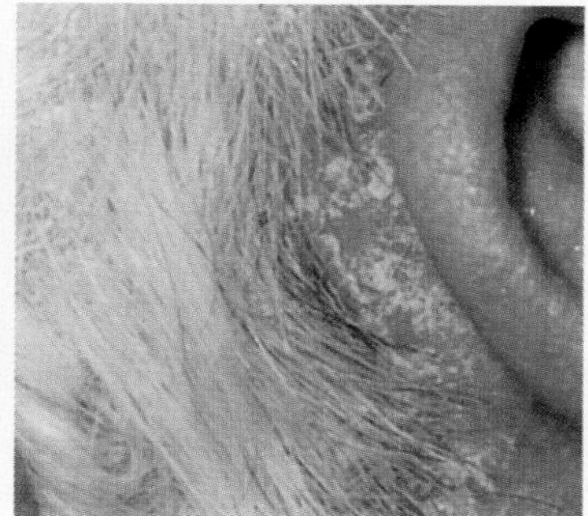 Stasis dermatitis in an early stage. (From Marks and DeLeo, 1992.)
KELOID Irregular-shaped, elevated, progressively enlarging scar; grows beyond the boundaries of the wound; caused by excessive collagen formation during healing	Keloid formation following surgery	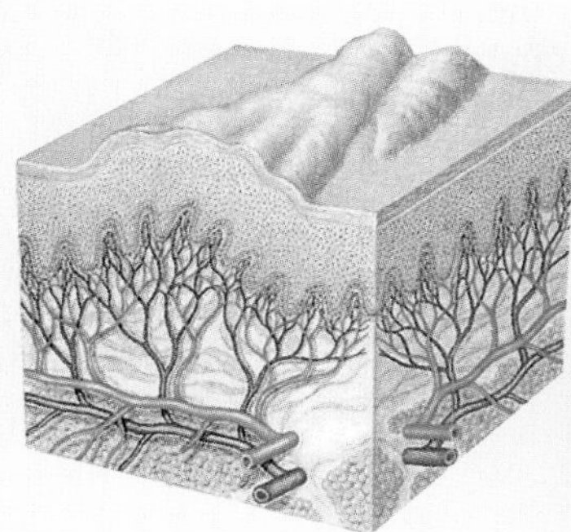	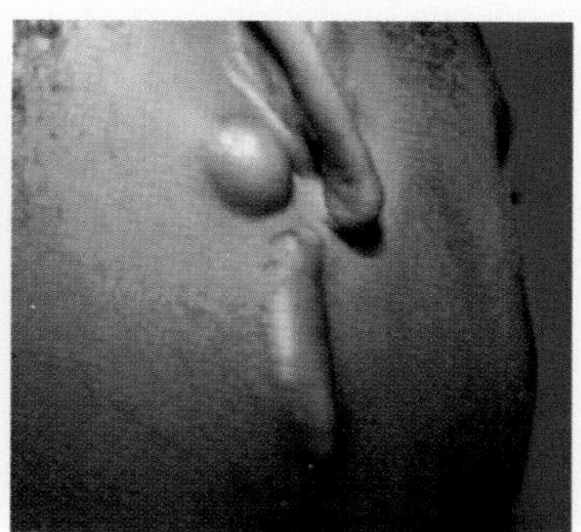 Keloid. (From Weston, Lane, and Morelli, 1996.)

Continued

Table 11-3 Secondary Skin Lesions—cont'd

SKIN LESIONS	EXAMPLES		
SCAR Thin to thick fibrous tissue that replaces normal skin following injury or laceration to the dermis	Healed wound or surgical incision	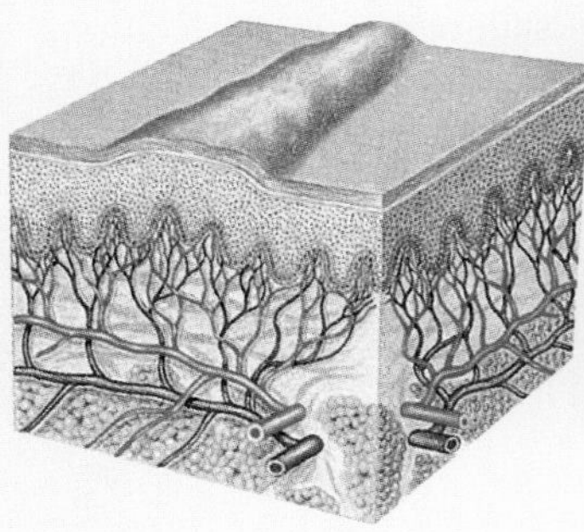	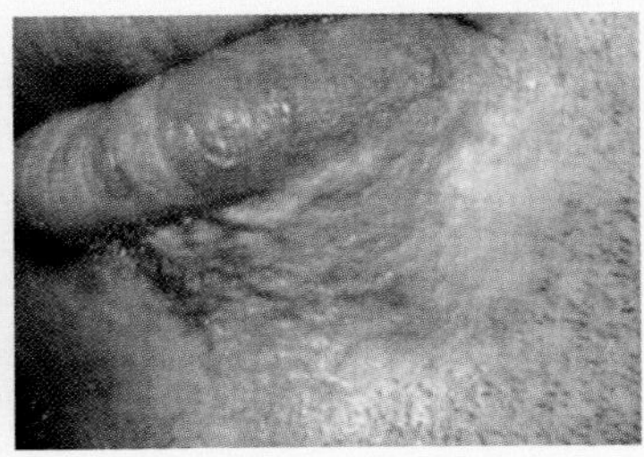 Hypertrophic scar. (From Goldman and Fitzpatrick, 1994.)
EXCORIATION Loss of the epidermis; linear hollowed-out crusted area	Abrasion or scratch, scabies	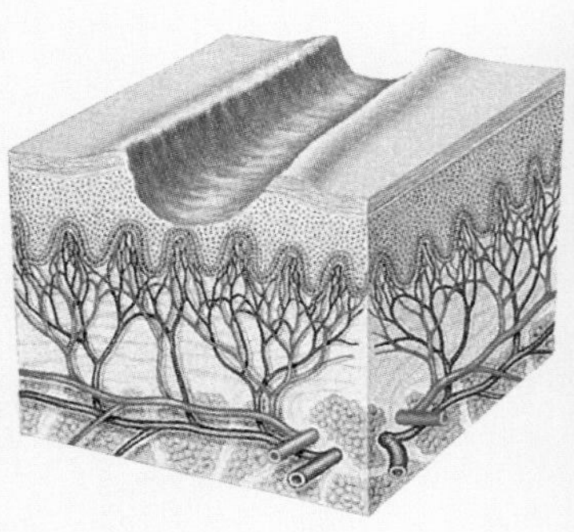	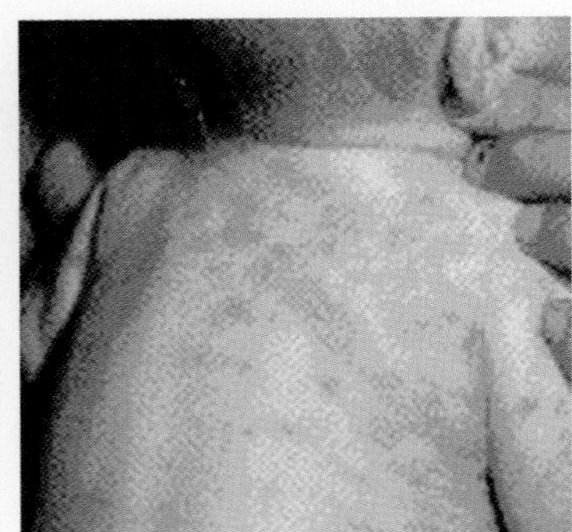 Scabies. (From Weston, Lane, and Morelli, 1996.)
FISSURE Linear crack or break from the epidermis to the dermis; may be moist or dry	Athlete's foot, cracks at the corner of the mouth, chapped hands, eczema, intertrigo labialis	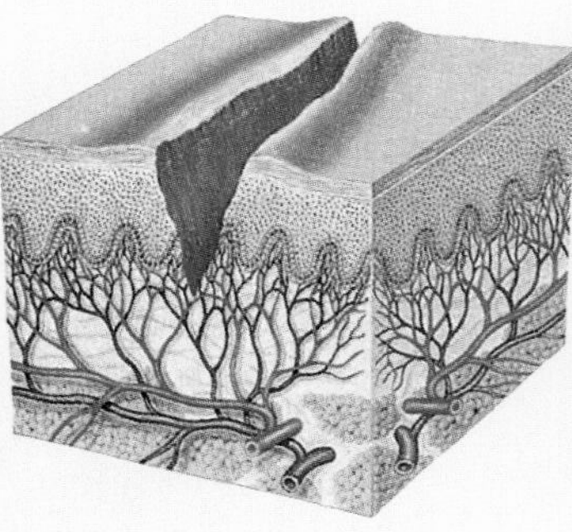	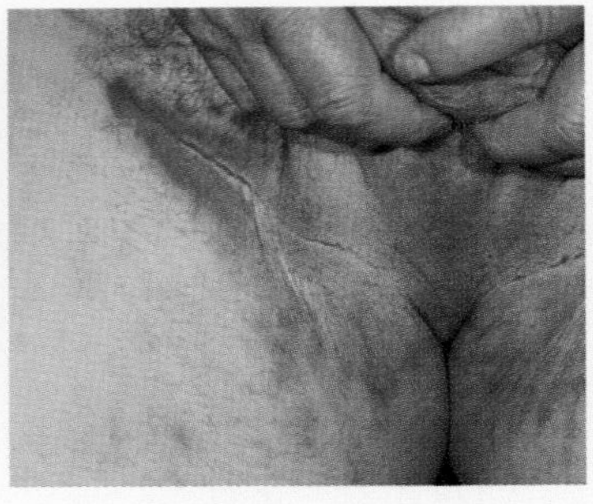 Fissure. (From Habif, 1996.)

Table 11-3 Secondary Skin Lesions—cont'd

SKIN LESIONS	EXAMPLES
EROSION	
Loss of part of the epidermis; depressed, moist, glistening; follows rupture of a vesicle or bulla	Varicella, variola after rupture, candidiasis, herpes simplex
ULCER	
Loss of epidermis and dermis; concave; varies in size	Decubiti, stasis ulcers, syphilis chancre
ATROPHY	
Thinning of the skin surface and loss of skin markings; skin appears translucent and paperlike	Aged skin, striae, discoid lupus erythematosus

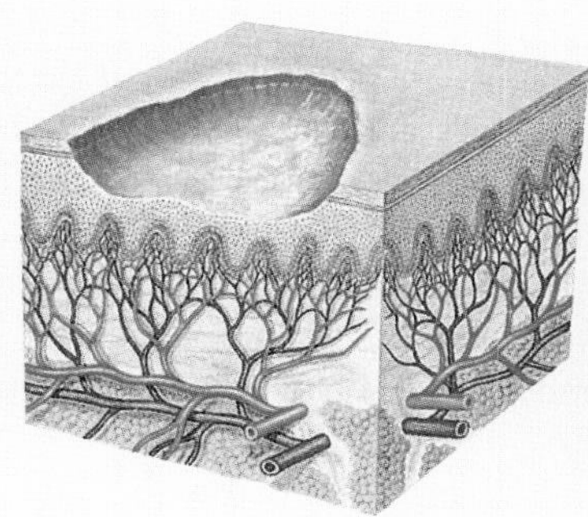

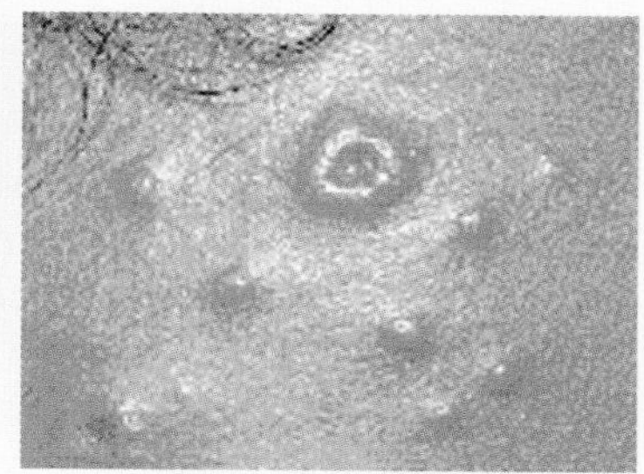

Erosion. (From Cohen, 1993.)

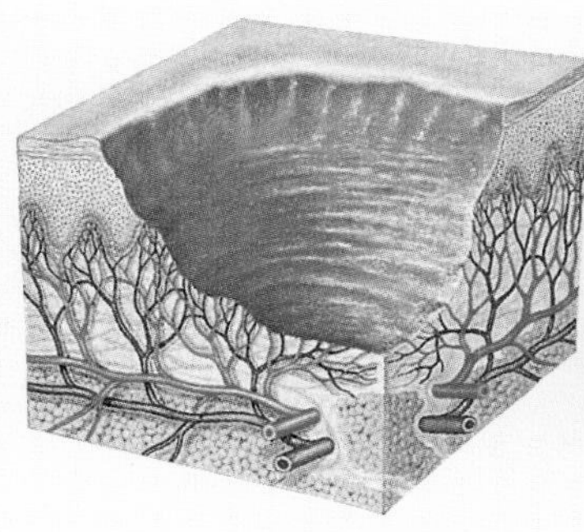

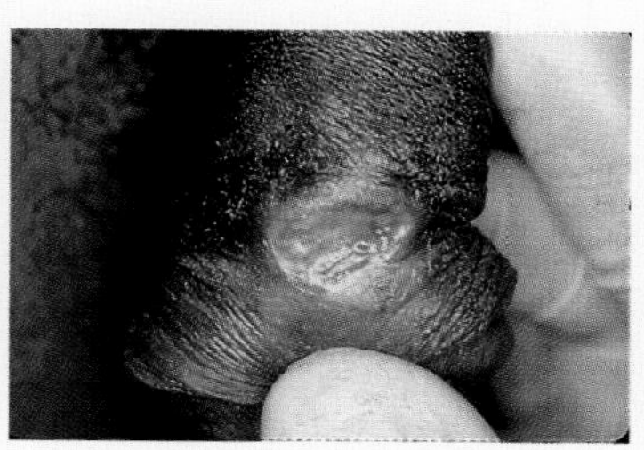

Ulcer caused by syphilis. (From Goldstein and Goldstein, 1997.)

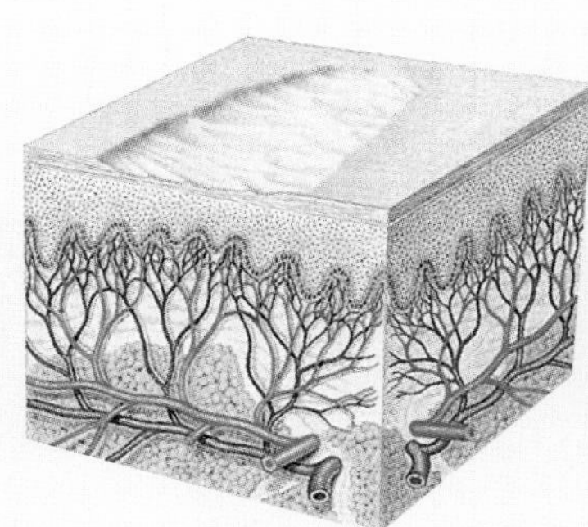

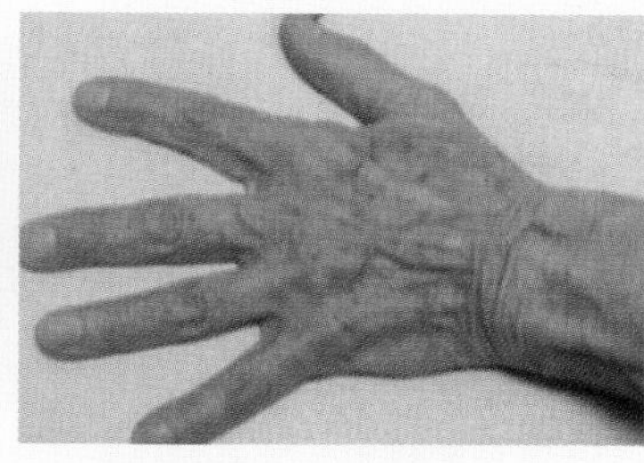

Aged skin. (From Seidel et al, 1999.)

PROCEDURES AND TECHNIQUES WITH NORMAL FINDINGS

➤**INSPECT and PALPATE the skin for vascular lesions.** Bruising on a bony prominence is generally considered to be a normal finding secondary to the activities of daily living. However, if bruising is noted over soft tissue areas of the body where no history of bumping or injury has occurred, or if there are multiple bruises on the body in various stages of healing, it may be considered abnormal and warrants further investigation. Possible causes such as physical abuse and indicators such as abnormal results of blood studies should be considered. Normal vascularity variations may include the following:

- *Nevus flammeus (port-wine stain).*
- *Telangiectasia:* A fine, irregular red line caused by permanent dilation of a group of superficial blood vessels.
- *Cherry angioma:* Small, slightly raised, bright red areas that appear on the face, neck, and trunk of the body. These increase in size and number with advanced age (Fig. 11-6).
- *Capillary hemangioma:* Red irregular patches caused by dilation capillaries within the dermal layer of the skin.

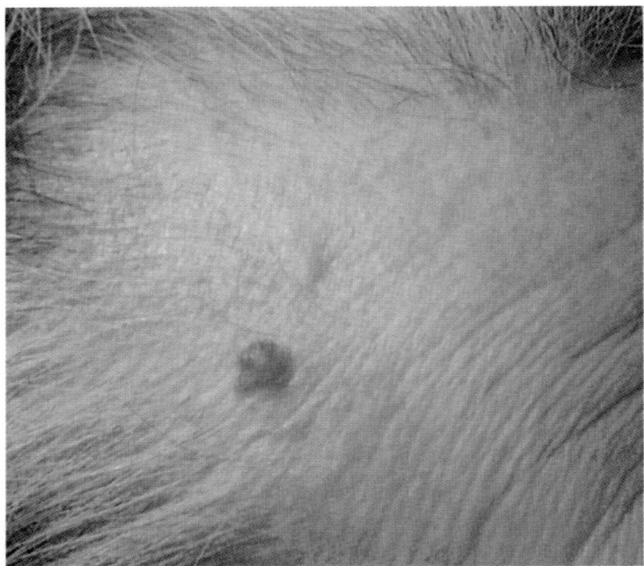

Fig. 11-6 Cherry angioma. (From Baran et al, 1991.)

ABNORMAL FINDINGS

■ Vascular abnormalities include such findings as the following:

- *Petechiae:* In light-skinned persons these appear as purple pinpoints. They are difficult to see on persons with dark skin except in the oral mucosa and conjunctiva. Petechiae will not disappear (blanch) with direct palpation (Fig. 11-5).
- *Ecchymoses (bruises):* In light-skinned persons these appear as purple to yellowish green areas; they are very difficult to see on dark skin except in the mouth or conjunctiva.
- *Purpura:* Brownish red or purple discolorations on the skin as a result of hemorrhage into the tissue or a disorder such as idiopathic thrombocytopenic purpura (ITP).
- *Spider angioma:* Small red central area with radiating spiderlike legs that blanch with pressure to the central body. This is most frequently caused by liver disease and vitamin B deficiency.

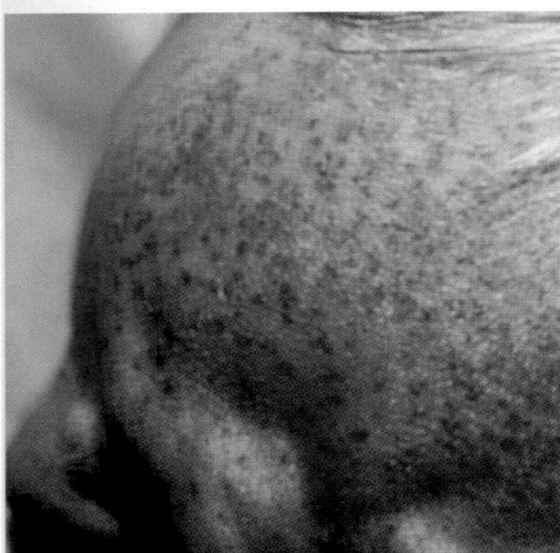

Fig. 11-5 Petechiae. (From Weston, Lane, and Morelli, 1996.)

PROCEDURES AND TECHNIQUES WITH NORMAL FINDINGS

➤**PALPATE the skin for texture, temperature, moisture, mobility, and turgor.**

Texture The skin should be smooth, soft, and intact, without cracking, flaking, or scaling. There should be no rough spots or calluses. Note bruises, scars, or lesions. Carefully examine the skin texture in body creases such as under breasts, under skin folds on the obese abdomen, and in the inguinal area. Specifically look for rashes, discoloration, or areas of maceration in these areas.

Temperature and Moisture The skin should be warm and dry without being hot. There should be minimal perspiration or oiliness.

Mobility and Turgor The skin should be assessed by picking up and slightly pinching the skin under the clavicle. The skin should move easily when lifted and should return to place immediately when released. The technique and normal skin turgor are shown in Fig. 11-8 (Fitzpatrick et al, 1999).

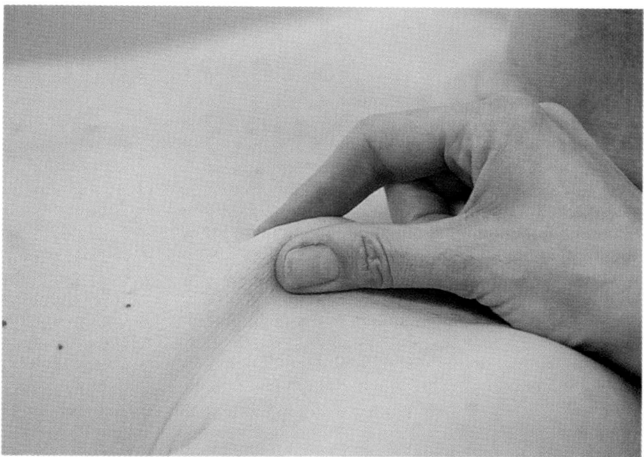

Fig. 11-8 Normal skin turgor.

ABNORMAL FINDINGS

■ Dryness, flaking, or cracking of the skin may occur secondary to environmental conditions or may be signs of systemic disease. (Increased perspiration may be associated with anxiety, environmental temperatures, body weight, or activity.) Poor skin turgor is shown in Fig. 11-7. This may be associated with dehydration or aging.

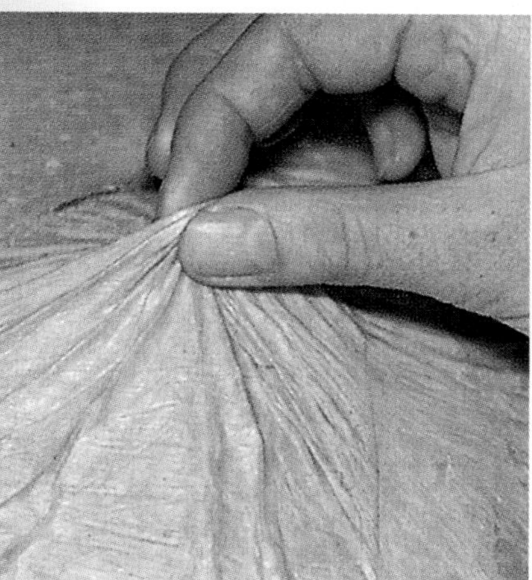

Fig. 11-7 Poor skin turgor. (From Kamal and Brocklehurst, 1991.)

PROCEDURES AND TECHNIQUES WITH NORMAL FINDINGS

HAIR

Although some characteristics of the hair may have been noted during the examination of the skin, take time to specifically examine the characteristics of all body hair. The areas of hair to be examined include the hair on the head and axillary, pubic, facial, and body hair.

➤**INSPECT and PALPATE the scalp and hair for surface characteristics, hair distribution, texture, quantity, and color.** The scalp should be smooth to palpation and should show no evidence of flaking, scaling, redness, or open lesions. The hair should be shiny and soft. The texture of the hair may be fine or coarse. Note the quantity and distribution of the hair for balding patterns and isolated areas of hair loss. If there are areas of isolated hair loss, note whether the hair shaft is broken off or whether it is absent completely. Men may show a gradual, symmetric hair loss on the scalp due to genetic disposition and elevated androgen levels.

ETHNIC & CULTURAL VARIATIONS

Hair texture varies widely across races. African Americans may have fine, thick, and very curly or kinky hair. Asian Americans, Pacific Islanders, American Indians, and Alaskan natives often have coarse, straight hair. African-American men often have curly facial hair that tends to ingrow, producing a condition known as "razor bumps." Body and facial hair is sparse or absent in many American Indians and Alaskan natives. Female balding patterns are frequently seen in American Indian women. Baldness is rare in American Indian men.

➤**INSPECT facial and body hair for hair distribution, quantity, and texture.** Examine the quantity and distribution of facial and body hair. Many men generally have noticeable hair present on the lower face, neck, nares, ears, chest, axilla, back, shoulders, arms, legs, and pubic region. The noticeable hair distribution in women is most commonly limited to the arms, legs, axillae, pubic region, and around the nipples. Women may also have fine or light-colored hair on the back, face, and shoulders. The women in some cultural groups may also have facial or chin hair. Note hair distribution patterns and areas of hair loss. Fine vellus hair covers the body, whereas coarser hair is found on the eyebrows and lashes, pubic region, axillary area, male beards, and to some extent on the arms and legs. The male pubic hair configuration is an upright triangle, with the hair commonly extending midline to the umbilicus. The female pubic hair configuration forms an inverse triangle; the hair may also extend midline to the umbilicus.

ABNORMAL FINDINGS

■ Hair is affected by a number of medical conditions. It becomes dull, coarse, and brittle with nutritional deficiencies and hypothyroidism; hyperthyroidism makes the hair texture fine (Fitzpatrick et al, 1999). Hair loss occurs with some anemic conditions and nutritional deficiencies. Alopecia (hair loss) may be due to a variety of causes, including exposure to chemicals, secondary to hair products and bleaching; hair loss secondary to scarring or radiation or secondary hair loss to antineoplastic agents; and syphilitic hair loss, a generalized thinning of the hair or mucous patches without hair. Asymmetric hair loss may indicate an underlying pathologic condition (see Fig. 11-64). Hair bleaching or coloring may cause the hair to become abnormally coarse and brittle. Lice or nits (eggs) may be found on the scalp at the base of the hair shaft (see Fig. 11-63).

■ Hair loss on the legs may indicate poor peripheral perfusion. Hirsutism (in women) is hair growth in a male distribution pattern with an increase of hair on the face, body, and pubic area. Hirsutism may be a sign of an underlying endocrine disorder (see Fig. 11-65). Pubic hair distribution in either the male or the female that does not follow the designated patterns may indicate a hormonal imbalance.

PROCEDURES AND TECHNIQUES WITH NORMAL FINDINGS

NAILS

➤**INSPECT and PALPATE the nails for shape, contour, consistency, color, thickness, and cleanliness.** Inspect the edges of the nails to determine if they are smooth and rounded. The curvature of the nail surface should be flat and slightly curved. In light-skinned individuals, nails are pink and blanch with pressure. Individuals with darker pigmented skin typically have nails that are yellow or brown, and vertical banded lines may appear (Fig. 11-9). The normal angle of the nail base is 160°. Inspect the nail surface itself to determine its smoothness. Note grooves, depressions, pitting, and ridges. Transverse grooves may be secondary to repeated injury to the nail. Examine the thickness of the nail itself. The nail should be smooth and have a uniform thickness. Finally, palpate the nail to ensure that the nail base feels firm and adheres to the nail bed.

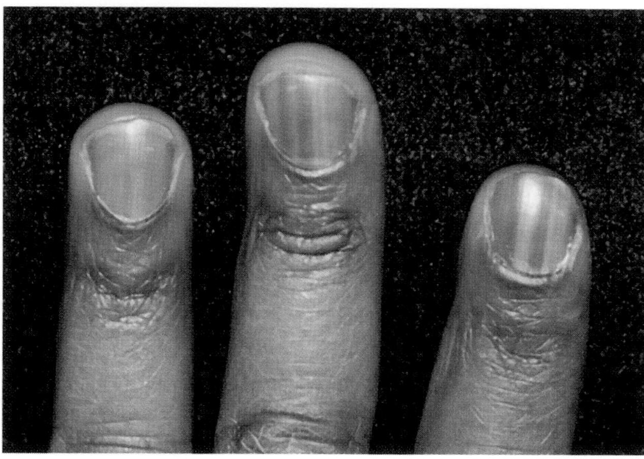

Fig. 11-9 Nail bed color of a dark-skinned person (pigmented bands occur as a normal finding in over 90% of African Americans). (From Habif, 1990.)

ABNORMAL FINDINGS

■ Clubbing is present when the angle of the nail base exceeds 160° (Baren and Tosti, 1999). Clubbing may be associated with respiratory or cardiovascular problems, cirrhosis, colitis, and thyroid disease (Fig. 11-10).

A thickening or hypertrophy of the nail is usually secondary to repeated trauma, fungal infection, or decreased vascular circulation. Thinning or brittleness of the nail may be secondary to poor peripheral circulation or inadequate nutrition.

Koilonychia (spoon nail) is present when the nail is thin and depressed and the lateral edges of the nail turn upward (Fig. 11-11). This finding may be congenital or may be associated with anemia.

Paronychia is an inflammation, swelling, and induration of the folds of the finger tissue near the base of the nail (Fig. 11-12). There is usually pain and tenderness associated with paronychia.

Lichen planus is an inflammation of the matrix of the nail, resulting in adherence of the proximal nail fold to the scarred matrix (Fig. 11-13).

Pitting of the nail is commonly associated with psoriasis. A minor degree of pitting may also be seen in persons with no other health care problems.

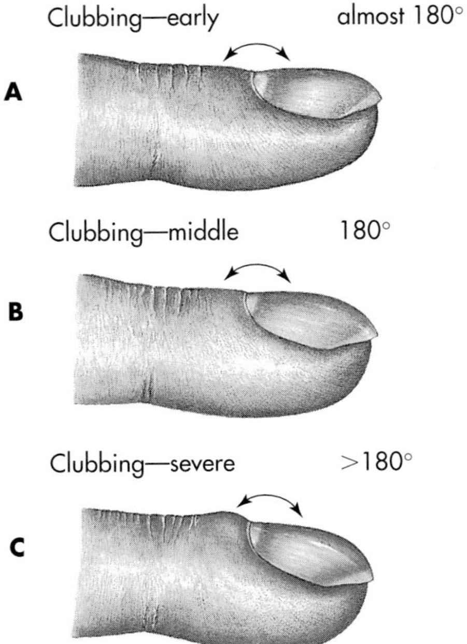

Fig. 11-10 Finger clubbing. **A,** Early clubbing—nail angle between 160 and 180°. **B,** Moderate clubbing—nail angle equals 180°. **C,** Severe clubbing—nail angle greater than 180°. (From Seidel et al, 1999.)

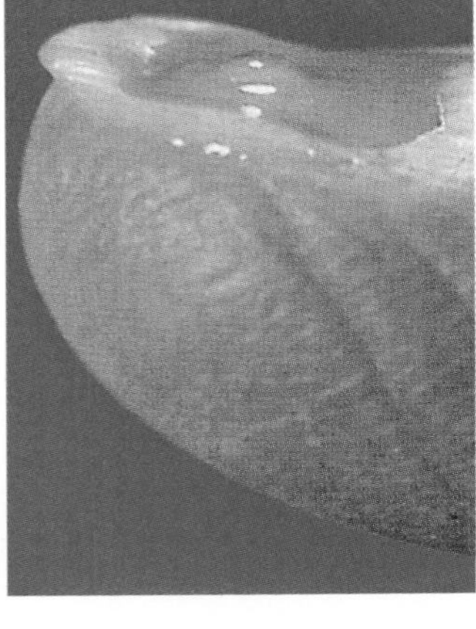

Fig. 11-11 Severe spooning with some thinning of the nail. (From Beaven and Brooks, 1994.)

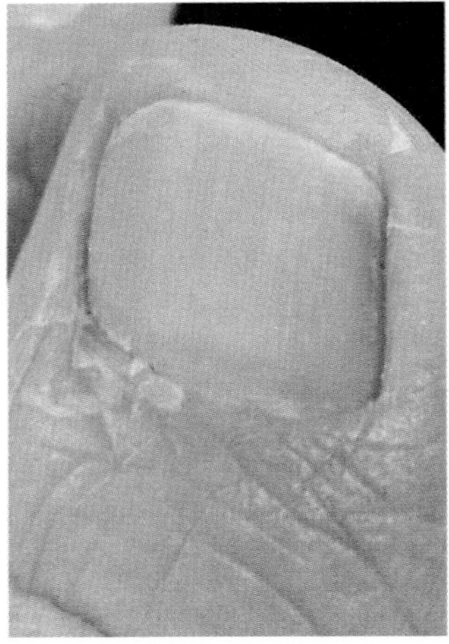

Fig. 11-12 Acute lateral paronychia. (From Beaven and Brooks, 1994.)

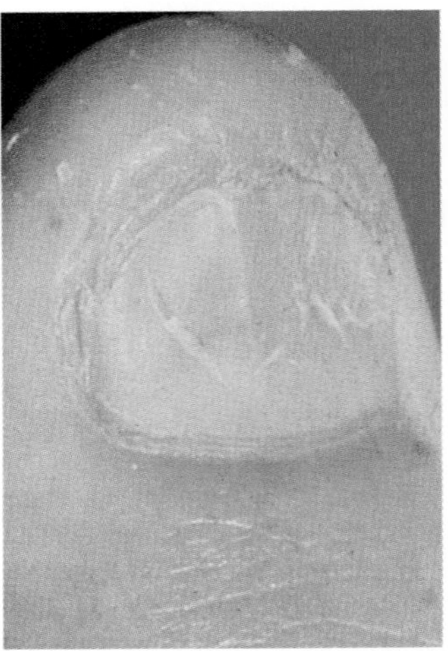

Fig. 11-13 Lichen planus. (From Beaven and Brooks, 1994.)

AGE-RELATED VARIATIONS

INFANTS

Anatomy and Physiology

The smooth texture of an infant's skin is due in part to its lack of exposure to the elements and in part to its lack of the coarser adult hairs, called terminal hairs. A newborn may have some desquamation, varying from flakiness to shedding of large strips of cornified epidermis. A white, waxy coating called vernix caseosa, a mixture of sebum and cornified epidermis, covers the newborn's body, and the shoulders and back may be covered with fine silky hair called lanugo, which is shed within 10 to 14 days after birth. The infant may be bald or have unusually thick scalp hair. In either case, the hair is usually shed within 2 to 3 months and is replaced by more permanent hair, which may or may not have the same color.

The newborn has ineffective temperature regulation. The subcutaneous fat layer is poorly developed in newborns, so they are subject to hypothermia. The eccrine sweat glands begin functioning after the first month of life, but will not be active until adolescence. Until then, the skin will have a less oily texture and a milder, inoffensive perspiration odor.

Health History

- Have there been changes in the skin color since birth? History of jaundice? If so, what day following birth? History of cyanosis? If so, what were the circumstances? Does the infant have any birthmarks?

  Rationale It is important to determine baseline information, as well as to identify signs that may indicate systemic problems.
- What is the infant eating? Breast milk? Formula? If formula, what type? Is the infant eating anything in addition to the formula? If yes, what?

  Rationale Formula or food allergies should be identified early and may be the cause of rashes.
- What type of diapers are used? Cloth diapers? Rubber pants? Disposable diapers? How do you normally clean the infant's bottom?

  Rationale A rash on the infant's buttocks may be due to poor hygiene or wet diapers that are left on the child for a long time. Simple skin irritation or a bacterial or fungal infection may result.
- Do you use powder on the diaper area? If so, what kind do you use?

  Rationale Some individuals use cornstarch as a baby powder. This should be avoided because cornstarch may foster the growth of monilia.
- What type of laundry detergent is used to wash the infant's clothing, cloth diapers, and blankets?

  Rationale If the infant has a rash under the clothing or diaper area, the examiner must inquire about a possible allergic reaction to laundry detergent.

Examination

Procedures and Techniques The techniques of the examination for the infant are the same as for the adult. To adequately examine the skin, the infant should be completely undressed. The examiner may want to keep the diaper in place until ready to examine the buttocks and genital area. Because many birthmarks and skin lesions may be in the diaper area, it is imperative that the diaper be removed at some point during skin examination. Care must also be taken to ensure that the infant remains warm during the examination period. Keeping the room warm and covering areas not being examined during the examination process will help to prevent excessive chilling. If the infant becomes chilled, the skin, hands, and feet may take on transient mottling (marked blotches or a marbled appearance).

Normal and Abnormal Findings

Skin. The skin color in the newborn is partially dependent on the amount of fat present. Preterm infants generally appear to be redder because they have less subcutaneous fat than do full-term infants. In addition, the infant may appear to have a red skin tone for a short period because of vasomotor instability. This color tends to fade within the first few days. Also, immediately following birth the neonate's lips, nail beds, and feet may be dusky or appear cyanotic. Once the newborn is adequately warmed, the dusky color should fade, and a well-oxygenated pink tone should reappear. Even dark-skinned newborns should have a dark pink tone, which is most evident on the palms of the hands and the soles of the feet.

Physiologic jaundice may be present in the newborn following the third or fourth day of life. The skin, mucous membranes, and sclera will appear to have a yellow tone. This generally normal phenomenon occurs in almost half of all newborns and is secondary to the increased number of red blood cells that hemolyze following birth.

Birthmarks in newborns may be a pigmentation variation or may be associated with a vascular variation.

- *Mongolian spot:* an irregularly shaped, darkened flat area over the sacral area and buttock (Fig. 11-14). They are most prevalent in African-American, Hispanic, American Indian, and Asian children and generally disappear by the time the child is 1 or 2 years of age.
- *Café-au-lait spot:* a large round or oval patch of light brown pigmentation that is generally present at birth

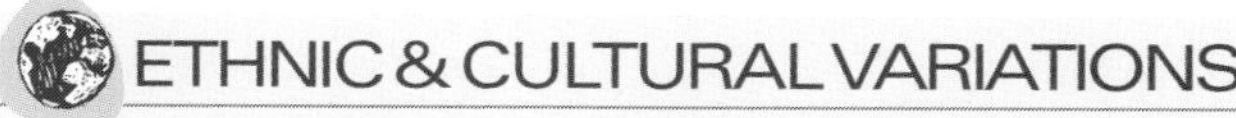

Initially, dark-skinned newborn infants have a light skin color. The child's actual skin color will take 2 to 3 months to develop. The nail beds and skin of the scrotum, however, are indicators of their full melanotic color (Seidel, 1999).

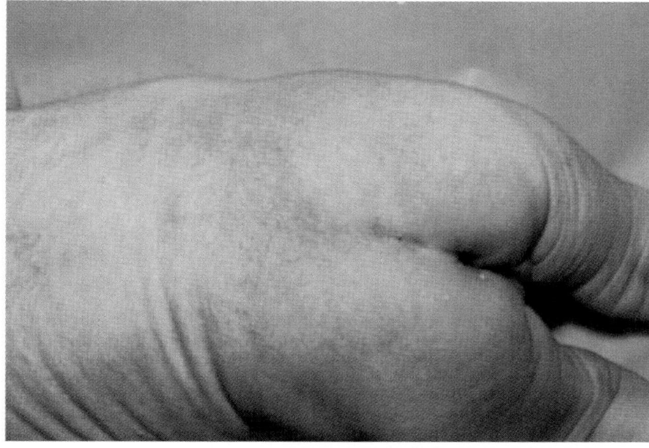

Fig. 11-14 Mongolian spot. (From Weston, Lane, and Morelli, 1996.)

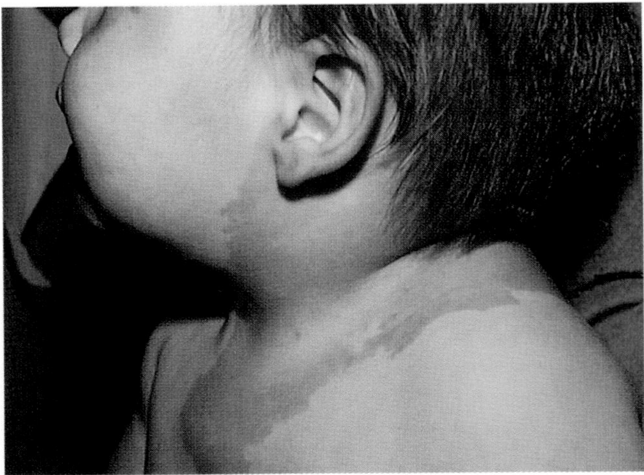

Fig. 11-15 Café au lait spot. (From Weston, Lane, and Morelli, 1996.)

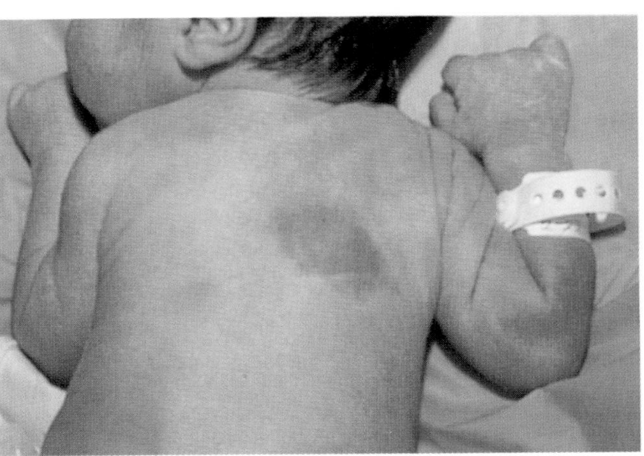

Fig. 11-17 Port-wine stain. (From Weston, Lane, and Morelli, 1996.)

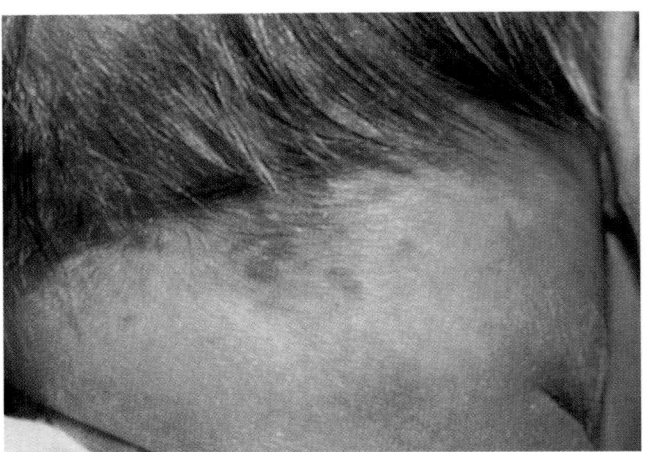

Fig. 11-16 Stork bite. (From Weston, Lane and Morelli, 1996.)

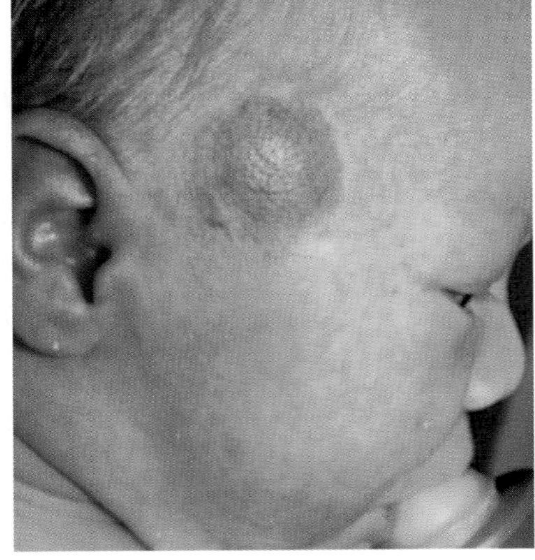

Fig. 11-18 Strawberry mark (hemangioma). (From Weston, Lane, and Morelli, 1996.)

(Fig. 11-15). Occasionally these spots may be associated with neurofibromatosis.

The skin of the neonate should be carefully examined for evidence of vascular-related birthmarks. These birthmarks may be either benign and within normal limits or considered to be deviations from normal. The most common normal vascular birthmark is a "stork bite."

- *Stork bite (telangiectasis or flat capillary hemangioma):* Small red or pink spot that is often seen on the back of the neck (Fig. 11-16). Stork bites will usually disappear by 5 years of age.

Vascular findings that should be considered deviations from normal include the following:

- *Port-wine stains (nevus flammeus):* Large, flat, bluish purple capillary areas (Fig. 11-17). They are most frequently found on the face along distribution of the fifth cranial nerve. Port-wine stains do not disappear spontaneously.
- *Strawberry mark (immature hemangioma):* Slightly raised, reddened areas with a sharp demarcation line (Fig. 11-18). They may be 2 to 3 cm in diameter and will usually disappear by 5 years of age.
- *Cavernous hemangioma:* A reddish blue round mass of blood vessels (Fig 11-19). They may continue to grow until the child reaches 10 to 15 months of age. Frequent reassessment should be conducted.

Common skin lesion findings include the following:

- *Milia:* Small, whitish papules that may be found on the cheeks, nose, chin, and forehead of newborns (Fig.

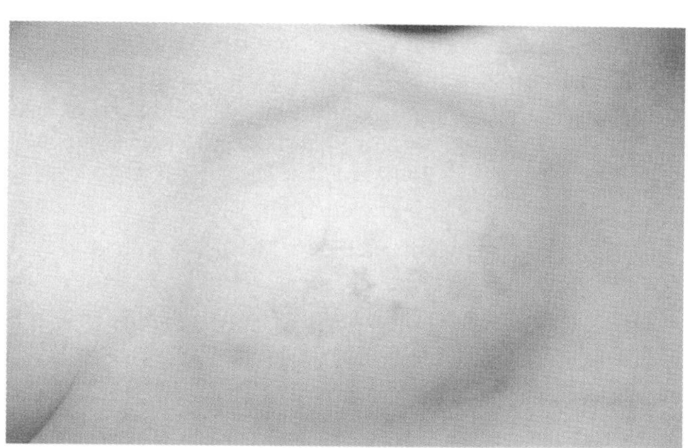

Fig. 11-19 Cavernous hemangioma. (From Cohen, 1993.)

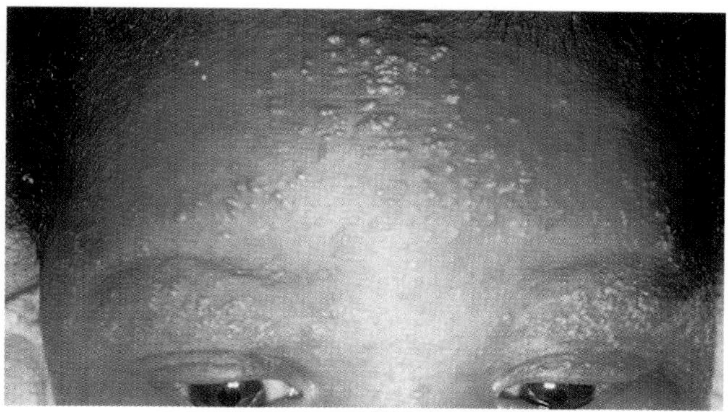

Fig. 11-20 Milia on the forehead of a newborn. (From Cohen, 1993.)

11-20). These are benign and generally disappear by the third week of life.

- *Erythema toxicum:* A very common rash among newborns (Fig. 11-21). It is a self-limited and benign rash of unknown etiology consisting of erythematous macules, papules, and pustules. The rash may appear anywhere on the body except the palms of the hands and the soles of the feet. Although it may be present at birth, it most commonly appears by the third or fourth day of life.
- *Diaper rashes:* These may be a benign reaction to damp skin or a contact reaction to the diaper, or they may be bacterial or fungal. If a rash is present, a careful history and possible cultures should be obtained.

Hair. Scalp hair on the newborn may be present or absent. If present, it is generally fine and soft. Seborrheic dermatitis (cradle cap) is a scaly crust that commonly appears on the scalp (see Fig. 11-37).

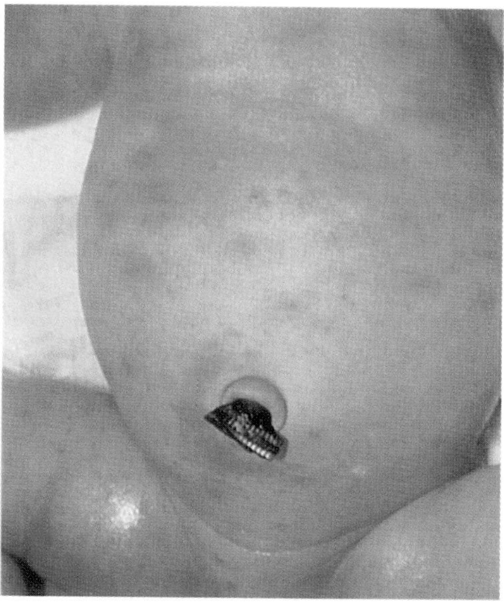

Fig. 11-21 Erythema toxicum on the trunk of an infant. (From Cohen, 1993.)

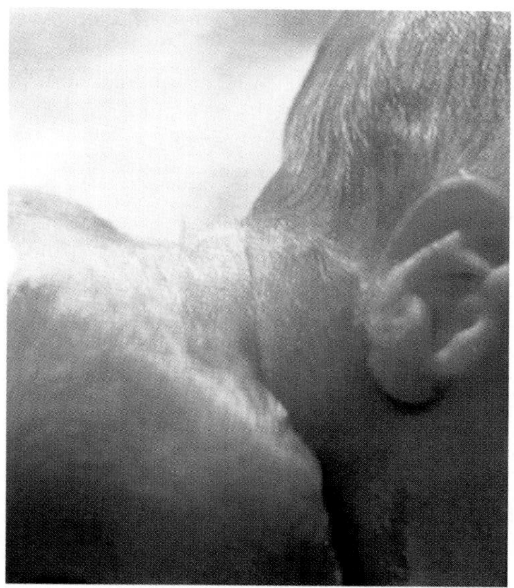

Fig. 11-22 Newborn silky body hair (lanugo). (From Zitelli and Davis, 1997.)

The newborn's skin may be covered with fine, soft, immature hair called lanugo hair (Fig. 11-22). This fine, soft hair may be found anywhere on the body but is most common on the scalp, ears, shoulders, and back. The lumbosacral area of the newborn should be carefully examined for evidence of tufts of hair. Hair in this area is suggestive of spina bifida or a sinus tract.

Nails. The nails of the newborn should be examined for presence and texture. Postterm infants may have long fingernails at birth.

CHILDREN

Health History

Many of the questions specific to this age group address rashes.

- If child is younger than 2 years, ask: Is the child still being introduced to new foods? If so, what foods have been introduced recently? Does your child have a rash? How soon afterward did the rash appear?

  Rationale The child may be having an allergic reaction to the new food.
- Does the child have allergies, hay fever, or asthma?

  Rationale Determine the relationship between possible allergens, such as food, pets, or drugs, and the symptoms.
- Has the child been exposed to other children with known diseases, rashes, or infections? If so, when and what?

  Rationale It is important to know the incubation period of common communicable diseases such as measles or chickenpox and the relationship of the child's symptoms with the known exposures, such as scabies.
- Does the child have a nail-biting habit? Chronic pulling or twisting of the hair? Rubbing of the head on the mattress, floor, or wall?

  Rationale Nervous habits such as nail biting, hair twisting, or hair rubbing are important to identify so that help may be sought.
- Is the child in day care, a nursery, or in school?

  Rationale The child may be at higher risk for infestations such as lice or scabies.

Examination

Procedures and Techniques Examine the skin of a young child with the child completely undressed. The examiner may want to have the child leave his or her underpants on during the skin examination. If the child is shy or modest, the examination of the skin in the genital area may be deferred until the actual examination of the buttocks and genitalia.

Normal and Abnormal Findings

Skin. It is important to assess a young child for evidence of bruising that may be inconsistent with the child's developmental level or bruising that may be in an unusual area. As the child becomes mobile, bruising is common on the lower legs and perhaps even the face. Bruising on other areas of the body (e.g., upper arms, back, buttocks, and abdomen) is abnormal and should be further examined. In addition to the location of bruising, it is equally important to note bruises that may be at different stages of healing. Bruising on the body in unusual areas or multiple bruises found at different stages of healing should be further investigated to rule out abuse (Giardino et al, 1997).

The most common lesions found in the young child are associated with communicable diseases and bacterial infections. The common problems and conditions seen in children are presented later in the chapter. These include the following:

- Herpes varicella (chickenpox)
- Rubella, rubeola, roseola
- Tinea corporis (ringworm)
- Impetigo
- Pediculosis corporis (body lice)
- Scabies

Dehydration must be evaluated in the ill young child. In addition to other clinical signs such as sunken eyes, dry mucous membranes, and decreased urinary output, it is important to evaluate the turgor of the skin. A child who is seriously dehydrated (more than 3% to 5% of body weight) will have skin that appears "tented" after the abdominal skin is pinched.

Hair. Common problems associated with the scalp and hair of the young child include alopecia, which may be secondary to hair pulling, twisting, or head rubbing; and lice, nits, and scabies, which are common problems for the young and school-age child. The young child should have very little body or facial hair.

Nails. Nail biting is an abnormal behavior and finding. Evidence of cyanosis of the nail bed or nail clubbing requires careful evaluation. These may indicate a cardiac problem or systemic disease such as cystic fibrosis.

ADOLESCENTS

Anatomy and Physiology

The apocrine sweat glands enlarge and become active during adolescence, and increased sebaceous gland activity, in response to increased hormone levels, heightens sebum production, leading to development of body odor and axillary perspiration. As a result, the teen will have oilier skin and possibly some acne. In response to increased androgen levels, the axillae and pubic areas of both males and females will develop coarse terminal hair; males will develop coarser facial hair as well.

Health History

- Do you have trouble with acne? If so, what have you done to treat it? Describe lotions, creams, medications, and other treatments used.

  Rationale Learning about the adolescent's self-care methods will not only assist in making recommendations for care, but also will provide insight into how the teen cares for himself or herself.

Examination

Procedures and Techniques Although the examination of the skin, hair, and nails is thought to be a benign and straightforward examination, special care must be taken when examining the adolescent. Because of maturational changes and body hair development, the client may want privacy. The examiner should provide adequate privacy and draping and should be sensitive to the client's concerns during the examination.

Normal and Abnormal Findings

Skin. There should be a continued evaluation of unusual bruising patterns (see discussion under the young children section). As the child becomes an adolescent, the skin un-

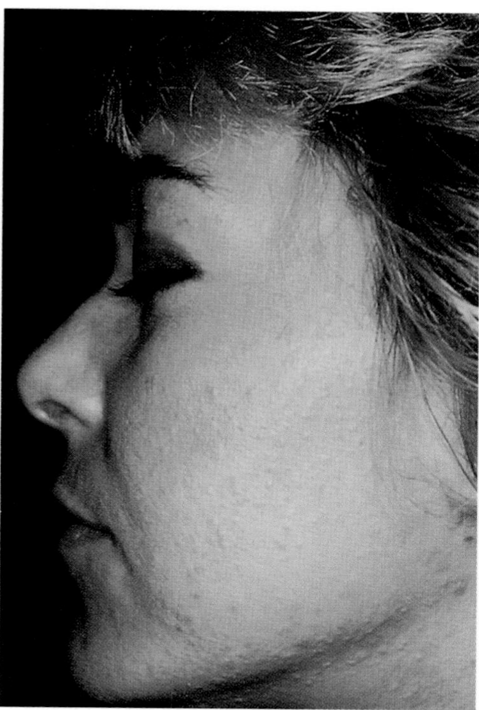

Fig. 11-23 Comedonal acne. Note closed comedones. (From Goldstein and Goldstein, 1997. Courtesy Department of Dermatology, Medical College of Georgia.)

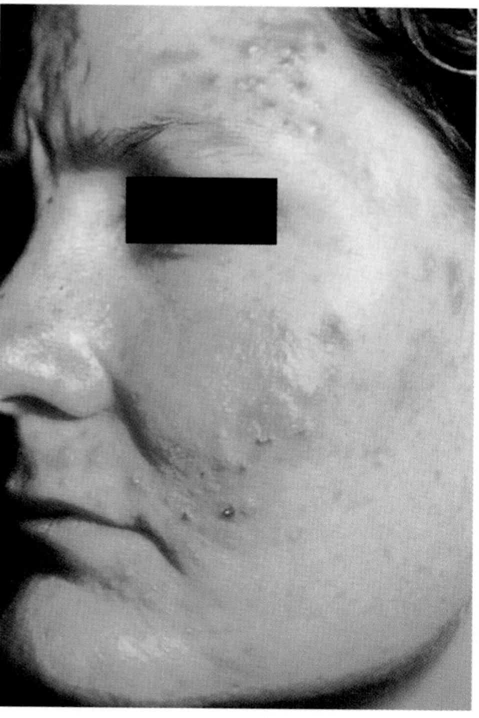

Fig 11-24 Severe acne. (From Goldstein and Goldstein, 1997. Courtesy Marshall Guill, MD.)

dergoes significant maturational development. The skin texture takes on more adult characteristics. In addition, the skin has increased perspiration, oiliness, and acne secondary to an increase in sebaceous gland activity.

The most common abnormal finding and concern for the adolescent is acne. Acne may appear in children as young as 7 to 8 years of age but peaks in adolescence at approximately 16 years of age. Although most acne appears on the face, it may also be prevalent on the chest, back, and shoulders. Acne may appear as blackheads (open comedones) or whiteheads (closed comedones) and is a common finding with this age group (Fig. 11-23) (Goldstein and Goldstein, 1999). Inflamed lesions of acne can be mild or severe. These lesions are painful and are concerning to the client because of the appearance (Fig. 11-24).

Hair. The presence and characteristics of facial hair in boys and body hair in both boys and girls changes significantly, and by the end of adolescence there is an adult hair distribution pattern (see Chapters 21 and 22). According to Tanner (1962):

- *Boys:* Pubic hair development in boys starts at about age 12 and continues until age 15.
- *Girls:* Pubic hair development in girls begins at about age 8 and continues until about age 13.

Nails. The examination and findings are the same as for the adult. Although persistent nail biting may be a habit, it may also be an abnormal or coping mechanism for dealing with stress. The nurse should take the time to evaluate why nail biting persists.

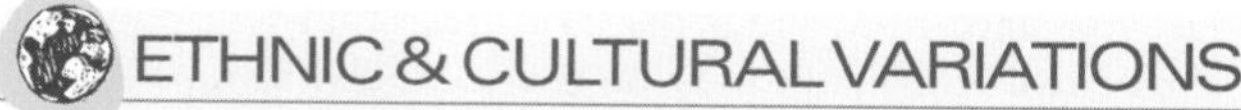

Light-skinned people wrinkle earlier than darker-skinned people. Brown or black hair grays much earlier in light-skinned people than in dark-skinned people. Graying hair is often not seen in American Indians and Alaskan natives until they reach their seventies.

OLDER ADULTS

Anatomy and Physiology

Older adults may notice that their skin is drier or that they seem to produce less perspiration. Both changes are due to decreased sebaceous and sweat gland activity. The thin, parchment-like appearance of the skin is caused by decreased dermal vascularity. Increased permeability of the epidermis results in a less efficient barrier of the stratum corneum.

Several factors contribute to the characteristic folding and wrinkled appearance of the skin in later life: the dermis loses elasticity, collagen, and mass (Matteson, 1997). Joints and bony prominences take on a sharp, angular appearance, and there is a deepening in the hollows of the thoracic, axillary, and supraclavicular regions. These changes are due to a decrease in cutaneous tissue.

A number of hormonal changes affect hair in various parts of the body. For instance, a decrease in melanin production tends to produce gray hair. Scalp, axillary, and pubic hair thin because of reduced hormonal functioning. Because the size of hair follicles also changes, there is a progressive transition of the coarse, terminal scalp hair into the finer, vellus hair. This causes the characteristic age-associated baldness in both men and women. The opposite change, from vellus to terminal, occurs in the hair of the nares and on the tragus of men's ears. Higher androgen-to-estrogen ratios cause women to produce increased coarse facial hair. Both genders experience a loss of hair from the trunk and extremities, axillary, and pubic areas. Decreased peripheral circulation slows nail growth. The nails also become thicker, brittle, hard, and yellowish; they also develop ridges and are prone to splitting into layers.

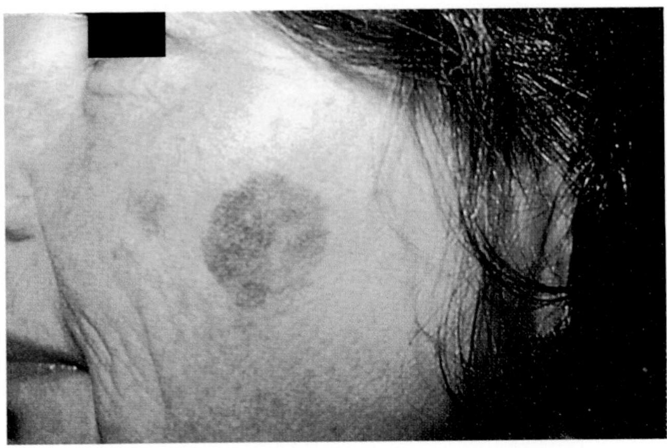

Fig. 11-25 Solar lentigo (liver spots). Brown macules that appear in chronically sun-exposed areas. (From Goldstein and Goldstein, 1997. Courtesy Department of Dermatology, University of North Carolina at Chapel Hil.)

Health History

- Has your skin changed as you have gotten older? If so, how? Have you noticed any changes in the way sores or lesions heal? If so, how has this changed?
  Rationale Healing may become slower with poor peripheral circulation or systemic diseases, such as diabetes mellitus or peripheral vascular disease.
- Do you have trouble cutting or clipping your fingernails or toenails? What type of instrument do you use? If you do have trouble, what do you usually do to care for yourself? Who clips your nails?
  Rationale The nails may thicken secondary to nutritional deficiency or fungal infection.
- Do you have multiple bruises or areas that will not heal?
  Rationale Bruising may be associated with falls and injuries or bleeding disorders.

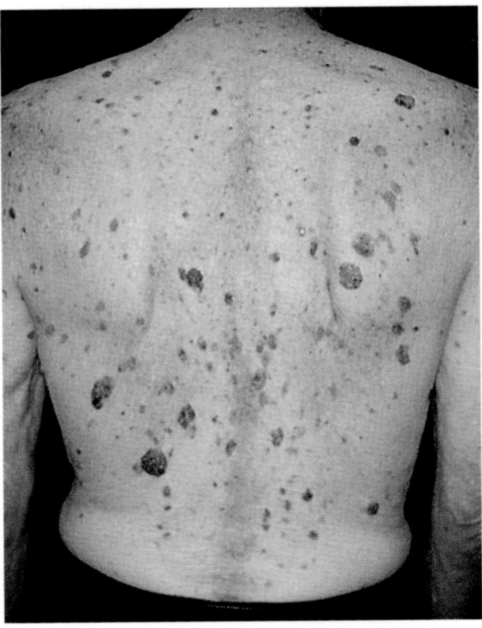

Fig. 11-26 Multiple seborrheic keratosis lesions on the trunk. (From Goldstein and Goldstein, 1997. Courtesy Department of Dermatology, Medical College of Georgia.)

Examination

Procedures and Techniques Because there are many physiologic skin changes with aging, the examiner must take special care when examining the skin, hair, and nails of the older adult and carefully correlate the client's history of the problem with the physical characteristics of the condition or lesion. Some changes are simply a normal aging process, whereas others may be indicative of a cancerous lesion or systemic disease. The examination techniques are the same as for the younger adult.

Normal and Abnormal Findings

Skin. Increased amount of pigmentation, especially in sun-exposed areas may be observed. Likewise, there may be isolated areas of hypopigmentation. Prolonged exposure to the sun may cause the skin to take on a thickened, ruddy appearance. Normal variations in the skin of the older adult include findings such as the following:

- *Solar lentigo (liver spots):* Irregularly shaped, flat, deeply pigmented macules that may appear on body surface areas having repeated exposure to the sun (Fig. 11-25).
- *Seborrheic keratoses:* Pigmented, raised, warty-appearing lesions that may appear on the face or trunk (Fig. 11-26). Care must be taken to differentiate these benign lesions from similarly appearing actinic keratoses, which are premalignant lesions.
- *Acrochordons (skin tags):* Small, soft tags of skin that generally appear on the neck and upper chest (Fig. 11-27). These tags may or may not be pigmented.
- *Sebaceous hyperplasia:* Yellowish, flattened papules that have a central depression (Fig. 11-28).

As the individual ages, the texture and characteristics of the skin change. Changes include (1) an increase in dryness and flaking of the skin, especially over the extremities; (2) thinning of the skin, which may take on a parchment-like appearance, especially over bony prominences, the dorsal

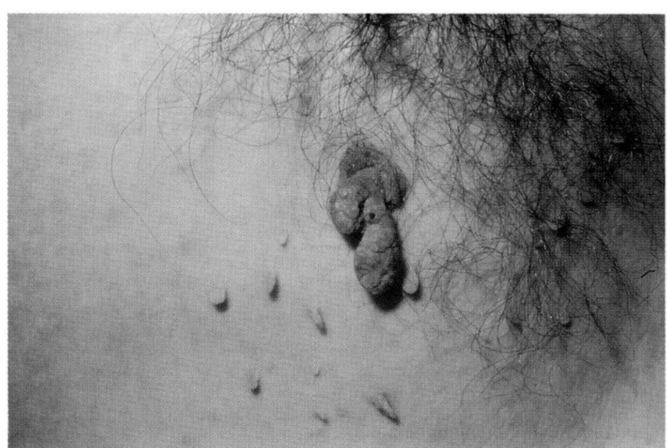

Fig. 11-27 Multiple skin tags. (From Goldstein and Goldstein, 1997. Courtesy Department of Dermatology, University of North Carolina at Chapel Hill.)

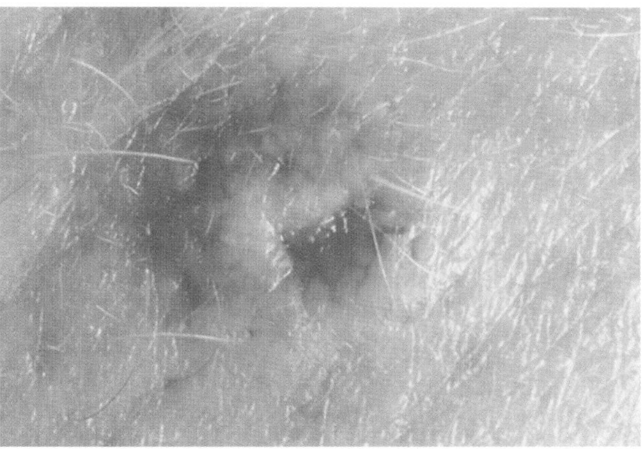

Fig. 11-28 Sebaceous hyperplasia. (From Habif, 1990.)

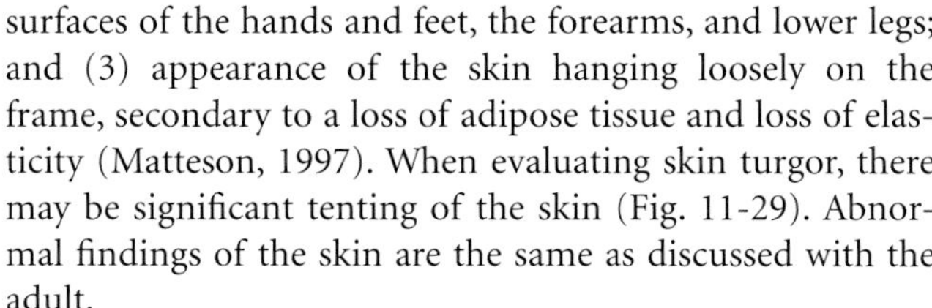

surfaces of the hands and feet, the forearms, and lower legs; and (3) appearance of the skin hanging loosely on the frame, secondary to a loss of adipose tissue and loss of elasticity (Matteson, 1997). When evaluating skin turgor, there may be significant tenting of the skin (Fig. 11-29). Abnormal findings of the skin are the same as discussed with the adult.

Hair. In the older adult, the hair of the head turns gray or white as the melanocytes cease to function. The hair may also become thin and change in texture. Symmetric balding may occur in men. Changes with aging include a decrease in the amount of body, pubic, and axillary hair. Men may have an increase in the amount and coarseness of nasal and eyebrow hair. Women may develop coarse facial hair.

Nails. Changes that occur with aging include thickening and increased brittleness of the nails. Both fingernails and toenails may become slightly deformed, lose their transparency, and may turn a yellowish color.

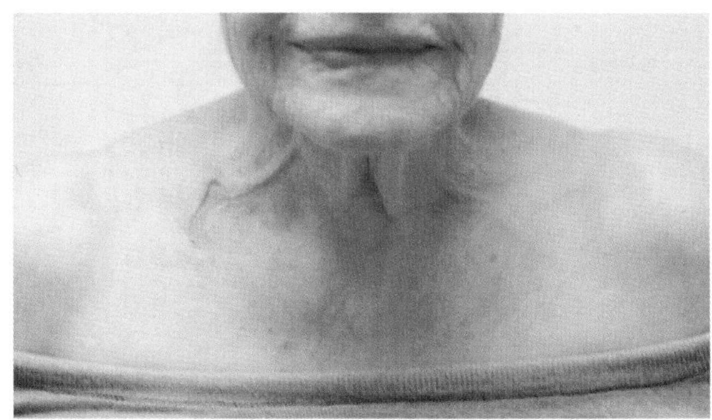

Fig. 11-29 Poor skin turgor with tenting in older adult. (From Seidel et al, 1999.)

CLIENTS WITH SITUATIONAL VARIATIONS

CLIENTS WITH LIMITED MOBILITY (HEMIPLEGIA, PARAPLEGIA, QUADRIPLEGIA)

Clients with limited mobility are at special risk for skin breakdown secondary to pressure and body fluid pooling. The nurse should carefully examine the client's skin, especially the areas of the body where there are bony prominences. The nurse may need assistance to move and turn the client so that a complete skin assessment may be performed.

In addition, clients who operate their own wheelchairs are at high risk for developing hand calluses. Therefore special care should be taken to examine the client's hands.

Normal and Abnormal Findings

Skin Carefully assess all contact and skin pressure points for clients who have limited mobility (Fig. 11-30). The examiner should expect areas to have initial pallor when pressure is applied, but when the pressure is removed, the skin tone should quickly become red and then return to its normal color. An abnormal response is prolonged blanching, indicating ischemia, or prolonged redness, indicating that the area is engorged with blood. The stages of actual tissue damage are as follows: Stage I, prolonged redness with unbroken skin; Stage II, partial-thickness skin loss appears as superficial abrasion, blister, or excoriation; Stage III, full-

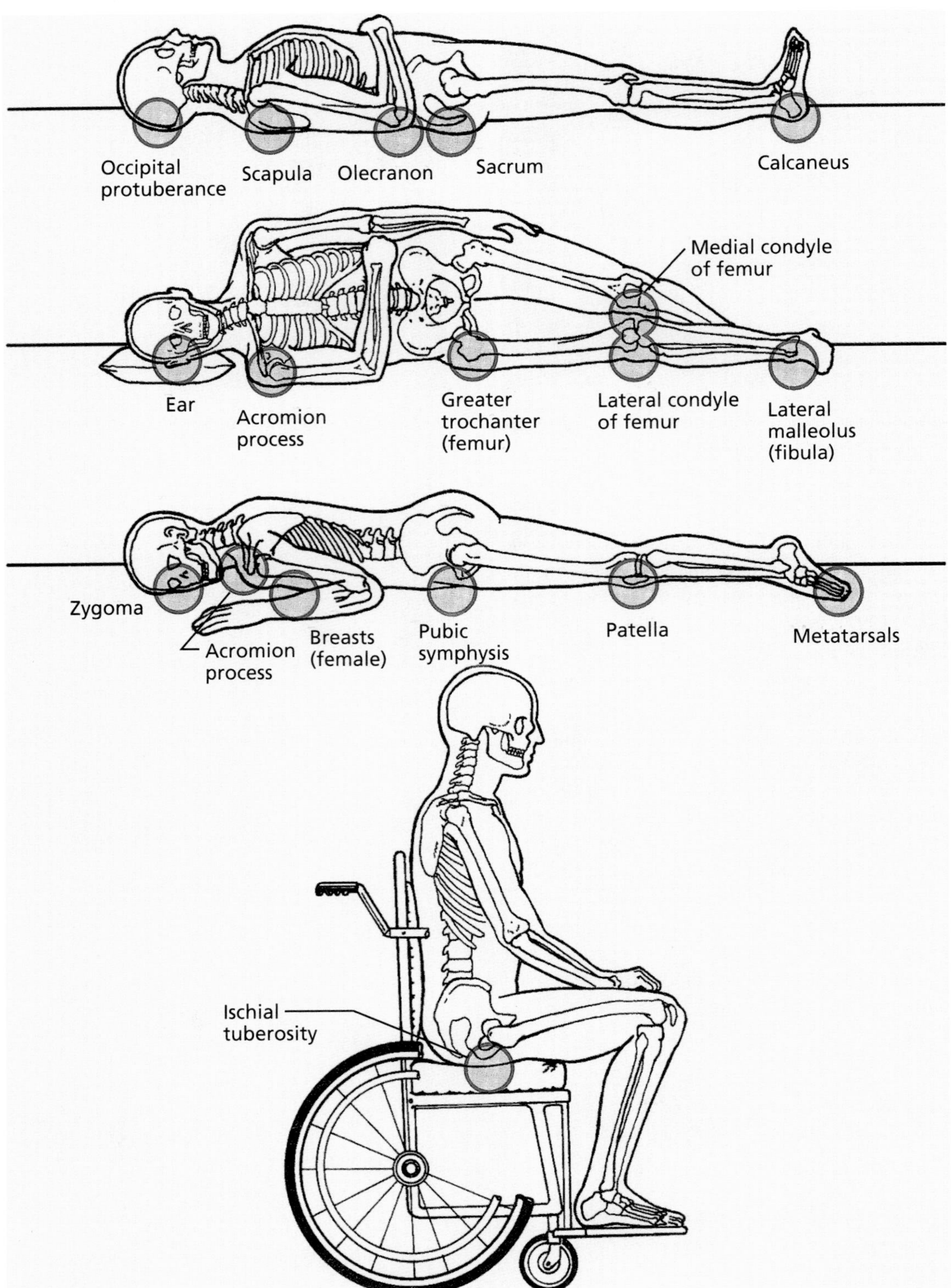

Fig. 11-30 Bony prominences vulnerable to pressure.

thickness skin loss with damage to the subcutaneous tissue; may note serosanguineous drainage; and Stage IV, full-thickness skin loss with invasion of deeper tissue into the muscle and/or bone (Lewis et al, 2000). The wound will appear as an open ulceration with purulent drainage and peripheral crusting (Fig. 11-31).

ETHNIC & CULTURAL VARIATIONS

A range of normal differences exists in the physical appearance of skin, hair, and nails. Skin color can range from white to deep brown with yellow, olive, copper, and red overtones. This color is often absent or diminished at birth, developing over months during infancy. Skin often retains its elasticity

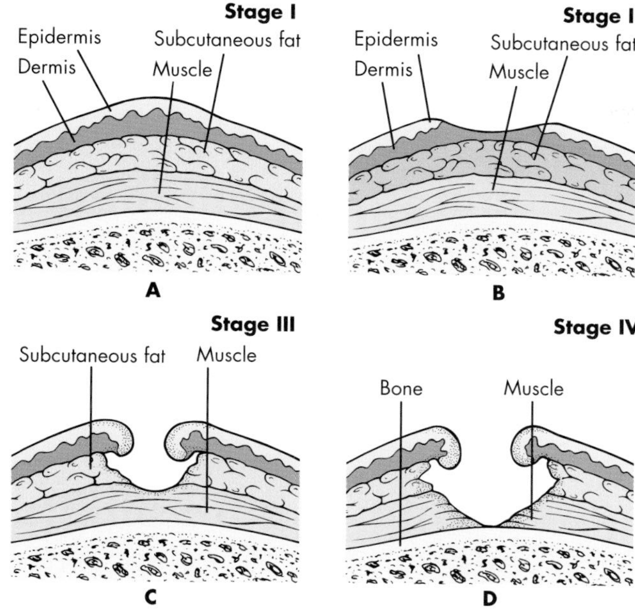

Fig. 11-31 Stages of pressure ulcers. **A,** Stage I. **B,** Stage II. **C,** Stage III. **D,** Stage IV. (From Lewis et al, 1996.)

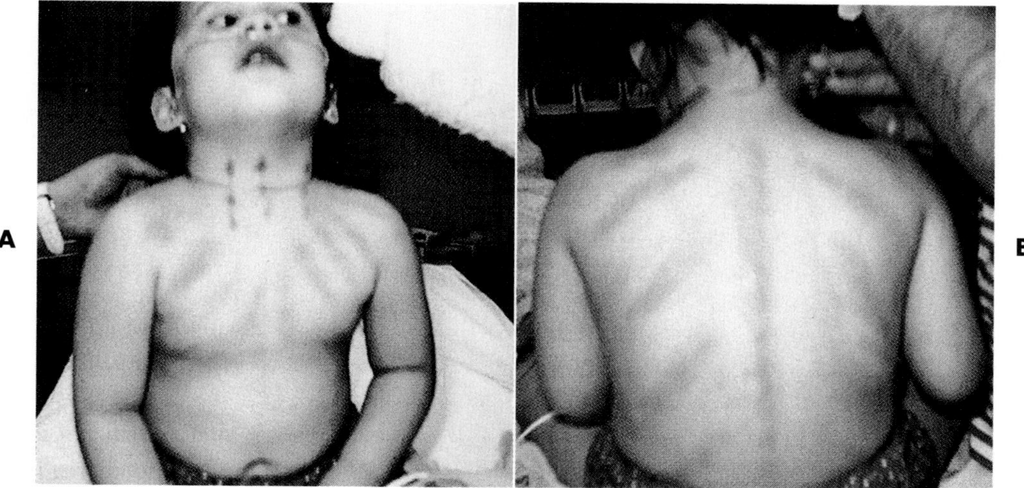

Fig. 11-32 Four-year-old South Asian girl with coining lesions along the rib cage on the front and back and on her neck. (From Monteleone, 1996.)

and tone longer and wrinkles later in the aging process in darker-skinned persons. Hair texture may range from fine to coarse, thin to thick, straight to kinky. Hair on the face and body may be absent or range from sparse to abundant. Brown and black hair gray earlier in light-skinned persons. Sweat glands have different distributions and produce various levels of salt concentrations on the skin. Nail color ranges from pink to dark brown, and pigment bands may be naturally present in darker-skinned persons.

Certain physical findings also vary by skin color. Cyanosis and pallor are easily observed on the skin of light-skinned persons, whereas these conditions are often seen only on the lips, tongue, or mucous membranes in dark-skinned persons. Jaundice and petechiae, although visible on light skin, are best seen in the oral mucosa and sclera/conjunctiva of those with darker skin. Bruising is often purple to yellowish green in light-skinned persons and purple to brownish black in dark-skinned persons. Inspection for pressure areas, which lead to decubitus, may require more careful scrutiny in those with darker skin.

Cultural practices may also affect findings when inspecting the skin. Practices such as coining or cupping may leave skin markings that are common in certain ethnic groups (Fig. 11-32). Various cultural groups are also at higher risk for certain disease processes, such as diabetes mellitus and peripheral vascular disease, that predispose them to skin complications. All of these factors should be considered when examining the skin, hair, and nails.

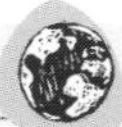

ETHNIC & CULTURAL VARIATIONS

Pressure areas in darker-skinned people are often harder to see in the early stages. Thus extra care should be taken when inspecting common pressure sites. Initially those with dark skin are likely to have a grayish or yellow-brown pallor at the pressure site that becomes purple, then returns to normal color when pressure is removed. A prolonged purple area may be seen as a beginning indication of actual tissue damage.

EXAMINATION SUMMARY

Skin, Hair, and Nails

PROCEDURE

Skin

- Inspect the skin for:
  Color
  Variations in skin color
- Inspect and palpate the skin for:
  Lesions
- Palpate the skin for:
  Texture
  Temperature
  Moisture
  Mobility
  Turgor

Hair

- Inspect and palpate the scalp and hair for:
  Surface characteristics
  Hair distribution
  Texture
  Quantity
  Color
- Inspect the facial and body hair for:
  Distribution
  Quantity
  Texture

Nails

- Inspect and palpate the nails for:
  Shape
  Contour
  Consistency
  Color
  Thickness
  Cleanliness

SUMMARY OF FINDINGS

Age Group	Normal Findings	Typical Variations	Findings Associated With Disorders
Infants and children	• *Skin:* Newborn skin may be red; physiologic jaundice common; vernix caseosa normal birth covering. • *Hair:* At birth, generalized lanugo suggests prematurity. • *Nails:* Newborn nails may need to be trimmed to prevent scratching.	• *Skin:* Primary irritant or eczematous dermatitis may cause localized lesions; roughness may be from clothing, coldness, or soap. Common lesions include mongolian spot, café-au-lait, stork bite, milia, diaper rash, and erythema toxicum.	• *Skin:* Newborn skin distortions suggest masses, nodules, or tumors; presence of patches, erythema, scaling, crusts, fissures, vesicles, lesions, and skin irregularities in children requires investigation.
Adolescents	• *Skin:* Adolescents prone to acne from hormonal changes. • *Hair:* Terminal hair develops at puberty.	• *Skin:* Perspiration may be from anxiety or obesity. • *Nails:* Nail hygiene is a clue about self-care and emotional and social levels.	• *Hair:* Fine or course hair and hair loss may be due to thyroid conditions.

Age Group	Normal Findings	Typical Variations	Findings Associated With Disorders
Adults	• *Skin:* Thinnest on eyelids; thickest on soles, palms, and elbows; color uniform, except sun-exposed areas; skin temperature symmetrical; texture smooth, soft, and even; skin is resilient. • *Hair:* Scalp hair shiny, smooth and resilient. • *Nails:* Nail color variations of pink; nail edges should be smooth and rounded.	• *Skin:* Calloused areas yellow; skin striae, freckles, birthmarks, nevi, and melasma may be present. • *Nails:* Nail shape and opacity vary; pigment deposits may be present in dark-skinned persons; darkened nails may be from antimalarial drug or shoe trauma; white spots in nail plate from mild trauma; peeling nails may occur with water exposure; longitudinal ridging and beading common.	• *Skin:* Freckling of buccal cavity, gums, and tongue in some dark-skinned persons; color hues best seen in sclera, mucosa, and nail beds; lips and gums are bluish in dark-skinned persons. Localized redness suggests inflammation; hemorrhage results from injury, steroids, or systemic disorders; fluid-filled lesions show red glow with transillumination. Generalized lesions may indicate systemic disorder, allergy, or genetic disorder. Annular patterns associated with pityriasis rosea, tinea corporis and cruris, and urticaria. Connective tissue diseases lead to changes in skin mobility. • *Hair:* Asymmetrical hair loss in males may indicate pathologic condition; female alopecia or female hirsutism in male hair patterns may indicate pathologic condition. • *Nails:* Yellow nails occur with psoriasis, fungal infections, and respiratory disease; darkened nails from *Candida* or hyperbilirubinemia; green-black nails caused by *Pseudomonas* or subungual hematoma. Nail depression and clubbing occur from systemic disease. Separation of nail plate from bed results from psoriasis and infections.
Older adults	• *Skin:* Becomes more transparent, pale, dry, and hyperpigmented with aging. • *Hair:* Becomes coarser with age. • *Nails:* Thicken with age.	• *Hair:* Grayness occurs from decrease in functioning melanocytes; balding patterns in men are genetically determined.	• *Skin:* Stasis dermatitis and solar keratosis are skin conditions that affect the elderly. • *Nails:* Cardiac disease influences nail conditions.

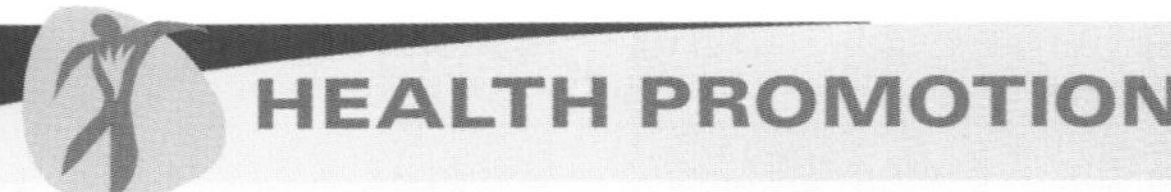

HEALTH PROMOTION

IMMUNIZATIONS

Clients of all ages should be taught about the benefits of immunizations and the lifetime schedules for immunizations. Adults, as well as children, should maintain current immunizations. Parents of young children should especially be encouraged to immunize their children against communicable diseases and taught to identify common skin lesions related to those diseases. See Table 2-7 for the age-specific immunization schedule.

SUN EXPOSURE AND PROTECTION

Clients of all ages should be taught about the need for careful protection of the skin with the use of sunscreens, avoidance of excessive exposure to the sun, and limited exposure to ionizing radiation. Sun exposure is intensified for clients living in sunny climates and those living near water or at high altitudes (e.g., mountains). Exposure to natural radiation from sunlight is linked directly to skin cancer, and there are approximately 400,000 cases of this type of cancer each year *(Healthy People 2010)*. Teach the client about the various strengths of available sunscreens and sunblocking creams and lotions. The use of sunblocking agents such as para-aminobenzoic acid (PABA) is recommended, since these agents can be chosen on the basis of skin type and sensitivity to burning. Instruct the client to use a sunscreen with a sun protection factor (SPF) of at least 15 (the SPF is shown on the bottle). Children and infants should have an even higher SPF level. All clients should be encouraged to wear hats.

SKIN CANCER

Young and older adults alike should be taught to perform skin self-assessment and to recognize the cardinal signs of skin changes that may be indicative of a malignancy.

SIGNS OF BASAL CELL CARCINOMA

Basal cell carcinoma is the most common type of cancer. One out of every four new cancers discovered is basal cell carcinoma, and one in eight Americans develops this type of skin cancer. The cause of 95% of all basal cell carcinomas is chronic overexposure to sunlight. That is why these lesions occur most frequently on exposed parts of the body—the face, ears, neck, scalp, shoulders, and back (see Fig. 11-54).

The most common signs of basal cell carcinoma are the following:

- A persistent, nonhealing, open sore that bleeds, oozes, or crusts and remains open for 3 or more weeks.
- A reddish patch or irritated area, usually on the chest, shoulders, or limbs, that may or may not itch or hurt.
- A smooth growth with an elevated, rolled border and indented center.
- A shiny bump or nodule that is pearly or translucent and that can be pink, red, white, tan, black, or brown.
- A scarlike area, white, yellow, or waxy, which often has poorly defined borders and loss of normal skin markings.

SIGNS OF MELANOMA

In the United States, the incidence of malignant melanoma is increasing at an alarming rate. The following signs may indicate the presence of a malignant melanoma (see Fig 11-56). Any one or more of the following changes occurring in a new or existing pigmented (tan or brown) area of the skin or in a mole may indicate the presence of a malignant melanoma:

- **Change in size:** especially sudden or continuous enlargement.
- **Change in color:** especially multiple shades of tan, brown, dark brown, black; the mixing of red, white, and blue; or the spreading of color from the edge into the surrounding skin.
- **Change in shape:** especially development of an irregular, notched border, which used to be regular.
- **Change in elevation:** especially the raising of a part of a pigmented area that used to be flat or only slightly elevated.
- **Change in surface:** especially scaliness, erosion, oozing, crusting, ulceration, or bleeding.
- **Changes in surrounding skin:** especially redness, swelling, or development of colored blemishes next to, but not part of the pigmented area.
- **Change in sensation:** especially itchiness, tenderness, or pain.
- **Change in consistency:** especially softening or hardening.

THE A, B, C, D EARLY SIGNS OF MELANOMA

A = Asymmetry
B = Border (notched, scalloped, or indistinct)
C = Color (uneven, variegated)
D = Diameter (usually larger than 6 mm)

INGROWN TOENAILS

These may in most cases be prevented if the nails are trimmed properly. The nail should be trimmed straight across, not curved around the toe.

COMMON PROBLEMS AND CONDITIONS

Skin, Hair, and Nails

SKIN

Dermatitis

The term *dermatitis* is used to describe a variety of superficial inflammatory conditions of the skin. These conditions can be acute or chronic.

Eczema

Eczema presents as erythematous papules and vesicles that may weep, ooze, and become crusted (Fig. 11-33). There is significant pruritus. The lesions are most prevalent on the scalp, forehead, cheeks, back of the knee, at the popliteal flexure, and on the arms, especially the antecubital flexure. Generally there is a family history of allergies. A chronic form of this disease is called atopic dermatitis.

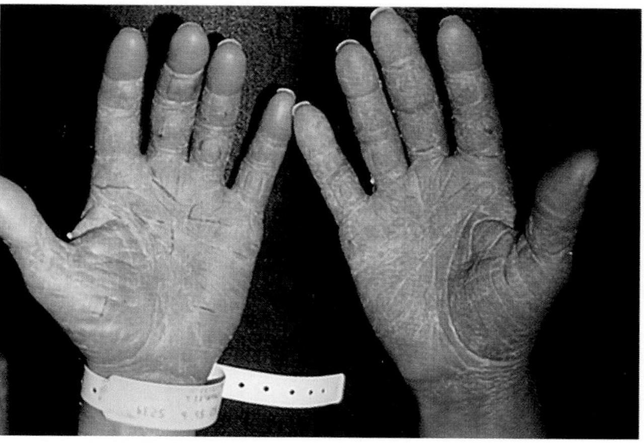

Fig. 11-33 Severe eczema of the hand. (From Hill, 1994.)

Contact Dermatitis

This is a local rash that may have secondary characteristics of swelling, wheals, urticaria, and sometimes papular vesicles or scales (Fig. 11-34). The dermatitis appears secondary to a contact or environmental irritant or allergy.

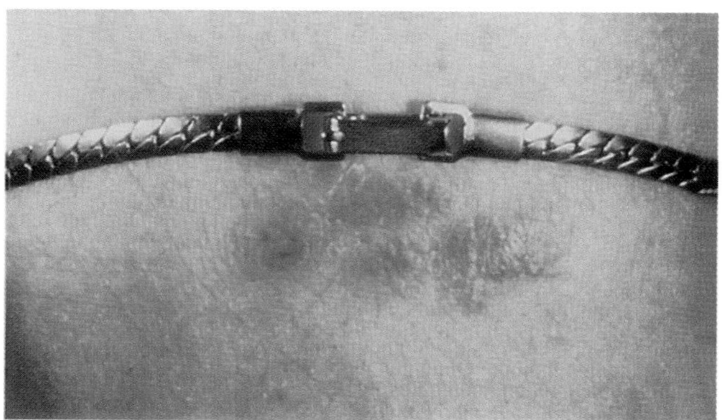

Fig. 11-34 Contact dermatitis. In this case, allergic reaction to nickel. (From Cohen, 1993.)

Stasis Dermatitis

Stasis dermatitis is an inflammation of the skin on the lower legs seen usually in the older adult. This condition typically appears as an area of brown pigmentation and areas of erythematous, scaling, and if advanced, areas of weeping patches (Fig. 11-35). The lesions are thought to be secondary to chronic edema and poor peripheral circulation. If left untreated, this eventually develops into a stasis ulcer.

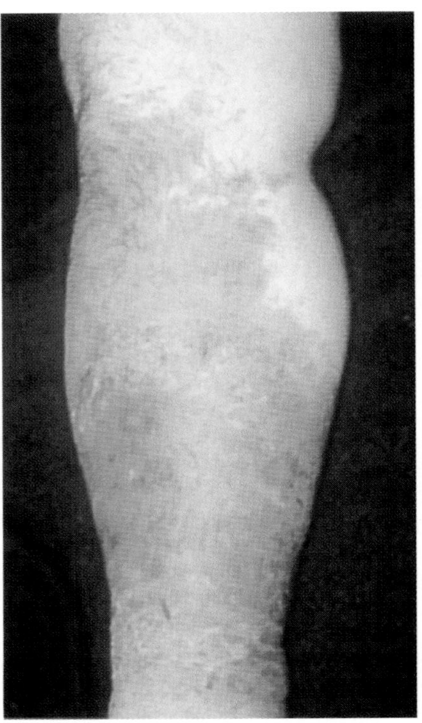

Fig. 11-35 Stasis dermatitis. (From Marks and DeLeo, 1992.)

Seborrheic Dermatitis

In adults, seborrheic dermatitis causes a dry or greasy scaly condition of the scalp (dandruff) but does not cause hair loss. In neonates, this condition is known as cradle cap. It is associated with a thick, scaly condition of the scalp and forehead (Fig. 11-36).

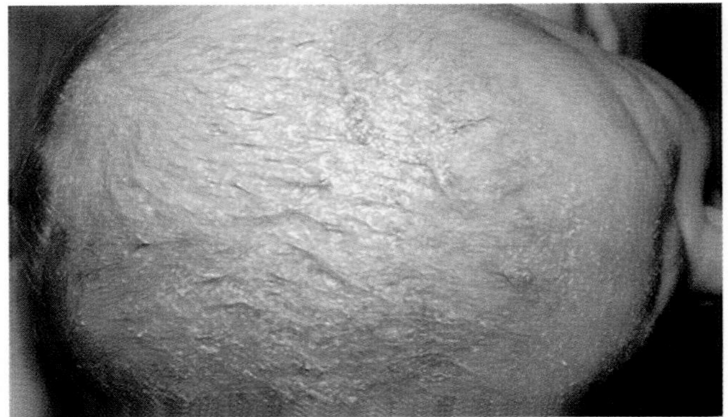

Fig. 11-36 Seborrheic dermatitis (cradle cap). (From Cohen, 1993.)

Psoriasis

This is a chronic recurrent condition that appears as well-circumscribed, scaly erythematous papules or plaques that may be a silver color on the surface (Fig. 11-37). Psoriasis appears most frequently on the elbows, knees, buttocks, lower back, and scalp.

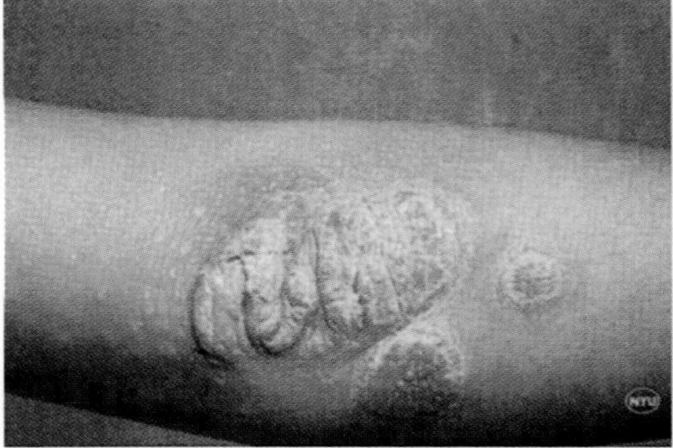

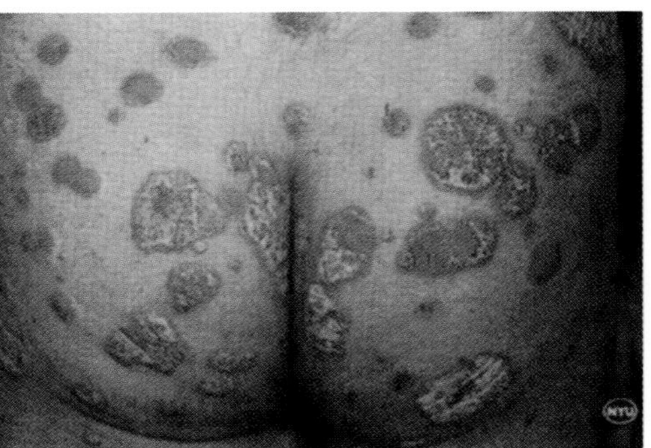

Fig. 11-37 Psoriasis on elbow and buttocks. (Courtesy American Academy of Dermatology and Institute for Dermatologic Communication and Education, Schaumburg, Ill.)

Pityriasis Rosea

Pityriasis rosea is a common, acute, self-limiting inflammatory disease of unknown origin (Fig. 11-38). It initially presents with a "herald patch," which is a single lesion, usually on the trunk, resembling tinea corporis. One to three weeks following the initial lesion, a generalized eruption of pale, erythematous and macular lesions occur on the trunk and extremities; occasionally, they will appear as vesicular lesions. The condition typically lasts for several weeks. The client generally feels well but may complain of mild itching. This condition is not infectious or contagious; however, because secondary syphilis may manifest with a similar-appearing rash, it is important to conduct serologic testing for individuals with pityriasis rosea.

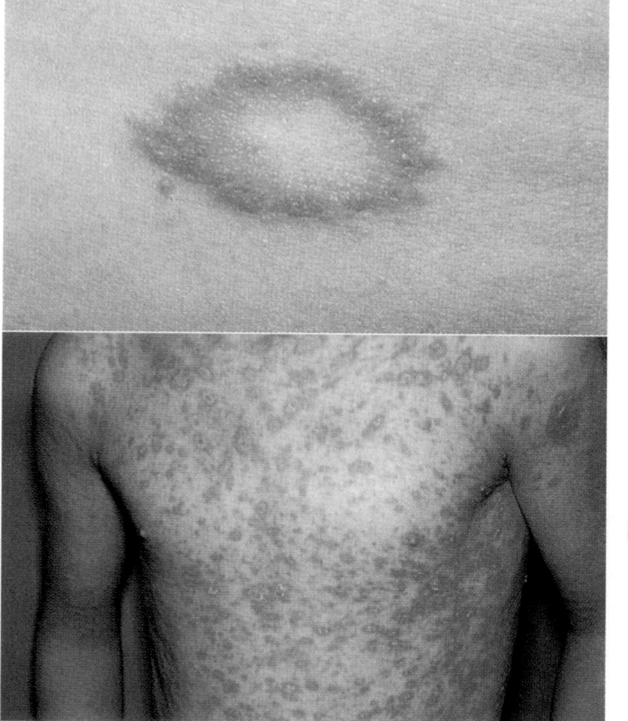

Fig. 11-38 Pityriasis rosea. **A,** Large herald patch shown on chest of a 10-year-old girl. **B,** Many oval lesions seen on the chest of a white teenager. (From Cohen, 1993.)

Lesions Caused by Viral Infection

Warts

Warts are caused by at least 60 types of human papillomavirus (HPV). There are many different types of warts occurring in many locations and in many sizes. They may appear at any age. Common warts (verrucae vulgaris) are firm, round- or irregular-shaped lesions that are light gray, yellow, or brownish black. They commonly appear on hands, fingers, elbows, and knees (Fig. 11-39). Plantar warts are found on the sole of the foot and are typically tender to pressure.

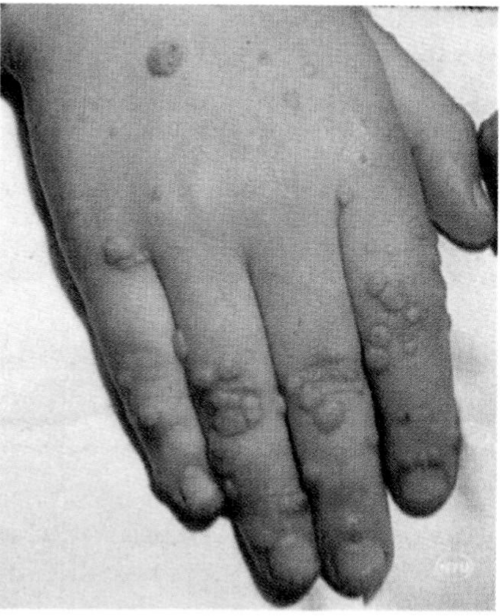

Fig. 11-39 Common warts on hand and fingers. (Courtesy American Academy of Dermatology and Institute for Dermatologic Communication and Education, Schaumburg, Ill.)

Herpes Simplex

Lesions caused by herpes simplex may appear on the upper lip (type 1) (Fig. 11-40) or on the genitalia (type 2). They start with a feeling of slight stinging and increased sensitivity. As the lesions erupt they move through maturational stages of vesicles, pustule, and finally crusting. (See Chapters 21 and 22 for herpes type 2.)

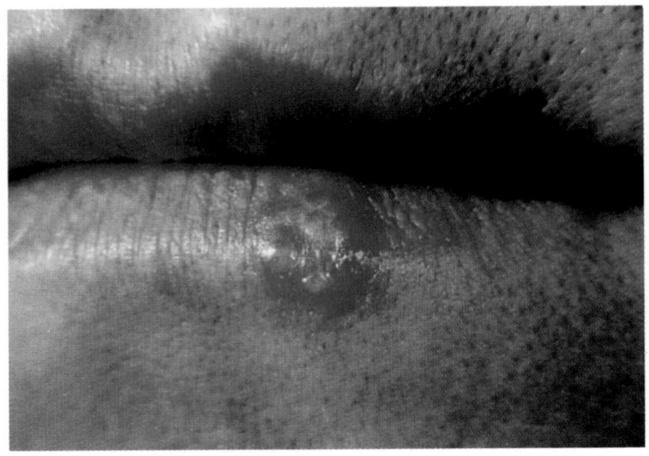

Fig. 11-40 Herpes simplex type 1 (cold sore). (From Grimes, 1991.)

Herpes Zoster (Shingles)

Herpes zoster is caused by the dormant virus of chickenpox. It appears as linearly grouped vesicles along a cutaneous sensory nerve line (Fig. 11-41). As the disease progresses, the vesicles turn into pustules, then crusts. This painful condition is generally unilateral and commonly appears on the trunk and face. Pain may precede lesion eruption by several days (Bjorgen, 1998).

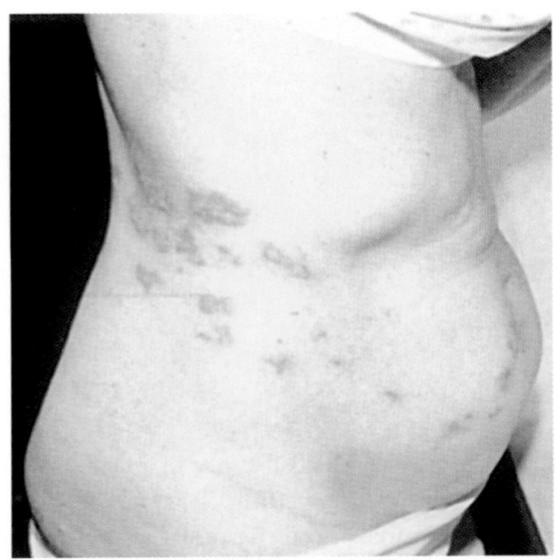

Fig. 11-41 Herpes zoster (shingles). (From Raj, 1992.)

Herpes Varicella (Chickenpox)

This is a highly communicable viral infection spread by droplets. Initially the lesions first appear on the trunk and then spread to the extremities and the face. Initially the lesions are macules, progress to papules, then vesicles, and finally the old vesicles become crusts. The lesions erupt in crops over a period of several days. For this reason, lesions in various stages are seen concurrently. The period of infectivity is from a few days before lesions appear until the final lesions have crusted—usually about 6 days after first lesions erupt (Fig. 11-42).

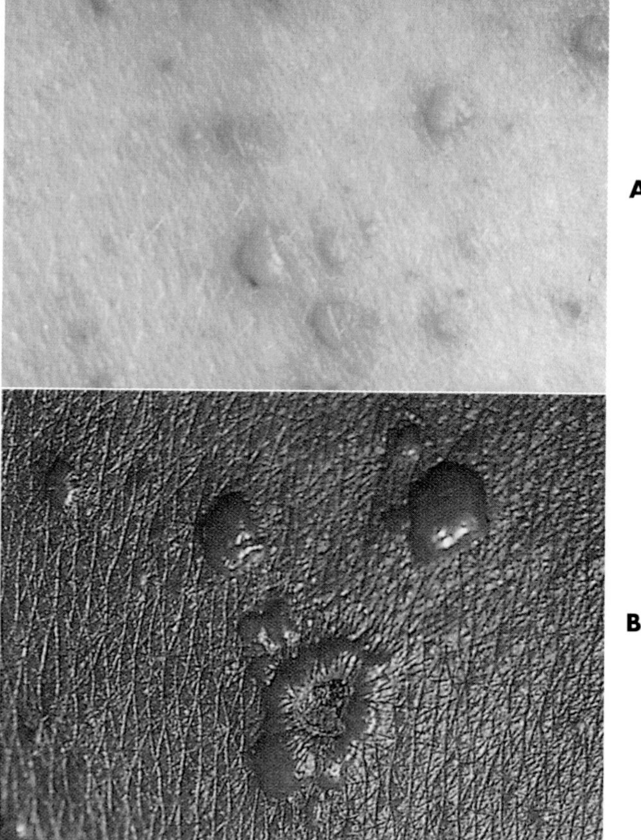

Fig. 11-42 Herpes varicella (chickenpox). Lesions in various stages of development, including red papules, vesicles, umbilicated vesicles, and crusts. **A,** Light-skinned person. **B,** Dark-skinned person. (From Farrar et al, 1992.)

Rubella (German Measles)

Rubella presents as a pink papular rash that generally starts on the face and then spreads to the trunk, arms, and legs (Fig. 11-43). Concurrent with the rash is the presence of lymphadenopathy. The rash typically lasts about 3 days.

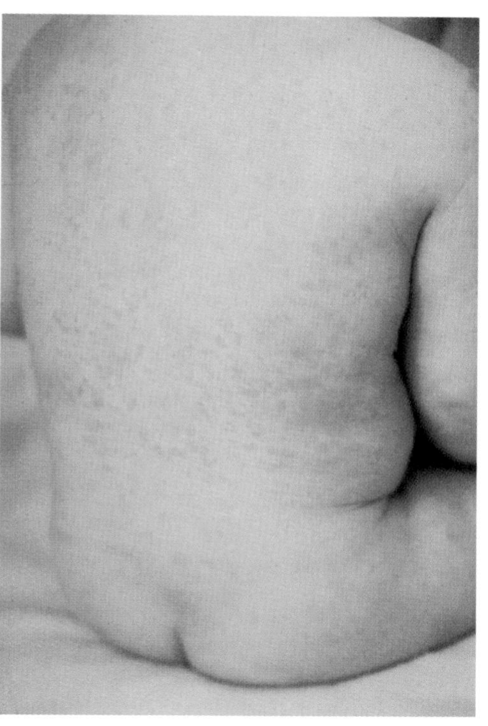

Fig. 11-43 Rubella (German measles). (From Grimes, 1991.)

Rubeola (Measles)

The initial symptoms of rubeola are fever and cough, followed by Koplik's spots in the mouth. A rash appears 3 to 4 days after the onset of symptoms. (See Fig. 14-32 in Chapter 14 to see Koplik's spots.) The rash is a red-purple, maculopapular, blotchy, nonblanching, slightly raised rash (Fig. 11-44). It generally starts behind the ears and spreads over the face, neck, trunk, arms, and legs.

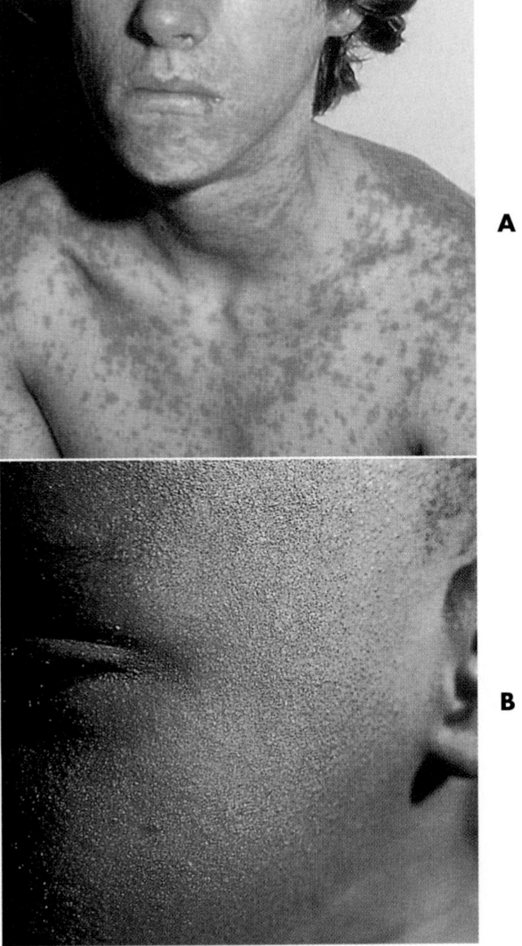

Fig. 11-44 Rubeola (measles). **A,** Blotchy, erythematous, blanching maculopapular eruption on a light-skinned woman. **B,** Slight follicular swelling on a dark-skinned child. (**A** From Cohen, 1993; **B** from Farrar et al, 1992.)

Lesions Caused by Fungal Infections

Tinea is a term used to identify a group of noncanididal fungal infections that can affect the skin, hair, and nails.

Tinea Corporis (Ringworm)

Tinea corporis appears as circular, well-demarcated lesions that tends to have a clear center (Fig. 11-45). These lesions appear on nonhairy parts of the body. They are hyperpigmented in light-colored skin and hypopigmented in dark-skinned persons.

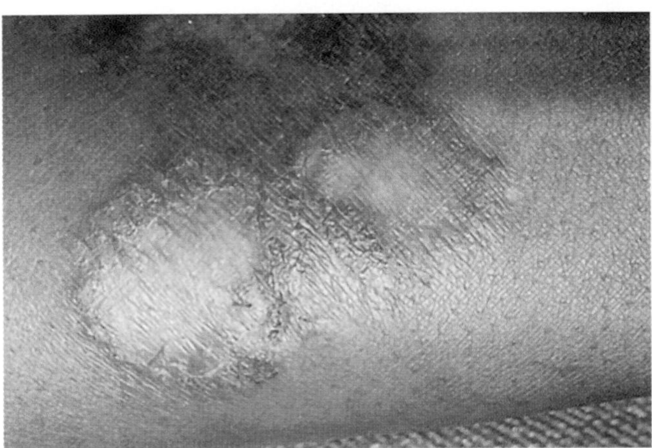

Fig. 11-45 Tinea corporis (ringworm). Classic presentation with central clearing. (From Hill, 1994.)

Tinea Pedis (Athlete's Foot)

Tinea pedis usually appears as small weeping vesicles between the toes and sometimes on the sole of the foot (Fig. 11-46). As the lesions develop, they may become scaly and hard and cause discomfort and itching.

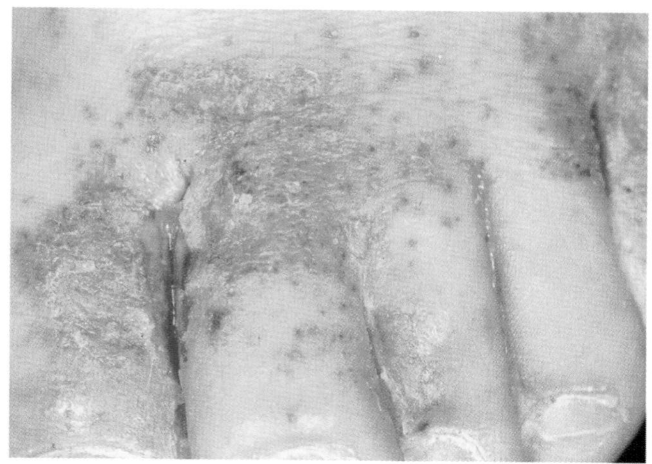

Fig. 11-46 Tinea pedis (athlete's foot). (From Habif, 1996.)

Candidiasis

This fungal infection is caused by *Candida albicans* and appears as a scalding red rash with sharply demarcated borders (Fig. 11-47). The area is generally a large patch but may have some loose scales. Common locations for the rash are the genitalia and inguinal area and along the gluteal folds. Urine, feces, heat, and moisture aggravate the problem.

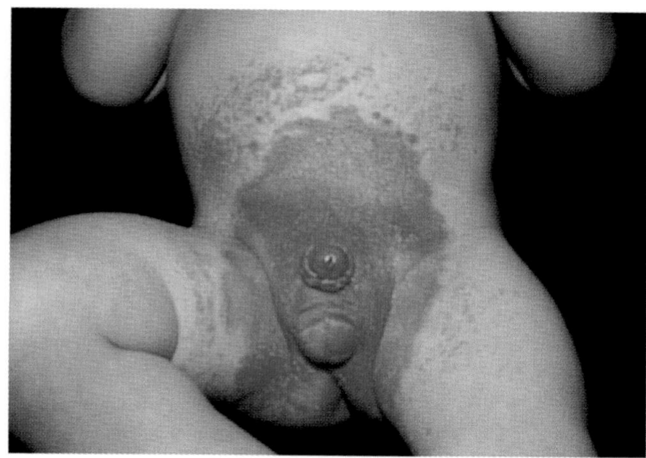

Fig. 11-47 Candidiasis. (From Weston, Lane, and Morelli, 1996.)

Lesions Caused by Bacterial Infections

Cellulitis

Cellulitis is an acute streptococcal or staphylococcal infection of the skin and subcutaneous tissue (Fig. 11-48). The skin is red, warm to the touch, tender, and appears to be indurated. There may be regional lymphangitic streaks and lymphadenopathy.

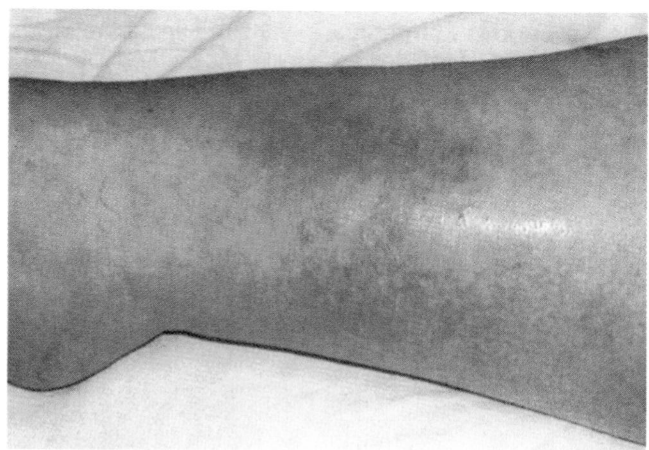

Fig. 11-48 Cellulitis to the lower leg.

Impetigo

This is a highly contagious bacterial infection caused by staphylococcal or streptococcal pathogens. It appears as an erythematous macule that becomes a vesicle or bulla and finally a honey-colored crust after the vesicles or bullas rupture (Fig. 11-49). This infection is most prevalent in infants and children.

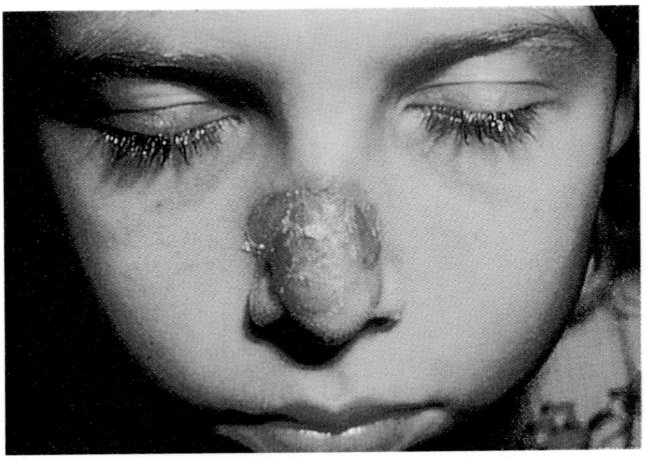

Fig. 11-49 Impetigo. (From Goldstein and Goldstein, 1997. Courtesy Department of Dermatology, University of North Carolina at Chapel Hill.)

Furuncle or Abscess (Boil)

A furuncle, also known as a boil, is a localized bacterial lesion caused by a staphylococcal pathogen. Initially it is a nodule surrounded by erythema and edema. As it progresses, it becomes a pustule; the center (or core) fills with a sanguineous purulent exudate. The skin around a furuncle is red, hot, and extremely tender (Fig. 11-50). Common locations for the lesions include the back of the neck and buttocks. An abscess is usually larger and deeper and has a variety of precipitating causes.

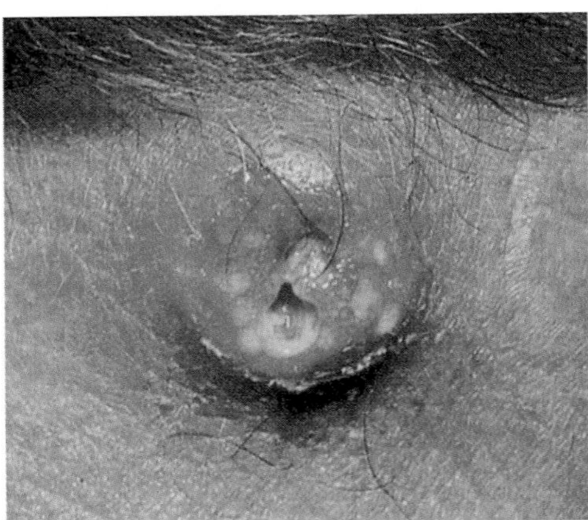

Fig. 11-50 Furuncle. (From Thompson et al, 1998. Courtesy James A. Tschen, MD, Baylor College of Medicine, Department of Dermatology, Houston, Texas.)

Folliculitis

This is an inflammation and infection of hair follicles. An acute lesion is characterized by a pustule surrounding the hair follicle (Fig. 11-51). A chronic condition can occur when deep hair follicles are infected—usually seen in bearded areas.

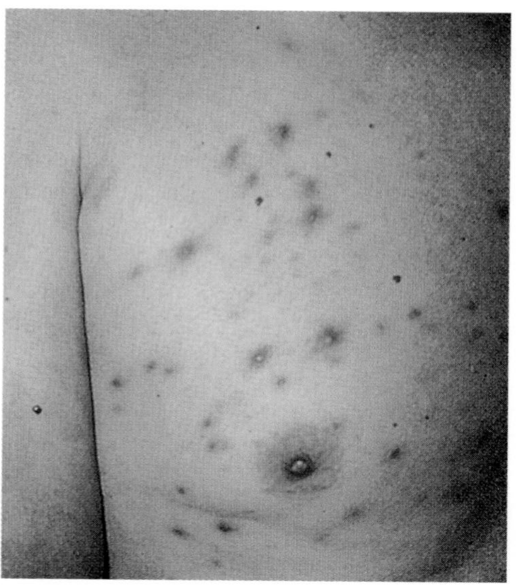

Fig. 11-51 Folliculitis. (From Goldstein and Goldstein, 1997. Courtesy Beverly Sanders, MD.)

Lesions Associated With Infestation

Scabies

Severe pruritus is the hallmark of scabies. It is a parasitic infection caused by *Sarcoptes scabiei.* The pruritus is caused by a hypersensitivity to the mite and its feces (Goldstein and Goldstein, 1997). Areas most commonly affected include the hands, wrists, axillae, genitalia, and inner aspects of the thigh (Fig. 11-52). The lesions are small papules, vesicles, and burrows that result from the mite entering the skin to lay eggs. The burrows appear as short irregular marks that look as if they were made by the end of a pencil.

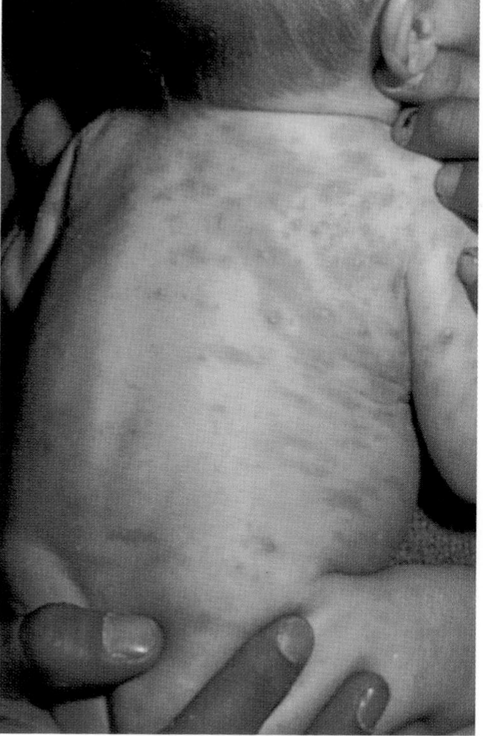

Fig. 11-52 Scabies in infant. Hundreds of lesions present. (From Weston, Lane and Morelli, 1996.)

Neoplasia

Kaposi's Sarcoma

Kaposi's sarcoma is a malignant neoplasm characterized by dark blue-purple macules, papules, nodules, and plaques (Fig. 11-53). It is most commonly seen on the legs, trunk, arms, neck, and head. The disease is most commonly seen in clients with acquired immunodeficiency syndrome (AIDS).

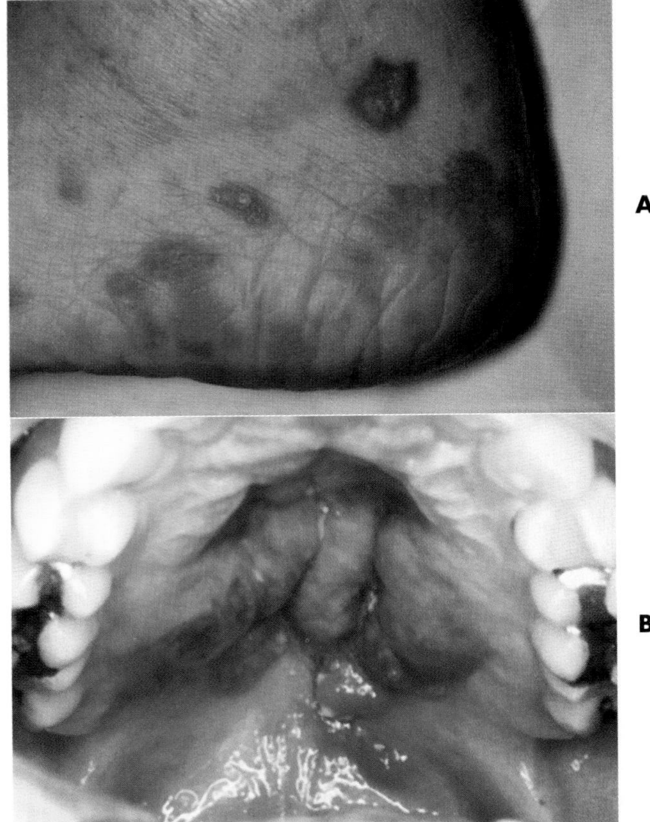

Fig. 11-53 **A,** Kaposi's sarcoma of the heel and lateral foot. **B,** Oral Kaposi's sarcoma. (**A** from Grimes et al, 1991; **B** courtesy Sol Silverman, Jr, DDS, University of California, San Francisco.)

Basal Cell Carcinoma

A malignant tumor of the skin, basal cell carcinoma is believed to arise from a hair follicle. This is the most common form of skin cancer and afflicts predominately people with light complexion. It is locally invasive and rarely metastasizes. The incidence increases with age and is more common in males than females (Leffel and Fitzgerald, 1999). The lesion has different forms but usually appears as a nodular pigmented lesion. It is most commonly found in areas that have had repeated exposure to the sun or ultraviolet light, such as the face (Fig. 11-54).

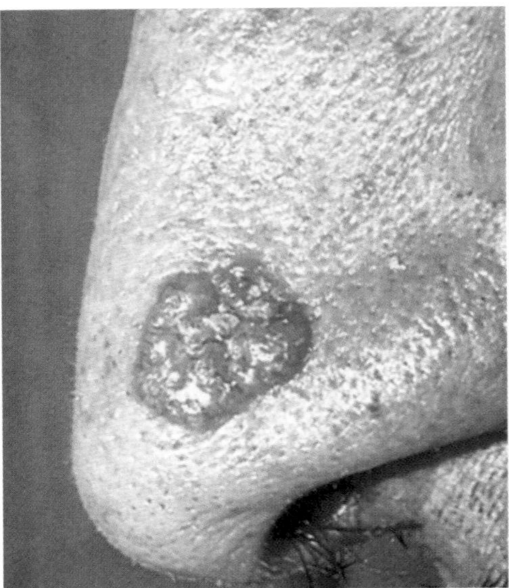

Fig. 11-54 Basal cell carcinoma. (From Thompson et al, 1993. Courtesy Gary Monheit, MD, University of Alabama at Birmingham School of Medicine.)

Squamous Cell Carcinoma

Squamous cell carcinoma appears as a red, scaly patch that has a sharply demarcated border (Fig. 11-55). The lesion is soft, mobile, and slightly elevated. As the tumor matures, a central ulcer may form with surrounding redness. The primary risk factors are sunlight and light pigmentation. Those most commonly affected are older individuals who have blue eyes and childhood freckling (Schwartz and Stroll, 1999). The most common areas for the lesion to appear include those areas exposed to excessive sun or ultraviolet light.

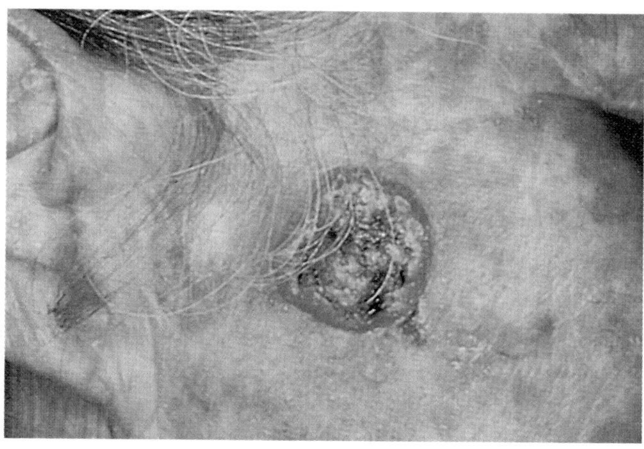

Fig. 11-55 Squamous cell carcinoma. (From Goldstein and Goldstein, 1997. Courtesy Department of Dermatology, Medical College of Georgia.)

Malignant Melanoma

Malignant melanoma lesions frequently grow from already present nevi (Fig. 11-56). The border of the melanoma is irregular, and the lesion may have a flaking or scaly texture. Its color may vary from brown to pink to purple, or it may have mixed pigmentation.

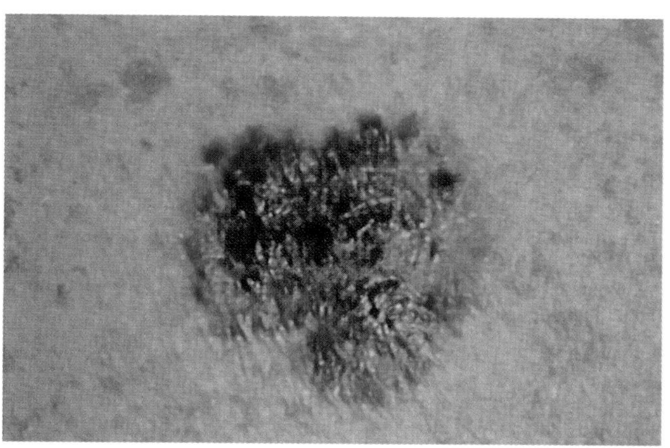

Fig. 11-56 Malignant melanoma. (From Hill, 1994.)

Hyperkeratosis

Clavus (Corn)

A corn is a flat or slightly raised, painful lesion that generally has a smooth, hard surface (Fig. 11-57). A "soft" corn is a whitish thickening commonly found between the fourth and fifth toes and is secondary to chronic pressure of a bony prominence against softer tissue. A "hard" corn is clearly demarcated and has a conical appearance. These usually occur secondary to chronic pressure from a shoe over a bony prominence.

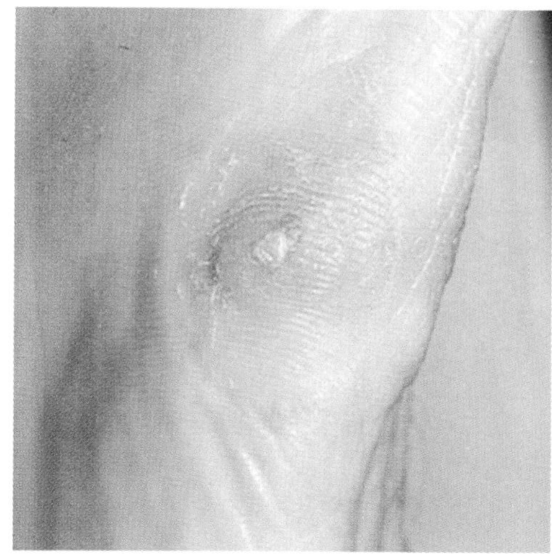

Fig. 11-57 Corn (clavus). (From White, 1994.)

Callus

A superficial "tough skin" nontender area on the hand or foot is referred to as a callus (Fig. 11-58). The area is well demarcated and develops secondary to repeated pressure or use.

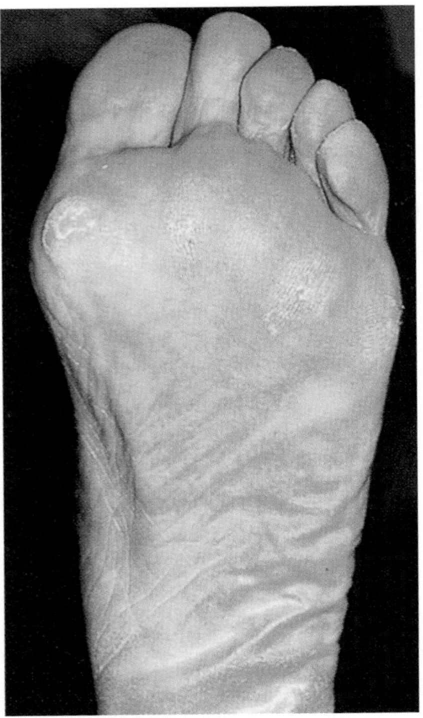

Fig. 11-58 Callus. (From Lawrence and Cox, 1993.)

Skin Lesions Caused by Abuse

Injuries to the skin are among the most common and most easily recognized signs of physical abuse. It is important to compare the type of injury or injuries to the history and to the developmental level of an infant or child. Injuries to the skin are generally recognized in three forms: bruises, bites, and burns.

Bruise

A bruise can indicate superficial injury or a deep injury such as injury to muscle or abdominal organs. Consider the location of bruises, appearance of bruise, pattern of bruises, and the type of mark made. Infants do not typically have bruises. Children between the ages of 2 and 5 may have bruises, but they usually appear on a bony prominence. Bruises on soft tissue are much less common. One can determine the age of a bruise by the appearance. A recent bruise 1 to 3 days old is purple to deep black in appearance. A bruise 3 to 6 days old is green to brown in color, whereas an older bruise 6 to 15 days old changes from green to tan to yellow and then fades. Look for a pattern in the bruise markings. Bruises associated with abuse may be caused by objects that leave distinctive patterns (Montelone, 1997) (Fig. 11-59).

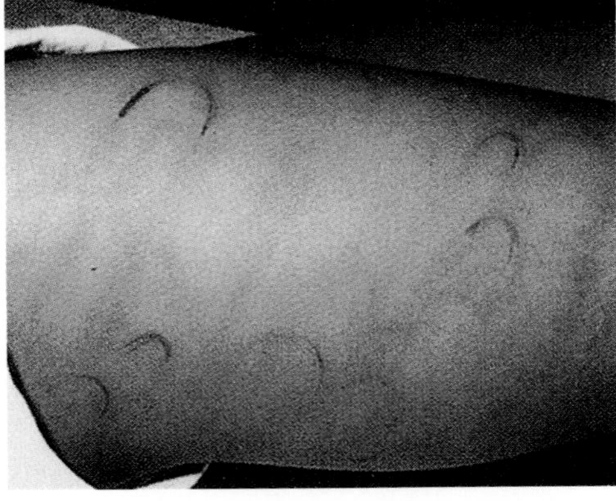

Fig. 11-59 Loop mark pattern of bruising caused by whipping with an electrical cord. (From Monteleone, 1996.)

Bites

Bites are always intentional and are a common injury associated with abuse (Fig. 11-60). Bite marks are ovoid with tooth imprints that may or may not break the skin. They may have a suck mark (bruising) in the middle. The size of the bite mark is important to note to determine the age of the person who may have left the mark (i.e., child versus adult). Bite marks on infants and children are frequently located on the genitals or buttocks (Montelone, 1997).

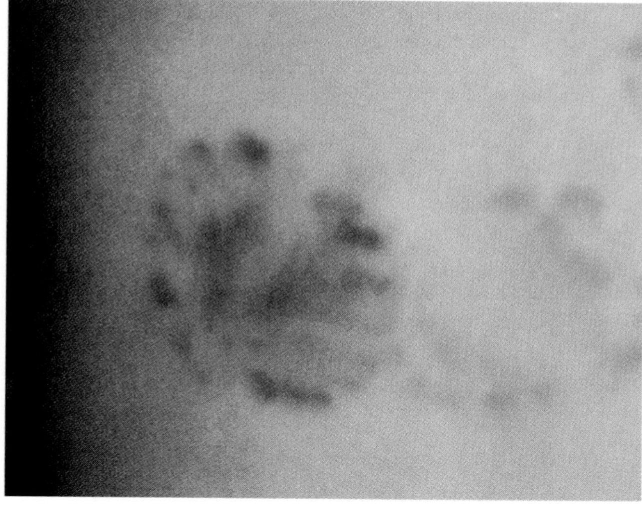

Fig. 11-60 Bite injury. (From Monteleone, 1996.)

Burns

Burns are frequently associated with abuse. The most common type is an immersion burn. This is easily recognizable by a "glove" or "stocking" burn pattern (a line of demarcation) where the child is immersed into scalding hot water. Look for this pattern on hands/arms; feet/legs and buttocks (Fig. 11-61). Another common type of burn associated with abuse is a contact burn—a burn caused by intentionally placing a hot object on the skin such as a cigarette, light bulb, lighter, or hot iron (Fig. 11-62). Intentional contact burns are easily recognizable because they literally leave a "branded pattern" on the skin. An accidental burn with an object typically leaves a glancing burn pattern with a non-uniform pattern (Giardino et al, 1997).

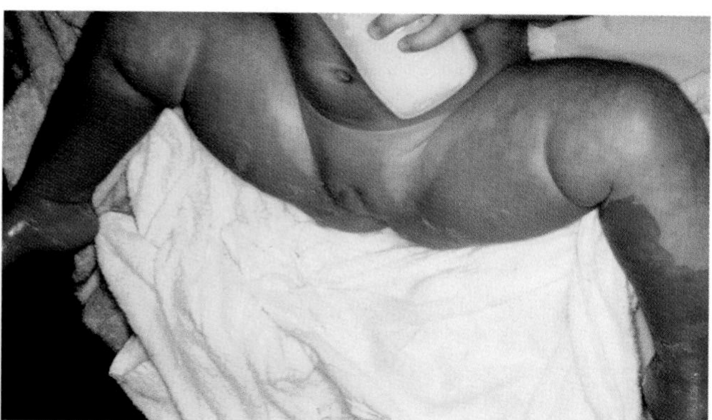

Fig. 11-61 Stocking burn patterns to perineum, thighs, legs, and feet. (From Zitelli and Davis, 1997; Courtesy Dr. Thomas Layton, Mercy Hospital, Pittsburgh, Penn.)

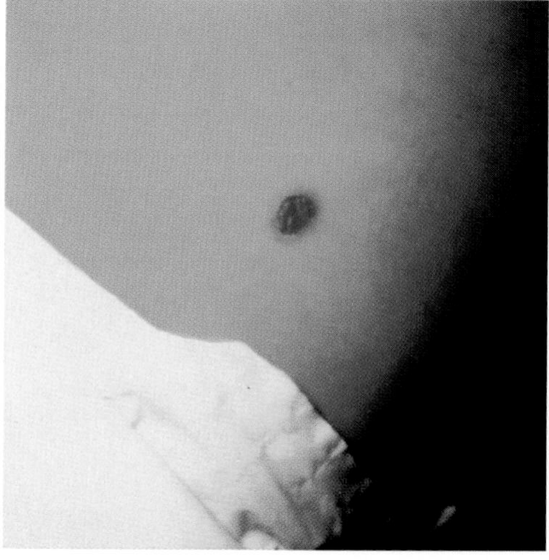

Fig. 11-62 Cigarette burn to a child's abdomen. (From Zitelli and Davis, 1997.)

Hair

Pediculosis (Lice)

Lice are parasites that may invade the scalp, body, or pubic hair regions (Fig. 11-63). The eggs (nits) are visible as small, white particles. The skin underlying the infested area may appear excoriated. Lice on the body are called pediculosis corporis, and pubic lice are called pediculosis pubis.

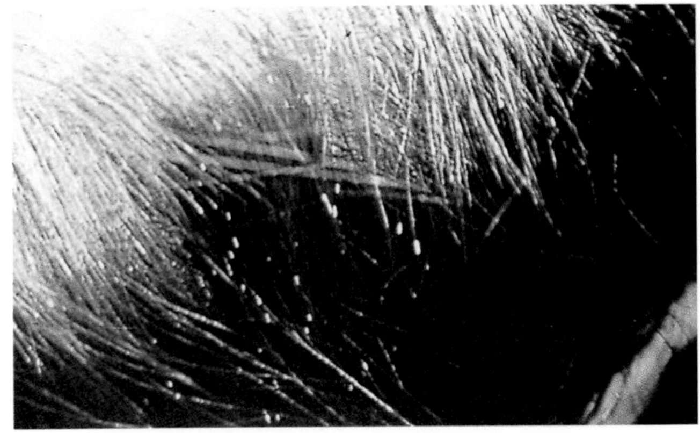

Fig. 11-63 Pediculosis (lice). The eggs, or nits, are visible attached to hair shafts. (From Farrar et al, 1992; Courtesy Dr. E. Sahn.)

Alopecia Areata

A sudden patchy loss of scalp or face hair is referred to as alopecia areata (Fig. 11-64). It is usually due to poorly developed and fragile hair shafts and will generally grow back within 3 to 4 months.

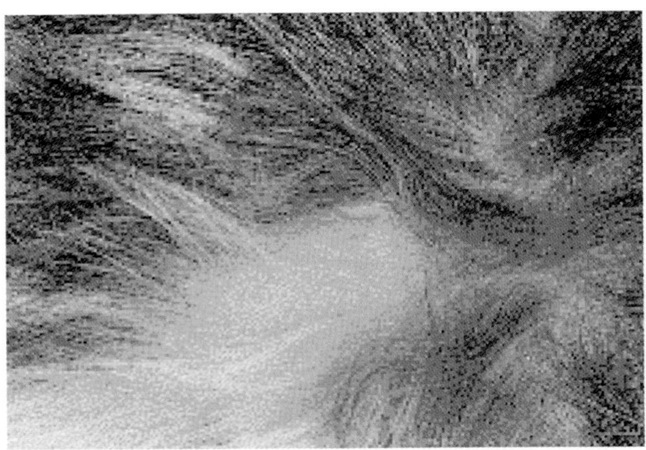

Fig. 11-64 Alopecia.

Hirsutism

This is a condition associated with an increase in the growth of facial, body, or pubic hair in women (Fig. 11-65). This condition has familial tendency and can be associated with endocrine disorders, menopause, and side effects of medications, especially corticosteroid or androgenic steroid therapy. The hair may take on a male distribution pattern and may or may not be associated with other signs of virilization.

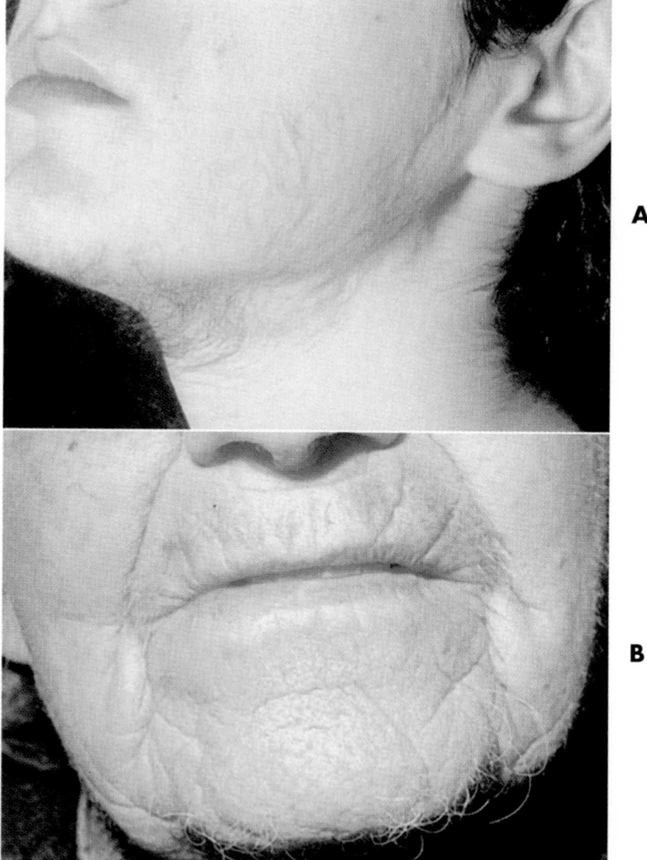

Fig. 11-65 Facial hirsutism. **A,** Hair growth on the jaw line and neck of a young woman. **B,** Hair growth on the chin of a postmenopausal woman. (From Baran et al, 1991.)

Nails

Leukonychia

In this condition, white spots may be seen in the nail plate (Fig. 11-66). The benign and transient lesions are generally secondary to minor trauma or manipulation of the cuticle.

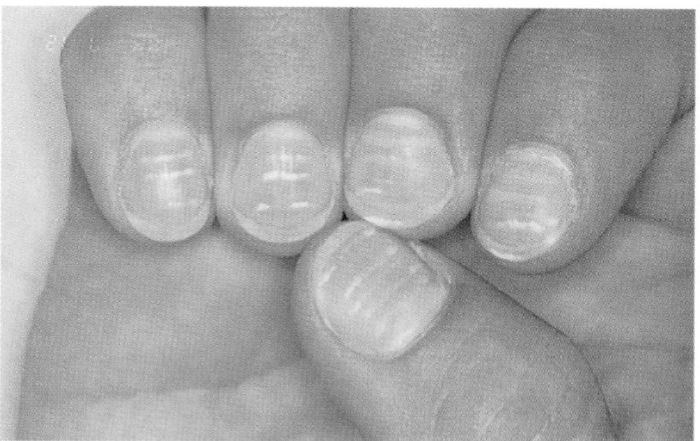

Fig. 11-66 Leukonychia punctata. Transverse white bands resulting from repeated minor trauma to the nail matrix. (From Baran et al, 1991.)

Tinea Unguium

This is a fungal infection of the fingernail (Fig. 11-67). The nail plate most commonly turns yellow or white as hyperkeratotic debris accumulates. As the problem progresses, the nail tends to separate from the nail bed, and the nail plate crumbles.

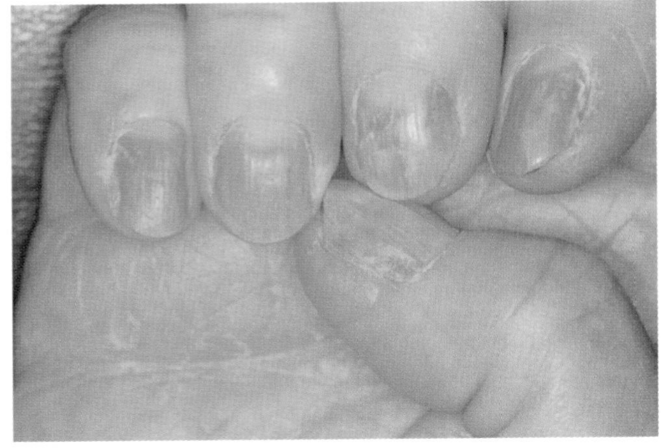

Fig. 11-67 Tinea unguium (fungal infection of the fingernail). (From Baran et al, 1991.)

Ingrown Toenail

This condition most commonly involves the great toe (Fig. 11-68). As the nail grows, it cuts into the lateral nail fold and actually grows into the dermis, causing pain, redness, and swelling.

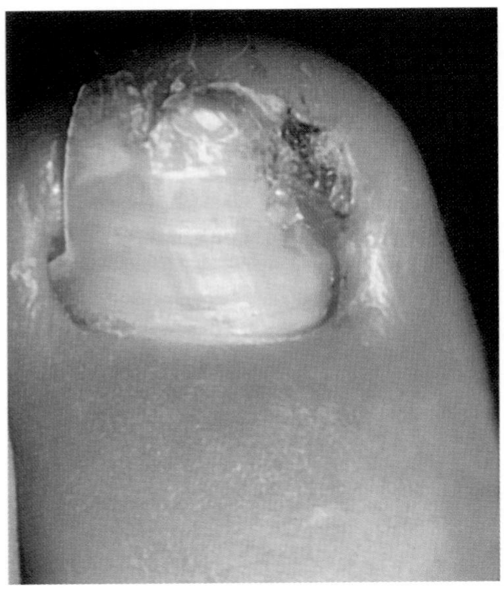

Fig. 11-68 Ingrown toenail. (From Baden, 1987.)

Beau's Lines

Beau's lines present as a groove or transverse depression running across the nail that occurs as a result of a stressor that temporary impairs nail formation (Fig. 11-69). Causative factors include trauma to the nail, illness, and toxic reaction. The groove first appears at the base of the nail by the cuticle and moves forward as the nail grows until it disappears.

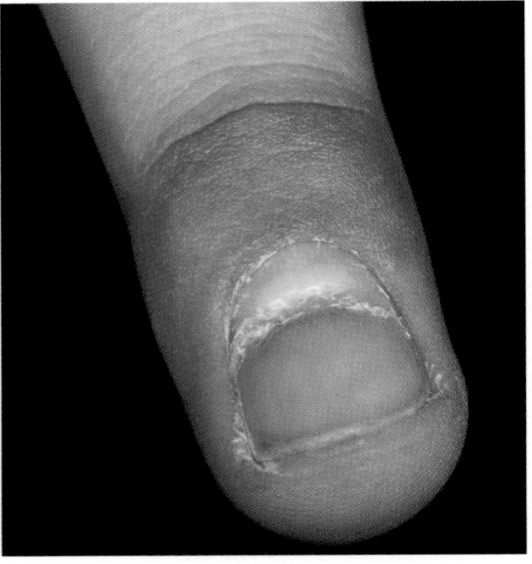

Fig. 11-69 Beau's lines. (From Habif, 1996.)

CLINICAL APPLICATION and CRITICAL THINKING

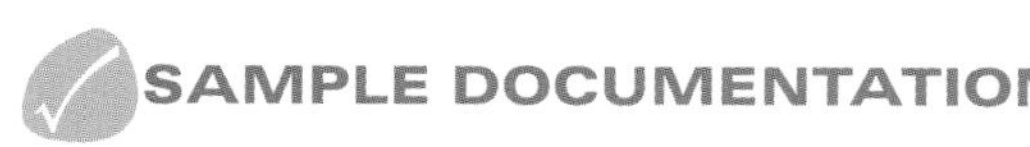

SAMPLE DOCUMENTATION

CASE 1

D.M. is healthy 8-year-old boy brought to the clinic by his mother. The chief complaint is "bad rash."

Subjective Data

Rash first noticed by mother 2 days ago; thinks rash is getting worse; child sent home from school. Mother states rash is "wet, sticky, and drains a lot." "He keeps touching it, but I don't think it really hurts him much, although he has not been eating or drinking much." Child is up-to-date on immunizations. Child states, "It is really itchy, but it only hurts a little. I don't want to go back to school with this because all the kids are making fun of me."

Objective Data

Vital signs: Temperature, 99.2° F (37.3° C); Pulse rate, 104; Respirations, 24.

Skin: Overall skin appearance is dry with olive skin color. Grouped lesions noted on face. Lesions are raised vesicles and pustules with erythematous bases around the mouth and extend up the left side of the nose and under the left eye. A clear yellow sticky exudate noted from the lesions; some exudate has dried into a crust. Lesions range in size from 1 to 2 cm.

Hair: Normal scalp and body hair distribution, texture, and quality. Scalp without lesions.

Nails: Fingernails intact without lesions; dirt under nails observed.

Medical Diagnosis

Impetigo

Functional Health Patterns Involved

- Nutrition–metabolic
- Self-perception–self-concept
- Cognitive–perceptual

Nursing Diagnosis and Collaborative Problems

- *Impaired skin integrity* related to inflammation of the dermis as manifested by:
  - Vesicles and pustules.
  - Lesions draining clear, yellow exudate.
- *Body image disturbance* related to concern of appearance as manifested by:
  - Statement that kids are "making fun of me."
- *Altered comfort:* pruritus related to skin lesions as manifested by:
  - Client's statement that "it's really itchy."
  - Mother's observation that child touches frequently.
- *Risk for infection transmission* related to contagious pathogen.
- *Risk for alteration in nutrition* related to loss of appetite.
- *Risk for fluid volume deficit* related to inadequate fluid intake and fever.
- *PC:* Infection related to contagious pathogen

CASE 2

M.L. is a 62-year-old white female whose chief complaint is a change in the appearance of a mole.

Subjective Data

M.L. states: "The mole on my forearm has changed in the way it looks. It has been present for the past 20 years. It has changed in color from light brown to purple and has grown from a small dot to an area that is now as big as my thumb." Noticed changes in the mole approximately 2 months ago. Read a pamphlet on skin cancer recently, is now "worried." Requests information regarding how to protect self from "skin problems." Has had no previous history of skin problems, changes in moles, or cancer; previously has been healthy and currently takes no medications; spends "lots of time in the sun, keeps a good tan year-round"; uses no sunblock or sunscreen lotion; no family history of cancer.

Objective Data

Skin: Warm, dry, dark tan skin tone of leathery appearance with evidence of tanning. No evidence of rash. Multiple light brown nevi noted on shoulders, back, and forearms. The nevus in question appears to be a 2-cm, bluish purple lesion with an irregular border. The lesion is slightly raised and has a rough, scaling texture. There is no evidence of flaking or oozing. No other nevi on the body has a similar appearance.

Hair: Gray, thinning scalp hair with normal distribution.

Nails: Fingernails and toenails intact and without lesions or deformity.

Functional Health Patterns Involved

- Health perception–health management
- Self-perception–self-concept
- Nutrition–metabolic

Medical Diagnosis

Rule out malignant melanoma

Nursing Diagnosis and Collaborative Problems

- *Impaired skin integrity* related to presence of the lesion secondary to sun exposure as manifested by:
  - Change in the mole created a disruption of the skin surface.
- *Anxiety* related to potential diagnosis of cancer as manifested by:
  - Client states she is "worried" with reassurance-seeking behavior.
- *Altered health maintenance* for skin protection related to inadequate knowledge or failure to assume responsibility for primary prevention as manifested by:
  - Lack of knowledge regarding basic health practices
- *Health-seeking behaviors:* desire for skin cancer prevention information.

CRITICAL THINKING QUESTIONS

1. Mr. Mason is a 72-year-old man who presents with a lesion on his cheek. He says it has been there for years, but his wife has been nagging him to "get it checked out in case it is cancer." After examination, the physician tells him it is a benign mole. However, the doctor also says he should "keep an eye on it." Before leaving, you teach Mr. Mason the warning signs to look for. What would you tell him?
2. Mrs. Tran brings her 3-year-old child to the pediatric clinic, informing the nurse that the child is red all over and cries frequently. The nurse notes a rash on the child's skin. What specific characteristics should be noted when examining and documenting a skin lesion?
3. A 9-month-old boy is brought to the emergency department by his mother and her boyfriend. The boyfriend tells the nurse, "The boy fell off the bed and hurt himself while I was baby-sitting." He indicated the injury occurred a couple of hours ago. The child has a large contusion approximately 1 ½ inches in diameter with swelling to the right mid-upper arm. The child also has older bruises to the legs and buttocks. What type of patterns or markings would be consistent with an injury from falling off a bed? What are some signs the nurse might assess for if concerned about child abuse?

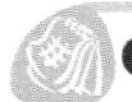

CASE STUDY

Dan Hillerman is a 38-year-old male paraplegic admitted to the hospital for unexplained weakness and depression. Listed below are data collected by the nurse during an interview and assessment.

Interview Data

Dan states he became a paraplegic 2 years ago after a motorcycle accident. He claims he is fully independent and needs no assistance. However, the past month or so he has felt weak and has had a loss of appetite. Normally he is able to transfer himself in and out of a wheelchair but admits that the last few weeks he has done very little activity. His mother and father keep telling him he is depressed, and this makes him feel very angry.

Examination Data

- **General survey:** Alert, very thin male with flat affect lying in a supine position. Height, 6′2″ (188 cm); Weight, 153 lb (69.5 kg). Slight foul-smelling odor noted.
- **Skin:** Skin color is pale. No evidence of bruising, no skin discoloration. Presence of skin breakdown over the left greater trochanter and over the sacrum.
- **Hair:** Full hair distribution on head with soft texture.
- *Abdomen:* Active bowel sounds. Abdomen soft, nondistended, nontender.
- **Musculoskeletal:** Paralysis, atrophy to both lower extremities; upper extremities fully functional.

1. What data deviate from normal findings, suggesting a need for further investigation?
2. What additional information should the nurse ask or assess for?
3. In what functional health patterns does data deviate from normal?
4. What nursing diagnosis and/or collaborative problems should be considered for this situation?

REMEMBER to check out your **companion CD-ROM**

12 Lymphatic System

www.mosby.com/MERLIN/wilson/assessment/

ANATOMY AND PHYSIOLOGY

Every tissue supplied by blood vessels has lymphatic vessels except for the central nervous system, the cornea, and the placenta. The lymphatic system is a special vascular system that provides immunity, phagocytizes foreign and abnormal cells, and collects interstitial fluid and returns it to the bloodstream. This system is made up of lymph fluid, the collecting ducts, and lymph tissue, which includes the lymph nodes, the spleen, the thymus, the tonsils, the adenoids, and Peyer's patches (Fig. 12-1). Lymph tissue is found within other parts of the body, such as mucosa of the stomach and the appendix, the bone marrow, and the lungs.

LYMPHATIC FLUID CIRCULATION

Lymphatic fluid is clear, composed mainly of water and a small amount of proteins, mostly albumin. As blood flows from arterioles into venules, fluid is forced out at the arterial capillary bed into the interstitial spaces, then into cells, and is finally reabsorbed by the venous capillaries. The fluid left in the interstitial spaces is absorbed by the lymph system and carried on to lymph nodes throughout the body (Fig. 12-2). Flow through lymph nodes is slow to allow the lymphocytes in the node to ingest and destroy foreign substances, thus preventing them from reentering the bloodstream. Finally, ducts from the lymph nodes empty into the subclavian veins. The right lymphatic duct drains fluid from the right side of the head and neck, right arm, and right chest into the right subclavian vein. The larger thoracic duct drains the rest of the body into the left subclavian vein (Fig. 12-3). The lymphatic system has no means of pumping this fluid; instead, it depends entirely on arterial pulsation, lymphatic vessel compression by the skeletal muscles, and smooth muscle contraction in the lymphatic vessels, lymph nodes, and collecting ducts.

LYMPHOCYTES

The important component of lymphatic fluid is its lymphocytes, since they are central to the body's immunity. There are two types of lymphocytes. The B lymphocytes produce specific antibodies (immunoglobulins) to provide humoral immunity. These immunoglobulins (IgA, IgD, IgE, IgG, and IgM) act by neutralizing bacterial toxins, neutralizing viruses, phagocytizing bacteria, and activating the inflammatory response. There are several types of T lymphocytes to provide cellular immunity, including cytotoxic, helper, and suppressor T cells, as well as cytokines. The functions of T lymphocytes are to kill cells infected by viruses, including tumors and transplanted tissue; activate the inflammatory response; and stimulate production of more B and T lymphocytes (McCance and Huether, 1998).

LYMPH NODES

Lymph nodes are tiny oval clumps of lymphatic tissue, usually occurring in groups along the blood vessels at numerous sites. Those located in subcutaneous connective tissue are called superficial nodes; those beneath the fascia of muscles or within various body cavities are called deep nodes. Deep nodes are not accessible to inspection or palpation. However, superficial nodes are accessible and become enlarged and tender, providing early signs of infection or inflammation.

Regional Nodes

Lymph nodes are widely distributed throughout the following regions.

Head In the head, the lymph nodes are categorized as follows: preauricular, postauricular (mastoid nodes), occipital, parotid, retropharyngeal (tonsillar), submandibular, submental, sublingual, suprahyoid, and thyrolinguofacial (Fig. 12-4). Table 12-1 contains the lymphatic drainage patterns for lymph nodes.

Neck The cervical nodes are named according to their relation to the sternocleidomastoid muscle and the neck's anterior and posterior triangles: anterior deep and superficial cervical; posterior cervical spinal nerve chain; posterior superficial cervical chain; anterior jugular and supraclavicular (Fig. 12-5).

The internal jugular chain of nodes is located beneath the sternocleidomastoid muscle.

Axilla There are five groups of lymph nodes in the axilla, draining upward and medially toward the main lymph-collecting channels. These nodes drain the breast, upper arm, and radial surface of the forearm. These are the lateral (brachial) axillary nodes; the posterior (subscapular) axillary nodes; the central axillary nodes; the anterior nodes; and subclavian (apical) axillary nodes (Fig. 12-6).

Breast Breast lymph vessels drain primarily into the axillary nodes. Lymph nodes receiving drainage from the

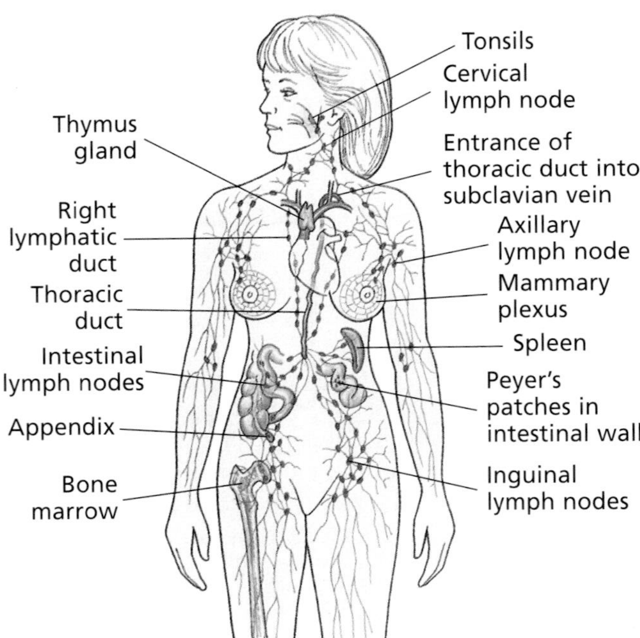

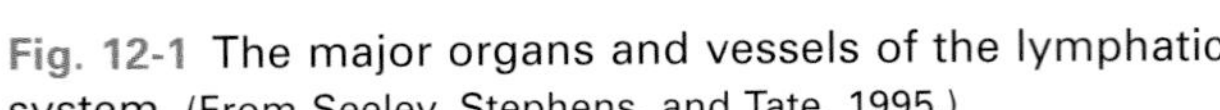

Fig. 12-1 The major organs and vessels of the lymphatic system. (From Seeley, Stephens, and Tate, 1995.)

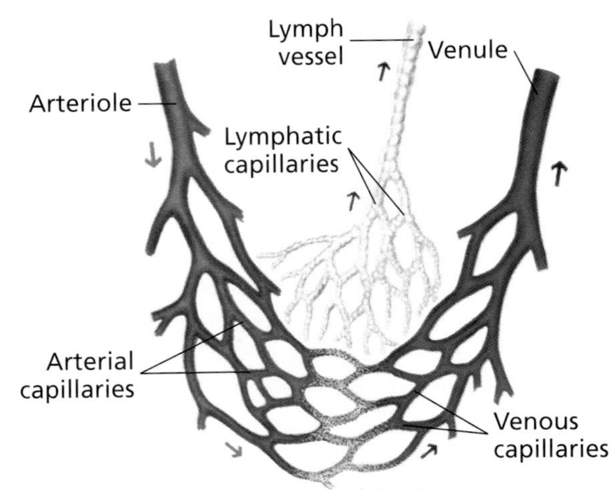

Fig. 12-2 Microcirculation involving blood, interstitial fluid, oxygen, and nutrients. (From Canobbio, 1990.)

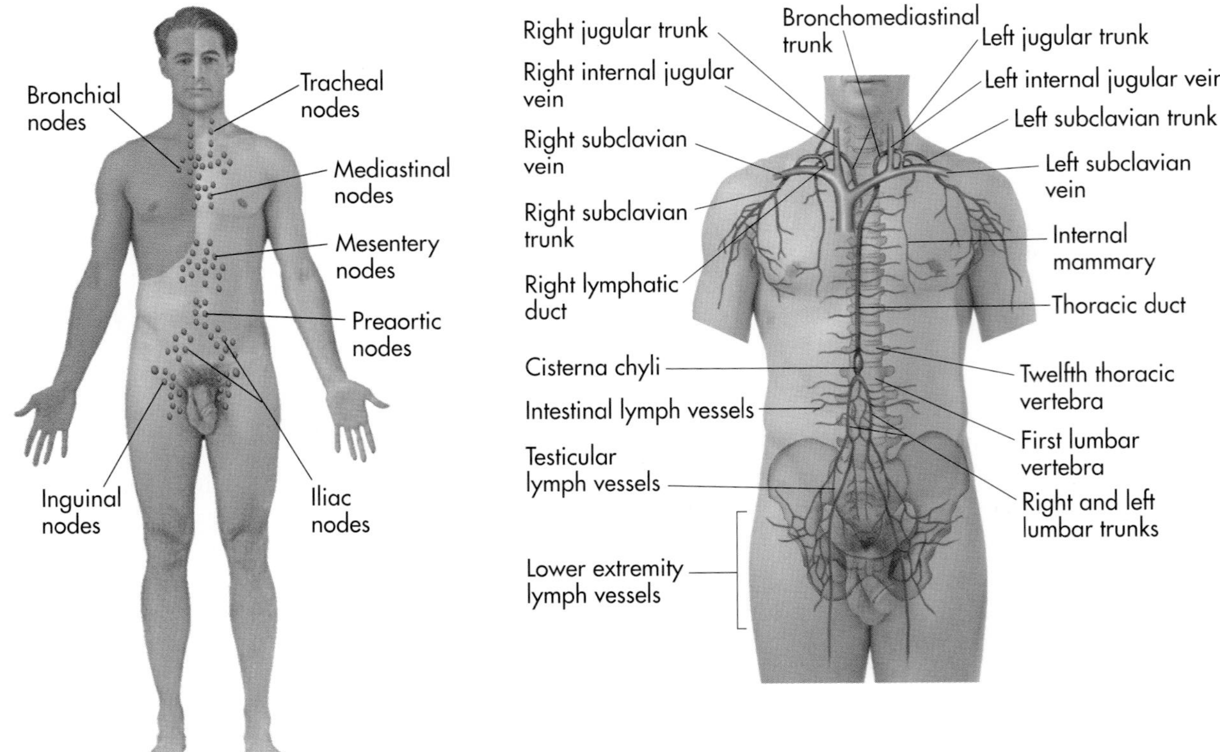

Fig. 12-3 Lymphatic drainage pathways. Shaded area of the body is drained via the right lymphatic duct, which is formed by the union of three vessels: right jugular trunk, right subclavian trunk, and right bronchomediastinal trunk. Lymph from the remainder of the body enters the venous system by way of the thoracic duct. (From Seidel et al, 1999.)

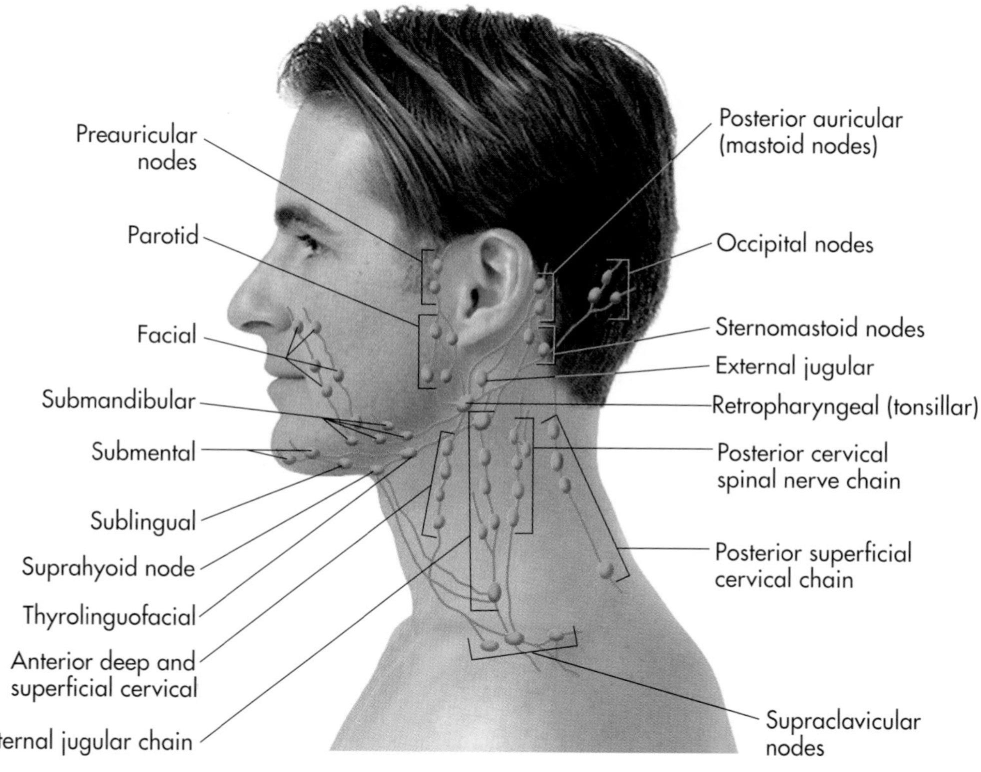

Fig. 12-4 Lymphatic drainage system of head and neck. If the group of nodes is referred to by another name, the second name appears in parentheses. (From Seidel et al, 1999.)

Table 12-1 Lymphatic Drainage Pattern

NODE	LOCATION	RECEIVES DRAINAGE FROM
HEAD		
Preauricular	In front of tragus of external ear	Scalp, external auditory canal, forehead or upper facial structures, lateral portion of eyelids
Postauricular (mastoid)	Behind ear on mastoid process	Parietal region of scalp, external auditory canal
Occipital	Midway between external occipital protuberance and mastoid process	Parietal region of scalp
Parotid	Near the jaw angle	Eyelids, frontotemporal skin, external auditory meatus, tympanic cavity
Retropharyngeal (tonsillar)	At angle of mandible	Tonsils, posterior palate, thyroid, floor of mouth
Submandibular	Halfway between angle and tip of mandible	Tongue, submaxillary glands, mucosa of lips and mouth
Submental	In midline behind tip of mandible	Tongue, mucosa of lips and mouth, floor of mouth
NECK		
Anterior cervical chain	Superficial to sternocleidomastoid muscle	Skin of neck, ear
Posterior cervical chain	Along anterior edge to trapezius muscle in the posterior triangle	Posterior scalp, thyroid, posterior skin of neck
Deep cervical chain	Under sternocleidomastoid muscle; includes four separate chains extending over larynx, thyroid gland, and trachea	Larynx, thyroid, trachea, ear, and upper part of esophagus
Supraclavicular	Deep in angle formed by sternocleido-mastoid muscle and clavicle	Upper abdomen, lungs, breast, arm
AXILLA		
Anterior	Along lateral border of pectoral muscle	Breast
Lateral (brachial)	Along upper surface of the arm	Breast
Posterior (subscapular)	Along border of scapula	Breast
Central	High and deep into the axilla	Breast
Subclavian (apical)	Below the midclavical	Breast
BREAST		
Mammary (Rotter's nodes)	Superior central breast	Superior breast
Internal mammary	Medial breast adjacent to sternal border	Medial breast
External mammary	Lateral breast	Lateral and posterior breast
ARM		
Epitrochlear	Depression above and posterior to medial condyle of humerus	Ulnar surface of forearm, fourth and fifth finger
GROIN		
Superior and inferior superficial inguinal	Over inguinal canal deep in groin	Upper and lower leg; vulva and lower third of vagina drain into inguinal nodes; penis and scrotal surface; nodes of the testes drain into the abdomen

Modified from Bowers AC, Thompson JM: *Clinical manual of health assessment,* ed 4, St. Louis, 1992, Mosby.

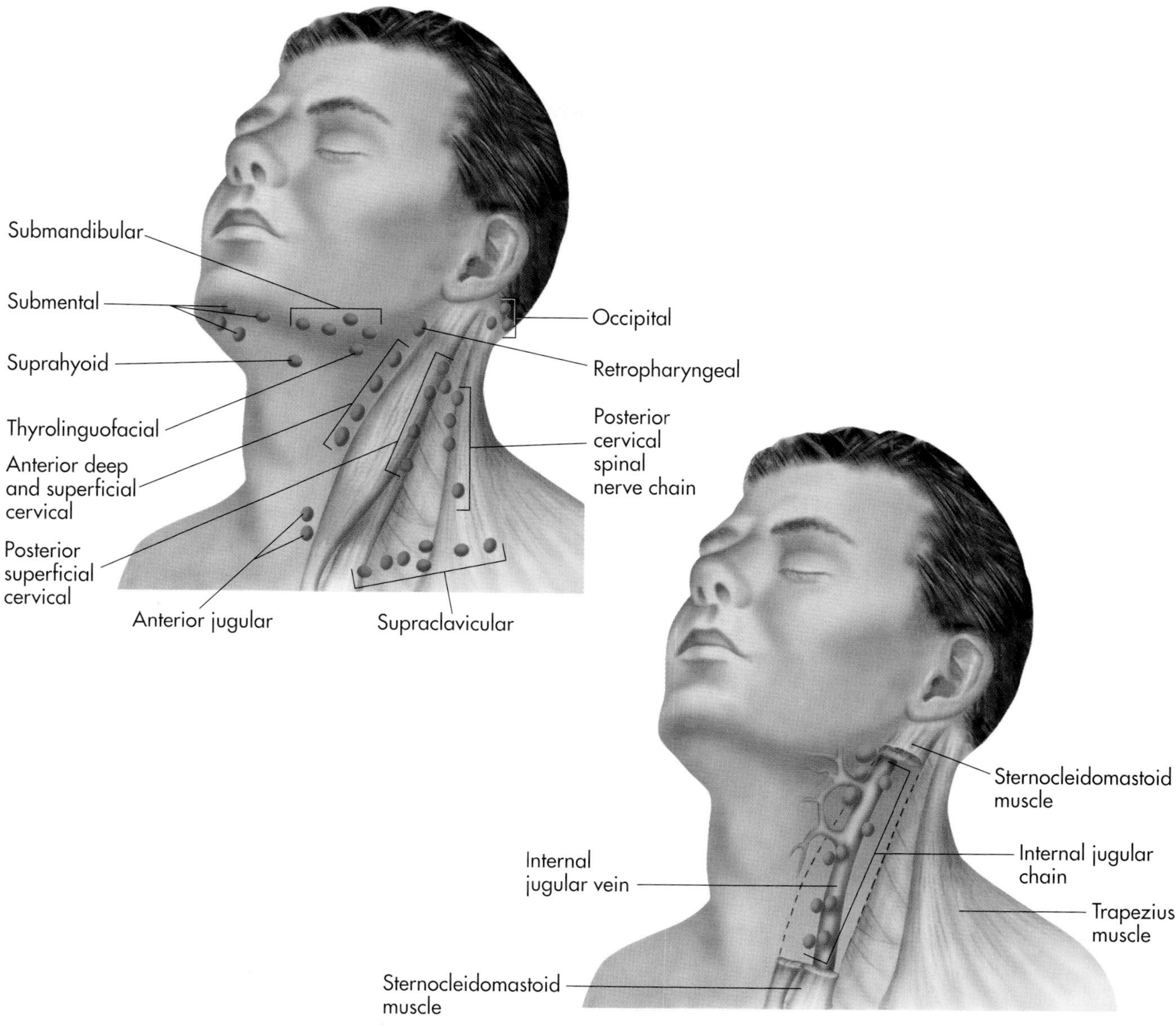

Fig. 12-5 Lymph nodes of the neck. Note their relationship to the sternocleidomastoid muscle. (From Seidel et al, 1999.)

breast include mammary (Rotter's nodes), internal mammary, and external mammary (Fig. 12-7).

Arm Only the epitrochlear nodes on the medial surface of the arm above the elbow are palpable (Fig. 12-8). This lymph node receives fluid via the radial, ulnar, and median lymph vessels.

Inguinal Area The superficial nodes in this area are divided into superior and inferior nodes; they receive most of the lymph drainage from the great and small saphenous lymphatic vessels in the legs. In men, lymph from the penile and scrotal surfaces drains to the inguinal nodes, but nodes of the testes drain into the abdomen (see Fig. 12-3).

Leg The posterior surface of the leg, behind the knee, houses the popliteal nodes, which receive lymph from the medial portion of the lower leg (Fig. 12-9).

THYMUS

The thymus is located behind the sternum in the superior mediastinum. This gland has its greatest importance in early life, when it produces T lymphocytes, the effector cells for cell-mediated immune reactions. With maturity into adulthood, the thymus atrophies with a loss of function.

SPLEEN

The spleen is a highly vascular organ about the size of a fist, situated in the upper left quadrant of the abdomen between the stomach and diaphragm. It is composed of two systems: the white pulp (consisting of lymphatic nodules and diffuse lymphatic tissue) and the red pulp (consisting of venous sinusoids). As a blood-forming organ early in life, the spleen stores red blood cells and destroys old ones, and filters the blood through its network of lymphocytes and macropha-

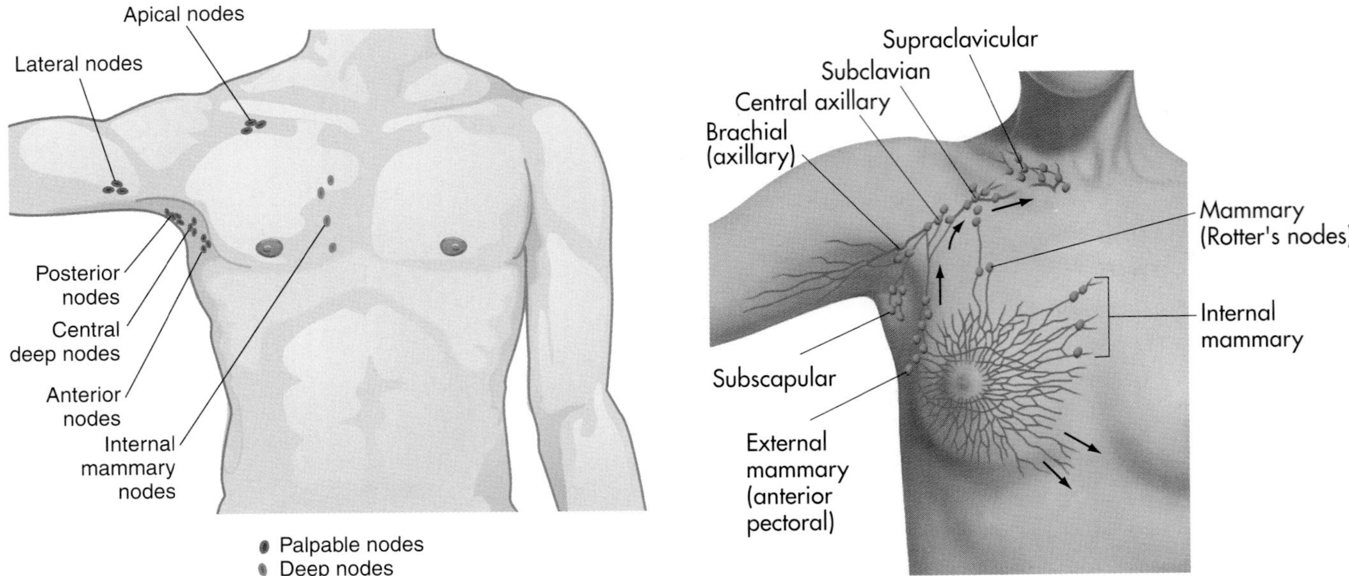

Fig. 12-6 Lymphatic drainage and lymph nodes of the axilla.

Fig. 12-7 Lymphatic drainage of breasts. (From Seidel et al, 1999.)

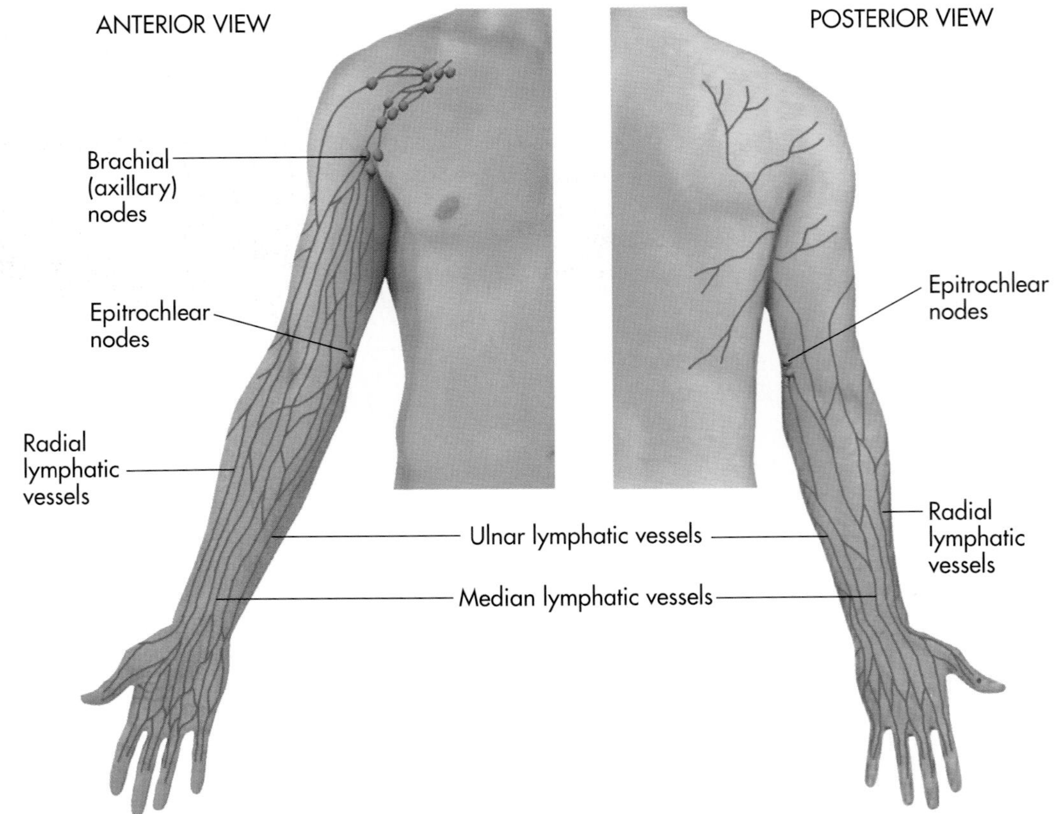

Fig. 12-8 System of deep and superficial collecting ducts, carrying lymph from upper extremity to subclavian lymphatic trunk. The only peripheral lymph center is the epitrochlear, which receives some of the collecting ducts from the pathway of the ulnar and radial nerves. (From Seidel et al, 1999.)

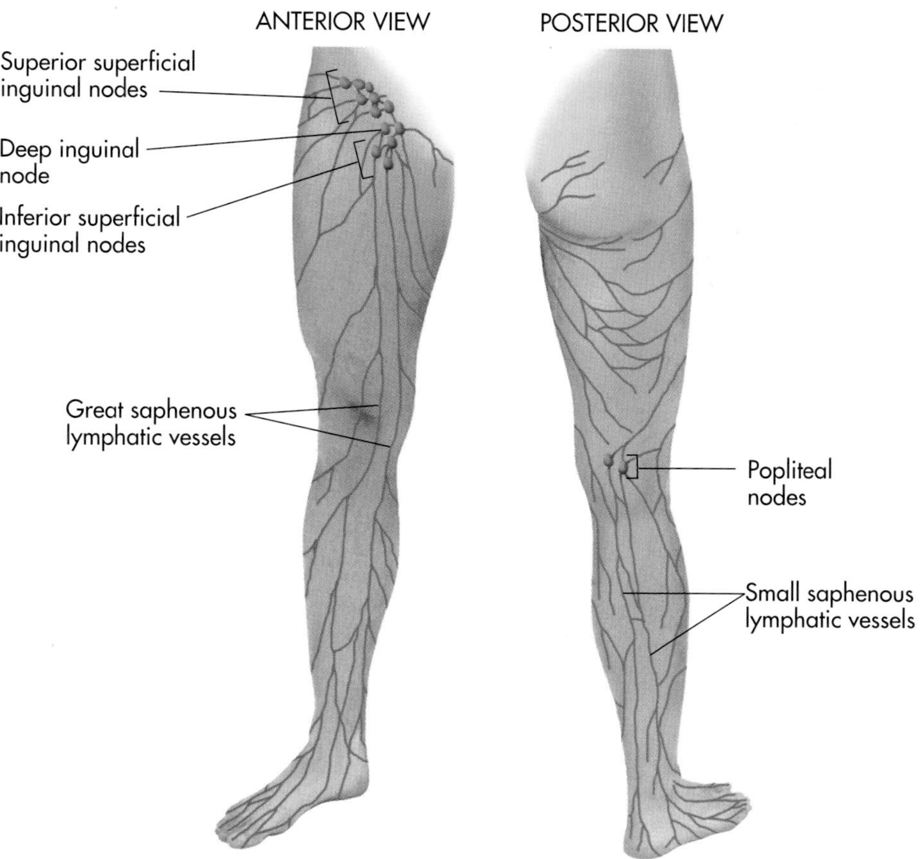

Fig. 12-9 Lymphatic drainage of lower extremity. (From Seidel et al, 1999.)

ges to provide immunity against microorganisms and abnormal and foreign cells.

TONSILS AND ADENOIDS

The oropharyngeal tonsils, more prominent in childhood than adulthood, are largely composed of lymphoid tissue with a mucous membrane. They are located between the palatine arches on either side of the larynx, below the base of the tongue. The nasopharyngeal tonsils, also called the adenoids, are located at the nasopharyngeal border. They can obstruct the nasopharyngeal passageway if they become enlarged as a result of infection.

PEYER'S PATCHES

Peyer's patches, groups of clustered lymphoid tissue, are referred to as gut-associated lymphoid tissue (GALT). They are present in the mucosa and submucosa of the small intestine, primarily the ileum.

HEALTH HISTORY

Lymphatic System

QUESTIONS	RATIONALE
PRESENT HEALTH STATUS	
➤ How would you describe your overall health?	■ Input from clients regarding their health status may provide data about the adequacy of their immune system.

QUESTIONS	RATIONALE
➤ What immunizations have you had? When did you have them? When was your last tetanus immunization?	■ Hepatitis B, tetanus, and flu vaccines are the primary immunizations for adults. Tetanus booster (Td) is recommended every 10 years.
➤ Do you have any chronic illnesses? (hepatitis, human immunodeficiency virus (HIV) infection, diabetes mellitus, malignancies, cardiac, renal)	■ Many chronic diseases impair the immune system function.
➤ Do you take any medications? If so, what do you take and how often?	■ There are many medications that cause immunosuppression, including chemotherapeutic agents to treat cancer and corticosteroid medications (e.g., prednisone or decadron) to treat a variety of inflammatory conditions.
➤ Do you use intravenous (IV) drugs? Have you in the past or do you now have multiple sexual partners? Have you had any blood transfusions? If so, when?	■ These questions are asked to determine the client's risk for HIV infection.
➤ Are you exposed to environmental radiation? Toxic chemicals? Infections?	■ These questions are asked to determine the client's risk factors for cancer and immune system impairment.
PAST MEDICAL HISTORY	
➤ Have you had any surgeries that involved removing lymph nodes (e.g., mastectomy)? What was the purpose of the surgery?	■ Surgery that removes lymph channels (e.g., as a part of a radical mastectomy) may result in lymphedema because the lymph no longer absorbs fluid from the interstitial spaces.
➤ Have you been diagnosed with a lymphoma (e.g., Hodgkin's disease)? If so, when? What treatment have you received?	■ Lymphoma is a neoplasm of the lymphoid tissue and is usually malignant. It is characterized by painless enlarged lymph nodes. Hodgkin's disease is a lymphoma characterized by painless, enlarged lymph nodes that is usually first evident in the cervical lymph nodes.
➤ Have you had any organ transplants? If so, when and what organ(s) were transplanted?	■ Clients who have organ transplants take immunosuppressive drugs to prevent organ rejection, which increases their risk for infection.
➤ Have you had any blood transfusions? If so, when?	■ Clients who have had blood transfusions have an increased risk of transmission of chronic infections such as hepatitis C.

QUESTIONS

RATIONALE

RISK FACTORS

COMMON RISK FACTORS ASSOCIATED WITH Lymphatic System Disorders

ACQUIRED IMMUNODEFICIENCY SYNDROME (AIDS)

Exposure to infected blood, vaginal secretions, semen, or breast milk by such actions as

a. Unsafe sexual practices—heterosexual or homosexual
b. Intravenous drug use
c. Occupational exposure

LEUKEMIA

Overexposure to ionizing radiation
Alkylating agents used to treat other cancer
Workers exposed to chemical agents such as benzene
Genetic factors with twins or siblings

HEPATITIS B

Unsafe sexual practices with person who is infected with hepatitis B
Unsafe sexual practices with more than one partner
Live in the same household with someone who has chronic hepatitis B
Have a job that involves contact with human blood
Have hemophilia

FAMILY HISTORY

➤ Is there a history of cancer in your family? If so, which family member(s) and what kind of cancer was diagnosed?

■ The client could have a genetic predisposition to cancer depending on the type. For example, with a positive history for breast cancer, the client's risk of developing cancer in the opposite breast is 5 times greater than that of the average population (Deters, 1999).

PROBLEM-BASED HISTORY

The most commonly reported problems related to the lymph system include infection, enlarged lymph nodes, and lymphedema. As with symptoms in all areas of health assessment, a symptom analysis is completed, which includes the location, quality, quantity, chronology, setting, associated manifestations, alleviating factors, and aggravating factors.

Infection

➤ Do you currently have or have you recently had an infection? Where is it? How long have you had it? Have you had a fever with this infection? What have you done to treat this infection? How effective has the treatment been?

■ Infections mobilize the immune system to defend the client. Areas of infection need to be examined for erythema, edema, warmth, pain, and involvement of regional lymph nodes.

➤ Do you have recurrent infections?

■ Recurrent infections may indicate an ineffective immune system and/or increased risk of infectious disease.

QUESTIONS | RATIONALE

Enlarged Lymph Nodes

➤ Have you noticed any "swollen glands"? If so, how long have you had them? Where have you noticed them (under your chin, along your lower jaw, in your neck, under your arm, at your elbow, in your leg, in your groin area)?

■ Swollen glands indicate activation of the immune system.

➤ What do they feel like? Are they hard? Soft? Tender? Warm? Are they red?

■ Enlarged glands from acute infection are soft, edematous, and tender, whereas those from chronic infections are round, rubbery, and mobile. In contrast, nodes involved in malignancies are hard and fixed (nonmobile) and often painless.

➤ Have you noticed any associated symptoms such as fatigue, pain, fever, or weight loss?

■ Ask about associated symptoms to help understand the scope of the problem. Fever is an indication of systemic effects of inflammation such as infection. Fatigue and weight loss may be associated with a chronic disease process.

Lymphedema

➤ Have you noticed any swelling of your arms or legs? If so, describe its location (unilateral or bilateral) and duration (intermittent or constant) and how long you have had it.

■ Unilateral edema of an extremity may be lymphedema caused by occlusion of (e.g., elephantiasis or trauma) or surgical removal of lymph channels (e.g., after mastectomy).

➤ Are there any associated symptoms with the swelling, such as warmth, redness, discoloration, or ulceration?

■ Warmth and redness may indicate an inflammatory process, whereas discoloration and ulceration may indicate ischemia.

➤ What have you done to treat the swelling? (Exercise, elevation, compression with support sleeve or stocking?) How successful has the treatment been?

■ Knowing success of previous treatment(s) helps in planning future therapy.

EXAMINATION

Equipment

- Centimeter ruler to measure enlarged nodes or alternatively estimate the size by comparing the node to the width of your finger
- Tape measure to document extent of edema of extremities

PROCEDURES AND TECHNIQUES WITH NORMAL FINDINGS | ABNORMAL FINDINGS

HEAD AND NECK

➤**INSPECT superficial lymph nodes for edema, erythema, and red streaks.** Superficial nodes should not be visible.

■ Infection of the head and throat may be indicated when nodes are palpable bilaterally and feel warm, tender, firm, but freely movable.

➤**PALPATE nodes for size, consistency, mobility, borders, tenderness, and warmth.** Location of nodes is shown in Fig. 12-4. Lymph nodes usually are not palpable.

PROCEDURES AND TECHNIQUES WITH NORMAL FINDINGS

Preauricular Nodes Begin with the preauricular nodes and palpate them, followed by the parotid, postauricular, occipital, retropharyngeal, submandibular, and submental nodes. Use a specific sequence so none is missed (Fig. 12-10). You may want to use both hands, one on each side of the neck, to compare the findings. However, the submental node is easier to palpate with one hand.

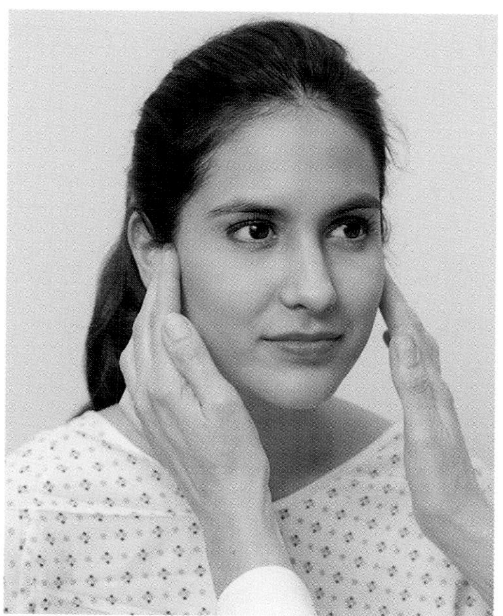

Fig. 12-10 Palpation of the preauricular nodes.

Anterior and Posterior Cervical Chain Examine the anterior and posterior cervical chain by tipping the client's head toward the side being examined, which relaxes these tissues. Palpate these nodes superficially first, then more deeply into soft tissues on either side of the sternocleidomastoid muscle (Fig. 12-11). The deep posterior cervical nodes are palpated at the anterior border of the trapezius muscle.

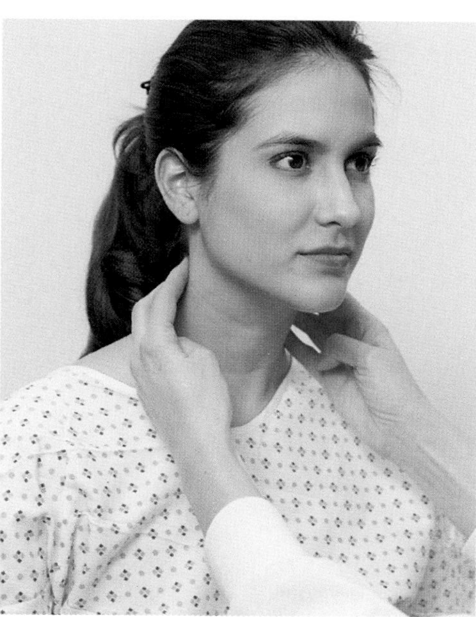

Fig. 12-11 Palpation of the posterior superficial cervical chain nodes.

ABNORMAL FINDINGS

- Malignancy may be indicated when nodes are unilateral, hard, discrete, asymmetric, fixed, and nontender. These nodes may be attached to underlying tissue.
- If nodes are enlarged and tender, check the structures they drain for the source of the problem. For example, an enlarged submental node may be caused by facial acne; an enlarged supraclavicular node may indicate a thoracic or abdominal pathologic condition such as carcinoma, lymphoma, sarcoidosis, HIV infection, syphilis, or tuberculosis.

PROCEDURES AND TECHNIQUES WITH NORMAL FINDINGS

Supraclavicular Nodes Palpate the supraclavicular nodes by having the client hunch the shoulders forward and flex the chin toward the side being examined, which makes the node more accessible (Fig. 12-12). An alternate approach is to palpate the supraclavicular nodes by standing behind the client. Place your fingers into the medial supraclavicular fossa, deep into the clavicle and adjacent to the sternocleidomastoid muscle. Instruct the client to take a deep breath while you press deeply behind the clavicles. As the client inspires, enlarged supraclavicular nodes will be felt.

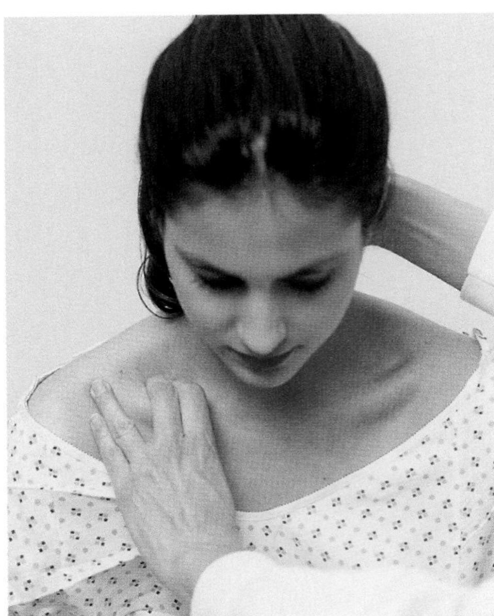

Fig. 12-12 Palpation of the supraclavicular nodes.

ABNORMAL FINDINGS

- Detection of supraclavicular nodes should always be considered cause for concern. These nodes are often sites of metastatic disease since they are at the end of several lymphatic ducts such as the thoracic duct.

PROCEDURES AND TECHNIQUES WITH NORMAL FINDINGS

AXILLARY AND BREAST AREAS

➤PALPATE axillary nodes for size, consistency, mobility, borders, tenderness, and warmth. Most of the lymph drainage from the breasts flows into axillary nodes. Palpable nodes are shown in Fig. 12-6. Support the client's arm on your contralateral arm or, alternatively, flex the client's elbow and lay the forearm across your arm (Fig. 12-13). Slightly cup the fingers of the examining hand and insert them high into the axilla using the pads of your fingers to feel the central nodes. Let the soft tissues roll between your fingers, the chest wall, and muscles as you palpate. Next move your fingers forward toward the lateral border of the pectoral muscle to feel the anterior nodes. From there, move across the armpit to palpate the posterior nodes along the border of the scapula. Then, move your fingers along the surface of the upper arm to palpate the lateral nodes. Finally, palpate between the midclavicle and the pectoral muscle for the subclavian nodes. For the ticklish client, use a firm, deliberate, yet gentle touch. Lymph nodes of the breast are normally not palpable.

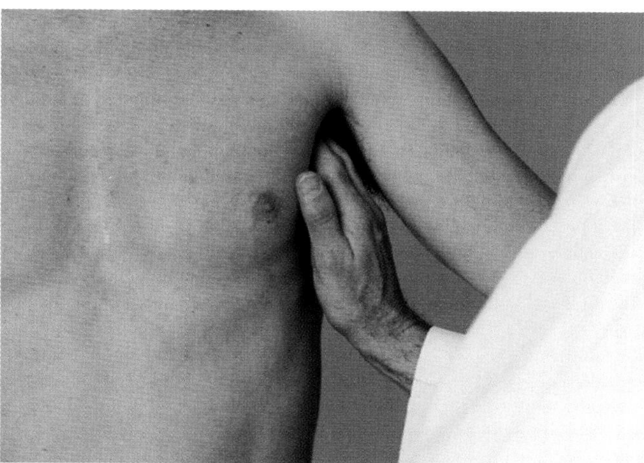

Fig. 12-13 Soft tissues of the axilla are gently rolled against the chest wall and the muscles surrounding the axilla. (From Seidel et al, 1999.)

ETHNIC & CULTURAL VARIATIONS

Modesty may be an issue for the client undergoing examination of the nodes in the breast or groin area. This may be a particularly sensitive issue for women in Asian, Hispanic, and American Indian or Alaskan native cultures and may be ameliorated by use of a female examiner and careful use of draping and privacy.

ABNORMAL FINDINGS

- Axillary nodes may be enlarged due to lymphatic drainage from the breast or arm or because of systemic disease. Infections of the fingers and hands, systemic syphilis, Hodgkin's disease, or breast cancer may result in enlarged axillary nodes.
- Enlarged nodes can be felt "popping" out from under the fingers.

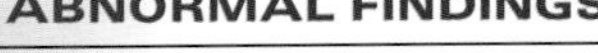

PROCEDURES AND TECHNIQUES WITH NORMAL FINDINGS

ABNORMAL FINDINGS

ARM

➤**PALPATE epitrochlear nodes for size, consistency, mobility, borders, tenderness, and warmth.** Flex the client's arm to a 90° angle and palpate below the elbow posterior to the medial condyle of the humerus (Fig. 12-14).

■ Enlargement and tenderness may be associated with infection of the ulnar aspect of the forearm and the fourth and fifth fingers.

GROIN

➤**PALPATE inguinal nodes for size, consistency, mobility, borders, tenderness, and warmth.** With the client in the supine position, lightly palpate with finger pads in the area just below the inguinal ligament and on the inner aspect of the thigh at the groin (Fig. 12-15). The inguinal nodes are small, mobile nodes, some of which may be nontender. It may not be possible to palpate them at all, but they should be smooth and soft if they can be felt. Moving inward toward the genitalia, you can locate the anatomy using the mnemonic NAVEL: **N,** nerve; **A,** artery; **V,** vein; **E,** empty space; **L,** lymph nodes.

■ Enlarged, tender, firm, warm, and freely movable nodes indicate an inflammatory process distal to these nodes, such as in the leg, vulva, penis, or scrotum.

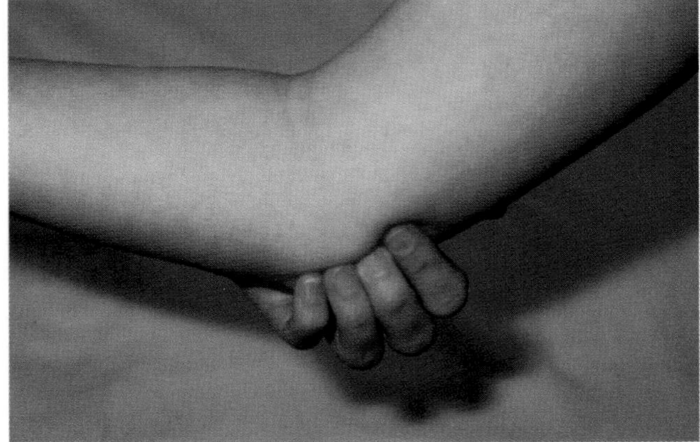

Fig. 12-14 Palpation for epitrochlear lymph nodes is performed in the depression above and posterior to the medial condyle of the humerus. (From Seidel et al, 1999.)

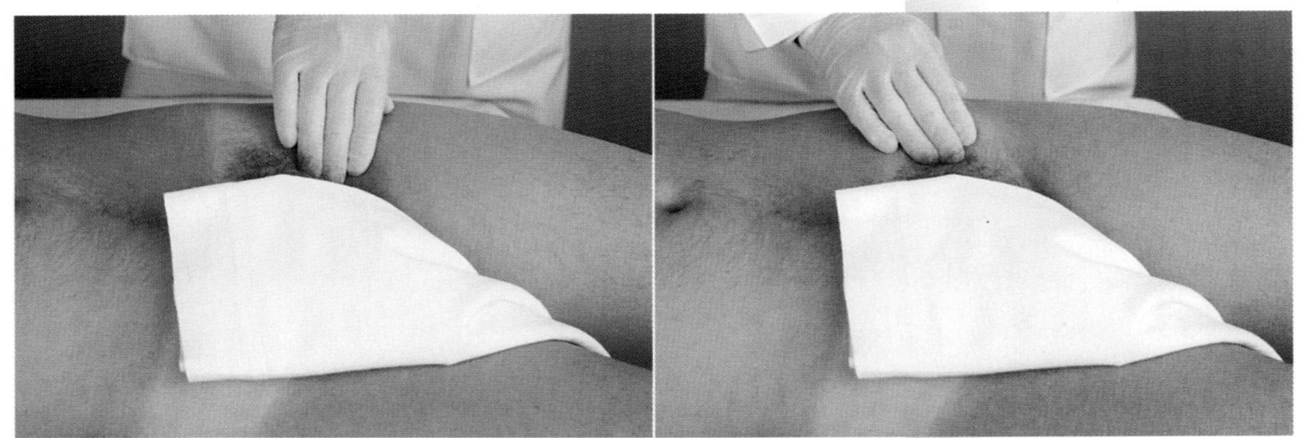

Fig. 12-15 **A,** Palpation of inferior superficial inguinal (femoral) lymph nodes. **B,** Palpation of superior superficial inguinal lymph nodes. (From Seidel et al, 1999.)

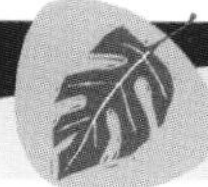

AGE-RELATED VARIATIONS

■ INFANTS

Anatomy and Physiology

At 20 weeks' gestation, the lymphoid system usually begins to develop, but the ability to produce immunoglobulins is not present for the first few months of life, making infants particularly susceptible to infection, especially bacterial infection. They do receive immunoglobulins (especially Ig G) from their mother to provide passive immunity until they are able to produce sufficient antibodies to protect themselves.

Health History

- What immunizations has your infant had?

  Rationale The immunizations to be completed by the end of the first year are three doses of hepatitis B; three doses of diphtheria, tetanus toxoid, and acellular pertussis (DTaP); three doses of *Haemophilus influenzae* type b; three doses of inactivated poliovirus (IPV); the first dose of measles, mumps, and rubella (MMR); and if desired, one dose of varicella (American Academy of Pediatrics, January-December 2000 immunization schedule. www.aap.org/family/parents/immunization.htm). The immunization schedule is found in Chapter 2.

Examination

Procedures and Techniques The examination of an infant is the same as for adults.

Normal and Abnormal Findings Normally the newborn's cervical and inguinal lymph nodes are not palpable. The breast tissue itself may be enlarged and secrete a milky substance in response to maternal estrogen, but this resolves over the first few days or weeks after birth. Abnormal findings include inguinal lymph nodes that may be enlarged due to diaper rash.

■ CHILDREN

Anatomy and Physiology

Lymph tissue increases during childhood, especially between 6 and 9 years. The palatine tonsils also reflect this same pattern. Like all lymph tissue, they are much larger in early childhood than after puberty.

Health History

- What immunizations has your child had?

  Rationale The immunizations to be completed between ages 1 and 10 years are fourth dose of diphtheria, tetanus toxoid, and acellular pertussis (DTaP); one dose of inactivated poliovirus (IPV); and second dose of measles, mumps, and rubella (MMR) (American Academy of Pediatrics, January-December 2000 immunization schedule, www.aap.org/family/parents/immunization.htm). The immunization schedule is found in Table 2-7.

Examination

Procedures and Techniques Assessment of the lymph system is the same in the child as in the adult. Often children are ticklish during assessment of lymph nodes, particularly in the neck and axilla. A firm palpation and assurance that you are not trying to tickle them is needed.

Normal and Abnormal Findings Normally lymph nodes up to 3 mm may be palpable in children and may reach 1 cm in the cervical and inguinal areas, but they are discrete, mobile, and nontender. The term "shotty" may be used to describe small, firm, and mobile nodes occurring as a normal variation in children. It is not unusual to find enlarged postauricular and occipital nodes in children under 2 years of age. Likewise, cervical and submandibular nodal enlargements are more frequent in older children. Thus the age of the client should be considered in your decision to further evaluate lymph node enlargement. Abnormal findings are tender, fixed nodes greater than 1 cm. Enlarged, tender nodes may occur after immunizations or upper respiratory infection (Wong et al, 1999).

■ ADOLESCENTS

Anatomy and Physiology

In puberty, lymph tissue regresses to adult levels.

Health History

- What immunizations has your adolescent had?

  Rationale The immunizations to be completed between ages 11 and 18 years are tetanus (Td) and second dose of measles, mumps, and rubella (MMR) if not received in childhood (Advisory Committee on Immunizations Practices, 1998). The immunization schedule is found in Table 2-7.

Examination

Procedures and Techniques Assessment of the lymph system is the same in the adolescent as in the adult.

Normal and Abnormal Findings Normally at puberty lymph tissue begins to atrophy so that nodes are no longer palpable. Abnormal findings are multiple discrete or matted nodes that are warm to the touch or in areas where the skin is erythematous.

■ OLDER ADULTS

Anatomy and Physiology

Lymph nodes may decrease in both size and number with advanced age. This results in an impaired ability to resist infection. The number of lymphocytes is not reduced; however, their function declines with age. The most significant change is the decline of T lymphocyte function due to thymus gland atrophy.

Health History

- Have you had an immunization against pneumococcal pneumonia?

Rationale The older the client, the higher the risk of death from pneumonia. Clients vaccinated prior to age 65 should receive this vaccine when they turn 65, if 5 years have passed since the first dose (Zanca, 1998).

- Have you had your annual influenza immunization?

Rationale Clients should receive influenza vaccine every autumn. Between 1972 and 1991, 90% of the deaths from pneumonia that resulted from influenza occurred in clients 65 years and older (Zanca, 1998).

Examination

Procedures and Techniques Assessment of the lymph system is the same in the older adult as in the younger adult.

Normal and Abnormal Findings As with younger adults, the lymph nodes are generally not palpable. The size of lymph nodes decreases with advancing age because of loss of lymphocyte function.

ETHNIC & CULTURAL VARIATIONS

IMMUNIZATIONS

Percentage of People Over 65 Who Reported Receiving Vaccines by Race/Ethnicity

Influenza vaccine	
White, non-Hispanic	67%
Black, non-Hispanic	50%
Hispanic	58%
Pneumococcal vaccine	
White, non-Hispanic	47%
Black, non-Hispanic	30%
Hispanic	34%

Data from Sepe S, November 1998

CLIENTS WITH SITUATIONAL VARIATIONS

CLIENTS WHO HAVE HAD A RADICAL MASTECTOMY

Examination

Normal and Abnormal Findings Surgical excision of malignant tissue may require the removal of surrounding lymph nodes to stage the cancer and prevent metastasis of the cancer to other sites. As a result, edema develops, called lymphedema, because lymph nodes are no longer present to drain fluid from the interstitial spaces. After a radical mastectomy, lymphedema may develop in the upper arm on the operative side. Clients with lymphedema should be carefully assessed for adequate peripheral circulation and range of motion. Lymphedema is further discussed under Common Problems and Conditions in this chapter.

CLIENTS TAKING IMMUNOSUPPRESSIVE THERAPY

Health History

- Are you taking medications to suppress your immune system? Have you been taught to stay away from family and friends who have infections, such as upper respiratory infections?

Rationale Immunosuppressed clients are at great risk for developing infections and should be separated from other clients who might be infectious. These clients include those who are taking large doses of corticosteroids to treat an autoimmune disease, inflammatory condition, or organ transplantation.

EXAMINATION SUMMARY

Lymphatic System

The lymphatic system is examined region by region during the examination of related body parts (head and neck, breast and axilla, arm, and groin).

PROCEDURE

Head and Neck (pp. 222-224)

- Inspect the superficial nodes for:
  Edema
  Erythema
  Red streaks
- Palpate nodes for:
  Size
  Consistency
  Mobility
  Borders
  Tenderness
  Warmth

Axillary and Breast Areas (p.225)

- Palpate nodes for:
  Size
  Consistency
  Mobility
  Borders
  Tenderness
  Warmth

Arm (p.225)

- Palpate nodes for:
  Size
  Consistency
  Mobility
  Borders
  Tenderness
  Warmth

Groin (p.226)

- Palpate nodes for:
  Size
  Consistency
  Mobility
  Borders
  Tenderness
  Warmth

SUMMARY OF FINDINGS

Age Group	Normal Findings	Typical Variations	Findings Associated With Disorders
Infants and children		• Lymph nodes up to 3 mm may be palpable in children and may reach 1 cm in the cervical and inguinal areas but are discrete, mobile, and nontender. These are called shotty and a normal variation in children. • Postauricular and occipital nodes may be enlarged in children under 2 years. • Cervical and submandibular nodes frequently enlarged in older children.	• Inguinal lymph nodes may be enlarged from a diaper rash. Enlarged preauricular nodes may indicate pharyngitis or otitis. • Excessively large palatine tonsils may cause nasopharyngeal obstruction. • Parotid node enlargement, anemia, thrombocytopenia, chronic diarrhea, and recurrent infections may indicate HIV/AIDS.

Age Group	Normal Findings	Typical Variations	Findings Associated With Disorders
Adolescents	• Lymph nodes palpable during childhood are no longer palpable.		• Pharyngitis with fever, malaise, and fatigue, as well as maculopapular rash with splenomegaly or hepatomegaly, may indicate Epstein-Barr virus mononucleosis. • Large, discrete, nontender, and firm- to-rubbery nodes may indicate Hodgkin's disease.
Adults	• Lymph nodes are not visible or palpable.	• Small, movable, discrete nodes < 1 cm may be detected.	• Palpable nodes, either fixed or matted, may indicate infection or malignancy. • Tender, warm, and enlarged nodes indicate infection. Site of infection indicated by which lymph nodes affected. Enlarged supraclavicular nodes indicate malignancy. • Chills, fever, night sweats, dyspnea, malaise, fatigue, oral lesions, weight loss, and lymphadenopathy may indicate HIV/AIDS.
Older adults	• Number and size of lymph nodes decrease.		• Fever, chills, productive cough, and headache may indicate pneumococcal pneumonia. Fever, myalgia, malaise, clear nasal discharge, sore throat, and nonproductive cough may indicate influenza.

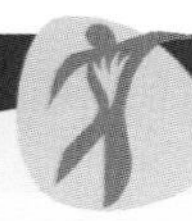

HEALTH PROMOTION

INFECTION

Risk factors that alter the host response to infectious agents include smoking, alcohol intake, dehydration, and inadequate dietary intake. You can reduce infections by maintaining a healthy immune system. This is accomplished by eliminating modifiable risk factors, eating a balanced diet, getting adequate sleep, and managing your stress.

Selecting your diet from the food pyramid provides all of the essential nutrients. Malnutrition alters the immune system. For example, deficits in vitamin A reduce the number of T lymphocytes, while deficits in vitamins B_6 and E reduce the antibody response to vaccines. Inadequate iron creates ineffective white blood cells. Insufficient zinc causes abnormalities in cellular and humoral immunity (Whitney, Cataldo, and Rolfes, 1998).

During periods of sleep, rest, relaxation, meditation, or visualization, potent immune-enhancing compounds are released, and many immune functions are increased (Snyder and Lindquist, 1998). They are also useful in reducing stress. The adrenal gland secretes more glucocorticoid (cortisol) than usual in response to stress as a protective mechanism. One action of prolonged stress, however, is extended release of cortisol, which interferes with immune and allergic responses. For example, cortisol decreases the number of lymphocytes, decreases the rate of antibody formation, and masks the signs of infection. Thus use of stress reduction techniques can help to lower cortisol levels, which improves immune system function.

COMMON PROBLEMS AND CONDITIONS

Lymphatic System

IMMUNE DEFICIENCY

Acquired Immunodeficiency Syndrome (AIDS)

The human immunodeficiency virus (HIV) causes a defect in helper T lymphocytes (CD4 positive levels). The result is progressive loss of immune competence with development of opportunistic infections, impairment of central nervous system, chronic wasting, and often malignancy. Common opportunistic infections associated with AIDS are *Pneumocystis carinii* pneumonia, cytomegalovirus (CMV), herpes simplex, herpes zoster, *Candida albicans, Cryptococcus* organisms, *Toxoplasma gondii, Cryptosporidium* organisms, and *Mycobacterium* tuberculosis. Malignancies often occur, especially Kaposi's sarcoma (Fig. 12-16) and non-Hodgkin's lymphoma. In children, although there is a prolonged clinical latency period, initial signs of AIDS may be parotid enlargement resembling mumps, anemia, thrombocytopenia, chronic diarrhea, and recurrent infections.

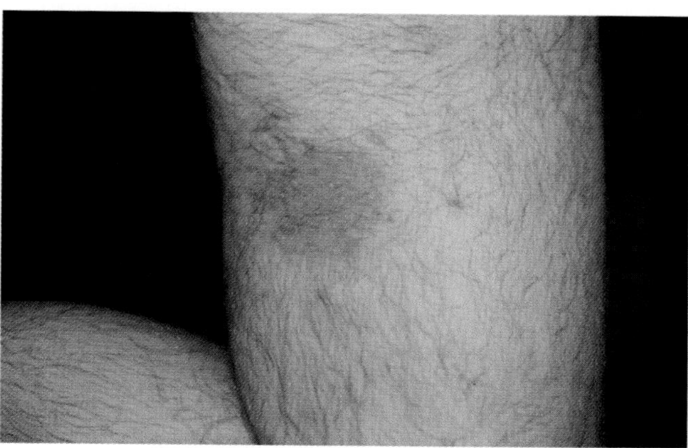

Fig. 12-16 Kaposi's sarcoma. The purple lesion commonly seen on the skin. (Courtesy Department of Dermatology, School of Medicine, University of Utah. From McCance and Huether, 1998.)

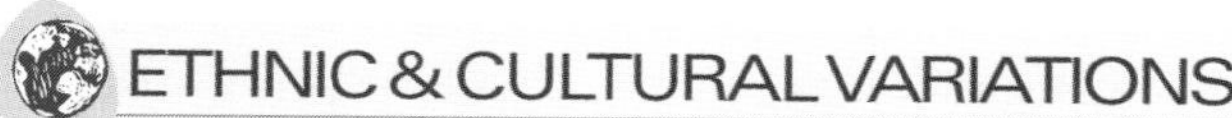

ETHNIC & CULTURAL VARIATIONS

THE HIV/AIDS EPIDEMIC IN MINORITIES IN THE UNITED STATES, 1997

- HIV prevalence was higher among non-Hispanic blacks than in other racial/ethnic groups in most populations surveyed.
- Non-Hispanic blacks and Hispanics accounted for 47% and 20%, respectively, of persons diagnosed with AIDS in 1997, the highest proportions thus far in the epidemic.
- From 1996 to 1997, AIDS incidence and deaths declined in all racial/ethnic populations.
- From 1996 to 1997, AIDS incidence and deaths declined 8% and 32%, respectively, in women (Data from www.cdc.gov.).

Lymphedema

Inadequate drainage from blocked or infected lymphatic channels or from surgical removal of lymph nodes causes an excessive collection of fluid in the interstitial spaces called lymphedema. Congenital lymphedema (Milroy's disease) is the hypoplasia and maldevelopment of the lymph system. Acquired lymphedema results from trauma to the ducts of regional lymph nodes (particularly axillary and inguinal) after surgery or metastasis. Lymphedema is nonpitting, and the overlying skin will eventually thicken and feel tougher than usual.

Malignant Neoplasms

Malignant neoplasms metastasize via the lymph tissue that drains from the primary site. The lymph node may be hard, fixed to surrounding tissue, and nontender. Malignant lymphomas, including Hodgkin's disease, cause lymph nodes to be large, discrete, nontender, and firm to rubbery. Enlarged nodes usually are unilateral and localized; however, chronic lymphocytic leukemia causes generalized lymphadenopathy (Fig. 12-17). Hodgkin's disease is a malignant lymphoma characterized by a painless, progressive enlargement of lymphoid tissue, usually first evident by the cervical lymph nodes, splenomegaly, and atypical macrophages. It occurs in adolescents and young adults as well as persons over 50 years of age.

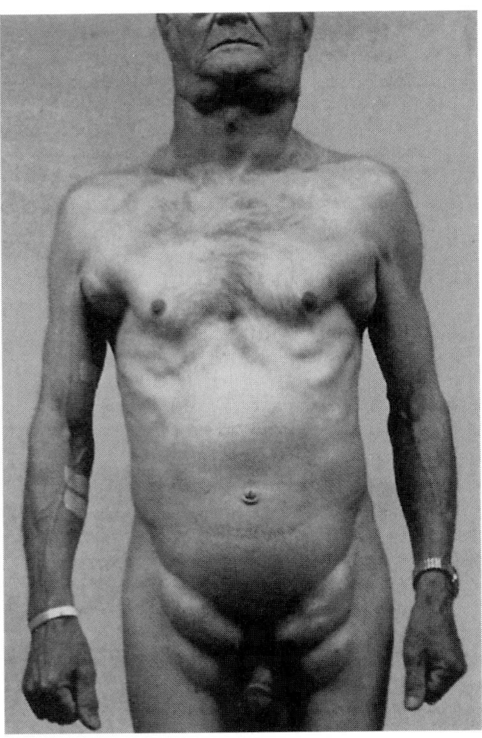

Fig. 12-17. Lymphadenopathy. Individual with lymphocytic leukemia with extreme but symmetric lymphadenopathy. (Courtesy Dr. A. R. Kagan, Los Angeles. From del Regato JA, Spjut HJ, Cox JD: *Ackerman and del Regato's cancer,* ed 6, St. Louis, 1985, Mosby.)

ACUTE INFLAMMATION

Epstein-Barr Virus Mononucleosis (Infectious Mononucleosis)

Mononucleosis occurs at any age but is most common in adolescents and young adults. It is spread person to person by the oropharyngeal route (by saliva). The incubation period is 4 to 6 weeks, and the period of communicability is prolonged; pharyngeal secretions may persist for a year after the illness. Initial signs and symptoms include pharyngitis with fever, malaise, and fatigue. Splenomegaly, hepatomegaly, and/or maculopapular rash may be noted. The affected nodes may be generalized but are more commonly palpated in the anterior and posterior cervical chains. The nodes vary in firmness and are generally discrete and occasionally tender.

Acute Lymphangitis

Inflammation of one or more lymphatic vessels usually results from an acute streptococcal infection of one of the extremities. Lymphangitis is characterized by fine red streaks extending from the infected area to the axilla or groin and by fever, chills, headache, and myalgia. Inspect and palpate distal to the inflammation for sites of infection, particularly interdigitally.

Acute Lymphadenitis

Inflammation of lymph nodes usually results from systemic neoplastic disease, bacterial infection, or other inflammatory condition. The involved nodes are enlarged, firm, and tender (Fig. 12-18). The surrounding tissue becomes edematous and skin appears erythematous, usually within 72 hours. The location of the affected node is indicative of the site or origin of disease. Other forms include actinomycotic adenitis resulting from dental disease and cat scratch disease or *Pasteurella multocida* infection at the site of a scratch or bite from a dog or cat.

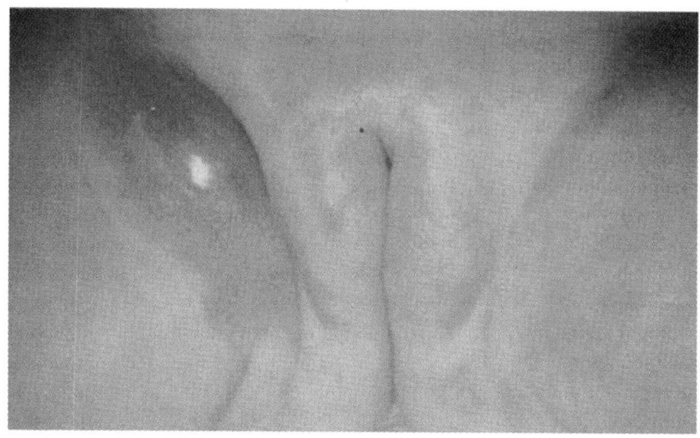

Fig. 12-18 Acute lymphadenitis. (From Zitelli and Davis, 1997.)

Streptococcal Pharyngitis

An inflammation of the pharynx and surrounding lymph tissue (tonsils) can be identified by firm, discrete, mobile, and tender anterior cervical nodes. Accompanying signs and symptoms include fever greater than 102.2° F (39° C), sore throat with dysphagia, and erythematous tonsils and pharynx with white or yellow exudate. (See Fig. 14-25 in Chapter 14: Nose, Paranasal Sinuses, Mouth, and Oropharynx.) This inflammation is commonly seen in school-age children.

CLINICAL APPLICATION and CRITICAL THINKING

SAMPLE DOCUMENTATION

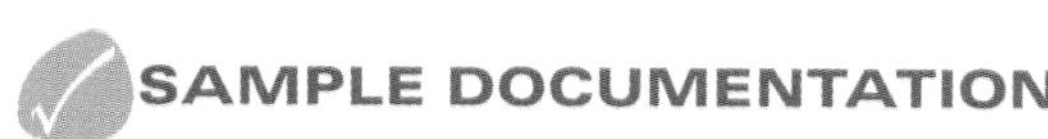

CASE 1

A 5-year-old Hispanic girl needs a physical examination before starting kindergarten. She is accompanied by her mother.

Subjective Data

Has no allergies and takes no medications on a regular basis; had diphtheria, tetanus, and acellular pertussis (DPaT), hepatitis B, and intramuscular poliovirus vaccines; last physical examination was 2 years ago. Mother not sure when physical examinations are necessary; does not have primary care provider. Child full-term vaginal delivery without complications. No hospitalizations; had chickenpox at age 3; has annual upper respiratory infection treated with over-the-counter drugs. No family history of cancer, hypertension, tuberculosis, or diabetes mellitus. Only child, attends day care while parents work. Review of systems noncontributory.

Objective Data

Temperature, 37° C (98.6° F); Pulse rate, 86 beats/min; Respiratory rate, 22/min; Blood pressure, 94/56 mm Hg.

Weight, 17 kg (37 lb); Height, 110 cm (43 inches).

Lymph system: Small (about 5 mm), firm, discrete, movable, nontender nodes postauricular and occipital bilaterally; nontender, shotty nodes along left superficial cervical chain; otherwise no nodes felt at supraclavicular, axillary, epitrochlear, or inguinal sites. Only lymph system is documented.

Functional Health Patterns Involved

Health perception–health management

Nursing Diagnosis and Collaborative Problems

- *Health-seeking behaviors:* interest in maintaining daughter's health.

CASE 2

Ms. Weiss is a 56-year-old woman who comes to the health clinic with a chief complaint of "swollen tender left arm."

Subjective Data

Client complains arm progressively swollen over the last couple of weeks; "heavy, dull feeling and uncomfortable." Had mastectomy 1 month ago for breast cancer. Distress regarding appearance, referring to self as "ugly." Fears cancer will spread if arm exercises performed. No other pertinent health history.

Objective Data

Temperature, 37.2° C (98.9° F); Pulse rate, 96 beats/min; Respiratory rate, 20/min; Blood pressure, 110/70 mm Hg.

56-year-old anxious female, cooperative and reliable. Avoids looking at the mastectomy site or left arm.

Chest: Well-healed incision over left chest—scar tissue present. Lungs clear bilaterally, respirations even, unlabored.

Upper extremities: Unilateral edema noted in left upper arm. Moves upper extremities well, some range-of-motion (ROM) limitation in left. Pulses palpable bilaterally. No pain with examination.

No enlarged axillary or breast nodes.

Functional Health Patterns Involved

- Health perception–health management
- Self-perception–self-concept
- Activity–exercise

Medical Diagnosis

Lymphedema

Nursing Diagnosis and Collaborative Problems

- *Ineffective management of therapeutic regime* related to mistrust as manifested by:
  - Fear that arm exercises would cause cancer to spread.
- *Body image disturbance* related to client's loss of body part and change in body appearance as manifested by:
  - Avoiding looking at arm and mastectomy incision site
  - Patient stating, "I look so ugly."
- *Risk for impaired physical mobility* related to edema.
- *Risk for infection* related to compromised circulation.
- *PC:* Left shoulder contracture.

CRITICAL THINKING QUESTIONS

1. During a physical examination of a 15-year-old girl you are palpating at the angle of the mandible on each side of her jaw. You note on the right a tender, warm lymph node that is enlarged (greater than 1 cm). (You are confident that this node is greater than 1 cm because it is wider than your little finger, which you know is about 1 cm in width.)
   a. Which node is it, and why is it enlarged?
   b. What additional data would you collect to determine the cause of this enlarged node?
2. You are examining a male toddler and find a small (<1 cm), firm, and mobile lymph node behind the right mastoid process. Later in the examination you palpate discrete and mobile nodes in the left groin.
   a. What are the names of these nodes, and why are they palpable?
   b. What additional data would you collect to interpret the meaning of these data?
3. How can you tell the difference between a lymph node that indicates inflammation and a lymph node that indicates malignancy?

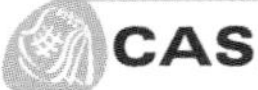

CASE STUDY

Mario is a 16-year-old boy complaining of fatigue and weakness. Listed below are data collected by the nurse during an interview and assessment.

Interview Data

Mario indicates he keeps a busy schedule with school, basketball, and work. He has always been a good student, but he seems to be having a harder time keeping up with everything. He feels he is beginning to let his family and friends down because fatigue and weakness are interfering with his performance at school and on the basketball court. He states that he gets out of breath easily, even with a little activity. Mario does not want to quit his job because he is saving for college. He denies changes in appetite or abdominal problems but reports that he thinks he sometimes has a fever.

Examination Data

- **General survey:** Alert, thin male. Height, 5′ 7″ (170 cm); Weight, 140 lb (63.6 kg); Blood pressure, 118/72 mm Hg; Pulse rate, 88 beats/min; Respiration rate, 18/min; Temperature, 37.8° C (100° F).
- **Skin:** Skin is warm, dry, turgor is elastic; overall color is pink. Maculopapular confluent rash noted on chest and back. No evidence of bruising; no skin discoloration.
- **Thorax:** Respirations are even and unlabored, clear to auscultation. Heart rate and rhythm regular.
- **Abdomen:** Bowel sounds auscultated × 4. Abdomen soft, nontender, and nondistended.
- **Musculoskeletal:** Moves all extremities, symmetric. Moves joints without tenderness.
- **Head and neck:** Enlarged and firm cervical lymph nodes and submandibular nodes. Supraclavicular nodes are also palpable.

1. What data deviate from normal findings, suggesting a need for further investigation?
2. What additional information should the nurse ask or assess for?
3. In what functional health patterns does data deviate from normal?
4. What nursing diagnosis and/or collaborative problems should be considered for this situation?

REMEMBER to check out your **companion CD-ROM**

13 Head and Neck

www.mosby.com/MERLIN/wilson/assessment/

ANATOMY AND PHYSIOLOGY

The bones of the head house and protect not only the brain and upper spinal cord, but also the components of the special senses of vision, hearing, smell, and taste.

The bones of the head are fused together and covered by the scalp. There are 6 bones: 1 frontal, 2 parietal, 2 temporal, and 1 occipital bone (Fig. 13-1). The face consists of 14 bones: 2 nasal, 2 nasal conchae, 1 frontal, 2 lacrimal, 1 sphenoid, 2 zygomatic, 1 ethmoid, 2 maxillae, and 1 movable mandible (Fig. 13-2).

The eyes, ears, nose, and mouth are basically symmetric; the facial muscles are innervated by cranial nerves V (trigeminal) and VII (facial). Facial expression is controlled through cranial nerve VII.

The neck is formed by the cervical vertebrae, which are supported by ligaments and by the sternocleidomastoid and trapezius muscles; these also give the neck its movement. This mobility is greatest at the level of C4-5 or C5-6.

Major structures of the neck include the sternocleidomastoid muscle, the hyoid bone, the thyroid cartilage, the cricoid cartilage, the thyroid gland, and the trachea. The right and left lobes of the thyroid gland are butterfly shaped and joined by the isthmus. The isthmus lies across the trachea under the cricoid cartilage and tucks behind the sternocleidomastoid muscle. The carotid artery and internal jugular vein lie deep and parallel to the anterior aspect of the sternocleidomastoid muscle. (Fig. 13-3, *A* and *B*).

The relationships of the neck muscles to each other and to adjacent bones create anatomic landmarks called triangles. The anterior triangle is formed by the medial borders of sternocleidomastoid muscles and the mandible. Inside this triangle lie the hyoid bone, cricoid cartilage, trachea, thyroid, and anterior cervical lymph nodes. The posterior triangle is formed by the trapezius and sternocleidomastoid muscles and the clavicle; it contains the posterior cervical lymph nodes (Fig. 13-4).

Lymph nodes of the head and neck occur in chains and clusters. Superficial nodes are located in subcutaneous connective tissue, and deeper nodes lie beneath the muscles (see Figs. 12-4 and 12-5). The deep cervical chain lies beneath the sternocleidomastoid muscles.

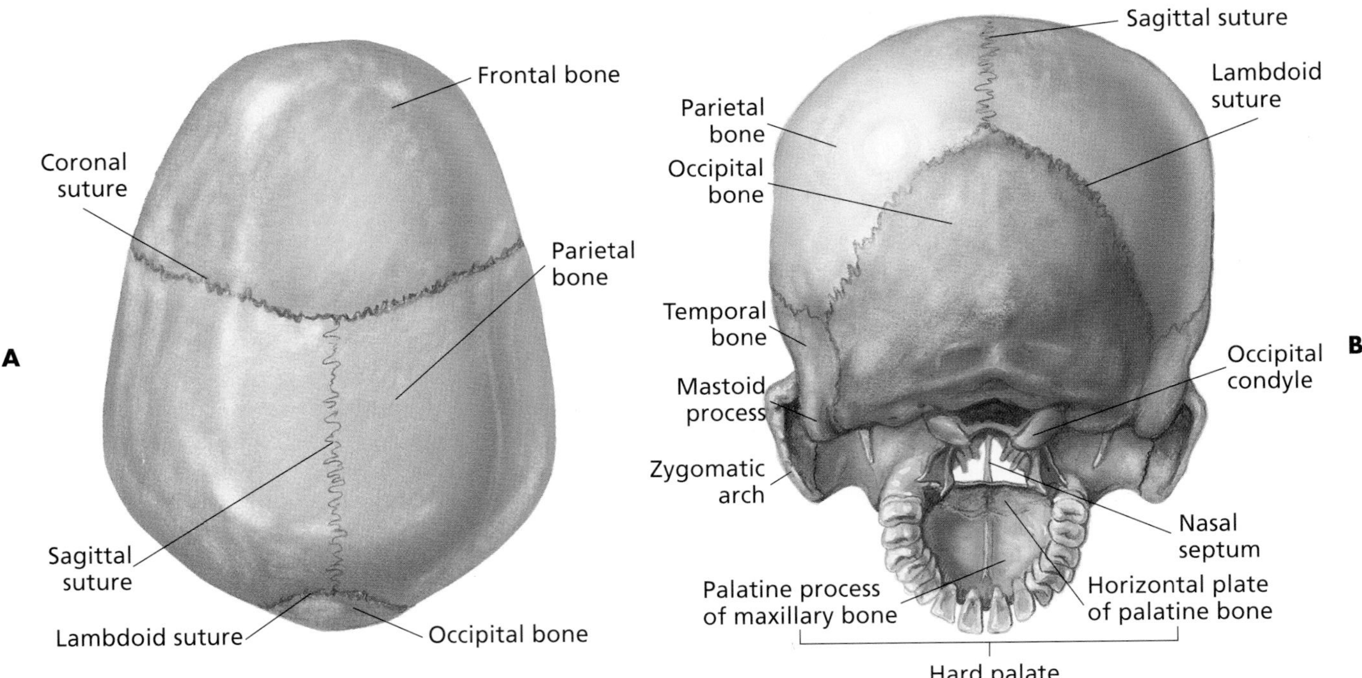

Fig. 13-1 **A,** Bones of the head as seen from the superior view. The two frontal bones that fused appear as one bone in the adult. **B,** Bones of the head as seen from the posterior view. (From Seeley, Stephens, and Tate, 1995.)

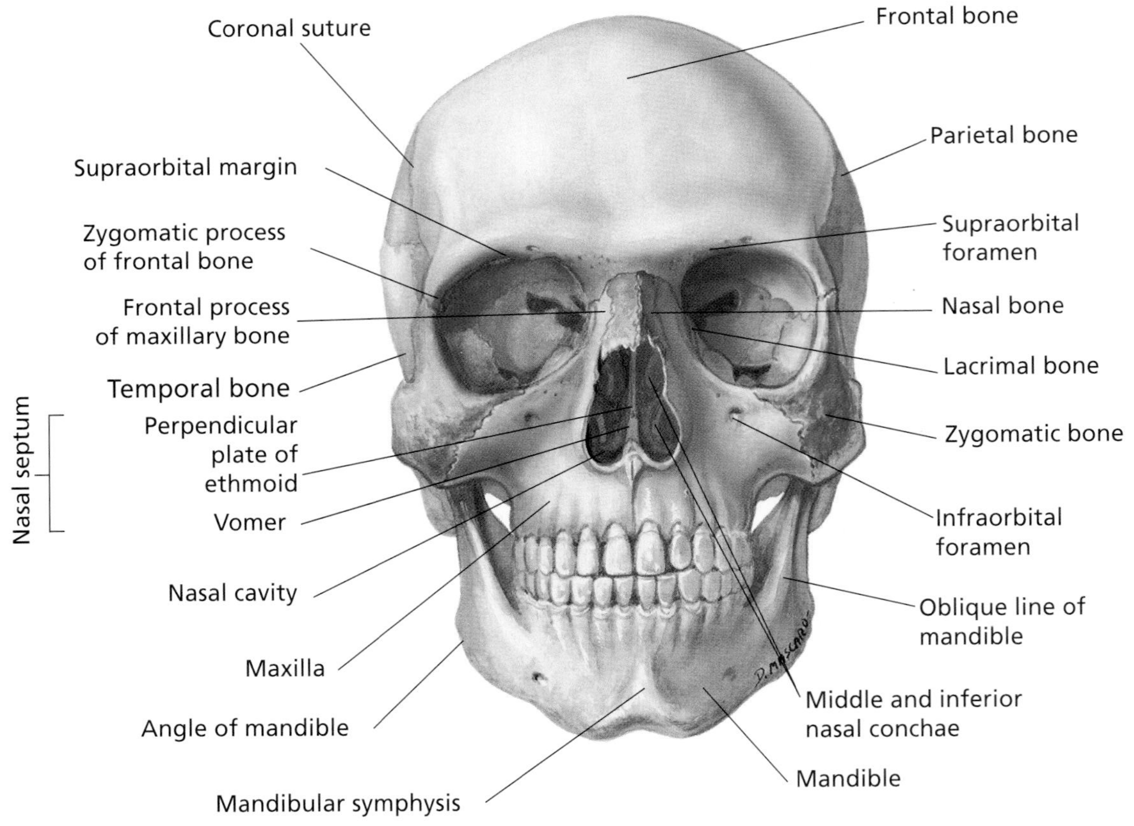

Fig. 13-2 Bones of the face. (From Seeley, Stephens, and Tate, 1995.)

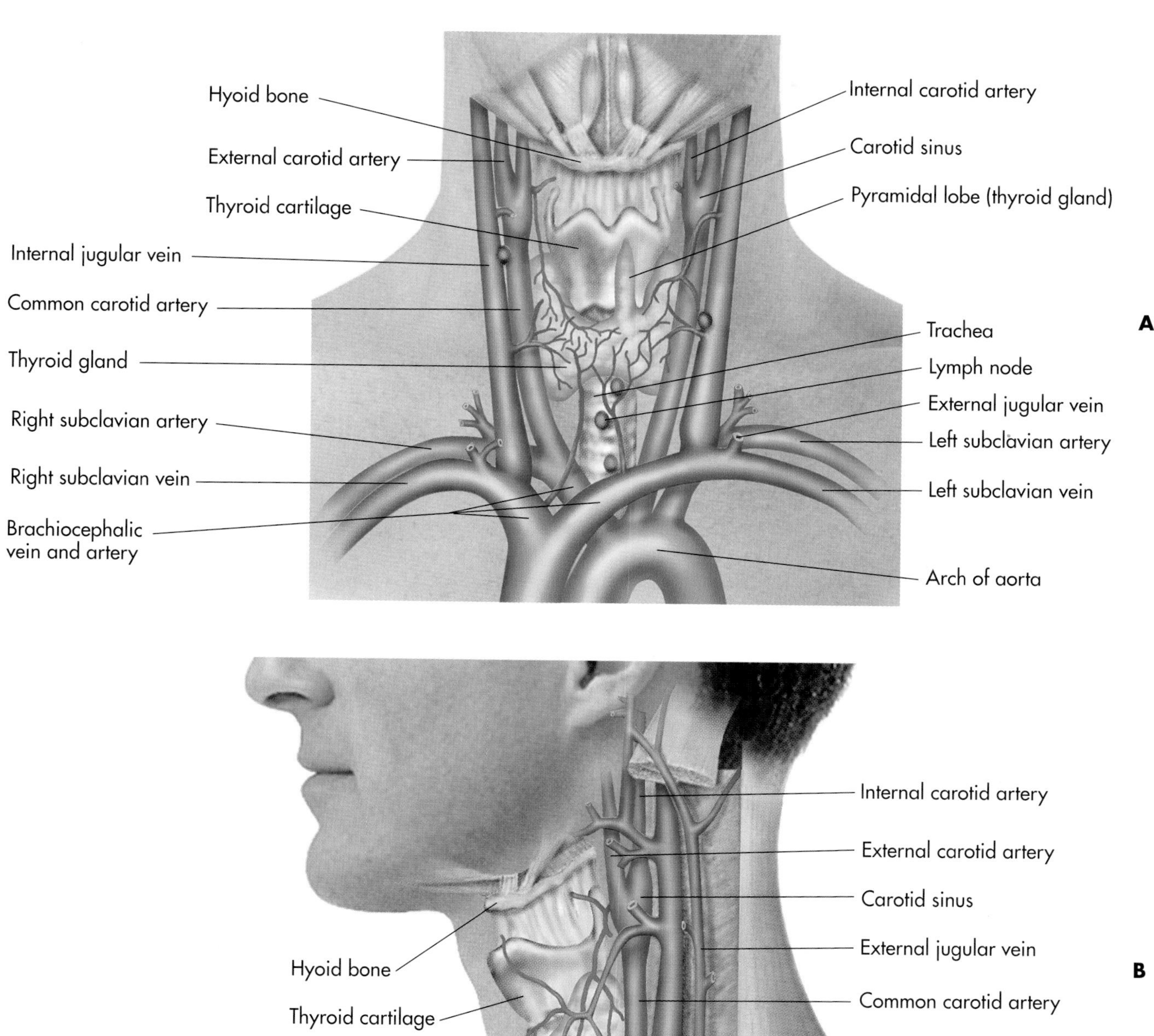

Fig. 13-3 Underlying structures of the neck. **A,** Anterior view. **B,** Lateral view. (From Seidel et al, 1999.)

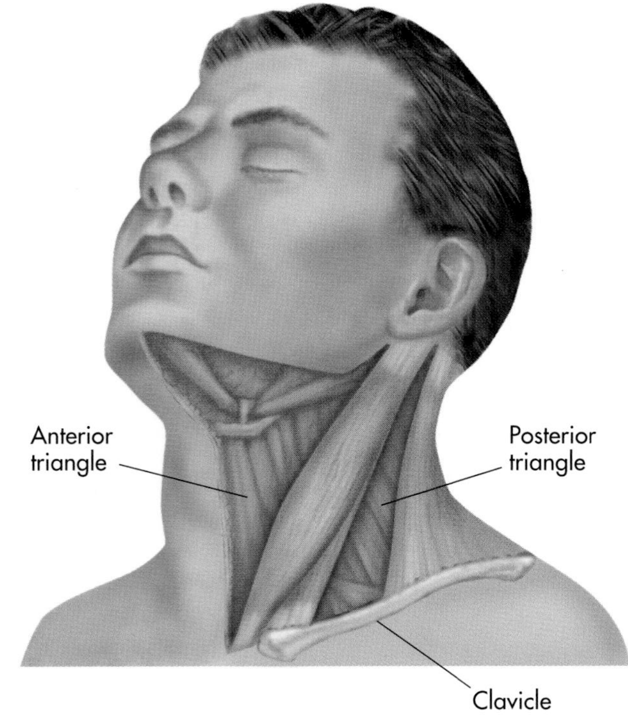

Fig. 13-4 Anterior and posterior triangles of the neck. (From Seidel et al, 1999.)

HEALTH HISTORY

Head and Neck

QUESTIONS	RATIONALE
PRESENT HEALTH STATUS	
➤ How would you describe the condition of your head and neck?	■ Input from clients may provide data about the health status of the head and neck.
➤ Have you noticed any changes in your head or neck? If yes, describe.	■ The client may have noticed a change that he or she does not think is a problem. This question allows you to screen clients for risk factors.
➤ Do you have any chronic diseases? (high blood pressure, diabetes, arthritis, myasthenia gravis, hyperthyroidism or hypothyroidism)	■ Chronic diseases may contribute to headaches, impaired neck range of motion, or impaired thyroid function.
➤ Do you take any medications? If so, what do you take and how often? When did you start taking this medicine?	■ Medications may have side effects that cause dizziness or headaches. Antihypertensives may cause dizziness. Oral contraceptives, estrogen preparations, or bronchodilators may actually cause headaches. It is important to assess the client's compliance with medications to ensure therapeutic effects.
➤ Do you wear your seat belt when in a car? Do you ride any vehicles that require a helmet? (bicycle, motorcycle) If so, do you wear a helmet?	■ These questions determine safety measures that the client uses and provide an opportunity for teaching if needed.

QUESTIONS

RATIONALE

➤ When was your last eye examination? Do you wear glasses or contact lenses?

■ Headaches can be caused by eye strain or an outdated prescription for eyeglasses or contact lenses.

PAST MEDICAL HISTORY

➤ Have you ever had surgery on your head, neck, or thyroid? If so, describe what happened, what surgical procedure was done, and when.

■ Surgery on the head, neck, or thyroid may lead to other questions you want to ask about any long-term effects of the operative procedure(s).

➤ Have you ever injured your head, neck, or thyroid? If so, describe the injury.

■ Note any predisposing factors, such as epilepsy or a seizure disorder, a blackout, poor vision, dizziness, cardiac irregularity, or light-headedness. Note also dangerous environmental conditions that may have led to the injury, such as wet floors, an unsecured throw rug, or getting up too fast.

➤ Did you lose consciousness following the injury? (It may be best if someone other than the client answers this question.) Do you remember what happened? Do you have difficulty with thinking or your memory? What were your symptoms following the injury? Did you have head or neck pain? A loss of consciousness? Blurred or double vision? Drainage from your nose or ears?

■ Determine what sequelae from a previous head injury are affecting the client now.

FAMILY HISTORY

➤ Has anyone in your family had thyroid disease? Type 1 diabetes mellitus? Myasthenia gravis? Rheumatoid arthritis?

■ Hyperthyroidism is an autoimmune disease that is associated with other autoimmune diseases such as those listed in the question.

➤ Does anyone in your family have high blood pressure? Does anyone in your family have migraine headaches?

■ There are genetic and environmental risk factors related to hypertension that may contribute to dizziness or headaches.

PROBLEM-BASED HISTORY

The most commonly reported problems related to the head and neck are headache; dizziness; neck pain, stiff neck, limited motion; neck mass; and thyroid disorders. As with symptoms in all areas of health assessment, a symptom analysis is completed, which includes location, quality, quantity, chronology, setting, associated manifestations, alleviating factors, and aggravating factors.

Headache

Everyone seems to have an occasional headache, so your questions should focus on headaches that are not usual or are debilitating to the client.

➤ Do you have frequent or severe headaches? How often do you have these headaches? Do they start gradually or suddenly? How long does the headache last?

■ Many times a headache may be a sign of stress. At other times, headaches may be a sign of chemical imbalance in the body or even a sign of a more serious pathologic condition.

➤ Where do they generally start? Forehead? Temples? Eye area? Nose and cheek? In the back of the neck at the base of the skull?

■ Sinus headaches may cause tenderness over frontal or maxillary sinuses. Tension headaches tend to be located in the front or back of the head, and migraine and cluster headaches are usually unilateral. Cluster headaches produce pain over the eye, temple, forehead, and cheek (Smith and Schumann, 1998).

QUESTIONS

RATIONALE

➤ When do you usually get the headache? Early morning? During the day? During the night? At work?

■ This question determines the pattern of the headache during the day that may help determine aggravating factors and causes.

➤ What is the pain like? Constant? Throbbing or pounding? Shooting? Dull or nagging ache? Sharp? How intense is the pain on a scale of 1 to 10 with 10 being the most pain you have ever had? Is there pressure over a single area or in general? Does it feel like a band around your head? Is it on one side or both? Is the headache aggravated with movement? Does it follow a pattern?

■ Tension headaches are described as viselike, migraine headaches produce throbbing pain, and cluster headaches cause a burning or stabbing feeling behind one eye.

■ Cluster headaches occur more than once a day and last for less than an hour to about 2 hours. They may follow this pattern for a couple of months and then disappear for months or years.

■ Migraine headaches may occur at periodic intervals and may last from a few hours to 1 to 3 days.

➤ What other associated symptoms do you have? Nausea? Vomiting? Diarrhea?
➤ Do you have blurred vision? Double vision (diplopia)? Sensitivity to light (photophobia)? Increased lacrimation? Nasal discharge?
➤ Do you have ringing in the ears (tinnitus)? Feelings of numbness (paresthesia)? If yes, is it always present or just sometimes?

■ These questions refer to associated symptoms of headache. Migraines may be accompanied by visual disturbances, nausea, and vomiting. Cluster headaches may occur with nasal stuffiness or discharge, red teary eyes, or drooping eyelids. Tension headaches occur with stress and anxiety.

➤ What factors do you feel may bring the headache on? Stress? Fatigue? Food additives? Sudden movement or exercise? Alcohol or medications? Weather? Allergies? Long periods without eating? Menstrual cycle? Do you have other health problems, such as a history of head injury or seizures? (Box 13-1 lists foods that trigger headaches.)

■ Illnesses that can precipitate headaches include hypertension, hypothyroidism, and vasculitis. Migraines are frequently associated with menstrual periods.

Box 13-1 Headache-Triggering Foods

- Alcohol: sulfites
- Avocado
- Bacon: nitrites
- Bananas
- Canned figs
- Chicken livers
- Chocolate
- Citrus fruits: lemon, lime, orange, grapefruit
- Herring
- Hot dogs
- Meats, processed: bologna, salami, pepperoni
- Monosodium glutamate (Chinese food)
- Nuts
- Onions
- Sunflower seeds
- Tea and coffee (caffeinated or decaffeinated)
- Yogurt

From Smith L, Schumann L: Differential diagnosis of headache, *J Am Acad Nurse Pract* 10(11):519, 1998.

➤ What do you usually do to treat the headache? Sleep? Take pain medication? If medication, what kind? Is the medication effective in relieving the pain? How often do you take the medication?

■ Knowing what brings relief may help in determining the cause of the headache. Rest can help relieve migraine headaches, whereas movement helps relieve cluster headaches.

QUESTIONS

RATIONALE

Dizziness

➤ Do you ever feel dizzy or light-headed, as though you cannot keep your balance and may fall? If so, when and how often does this occur? How long does the dizziness last?

■ First, ask the client to define what he or she means when reporting a history of dizziness. Dizziness is a feeling of faintness that is felt from within the client due to inadequate blood and oxygen to the brain. By contrast, vertigo is a sensation from outside when the client complains that the environment is whirling around. Vertigo is caused by inner ear disorders such as Meniere's disease (Barrett, 1998).

➤ What do you do when the dizziness occurs? What decreases the dizziness? What makes the dizziness worse? Does it interfere with your activities of daily living?

■ These questions complete the symptom analysis. Knowing the effect on activities of daily living (ADLs) helps to know the extent to which the dizziness is interfering with the client's life and the frequency of the problem.

➤ Does the dizziness ever occur when you are driving the car or operating machinery? Have you ever fallen as a result of the dizziness?

■ It is important to ensure client safety and to inquire whether the client is at risk during periods of dizziness.

Neck Pain, Stiff Neck, or Limited Motion

➤ Do you have any neck pain? When did you first notice it? In what part of your neck did you experience the pain? What do you think caused the pain?
➤ If there has been no injury, ask: Have you been ill? Do you have a fever? A rash? A headache?
➤ Does the pain radiate to the arm, shoulders, hands? Down the back? Do you have any tingling or numbness of the neck, shoulders, arms, or hands? How would you rate the pain severity on a scale of 1 to 10?
➤ Is there a limitation of movement or pain with movement? Is the pain relieved by movement? What changes have you made in your daily activities because of the pain? Are you able to drive safely, work, do housework, sleep, look down when going down stairs? Does the pain or stiffness keep you from sleeping or working?

■ It is important to differentiate between neck pain and stiffness caused by sudden injury, the slow onset of pain resulting from stress and strain, and neck pain and stiffness secondary to systemic illness. Stiffness that begins suddenly and is accompanied by fever and headache may indicate meningeal inflammation. Likewise, a myocardial infarction may cause radiating pain up into the neck and even the jaw.

➤ What makes the pain worse?

■ Pain and tension may create a cycle of further pain and tension, thereby increasing anxiety and causing related problems.

➤ What makes the pain better? What have you done to alleviate the pain or stiffness? Medications? Applying heat or cold? Physical therapy?

■ Evaluating previous treatment methods helps in planning therapy for the current problem.

Neck Mass

➤ When did you first notice a lump (mass) in your neck? Where is it located? What does it feel like?
➤ Has it changed in size? If so, how?
➤ What have you done to treat the mass? How effective is the treatment?
➤ Have you had a recent ear infection? An infection of a tooth or in your mouth? A sore throat? Fever?

■ If the mass has had a sudden onset and is painful and the client reports a history of infection or fever, the mass is most likely enlarged lymph nodes. If, on the other hand, the mass is midline in position and has been slowly growing or has been present for months, it is more likely to be a neoplasm, cyst, or goiter.

➤ Have you had any hoarseness of your voice since you first noticed the mass?

■ Hoarseness in association with an enlarged thyroid may indicate a tumor involving the laryngeal nerve.

QUESTIONS

RATIONALE

Thyroid Disorders

➤ Have you been feeling moody, maybe irritable or nervous? Have you had increased energy, decreased energy, or lethargy? Has your sleep pattern changed? When did you notice the changes?

■ Hyperthyroidism increases the body's metabolism, whereas hypothyroidism decreases metabolism. A determination must be confirmed by thyroid-stimulating hormone (TSH), triiodothyronine (T_3), and thyroxine (T_4) laboratory studies.

➤ Are you more sensitive to hot and cold? Are you wearing more or less clothing than the rest of your family? When did you notice these changes?

➤ Have you recently lost more hair than usual? Have your nails become brittle, or has your skin texture changed? When did you notice these changes?

➤ Have you experienced changes in appetite, weight loss, or bowel habits? When did you notice changes?

➤ For female clients: Has the flow of your menstrual cycle changed? When did you notice this change?

■ Hyperthyroidism (Graves' disease) causes insomnia; irritability; nervousness; fatigue; thin, brittle hair; increase in appetite; weight loss; diarrhea; palpitations; exertional dyspnea; tremor; and a feeling of being hot (Scripture, 1998). Hypothyroidism causes drowsiness; depression; thick, brittle nails; decrease in appetite; weight gain; constipation; increased sensitivity to cold; and amenorrhea.

➤ Do you feel that your pulse is racing (tachycardia) or that your heart pounds (palpitations)? How often does this occur? When did you first notice it? Do you have chest pain when the racing occurs?

■ Increased thyroid function causes an increase in metabolism and tachycardia.

➤ Have you had difficulty buttoning the collar of your shirt? Does your neck seem to be larger or swollen? When did you notice this change?

■ An enlarged thyroid may cause subtle neck swelling that may be noticed as a tight collar.

RISK FACTORS

COMMON RISK FACTORS ASSOCIATED WITH Head and Neck Disorders

TENSION HEADACHES

Anxiety
Poor dental hygiene contributing to infected teeth or gums
Lack of adequate stress reduction (e.g., exercise, relaxation, visual imagery)

MIGRAINE HEADACHES

Perfectionistic tendencies
Fatigue
Bright lights
Excessive smoking
Alcohol
Trigger foods such as chocolate, cheeses, citrus fruits, coffee, pork, or dairy products
Lack of adequate stress reduction

HEAD INJURY

Alcohol abuse
Drug abuse
Careless driving
Failure to wear seat belts
Failure to wear helmet when riding bicycle or motorcycle or when roller blading
Firearms

THYROID CANCER

Previous radiation exposure of the head and neck
Females have more nodules, men have higher incidence of malignancy
Family history of thyroid cancer

EXAMINATION

Examination of the head and neck may be organized in numerous ways. The focus of this chapter is only on the head and neck. The discussion of assessment of skin, hair, eyes, ears, nose, mouth, lymphatics, and pulses of the head and neck are described in the chapters listed below:

Skin and hair: Chapter 11
Lymphatic system: Chapter 12
Nose and mouth: Chapter 14
Ears: Chapter 15
Eyes: Chapter 16
Vascular system: Chapter 18

Equipment

- A glass of water for the thyroid examination
- Gloves optional for scalp assessment

PROCEDURES AND TECHNIQUES WITH NORMAL FINDINGS

HEAD

➤**INSPECT the client's face for characteristics of facial features and appropriateness of facial expression.** The client should be alert and responsive.

➤**INSPECT and PALPATE the skull to assess contour, tenderness, and intactness.** Palpate the skull from front to back using a gentle rotary motion. Inspect temporal arteries for redness and palpate for tenderness. Note areas of tenderness, marked protrusions, or lumps. The skull should be symmetric and should feel firm without tenderness. The frontal, parietal, and bilateral occipital prominences may be felt. *Examination gloves should be worn if the client has scalp lesions, injury, or poor hygiene.*

Normocephalic is the term designating that the skull is symmetric and is appropriately proportioned for the size of the body.

➤**INSPECT and PALPATE the bony structures of the face and jaw, noting size, symmetry, intactness, and tenderness.** The eyebrows, palpebral fissures, nasolabial folds, and sides of the mouth should be symmetric (Fig. 13-5). (Assessment of sinuses is found in Chapter 14.) The facial bones should be symmetric and appear proportionate to the size of the head.

CULTURAL NOTE

Many Asian cultures believe that the soul resides in the individual's head. The examiner should therefore ask permission before examining the head (Kneisl and Hutchinson, 1988).

ABNORMAL FINDINGS

- Note evidence of pain, coarse facial hair (in women), or asymmetry or abnormality in the client's face.
- Lumps, marked protrusions, or tenderness should be differentiated to determine if they are on the scalp or actually part of the skull. Depressions or unevenness of the skull may occur secondary to skull injury. Tender or hardened temporal arteries with redness over the temporal region suggest temporal arteritis may cause the headache (Smith and Schumann, 1998).
- *Microcephaly* is an abnormally small head.
- *Macrocephaly* is an abnormally large head.
- Abnormal facial structures include prominent eyes (exophthalmos), pallor, uneven skin pigmentation, swelling, and abnormal facial movements (tics).

PROCEDURES AND TECHNIQUES WITH NORMAL FINDINGS

ABNORMAL FINDINGS

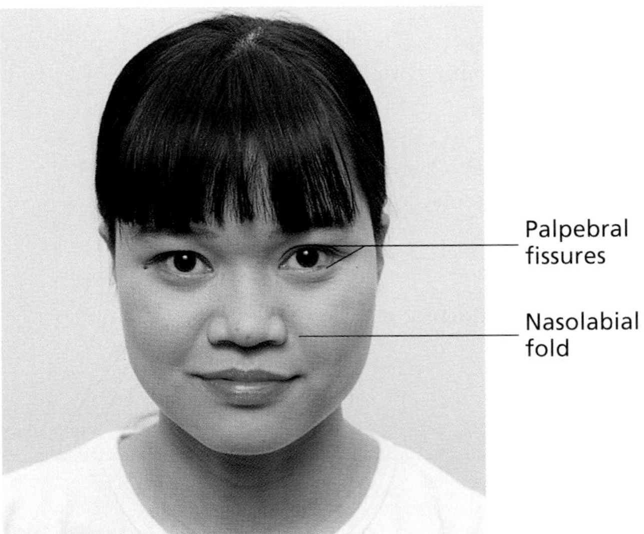

Fig. 13-5 Symmetry of eyebrows, palpebral fissures, nasolabial folds, and the corners of the mouth are normal findings.

NECK

➤**INSPECT the neck for positioning in relation to the head and positioning of the trachea.** The neck should be centered, and the trapezius and sternocleidomastoid muscles should be bilaterally symmetric (Fig. 13-6). Inspect the midline position of the trachea.

■ Note rhythmic movements or tremor of the neck and head. Observe also for tics or spasms. Tracheal deviation suggests displacement by a mass in the chest.

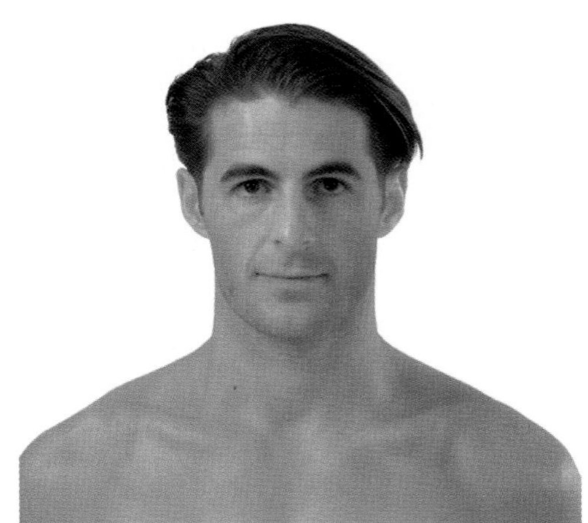

Fig. 13-6 Bilateral symmetry of the neck muscles.

PROCEDURES AND TECHNIQUES WITH NORMAL FINDINGS

➤INSPECT the neck for range of motion (ROM). Ask the client to do the following:

- Move the chin to the chest. Movement should be 45°.
- Move the head back so that the chin points toward the ceiling. Movement should be 55°.
- Move the head side to side so the ear moves close to the shoulder. Note: Remind the client to hold the shoulders stationary during the performance of ROM of the head and neck. "Bend your head to your shoulder; do not raise the shoulder to meet the head. Do not force range of motion beyond the range of comfort." Movement should be 40°.
- Rotate the head laterally to the right and then to the left. Rotation should be 70° in both directions. All movements should be controlled and smooth.

➤PALPATE the neck for positioning of the anatomic structures. Palpate the neck and trachea just above the suprasternal notch (see Fig. 14-3). Palpate for the tracheal rings, cricoid cartilage, and thyroid cartilage. All structures should be midline and nontender.

THYROID

➤INSPECT the anterior neck to visualize the thyroid. Instruct the client to raise the chin up as if drinking from a glass and then swallow. The thyroid gland may not be clearly visualized. The lobes of the gland may be seen as a slightly thickening as the client swallows. Characteristics of thyroid nodules are listed in Box 13-2.

Box 13-2 Characteristics of Thyroid Nodules

BENIGN THYROID NODULES	MALIGNANT THYROID NODULES
• Adult onset	• Adult onset
• Prevalent in females	• Prevalent in males
• Family history of benign thyroid disease	• History of multiple x-ray examinations
• Slow growth of nodule	• No family history of thyroid problems
• No change in voice	• Rapid growth of nodule
• More than one nodule	• Voice change (hoarseness)
• No lymphatic involvement	• Generally only one nodule
	• May have lymph node involvement

ABNORMAL FINDINGS

■ Limited ROM or pain during movement may indicate either a systemic infection with meningeal irritation, a musculoskeletal problem such as muscle spasm, or degenerative vertebral disks.

■ Note pain or weakness of muscles or tremors. Note if the client complains of pain throughout the movement or at particular points.

■ Abnormalities include tenderness upon palpation or location of the structures away from the midline position.

■ A goiter may be seen as a fullness in the neck (Fig. 13-7).

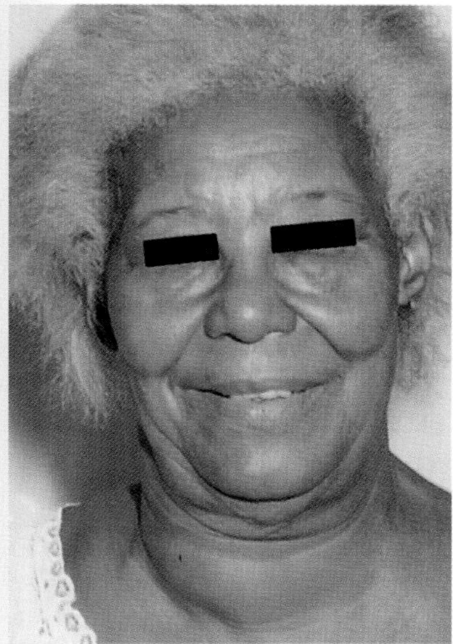

Fig. 13-7 A goiter is a palpable or visible enlargement of the thyroid gland. (From Bingham, Hawke, and Kwok, 1992.)

PROCEDURES AND TECHNIQUES WITH NORMAL FINDINGS

ABNORMAL FINDINGS

❖ ➤**PALPATE the thyroid gland for size, shape, consistency, tenderness, and presence of nodules.** The normal thyroid gland is approximately the size of your thumb pad. The right lobe of the thyroid may be 25% larger than the left. If the thyroid gland is enlarged, use the bell of the stethoscope to auscultate the thyroid for vascular sounds (see Chapter 18).

Caution: Your fingernails should be well trimmed. The palpation of the thyroid may be done by either an anterior or posterior approach. The technique used is the choice of the examiner. Use a gentle touch to palpate the thyroid. Nodules and asymmetric position will be more difficult to feel if the pressure is too hard. In either technique the client should flex the neck slightly forward and toward the side being examined to relax the sternocleidomastoid muscle.

Posterior Approach (Fig. 13-8). Stand behind the client. Have the client sit straight with the head slightly flexed. Instruct the client to take a sip of water from the glass and hold the water in the mouth until instructed to swallow. Reach from behind around the client's neck and place your fingers on either side of the trachea below the cricoid cartilage. Use two fingers of the left hand to push the trachea to the right. Instruct the client to swallow while using the finger pads of your right hand to feel for the right lobe of the thyroid gland, the right sternocleidomastoid muscle, and the trachea. Then have the client take and hold another sip of water. Repeat the technique using the right hand to push the trachea to the left. Instruct the client to swallow while your left hand feels for the left lobe of the thyroid.

Anterior Approach (Fig. 13-9). You should be standing in front of the client. Ask the client to take a sip of water from the glass and hold the water in the mouth until instructed to swallow. Ask the client to sit up straight, then bend the head slightly forward and to the right. Push the client's trachea to the right with your left thumb. Locate the thyroid gland below the cricoid process. Instruct the client to swallow the sip of water. As the sip of water is swallowed, the client's displaced right thyroid lobe may be palpated between the sternocleidomastoid muscle and the trachea by the finger pads of your left index and middle fingers. After the right lobe is evaluated, instruct the client to take another sip of water and hold it. Use the same examination techniques with reversed hand position to examine the left thyroid lobe.

The thyroid gland, if felt, should feel smooth and soft, and the gland should move freely during swallowing. The right side is frequently slightly larger than the left.

■ A tender thyroid may be an indication of acute infection. The presence of nodules or swelling may indicate a thyroid tumor or goiter. A vascular bruit, indicating a hypermetabolic state, sounds like a soft rushing sound.

PROCEDURES AND TECHNIQUES WITH NORMAL FINDINGS

ABNORMAL FINDINGS

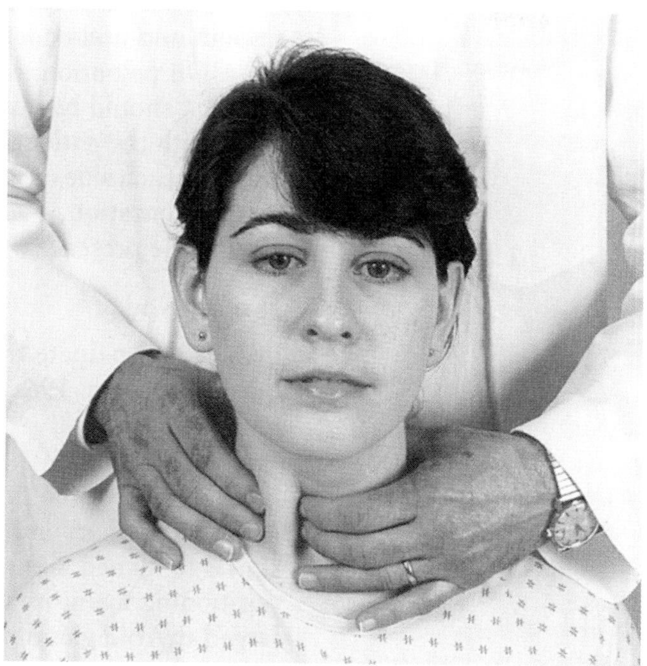

Fig. 13-8 Posterior approach for palpating the thyroid. (From Seidel et al, 1999.)

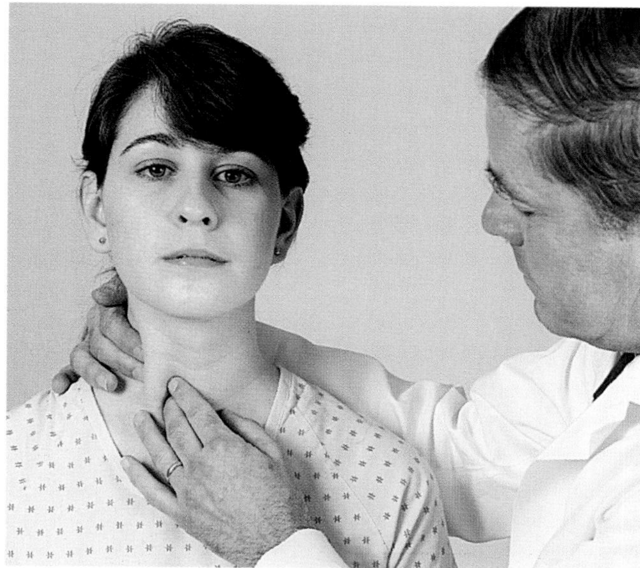

Fig. 13-9 Anterior approach for palpating the thyroid. (From Seidel et al, 1999.)

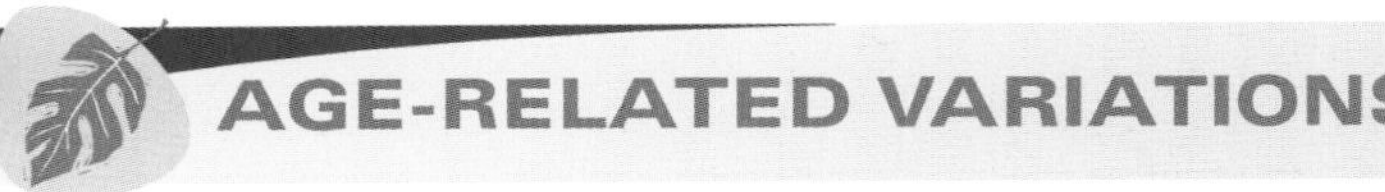

AGE-RELATED VARIATIONS

■ INFANTS

Anatomy and Physiology

The cranial bones are soft and separated by the frontal, sagittal, coronal, and lambdoid sutures at birth; these intersect at membranous spaces called anterior and posterior fontanels, which permit expansion of the skull to accommodate brain growth (Fig. 13-10). Ossification of the sutures begins at about 6 years of age when brain growth is completed; it is not finished until adulthood. However, the fontanels ossify earlier, the posterior fontanel closing by 2 months, and the anterior fontanel closing by 24 months. Passage through the vaginal canal at birth may temporarily alter the shape of the newborn skull as cranial bones overlap or move to new positions. Within days the skull resumes its appropriate shape and size. The infant should be able to turn his or her head from side to side by 2 weeks of age. Head control should be gained by 3 to 4 months of age.

Health History

- Did the mother use alcohol or recreational drugs while she was pregnant? How much, how often?

  Rationale These substances increase the risk for developmental, emotional, and neurologic impairment, including fetal alcohol syndrome.
- Was the delivery vaginal or by cesarean section? Were forceps used? Were there any problems?

  Rationale The use of forceps can increase the risk of caput succedaneum, cephalhematoma, and Bell's palsy.
- Have you noticed any depression or bulging over the infant's "soft spots" (fontanels)?

  Rationale A sunken fontanel may be a sign of dehydration. A swollen or bulging fontanel may be a sign of increased cerebral swelling consistent with infection. The fontanel may also appear full or bulging when the infant cries.

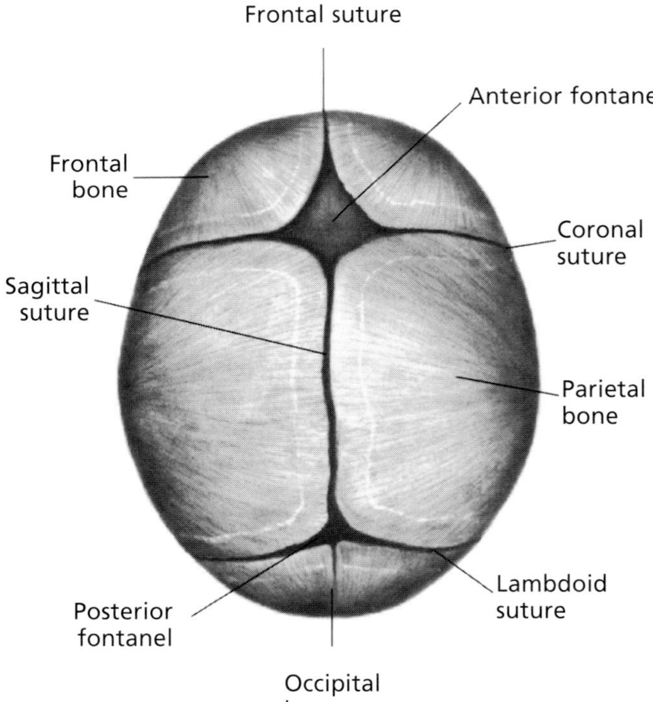

Fig. 13-10 Sutures and fontanels on the infant skull. (From Wong et al, 1999.)

Examination

Equipment Tape measure to determine head circumference.

Procedures and techniques. The circumference of the skull is determined using a tape measure wrapped snugly around the infant's head at the largest circumference, usually just above the eyebrows, pinna of the ears, and the occipital prominence at the back of the skull. Inspect the infant's head for shape and contour. Palpate the anterior and posterior fontanels for fullness and measure for size. To do this, the infant should be held in a sitting position and not be crying. If the infant is lying down or crying, a false fullness may be felt. It is important to assess the infant's head until the child reaches age 2, when the anterior fontanel usually closes. Monitoring the head circumference allows detection of growth abnormalities, either larger or smaller than expected.

❖ If the infant's fontanels are full or the infant has a rapidly increasing head circumference, transillumination of the skull may be performed. To do this, darken the room and wait for at least 1 minute to allow your eyes to adjust to the dark. Place a transilluminator or penlight firmly against the

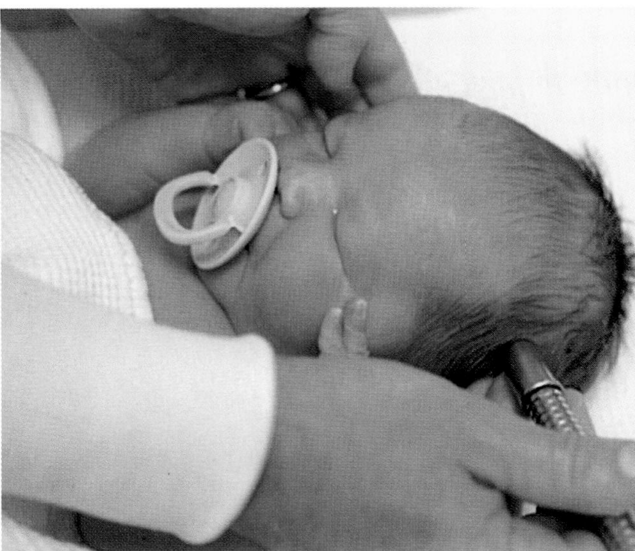

Fig. 13-11 Transillumination of the infant's scalp. (From Seidel et al, 1999.)

infant's skull so that no light escapes (Fig. 13-11). Start the assessment at the midline position of the infant's frontal region and repeat the procedure at 1-inch increments over the entire head. You should expect to see a ring of light around the light extending out 1 to 2 cm. The ring of light should be symmetric and even around the transilluminator. If the ring of light is asymmetric or extends beyond 2 cm, excess fluid or decreased brain tissue in the skull should be suspected.

Begin the infant's neck examination by lifting the infant's shoulders off the examining table by lifting the infant by the arms. Permit the infant's head to lag back and inspect the infant's neck for a midline trachea, abnormal skin folds, and generalized neck enlargement. Palpate the neck for tone, presence of masses, and enlarged lymph nodes. Because the infant's neck is short and thick, the examination of the thyroid is extremely difficult.

Normal and abnormal findings. Normally the skull diameter usually measures approximately 2 cm greater than the infant's chest diameter. The infant's head circumference should be measured at each visit and plotted on a growth chart. Box 13-3 contains growth rates. The normal head circumference of the infant should measure between 27 and 32 cm (Fig. 13-12). Molding is a common finding of the neonate when the cranial bones actually override each other. The molding is secondary to the head passing through the birth canal and generally lasts less than a week. The fontanels should have a slight depression, feel soft, and may have a slight pulsation. The anterior fontanel in infants less than 6 months of age should not exceed 4 to 5 cm. It should get progressively smaller as the child gets older and should be completely closed by the time the infant reaches 18 to 24 months of age. The infant's posterior fontanel may or may not be palpable at birth. If it is palpable, it should measure no more than 1 cm, and it should close by 2 months of age.

Abnormal findings include a deeply depressed fontanel, which may be an indication of dehydration. A bulging fontanel, dilated scalp veins, and enlarged head circumference may indicate hydrocephalus. A common finding in newborns is a *cephalhematoma.* This is a subperiosteal hematoma under the scalp that occurs secondary to birth trauma. The area, which appears as a soft, well-defined swelling over the cranial bone, generally is reabsorbed within the first month of life. The hematoma does not cross suture lines.

If the infant's neck is proportionately short or has webbing (loose, fanlike skin folds), the infant should be evaluated for congenital abnormalities such as Down or Turner's syndromes. If an enlargement of the infant's anterior neck is palpated, the infant should be referred to a physician for further evaluation.

Box 13-3 Head Circumference Growth Rates

Full-term newborn to 3 months	2.0 cm/month
3 to 6 months	1.0 cm/month
6 months to 1 year	0.5 cm/month

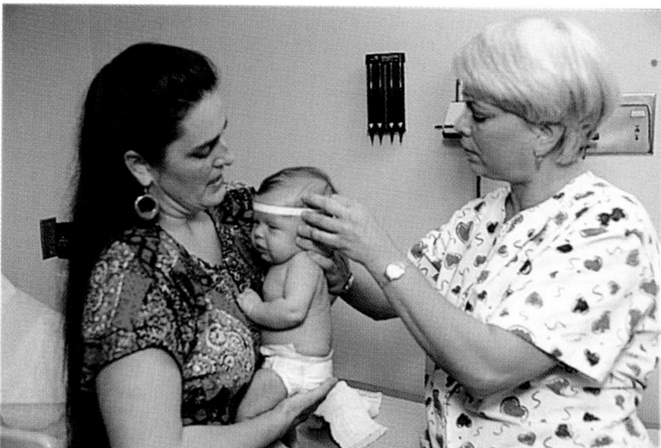

Fig. 13-12 Measuring skull circumference in an infant.

■ CHILDREN

Anatomy and Physiology

The anatomy and physiology for the child is the same as for the adult.

Health History

- Is the child growing and developing as other children his or her age? Is the child's neck growing along with the body?

  Rationale Delay in achieving developmental milestones may indicate some type of developmental or congenital problem. Many times problems will not be identified in young children until they show indications of developmental delay.

- Have you noticed any swelling of the child's neck, or has the child complained of any neck stiffness? If so, does the child have any other signs of infection or illness? Fever? Sore throat? Crying with neck movement? Swollen glands?

  Rationale The most common reason for a stiff neck or swollen glands in the child is either a localized or systemic infection.

- Does the child have headaches? If so, how often and how severe? Does the child ever have to stay home from school because of the headache? Does the child have allergies? How is his or her appetite? How many hours of sleep does

CULTURAL NOTE

American Indian and Alaskan native infants may be secured to traditional cradle boards from birth, which may cause a cosmetic flattening of the posterior skull.

the child get at night and with naps? Has the child ever had a medical evaluation for the headaches? When was the child's last eye examination?

Rationale These questions narrow the potential causes of headache for this client. Headaches may be due to many factors, including inadequate sleep, poor nutrition, eye strain, stress, and allergies. Migraine headaches also are common in children 5 to 6 years of age. Tension headaches can occur in children ages 8 to 12 (Uphold and Graham, 1997).

- Ask the child: Do you have a bicycle helmet? If so, ask: Do you wear it when you ride your bicycle? If so, how often—always or occasionally? Do you wear a helmet or head protection when you roller blade or play other high-risk sports?

Rationale Head injury in children is a leading cause of death and disability. Determine whether the child owns a helmet. If not, provide resource material. If the child does own a helmet but does not wear it, determine the causative factors.

Examination

Procedures and Techniques Examination of a child's head and neck is similar to that of the adult. The child's fontanels should continue to be evaluated at each assessment visit until they are closed, by at least age 2.

The thyroid of the child may be assessed using the same techniques as for the adult. The challenge is to encourage the child to sit still and swallow the water as described so that an adequate evaluation may be done. If the child is not able to cooperate, the thyroid examination may be deferred.

Normal and Abnormal Findings Findings are similar to those for the adult.

■ OLDER ADULTS

Anatomy and Physiology

The rate of thyroxine (T_4) production gradually decreases, but tissue utilization of T_4 declines as well so that thyroid function remains adequate throughout life. The size of the thyroid decreases due to atrophy (Lueckenotte, 1994). The client may have increased concave cervical curvature, causing the positioning of the head in a forward and downward position.

Health History

In addition to the questions in the adult section, ask the following:

- Do you have episodes of dizziness? How long has it been going on? When does it most generally occur?

Rationale Risk of impaired blood flow to the brain increases with age.

- Does your dizziness interfere with your daily activities? Have you fallen because you lost your balance?

Rationale Determine the extent to which dizziness alters activities of daily living and assess for risk for falls.

Examination

Procedures and Techniques Assess range of motion of the neck with one movement at a time, rather than a full rotation of the neck to avoid causing dizziness on movement. Note any pain, crepitus, dizziness, or limited movement. The technique of examining the thyroid is the same as for the younger adult.

Normal and Abnormal Findings A stiff neck in the older adult may indicate cervical arthritis (Smith and Schmann, 1998).

EXAMINATION SUMMARY

Head and Neck

HEAD (pp. 243-244)

- Inspect the head for:
  Facial features
  Appropriateness of facial expression
- Inspect and palpate the skull for:
  Contour and intactness
  Tenderness
- Inspect and palpate the face and jaw for:
  Size
  Symmetry
  Intactness
  Tenderness

NECK (pp. 244-245)

- Inspect the neck for:
  Positioning in relation to the head
  Midline position of trachea
  Range of motion
- Palpate the neck for:
  Positioning of the anatomic structures of the neck

THYROID (pp. 245-247)

- Inspect anterior neck to visualize thyroid
- Palpate the thyroid for:
  Size
  Shape
  Consistency
  Tenderness
  Presence of nodules or enlargement

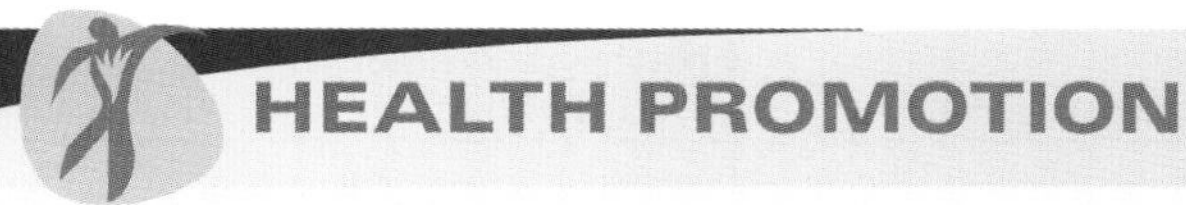

HEALTH PROMOTION

IODINE IN THE DIET

To prevent goiter, the diet should contain iodine in some manner. Many areas of the United States have iodine in the ground. Subsequently, the individual has an adequate iodine intake secondary to the foods grown locally and eaten. Other areas of the country have little iodine in the earth. Individuals living in these areas should supplement their diet with iodine. This may be done easily and inexpensively by using iodized salt.

CONGENITAL HYPOTHYROIDISM

The American Academy of Pediatrics and the American Thyroid Association recommend that all neonates be screened for congenital hypothyroidism during the first week of life. Congenital hypothyroidism occurs each year in about one of every 3500 to 4000 newborns. Because many cases go undiagnosed and do not receive prompt treatment they develop irreversible mental retardation and a variety of neuropsychologic deficits comprising the syndrome of cretinism (Wong et al, 1999).

THYROID CANCER

It is estimated that in the United States, each year 11,300 individuals are diagnosed with thyroid cancer and an additional 1000 people die from thyroid cancer. Individuals who require careful screening include people with a neck mass, hoarseness, a history of multiple endocrine neoplasia syndrome, and multiple exposure to upper body radiation since childhood. Palpation of the thyroid remains the routine screening examination for adults. More invasive screening procedures such as ultrasonography or needle aspiration are reserved for individuals with nodular disease or goiter.

SUMMARY OF FINDINGS

Age Group	Normal Findings	Typical Variations	Findings Associated With Disorders
Infants and children	Facial features symmetric. Anterior fontanel 4-5 cm in diameter and closes at 24 months.	Molding occurs when cranial bones override each other, lasts < 1 week.	Cephalhematoma occurs from birth injury. Contraction of sternocleidomastoid muscle from birth injury or later trauma may be torticollis. Hydrocephalus is associated with dilated veins over scalp, bulging fontanel, and enlarged head circumference. Short neck or loose, fanlike skin folds may indicate Down or Turner's syndromes. Large ring of light during transillumination $>$1-2 cm may indicate excess fluid or decreased brain tissue.
Adolescents	Same as for adult.	Same as for adult.	Same as adult.
Adult	Skull symmetric and firm. Face and jaw symmetric. Trachea midline. Thyroid, smooth, soft, movable, not visible, not enlarged.	Right lobe of thyroid 25% larger than left.	Headache may be migraine, cluster, or tension. Prominent eyes and puffy face suggest hyperthyroidism. Goiter seen or palpated. Fine or coarse hair may indicate thyroid disease.

Age Group	Normal Findings	Typical Variations	Findings Associated With Disorders
	Full range of motion of neck.		Limited range of motion of neck may indicate systemic infection or musculoskeletal problem, e.g., spasms, degenerative vertebral disks. Tracheal deviation suggests displacement by mass in chest.
Older adults	Size of thyroid decreases. Concave cervical curvature causes head to be in a forward and downward position.		Dizziness may be due to cardiovascular or neuromuscular problems. Neck range of motion may be limited due to arthritis, degenerative cervical disk changes.

COMMON PROBLEMS AND CONDITIONS

Head and Neck

HEAD

Vascular Headaches

Migraine Headache

These vascular headaches generally begin in childhood, adolescence, or early adult life. They are frequently familial and occur in approximately 5% of the general population. Women are twice as likely as men to have migraines. Young women are most susceptible. The frequency of the headaches generally decreases with advancing age. The headache generally starts with an aura caused by a vasospasm of intracranial arteries and is described as throbbing unilateral pain. Accompanying signs may include feelings of depression, restlessness or irritability, photophobia, and nausea or vomiting. The headache may last 2 to 72 hours.

Cluster Headache

These vascular headaches are characterized by intense episodes of excruciating unilateral pain. Cluster headaches last from 1/2 to 1 hour but may repeat over a period of days or weeks. Pain is described as burning or stabbing behind one eye. They may be accompanied by unilateral ptosis, ipsilateral lacrimation, nasal stuffiness and drainage. The only prodromal sign may be slight nausea. Cluster headaches are 4 times more common in men and generally occur in the third or fourth decade of life.

Tension Headache

Muscle Contraction Headache

This tension headache is the most common type for persons 20 to 40 years of age. It is usually bilateral and may be diffuse or confined to the frontal, temporal, parietal, or occipital area. The onset may be very gradual and may last for several days. The headache may be accompanied by contraction of the skeletal muscles of the face, jaw, and neck. Clients frequently describe this headache as feeling as if a tight band was around their head, causing pain.

Traumatic Headache

This tension headache occurs secondary to a head injury or concussion. It is characterized by a dull, generalized head pain. Accompanying symptoms may be a lack of ability to concentrate, giddiness, or dizziness.

Hydrocephalus

Hydrocephalus is abnormal accumulation of cerebrospinal fluid (CSF) that may develop from infancy to adulthood. In infants there is an obstruction of the drainage of CSF in the head (Fig. 13-13). Because of this drainage problem, fluid accumulates, causing an increase in intracranial pressure and actual enlargement of the head. As the head enlarges, the facial features appear small in proportion to the cranium, the fontanels may bulge, and scalp veins dilate. In adults the hydrocephalus may be caused by obstruction of CSF as well as increased production or impaired absorption of CSF. In adults the signs of increased intracranial pressure are noted.

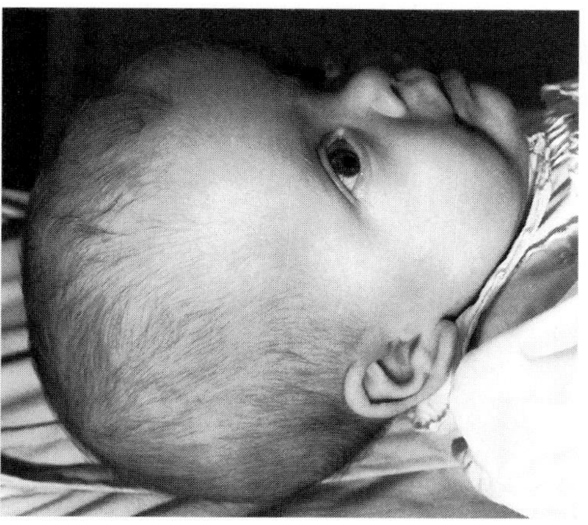

Fig. 13-13 Three-month-old child with enlarged head caused by hydrocephalus. (From McCullough, 1989.)

Microcephaly

This congenital anomaly is characterized by an abnormally small head in relation to the rest of the body and by the underdevelopment of the brain, resulting in some degree of mental retardation. Facial features are generally normal. This disorder may be caused by an autosomal recessive disorder, a chromosomal abnormality, or a toxic stimulus such as radiation, chemical agents, or maternal infection, particularly during the third trimester.

Macrocephaly

This congenital anomaly is characterized by an abnormally large head and brain in relation to the rest of the body, resulting in some degree of mental and growth retardation. This disorder may be caused by a defect in embryonic development or degenerative disease. In macrocephaly there is symmetric overgrowth of the head without an increase in CSF or intracranial pressure, which distinguishes it from hydrocephalus.

NECK

Torticollis (Wry Neck)

The client's head is tilted and twisted toward the sternocleidomastoid muscle due to the muscle contraction on this side of the neck (Fig. 13-14). It is often the result of injury during the birth process. Torticollis may also occur in older children and adults secondary to neck injury, muscle spasms, infections, or drug ingestion.

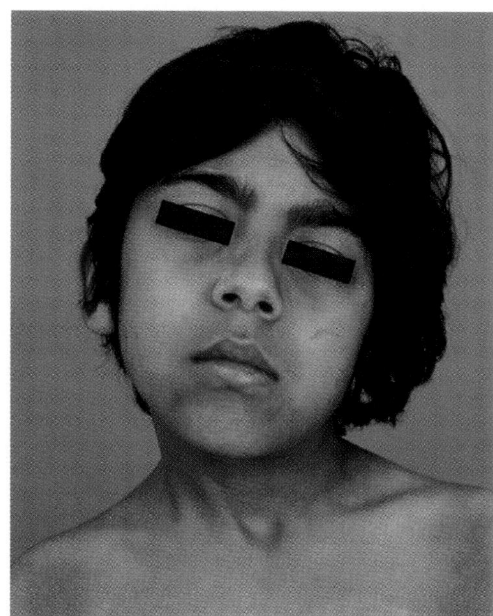

Fig. 13-14 Torticollis (wry neck). Child has tilt of the head to the left. Underlying problem was an inflammatory mass in the left parapharyngeal space. (From Bingham, Hawke, and Kwok, 1992.)

Hyperthyroidism

Excessive thyroid hormone at the cellular level causes signs and symptoms in many body systems. The signs and symptoms reflect the increased metabolism so that clients seem to be "going at top speed" or " moving fast forward." Graves' disease is characterized by one or more of the following: increased secretion of the thyroid gland, enlargement of the gland, and exophthalmos (Fig. 13-15). The disease is 5 times more common in women than men, occurs most frequently between 20 and 40 years of age, and often arises after an infection or physical or emotional stress. Typical signs and symptoms of hyperthyroidism are contrasted with those of hypothyroidism in Box 13-4.

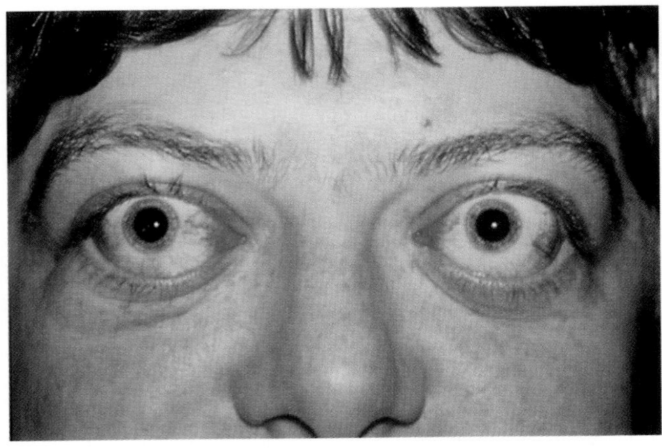

Fig. 13-15 Graves' disease. Client shows characteristic features of endocrine orbitopathy, with peculiar stare produced by retraction of the upper eyelid and the unnatural degree of separation between the margins of the two eyelids. (From Bingham, Hawke, and Kwok, 1992.)

Hypothyroidism

Decreased activity of the thyroid gland is caused by removal of part or all of the thyroid gland, by decreased secretion of thyroid-releasing hormone from the hypothalamus, or atrophy of the thyroid gland. The signs and symptoms reflect the decreased metabolism so that clients seem to be "in slow motion." Typical signs and symptoms of hypothyroidism are contrasted with those of hyperthyroidism in Box 13-4.

Box 13-4 Signs and Symptoms of Hyperthyroidism and Hypothyroidism

BODY SYSTEM	HYPERTHYROIDISM (HIGH METABOLISM)	HYPOTHYROIDISM (SLOW METABOLISM)
General	Intolerant of heat Insomnia	Intolerant of cold, fatigue Lethargy
Eyes	Prominence of eyeballs Elevation of upper eyelid	
Cardiovascular	Tachycardia, palpitations	Bradycardia
Respiratory	Exertional dyspnea	Dyspnea
Gastrointestinal	Increased appetite Weight loss Diarrhea	Decreased appetite Weight gain Constipation
Musculoskeletal	Tremor, muscle weakness	Muscle aching, stiffness Slow movement, slow reflexes
Neurologic	Restless, short attention span Emotional lability	Confused; slow speech; memory loss; night blindness; slow, clumsy movements
Reproductive	Amenorrhea, impotence, decreased libido	Heavier menses, impotence, decreased libido
Skin	Hair fine, soft, straight; temporary hair loss; increased perspiration; warm skin	Dry, flaky skin; dry, brittle hair; reduced growth of nails and hair; slow wound healing; cool skin

Data from McCance KL, Huether SE: *Pathophysiology: the biologic basis for disease in adults and children,* ed 3, St Louis, 1998, Mosby; and Swartz MH: *Pocket companion for textbook of physical diagnosis,* ed 3, Philadelphia, 1998, WB Saunders.

CLINICAL APPLICATION and CRITICAL THINKING

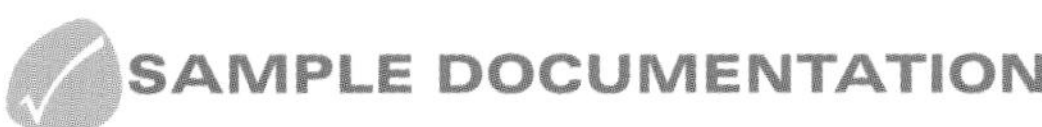

SAMPLE DOCUMENTATION

CASE 1

A 4-month-old boy is brought to the clinic by his mother for a well-baby checkup and immunizations.

Subjective Data

Mother reports infant healthy at birth, weighing 6 lb 10 oz (3 kg); infant holds head up from prone position and has adequate head control; mother concerned that infant's head is "too big"; difficult to pull his shirts over his head.

Objective Data

Alert, active, healthy-appearing male infant accompanied by mother.
Length: 24″ (61 cm).
Weight: 6 lb 10 oz (3 kg).
Head: Lifts head from prone position with ease, turns side to side; skull contour smooth, without depressions; sagittal and coronal suture lines palpable; anterior fontanel 2 in (5 cm); posterior fontanel not palpable; head circumference 15 in (38 cm), chest circumference 12 in (30.5 cm). (Note: at 3 months head circumference 14.5 in [37 cm].)
Neck: Full range of motion, no deformities noted, thyroid not palpable.
Denver II appropriate for age.

Functional Health Pattern Involved

- Health promotion–health maintenance

Nursing Diagnosis and Collaborative Problems

- *Health-seeking behaviors:* well-baby checkup
- *Anxiety and knowledge deficit* related to normal head size and growth of infants as evidenced by:
  - Mother's concern about size of infant's head and difficulty putting shirts over infant's head.

CASE 2

Esther Martinez is a 38-year-old Hispanic woman with complaints of fatigue and weight gain.

Subjective Data

Complains of 2-month gradual onset of fatigue, inability to stay warm, constipation, and feeling of facial puffiness; denies similar feeling in the past; reports dry skin despite daily use of moisturizer. Concerned about thinning hair and menses heavier than usual. Reports gaining 18 lb (8 kg) over last 4 months; uncomfortable with her looks. Reports no other problems; denies thyroid testing in past.

Objective Data

Alert, cooperative woman in no acute distress.
Head: Normocephalic with no lesions, or injury; hair thin, fine, brittle, and dull in color.
Neck: Supple with full range of motion; thyroid—goiter palpated.
Skin: Dry flaking skin, inelastic texture. No lesions noted.

Functional Health Patterns Involved

- Nutrition–metabolic
- Elimination
- Self-perception–self-concept

Medical Diagnosis

Hypothyroidism

Nursing Diagnosis and Collaborative Problems

- *Fatigue* related to reduced metabolic rate and blood loss as evidenced by:
  - Expressed fatigue
  - Weight gain
  - Heavy menses
  - Goiter
- *Constipation* related to decreased peristalsis as evidenced by:
  - Report of constipation
- *Body image disturbance* related to changes in physical appearance as manifested by:
  - Verbalized concern over changes in appearance: facial puffiness; weight gain; dry skin; thinning, brittle, dull hair.
- *PC:* Decreased metabolic function.

CRITICAL THINKING QUESTIONS

1. You see on the outpatient schedule of client visits that a 35-year-old woman is coming in with the chief complaint of headache. Before you meet this client you need to distinguish among the different kinds of headaches. What distinguishes migraine from cluster from tension headaches?
2. You are examining a 4-month-old infant. While the infant is supine, you detect that the anterior fontanel is bulging during palpation of the skull. The infant has an otherwise normal examination. What additional data do you need to seek before concluding the meaning of your findings?

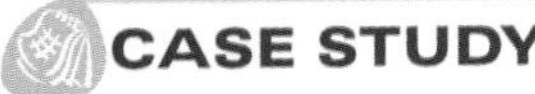

CASE STUDY

Rob is a 44-year-old carpenter who came to the emergency department complaining of a severe headache. Listed below are data collected by the examiner.

Interview Data

When the examiner attempts to ask Rob about the headache, he cries out, "I can't take this any more—it hurts too much." His wife says that Rob has been getting these headaches a couple times a day for the last week, sometimes at night, so she has not been sleeping well. She indicates that he had headaches like these about a year ago and that they lasted about a month. When Rob is asked if he experiences nausea or sensitivity to light, he replies, "No, I just get a stuffy nose." His wife says that Rob is constantly worried about whether—and when—the headache will come back because "We don't know what is causing them, and nothing seems to help them go away." She says Rob feels as though all he can do is hold his head and pray that the pain will stop.

Examination Data

- **General survey:** Alert, well-nourished male of average weight, in moderate distress. He is unable to lie still and paces the floor holding his left eye and forehead.
- **Head and neck:** Skull is intact, with no lumps, depressions, or tenderness. Facial structures symmetric. Head is centered on the neck; trachea is midline. Thyroid is in midline, soft, and normal size.

1. What data deviate from normal findings, suggesting a need for further investigation?
2. What additional information should the nurse ask or assess for?
3. In what functional health patterns does data deviate from normal?
4. What nursing diagnoses and/or collaborative problems should be considered for this situation?

REMEMBER to check out your **companion CD-ROM**

14 Nose, Paranasal Sinuses, Mouth, and Oropharynx

www.mosby.com/MERLIN/wilson/assessment/

ANATOMY AND PHYSIOLOGY

NOSE AND PARANASAL SINUSES

Besides serving as a passageway for inspired and expired air, the nose also humidifies, filters, and warms air before it enters the lungs. Other functions of the nose include identifying odors and giving resonance to laryngeal sounds. The paranasal sinuses are air-filled cavities that make the skull lighter and perform the same functions as the nose.

The upper third of the nose is encased in bone, which attaches to the frontal bone (Fig. 14-1). The bone extends to the lower two thirds of the nose, which is composed of cartilage. The septal cartilage maintains the shape of the nose and separates the nares (nostrils), which maintain an open passage for air. The interior of the nose—the nasal cavity—is lined with highly vascular mucous membranes containing cilia (nasal hairs) that trap airborne particles and prevent them from reaching the lungs. The lateral walls of the nasal cavity are lined with the inferior, middle, and superior turbinates, which contain openings, or meatus. The inferior meatus drains tears from the nasolacrimal duct, the middle meatus serves as an outlet for sinus drainage from the frontal, maxillary, and anterior ethmoid sinuses, and the superior meatus drains the posterior ethmoid sinus (Fig. 14-2).

The paranasal sinuses extend out of the nasal cavities through narrow openings into the skull bones to form bilateral (paired), air-filled pockets. They are lined with mucous membranes and cilia that move secretions along excretory pathways. The sphenoid, frontal, ethmoid, and maxillary sinuses constitute the paranasal sinuses in the adult (Fig. 14-3). The frontal sinuses are in the frontal bone superior to the nasal cavities. The ethmoid sinuses lie behind the frontal sinuses and near the superior portion of the nasal cavity. The sphenoid sinuses are deep in the skull behind the ethmoid sinuses.

MOUTH

The mouth contains the tongue, which has hundreds of taste buds (papillae) on its dorsal surface (Fig. 14-4, *A*). The taste buds distinguish sweet, sour, bitter, and salty tastes. The ventral surface is smooth and very vascular (Fig. 14-4, *B*). Three pair of salivary glands—the parotid, submandibular, and sublingual—release saliva through small openings (ducts) in response to the presence of food particles to begin the process of digestion (Fig. 14-5). The parotid glands, the largest salivary glands, lie anterior to the ears, immediately above the mandibular angle. Stensen's ducts (parotid gland openings) are visible on both sides of the cheek adjacent to the second molars. The submandibular glands are tucked under the mandible and lie approximately midway between the chin and the posterior mandibular angle. Wharton's ducts, the openings for the submandibular glands, are visible on either side of the lingual frenulum under the tongue. The sublingual glands, the smallest salivary glands, lie on the floor of the mouth. Each gland drains through 10 to 12 small ducts located on either side of the lingual frenulum behind the Wharton's ducts. Ducts that drain the sublingual glands are not visible. The adult has 32 teeth, which are tightly encased in mucous membrane-covered, fibrous gum tissue and rooted in the alveolar ridges of the maxilla and mandible (Fig. 14-6).

OROPHARYNX

The oropharynx includes the structures at the back of the mouth that are visible on examination: the uvula, the anterior and posterior pillars, the tonsils, and the posterior pharyngeal wall (see Fig. 14-4, *A*). The uvula is suspended, midline, from the soft palate, which extends out to either side to form the anterior pillar. The tonsils are tucked between the anterior and posterior pillars and may be atrophied in adults to the point of being barely visible. The posterior pharyngeal wall is visible when the tongue is extended and depressed. This wall is highly vascular and may show color variations of red and pink because of the presence of small vessels and lymphoid tissue. The epiglottis, a cartilaginous structure that protects the laryngeal opening, sometimes projects into the pharyngeal area and is visible as the tongue is depressed.

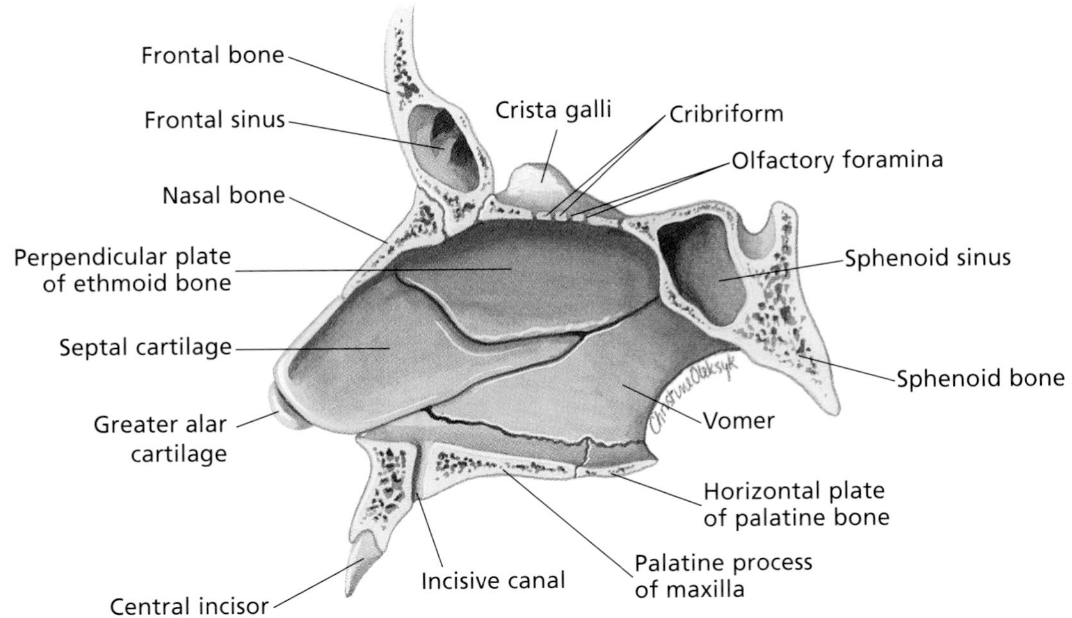

Fig. 14-1 Bones of the nasal cavity. (From Seeley, Stephens, and Tate, 1995.)

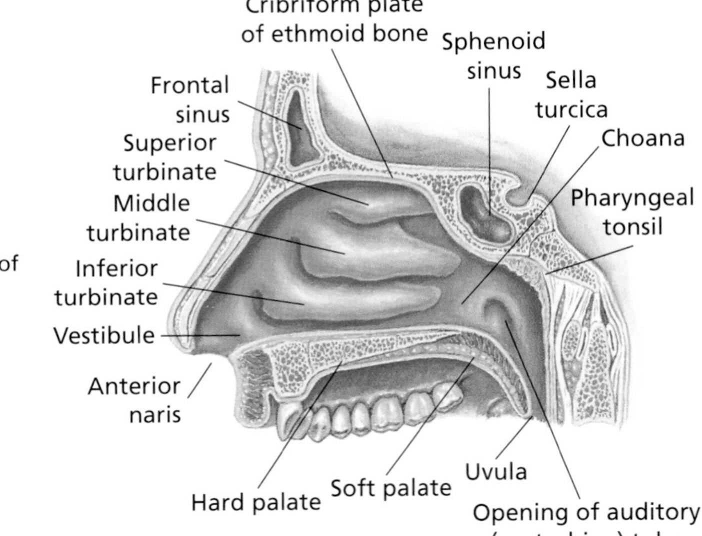

Fig. 14-2 Cross-sectional view of the anatomic structures of the nose and nasopharynx. (From Seidel et al, 1999.)

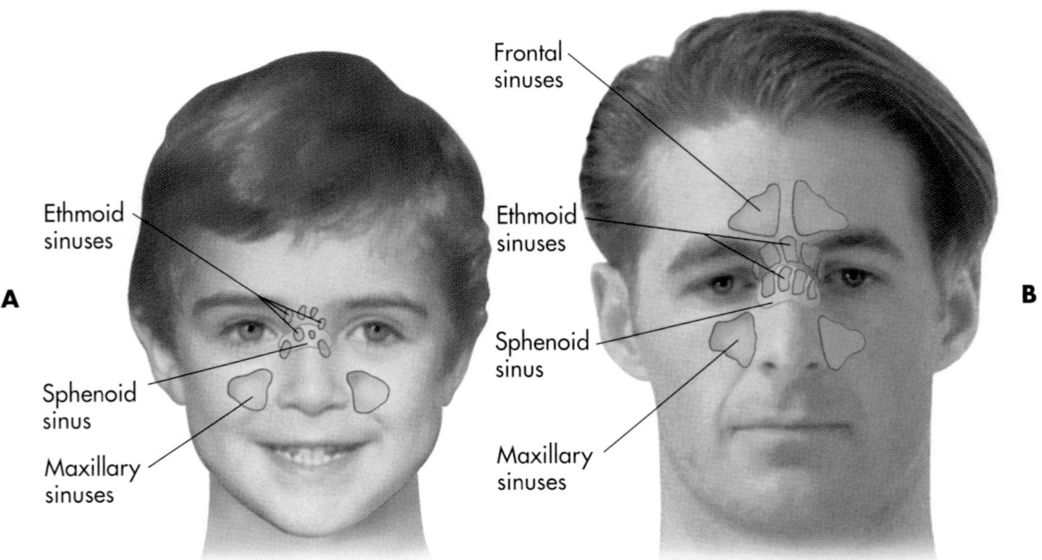

Fig. 14-3 Anterior view of paranasal sinuses. **A,** Six-year old child. **B,** Adult. (From Seidel et al, 1999.)

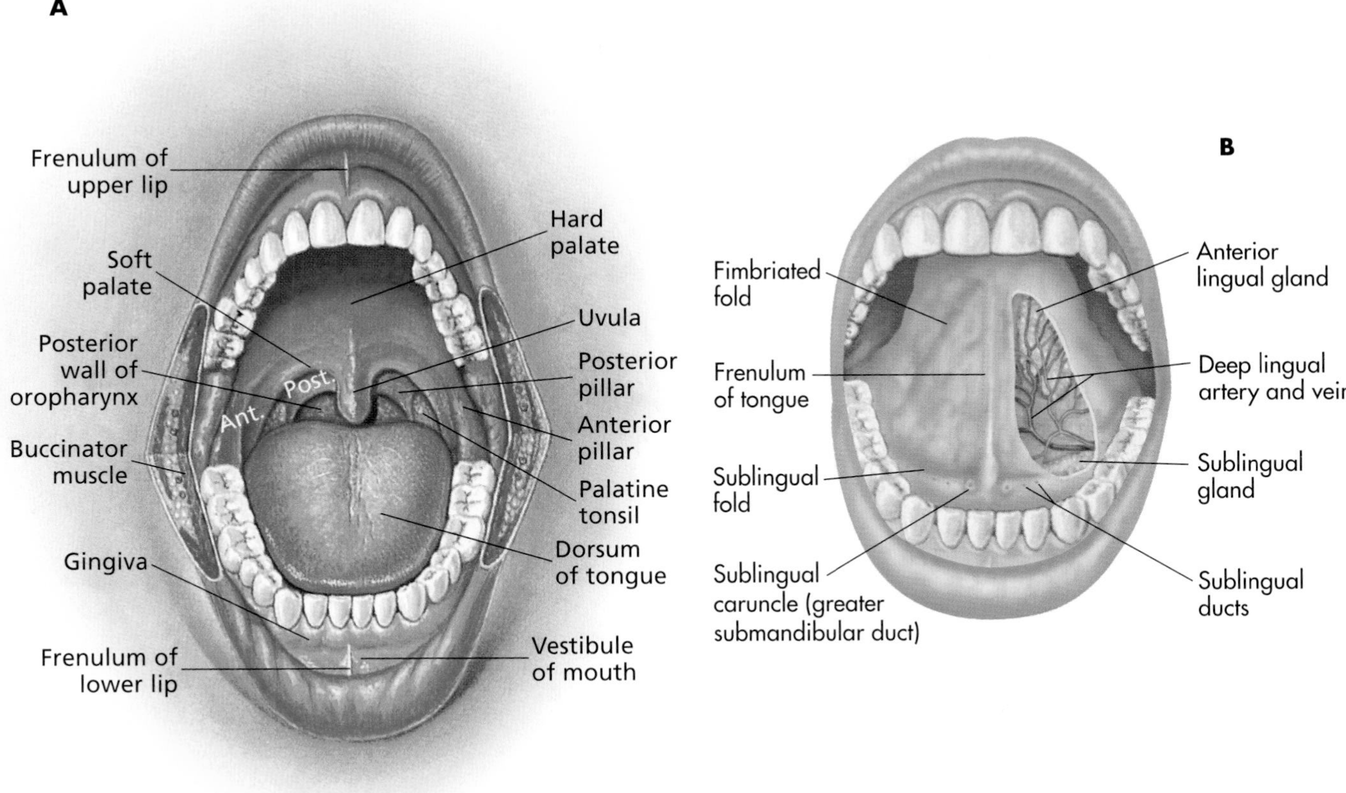

Fig. 14-4 **A,** Dorsal. **B,** Ventral surfaces of the tongue. (From Seidel et al, 1999.)

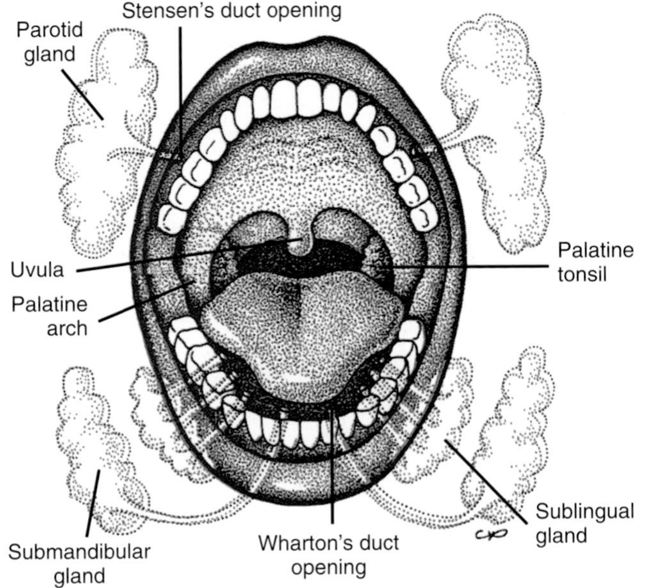

Fig. 14-5 Position of the major salivary glands. (From Barkauskas et al, 1998.)

ETHNIC & CULTURAL VARIATIONS

About 30% of Asian Americans, 15% of American Indians/Alaskan natives, and 10% of whites have agenesis of the third molar, displaying a pattern of 28 teeth as adults. This pattern is rare in African Americans.

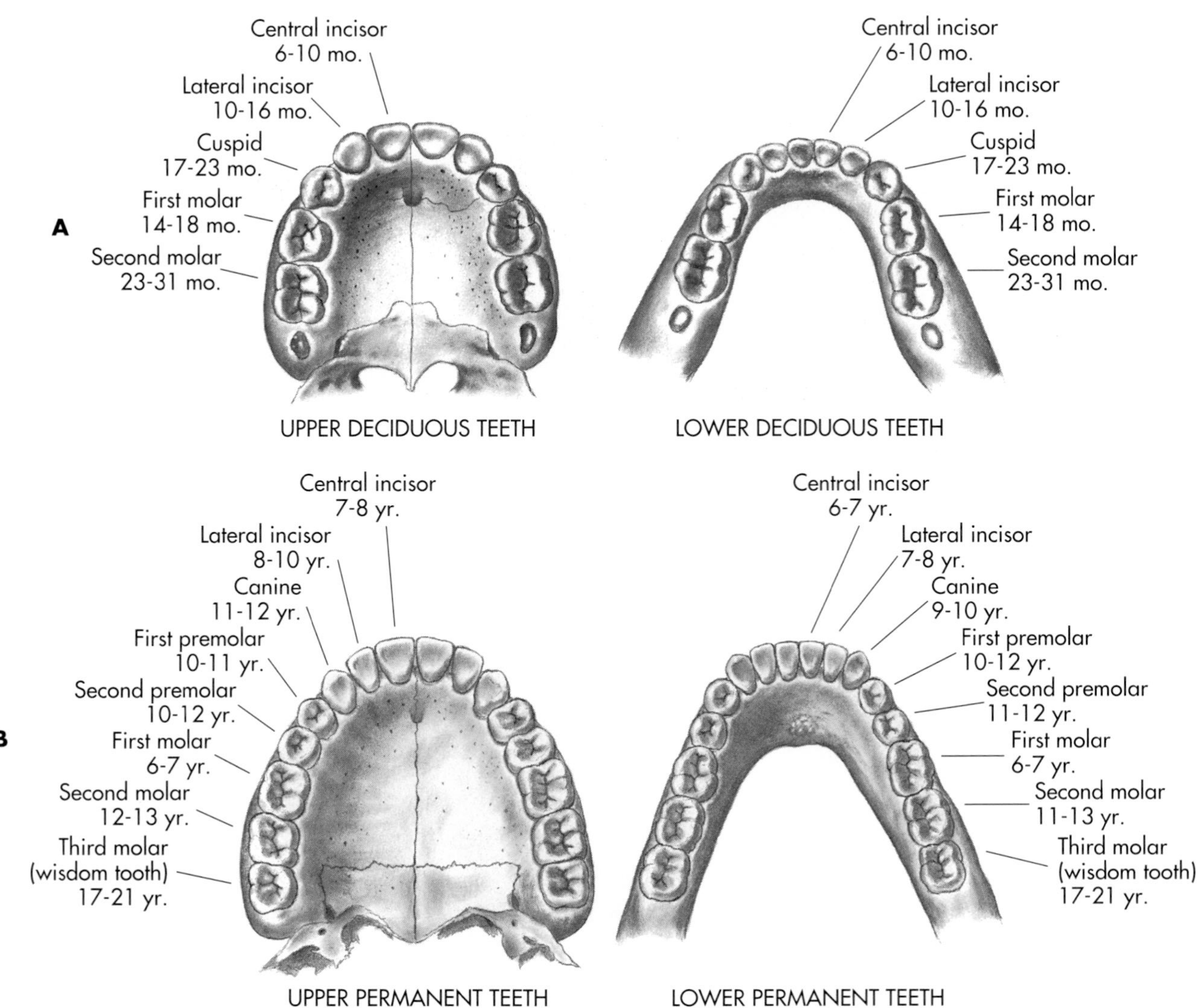

Fig. 14-6 **A,** Dentition of deciduous teeth and their sequence of eruption. **B,** Dentition of permanent teeth and their sequence of eruption. (From Seidel et al, 1999.)

HEALTH HISTORY

Nose, Paranasal Sinuses, Mouth, and Oropharynx

QUESTIONS	RATIONALE
PRESENT HEALTH STATUS	
➤ How would you describe the condition of your nose, sinuses, and mouth?	■ Input from clients may provide data about the health status of the nose, sinuses, mouth, and oropharynx.
➤ Have you noticed any changes in breathing through your nose or your mouth?	■ Ask clients if they have noticed changes as opposed to asking them if they have any problems.

QUESTIONS	RATIONALE
➤ Do you have any chronic illnesses?	■ Chronic diseases may contribute to such conditions as nasal polyps, which occur with cystic fibrosis or allergic rhinitis; mouth lesions, which occur with herpes simplex; or dysphagia, which may occur after a stroke.
➤ Do you take any medications? If so, what are you taking and how often? When did you start taking the medications?	■ Medications may have side effects on these systems, such as dry mouth. It is important to assess the client's compliance with prescription and nonprescription medications to ensure therapeutic effects.
➤ How often do you brush your teeth? Do you use dental floss? Do you use toothpaste?	■ These questions assess for proper dental care and provide an opportunity to remind client, if needed, of its importance. It determines the client's normal dental care patterns so that health teaching may be provided. If the client has dental or gum problems, a dental referral should be made.
➤ Do you have dentures? Bridges? Other dental appliances? If the client has dentures: How long have you had this set? How do you care for them? How well do they fit?	■ These questions assess for proper care of dental appliances and determine if they are functioning as intended. If the client wears dentures and reports difficulty with the fitting of the dentures or difficulty with chewing or sore gums, a dental referral should be made.
➤ When was your last visit to the dentist?	■ Counseling clients to obtain dental care on a regular basis is recommended based on evidence of risk reduction from such visits when combined with regular oral hygiene (U.S. Preventive Services Task Force, 1996).

ETHNIC & CULTURAL VARIATIONS

In a study of oral health of African Americans and whites in a large metropolitan city, a group of dentists interviewed 787 subjects and performed oral examinations of 577 subjects. Better dental health was found in African Americans who flossed their teeth, had annual dental examinations, and did not smoke. In the white sample better dental health was found among those who had annual dental examinations. No difference was found for those who brushed or flossed or smoked. There were no differences between men and women in either group (Lang P et al, http://nformatics.dent.umich.edu/health/research/abstract).

QUESTIONS	RATIONALE
➤ Have you been told frequently that you have bad breath? If so, is it just in the morning, or does it continue even after you have brushed your teeth?	■ Bad breath (halitosis) is expected upon first awakening in the morning from bacteria in the mouth, but further evaluation is needed for halitosis that continues after oral hygiene.
➤ Do you smoke? If so, what do you smoke (pipe, cigarettes, or cigars) and how much? Do you use smokeless tobacco? If so, how long have you used it?	■ Smoking is a risk factor for mouth cancer, particularly smokeless tobacco that has contact with the oral mucous membranes.

QUESTIONS | RATIONALE

PAST MEDICAL HISTORY

➤ Have you ever had nasal surgery? If so, when and for what? Have you ever had an injury to your nose? If so, what?

■ Nasal surgery may change the anatomy of the nose that you would note on examination. Nasal surgery may be done to correct airway obstruction that may be secondary to trauma-induced blockage of nasal passage or to remove nasal polyps caused by chronic allergic rhinitis or cystic fibrosis.

FAMILY HISTORY

➤ Is there a history of seasonal allergies in your family?

■ Family history for allergies is a risk factor for allergic rhinitis (Brown, Parker, and Stegbauer, 1999).

PROBLEM-BASED HISTORY

The most commonly reported problems related to the nose, paranasal sinuses, mouth, and oropharynx are nasal discharge, sinus congestion, nosebleed, snoring, mouth pain, difficulty swallowing, sore throat, and hoarseness or voice change. As with symptoms in all areas of health assessment, a symptom analysis is completed, which includes location, quality, quantity, chronology, setting, associated manifestations, alleviating factors, and aggravating factors.

Nasal Discharge

➤ Do you have any nasal discharge or runny nose? If so, how often? Occasionally or constantly? How would you describe the discharge? What color is the discharge? Is it watery, thick, or bloody? Is it foul smelling? Is it on one side of your nose or both? Are there any symptoms associated with the discharge? Headache? Chronic postnasal drip? Coughing? Fever? Does anything make the discharge worse? If so, what?

■ A thick or purulent green or yellow discharge results most commonly from a bacterial infection. A bloody discharge may result from a neoplasm, trauma, or an opportunistic infection such as a fungal disease. A foul-smelling discharge, especially unilateral discharge, is most commonly associated with a foreign body or chronic sinusitis. A clear, watery discharge from the nose secondary to a head injury may be indicative of cerebrospinal fluid leakage.

➤ If you have clear drainage, is it from allergies? If so, allergies to what? When do these symptoms occur? How long do they last? Do you have any other symptoms associated with the allergies? Itching, swelling, or discharge from eyes? Wheezing? Postnasal drip? Coughing? Changes in taste or smell? What makes the allergies worse?

■ Allergies are a common cause of nasal discharge. A thin, watery discharge is generally due to excess mucus production resulting from a viral infection or allergy. Associated symptoms are consistent with allergic rhinitis (Brown, Parker, and Stegbauer, 1999).

➤ Does anything decrease the discharge? What do you do to treat the discharge? Do you use nose drops or a nasal spray? If so, what kind and how often? How effective is the treatment?

■ Determining what has been used successfully in the past may guide current treatment strategies. If the client uses nasal spray other than normal saline, alert him or her that it should be used for only 3 to 5 days to avoid causing rebound congestion.

QUESTIONS

RATIONALE

Sinus Congestion

➤ Are your sinuses congested? If yes, when did the congestion start? How long does it last? Do you have any symptoms associated with the congestion? Do you have any pain over your sinus areas (e.g., face, around eyes, forehead)? What makes the congestion worse?

■ Sinus congestion or infection causes referred pain around the eyes and to the front teeth. Trauma to the face may cause an alteration to the normal facial structures and may cause sinus obstruction, which in turn may promote the growth of organisms leading to infection. A deviated septum or foreign body in the nose may also cause obstruction.

➤ What makes the congestion better? What do you do to treat the sinus congestion? How effective is the treatment?

■ Determining what has been used successfully in the past may guide current treatment strategies.

Nosebleed (Epistaxis)

➤ Do you have nosebleeds? If yes, how often? How long does the nosebleed last? Is the blood thin or clotted? Does it come from just one side or both? What makes the nosebleed worse? Are the membranes inside your nose dry? Do you snort cocaine?

■ Epistaxis may occur secondary to trauma, chronic sinusitis, malignancy, or a bleeding disorder. While the most common causes of epistaxis are nose picking or friable membranes secondary to dryness, it may also result from cocaine abuse.

➤ What makes the nosebleed better? How do you treat your nosebleeds? How effective is the treatment?

■ Determining what has been used successfully in the past may guide current treatment strategies. This question also provides an opportunity to teach how to stop nosebleeds, if indicated.

Snoring

➤ Does your sleeping partner complain about your loud snoring? Do you wake up during the night gasping or choking? Do you feel confused when you awaken in the morning? Do you have a headache when you awaken? Do you get sleepy during the day (Yantis, 1999)?

■ These are risk factors for sleep apnea and need further evaluation. If risk factors are confirmed, a referral to a health care provider for treatment may be indicated.

Mouth Pain

➤ Do you have pain in your mouth? If yes, describe where it is and how intense the pain is, using a pain scale of 1 to 10. How long has the pain been present? Is the pain intermittent or constant? Does the pain interfere with eating? What seems to start the pain? What makes it worse? Are you currently having gum or teeth problems? If yes, describe them. Are you able to eat/chew all types of foods?

■ Mouth pain may be secondary to dental problems or gingival disease. It is important to take a careful dental history.

➤ Do you have any sores in your mouth or on your lips? Are they painful? If yes, have you ever had a sore like this before? How long has it been present? What have you done to treat it? Have you noticed any odor from your mouth?

■ Mouth lesions may have benign causes, such as trauma from a toothbrush or food, or they may be a sign of an infection, immunologic problem, or cancer.

➤ Are there any other sores anywhere else on your body, such as in the vagina? In the urethra? On the penis? In the anus? Do you have a history of venereal disease?

■ Sexually transmitted infections such as herpes may be transmitted through oral sex.

➤ Do the sores in your mouth heal within a 2-week period? Are there areas in your mouth that bleed easily without a known cause? Do you have swelling, lumps, or thickened areas in your mouth? Have you had difficulty in chewing, swallowing, or moving your tongue or jaw? Do you have a feeling of discomfort in your throat?

■ These are early warning symptoms of oral cancer (Shugars and Patton, 1997).

QUESTIONS | **RATIONALE**

Difficulty Swallowing (Dysphagia)

➤ Do you have pain or difficulty when swallowing? If yes, how often does this occur? Does it occur with liquids (including saliva), solids, or tablets? Did the difficulty in swallowing occur suddenly or progressively? What makes swallowing worse? Do you have frequent throat infections? Do you choke while trying to swallow? Have you been drooling? What do you do to relieve the swallowing difficulty?

■ Throat pain or difficulty swallowing may be secondary to infection, a foreign body, an inflammatory process, or a neurologic disorder such as a stroke. If unable to swallow his or her own oral saliva or liquids, the client will be unable to swallow solids and tablets safely. A sudden onset of drooling or difficulty swallowing is a medical emergency due to the concern for aspiration or choking.

Sore Throat

➤ How frequently do you get sore throats? Is your throat sore now? If yes, how long has it felt that way? Describe what it feels like—a lump, burning, scratchy? Does it hurt to swallow? Is it worse when you get up in the morning? Do you notice that you are breathing from your mouth? If so, is it because you are having difficulty breathing through your nose? Is your sore throat associated with fever, cough, fatigue, headache, postnasal drip, or hoarseness?

■ A sore throat may have many causes, from nasal congestion or sinus drainage to an infection or allergy. A careful history will help to determine the cause of the complaint.

■ Postnasal drip may cause early morning sore throat or a cough on lying down. The maxillary sinuses do not drain when the client is upright, but they do drain when the client lies down. Nasal congestion that requires mouth breathing during the night may cause a sore throat in the morning.

➤ Are others in your home ill or just recovered from a sore throat or cold? Do you inhale dust or fumes at work? Is the air in your home or office dry? Are you hoarse?

■ This question determines environmental factors that may contribute to sore throat and whether the sore throat may be communicable.

➤ What makes your sore throat feel better? How have you been treating it? How effective was the treatment?

■ Determining what has been used successfully in the past may guide current treatment strategies.

Hoarseness or Voice Change

➤ How long have you had this hoarseness or voice change? Is it constant, or does it come and go? Do you feel as though you have to clear your throat a lot? What makes the hoarseness worse? Does the weather affect your voice? Does your voice seem different from what you consider normal (weak, husky, higher, lower)? Do you feel that the hoarseness or voice change is associated with a cold or sore throat?

■ Common causes of hoarseness or a voice change are overuse of the voice and laryngeal irritation secondary to smoking. Hoarseness that cannot be traced to an irritation or specific cause should be evaluated for possible neoplastic involvement.

➤ What makes the hoarseness better? How have you treated it? How effective has the treatment been?

■ Determining what has been used successfully in the past may guide current treatment strategies.

EXAMINATION

Equipment

- Examination gloves to wear when inspecting and palpating the tongue
- Penlight to inspect the oropharynx; may be used instead of transilluminator to transmit light through the sinuses
- Otoscope with broad-tipped nasal speculum or nasal speculum to inspect the nasal mucosa
- Transilluminator to transmit light through sinuses
- Tongue blade to inspect the mouth and oropharynx and to determine presence of gag reflex
- 4 × 4 gauze pad to grasp tongue

PROCEDURES AND TECHNIQUES WITH NORMAL FINDINGS

ABNORMAL FINDINGS

NOSE AND PARANASAL SINUSES

➤**INSPECT and PALPATE the nose for general appearance, symmetry, patency, discharge, and tenderness.** The skin should be smooth and intact, with the color matching the rest of the face. The nose should appear symmetric and midline. The nostrils should be symmetric, dry (no crusting), and not flaring or narrowed.

■ Lesions or a warty appearance, redness, or discoloration may be signs of a systemic illness.

Increased vascularity with many small new blood vessels may indicate liver disease.

Marked asymmetry may be noted secondary to injury.

Narrowing of the nostrils when the client inhales may be associated with chronic obstruction that may necessitate mouth breathing.

➤**INSPECT nasal discharge for character (watery, mucoid, purulent, bloody, etc.) and amount.**

■ Swelling, hypertrophy, nasal discharge, or crusting may all be signs of infection or allergy.

Watery, unilateral nasal discharge following a history of head injury may be indicative of skull fracture. Likewise, unilateral, purulent, thick nasal drainage may indicate a foreign body.

➤**ASSESS the nose for patency. Apply pressure to one side of the nose; ask the client to close his or her mouth and sniff through the opposite side; repeat on the opposite side.** There should be noiseless, free exchange of air on each side.

■ Noisy or obstructed breathing may occur secondary to nasal congestion, trauma to the nasal passage, polyps, or allergies.

➤**PALPATE the external nose to be sure it is firm and not tender.**

■ Instability or tenderness from trauma or inflammation may be noted on palpation. Presence of masses may be observed.

➤**EVALUATE the olfactory nerve (cranial nerve I) for intactness.** Ask the client to close his or her eyes and mouth. Hold one nostril closed at a time, then hold an aromatic substance (such as coffee or lemon extract) under the nostril. Repeat with the other nostril. The client should be able to identify the smell. (This procedure may be deferred until the neurologic examination.)

■ Allergic rhinitis, inflammation of the mucous membranes, and excessive smoking may interfere with the sense of smell. Anosmia, the loss of sense of smell or inability to identify odors, can be caused by trauma to the diencephalon affecting the olfactory tracts (Seidel et al, 1999).

PROCEDURES AND TECHNIQUES WITH NORMAL FINDINGS

➤INSPECT the internal nasal cavity for patency. Use a nasal speculum and a good light source. Hold the speculum in the palm of the hand and use your index finger to stabilize the speculum against the side of the nose. Insert the speculum slowly and cautiously about 1 cm and spread the outer naris as much as possible without causing pain or discomfort. Use your other hand to hold the light source (Fig. 14-7). (Alternatively, an otoscope with a nasal speculum attached may be used for the examination.) Chapter 5 includes a photograph of a nasal speculum (see Fig. 5-11).

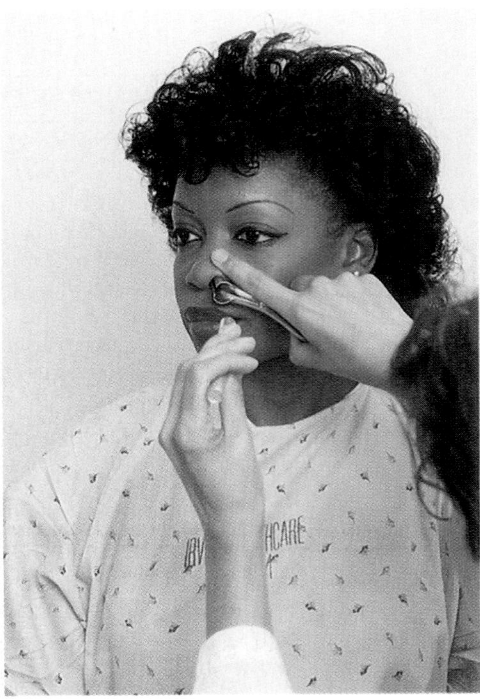

Fig. 14-7 Hold the speculum in the palm of the hand and use your index finger to stabilize the speculum.

The nares are inspected for two reasons. The first is to observe the nasal septum for deviation. Deviation is not an important finding unless the client complains of a decreased air flow through the nares. If breathing through the nares is a problem, then the finding is significant. The second is to evaluate the turbinates and nasal mucosa. Observe the following:

1. With the client's head erect: Note floor of the nose, inferior turbinate, nasal hairs, and mucosa, which should be slightly darker red than oral mucosa. Also note the vascular area on the medial side of the septum in the lower third of the nasal cavity (Kiesselbach's area) (Fig. 14-8). (Most nosebleeds occur from Kiesselbach's area.) The client's nasal septum should be straight and midline. There should be no perforations, bleeding, or crusting.
2. Client's head back: Observe the middle meatus and middle turbinate. The turbinates should be the same color as surrounding tissue, which is deep pink.

ABNORMAL FINDINGS

- Deviated nasal septum with a decrease in turbulent air flow should be considered abnormal.
- Sinus drainage or masses may be observed.
- Turbinates may appear pale pink or bluish gray and edematous, indicating an allergic response. Increased redness may occur secondary to infection, whereas localized redness and swelling in the vestibule may indicate a furuncle or localized infection.
- A rounded, elongated mass projecting into the nasal cavity may be a polyp. Nasal polyps are benign growths that may occur secondary to chronic allergies or systemic diseases such as cystic fibrosis.

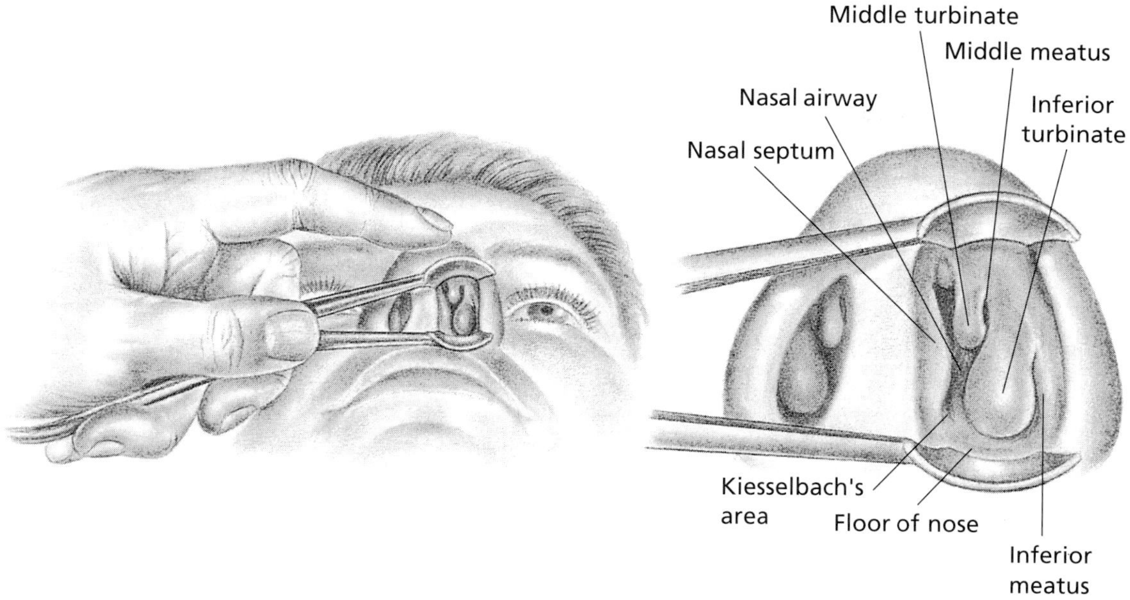

Fig. 14-8 View of the nasal mucosa through the nasal speculum. (From Seidel et al, 1999.)

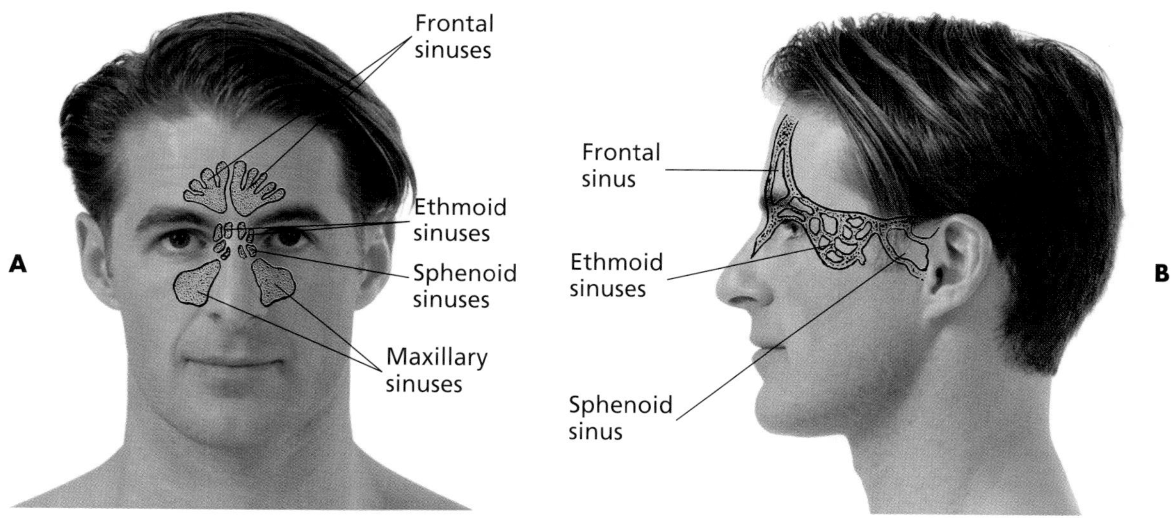

Fig. 14-9 Paranasal sinuses. **A,** Front view. **B,** Side view.

PROCEDURES AND TECHNIQUES WITH NORMAL FINDINGS

➤**PALPATE the frontal and maxillary paranasal sinus areas for tenderness or bogginess (wetness or sponginess) (Fig. 14-9).** To assess the frontal sinuses, press upward with your thumbs over the sinus areas above the eyebrows. (CAUTION: Do not press directly over the eyeballs.) To assess the maxillary sinuses, press in the same manner over the sinus areas below the cheekbones.

ABNORMAL FINDINGS

■ The appearance of swelling, bogginess (wetness, sponginess), or tenderness on palpation may indicate sinus congestion or infection.

PROCEDURES AND TECHNIQUES WITH NORMAL FINDINGS

ABNORMAL FINDINGS

❖ ➤**TRANSILLUMINATE the sinus area if the client complains of sinus pain or shows signs of sinus congestion, perform transillumination of the sinus area.** To do this:

1. Darken the room. Use a sinus transilluminator or small bright penlight.
2. Transilluminate the maxillary sinuses by placing the source of light lateral to the nose, just beneath the medial aspect of the eye. Look through the client's open mouth for illumination of the hard palate (Fig. 14-10).

■ An absence of a glow during transillumination of the sinuses may indicate that the sinus is congested and is filled with secretions or that the sinus has never developed.

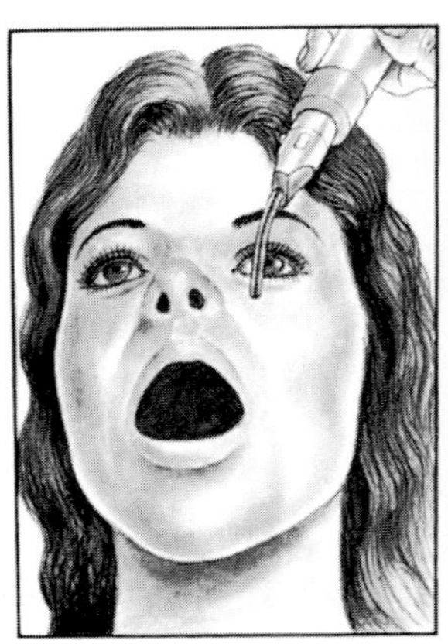
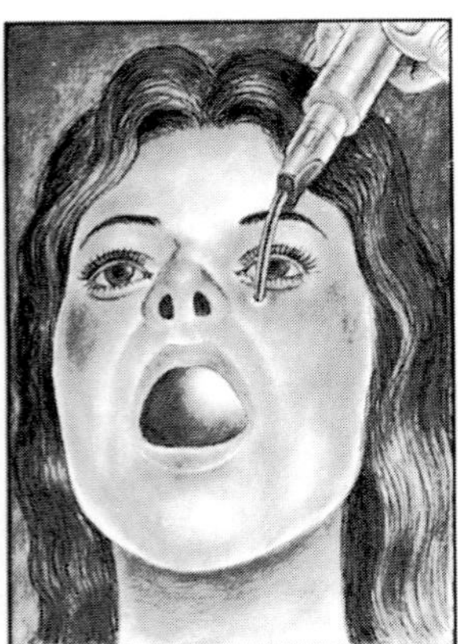

Fig. 14-10 Transillumination of the maxillary sinuses.

3. Transilluminate the frontal sinuses by placing the light source against the medial aspect of each supraorbital rim. Look for a dim red glow as light is transmitted above the eyebrows (Fig. 14-11).

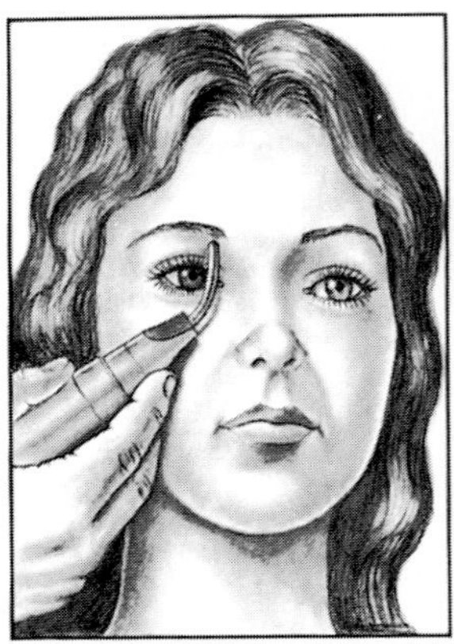
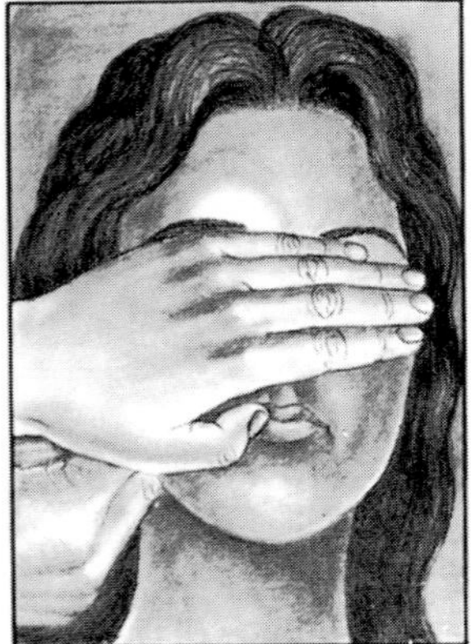

Fig. 14-11 Transillumination of the frontal sinuses.

MOUTH AND OROPHARYNX

➤**PALPATE the temporomandibular joint for movement, tenderness or discomfort.** Place two fingers in front of each ear and ask the client to slowly open and close the mouth and move the lower jaw from side to side (Fig. 14-12). The jaw should move smoothly, opening 1 ⅓ to 1 ¾ inches (3.5 to 4.5 cm). Note presence of tenderness, crepitus, clicking, or referred pain with jaw movement on either one or both sides.

■ A limited excursion (range of motion less than normal) is abnormal. Complaints of tenderness or referred pain, crepitus, or clicking, especially on closure of the jaw, may indicate temporomandibular joint (TMJ) disease.

PROCEDURES AND TECHNIQUES WITH NORMAL FINDINGS

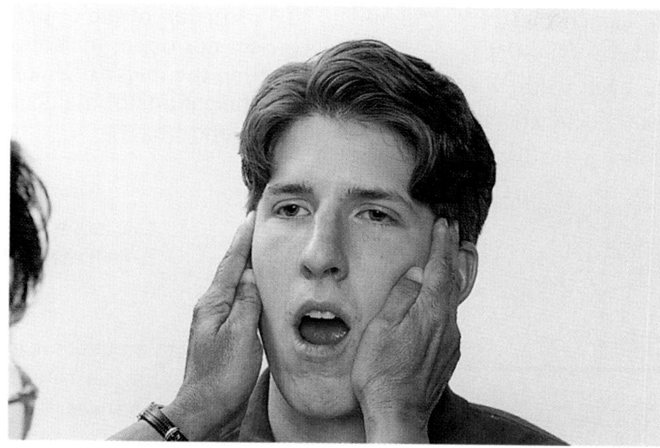

Fig. 14-12 Position fingers in front of each ear in preparation for examination of the temporomandibular joint (TMJ).

➤**INSPECT the lips for color, symmetry, moisture, and texture.** Lips should appear pink and symmetric both vertically and laterally. The lips should be smooth and moist and have slight vertical linear markings. There should be a distinct border between the lips and the facial skin (vermillion border), and should not be interrupted by lesions.

ETHNIC & CULTURAL VARIATIONS

Dimpling or lip pits are a normal variation found in the commissure of the lips, occurring in about 20% of African Americans, 12% of whites, and 7% of Asian Americans. Lips may have a natural blue tone in darker-skinned individuals.

ABNORMAL FINDINGS

- Pale lips may be indicative of anemia or shock. Cyanotic-colored lips and circumoral cyanosis may indicate lack of adequately oxygenated blood flow related to cardiovascular or respiratory problems or hypothermia. Reddened or cherry-colored lips may indicate carbon monoxide poisoning.
- Dry, flaking, or cracked lips may be caused by dehydration; chapping may be secondary to dry air or wind or excessive lip licking or dehydration. Cracks and redness in the corners of the mouth may be caused by vitamin B_2 (riboflavin) or B_6 (pyridoxine) deficiencies (Whitney, Cataldo, and Rolfes, 1998).
- Infection or allergy may cause swelling of the lips. Lesions, plaques, vesicles, nodules, or ulcerations may be signs of infection, irritation (such as lip biting), or skin cancer (Fig. 14-13).

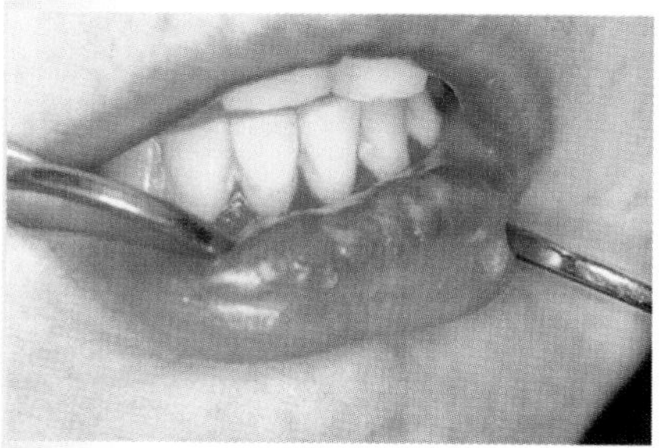

Fig. 14-13 Ulceration of the lower lip. (From Tyldesley, 1994.)

PROCEDURES AND TECHNIQUES WITH NORMAL FINDINGS

➤**INSPECT the teeth for alignment.** Ask the client to clench the teeth and smile. (Showing the teeth and smiling partially tests cranial nerve VII—the facial nerve). The upper back teeth should rest directly on the lower back teeth, with the upper incisors slightly overriding the lower ones. The teeth should be evenly spaced.

ETHNIC & CULTURAL VARIATIONS

Whites have the smallest teeth.
African Americans have somewhat larger teeth.
Asians and American Indians have the largest teeth.

➤**INSPECT the teeth for number, color, and surface characteristics.** There should be 32 teeth, which should be white, yellow, or gray and have smooth edges. During the examination, note notching, caries, and missing teeth. The characteristics of the teeth may have racial variations.

ABNORMAL FINDINGS

■ Protrusion of the upper or lower incisors or upper incisors that do not overlap the lower ones on closure are indications of malocclusion (Fig. 14-14 and Box 14-1).

Box 14-1 Classes of Malocclusion

CLASS I

Molars have customary relationship, but the line of occlusion is incorrect because of malpositioned teeth from rotations or other causes.

CLASS II

Lower molars are distally positioned in relation to the upper molars; the line of occlusion may or may not be correct.

CLASS III

Lower molars are medially positioned in relation to the upper molars; the line of occlusion may or may not be correct.

(From Seidel HM et al: *Mosby's guide to physical examination,* ed 4, St. Louis, 1999, Mosby.)

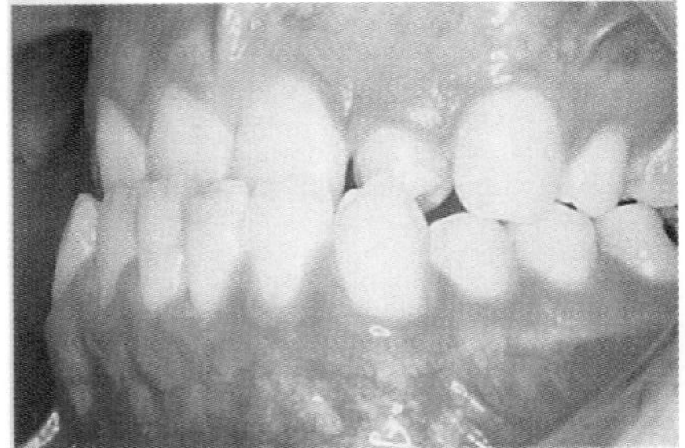

Fig. 14-14 Class III malocclusion. (From Scully and Welbury, 1994.)

PROCEDURES AND TECHNIQUES WITH NORMAL FINDINGS

➤PALPATE the teeth for stability. Wearing examining gloves, attempt to move the teeth with your fingers. The teeth should be firmly anchored and should move little if at all.

➤NOTE the odor of the breath. Normally the mouth should have a slightly sweet odor or no odor at all. Ask the client close his or her mouth.

➤INSPECT and PALPATE the inner lips and gums for integrity, tenderness, color, and moisture (wear examining gloves). Ask the client to remove any dental appliances. Have him or her open the mouth slightly so you can inspect and palpate the inner lips and upper and lower gingivobuccal fornices. Palpate the gums for lesions, thickening, tenderness, or masses. The gingiva, the gum line around the base of the teeth, should have a pink, moist appearance with a clearly defined margin at each tooth. The gum line beneath dentures should be free of inflammation, swelling, or bleeding.

ABNORMAL FINDINGS

- Missing teeth may occur secondary to tooth extraction or trauma.
- Darkened or stained teeth may occur secondary to coffee, medications, poor dental care, or frequent vomiting by one who has bulimia.
- Presence of debris, especially at the gum line, usually occurs because of poor dental habits.
- Excessively exposed tooth neck with receding gums may occur secondary to aging or gingival disease. Gingivitis and edema can develop into advanced periodontal disease, with erosion of gum tissue, destruction of underlying bone, and loosening of the teeth. slightly sweet odor or no odor at all. Ask the client close his or her mouth.
- Marked movement of the teeth or loose teeth may be secondary to either periodontal disease or trauma.
- An acetone odor on the breath may indicate diabetic ketoacidosis.
- A fetid odor may occur secondary to gum disease, caries, poor dental care, or sinusitis.
- Color changes of the gums to pale, cyanotic, or red may indicate systemic problems.
- Bleeding of the gums may occur secondary to systemic disease such as vitamin C or K deficiency or gingival gum disease.
- Other specific changes of the gums may be indicative of specific problems. For example, a blue-black line along the gum margin may indicate chronic lead or bismuth poisoning.
- Thickening or masses may indicate gingival disease secondary to Dilantin therapy (Fig. 14-15).

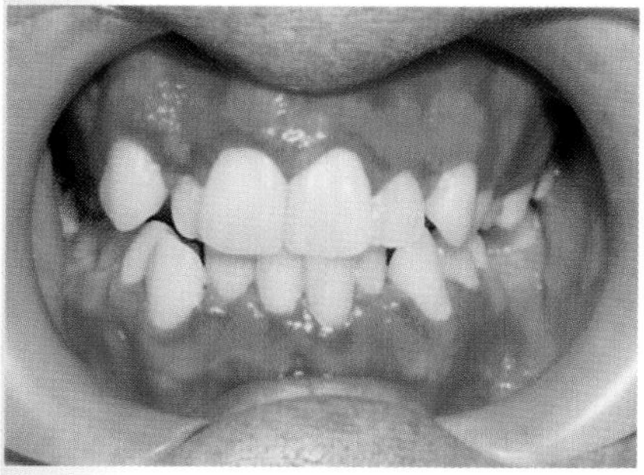

Fig. 14-15 Enlargement of the gums. (From Bingham, Hawke, and Kwok, 1992.)

PROCEDURES AND TECHNIQUES WITH NORMAL FINDINGS

➤**For clients who wear dentures, observe for any pressure areas or ulcerations.**

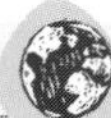

ETHNIC & CULTURAL VARIATIONS

Dark-skinned people may have a patchy brown pigmentation of the gums. There may be a dark melanotic line along the gingival margin.

➤**INSPECT the buccal mucosa, anterior and posterior pillars, and Stensen's duct for color and symmetry.** Ask the client to open the mouth widely to allow you to inspect the buccal mucosa using a penlight and tongue blade. Inspect the anterior and posterior pillars. Note the color of the mucosa and the symmetry of the pillars. The color of the tissue should be pale coral or pink with slight vascularity. Stensen's duct (the parotid duct) should be inspected using a tongue blade to gently pull the buccal mucosa away from the second molar to visualize a slightly elevated pinpoint red marking (see Fig. 14-5). The buccal mucosa should be smooth, with a transverse occlusion line appearing adjacent to where teeth meet. Clear saliva should cover the surface.

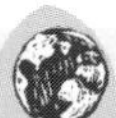

ETHNIC & CULTURAL VARIATIONS

Darker-skinned persons often have darker oral pigmentation. This pigmentation increases with age and may also be seen in older, fair-skinned adults. A gray-white, benign lesion of the buccal mucosa called leukoedema occurs in 70% to 90% of dark-skinned persons and 40% of those with fair-skin. This finding also increases with age.

➤**INSPECT the tongue for movement, color, ulceration, and surface characteristics.** Ask the client to stick out his or her tongue. (This maneuver also tests cranial nerve XII—the hypoglossal nerve). The forward thrust should be smooth and symmetric, and the tongue itself should appear symmetric. The tongue should be pink and moist with a glistening surface dorsally and laterally. The surface may appear slightly rough due to the papillae on the dorsal surface of the tongue. During the inspection, note any swelling or variation in size, color, coating, or ulceration.

➤**PALPATE the tongue for irregularities.** Following inspection, put on examination gloves, grasp the tongue with a 4 × 4 inch gauze pad, and palpate all sides for texture (Fig. 14-16). The tongue should feel relatively smooth and even. Papillae create slight roughness on the dorsum of the tongue. During the palpation, note any lumps, nodules, or areas of thickening. Note: After putting on the gloves, wash your hands with water to remove any powder coating before putting your hands in the client's mouth.

ABNORMAL FINDINGS

- For clients who wear dentures: gum tenderness, lesions, or thickening may indicate dentures that do not fit.

- Aphthous ulcers on the buccal mucosa appear as white, round, or oval ulcerative lesions with a red halo.
- White patches or plaques may indicate leukoplakia.
- Excessively dry mouth or excessive salivation may indicate salivary gland blockage or may occur secondary to medications, dehydration, or stress.

- Atrophy of the tongue on one side or deviation of the tongue may be a sign of a neurologic disorder.
- A smooth or beefy-colored, red, swollen tongue with a slick appearance may indicate folate, vitamin B_2 (riboflavin), B_3 (niacin), B_6 (pyridoxine), or B_{12} (cobalamin) deficiency (Whitney, Cataldo, and Rolfes,1998).
- A hairy tongue with yellow-brown to black elongated papillae may occur secondary to antibiotic therapy for superinfection or pipe smoking.
- An enlarged tongue may be seen in clients with mental retardation or hypothyroidism.

- Lumps, nodules, or masses may indicate local or systemic disease or cancerous lesions.

PROCEDURES AND TECHNIQUES WITH NORMAL FINDINGS

ABNORMAL FINDINGS

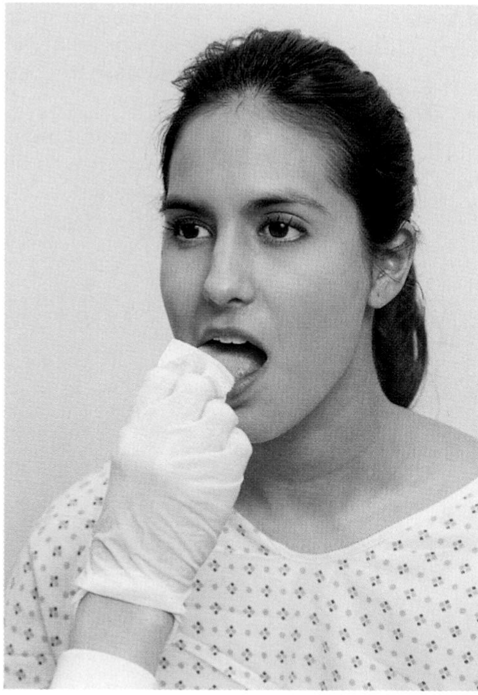

Fig. 14-16 Grasp the tongue with a 4 × 4 inch gauze pad.

➤**INSPECT the lateral surfaces of the tongue for lesions.** Pull the tongue to either side. If lesions are noted, scrape the area with a tongue blade to differentiate between food particles and actual mouth lesions.

Ask the client to raise the tongue to the roof of the mouth. Inspect and palpate the ventral surface and floor of the mouth. It should be pale coral, or pink, with the frenulum centered and the submandibular (also called submaxillary) duct on either side of the frenulum. The sublingual duct openings are visible laterally and slightly posterior to the submandibular ducts (see Fig. 14-5).

■ Leukoplakia is a whitish lesion that may not be scraped off by a tongue blade. Oral candidiasis is similar in appearance.

■ Abnormalities include discoloration, ulceration, masses, or other lesions.

➤**INSPECT the palate and uvula for texture, color, and surface characteristics.** Instruct the client to tilt his or her head back so that the palate and uvula may be inspected. The hard palate should be smooth, pale, and immovable with irregular transverse rugae. The soft palate and uvula should be smooth and pink, with the uvula in a midline position.

■ Nodules that are noted on the palate that are not at the midline may indicate a tumor. Other systemic diseases such as human immunodeficiency virus (HIV) infections may show oral lesions, such as Kaposi's sarcoma on both the hard and soft palates.

■ Opportunistic infections such as candidiasis may occur when an individual has been on antibiotics or is immunosuppressed.

ETHNIC & CULTURAL VARIATIONS

A split uvula have been reported as occurring in about 10% of Asians and 18% of some American Indian groups (Giger and Davidhizar, 1995).

➤**INSPECT the movement of the soft palate.** Instruct the client to say "ah." (If necessary, depress the tongue with a tongue blade.) (This tests the vagus cranial nerve.) Observe if the soft palate rises symmetrically with the uvula remaining in the midline position. (This tests both cranial nerves IX and X—the glossopharyngeal and vagus nerves).

■ Failure of the soft palate to rise bilaterally, as well as uvula deviation during vocalization, may indicate a neurologic problem such as a stroke that impairs functioning of the vagus or glossopharyngeal nerve. Swallowing may be difficult for these clients.

PROCEDURES AND TECHNIQUES WITH NORMAL FINDINGS

ABNORMAL FINDINGS

➤INSPECT the posterior wall of the pharynx for color and surface characteristics. With the client's mouth wide open and a tongue blade holding the tongue down, examine the posterior wall of the pharynx (Fig. 14-17). The tissue should be smooth and have a glistening pink coloration. There may be small irregular spots of small blood vessels.

- Exudate or mucoid film on the posterior pharynx may be present secondary to postnasal drip or infection.
- A grayish tinge to the membrane may occur with allergies or diphtheria.

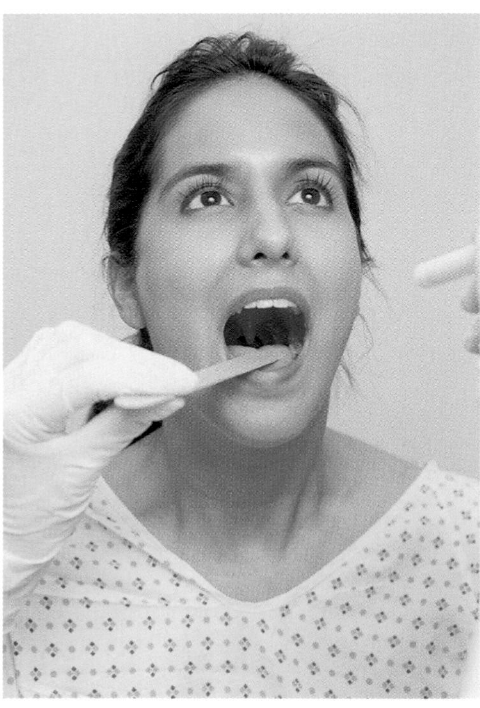

Fig. 14-17 Displace the tongue with a tongue depressor for inspection of the pharynx.

➤INSPECT the tonsils for texture and color. The tonsils extend beyond the posterior pillars. The tonsils should appear slightly pink with an irregular surface.

- Swollen, reddened tonsils with or without exudate may be indicative of infection. Tonsil swelling ranges from 1+ (slightly swollen) to 4+ (kissing tonsils).

AGE-RELATED VARIATIONS

■ INFANTS

Anatomy and Physiology

Although the maxillary and ethmoid sinuses are present at birth, they are very small and cannot be examined until the child is much older; the sphenoid sinus is a tiny cavity at birth that is not fully developed until puberty.

By the time the infant is 3 months old, the infant drools because salivation has increased. Salivation normally increases in children between 3 months and 2 years of age. The infant continues to drool until he or she learns to swallow the saliva. In the third month of fetal development, deciduous teeth begin to calcify. When each tooth has enough calcification to withstand chewing, it erupts to the surface. The 20 deciduous teeth usually appear between 6 and 24 months of age (see Fig. 14-6). The permanent teeth begin forming in the jaw by 6 months of age (Seidel et al, 1999).

Health History

- Did the infant's mother have a history of maternal infection, alcohol or drug use, irradiation, hypertension, or diabetes during pregnancy?

  Rationale Maternal infection or substance abuse during pregnancy may lead to congenital defects or infections.
- Were any abnormalities present at the infant's birth? If so, what were they? Has the infant undergone repair for problems such as cleft lip or cleft palate?

  Rationale Identifying problems early can help in providing treatment and follow-up care.

Examination

The examination of the nose and mouth is straightforward; the problem arises when the infant is uncooperative or unable to hold still. The infant must be carefully and securely restrained by a parent or other adult who acts as a "holder" to ensure the infant's safety and to permit the full viewing of the examination area. The restraining is usually done with the infant in a supine position, with the arms extended securely above the infant's head (Fig. 14-18). The holder will then be able to secure both the infant's arms and head. A second holder or the examiner may need to immobilize the infant's lower extremities.

Procedures and Techniques The infant's nose is small and difficult to examine. Do not attempt to insert a speculum into the nares. Inspect the inside of the nose by tilting the infant's head back and shining a light into the nares. Determine the nares' patency by holding one nostril closed and then the other one. If an infant has nasal congestion, suction the nares with a bulb syringe or small-lumen catheter.

Inspect the infant's mouth for integrity, especially hard palate, and for absence of congenital abnormalities such as cleft lip. The examination of the lips may show evidence of a sucking callus. This should disappear after the first few weeks of life. It is generally possible to examine the infant's mouth while the infant is crying. Palpate the buccal mucosa and gums using a gloved hand and a light source. While your finger is in the infant's mouth, check the strength of the infant's suck.

Normal and Abnormal Findings Normally you expect to find that the base of the nose is appropriate to the size of the face. You may find milia across the infant's nose. The infant's nares have only minimal movement with breathing.

The buccal mucosa should appear pink, moist, and smooth. The infant's gums should appear smooth and full. Other normal findings may include the presence of small white epithelial cells on the palate or gums. These are called Bohn's nodules or Epstein's pearls (Fig. 14-19). The infant's tongue should be appropriate to the size of the mouth and fit well into the floor of the mouth. The infant should have a strong suck with the tongue pushing upward against your finger.

Abnormal findings include nasal flaring, which may be seen if the infant has respiratory distress. Because infants are obligatory nose breathers, any obstruction of the nares secondary to a congenital abnormality such as choanal atresia (occlusion between pharynx and nose), foreign body, or nasal secretions will cause the infant to be irritable or distressed.

If whitish patches are seen along the mucosa, scrape the area with a tongue blade to differentiate between a lesion and milk deposits. Patches that do not scrape clean may indicate candidiasis (thrush). Occasionally, a natal loose tooth may be found. These teeth should be removed to prevent possible aspiration. Macroglossia (excessive tongue size) may be a sign of Down syndrome or congenital hypothyroidism.

■ CHILDREN

Anatomy and Physiology

The frontal sinuses are absent (see Fig. 14-3) until 7 to 8 years of age. The roots of the deciduous teeth are reabsorbed by pressure from the permanent teeth until the crown is shed. The permanent teeth begin to erupt when the

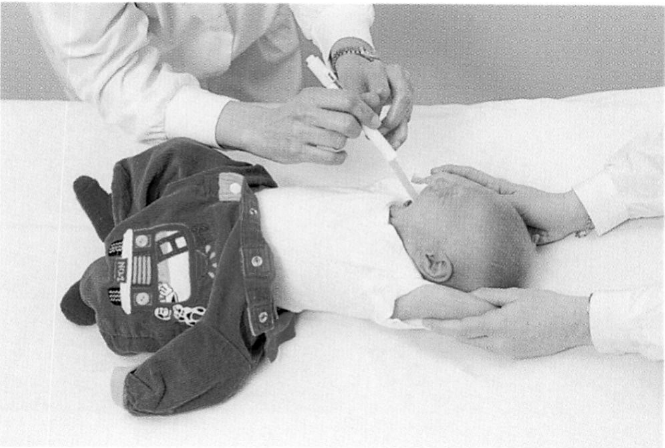

Fig. 14-18 Positioning of infant for examination of nose and mouth.

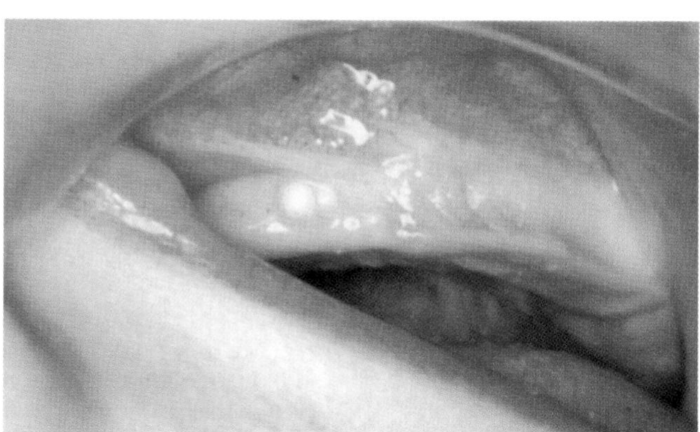

Fig. 14-19 Epstein's pearls (gingival cysts) in an infant. (From Scully and Welbury, 1994.)

child reaches about the age of 6 and continue until about age 18, when the third molars, or wisdom teeth, erupt (see Fig. 14-6) (Seidel et al, 1999).

Health History

Young Child

- Are the child's teeth erupting? If so, when did this start, and what teeth does he or she have?

  Rationale A delay in tooth eruption may be associated with calcium or vitamin D deficiencies or congenital disorders such as Down syndrome.
- Does your child tend to put objects in his or her nose? Have you noticed any unilateral nose drainage or odor from the nose?

  Rationale Foul-smelling unilateral nasal drainage may be an indication of an object obstructing the nose.
- Is the child using a bottle? If so, how often? Does he or she go to bed with a bottle? Does the child have any caries?

  Rationale Dental problems and caries may be related to the child taking a bottle to bed, leaving milk on or around the teeth overnight.
- Does the child suck his or her thumb or use a pacifier?

  Rationale Thumb sucking or using a pacifier should be a concern only if the child's secondary teeth are present.
- Does the child have any mouth infections or sores in the mouth such as thrush? If so, how often do they occur? Does the child seem to have sore throats or colds often? How often? How are these treated? Has he or she had streptococcal throat?

  Rationale Frequent colds and sore throats may be common, but should be evaluated because of risk related to causing hearing problems and preventing them by treating allergies.
- Do you brush your child's teeth? Has the child seen a dentist? If so, how often? Do you use fluoridated water or a fluoride supplement?

  Rationale A caregiver should brush the child's teeth as soon as they are present, using toothpaste. By the age of 3, the child should see a dentist. Good dental hygiene starts at a young age and serves as a preventive health habit later.

Older Child

Questions for the older child should include those for the younger child but should also focus on the characteristics of the teeth and dental habits and care.

- How does the child care for his or her teeth each day? Brushing and flossing habits? How often does the child see a dentist? Does the child have a habit of grinding his or her teeth (bruxism)? If so, when does this happen (night, day, or both)? Do the child's teeth appear straight? If not, are there plans for correction?

  Rationale Parents need to monitor the dental hygiene practices of their children to be sure that a complete job of brushing is done. Role modeling is an effective strategy to use.

Examination

Procedures and Techniques A toddler or young child will probably tolerate the mouth and nose examination better while sitting on the parent's lap. Have the child sit on the adult's lap with his or her back to the parent. The parent may then immobilize the child's legs by placing them between the adult's legs. The parent then has both hands free. One hand should be used to reach around the child's body to restrain the child's arms and chest. The other hand may be used to assist the nurse by immobilizing the child's head (Fig. 14-20). Once the child becomes too large for the parent's lap, the examination is best performed with the child in a supine position on the examination table. Care must always be taken to prevent the child from making a sudden movement during the examination.

Regardless of the immobilization technique used, time should also be taken to try to gain the cooperation of the child. Once the child is old enough to understand and is curious about what is happening, the examiner should also take the time to engage the child. Move slowly and permit the child to handle the equipment, and assure the child that the intent is not to hurt. The actual examination procedure may start by permitting the child to play with the tongue blade and to ask the young child to show his or her teeth or play smiling and "ah" games. This is generally nonthreatening and may lead the way to cooperation. There is no guarantee that these methods will work with all children. It may be helpful to divide the examination into two phases and work them into the rest of the examination at different points. If all else fails and the child is uncooperative, the child must be immobilized by a "holder" to ensure the child's safety. A sudden move by the child could result in injury.

The young child's nose should be assessed in the same manner as the infant's. Inspect the child's external nose for a transverse crease. The child's head should be tilted backward, and the light should be shone into the nares. Use your thumb on the tip of the nose to improve visualization. If vi-

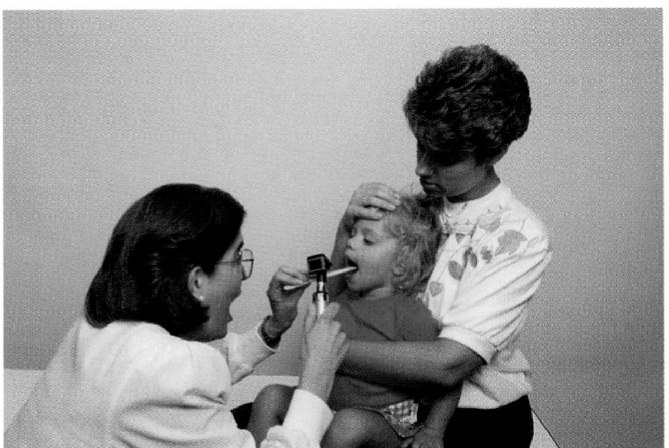

Fig. 14-20 Technique for immobilizing a young child's head before examination.

sualization of a larger area is needed, use the otoscope with a large speculum. The examination of the child's sinuses should become part of the examination after approximately age 7 to 8. There is a wide age variation in the development of the sinuses.

Inspect the child's lips for appearance. Inspect the oral cavity and buccal mucosa for color, moisture, and surface characteristics. Examine the teeth, noting eruption sequence and timing. Also note the condition and the positioning of the teeth, as well as the health of the teeth and the presence of debris around the teeth or gum line. Note the characteristics and size of the tongue.

Normal and Abnormal Findings Normal findings include buccal mucosa that is pink, moist, and without lesions. The child's tonsils are larger than an adult's but should not interfere with swallowing or breathing. Tooth eruption depends on the age of the child.

Abnormal findings include the presence of a transverse crease at the bridge of the nose called an "allergic salute," which occurs when a child has a frequent runny nose or allergies and wipes the nose with an upward sweep of the palm of the hand. If the child has unilateral nasal obstruction or has an odor from the nose, carefully evaluate the nares for a possible foreign body.

Dryness, flaking, or cracking corners of the mouth, if present, may indicate excess licking of the lips, vitamin deficiency, or infection such as impetigo. An excessively dry mouth may indicate dehydration or fever. Excessive salivation may indicate gingivostomatitis or multiple dental caries. Drooling after 12 months of age may be indicative of a neurologic disorder.

Flattened edges on the teeth may indicate teeth grinding (bruxism). Darkened, brown, or black teeth may indicate decay or oral iron therapy. Mottled or pitted teeth may result from tetracycline therapy during tooth development. A strawberry-colored tongue, along with other clinical signs, may be indicative of scarlet fever. If the mouth has a fetid or musty smell, further investigation should be made regarding hygiene practices, local or systemic infections, or sinusitis.

The child's tonsils should be dark pink and without vertical reddened lines, general redness, swelling, or exudate. The tonsils grow to their maximum size between 2 and 6 years of age and have the maximum potential to obstruct the child's airway during this time. Lesions such as Koplik's spots (as seen in measles) or candidiasis (thrush) may be observed.

■ OLDER ADULTS

Anatomy and Physiology

The nose becomes larger and more prominent because of unabated cartilage formation. The granular lining on the lips and cheeks becomes more prominent. The older adult's buccal mucosa may appear thin and less vascular than the younger adult's. There may also be a decrease in saliva secondary to medications. The gingival tissue is less elastic and more vulnerable to injury. Because of gingival recession, the root surfaces of the teeth are exposed to caries formation. As teeth lose their translucency, they darken and become worn from long use. Other effects of the aging process include tooth enamel erosion and slow deterioration from years of vigorous brushing. The tongue becomes more fissured. The older adult may have altered motor function of the tongue, leading to problems with swallowing. After the age of 45, the papillae on the lateral edges of the tongue gradually atrophy and the number of papillae and taste buds drop in general. As a result, taste perception may be diminished. The older adult's body heals more slowly, thereby leading to a higher risk of infection of the oral cavity.

Health History

- Are you currently taking medications that make your mouth dry (xerostomia)? Is your nose dry? If so, what do you do about the dryness?

  Rationale A side effect of many medications is a dry mouth, which may be relieved with fluids.
- If you have had a loss of teeth or you have dentures that do not fit well, does this interfere with your eating or chewing? Are you able to chew the foods that you want to?

  Rationale Ill-fitting dentures contribute to mouth pain and altered nutritional intake.

Examination

Procedures and Techniques Clients with dentures or dental appliances may be sensitive to having their oral cavity examined, especially if dentures or appliance are removed. Be aware of the client's sensitivity but reassure the client that a full examination of the gums is necessary to ensure that no problems are present. The examination of older adults proceeds as for adults.

Normal and Abnormal Findings Abnormal findings include loss of elasticity of joint ligaments, such as the temporomandibular joint, which may dislocate when the mouth is opened widely. Care should therefore be taken during the mouth examination to not cause undue stress on the mouth.

The surface of the lips may be marked with deep wrinkling and fissures at the corner of the mouth (perlèche) associated with an inflammatory response to severe overclosure or vitamin deficiency. The older client is at higher risk for squamous cell carcinoma of the lip, especially if the client has been a longtime pipe smoker. Aging changes cause the gum line to recede secondary to bone degeneration, causing the teeth to appear longer. The gums may become more friable and bleed with slight pressure.

The teeth may become darkened or stained. Many older adults may become edentulous or have caps or bridges. Dental occlusion surfaces may be markedly worn down. Malocclusion of the teeth may be common secondary to the migration of teeth after tooth extraction.

RISK FACTORS

COMMON RISK FACTORS ASSOCIATED WITH
Oral Cancer

MODIFIABLE RISK FACTORS

Lifestyle: Smoking cigarettes, cigars; chewing tobacco, snuff; excessive alcohol consumption
Using tobacco and alcohol together—much greater risk than using either substance alone
Excessive exposure to sunlight
Dietary deficiency in vitamins A, C, and E
Diet high in salted and smoked meats, fats, and oils

NONMODIFIABLE RISK FACTORS

Gender: Rate for men twice that for women
Race: African American
Age: Greater than 40 years; with peak in persons age 64 to 74 years
Peak between ages 54 and 64 for African Americans
Previously diagnosed cancer

Modified from *Art@tambcd.edu,* 1996; Shugars D, Patton L: Detecting, diagnosing, and preventing oral cancer, *Nurse Pract* 22(6):105, 1997.

EXAMINATION SUMMARY

Nose, Paranasal Sinuses, Mouth, and Oropharynx

NOSE AND PARANASAL SINUSES
(pp. 265-268)

- Inspect and palpate the nose for:
  General appearance and symmetry
  Patency
  Discharge
  Tenderness
- Assess the nose for:
  Patency
- Evaluate the olfactory nerve for:
  Intactness
- Inspect the internal nasal cavity for:
  Patency
- Palpate the paranasal sinuses for:
  Tenderness or bogginess

MOUTH AND OROPHARYNX
(pp. 268-274)

- Palpate the temporomandibular joint for:
  Movement
  Tenderness
  Discomfort
- Inspect the lips for:
  Color
  Symmetry
  Moisture and texture
- Inspect teeth for:
  Alignment
  Number

MOUTH AND OROPHARYNX—cont'd

  Color
  Surface characteristics
- Palpate the teeth for:
  Stability
- Note breath for:
  Odor
- Inspect and palpate lips and gums for:
  Integrity
  Tenderness
  Color and moisture
- Inspect the oral cavity and buccal mucosa for:
  Color
  Symmetry
  Texture
- Inspect and palpate the tongue for:
  Movement
  Color
  Lesions
  Surface characteristics
- Inspect the hard and soft palates and uvula for:
  Texture
  Color
  Surface characteristics
- Inspect soft palate for:
  Movement
- Inspect the posterior pharynx for:
  Color and surface characteristics
- Inspect tonsils for:
  Texture and color

SUMMARY OF FINDINGS

Age Group	Normal Findings	Typical Variations	Findings Associated With Disorders
Infants and children		• Epstein's pearls may be present on gums.	• *Mouth:* Natal teeth may be found; white patches on buccal mucosa may indicate thrush.
Adolescents	• Same as for adult.	• Same as for adult.	• Same as the adult.
Adult	• *Nose:* Skin smooth and intact; nose firm and patent; olfactory function intact. • *Sinuses:* Not palpable. • *Temporomandibular joint:* Moves without discomfort. • *Lips:* Pink, symmetric, moist. • *Teeth:* 32 present; white, yellow, or gray. • *Gums:* Pink, moist. • *Buccal mucosa:* Pink, moist. • *Stensen's and Wharton's ducts:* Patent and smooth. • *Tongue:* Symmetric, pink, moist. • *Mouth:* Ventral surface and floor of mouth pale coral or pink, with frenulum in center; hard palate is smooth, pale, and immovable. • *Uvula:* Moves symmetrically. • *Tonsils:* Pink with irregular surface.	• *Tongue:* Geographic tongue is pattern of irregular papillae lengths. • *Pharynx:* Yellow film typical of postnasal drip. • *Tonsils:* May have been surgically removed.	• *Nose:* Swelling and nasal discharge are signs of infection or allergy. Deviated septum with a decrease in air flow is abnormal. Turbinates may be pale or bluish gray and edematous from allergic response. Nasal polyps are found in chronic allergic rhinitis and cystic fibrosis. • *Mouth:* Deep mouth fissures may be riboflavin or pyridoxine deficiency; ulcer, nodule, or white patches in mouth suggest cancer. • *Lips:* Pallor suggests anemia; cynanosis of lips suggests poor oxygenation. • *Gums:* Bleeding or swollen gums suggest periodontal disease; bleeding gums may indicate Vitamin C or K deficiency or gum disease. • *Uvula:* No movement indicates vagus nerve paralysis.
Older adults	• *Tongue:* After age 45, papillae on lateral edges of tongue atrophy; taste perception decreases. • *Gingival tissue:* Becomes less elastic. • *Buccal mucosa:* Becomes thinner and less vascular.	• Remove dentures or dental appliances to inspect and palpate the gums.	• *Mouth:* Dry mouth may be caused by medication side effects or dehydration. • *Gums:* May be more friable and bleed easily. • *Lips:* Lesions may be squamous cell carcinoma.

HEALTH PROMOTION

DENTAL CARE

All clients, regardless of age, should be encouraged to visit a dentist on a regular basis. Dental visits should begin between 2 and 3 years of age. In addition, clients should be encouraged to use dental floss and regular brushing. Flossing on a regular basis reduces the risk of periodontal disease (U.S. Preventive Task Force, 1996).

Parents should be taught that young children who take

the bottle to bed and suck on the nipple during the night are at higher risk of developing dental caries of the primary teeth. This is especially true if the bottle contains an acidic or cariogenic beverage (fruit juice, milk, or formula). Parents should also be taught that, if their young children have caries of the baby teeth, they should not ignore the problem but should seek dental evaluation. Infection or caries of the primary teeth may affect the secondary teeth.

Parents should be taught to start brushing the child's teeth as soon as they erupt. This not only teaches the child good dental care but is also a preventive dental practice. It is necessary for the young child to use toothpaste.

Fluoride is also an important factor in reducing dental caries, especially in children. Clients living in areas where there is no fluoride in the water should be referred for dental evaluation and supplemental fluoride treatments.

NOSE SPRAYS

Nose sprays may be very effective in relieving nasal congestion. If used for a long period or routinely, they may indeed cause a "rebound" effect and actually make the nasal congestion problem worse. Clients should therefore be advised to use nose sprays only occasionally. Nose sprays should not be used for more than 5 consecutive days.

NASAL FOREIGN BODIES

Parents should be advised that young children are curious about small objects and may push them up their nose. This may include small objects such as peanuts, corn, beads, or rocks. Children should not be left alone with any small object that may cause them to choke or objects that are smaller than the child's little finger.

COMMON PROBLEMS AND CONDITIONS

Nose, Paranasal Sinuses, Mouth, and Oropharynx

NOSE

Nasal Polyps

Smooth, pale gray tissue enlargements in the nasal cavity are polyps that occur most commonly in clients with chronic allergic rhinitis (Fig. 14-21). These nontender growths may become so large that they actually obstruct the nasal passage. They also are seen in clients with cystic fibrosis.

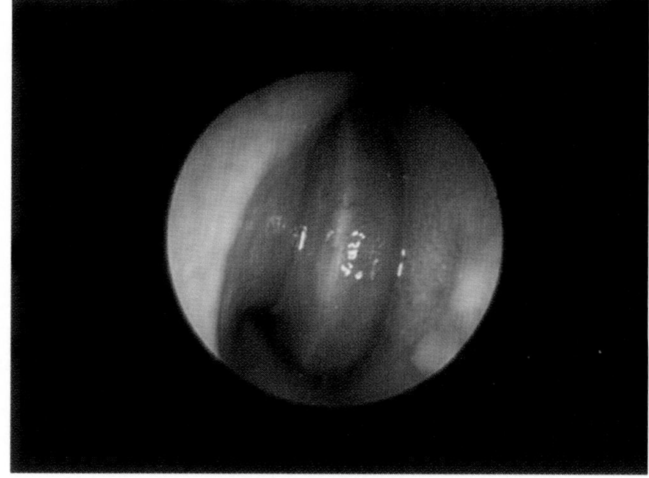

Fig. 14-21 A simple benign nasal polyp *(center)*. It is smooth, semitranslucent, and gray. (From Bingham, Hawke, and Kwok, 1992.)

LIPS, MOUTH, AND OROPHARYNX

Herpes Simplex Type 1 (cold sore)

This common viral infection of the lip may occur secondary to fever, colds, allergy, or trauma to the lip (Fig. 14-22). Like other herpes type of lesions, the lesion stages progress from a cluster of clear vesicles, to pustules, and finally crusts.

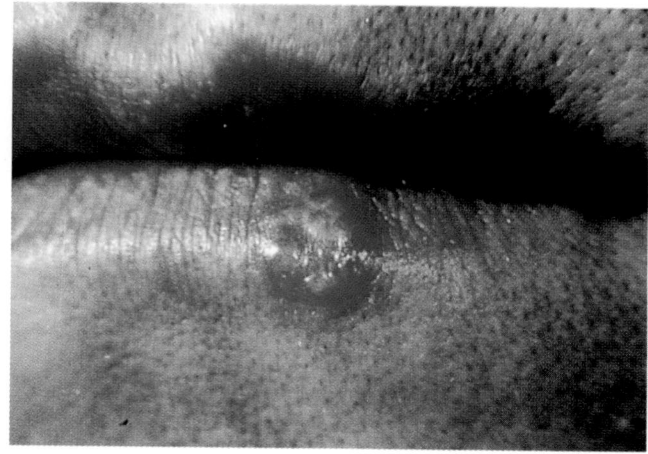

Fig. 14-22 Herpes simplex lesion (cold sore) of lower lip. (From Grimes, 1994.)

Squamous Cell Carcinoma of the Lip

This is a slow-growing malignant tumor of squamous epithelium that appears as ulcerated sores of the lip (Fig. 14-23). It may also be seen on the floor of the mouth or the lateral border of the tongue. The lesion is usually indurated and has a raised irregular border and an erythematous base.

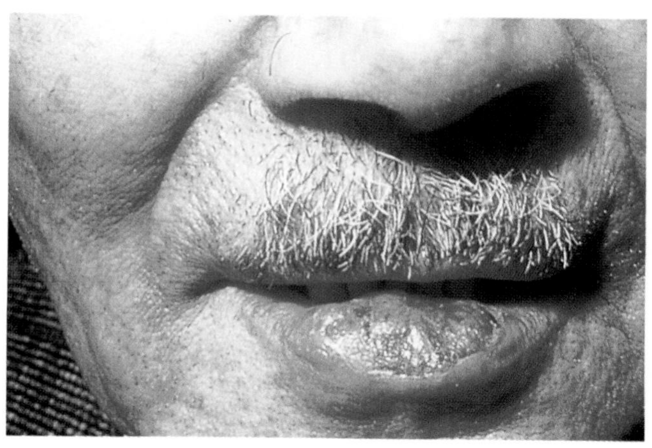

Fig. 14-23 Squamous cell carcinoma. (From Hill, 1994.)

RISK FACTORS

HIGH- AND LOW-RISK SITES FOR Oral Cancer

HIGH-RISK SITES	LOW-RISK SITES
Soft palate	Hard palate
Anterior tonsillar pillar	Posterior tonsillar pillar
Tongue (ventral surface)	Tongue (dorsal surface)
Base of tongue	Uvula
Floor of mouth	Tonsil
Mandibular gingiva	Buccal mucosa
Lower lip	Upper lip

Modified from Shugars D, Patton L: Detecting, diagnosing, and preventing oral cancer, 1997. *Nurse Pract* 22(6)105, 1999.

Cleft Lip

When the maxillary and median processes do not close, this congenital abnormality occurs, involving only the upper lip or both the lip and the hard palate (Fig. 14-24).

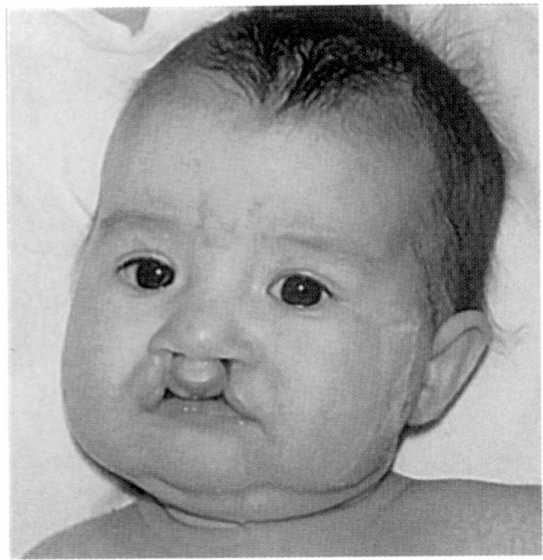

Fig. 14-24 Bilateral cleft lip in an infant. (From Scully and Welbury, 1994.)

Tonsillitis

Infection or inflammation of the tonsils frequently is caused by streptococcal infection. Symptoms include severe sore throat, headache, and malaise. Signs include temperature above 38.3° C (101° F) and enlarged anterior cervical and tonsillar lymph nodes. White or yellow exudate may be seen on tonsils or oropharynx (Fig. 14-25). Tonsillitis is commonly seen in 21% to 50% of school-age children but rarely in children under 3 years old (Wong et al, 1999).

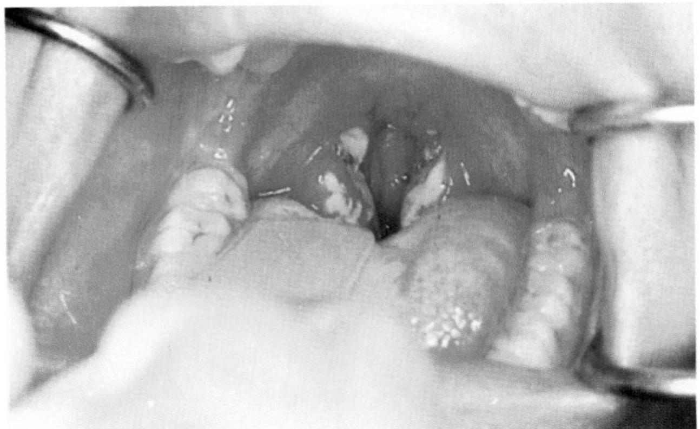

Fig. 14-25 Tonsillitis and pharyngitis. (Courtesy Dr. Edward L Applebaum, Head–Department of Otolaryngology. University of Illinois Medical Center. From Wong et al, 1999.)

TEETH AND GUMS

Advanced Pyorrhea

Gingivitis and edema can develop into advanced pyorrhea, a purulent inflammation of tissues surrounding the teeth. Erosion of the gum tissue, destruction of underlying bone, and loosening of the teeth may result from this inflammation (Fig. 14-26).

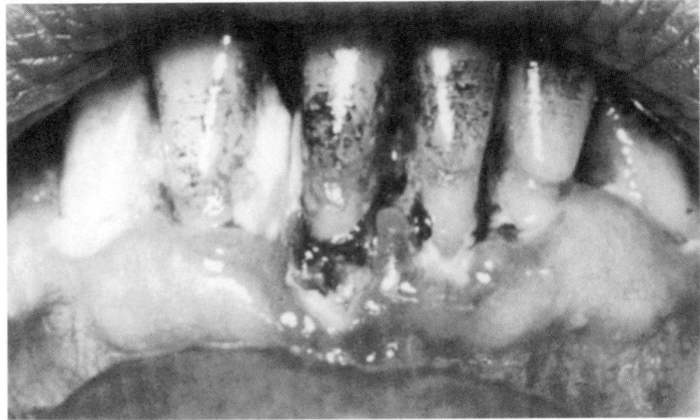

Fig. 14-26 Advanced pyorrhea. (From DeWeese et al, 1988.)

TONGUE

Hairy Tongue

The term of this disorder describes how the tongue feels to clients. There are blackish, painful lesions felt on top of the tongue (Fig. 14-27). These are reported as feeling like a "hairy" sensation. There is usually a history of excessive antibiotic use, excessive use of mouthwash, smoking, or alcohol consumption.

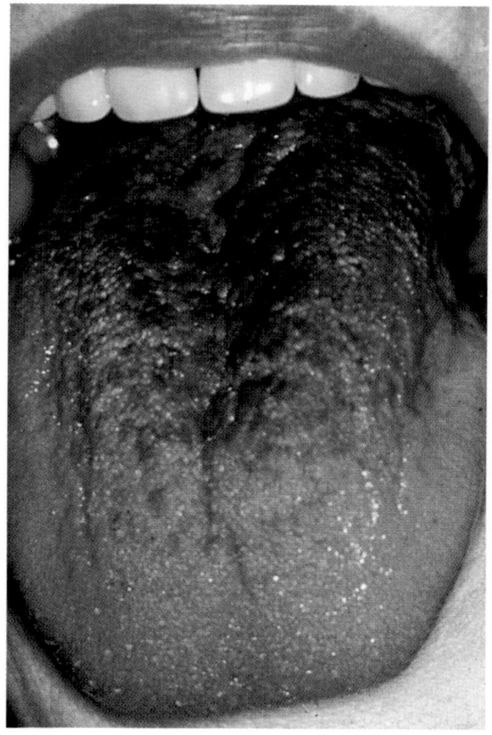

Fig. 14-27 Hairy tongue. (From Dunlap and Barker, 1991.)

BUCCAL MUCOSA

Candidiasis (Thrush)

Monilial infection is another name for this disorder. It appears on the tongue, buccal mucosa, or posterior pharynx as a whitish, cheesy patch resembling milk curd (Fig. 14-28). If the membrane is peeled off, a raw, bleeding, erythematous area results. Thrush is commonly seen in infants but in adults is seen primarily in individuals who are chronically debilitated, in clients who are immunosuppressed, persons with HIV or acquired immunodeficiency syndrome (AIDS), or those who have been on antibiotic therapy.

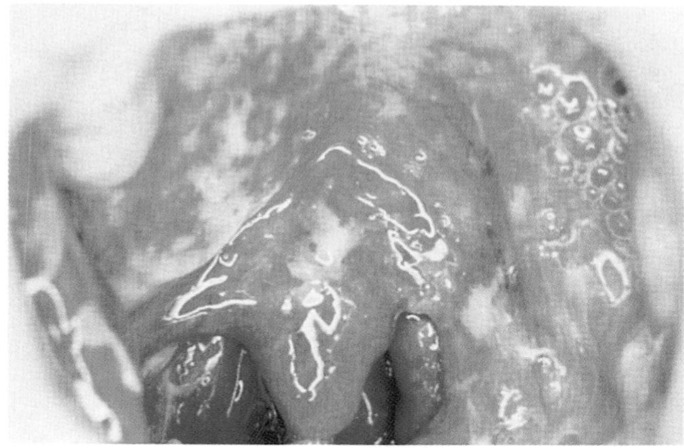

Fig. 14-28 Candidiasis (thrush). (From Sigler and Schuring, 1993.)

Aphthous Ulcer (Canker Sore)

These painful lesions appear commonly on the buccal mucosa (Fig. 14-29). They may also appear on the lips, tip and sides of tongue, or palate. They appear as white, round, or oval ulcerative lesions with a red halo. Ulcers may last up to two weeks; the etiology is unknown.

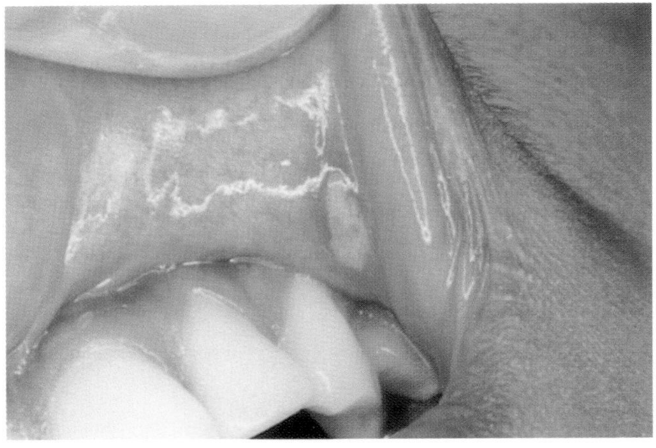

Fig. 14-29 A small aphthous ulcer (canker sore) on the lower lip. (From Bingham, Hawke, and Kwok, 1992.)

Leukoplakia

This painless white lesion on the inside of the cheek, tongue, lower lip, or floor of the mouth (Fig. 14-30, *A* and *B*) is hyperkeratinized and cannot be scraped off. Leukoplakia is linked to smoking, AIDS, alcoholism, and chewing tobacco.

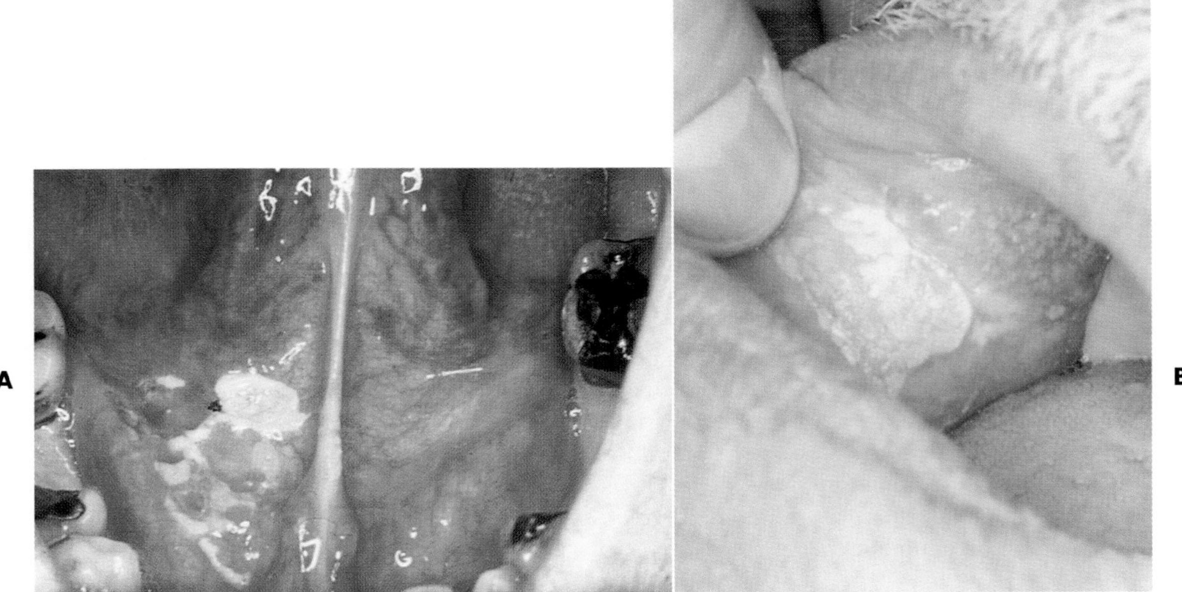

Fig. 14-30 Leukoplakia. (**A** from Dunlap and Barker, 1991; **B** from Bingham, Hawke, and Kwok, 1992.)

Oral Kaposi's Sarcoma

This malignancy is seen in persons with AIDS and appears as incompletely formed blood vessels in the mouth (Fig. 14-31). These vessels form lesions of various shades and sizes as the blood escapes into tissues in response to the malignant tumor of the membrane.

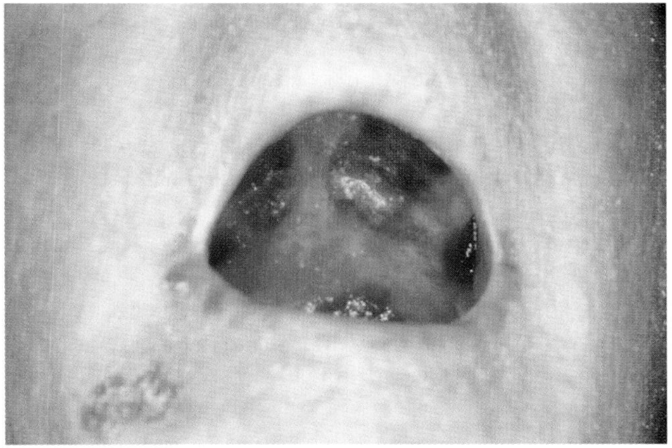

Fig. 14-31 The bluish raised lesion seen on the palate of this client who has AIDS is Kaposi's sarcoma. (From Bingham, Hawke, and Kwok, 1992.)

Koplik's Spots

A classic diagnostic finding of measles is Koplik's spots (Fig. 14-32). They appear on the buccal mucosa as small bluish white areas with irregular borders.

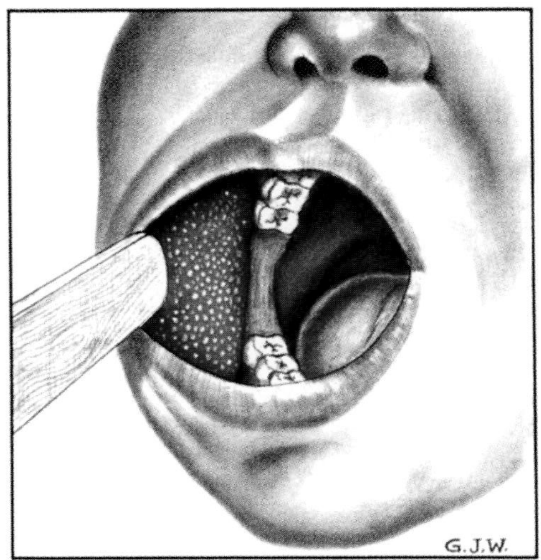

Fig. 14-32 Koplik's spots on the buccal mucosa. (From Wong et al, 1999.)

CLINICAL APPLICATION and CRITICAL THINKING

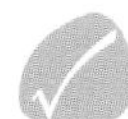

SAMPLE DOCUMENTATION

CASE 1

Hershel is a 19-month-old boy brought to the clinic by his mother with the chief complaint of nasal discharge and odor about the head.

Subjective Data

Mother reports 4-day history of yellow nasal discharge; child very fussy. No history of illness, fever, congestion, rash, or nausea or vomiting. Slow onset of bilateral nasal stuffiness and discharge and increasing foul odor about child's head; child sits in high chair, feeds self finger food; child snacks on peanuts, cheerios, raisins, and crackers while playing.

Objective Data

Tympanic temperature, 37.3° C (99.1° F).

Healthy-appearing, playful male child actively exploring examining room.

Nose: Bilateral purulent, yellow nasal discharge; internal nasal examination—small swollen, foul-smelling raisin in left nostril; right nostril clear.

Mouth: Lips pink, no lesions; 18 primary teeth, all intact; oral cavity and buccal mucosa pink without lesions; posterior pharynx pink with large tonsils visualized behind posterior pillar; tonsils without exudate or lesions.

Respiratory: Bilaterally equal breath sounds; no acute respiratory distress.

Functional Health Pattern Involved

Health promotion–health maintenance

Medical Diagnosis

Foreign body—left naris

Nursing Diagnosis and Collaborative Problems

- *Altered health maintenance* related to lack of education about age-related factors as manifested by:
  - Mother reports child given peanuts, raisins for snacks
  - Raisin found in left naris.
- *Risk for injury* related to lack of education about age-related factors.

CASE 2

M.M. is a 42-year-old woman with the chief complaint of jaw pain and clicking when she chews.

Subjective Data

M.M. reports that approximately 2 months ago, when she was eating, she felt a catch and pain in the jaw and was unable to close her mouth; during the following 30-to-40 minute period, the "locking" eased, and she was able to close her mouth; however, the pain continued. Since that time, increased jaw pain during chewing, with pain radiating to left ear; reports "clicking" sensation and sound when attempting to chew. Attempted to relieve pain with aspirin and ibuprofen without success. Delayed seeking health care because of a busy schedule and stressful job; could not find the time for evaluation.

Has been on a liquid diet since the problem began; decreased weight from 132 lb (60 kg) to 115 lb (52 kg). Infrequent hard stools; last bowel movement 2 days ago; normal bowel pattern—daily passage of soft, formed, brown stool.

Objective Data

Height: 5′5″ (165 cm); Weight 115 lbs (52 kg).

Healthy-appearing female in no acute distress.

Mouth: Able to open and close widely with slight pain on left side, radiating to ear.

Teeth: Align correctly upon closing mouth and clenching teeth; no evidence of malocclusion.

TMJ: Complains of left-side jaw tenderness with palpation of TMJ as client opens mouth; crepitation with clicking felt at left TMJ with opening and closing jaw.

Remaining mouth examination not remarkable.

Functional Health Patterns Involved:

- Nutrition–metabolic
- Elimination
- Cognitive–perceptual

Medical Diagnosis

Temporomandibular joint syndrome

Nursing Diagnosis and Collaborative Problems

- *Pain* related to temporomandibular joint dysfunction as manifested by:
  - Increased jaw pain; clicking sensation with chewing.
- *Altered nutrition: less than body requirements* related to inadequate food intake secondary to painful chewing as manifested by:
  - Weight loss of 17 lb in 2 months.
- *Constipation* related to decreased oral intake as manifested by:
  - Decreased frequency of bowel elimination.
  - Passage of small hard stools.
- *Risk for fluid volume deficit* related to insufficient oral intake.

CRITICAL THINKING QUESTIONS

1. A 42-year-old woman complains of constant nasal congestion for about a month. She tells you that she has been treating her symptoms with a nasal decongestant spray, but it doesn't seem to help very much. What kind of client teaching is appropriate in this situation?
2. A 54-year-old man complains of chronic hoarseness. Since hoarseness is considered a "possible warning" of laryngeal cancer, what clues can the nurse look for that might help differentiate hoarseness due to malignancy versus another cause?
3. A young mother brings in her 6-month-old baby to the clinic for a well-baby visit and immunizations. She shares with the nurse that her grandmother told her it was bad for the baby to go to bed at night with a bottle and that she needs to take care of the baby's teeth. The mother wants to know if what her grandmother says is true, and if so, how she should take care of the baby's teeth without hurting the baby. What information should be shared with the mother?

CASE STUDY

Jack Ruff is a 61-year-old man who complains of a burning in his mouth that is getting worse. Listed below are data collected by the nurse during an interview and examination.

Interview Data

Mr. Ruff tells the nurse, "My friend Hal looked at my mouth and told me I better go get checked 'cause he says I might have cancer." He adds, "I don't want no cancer growing in my mouth. I've seen what they do to people with mouth cancer. They cut the tongue out and leave scars on the neck." Mr. Ruff reports he went to the dentist last year for this problem and was told he had a canker sore. He was advised at that time to put a topical cream on it. He has been using the cream all along, but the spot is not going away. Mr. Ruff reports he has been a smoker for about 40 years, but that it has never caused him any problems.

Examination Data

- **General survey:** Alert, thin male in no obvious distress.
- **Head and neck:** Skull is firm, symmetric, and nontender. Facial bones are symmetric and appear appropriate for size of head; the trachea is midline. Thyroid is in midline position and of normal size. Submandibular, submental, retropharyngeal, and deep cervical chain lymph nodes palpable and somewhat tender.
- **Mouth and oropharynx:** Teeth are in good condition; 28 teeth present; 4 third molars have been removed. Teeth stained yellow, consistent with cigarette use. Multiple whitish spots are seen inside the cheek and internal lower lip; nontender, cannot be scraped off. Large yellow and black raised lesion with an irregular border noted on the floor of the mouth, underneath the tongue.

1. What data deviate from normal findings, suggesting a need for further investigation?
2. What additional information should the nurse ask or assess for?
3. In what functional health patterns does data deviate from normal?
4. What nursing diagnosis and/or collaborative problems should be considered for this situation?

REMEMBER to check out your companion CD-ROM

15 Ears and Auditory System

www.mosby.com/MERLIN/wilson/assessment/

ANATOMY AND PHYSIOLOGY

The ear is a sensory organ that functions in both equilibrium (balance) and hearing. It is divided into three sections: the external ear, the middle ear, and the inner ear.

EXTERNAL EAR

The external ear is made up of the auricle (pinna) and the external auditory ear canal. The auricle is composed of cartilage and skin. The helix is the prominent outer rim; the concha is the deep cavity in front of the external auditory meatus (Fig. 15-1).

The adult's external ear canal is approximately 2.5 cm in length and is configured as an S-shaped pathway leading from the outer ear to the tympanic membrane (Fig. 15-2). The external ear canal is lined with skin and lubricated with cerumen, which is secreted by sebaceous glands in the canal. This area is rather sensitive. The underlying structures of the distal half of the external ear and the proximal half of the canal are cartilage and bone, respectively.

The external ear is separated from the middle ear by the shiny, translucent, pearl-gray tympanic membrane, made up of layers of skin, fibrous tissue, and mucous membrane (Fig. 15-3). This membrane covers the proximal end of the auditory canal. The tympanic membrane is pulled inward at its center by one of the ossicles of the middle ear, called the malleus. Most of the tympanic membrane is taut and is known as the pars tensa; a smaller, less taut part is the pars flaccida, and the dense fibrous ring around the membrane is the annulus. The cone of light may be seen downward and anteriorly. The tympanic membrane is translucent, permitting visualization of the middle ear cavity.

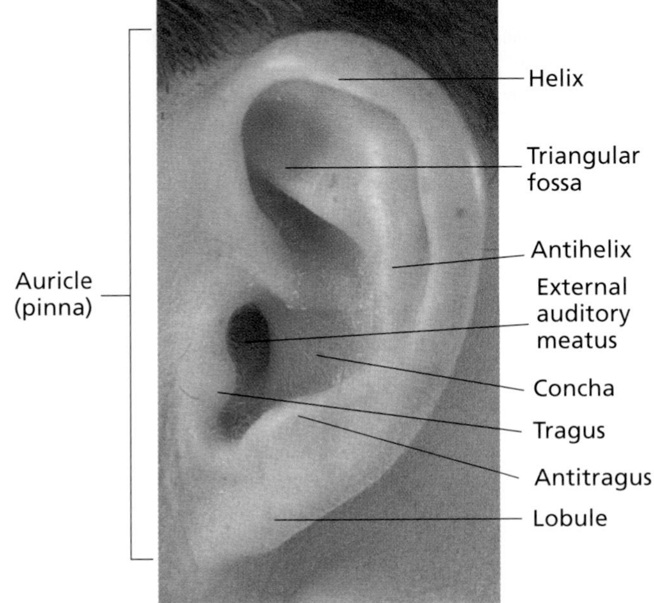

Fig. 15-1 Anatomic structure of the auricle (pinna). The helix is the prominent outer rim, whereas the antihelix is the area parallel and anterior to the helix. The concha is the deep cavity containing the auditory canal meatus. The tragus is the protuberance lying anterior to the auditory canal meatus, and the antitragus is the protuberance on the antihelix opposite the tragus. The lobule is the soft lobe on the bottom of the auricle.

MIDDLE EAR

The middle ear is an air-filled cavity that transmits sound by way of the three tiny bones that make up the ossicles—the malleus, incus, and stapes (Fig. 15-4). The malleus may actually be visualized through the tympanic membrane. Lying between the nasopharynx and the middle ear is a cartilaginous passage, the eustachian tube, which opens briefly during yawning, swallowing, or sneezing to equalize the pressure of the middle ear to the atmosphere.

INNER EAR

The inner ear is a curved cavity inside a bony labyrinth consisting of the vestibule, the semicircular canals, and the cochlea. The vestibule and the semicircular canals make up the organs that coordinate equilibrium. The cochlea is a coiled structure containing the organ of Corti, which transmits sound impulses to the acoustic cranial nerve (VIII) (see Fig. 15-2).

HEARING

Hearing occurs when sound waves enter the external auditory ear canal and strike the tympanic membrane. The membrane begins to vibrate, which then causes the ossicles behind the tympanic membrane to vibrate. The vibrations then travel via the fluid of the cochlea to the hair cells of the organ of Corti. When the delicate hair cells of the organ of Corti are set into motion, cranial nerve VIII is stimulated. The sound wave impulses from the cranial nerve are transmitted to the temporal lobe of the brain for interpretation.

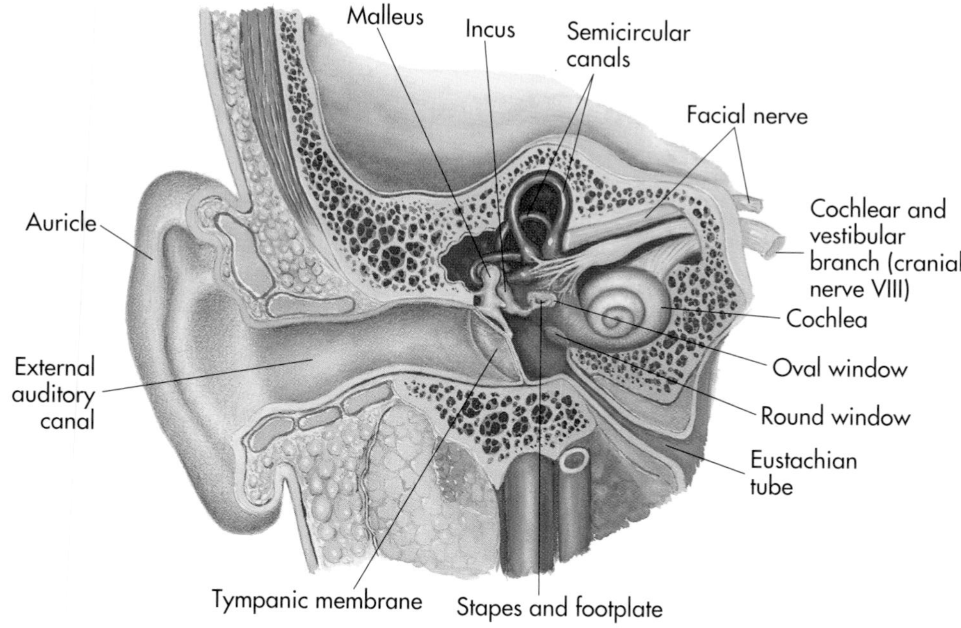

Fig. 15-2 Anatomy of the ear showing outer ear, external auditory canal, tympanic membrane, and structures of the middle and inner ear. (From Seidel et al, 1999.)

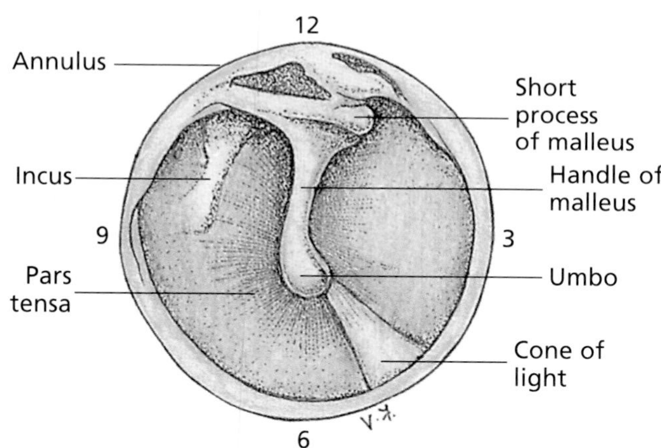

Fig. 15-3 Landmarks of tympanic membrane with "clock" superimposed (right ear). (From Potter and Perry, 1991.)

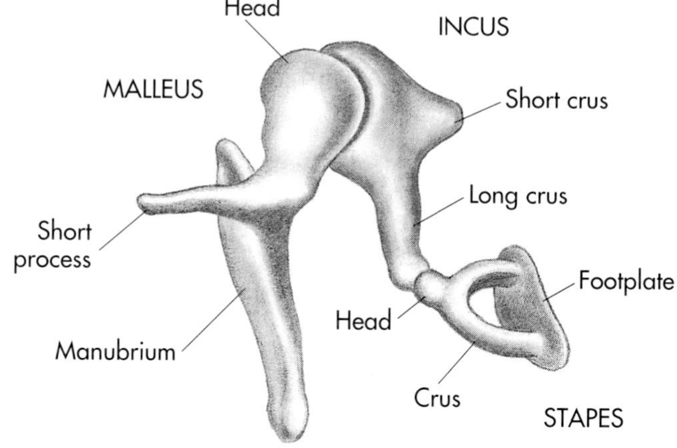

Fig. 15-4 Ossicles of the middle ear showing structures of the malleus, incus, and stapes. (From Thompson et al, 1997.)

RISK FACTORS

COMMON RISK FACTORS ASSOCIATED WITH Hearing Loss

Health history
- Family history of hereditary childhood sensorineural hearing loss
- Congenital or perinatal hearing loss risk factors (see box on p. 305)
- Multiple incidences of otitis media

Environmental—repeated exposure to constant loud noise (>80 dB)
- Workplace—working around heavy machinery
- Home—noises in home, noises near home (airport, construction)
- Recreation—listening to loud music, going to rock concerts

Ototoxic medications
- Aminoglycocide antibiotics
- Salicylates
- Furosemide

HEALTH HISTORY

Ears and Auditory System

QUESTIONS	RATIONALE

PRESENT HEALTH STATUS

➤ How would you describe the condition of your ears?

■ Assess the client's perception of his or her hearing and condition of ears.

➤ Have you noticed any changes in the way your ears feel or function?

■ Ask the client if he or she has noticed changes as opposed to asking them if they have any problems. A client may have an ear or hearing condition yet may not be aware of it or may not consider it a problem.

➤ Do you have any chronic illnesses or conditions?

■ Some chronic diseases can affect ear function (hypertension, diabetes, or nephritis).

➤ Are you currently taking any medications? If so, what are you taking, and when did you start taking the medications? Have you noticed any problems related to hearing or balance since you have been taking the medications?

■ Some medications are ototoxic and cause a side effect of vertigo, dizziness, or tinnitus. If the client reports such symptoms and also relays a history of being on an ototoxic medication, the client should be referred for medical reevaluation.

➤ Have you ever had your hearing tested? If so, when was it done and for what reason?

■ It is important to determine if baseline hearing testing has been performed.

➤ Do you currently wear a hearing aid? If so, for how long? Do you feel your hearing aid helps you hear adequately?

■ Many individuals wear a hearing aid. They may or may not hear well with the hearing aid.

➤ Are you exposed to loud noises at work or at home? If so, describe. Do you wear a hearing protection device or earplugs? If so, do you wear it all of the time or just occasionally? Do the earplugs or headset help reduce the environmental noise? How long have you worked in such an environment? Do you listen to loud music or attend music concerts where the volume of music is loud?

■ Assessment of environmental risk factors that can contribute to hearing loss is an important component of a health history. Repeated and prolonged exposure to loud noise either at work, home, or in the community may lead to hearing loss. Examples of known high-volume noise areas include airports, busy traffic areas, factories, heavy machinery, and construction sites. If any person, regardless of age, provides a history of hearing loss and environmental exposure to loud noise, he or she should be referred for further testing (Lusk, 1997).

QUESTIONS | **RATIONALE**

➤ How do you clean your ears? Do you stick anything such as a cotton-tipped applicator in your ears to clean them?

■ Assess potential injury to the ear from aggressive cleaning. Cleaning of the ears with a cotton-tipped applicator may cause cerumen to be impacted against the tympanic membrane. This impaction, in turn, may cause hearing loss.

PAST MEDICAL HISTORY

➤ In the past, have you had problems with multiple ear infections? If so, did this occur during childhood? Adulthood? How was the problem treated?

■ Establish baseline information for persons with chronic ear infection disease. A history of chronic ear infections or problems may shed light on current problems.

➤ In the past, have you had any problems with your hearing or balance? If so, describe.

■ A brief general history about the ears and hearing should provide good information that may then be used during the assessment of specific problems.

➤ Have you ever had surgery on your ears? If so, when and for what? Did it help?

■ Knowledge of past ear surgery may provide information that may be applied to symptoms or complaints.

➤ Have you ever been struck in the ear or had an injury to your ear? If so, describe when and what happened. Was there any type of discharge or bleeding from your ear following the injury?

■ Ear injuries, either recent or past, may also provide information that may be applied to a client's ear symptoms or complaints. Bleeding or discharge from the ear following an injury may be a sign of basilar skull fracture or a ruptured tympanic membrane.

FAMILY HISTORY

➤ Has anyone in your family experienced hearing loss or been diagnosed with Ménière's disease?

■ Family history of hearing loss or Ménière's disease is significant.

PROBLEM-BASED HISTORY

The most commonly reported problems related to the ears include pain/discomfort, hearing loss, ringing in the ears (tinnitus), and vertigo. As with symptoms in all areas of health assessment, a symptom analysis is completed, which includes the location, quality, quantity, chronology, setting, associated manifestations, alleviating factors, and aggravating factors (see Box 4-2 in Chapter 4).

QUESTIONS | **RATIONALE**

Earache (Box 15-1)

Box 15-1 Focus on Pain—Earache

The medical term for ear pain or earache is *otalgia.* Otalgia can be primary (pain caused by a disorder within the ear) or referred (pain caused by a disorder outside of the ear). Clues regarding the cause of the pain can be gained from taking a careful history—specifically ask the client what events may have triggered the pain. A recent history considered significant which may explain the onset of ear pain include:

- Infection to the upper respiratory tract (viral or bacterial)
- Injury or trauma to the head
- Exposure to a loud noise
- Stress (which leads to grinding teeth)
- Airplane travel

Data from Black JM, Matassarin-Jacobs E: *Medical-surgical nursing: Clinical management for continuity of care,* ed 5, Philadelphia, 1997, Saunders.

➤ How long have you had an earache? Describe the location of the pain—on the outside part of the ear? Inside your ear? Deep in your head?

■ Determine the onset and location of the pain. Ear pain can be unilateral or bilateral; it can be internal or external. Ear pain can also be referred from a problem in the mouth, sinuses, or throat. Likewise, an infection may migrate from a primary site outside the ears into the middle ear.

➤ Is the pain constant, or does it come and go? If it comes and goes, how often does it occur, and how long does it last?

■ Determine the duration of the pain. If the pain is intermittent, explore possible triggering mechanisms.

➤ What does the pain feel like? (Sharp, dull, aching, pounding?) Does it hurt just when you pull on or touch your ear, or does it ache without touching? Does the pain change when you change your position, such as lying down?

■ Description of the pain may help determine the cause. Pain caused by an ear infection involving the external ear or ear canal increases with movement of the ear; pain caused by otitis media does not change with manipulation of the ear.

➤ On a scale of 1 to 10, how would you rate the intensity of your ear pain?

■ A pain scale helps the nurse understand the severity of the pain the client is experiencing.

➤ Is there any discharge from your ear? If yes, what does it look like (clear, purulent, bloody)? Does the discharge have an odor?

■ A description of the discharge may help determine the problem.

➤ Have you done anything to try to stop the pain? If yes, has this been effective?

■ Always explore self-care activities, including medications and home remedies, as this may affect how the health care provider treats the problem.

➤ Do you have a cold or any problems or infections in your mouth, teeth, sinuses, or throat?

■ An infection may migrate from a primary site outside the ears into the middle ear.

Itching of the Ears

➤ When did you start having itching of your ears? Where do you noticing the itching? (One ear? Both ears? Inside the ear? Outside the ear?)

■ Determine onset and location of the problem.

➤ Is the itching constant or does it come and go? If it comes and goes, how often does it occur, and how long does it last?

■ Try to establish a pattern to the itching. This may provide clues to the cause.

QUESTIONS | **RATIONALE**

➤ How do you clean your ears? Do you put any cleaning solution in your ears?

■ Itching in the ears may be caused by improper cleaning techniques such as introduction of soap into the external canal that is not properly rinsed, or irritating the canal with aggressive cleaning.

➤ Have you been swimming recently? If so, when? How often do you swim?

■ Itching in the ears may occur secondary to dry skin in the external canal or an infection in the external canal of the ear, such as swimmer's ear (external otitis).

Ringing in the Ears (Tinnitus)

➤ Describe the noise that you are hearing. Is it ringing, hissing, crackling, or buzzing? If so, when did it start?

■ Ringing of the ears (tinnitus) is a sensation or sound heard only by the affected individual. It can present differently with a variety of sounds or sensations.

➤ Does it occur all of the time, or does it come and go? If it comes and goes, does it occur with certain activities or at the same time of day, such as at night?

■ Establish the pattern of the symptom; this may provide clues to determine the cause of the problem.

➤ Are you currently taking any medications? If so, what are you taking, and when did you start taking the medications? Have you taken the same medication in the past? If so, did it cause any similar problems, such as ringing in the ears?

■ Tinnitus may occur secondary to medications that are ototoxic, such as acetylsalicylic acid (aspirin), quinine, streptomycin, neomycin, gentamicin, furosemide (Lasix), indomethacin (Indocin), or nitrofurantoin.

➤ Have you noticed any other symptoms?

■ Other symptoms may include hearing loss, vertigo, or dizziness.

➤ What have you done to treat the problem? Has it been effective?

■ Explore self-treatment measures and the degree of effectiveness as this may guide further treatment measures.

Hearing Loss

➤ How long have you had the feeling that you are having trouble hearing? Has it occurred suddenly, or has it gradually become worse?

■ Establish onset of problem. It is important to assess if hearing loss has occurred suddenly or over time. A sudden hearing loss in one or both ears that is not associated with an ear infection or upper respiratory infection requires further evaluation. Hearing loss associated with aging (presbycusis) occurs gradually over time and increases with advancing age, particularly at high frequencies.

➤ What type of sounds or tones do you have difficulty hearing? Is there a certain pitch you have trouble hearing, such as conversation on the telephone or an alarm clock ringing? Do people tell you that they have to "shout" for you to hear them?

■ Hearing loss typically first affects high-frequency hearing.

➤ Have you noticed other symptoms associated with the hearing loss?

■ Explore other symptoms such as fevers, headaches, visual changes, etc.

QUESTIONS

➤ To what degree does your hearing loss bother you? Does it interfere in your activities of daily living, such as causing a problem on the job or during telephone conversations? What do you do to cope with your hearing difficulty? Do you find yourself not going out or being with your friends because you have difficulty hearing?

➤ Do you wear a hearing corrective device (e.g., hearing aid)? If so, how long have you worn it? Does it help? Do you wear it all of the time? If not, why not? Do you have any problem with upkeep, cleaning, or changing the batteries?

Dizziness and Vertigo

➤ Do you feel a sensation of faintness (dizziness) or a whirling motion sensation (vertigo)? If so, describe the sensation you are experiencing (Box 15-2).

Box 15-2 Vertigo Versus Dizziness

VERTIGO

The sensation of whirling motion when the client feels himself or herself in motion or the room is spinning. It is a dysfunction of the labyrinth.

DIZZINESS

A sensation of faintness or inability to maintain normal balance in a standing or seated position.

➤ When did the problem start? Does it bother you all of the time, or does the problem come and go?

➤ If the problem comes and goes, do you notice if it occurs at certain times, such as when lying down, standing up, or bending over? Describe.

➤ Have you noticed any other symptoms, such as nausea, vomiting, or visual changes?

➤ Does the problem interfere with your daily activities? Are you able to function adequately? Are you able to drive or go up and down stairs?

RATIONALE

■ Hearing loss may cause individuals to withdraw or become isolated because they cannot hear or because they are embarrassed. This may lead to reduced interpersonal communication, depression, reduced mobility, and exacerbation of coexisting psychiatric conditions.

■ Some clients have hearing devices but do not use them because of the extraneous noise they cause or because the batteries are nonfunctional. If the client has a hearing device but does not wear it, try to determine why.

■ Vertigo may occur secondary to an internal ear problem such as Ménière's disease or medications.

■ Establish the onset and pattern of the problem.

■ Explore for contributing factors to the symptoms.

■ Assess for the presence of associated symptoms.

■ If the client reports dizziness or vertigo as a problem, he or she should be advised about the potential hazard of driving or operating machinery.

EXAMINATION

Equipment

- Otoscope with clean reusable or disposable speculum to visualize the tympanic membrane
- Pneumatic bulb attachment for the otoscope to observe fluctuation of the tympanic membrane
- Tuning forks—500 and 1000 Hz to evaluate hearing frequencies

PROCEDURES AND TECHNIQUES WITH NORMAL FINDINGS

EAR

➤**INSPECT the ears for alignment and position on the head in relation to the outer canthus of the eyes.** The pinna of the ear should align directly with the outer canthus of the eye and be angled no more than 10° from a vertical position (Fig. 15-5).

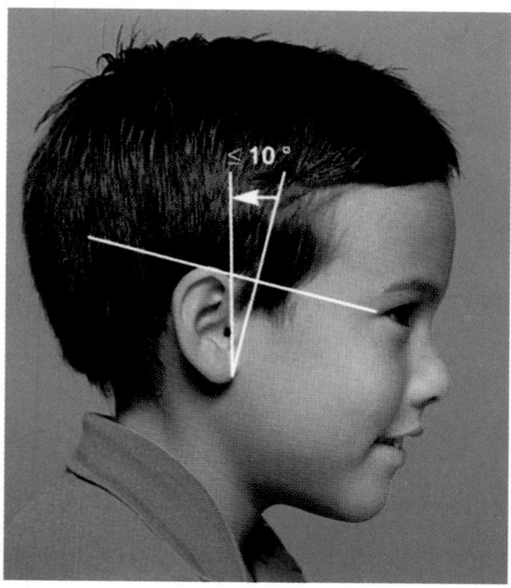

Fig. 15-5 Normal ear position and alignment. (From Wong et al, 1999.)

➤**INSPECT both external ears for size, shape, symmetry, skin color, uniformity, and skin intactness.** The skin should be an even skin tone, with color about the same skin tone as that noted on the face. The color should be uniform throughout. There should be no lesions. A small, painless nodule, called a darwinian tubercle, is a normal deviation and may be noted at the helix of the ear (Fig. 15-6).

ABNORMAL FINDINGS

■ Low-set ears (the pinna is located below the external corner of the eye) or ears that are misaligned (the ear is angled more than 10° from a vertical position) should be considered abnormal. Low-set ears are seen in persons with congenital diseases such as Down syndrome or renal disorder.

■ Abnormal findings include the following:
-*Ear size:* If the ears are smaller than 4 cm in length, they are referred to as microtia ears. Likewise, if the ears are larger than 10 cm in length, they are referred to as macrotia ears.

PROCEDURES AND TECHNIQUES WITH NORMAL FINDINGS

The shape of the earlobes should be noted; three variations are common (Fig. 15-7). If the ears are pierced, note the skin around the piercing for skin intactness, swelling, discharge, or lesions.

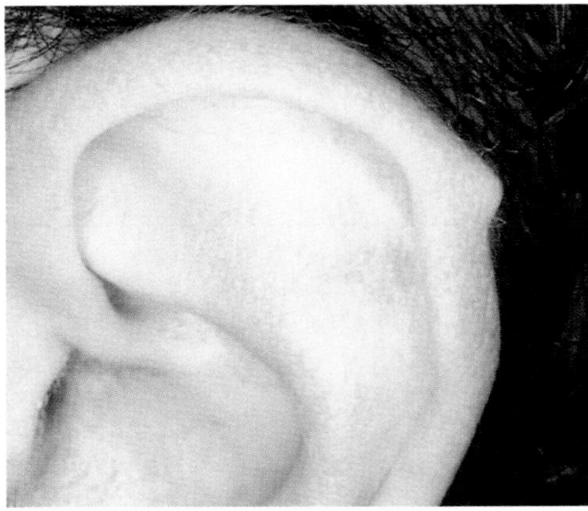

Fig. 15-6 A darwinian tubercle. (From Bingham, Hawke, and Kwok, 1992.)

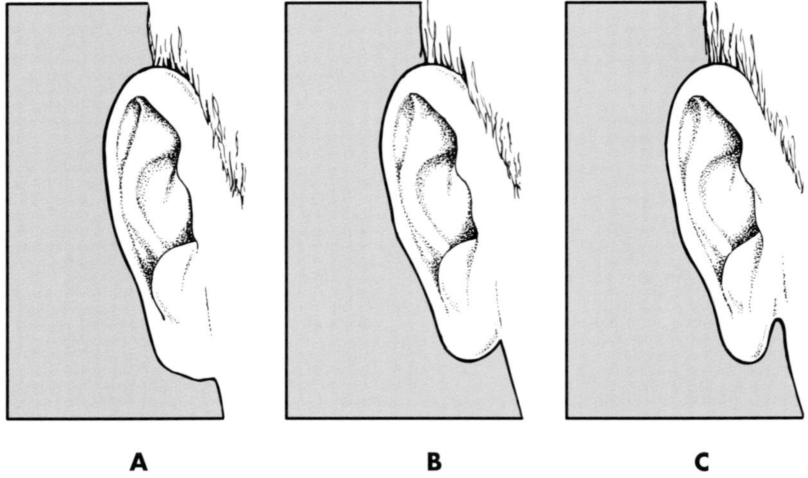

Fig. 15-7 The three common shapes of earlobes. **A,** Soldered. **B,** Attached. **C,** Free. (From Seidel et al, 1999.)

➤**INSPECT the external auditory canal for discharge or lesions.** There should be no lesions or discharge.

➤**PALPATE both external ears and mastoid areas behind the ears for tenderness, swelling, or nodules.** The upper part of the ear should be firm and flexible; the ear lobe should be soft. All areas should be without tenderness or swelling. Gently pull on the helix of the ear to determine if there is any discomfort or pain. There should be none. (Note: If the client complains of a painful ear, always examine the unaffected ear first.)

ABNORMAL FINDINGS

- *Ear shape:* Abnormal findings include lesions or deformities of the external ear, such as nodules, tophi (see Common Problems and Conditions, later in this chapter), sebaceous cysts, or cauliflower ear, which may occur secondary to injury.
- *Ear color:* The color of the ears may change with certain conditions. For example, blueness may indicate cyanosis; redness may indicate flushing, warming after exposure to cold, or vasomotor instability; and pallor may indicate frostbite.
- *Ear swelling or lesions:* These findings with or without discharge may indicate infection.

■ Discharge-clear, purulent, crusty, or bloody—from the ear should be considered abnormal. A bloody or clear discharge from the ear accompanied by a history of head injury should lead to suspicion of possible skull fracture. A purulent or crusty discharge may indicate infection of the external canal, a foreign body, or, if the tympanic membrane has ruptured, infection of middle ear.

■ Tenderness of the mastoid area may indicate mastoiditis. Pain when the helix of the ear is pulled may indicate external ear canal infection.

PROCEDURES AND TECHNIQUES WITH NORMAL FINDINGS

AUDITORY CANAL AND TYMPANIC MEMBRANE

❖ ➤**INSPECT the external auditory canal using an otoscope for tissue swelling or redness, discharge, and cerumen.** If you have a choice of speculum size, always choose the largest speculum that will comfortably fit into the external auditory meatus. To use the otoscope, grasp the pinna of the adult client's ear with one hand and gently pull the helix upward and slightly toward the back of the head (Fig. 15-8). This straightens the S-shaped curve of the auditory canal.

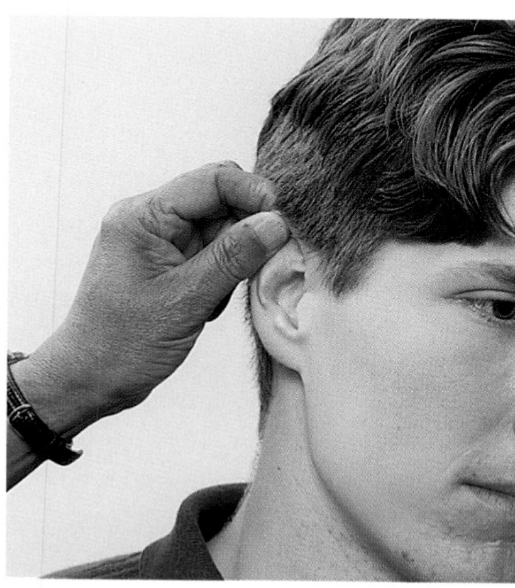

Fig. 15-8 Pull the client's helix upward and slightly toward the back of the head.

With the other hand, gently position the lighted speculum of the otoscope into the client's external auditory canal. Hold the otoscope upside down in the palm of your hand. Rest the back of your hand against the client's temple area to steady the positioning of the otoscope (Fig. 15-9). (An alternative way to hold the otoscope is to hold the handle downward and immobilize the positioning of the speculum by placing the index finger of the hand holding the handle of the otoscope on the client's face.)

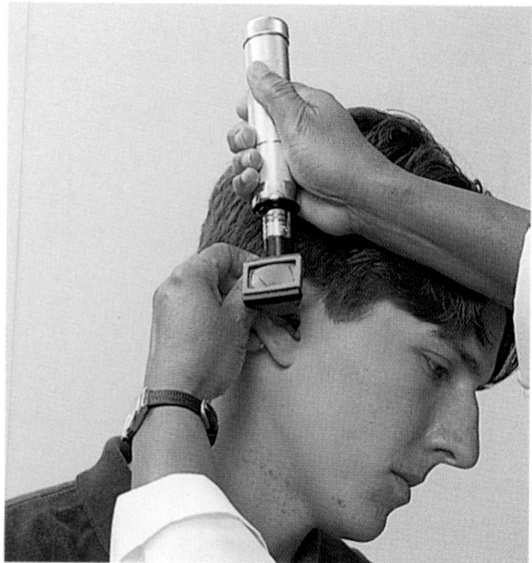

Fig. 15-9 Holding the otoscope "upside down," rest the back of your hand against the client's temple area to steady the otoscope.

ABNORMAL FINDINGS

■ Redness and swelling of the external auditory canal may be an indication of otitis externa. The infection may cause the canal to become swollen and completely closed. Purulent discharge from the auditory canal may occur secondary to otitis externa or, if the tympanic membrane is ruptured, it may be drainage from behind the eardrum. Clear fluid or frank bloody drainage from the auditory canal following a head injury may indicate a basilar skull fracture. To confirm that clear fluid drainage is indeed cerebrospinal fluid, test the drainage with a glucose test strip. Cerebrospinal fluid will test positive for glucose. Other abnormal findings in the auditory canal include the presence of foreign bodies, polyps, exostosis, and furuncles (see photographs in Common Problems and Conditions, later in this chapter).

PROCEDURES AND TECHNIQUES WITH NORMAL FINDINGS

ABNORMAL FINDINGS

Do not release the hand holding the pinna. There must be continuous traction on the pinna throughout the examination of the auditory canal and the tympanic membrane. Watch the insertion of the otoscope as it is placed in the canal, and then look through the lens of the otoscope. Insert the speculum 1.0 to 1.5 cm (½ inch). Be careful not to insert the otoscope speculum into the canal too far. If the speculum touches the bony section of the canal (inner two thirds of the canal), there may be a sensation of pain. If you are unable to see anything but canal walls, reposition the client's head, apply more traction on the pinna, and reangle the otoscope toward the nose.

Once the otoscope is properly positioned, note any evidence of tissue swelling, redness, or discharge along the walls of the canal. Note the amount, color, and characteristics of cerumen. Some cerumen almost always is in the canal, but it should not occlude the canal or obscure the visualization of the tympanic membrane (Fig. 15-10). If this has occurred, the cerumen must be removed before examination can continue (Box 15-3). Note the characteristics of the cerumen. The color may be black, brown, dark red, creamy, to brown-gray. The texture ranges from moist, to dry and flaky, to hard. There should be no odor.

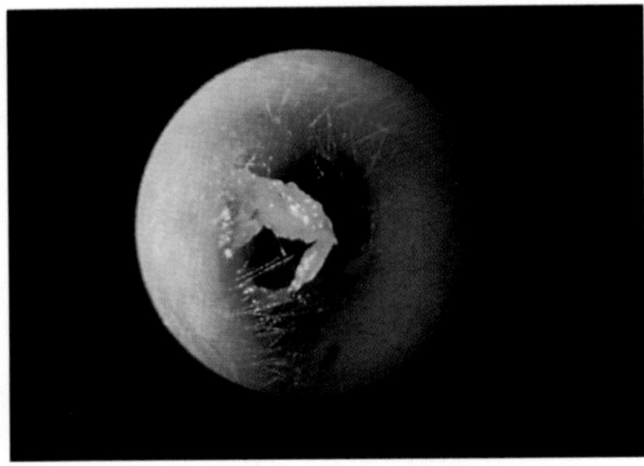

Fig. 15-10 Normal piece of cerumen (earwax) in the external meatus. (From Bingham, Hawke, and Kwok, 1992.)

Box 15-3 Removing Cerumen from Auditory Canal

To remove cerumen from the auditory canal, the examiner may first fill the canal with a cerumen-softening agent. Block the opening of the canal with a cotton ball and wait 5 to 10 minutes. The cerumen may then be easily removed from the canal by irrigating the canal with warm water. Some examiners prefer to remove the cerumen with a cerumen spoon. This technique requires skill so as not to scrape the walls of the canal or injure the tympanic membrane.

CAUTION: *Do not use water irrigation of the canal if any of the following are suspected: otitis externa, tympanic membrane perforation, or myringotomy tubes in place.*

ETHNIC & CULTURAL VARIATIONS

White and dark-skinned races have cerumen that is moist, sticky, and dark. *Asians, American Indians, and Alaskan natives* have cerumen that is generally sparse, dry, flaky, and lighter.

PROCEDURES AND TECHNIQUES WITH NORMAL FINDINGS

❖ ➤**INSPECT the tympanic membrane for landmarks, color, contour, translucence, and fluctuation.** First, locate all landmarks (umbo, handle of the malleus, and light reflex). Next, note the color of the TM, the contour (bulging or retracted), and any indications of perforation. You may need to slightly adjust the light source so that the entire membrane can be evaluated. The TM should be a translucent, pearly-gray color; it should be neither bulging nor retracted, and have no perforations. A cone of light reflex should be prominently noted in the lower anterior quadrant of the drum. (Fig. 15-11).

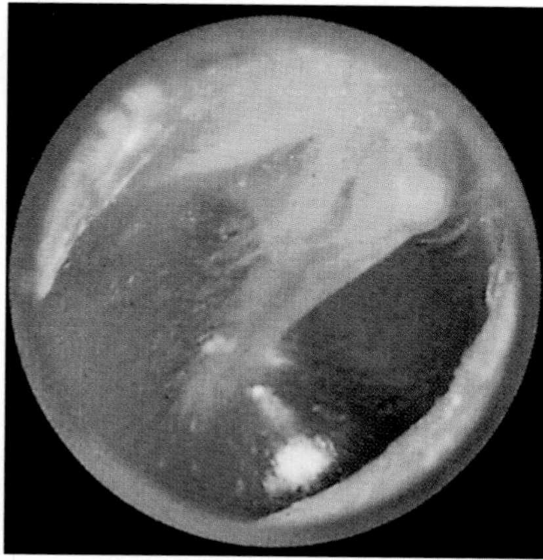

Fig. 15-11 Normal appearance of a tympanic membrane. (Courtesy Dr. Richard A Buckingham, Clinical Professor, Otolaryngology, Abraham Lincoln School of Medicine, University of Illinois, Chicago, Ill. From Barkauskas et al, 1998.)

The fluctuation of the tympanic membrane (TM) (which is a further evaluation to determine if the TM is retracted or bulging) may be done by attaching a pneumatic bulb to the otoscope. To perform this procedure, make sure that the speculum is fully inserted into the canal and that the speculum is large enough to completely occlude the canal. Gently squeeze the bulb so that puffs of air are transmitted to the TM. A normal response is that the TM itself will slightly fluctuate with the puffs of air. This procedure can be performed with any age group, but is most commonly done when examining infants and young children because infants and young children are unable to provide a history regarding the pain they are experiencing the way that older children and adults are able to.

ABNORMAL FINDINGS

■ Absence or distortion of the landmarks on the TM should be considered abnormal.

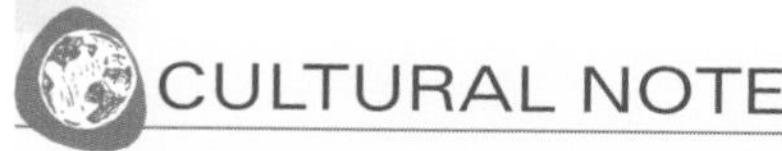

CULTURAL NOTE

American Indian, Alaskan native, and Pacific Islander children have the highest rates of otitis media in the world. African-American children have the lowest incidence.

Variations in the color and characteristics of the TM indicating an abnormality include the following:

- *Yellow/amber:* Serous fluid in the middle ear, which may indicate serous otitis media or chronicotitis media with air bubbles.
- *Redness:* Infection in the middle ear, such as acute purulent otitis media.
- *Chalky white:* Infection in the middle ear, such as otitis media.
- *Blue or deep red:* Blood behind the TM, which may have occurred secondary to injury.
- *Red streaks:* Injected/increased vascularization may be due to allergy.
- *Dullness:* Fibrosis or scarring of the TM secondary to repeated infections.
- *White flecks/plaques:* Healed inflammation of the TM.
- *Air bubbles or a fluid level:* Indicates serous fluid in the middle ear.
- *Perforation of TM* (Fig. 15-12).

Abnormal variations in the mobility of the TM include the following:

- *Bulging of TM with no mobility:* Indicates pus or fluid behind the TM.
- *Retraction of TM with no mobility or mobility of the TM with negative pressure only:* Indicates obstruction of the eustachian tube.
- *Increased mobility of only one part of the TM:* Indicates an area of healed TM perforation.

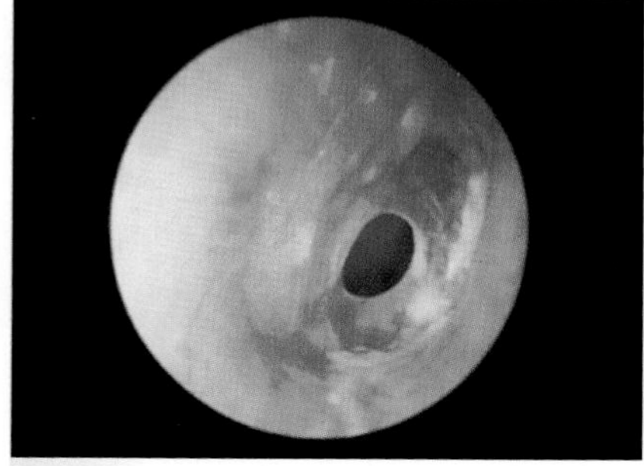

Fig. 15-12 Perforated tympanic membrane. (From Bingham, Hawke, and Kwok, 1992.)

PROCEDURES AND TECHNIQUES WITH NORMAL FINDINGS

ABNORMAL FINDINGS

HEARING

➤**ASSESS client's responses to questions.** As you conduct the history and perform the hearing assessment, watch the client's response. A client's ability to engage in conversation is considered a normal finding.

■ Subtle indications of hearing loss include such signs as the following:
-Asking you to repeat the question.
-Repeated misunderstanding of the questions you ask.
-Garbled speech sounds with word distortion.
-Leaning forward, tilting head, frowning, and seeming to watch your lips as you speak.
-Speaking in a loud voice that may be monotone.

➤**TEST the acoustic cranial nerve (VIII) to evaluate auditory function. The following tests are used for screening only and should not be considered diagnostic of a hearing problem.**

Whispered Voice Test This is considered the best among simple tests to identify clients with hearing loss in an office or clinic setting (Eckhoff et al, 1996). Stand 1 to 2 feet in front of or to the side of the client. Instruct the client to cover one ear with his or her hand so that one ear may be tested at a time. Shield your mouth so that the client cannot read your lips. Softly whisper several monosyllabic (e.g., ball, chair, cat) and disyllabic (e.g., streetcar, baseball, highchair) words. The client should be able to hear at least 50% of all words whispered. Repeat the procedure with the other ear. A variance in results can occur between examiners due to loudness of whispering. It is important to be aware of the volume of the whispers during the screening (Eeckhoff et al, 1996).

■ It should be considered abnormal if the client cannot repeat at least 50% of the spoken words. Consider each ear separately.

Finger-Rubbing Test A gross hearing test may be done by holding your hand 3 to 4 inches from the client's ear and briskly rubbing your index finger against your thumb. The client should be able to hear the noise generated by rubbing the fingers together. Repeat the technique with the other ear.

■ Clients with a high-frequency hearing loss may not be able to hear the noise generated by your fingers. Consider each ear separately.

Rinne Test This test uses a tuning fork to compare air conduction (AC) to bone conduction (BC). The AC route through the ear canal is a more sensitive route. To activate the tuning fork, hold it by the base stem and softly strike the forked section against the back of your hand. (If you strike the fork too hard, the tone is too loud and it will take a long time to fade out.) Place the base of the tuning fork directly on the client's mastoid process (Fig. 15-13, *A*). Begin timing

■ Consider the test abnormal when the sound is heard longer by bone conduction than air conduction or when AC is not twice as long as BC.

A

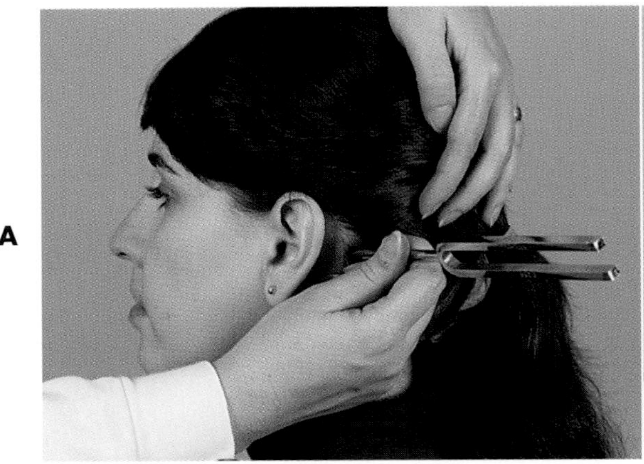

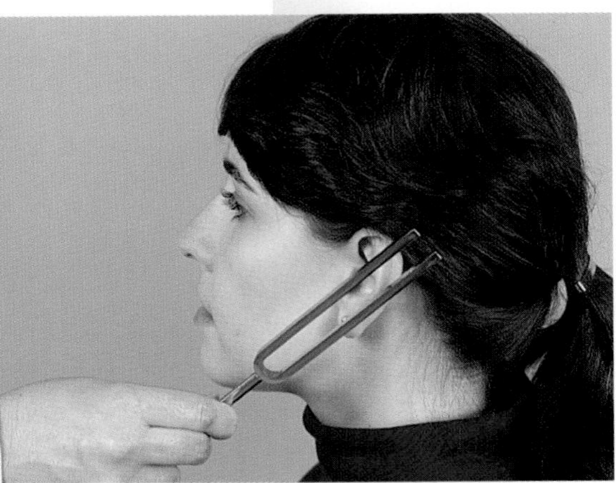

B

Fig. 15-13 Rinne test. **A,** The tuning fork is placed on the mastoid bone for bone conduction. **B,** The tuning fork is placed in front of the ear for air conduction. (From Seidel et al, 1999.)

PROCEDURES AND TECHNIQUES WITH NORMAL FINDINGS

by counting the seconds. The client should be able to hear the tone. Instruct the client to tell you when the tone can no longer be heard. At that time, note the number of seconds counted; quickly remove the fork from the mastoid process, invert the fork, and hold the vibrating section of the tuning fork in front of the client's ear (Fig. 15-13, *B*). Begin timing again. The client should be able to hear the tone again. Instruct the client to tell you when the vibration is no longer heard. Note the time. The tone heard in front of the ear should last twice as long as the tone heard when the fork was on the mastoid process (AC > BC [2:1]) (Fig. 15-15). This is the normal, or positive, response. Repeat the test with the other ear.

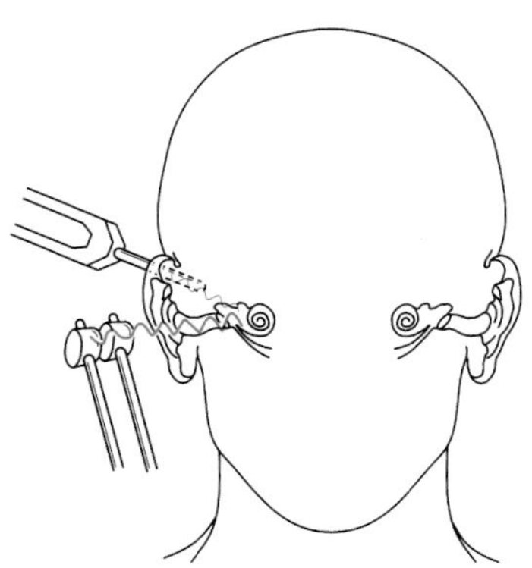

Fig. 15-15. Illustration depicting expected client perception of hearing with Rinne test. Air conduction is twice as long as bone conduction. (From Barkauskas et al, 1998.)

ABNORMAL FINDINGS

- Clients with conductive hearing loss will have bone conduction longer than air conduction in the affected ear (Fig. 15-14, *A*).
- Clients with sensorineural hearing loss will have air conduction longer than bone conduction in the affected ear, but it will be less than 2:1 ratio (Fig. 15-14, *B*).

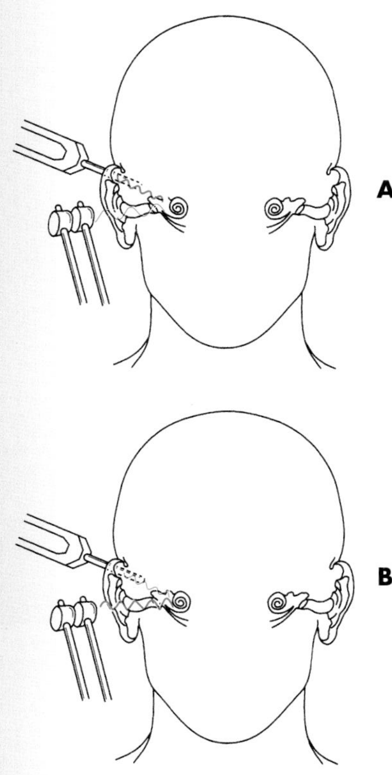

Fig. 15-14. **A,** Client with conduction loss will hear bone conduction longer than air conduction (BC > AC). **B,** Client with sensorineural loss will hear air conduction longer than bone conduction (AC > BC), but duration is less than 2:1. (From Barkauskas et al, 1998.)

PROCEDURES AND TECHNIQUES WITH NORMAL FINDINGS

Weber's Test This test assesses bone conduction by testing the lateralization of sounds. Softly strike the tuning fork and place it on the midline of the client's skull (Fig. 15-16). The client should hear the tone equally in both ears (Fig. 15-17).

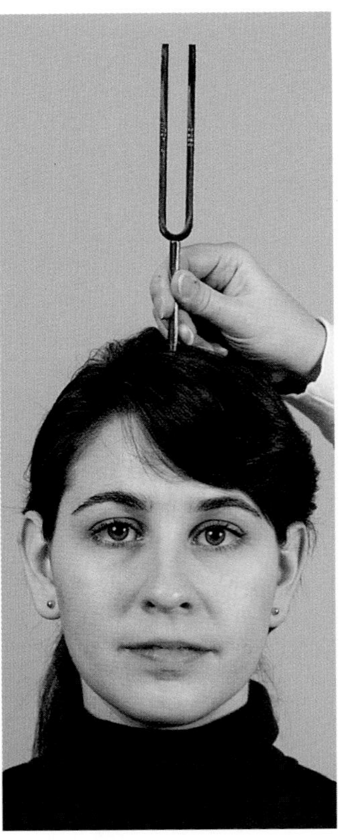

Fig. 15-16 Weber's test. The tuning fork is placed on the midline of the skull. (From Seidel et al, 1999.)

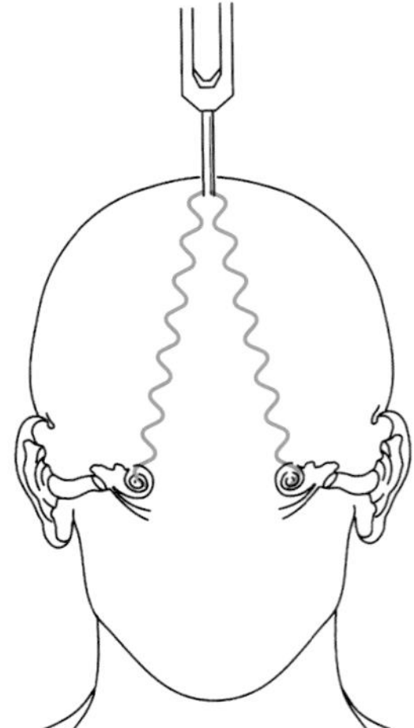

Fig. 15-17 Illustration depicting expected (normal) client perception of hearing with Weber's test; sound is heard equally well in both ears. (From Barkauskas et al, 1998.)

ABNORMAL FINDINGS

■ When the sound lateralizes to one side and the client hears the tone better in one ear than the other, the test should be considered abnormal.
- Clients with conductive hearing loss will have a lateralization of sound to the deaf ear (Fig. 15-18, *A*).
- Clients with sensorineural hearing loss will have lateralization of sound to the better ear (Fig. 15-18, *B*).

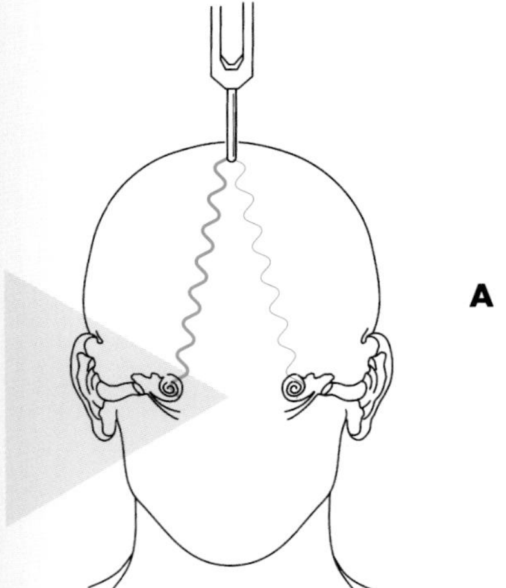

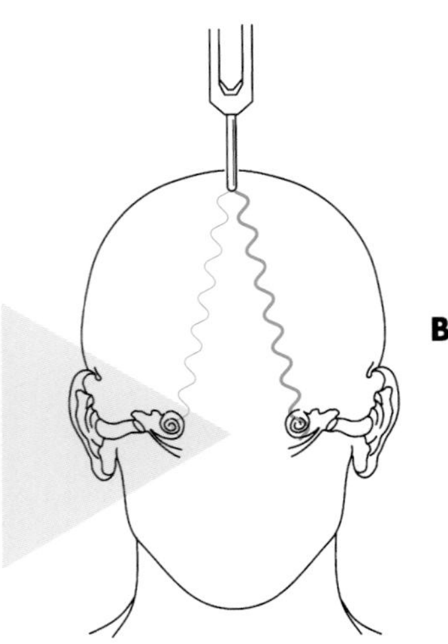

Fig. 15-18 **A,** Client with conduction loss; sound lateralizes to the defective ear *(shaded area)* because the sound transmits through the bone rather than air. **B,** Client with sensorineural loss; sound lateralizes to the unaffected ear. (From Barkauskas et al, 1998.)

PROCEDURES AND TECHNIQUES WITH NORMAL FINDINGS

➤TEST the acoustic cranial nerve (VIII) to evaluate vestibular function. Romberg's test assesses the ability of the vestibular apparatus in the inner ear to help maintain standing balance. To evaluate it, ask the client to stand in front of you and facing you. Instruct the client to stand with his or her feet together, arms at the side, and eyes closed. Wait 20 seconds and watch the client's swaying and ability to maintain balance. The client may sway slightly but should be able to maintain the balance without stepping sideways (Fig. 15-19). (Stay close to the client to offer balance support if necessary.)

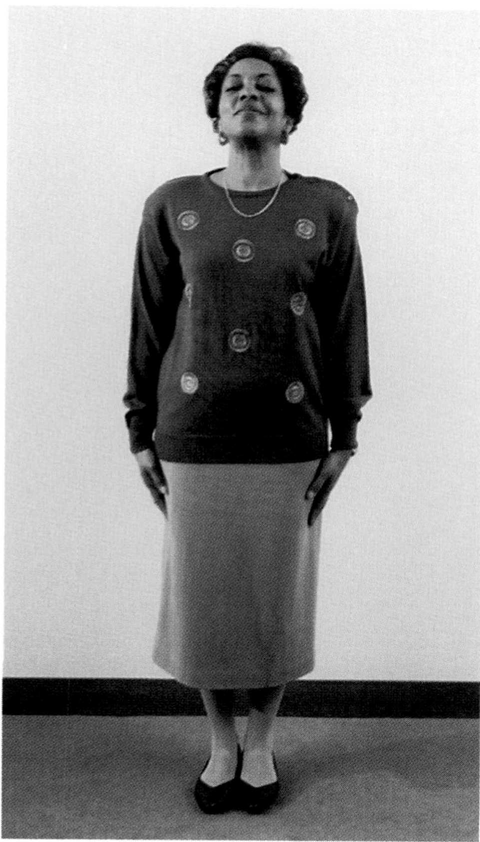

Fig. 15-19 Romberg's test evaluates client's balance. Offer balance support to the client if necessary to prevent falls. (From Sigler and Schuring, 1993.)

ABNORMAL FINDINGS

■ If the client is unable to maintain his or her position, steps sideways, or widens the base of support, the test should be considered abnormal, or positive. A positive finding suggests an inner ear or cerebellar problem.

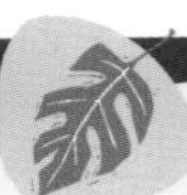

AGE-RELATED VARIATIONS

INFANTS

Anatomy and Physiology

The inner ear develops during the first trimester of pregnancy; an insult to the fetus during that time may impair hearing. The infant's eustachian tube is wider and, at the same time, shorter and more horizontal than the adult's. Unfortunately, this makes the infant prone to ear infection because pathogens easily migrate from the nasopharynx to the middle ear.

Health History

Questions asked to the parent of an infant help to rule out the presence of hearing disability.

- Does the infant jump, startle, or cry when there is a bang or loud noise? Does the older infant turn his or her head toward a noise?

  Rationale Infants should respond to noise in the environment. The parent may be the first to notice that the infant does not respond to noise.

- Did the mother have any viral infections while pregnant, such as syphilis or meningitis? Any x-ray examinations while pregnant? Did the mother drink alcohol or smoke tobacco while pregnant? If so, how much? Did the mother have diabetes or high blood pressure while pregnant?

  Rationale A prenatal history may also provide information about infants at risk for hearing impairment.

- How much did the infant weigh at birth? Were there any congenital infections following birth, such as rubella or meningitis? Were any congenital defects noted at birth, such as cleft palate or malformations of the face or head? Was there any birth trauma or perinatal asphyxia? Was the baby jaundiced? Did the baby have high bilirubin levels following birth? Was the baby premature or in the newborn intensive care unit following birth?

  Rationale Infants at risk for hearing impairment should be identified.

Examination

Procedures and Techniques Congenital abnormalities may be found with careful examination of a newborn infant's ears. Examine the shape and position of the ears the same way as previously described for the adult.

Examine the auditory canal and tympanic membrane. To ensure safety, the infant must be securely immobilized during this part of the examination. The infant may be placed

RISK FACTORS

COMMON RISK FACTORS ASSOCIATED WITH Congenital or Perinatal Hearing Loss

- Family history of hereditary childhood sensorineural hearing loss
- Preterm infants
- Infants born weighing less than 1500 g
- Congenital perinatal infection involving herpes, syphilis, rubella, cytomegaloviris, or toxoplasmosis
- Congenital malformations such as cleft palate and abnormal pinna
- Perinatal infection such as bacterial meningitis
- Hyperbilirubinemia requiring blood transfusion
- Perinatal asphyxia
  - Apgar scores of 0 to 4 at 1 minute or 0 to 6 at 5 minutes
  - Absence of spontaneous respiration for 10 minutes
- Administration of ototoxic medications

Data from U.S. Preventive Task Force: *Guide to clinical preventive services,* ed 2, Baltimore, Md, 1996, Williams & Wilkins.

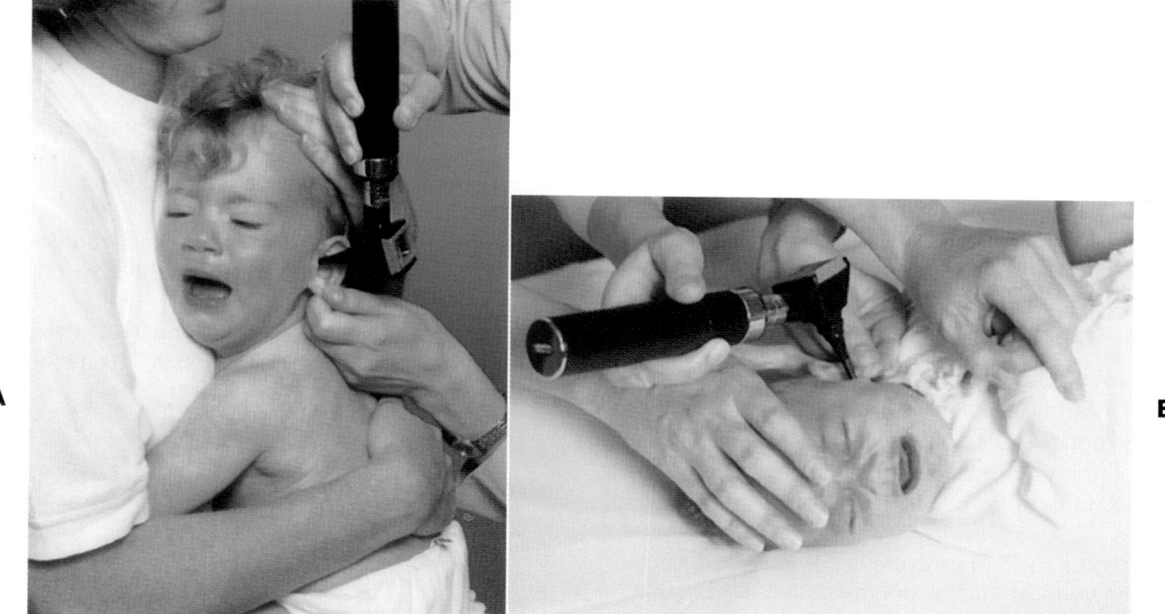

Fig. 15-20 Immobilization of young child or infant during otoscopic examination. Note that lower portion of pinna of ear is pulled down and slightly backward. **A,** Prone position. **B,** Supine position. (From Wong et al, 1999.)

in either a prone or supine position. For prone position, instruct the "holder" to secure the infant's arms down at the side with one hand and turn and hold the infant's head to one side with the other hand (Fig. 15-20, *A*). You must have both hands free to hold the helix of the ear and maneuver the otoscope. If supine, have a "holder" secure the infant's arms down at the sides with one hand and turn and immobilize the head to one side with the other (Fig. 15-20, *B*).

To optimize visualization of the ear canal and tympanic membrane, you must alter the method of holding the auricle of the ear. For infants and children up to age 3 years, grasp the lower portion of the pinna and apply gentle traction down and slightly backward (as opposed to pulling the pinna of the ear up and back for the adult). This maneuver straightens the canal of the ear. A simple hearing screening should also be included with the examination. Gross screening of the newborn's ability to hear may be conducted by eliciting a loud noise (e.g., clapping hands or ringing bell) and observing the infant's body movement, startle response, or cry in response to the auditory stimuli.

Normal and Abnormal Findings The external ear should be well formed, appear smooth and intact, and have no skin tags or other formations. Low-set ears or ears with angulation greater than 10° may be an indication of a congenital problem such as Down syndrome. The TM of the infant may be difficult to visualize because it is more horizontal. The TM may appear slightly reddened secondary to crying. Also, because the TM does not become conical for several months, the light reflex may appear diffuse. By age 6 months, the infant's TM takes on an adult type of appearance and is easier to visualize and examine.

By age 4 to 6 months the infant should turn the head toward the source of the sound, should respond to the parent's voice, and should respond to music toys. By 6 to 10 months the child should respond to his or her name and follow sounds. Abnormal responses should be confirmed by repeat testing. Referral for ongoing audiologic assessment is encouraged for infants with abnormal responses and for many high-risk infants (U.S. Preventive Services Task Force, 1996).

CHILDREN

Anatomy and Physiology

As the child grows, ear infections usually become less frequent because the eustachian tube lengthens and its pharyngeal orifice moves inferiorly. However, with the growth of lymphatic tissue, specifically the adenoids, the eustachian tube may become occluded, interfering with aeration of the middle ear.

Health History

Younger Children

- Does the child behave in any way that indicates that there may be a hearing problem, such as not babbling by 6 months or not reacting to loud or strange noises, no attempts at communicative speech by 15 months, not seeming to communicate or be attentive to peers of the same age?

  Rationale If a hearing problem is not identified at infancy, it may be identified when the parent notices that the young child is not making noises or talking like other children of a similar age.
- If the child is talking, at what age did the talking begin? How difficult is it for you to understand the child's language?

  Rationale If the child has a hearing problem, he or she will not be able to imitate sounds or words. Language development is significantly affected by hearing impairment (Mannina, 1997).
- Have you ever had your child's hearing tested? If so, at what age and for what reason? What were the results?

  Rationale Collect baseline information.
- Does the child have frequent ear infections? If so, how old was the child with the first infection? How many ear infections has the child had during the past 6 months? What has been done to treat these infections? Are the infections increasing in frequency or severity?

  Rationale If the child has more than two or three ear infections (otitis media) each year, the child is said to be "otitis-prone." Chronic ear infections may be associated with delays in language development (Mannina, 1997).
- If otitis media is suspected, ask: Does the child seem to pull at the ears? If so, which one?

  Rationale Children suffering from an ear infection are frequently observed to pull at their ear.
- Has the child ever had ear surgery, such as having tubes placed in the ears?

  Rationale The placement of tubes in the ears (myringotomy) is generally an indication that the child has had numerous ear infections. The tubes are placed as a method to prevent recurrent infections.

Older Children

- Do you swim? If so, does the water ever bother your ears? Do you wear earplugs?

  Rationale Frequent swimming may put the susceptible child at greater risk for external ear canal infections.
- Do you have any trouble hearing things that you think you should hear? Do you have trouble hearing the teacher at school?

  Rationale Hearing loss in the school-age child may occur secondary to otitis media with middle ear effusion and is usually self-limiting. A second common cause of hearing difficulty in the child is the build-up of cerumen in the external ear canal.
- Ask the caregiver: Does the child have trouble learning or engage in disruptive behavior in school, or does the child act withdrawn?

  Rationale Academic progress may be affected by chronic otitis media (Mannina, 1997). Disruptive behavior may be a result of a sensory deficit.

Examination

Procedures and Techniques The biggest challenge to examining the ears of the young child is immobilization. Immobilize the child in either the supine or prone position as discussed previously. Inadequate immobilization can result in pain to the child and also may cause injury to the ear canal itself. If the child is fearful, screaming, or uncooperative, the examiner should place his or her hand against the head of the child to protect the ear canal from sudden movement or jolt (E.S. Miola, 1994). Because the otoscope examination may be perceived as traumatic by the young child, it may be deferred until the very last procedure of the entire examination. If the child becomes upset during the examination, be sure to quickly return the child to the parent for comforting.

As the child becomes older, the examiner should take the time to elicit the child's cooperation during the examination. If time is taken, and the child is reassured, the examination should not be traumatic. Nevertheless, if the examiner has any question regarding the child's ability to hold perfectly still during the otoscope examination, the parent or adult who is with the child should assist in immobilizing the child to ensure the child's safety.

The procedure for examination proceeds similarly as previously discussed for the adult. If the child is less than 3 years of age, the pinna of the ear should be pulled down during the examination as described for the infant. If the child is older, the pinna should be pulled up and backward as for the adult. Routine hearing screening of asymptomatic children beyond 3 years of age is not recommended (U.S. Preventive Services Task Force, 1996).

Normal and Abnormal Findings The findings of the examination do not differ significantly from the adult. Young children are at risk for insertion of foreign bodies into their ears. All children presenting with suspect history should be carefully examined.

A common, normal variation of the TM is the presence of myringotomy tubes (Fig. 15-21). These are small polyethylene tubes surgically placed through the tympanic membrane to relieve middle ear pressure and to permit drainage of fluid or material collected behind the TM. They

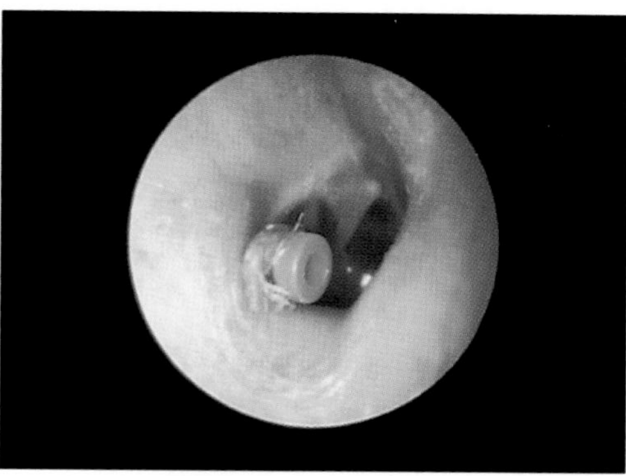

Fig. 15-21 Tympanotomy tube protruding from the right tympanic membrane. (From Bingham, Hawke, and Kwok, 1992.)

are most commonly put in the ears of young children because of recurrent ear infections. Usually they will spontaneously work their way out of the TM within 6 to 12 months after insertion.

The pneumatic bulb is frequently used with young and older children to evaluate fluctuation (mobility) of the TM. Review the adult section for the procedure and anticipated findings.

Hearing evaluation of the young child may be necessary if the parent or examiner perceives that the child has some type of lag related to the child's developmental milestones. Behavioral manifestations that may indicate hearing impairment include delay in verbalization skills; speech that is monotone, garbled, or difficult to understand; inattentiveness during conversation; facial expressions that appear strained or puzzled; withdrawal and lack of interaction with others; asking "What?" a lot or asking for statements to be repeated; or having frequent earaches.

ADOLESCENTS

Health History

- Do you participate in contact sports? If so, which ones? How often? What kind of head protection is used?
  Rationale Adolescents participating in contact sports such as wrestling, boxing, football, rugby, or soccer should be carefully assessed and educated about ear protection and injury prevention.
- Do you listen to loud music or go places where there is loud noise, such as a concert? If so, does the noise hurt your ears? How often do you listen to loud music?
  Rationale Repeated exposure to loud noise, such as music concerts, starting this early in life places the individual at risk for long-term, nonreversible hearing loss. Risk education may be indicated.

Examination

Procedures and Techniques The procedure for examination is the same as the adult. If the adolescent is at risk for hearing injury due to noise or injury and has not had a baseline test, testing may be warranted.

Box 15-4 Hearing Loss Statistics in Middle-Age Adults, Older Adults, and Old-Old Adults

Middle-age adults (51 to 65 years of age)—25% of population in this age group have early changes in hearing loss that may go unnoticed.

Older adults (65 to 85 years of age)—33% of population in this age group have documented hearing loss.

Old-old adults (85 years and older)—50% of population in this age group have documented hearing loss.

Data from U.S. Preventive Services Task Force: *Guide to clinical preventive services,* ed 2, Baltimore, Md, 1996, Williams & Wilkens.

Normal and Abnormal Findings The findings are the same as those for the adult.

OLDER ADULTS

Anatomy and Physiology

An almost inevitable consequence of advancing age is some degree of hearing loss. Generally speaking, the older the individual, the more structural and functional changes occur. This is reflected by statistics of individuals with hearing loss by age groups (Box 15-4). As the individual ages, the cartilage formation may make the auricle larger and more prominent. A decrease in active sebaceous glands causes the cerumen to become very dry, and this dry cerumen may completely obstruct the external auditory canal. As a result, hearing is diminished. In addition, the tympanic membrane becomes more translucent and sclerotic, causing conductive hearing loss.

As the hair cells in the organ of Corti begin to degenerate, hearing tends to deteriorate, usually after the age of 50. The stria vascularis, a network of capillaries that secrete endolymph and promote sensitization of hair cells in the cochlea, may atrophy with age, contributing to hearing loss. In addition, sensorineural hearing loss first occurs with high-frequency sounds and then progresses to lower-frequency tones. An excess deposition of bone cells along the ossicle chain can cause fixation of the stapes in the oval window; as a result, hearing further deteriorates.

Health History

Older adults face a gradual loss of hearing due to sensorineural changes of the organ of Corti. The questions already presented in the adult section related to hearing loss, ototoxic medications, and hearing aids should be asked. In addition, a careful history should be taken regarding dizziness and balance, which may have a root cause in the inner ears and put the client at risk for falling and injury.

Examination

Procedures and Techniques Examination of the older adult should proceed as previously discussed with adults. While obtaining a history, the examiner should specifically observe for subtle indications of hearing loss as described previously. If the client wears a hearing device, the ear should be carefully examined, and assessed for any skin irritation or sores that may be secondary to the molded device.

Normal and Abnormal Findings Physical characteristics of the older adult that are slightly different from those of the younger adult include pendulous and linear wrinkling to the earlobes; there may be the presence of or an increase in wiry hair in the opening of the auditory canal; and the tympanic membrane may appear whiter, opaque, and thickened. If the client wears a hearing device, there is an increased likelihood of cerumen impaction.

CLIENTS WITH SITUATIONAL VARIATIONS

CLIENTS WITH IMPAIRED HEARING

Health History

To obtain a history of an individual with hearing impairment, first determine to what degree the client can or cannot hear. Hearing loss spans a continuum from diminished auditory acuity to profound deafness. Knowing what type of hearing loss the client has will help to determine your approach. An adult client who has been deaf since birth may have very different coping and communicating skills from a client who suddenly lost hearing secondary to an injury or an older adult who just can no longer hear well. Inquire specifically about the reason for and type of hearing loss; the length of time that the client has had a hearing loss; adaptation to the hearing loss; most common methods of communication; difficulties with communication if any; and knowledge of services and resources for individuals with hearing impairment.

If the client is profoundly deaf and communicates by sign language, and you do not sign, it is best to arrange the client's examination so that someone can be with the client who both signs and speaks. If the client reads lips and can speak, then you may be able to communicate. If, on the other hand, the client reads lips but cannot speak, an interpreter is again required. While communication may be done by writing questions and answers back and forth, it is a laborious task and not desirable. If you are interacting with a client who reads lips, or a client who has diminished hearing, remember to speak slowly and distinctly and to face the client directly so that he or she can see your face.

Examination

❖ Examination of hearing requires referral to a health care provider proficient in evaluation of hearing loss. Hearing loss can occur in low, medium, or high frequencies or in a combination. Hearing is measured in decibels (dB). A decibel is a ratio that compares the relationship between two sound intensities. Hearing loss is also classified by the decibel level as recorded on an audiogram. Hearing loss measurements are as follows:

0-25 dB	Normal hearing range
30 dB	Mild hearing impairment
31-55 dB	Moderate hearing impairment
56-70 dB	Moderate to severe hearing impairment
70-90 dB	Severe hearing impairment
$>$ 90 dB	Profoundly deaf

(Goldblum and Collier, 1996.)

EXAMINATION SUMMARY

Ears and Auditory System

Procedure

External Ear

- Inspect both external ears for:
  Alignment and position
  Size
  Shape
  Symmetry
  Skin color
  Uniformity
  Skin intactness
- Inspect external auditory canal for:
  Discharge or lesions
- Palpate both external ears and mastoid areas for:
  Tenderness, swelling, or nodules

Auditory Canal and Tympanic Membrane

- Inspect the external auditory canal for:
  Tissue swelling or redness
  Discharge
  Cerumen (amount and characteristics).
- ❖ Inspect the tympanic membrane for:
  Landmarks
  Color
  Contour
  Translucence
  Fluctuation of membrane (if appropriate)

Hearing

- Assess client's response to questions.
- Test acoustic cranial nerve (VIII) to evaluate auditory function:
  Whispered voice test
  Finger-rubbing test
  Rinne test
  Weber's test
- Test acoustic cranial nerve (VIII) to evaluate vestibular function:
  Romberg's test

SUMMARY OF FINDINGS

Age Group	Normal Findings	Typical Variations	Findings Associated With Disorders
Infants and children	• *Eustachian tube:* Wide and short in infant. • *Hearing test:* Responds to noise with startle reflex or turning head toward noise.	• *Tympanic membrane:* May appear red if child has been crying. • *Cone of light reflex:* May appear diffuse before 6 months of age.	• Foreign objects in ear canal. • Otitis media. • Does not respond to noise.
Adolescents	• Same as for adult.	• Same as for adult.	• Hearing loss most commonly associated with exposure to loud noise.
Adult	• *Pinna of ear:* Should align with the outer canthus of eye; angled no more than 10° from vertical position. • *Auricle of ear:* Same color as facial skin. • *Tympanic membrane:* Translucent with bony landmarks and cone of light apparent. • *Hearing tests:* Hears well. • *Romberg's test:* Maintains balance with eyes closed.	• Darwinian tubercle. • *Cerumen:* Color black, brown, dark red, creamy, or brown-gray; texture ranges from moist to dry.	• *Ears:* Low-set ears; lesions on ears; discharge from ears. • *External ear canal:* Redness/swelling. • *Tympanic membrane:* Appears yellow, red, chalky white, blue, has red streaks. • Hearing loss. • *Balance:* Unable to maintain with eyes closed.
Older adults	• Hearing starts to deteriorate from hair cell degeneration in organ of Corti and cochlea.	• Sclerotic changes in tympanic membrane. • Conductive hearing loss.	• Presbycusis caused by changes in inner ear or nerve.

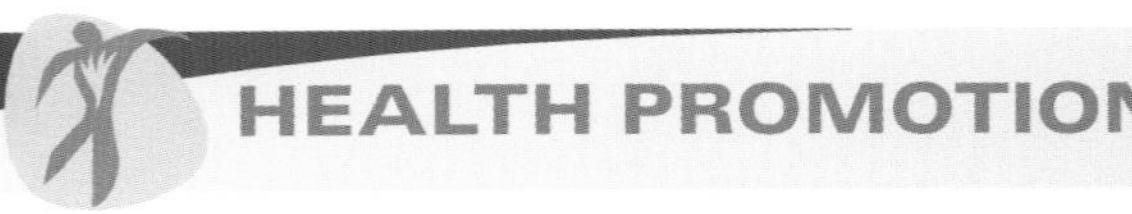

HEALTH PROMOTION

PROTECTION FROM NOISE

Repeated exposure to an excess of constant loud noise (>80 dB) in the work place, at home, or during recreational activities is the major cause of permanent hearing loss. Table 15-1 lists common representative sounds and their decibel levels.

The National Institute for Occupational Safety and Health (NIOSH) estimates that 30 million workers are exposed to hazardous levels of noise (NIOSH, 1996). Although most occupational workplaces have noise-level thresholds above which earplugs or ear protectors must be worn, farms and agricultural settings have virtually no regulations. Thus one occupational group that has a high incidence of hearing loss are farmers and agricultural workers who operate farm machinery. Children and adolescents are another group at high risk for repeated hazardous noise exposure. Music and rock concerts are known for loud music in a confined space. Persons living near airports are passively exposed to loud noises every day, and even though they may "tune them out," the chronic repeated noise may affect their hearing over time.

Teach clients and their families to be aware of hazardous noise levels and then to either limit their exposure to such noise or consistently wear protective earplugs or ear protectors (also called noise defenders). Teach clients to monitor the presence of noise. One way to monitor noise is to listen for a ringing in the ears. If the ears are ringing from noise, ear damage and hearing loss may occur. The best noise defender is one that is comfortable to wear. Different types of noise defenders are available, made from various materials, including sponge rubber, soft rubber, dense cotton, and molded materials. The client should be advised to try several different types. The one that is most comfortable and blocks the greatest amount of noise will be the one that the client will most likely consistently wear.

Table 15-1 Noise Levels

DECIBELS (dB)	REPRESENTATIVE SOUND
0	Softest sound normal ear can hear
10	Heartbeat, rustling of leaves
20	Whisper from 5 feet (1.5 m)
30-40	Normal conversation
60	Noise in average restaurant
17-80	Street noises
80	Loud radio in home
90-100	Train
120	Thunder, rock music
140	Jet airplane during takeoff
>140	Pain threshold

If the client is repeatedly exposed to very loud noises, earmuffs are the only defender that will protect the ears. Earmuffs also vary in type. Under rare circumstances, both ear canal noise defenders and earmuffs may be warranted.

Routine Hearing Screening and Examination

Screening for hearing impairment is routinely done only for certain population groups. All high-risk neonates (see Box 15-4) should be screened prior to discharge from the hospital at birth. If not tested during the birth admission, they should be screened by age 3 months (U.S. Preventive Services Task Force, 1996). Routine screening for other children is not indicated unless conditions exist that suggest a possible hearing impairment. Delayed or difficult language development, learning disabilities, or behavior problems may warrant screening. Screening of asymptomatic adolescents and adults is not necessary except those who are exposed regularly to excessive noise. Screening of workers exposed to excessive occupational noise should be performed in the context of existing work-site programs and guidelines. Older adults should be periodically evaluated to determine changes in their hearing status.

Cleaning of the Ears

Cerumen (earwax) is healthy and serves to actually clean the ears. The sticky nature of the cerumen catches foreign debris in the ear. Most of the time, the ear canals are self-cleaning due to the migration of the wax. If cerumen accumulates and actually blocks the canal, hearing is impaired and the canal must be cleaned.

There are three methods to clean the cerumen from the ear canal. The first is to carefully use a cotton swab. Only the cotton portion should be placed in the ear. Once it is in place, rotate the swab to clean the distal portion of the ear canal. Caution is necessary because if the applicator is inserted too far in the canal, or if the arm is bumped while the applicator is in the ear, damage to the ear canal and tympanic membrane may result. Also, the cotton swab may actually push the cerumen deeper into the canal, causing cerumen impaction.

The second method of cleaning the ear canal is to irrigate the canal with water, using a rubber ear syringe. With this method, use warm water and vigorously but carefully flush the ear. The water will run quickly in and out, so be sure to position the head over a sink or basin. Warn the client that a lot of noise will be generated as water is forced into the ear. If the water is too warm or too cold, temporary dizziness may result. If irrigation causes pain, stop immediately; the tympanic membrane may be ruptured.

The third method to remove excessive cerumen is to instill ear drops that soften and remove the cerumen.

Frequently drops alone are not adequate to clean the wax, especially if there is a large amount of cerumen deep in the canal. In this case, it may be more effective to use a combination of softening drops and warm water irrigation. If this is done, it is best to place the ear drops in the ear canal and plug the ear canal with a cotton ball for 5 to 10 minutes, then irrigate as described above. This combination is usually very successful.

FOREIGN BODIES IN THE EAR

Young children are notorious for putting everything they can find into their mouths, noses, and sometimes ears. Parents must be taught about the hazards of small children having access to objects small enough to be placed in the ear. Parents should also be advised that if a foreign body in the ear is suspected, they should *not* attempt to remove it at home by themselves; rather they should take the child to a health care provider for foreign body removal.

Reasons to avoid removal of a foreign body at home are numerous and include the following: (1) the object may be pushed further into the ear canal; (2) any object the parent may use to "get the object out of the ear" may actually damage the wall of the ear canal, setting up the possibility of a secondary infection; (3) if the parent does not adequately immobilize the child, the child may jerk during the parent's attempt to remove the object and further injure the ear from the sudden movement; and finally, (4) should the parent believe that the foreign body can be flushed out with water without knowing exactly what the foreign body is, further problems may develop. If the object is a food substance such as a bean or a piece of corn, the object may swell in the ear canal.

Foreign bodies that may be a problem for persons of all ages are insects. All persons should be advised about this risk, especially if they spend a lot of time outdoors. If a bug crawls into the ear, the individual will experience a great deal of noise and potentially pain from the insect movement within the ear. This will continue until the bug is killed or removed. One safe way to kill the creature is to suffocate it by placing some mineral oil in the ear canal. Advise individuals to go to a health care provider for insect removal to ensure that the insect is removed correctly and to ensure that the ear canal has not been damaged by the insect.

COMMON PROBLEMS AND CONDITIONS

Ears and Auditory System

EXTERNAL EAR

Hematoma

An acute hematoma of the auricle is most commonly caused by direct trauma (Fig. 15-22). This trauma could be caused by a contact sport (such as football, rugby, wrestling) or a blow to the side of the head (trauma from a motor vehicle accident, or assault). It is important to note that when observed in infants and young children, child abuse should be suspected (Monteleone, 1996). Repeated injury results in cauliflower ear.

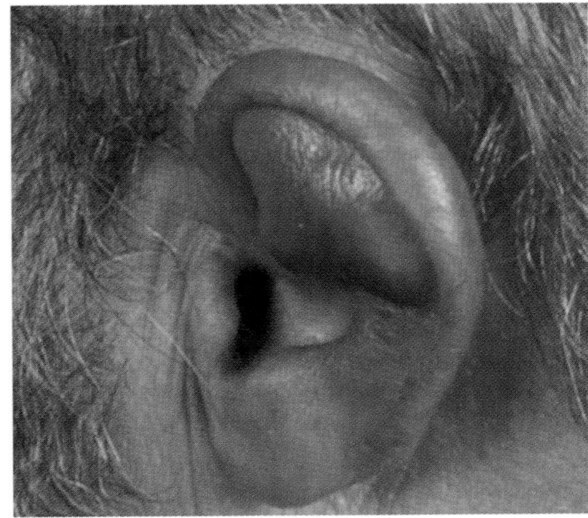

Fig. 15-22 Hematoma to pinna. (From Bingham, Hawke, and Kwok, 1992.)

Cauliflower Ear

A cauliflower ear (Fig. 15-23) is a thickened, disfigured auricle resulting from repeated episodes of minor or major blunt trauma. When observed in infants and young children, child abuse should be suspected (Montelone, 1996).

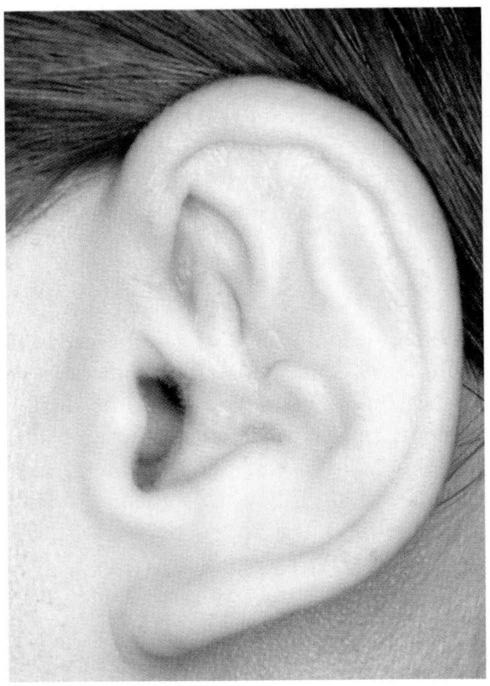

Fig. 15-23 Cauliflower ear. Note loss of definition in the finely sculpted cartilage. (From Bingham, Hawke, and Kwok, 1992.)

Sebaceous Cyst

A sebaceous cyst of the ear presents as a nodule usually found behind the earlobe in the postauricular fold. If it becomes infected, this becomes a very painful condition (Fig. 15-24).

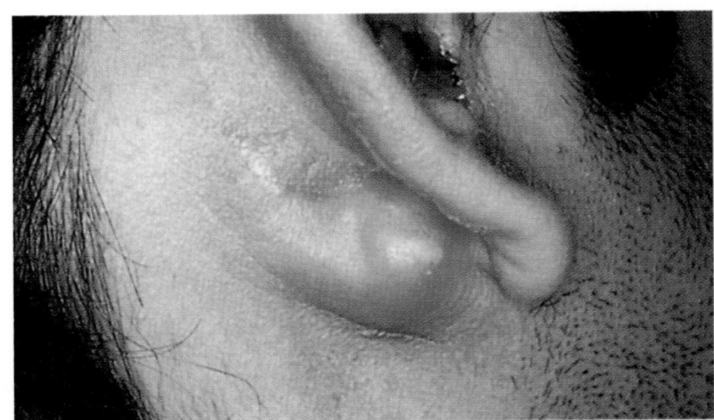

Fig. 15-24 Sebaceous cyst. (From Bingham, Hawke, and Kwok, 1992.)

Tophi

Tophi are small, hard, whitish yellow, nontender nodules in or near the helix of the ear (Fig. 15-25). They contain uric acid crystals and are a sign of gout.

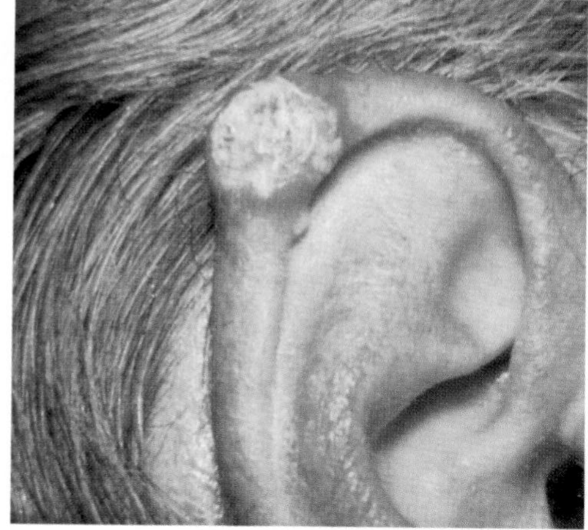

Fig. 15-25 Tophus of the pinna. (From Sigler and Schuring, 1993.)

AUDITORY CANAL

Excessive Cerumen

Cerumen is normally found in the ear and does not usually create a problem. However, if excessive amounts of cerumen is present in the ear, it may become impacted and occlude the entire ear canal (Fig. 15-26). If the entire canal is blocked, the client will feel a sense of fullness in the ear and experience decreased hearing.

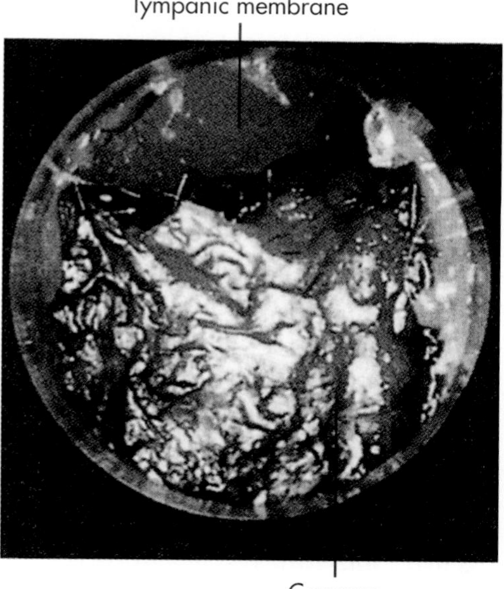

Fig. 15-26 Excessive earwax in the external auditory canal. (Courtesy Dr. Richard A. Buckingham, Clinical Professor, Otolaryngology, Abraham Lincoln School of Medicine, University of Illinois, Chicago, Ill. From Barkauskas et al, 1998.)

Foreign Body

A foreign body within the ear is most frequently seen in children, although it may occur in all age groups. A foreign body can be any small object such as a small stone, a small part of a toy, or even an insect. If the object is not removed, it may set up a secondary infection. This is especially true if the item is a food substance, such as a raisin or a kernel of corn (Fig. 15-27).

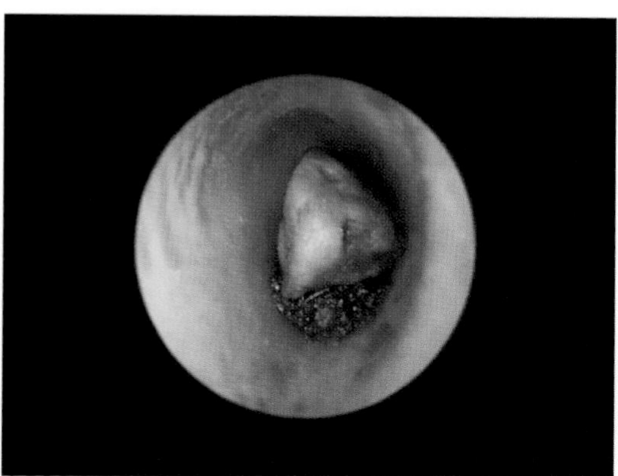

Fig. 15-27 Client inserted a small stone into the deep part of the external ear canal. It is lying against the tympanic membrane. (From Bingham, Hawke, and Kwok, 1992.)

Otitis Externa (Swimmer's Ear)

Swimmer's ear is a bacterial or fungal infection of the external ear canal that occurs secondary to tissue injury or a moist environment such as swimming (Fig. 15-28). The tissue appears red and swollen and may obscure the tympanic membrane.

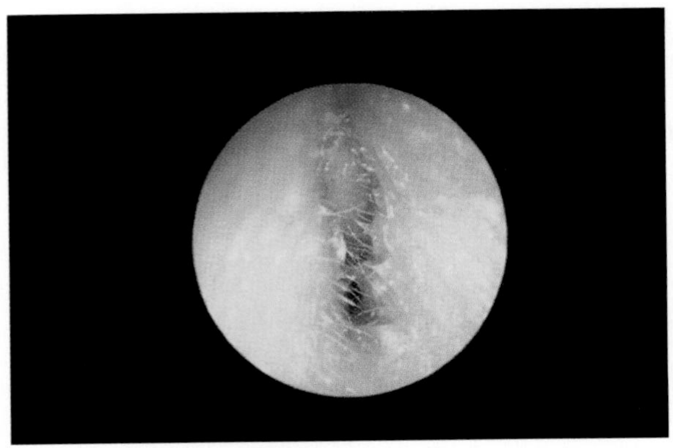

Fig. 15-28 Acute external otitis (swimmer's ear). (From Bingham, Hawke, and Kwok, 1992.)

Polyp

Polyps are a sign of possible chronic ear disease arising from tissue within the auditory canal (Fig. 15-29). The tissue enlarges, becomes reddened, and bleeds easily. There is also an associated purulent discharge.

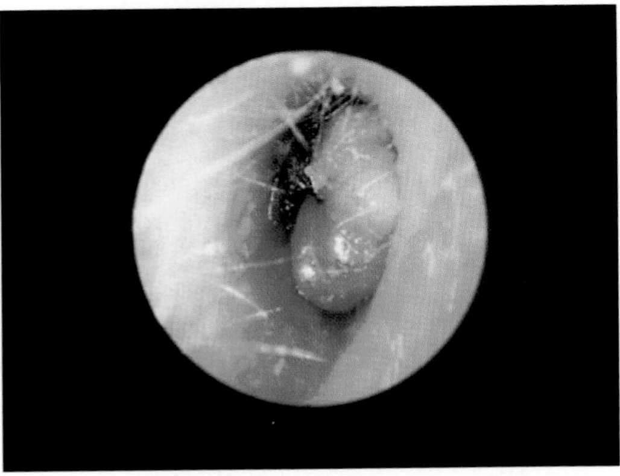

Fig. 15-29 Large solitary osteoma of the external auditory meatus, which is blocking and trapping earwax (to the left and behind the osteoma). (From Bingham, Hawke, and Kwok, 1992.)

TYMPANIC MEMBRANE/MIDDLE EAR

Bacterial Otitis Media

Bacterial otitis media is an infection of the middle ear (Fig. 15-30). The tympanic membrane often appears red, thickened, and bulging. There is accompanying fever and earache. There may be conductive hearing loss and a feeling that the ear is blocked. This commonly occurs in the pediatric population.

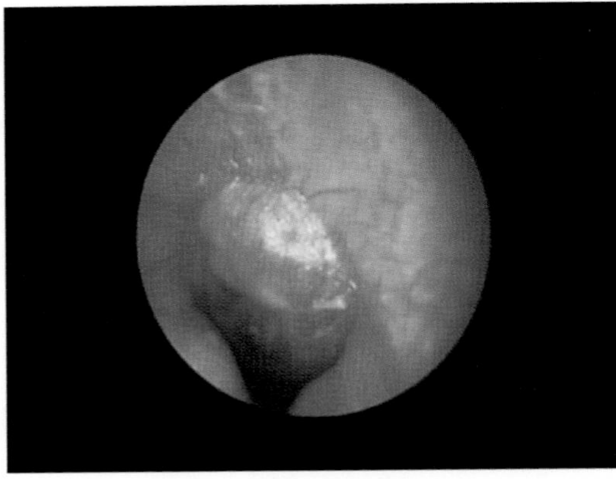

Fig. 15-30 Acute otitis media with redness and edematous swelling of the pars flaccida, shown in the central part of the illustration (left ear). (From Bingham, Hawke, and Kwok, 1992.)

Secretory Otitis Media (Serous Otitis Media)

This is an accumulation of serous fluid in the middle ear, secondary to an obstruction or dysfunction of the eustachian tube (Fig. 15-31). The cause ranges from allergies to enlarged lymphoid tissue blocking the eustachian tubes. The tympanic membrane may be retracted and yellow, and air bubbles may be seen. The client may complain of a crackling sound when yawning or swallowing.

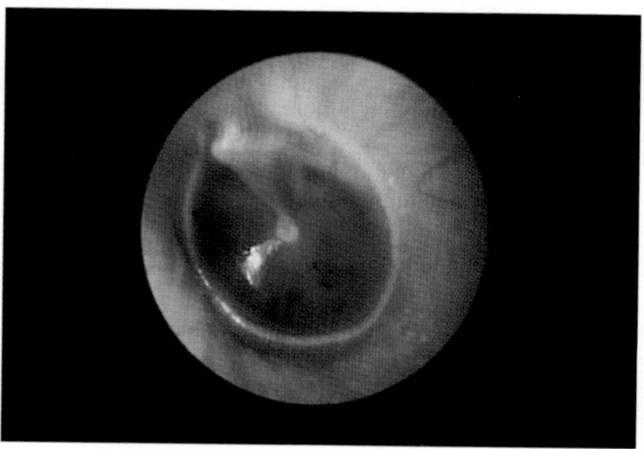

Fig. 15-31 Secretory otitis media. The tympanic membrane is markedly retracted and produces a foreshortened appearance to the handle of the malleus. (From Bingham, Hawke, and Kwok, 1992.)

Perforation of the Tympanic Membrane

Perforation of the tympanic membrane may occur if acute otitis media is left untreated. The rupture releases pressure and permits drainage of the infectious substance built up behind the tympanic membrane (Fig. 15-32). Perforation may also occur secondary to a blow to the head or penetration of the ear canal by a foreign body.

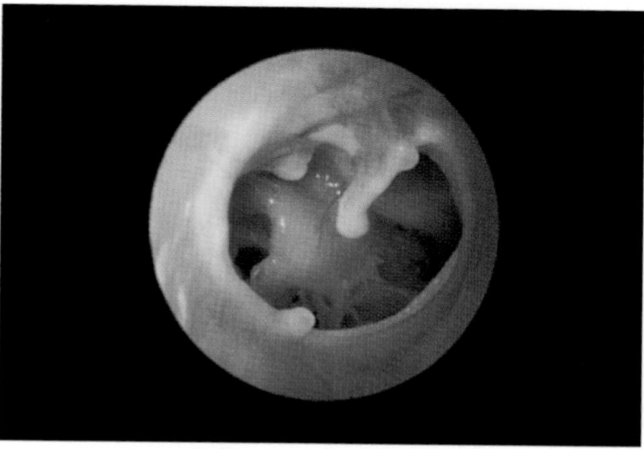

Fig. 15-32 Right tympanic membrane has a total perforation. The long process of the incus and its articulation with the head of the stapes and stapedius tendon can be seen through the perforation. (From Bingham, Hawke, and Kwok, 1992.)

HEARING LOSS

Conductive Hearing Loss

Hearing loss caused by the interference of air conduction to the middle ear is referred to as conductive hearing loss. Common causes include foreign bodies, cerumen build-up, tumors or polyps in the canal, and infection such as otitis media (Lindblade and McDonald, 1995).

Sensorineural Hearing Loss

Hearing loss caused by structural changes or disorders of the inner ear or auditory nerve are categorized as sensorineural hearing loss. Presbycusis is the most common cause of sensorineural hearing loss in the elderly and can be caused by atrophy and deterioration of the cells in the cochlea or atrophy, degeneration, and stiffening of cochlear motion. Presbycusis usually presents as a gradual and progressive bilateral deafness with a loss of high-pitched tones (Lindblade and McDonald, 1995).

VESTIBULAR FUNCTION

Ménière's Disease

Ménière's disease affects the vestibular labyrinth, which, over time, leads to profound sensorineural hearing loss. The disease progresses in steps from a sensation of fullness in the ear with slight hearing loss to ringing in the ears (tinnitus) to, finally, disabling vertigo.

CLINICAL APPLICATION and CRITICAL THINKING

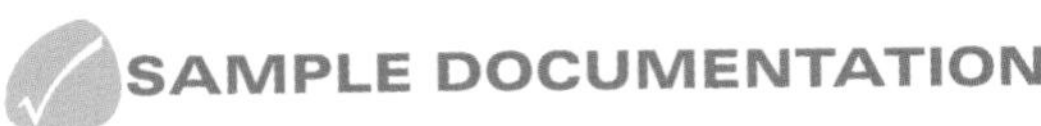

SAMPLE DOCUMENTATION

CASE 1

L.K. is a 56-year-old man who comes to the clinic with a complaint of "funny growths" on his ears.

Subjective Data

Reports 1 month ago noticed small, hard, yellowish white bumps on top of left ear; 2 weeks later noticed same type of growth on right ear; reports he has tried to pick the growths off his ears with his fingernails "until they bleed"; client verbalizes concern.

Does not report recent illness or infection; does not report medical problems, except recent aching and swelling of big toe joints—tested for gout and told uric acid level elevated; reports being given dietary instruction and "some type of medication" for discomfort in toes; since then, aching and swelling of great toe has subsided.

Does not report earaches, ear discharge, hearing loss, tinnitus, or vertigo.

Reports not following special diet received—diet includes foods he does not eat; states will continue to eat what he has always eaten.

Objective Data

Weight, 246 lb (111.6 kg).

Alert male.

Ears: External ears smooth, even color; multiple small (0.5 cm), whitish yellow, nontender nodules on helix and antihelix of both ears; no drainage from nodules.

Auditory canal: Clear with small amount of cerumen seen bilaterally.

Tympanic membranes: Pearly gray bilaterally; light reflex and all landmarks clearly visualized.

Hearing and vestibular function not tested.

Functional Health Patterns Involved

- Health perception–health management
- Nutrition–metabolic
- Self-perception–self-concept

Medical Diagnosis

Gout; bilateral tophus of pinna

Nursing Diagnosis and Collaborative Problems

- *Anxiety* (mild) related to nodules on ears as manifested by:
  - Verbalized concern about nodules on ears.
- *Ineffective management of therapeutic regimen* related to difficulty following prescribed diet as manifested by:
  - Reports not following special diet received.
  - Diet includes foods he does not eat.
  - Worsening of symptoms.
- *Risk for infection* related to skin integrity disruption associated with picking at lesions with fingernails.

CASE 2

M.J. is a 76-year-old man who presents with a complaint of ringing in the ears and hearing loss.

Subjective Data

Client describes gradual and progressive hearing loss and ringing in ears. Symptoms first noted 6 months ago; complains of decreased ability to hear television and general conversation. Reports recent problem conversing with wife and other family members; finds ringing in ears annoying and "uncomfortable"; makes him feel irritable; avoids interactions because he feels "embarrassed." Denies pain in ears, dizziness, or vertigo. Takes no medications—describes health as excellent.

Objective Data

Ear alignment and position: Appropriate bilaterally.

Lesions or swelling: None noted.

Skin color: Consistent with skin on face.

Otoscopic examination for right and left ear: Auditory canal without redness or discharge; no obstructions; TM visualized, pearly gray without perforations—cone of light noted.

Whispered voice test: 10% right ear; 40% left ear.

Rinne test: AC = BC in right ear.

Weber's test: Lateralization to left.

Romberg's test: Negative.

Functional Health Patterns Involved

- Health-perception–health-management
- Cognitive–perceptual
- Self-perception–self-concept
- Role–relationship

Medical Diagnosis

Presbycusis

Nursing Diagnosis and Collaborative Problems

Altered comfort related to perceived discomfort as manifested by:
- Complaints of ringing in ears.
- Finds ringing uncomfortable and annoying.

Self-esteem disturbance related to withdrawing from social contacts as manifested by:
- Statements of feeling embarrassed regarding hearing loss.
- Avoidance of social interaction.

Impaired verbal communication related to effects of hearing loss as manifested by:
- Verbalizes difficulty conversing with wife and other family members.

Risk for social isolation related to avoidance of interactions with others.

Risk for injury related to impaired sensory function.

CRITICAL THINKING QUESTIONS

1. A client at a health fair asks you, "What is the best way to clean ears?" What information could you share with this client?
2. You are asked to test the acoustic nerve (cranial nerve VIII) to evaluate auditory and vestibular function of a client. List the screening tests you could perform that would help you determine any need for further evaluation.
3. While inspecting the tympanic membrane, it is assessed for fluctuation. Why is this done, how is this done, and what do the results tell the examiner?
4. A mother brings her 6-month-old infant to the clinic and tells the examiner, "She has had a fever all night and has been crying for the last hour." The nurse looks in the baby's ears and notes that the tympanic membrane is red. How can the nurse differentiate redness caused by otitis media from redness caused by crying?

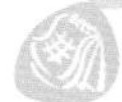

CASE STUDY

Trudy is a 5-year-old American Indian girl who was brought to the clinic by her mother. Listed below are data collected by the nurse during an interview and assessment.

Interview Data

The mother tells the examiner, "Trudy has been complaining of ear pain. She has been very hot and crying frequently." She adds, "I wanted to bring Trudy to the clinic yesterday, but my grandmother told me I shouldn't." Trudy's mother continues, telling the examiner, "Trudy has been treated many times for this problem over the last several years by the medicine man. Last night I saw drainage from Trudy's ears. Grandmother told me this was a sign that the illness was being chased from the body. I did not know what it was, but I felt scared." The mother indicates that Trudy knows English, but that the girl has never really talked very much.

Examination Data

- **General survey:** Small-for-age 5-year-old girl; quiet, flat affect. Does not look at the examiner; does not interact with the mother or the examiner.
- **External ear examination:** Typical position of ears bilaterally. Left ear pinna red. Dried bloody drainage noted on left external ear and in left external canal. Cries when left ear is touched. Right ear unremarkable.
- **Internal canal and tympanic membrane:** Dried drainage noted in left ear canal. TM perforated. Right ear unremarkable.
- **Hearing examination:** Whisper test in right ear = 80%; whisper test in left ear = 0%. Weber's test: hears tuning fork in right ear.

1. What data deviate from normal findings, suggesting a need for further investigation?
2. What additional information should the nurse ask or assess for?
3. In what functional health patterns does data deviate from normal?
4. What nursing diagnosis and/or collaborative problems should be considered for this situation?

REMEMBER to check out your companion CD-ROM

16 Eyes and Visual System

www.mosby.com/MERLIN/wilson/assessment/

ANATOMY AND PHYSIOLOGY

As one of the sensory organs, the eye transmits visual stimuli to the brain for interpretation via the optic nerve (cranial nerve II). The bony orbit that is lined with fatty tissue protects the eye. Additional protection is provided by the corneal or blink reflex that keeps out foreign objects and spreads tears over the surface of the eyeball.

EXTERNAL OCULAR STRUCTURES

The external eye is composed of the eyebrows, eyelids, eyelashes, conjunctivae, and lacrimal glands. The opening between the eyelids is called the palpebral fissure. The eyelashes curve outward from the lid margins, filtering out dirt. Two different thin, transparent mucous membranes called conjunctivae lie between the eyelids and the eyeball. The bulbar conjunctiva covers the scleral surface of the eyeballs. The palpebral conjunctiva lines the eyelids and contains blood vessels, nerves, hair follicles, and sebaceous glands. One of the sebaceous glands, the meibomian gland, secretes an oily lubricating substance that appears as vertical yellow striations in the palpebral conjunctiva. Secretions from these glands lubricate the lids, prevent excessive evaporation of tears, and provide an airtight seal when the lids are closed (Fig. 16-1).

Tears are formed by the lacrimal glands in the anterior lateral fossa of the orbit. They combine with sebaceous secretions to maintain a constant film over the cornea (see Fig. 16-1). In the inner (or medial) canthus, small openings called the upper and lower lacrimal puncta drain tears from the eyeball surface into the nasolacrimal ducts.

EYE MOVEMENT

The movement of the eye is provided by six extraocular muscles and three cranial nerves. The medial, inferior, and superior rectus muscles, as well as the inferior oblique muscle, control the following eye movement directions: upward outer, lower outer, upward inner, and medial eye movements. These muscles are guided by the oculomotor nerve (cranial nerve III). The superior oblique muscle controls lower medial movement, innervated by the trochlear nerve (cranial nerve IV). The lateral rectus muscle controls lateral eye movement, innervated by the abducens nerve (cranial nerve VI) (Fig. 16-2).

GLOBE OF THE EYE

The globe of the eye is surrounded by three separate layers. The outer layer is the sclera, which is the tough, fibrous layer, sometimes called the "white" of the eye. The sclera merges with the cornea in front of the globe at a junction called the limbus. The cornea covers the iris and the pupil. It is transparent, avascular, and richly innervated with sensory nerves via the ophthalmic branch of the trigeminal nerve (cranial nerve V). The constant wash of tears provides the cornea with its oxygen supply and protects its surface from drying. An important corneal function is to allow light transmission through the lens to the retina (Figs. 16-1 and 16-3).

The middle layer, called the uvea, consists of the choroid posteriorly and the ciliary body and iris anteriorly. The choroid layer is highly vascular and supplies the retina with blood. The iris is a circular, muscular membrane that regulates pupil dilation and constriction via the oculomotor nerve (cranial nerve III). The central aperture of the iris, the pupil, admits light to the retina. The ciliary body has two functions: it adjusts the shape of the lens to accommodate vision at varying distances, and it produces aqueous humor (Fig. 16-4). The transparent aqueous humor, which fills the space between the cornea and lens, is secreted by the ciliary epithelium in the posterior chamber. The aqueous humor flows between the lens and the iris and is then reabsorbed by the trabecular meshwork (Fig. 16-5). This meshwork lies at the angle where the iris and cornea merge and encircles the anterior chamber. The trabecular meshwork filters the aqueous humor before it enters the canal of Schlemm and then flows into the anterior ciliary veins. The aqueous humor helps to maintain the intraocular pressure and metabolism of the lens and posterior cornea. The transparent lens attaches to the ciliary body by suspensory ligaments. The lens alters its shape for visual clarity when the eyes are viewing an object at close range.

Finally, the inner layer of the eyes, the retina, serves as an extension of the central nervous system. This transparent layer has photoreceptor cells, called rods and cones, scattered throughout its surface. As the name photoreceptor suggests, these cells perceive images and colors in response to varying light stimuli. Rods respond to low levels of light and cones to higher levels of light. These rods and cones, although scattered throughout the retina, are not at all evenly distributed. The macula lutea, a pigmented area about 4.5

mm in diameter, is densely packed peripherally with rods. At the same time, the fovea centralis, a small depression in the center of the macula lutea on the posterior wall of the retina, contains no rods but is densely packed with cones. Visual acuity is sharpest in this area in higher levels of light.

Perforating the retina is the optic disc, which is the head of the optic nerve (cranial nerve II). It contains no rods or cones, causing a small blind spot located about 15° laterally from the center of vision. The optic disc is where the central retinal artery and central vein bifurcate, emerge, and feed into smaller branches throughout the retinal surface (see Fig. 16-17 on p. 335).

VISION

Rods and cones in the retina perceive images and colors in response to varying light stimuli. The lenses are constantly adjusting to stimuli at different distances by accommodation. For example, the normally flat lens becomes thicker and more convex to accommodate near objects. Through lens accommodation, an image is focused on the retina.

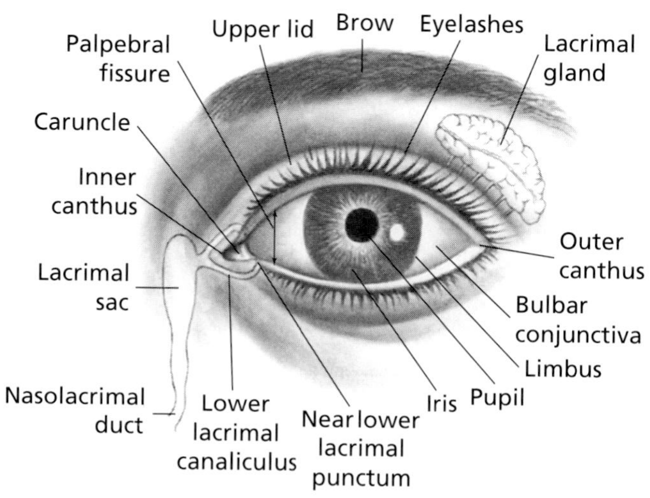

Fig. 16-1 Visible surface of eye. (From Thompson et al, 1997.)

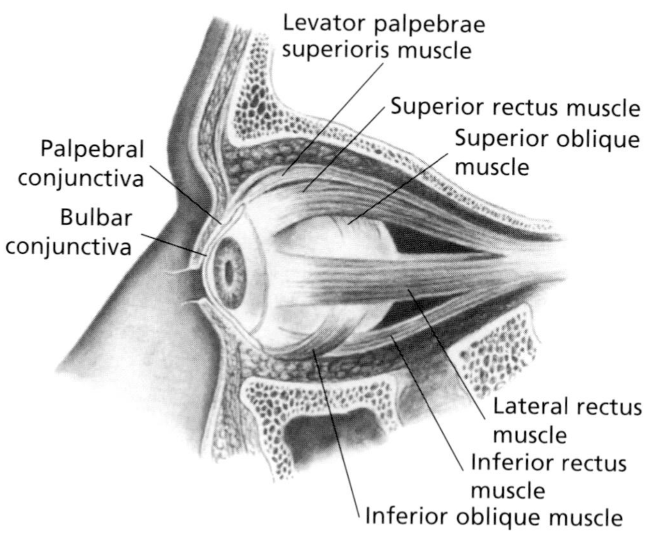

Fig. 16-2 Diagrammatic section of orbit. (From Thompson et al, 1997.)

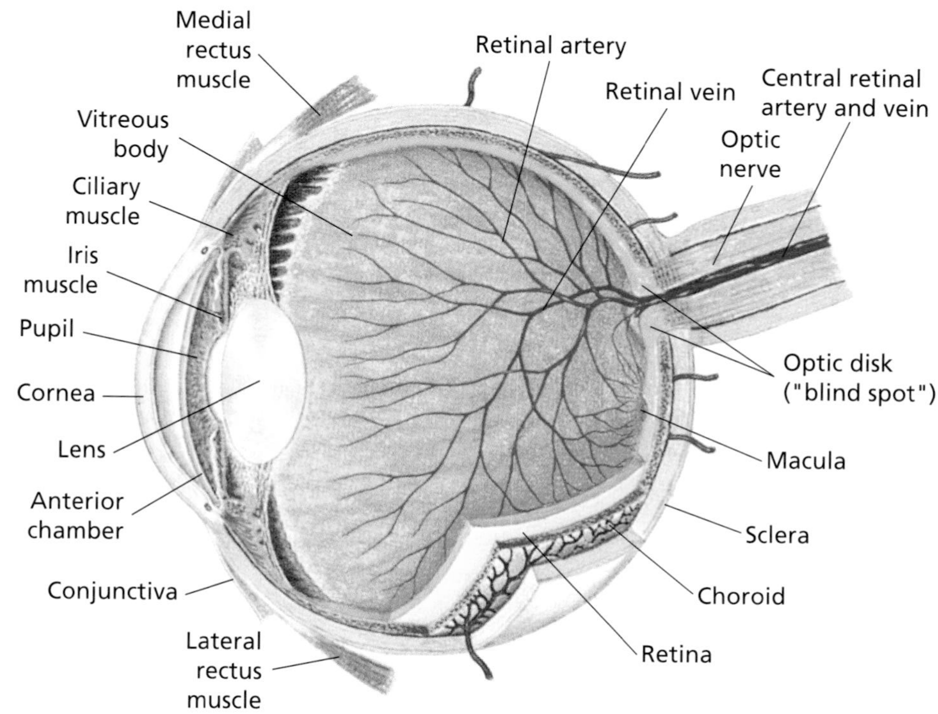

Fig. 16-3 Anatomy of the human eye. (From Seidel et al, 1999.)

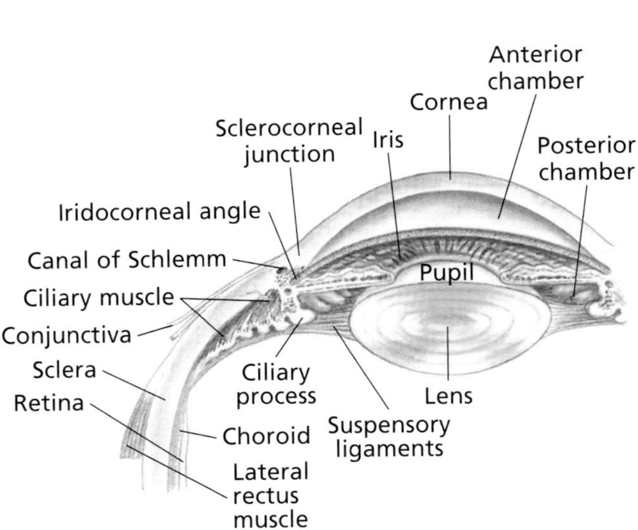

Fig. 16-4 Close-up view of ciliary body, zonules, lens, and anterior and posterior chambers. (From Thompson et al, 1997.)

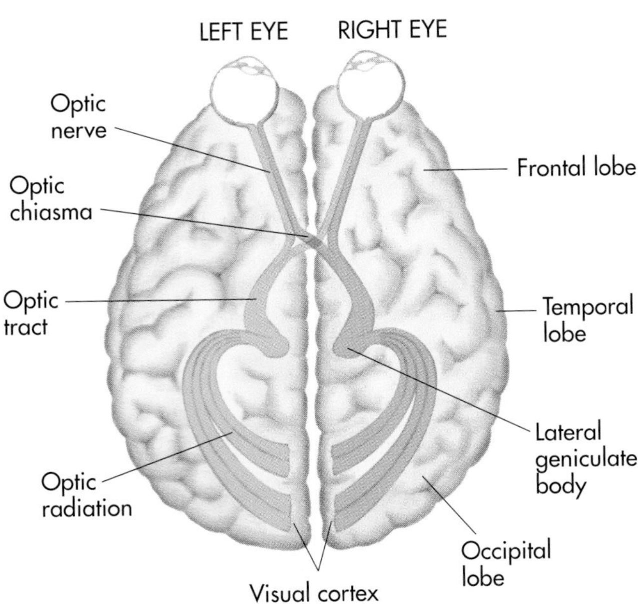

Fig. 16-6 Visual pathway. (From Thompson et al, 1997.)

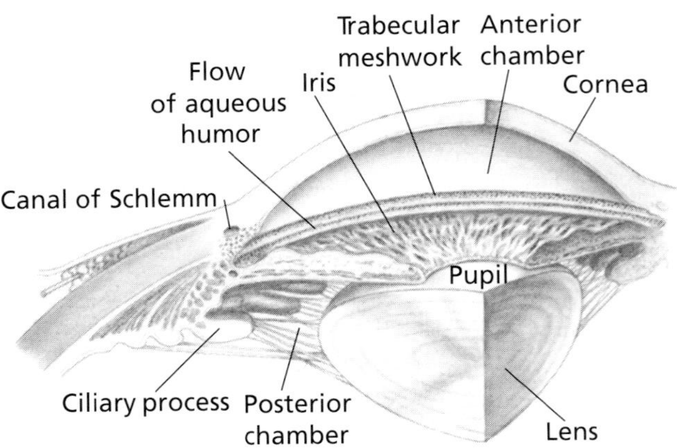

Fig. 16-5 Close-up view of trabecular meshwork and flow of aqueous humor. (From Thompson et al, 1997.)

Nerve impulses then are transmitted along the optic nerve and optic tract, reaching the optic cortex for interpretation. Objects in the visual field stimulate the opposite side of the retina. When nerve fibers pass into the optic nerve, the nasal and temporal fibers are separate within the sheath. The nerves merge at the optic chiasm, and the nasal fibers cross over to the opposite optic tract. Optic tracts emerging from the optic chiasm encircle the hypothalamus and terminate in the lateral geniculate bodies in the temporal lobes. From there, optic impulses are transmitted via visual nerve fibers to the occipital lobe of each cerebral hemisphere (Fig. 16-6).

HEALTH HISTORY

Eyes and Visual System

QUESTIONS	RATIONALE
PRESENT HEALTH STATUS	
➤ How would you describe your vision?	■ Assess the client's perception of his or her vision.
➤ Have you noticed any changes in your vision?	■ Ask the client if he or she has noticed a change rather than a problem with vision. A client may have a vision change yet not consider it a problem to report.

QUESTIONS

RATIONALE

➤ Have you had your eyes examined? If yes, when was the last examination? What was the outcome of that examination? Have you been tested for glaucoma?

■ There are no recommendations for visual screening for adults. Glaucoma screening is recommended for African Americans over age 40, whites over age 65, those with a family history, with diabetes, and with severe myopia because they are at increased risk (U.S. Preventive Services Task Force, 1996).

➤ Do you have any chronic illnesses or conditions? Diabetes mellitus? Hypertension?

■ Cardiovascular disease, diabetes, hypertension, and obesity are risk factors for glaucoma (Vader, 1997). Hypertension and diabetes also can cause retinopathy (see Figs. 16-36 to 16-39 on pp. 353-354).

➤ Are you taking any medications? If yes, what are you taking, and when did you start taking them?

■ Many prescription drugs affect the eyes (e.g., insulin, corticosteroids, oral hypoglycemics, and thyroid hormone). Over-the-counter drugs such as antihistamines and decongestants can dry out the eyes (Vader, 1997). Parasympatholytics and sympathomimetics dilate the pupil. Adverse reactions of drugs may cause myopia, blurred vision, or light sensitivity.

➤ Do you use eyedrops? For what reason? What kind of drops? How many drops? How often?

■ Eyedrops are medications that may affect eye function. Natural tears may be used to treat dry eyes.

➤ Do you wear contact lenses or glasses? When were they prescribed? For what problem? Are the contact lenses soft, hard, or extended wear? How long do you wear them each day? Do you ever sleep with contact lenses in place? How often do you clean your glasses? Your contact lenses? How do you clean them?

■ Clients who answer yes to these questions should have answered yes to the question about periodic eye examination. Determine if client knows how to care for eyewear. Contacts left in longer than intended can cause corneal abrasions.

➤ Do you wear sunglasses when in the sunlight?

■ Sunglasses are important to protect the eyes from ultraviolet light rays to prevent risk of glaucoma.

➤ Do you wear protective eyewear when playing sports such as racquetball?

■ The client may need to be reminded of the importance of preventing eye trauma from sports injuries.

➤ Does your job involve risks for your vision? For example, are there sparks or flying bits of metal that could injure your eyes? If yes, what actions do you take to protect your eyes? Do you use safety goggles?

■ Clients need to protect their eyes in the work environment, if needed. Regulatory agencies such as the Occupational Safety and Health Administration (OSHA) have developed guidelines and regulations to reduce eye injuries in the work environment.

PAST MEDICAL HISTORY

➤ In the past, have you had any problems with your eyes or your vision?

■ Past problems with the eye, such as infections, may recur and may help explain current visual problems.

➤ Have you ever had any surgery on your eyes? If yes, what procedure was done, when was it, and what was the outcome of the surgery? Have you ever had an injury or trauma to the eyes?

■ Incidence of injury or surgery may provide additional information about possible eye or visual problems.

QUESTIONS

RATIONALE

RISK FACTORS

COMMON RISK FACTORS ASSOCIATED WITH Eye and Visual System Disorders

CATARACTS

Viral infection during uterine growth—congenital cataracts
Prolonged exposure to ultraviolet light
Eye trauma
Diabetes mellitus
Smoking
Alcohol use
Increasing age

TRANSIENT INCREASES IN INTRAOCULAR PRESSURE

Smoking
Ingestion of alcohol
Illicit drugs
Corticosteroid drugs

GLAUCOMA

Hypertension
Cardiovascular disease
Diabetes mellitus
Obesity

BLINDNESS

Diabetes mellitus
Hypertension
Glaucoma
Eye injury

FAMILY HISTORY

➤ Does anyone in your family have cataracts? Glaucoma? Diabetes mellitus? Nearsightedness (myopia)? Farsightedness (hyperopia)? Migraine headaches?

■ All these conditions have familial tendencies, and all may affect vision. If there is a positive answer to any of these conditions, the client's risk of developing them increases.

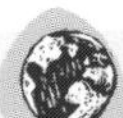

ETHNIC & CULTURAL VARIATIONS

Glaucoma is a leading cause of blindness among African Americans. The prevalence among African Americans is 15 times higher than in whites. There is no explanation for this discrepancy (Astle and Allen, 1999).

PROBLEM-BASED HISTORY

The principal areas to be investigated during the history relating to the eyes and visual system are difficulty with vision, pain, redness and/or edema, and watering or discharge. As with symptoms in all areas of health assessment, a symptom analysis is completed, which includes location, quality, quantity, chronology, setting, associated manifestations, alleviating factors, and aggravating factors.

Difficulty With Vision

➤ What type of difficulty are you having with vision? When did it begin? Did it begin suddenly or gradually? Does the problem affect one eye or both? Is it constant, or does it come and go? How would you describe it—blurring? Cloudiness? Images out of focus? Spots (floaters) in front of your eyes?

■ The client's description is essential in determining the cause of the visual difficulty. Note that a sudden onset of visual symptoms, which may indicate a detached retina, requires an emergency referral. Floaters in eyes reported by clients usually are not significant. Involvement of both eyes tends to indicate a systemic problem, whereas involvement of one eye is a local problem.

QUESTIONS	RATIONALE
➤ Have you ever seen a halo or multicolored ring around objects or lights?	■ Halos surrounding lights may indicate acute narrow-angle glaucoma or digoxin toxicity.
➤ Have you noticed a "blind spot"? Does it move as you shift your gaze? Do you feel your peripheral vision has decreased?	■ A blind spot surrounded by an area of normal or decreased vision (a scotoma) occurs in glaucoma and with optic nerve and visual pathway disorders.
➤ Do you have difficulty seeing at night?	■ Night blindness can occur in optic atrophy, glaucoma, or vitamin A deficiency.
➤ Do your eyes cross? When does this occur? When they are tired?	■ Crossed eyes may indicate strabismus.
➤ Do you have double vision? When does it occur? Does it occur continuously or intermittently? Does it occur when you have one eye or both eyes open?	■ Diplopia, the perception of two images of a single object, may indicate defective function of the extraocular muscles or a disorder of the nerves that innervate these muscles.
➤ What makes the your vision worse? What treatment have you tried for the vision difficulty? How effective was the treatment?	■ Determining what therapies have been used successfully or unsuccessfully helps in understanding the problem and guiding current treatment strategies.
➤ Have your vision problems interfered with your daily life? Describe how this has happened. Do you require books with large print, or those on audiotape, or those in braille?	■ Determine the impact this visual difficulty has had on the client's quality of life and evaluate the adjustments the client has made to lifestyle and routines.
➤ Are you concerned that you may not be able to see someday?	■ Assess the client's attitudes and fears concerning blindness.
Pain	
➤ Do you have pain in your eye(s)? When did it start? Did it begin suddenly or gradually? Where do you feel the pain?	■ Sudden onset of eye pain may be from a detached retina and requires immediate medical care. Refer the client to a health care provider who can evaluate the pain further.
➤ Describe the pain. Is it sharp? Dull? Throbbing? Burning? Itching? How intense is the pain on a scale of 1 to 10?	■ Although some common eye diseases cause no pain, any complaint of pain should be noted and investigated.
➤ What do you think is causing the pain? Do you feel that there is a something in your eye? Headache?	■ Clients often can feel a foreign object in their eyes; they also may have tearing, redness, and photophobia as a result.
➤ What makes the pain worse? What makes the pain better? How have you treated the pain? How effective was the treatment?	■ Determining what therapies have been used successfully or unsuccessfully helps in understanding the problem and guiding current treatment strategies.

QUESTIONS

RATIONALE

Redness and/or Edema

➤ Have you noticed any redness or swelling in the eye area? If yes, describe it. How long have your eyes been red? Is this associated with any sport you may be involved in? Do you have allergies? Does anyone else with whom you are in close contact have a similar redness?

■ Allergies may cause seasonal redness, swelling, or excessive tearing.

■ Chlorine from pools may cause redness.

■ Trauma to the eye in sport-related or other accidents can cause redness.

■ Redness can be caused by infection. If others close to the client have the same symptoms, it could be a contagious infection.

➤ What makes the redness or edema worse? What makes it better? What treatment have you tried? How effective was the treatment?

■ Determining what therapies have been used successfully or unsuccessfully helps in understanding the problem and guiding current treatment strategies.

Watering or Discharge

➤ Do you have watering or excessive tearing? When does it occur? Does it occur in one eye or both? Does your eye itch or hurt? Do your eyes feel strained or tired when they water?

■ Tearing (lacrimation) and excessive tearing (epiphora) can be caused by irritating substances or allergies. Unilateral watering may be a blocked lacrimal duct. Eye strain or fatigue can produce tearing.

➤ Have you noticed a discharge or matter in the eyes? Does it occur only in the morning? Is it hard to open your eyes in the morning because of the discharge? How do you remove the matter?

■ Thick yellow or green discharge is abnormal. Crusts can form overnight and make the eyes difficult to open. This can be caused by allergies. Hygiene practices and cross-contamination control should be evaluated.

➤ What have you done to treat the watering or discharge? How effective was the treatment?

■ Determining what therapies have been used successfully or unsuccessfully helps in understanding the problem and guiding current treatment strategies.

EXAMINATION

Equipment

- Snellen's chart or "E" chart to assess far vision (20 feet)
- Hand-held near-vision screener (Rosenbaum or Jaeger) to assess near vision (14 inches)
- Cover card (opaque) for the cover-uncover test to assess for deviation of gaze
- Penlight to assess pupillary reaction to light and corneal light reflex
- Ophthalmoscope to inspect the red reflex and optic disk

PROCEDURES AND TECHNIQUES WITH NORMAL FINDINGS

VISION

➤TEST visual acuity and be alert for any outward cues indicating any difficulty with vision. Assess distant visual acuity using Snellen's chart (see Fig. 5-13, *A* on p. 71). This tests the function of the optic nerve (cranial nerve II).

Place Snellen's chart on the wall in a well-lighted room. The client may sit or stand about 20 feet (6 m) from the chart. If a client wears contact lenses or glasses, he or she should leave them in place unless they are for reading only. Reading glasses are intended for near vision, rather than distance, and they magnify letters.

Have the client cover one eye with an opaque card and read the line of smallest letters possible. Next, ask the client to read any letters possible on the line below the one just read for a further assessment. Test the other eye using the same procedure. The reading pattern should be smooth and without hesitation. Eyes should remain open without squinting. Record whether the client wore glasses or contact lenses. Document the line read completely by the client, using the fraction printed at the end of the line.

A finding of 20/30 means the client can read at 20 feet what a person with normal vision can read at 30 feet. If the client can read all the letters in the 20/30 line and two letters in the 20/20 line, document the finding as 20/30 +2.

Next, ask the client to use both eyes to distinguish which of the two horizontal lines is longer to assess perception. Finally, ask him or her to name the colors of the two horizontal lines to document red and green color perception.

Note: Use the "E" chart for the client who cannot read letters. This can be a very sensitive area for adults who do not know how to read. You may show both eye charts to the client and ask which one would be easier to use. The client is asked to indicate the direction in which the *E* points (see Fig. 5-7, *B* on p. 71). Repeat the procedure with the other eye.

Assess near vision for people over 40 years of age or for those who feel they have difficulty reading. Ask the client to cover one eye and hold a Jaeger or Rosenbaum card or a newspaper at about 14 inches and to read the smallest line possible (Fig. 16-7). Repeat the assessment covering the other eye. NOTE: Myopic (nearsighted) people may be able to read at a normal distance if they remove their glasses. This will be reported as a change in vision because formerly they were able to read while wearing their glasses. Visual acuity is documented using the abbreviations for Latin words that designate right eye, left eye, and both eyes as shown Box 16-1.

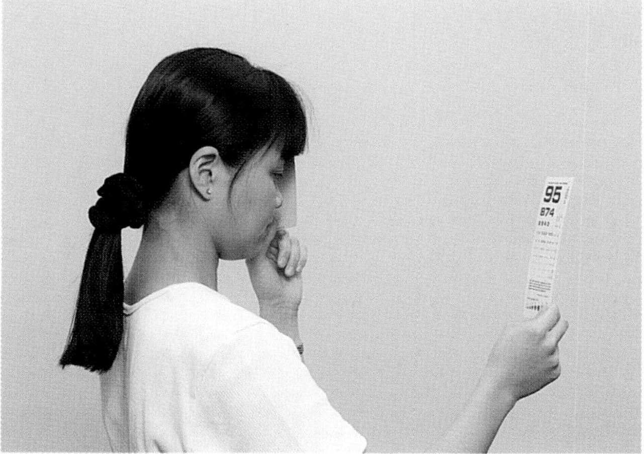

Fig. 16-7 Assessing a client's near vision with the Rosenbaum chart.

ABNORMAL FINDINGS

- Note any hesitancy, squinting, leaning forward, or misreading of letters. Blinking or facial expressions indicating that the client is struggling should be noted also. These signal difficulties in perceiving the letters and a possible visual problem that needs a referral to an optometrist or ophthalmologist.
- Criterion for legal blindness is 20/200.
- Note that the larger the denominator, the poorer the vision. If vision is poorer than 20/30, refer the client to an ophthalmologist or optometrist. Impaired vision may be caused by refractive error, opacity of the lens, cornea, or vitreous, or a retinal or optic pathway disorder.
- Clients who cannot distinguish colors on Snellen's chart need further assessment. Ishihara's test consists of a series of polychromatic cards that have numbers and patterns embedded in different colors. A color-blind client may not be able to identify the embedded figures.
- With age, there is a tendency for the eyes to lose their ability to perform accommodation; this tendency is known as presbyopia. As a result, the client will need to move the card farther away to see it clearly.

PROCEDURES AND TECHNIQUES WITH NORMAL FINDINGS

ABNORMAL FINDINGS

Box 16-1 Abbreviations Used in Eye Assessment

O.S.: oculus sinister (left eye)
O.D.: oculus dexter (right eye)
O.U.: oculus uterque (each eye)

➤**ASSESS visual fields for peripheral vision using the confrontation test.** The confrontation test assesses the optic nerve (cranial nerve II) function. The examiner faces the client, standing or sitting at a distance of 2 to 3 feet (60 to 90 cm).

1. Have the client cover one eye with an opaque card as you cover your own eye directly opposite the client's covered eye. (NOTE: This test assumes that the examiner has normal peripheral visual fields.) Ask the client to look directly at you.
2. Hold a pencil or use your finger and extend it to the farthest periphery.
3. Gradually bring the object close to the midline (equal distance between you and the client).
4. Ask the client to report when he or she first sees the object; you should see the object at the same time. Slowly move the object inward from the periphery in four directions as if following the outline of an imaginary glass bowl over the client's head. Move your fingers anteriorly (from above the head down into field of vision); inferiorly (from upper chest up toward field of vision), temporally (move in laterally from behind the client's ear into field of vision), and nasally (move medially into the field of vision) (Fig. 16-8). Estimate the angle between the anteroposterior axis of the eye and the peripheral axis when the pencil or finger is first seen. Normal values are 50° anteriorly, 70° inferiorly, 90° temporally, and 60° nasally. The temporal value is greater than the nasal value because of the position of the opaque card covering one of the eyes.

■ If the client cannot see the pencil or finger at the same time that you see it, peripheral field loss is suspected. Refer the client to an eye care specialist for more precise testing.

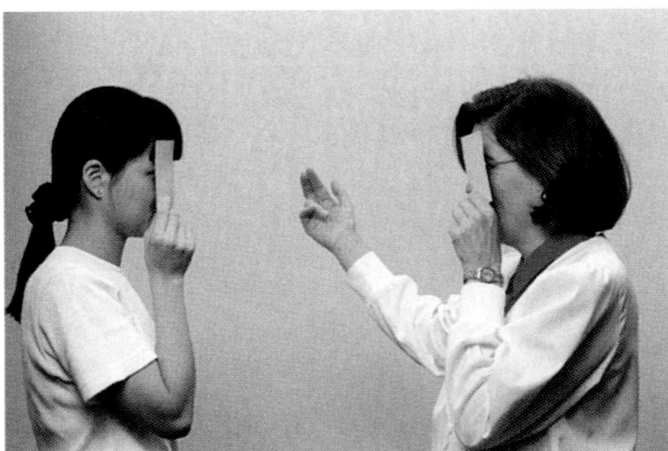

Fig. 16-8 Assessing a client's peripheral vision nasally by moving object medially into the field of vision.

PROCEDURES AND TECHNIQUES WITH NORMAL FINDINGS

➤INSPECT extraocular muscles for movement. Inspect eye movement in the six cardinal fields of gaze (oculomotor [cranial nerve III], trochlear [cranial nerve IV], and abducens nerve [cranial nerve VI]), as follows (Fig. 16-9):

1. Have the client look directly at you.
2. Position your finger or object about 10 to 12 inches from the client's nose. Ask the client to keep the head still and use the eyes only to follow your finger or an object in your hand.
3. Move the object from its center position to upper outer extreme, hold there, move back to center, to lower inner extreme, and hold there.
4. Move the object to temporal-nasal extremes, holding there momentarily.
5. Move the object to opposite upper outer extreme and back to opposite lower inner extreme.

Normally there will be parallel tracking of the object with both eyes. Mild nystagmus at extreme lateral gaze is also normal.

NOTE: An alternative method to steps 3 to 5 above is to move your finger slowly in a circle to each of the six directions. Stop in each position so that client can hold the gaze briefly before moving to the next position.

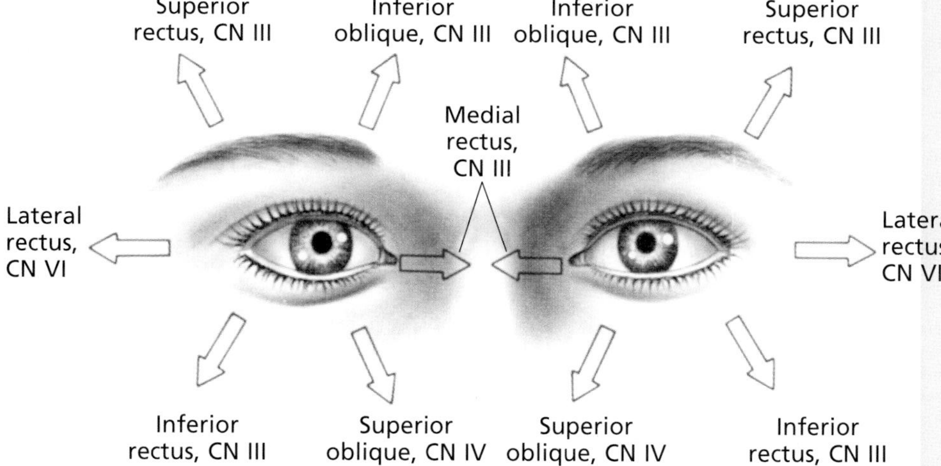

Fig. 16-9 The six cardinal fields of gaze. (From Seidel et al, 1999.)

ABNORMAL FINDINGS

- Eye movement that is not parallel indicates an extraocular muscle weakness or dysfunction of cranial nerve III, IV, or VI.
- Note any nystagmus other than that considered normal, especially on lateral gaze. (*Nystagmus* is involuntary movement of the eyeball in a horizontal, vertical, rotary, or mixed direction.)
- *Esotropia*—inward (nasal) deviation of the eye.
- *Exotropia*—outward (temporal) deviation of the eye.

PROCEDURES AND TECHNIQUES WITH NORMAL FINDINGS

➤INSPECT the corneal light reflex for symmetry (Hirschberg test). Ask the client to stare straight ahead with both eyes open. Shine a penlight toward the bridge of the nose at a distance of 12 to 15 inches (30 to 38 cm). Light reflections should appear symmetrically in both corneas (Fig. 16-10). When an imbalance is found in the corneal light reflex, perform the cover-uncover test.

To perform the cover-uncover test, ask the client to stare straight ahead at your nose even though the gaze may be interrupted.

1. Cover one of the client's eyes with the opaque card. Observe the uncovered eye for any deviation or movement from a steady, fixed gaze.
2. Remove the card from the eye and observe if the just-uncovered eye moves to try to focus. It should not move.
3. Repeat steps 1 and 2 with the other eye.

For example, cover the left eye (Fig. 16-11) and observe the right eye for movement; it should not move. Uncover the left eye and observe it for movement; it should not move when it is uncovered.

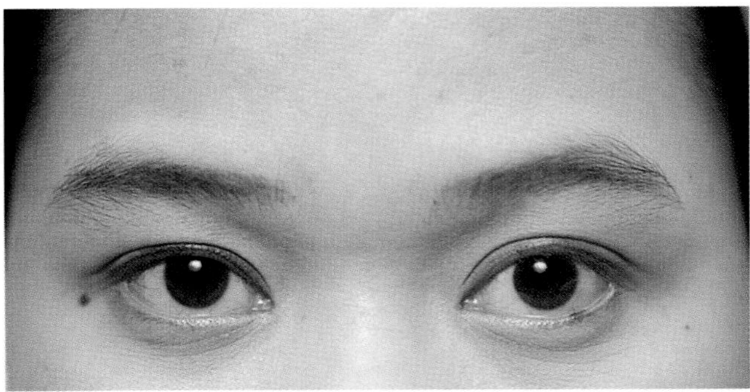

Fig. 16-10 Testing the corneal light reflex. Symmetric light reflections in both corneas is a normal finding.

ABNORMAL FINDINGS

- If light reflections appear at different spots in each eye (asymmetrically), this may indicate weak extraocular muscles.
- If the uncovered eye moves to focus, it is the weaker eye and strabismus is present.
- If the just-uncovered eye moves to focus, it is the weak eye because it relaxed while being covered, indicating strabismus.
- Pupil abnormalities: See Table 16-2 on p. 349.

A

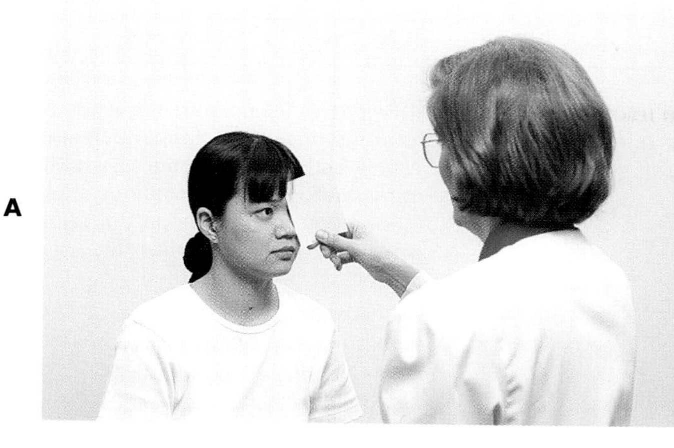

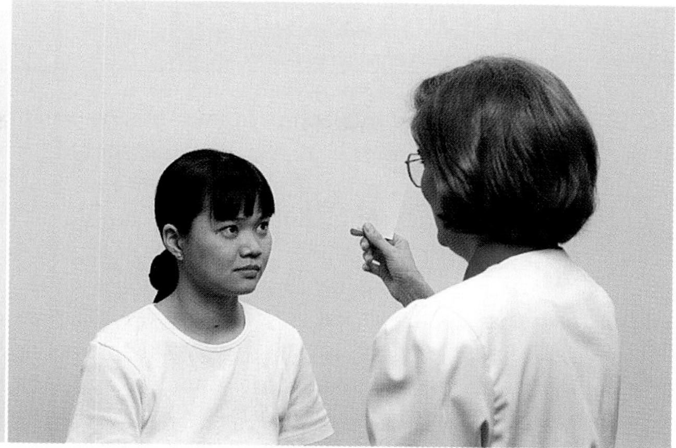

B

C

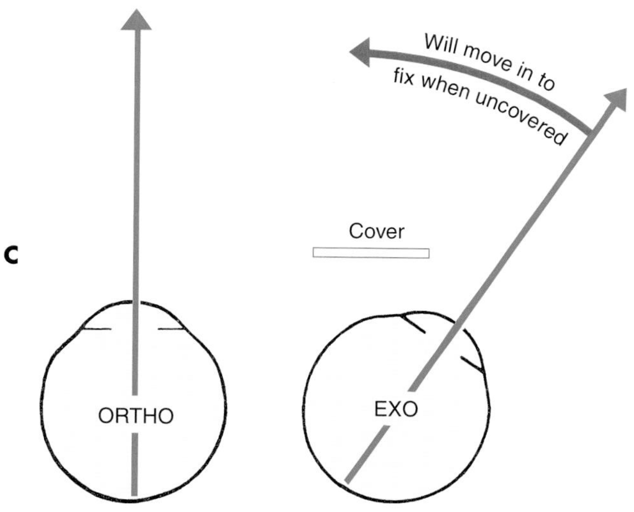

Fig. 16-11 The cover-uncover test is used to evaluate function of eye muscles. **A,** Left eye covered, observe right eye. **B,** Left eye uncovered, observe it for movement. **C,** Exophoria, the right eye shifted from right to center when the eye uncovered. (**C** from Prior, Silberstein, and Stang, 1981.)

PROCEDURES AND TECHNIQUES WITH NORMAL FINDINGS	ABNORMAL FINDINGS

EXTERNAL OCULAR STRUCTURES

➤INSPECT the eyebrows for hair distribution, underlying skin, and symmetry. Skin should be intact and eyebrows symmetric. Note whether the eyebrow extends over the eye.

■ Flakiness, loss of hair, scaling, and unequal alignment of movement should not be seen. Loss of the lateral one third of the eyebrow occurs in hypothyroidism.

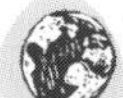

ETHNIC & CULTURAL VARIATIONS

The palpebral fissures are horizontal in non-Asians, whereas Asians normally have an upward slant to the palpebral fissures (Fig. 16-12.)

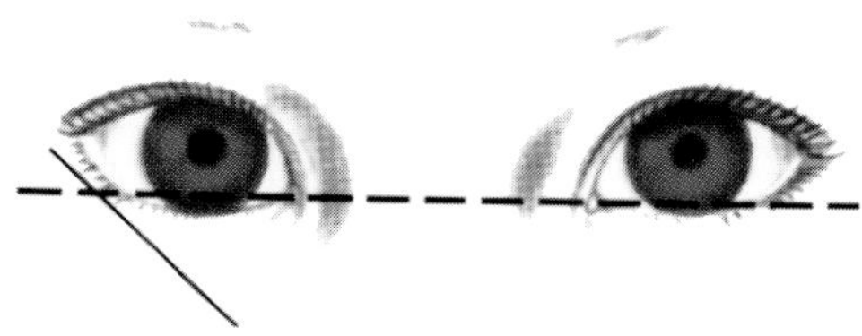

Fig. 16-12 Narrowed and upwardly slanting palpebral fissures are a normal finding in Asians. (From Wong et al, 1999.)

PROCEDURES AND TECHNIQUES WITH NORMAL FINDINGS

➤**INSPECT the eyelids and eyelashes for symmetry, position, closure, blinking, discharge, and color.** Palpebral fissures should be bilaterally equal. The upper lid margins should cover part of the iris but not the pupil. The lower lid generally covers to just below the limbus. Lid closure should be complete, with smooth, easy motion. Blinking should generally consist of frequent, bilateral, involuntary movements, averaging 15 to 20 blinks per minute. Lid margins should fit flush against the eyeball surfaces, and eyelashes should be equally distributed and curled slightly outward. The color of the lids should correspond to skin color, and margins should be pale pink.

ETHNIC & CULTURAL VARIATIONS

For white clients, the eyeball does not protrude beyond the supraorbital ridge of the frontal bone. For African-American clients, the eyeball may protrude slightly beyond the supraorbital ridge.

➤**INSPECT and PALPATE the globe in the bony socket for position and indentation.** Ask the client to look down with lids closed so that you will not palpate the cornea. Gently palpate the eyeball; it should indent with slight pressure. Palpate the lower orbital rim near the inner canthus. This pressure slightly everts the lower lid.

➤**INSPECT the lacrimal puncta for color, moisture, discharge, tenderness, and nodules.** Puncta are seen as small elevations on the nasal side of the upper and lower lid margins. Mucosa should be pink and intact despite pressure. Eyes should be moist, without excessive tears. Gently palpate the upper and lower lids for tenderness or nodules.

ABNORMAL FINDINGS

- Palpebral fissures are asymmetrically positioned. Sclera is visible between the upper lid and iris in hyperthyroid exophthalmos. The lid of either eye covers part of pupil, causing ptosis, which may be congenital or acquired.
- Closure of the lid that is incomplete or accomplished only with pain or difficulty may occur with infections.
- Edema of the lid may occur with trauma or infection.
- The presence of lesions, nodules, redness, flaking, crusting, excessive tearing, or discharge should be documented. Note lid deformity and whether lashes are absent or turned in.
- Red, edematous eyelids may indicate infection, for example, sty (hordeolum, see Fig.16-26), orinflammation, for example, meibomian cyst (chalazion, see Fig. 16-25).
- Asymmetric placement of the globe should be noted. Note whether the placement is too far forward (exophthalmos, see Fig.16-23) or backward (enophthalmos, see Fig.16-22).
- An eyeball that is firm may occur in glaucoma.
- Lacrimal puncta that are clogged with mucus or dirt cause inflammation (dacryocystitis). Fluid or purulent material may be discharged from the puncta in response to pressure. Excessive tearing (epiphora) may be caused by blockage of nasolacrimal duct. Tenderness, nodules, or irregularities should be noted.

PROCEDURES AND TECHNIQUES WITH NORMAL FINDINGS

➤**INSPECT the bulbar conjunctiva for color and clarity.** Ask the client to look up. Gently separate the lids widely with the thumb and index finger, exerting pressure over the bony orbit surrounding the eye. Have the client look up, down, and to each side. The bulbar conjunctiva should be clear, possibly with tiny red vessels.

Pull down and evert the lower lid; ask the client to look up. The palpebral conjunctiva should be opaque, pink, and vascular (Fig. 16-13).

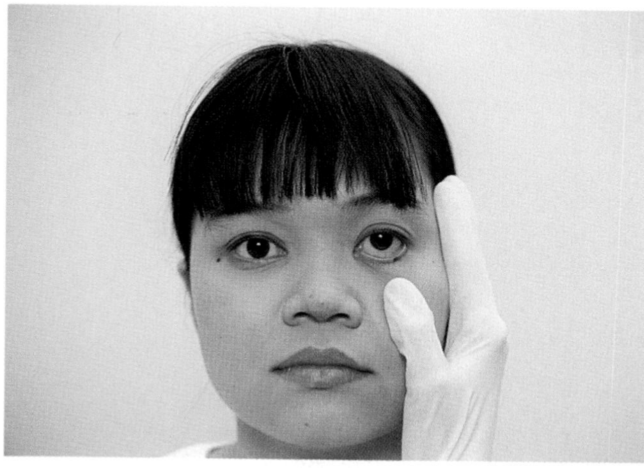

Fig. 16-13 To inspect the palpebral conjunctiva, gently pull down and evert the lower eyelid.

Eversion of the Upper Lid Although not a part of routine screening, eversion of the upper eyelid is used when you must inspect the conjunctiva of the upper lid, such as when clients complain of eye pain or a foreign body is suspected. To ensure the client's cooperation, explain the procedure before performing it (Fig. 16-14).

1. Ask client to look down but keep eyes slightly open; this relaxes the levator muscle of the eyelid.
2. Don examination gloves.
3. Gently grasp the upper eyelashes and pull gently downward. Do not pull the lashes outward or upward, causing muscle contraction.
4. Place a cotton-tipped applicator stick about 1 cm above the upper lid margin and push gently down with the applicator while still holding the lashes to evert the lid.
5. Hold the lashes of the everted lid against the upper ridge of the bony orbit, just below the eyebrow but not pushing against the eyeball.
6. Examine the lid for swelling, infection, or foreign bodies.
7. Return the lid to normal by moving the lashes slightly forward and asking the client to look up and then blink. The lid returns easily to normal position.

ABNORMAL FINDINGS

■ Red and congested conjunctiva may indicate conjunctivitis. A sharply defined area of blood adjacent to normal-appearing conjunctiva may indicate subconjunctival hemorrhage.

■ Lesions, nodules, or foreign bodies should be noted.

■ Pale conjunctiva occurs in anemia. Observe for discharge and crusting. Note any tissue growth of bulbar conjunctiva from the periphery toward the corneal center (pterygium, see Fig. 16-28).

■ Swelling, presence of a foreign body, and redness should be noted, with the client referred for further examination.

PROCEDURES AND TECHNIQUES WITH NORMAL FINDINGS

ABNORMAL FINDINGS

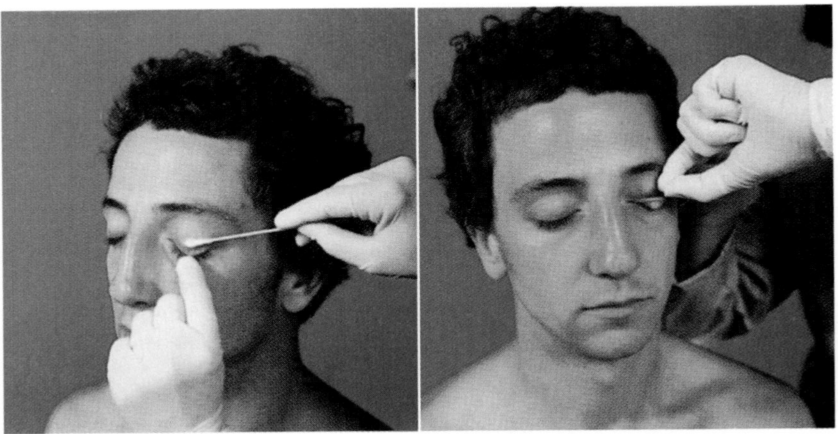

Fig. 16-14 Everting upper eyelid. (From Barkauskas et al, 1998.)

GLOBE OF THE EYE

➤**INSPECT the sclera for color and clarity.** Sclera should be white and moist.

■ Yellow sclera may indicate jaundice.

ETHNIC & CULTURAL VARIATIONS

The sclera appears white except in darker-skinned clients, in whom it is normally a darker shade. Tiny black dots of pigmentation may be present near the limbus in dark-skinned individuals. In light-skinned individuals, there may be a slight yellow cast.

➤**INSPECT the cornea for transparency and surface characteristics.** Use oblique lighting and slowly move the light reflection over the corneal surface. Observe for transparent quality and a smooth surface that is clear and shiny.

Test the corneal reflex ONLY in selected cases, such as unconscious clients. Lightly touch the cornea with cotton. The lids of both eyes blink when either cornea is touched. This reflex tests the sensory reception of the ophthalmic branch of the trigeminal nerve (cranial nerve V) and the motor branch of the facial nerve (cranial nerve VII) which creates a blink.

■ Note opacities, irregularities in light reflections, lesions, abrasions, or foreign bodies. Especially note any white opaque ring encircling the limbus, called corneal arcus. The arc is composed of lipids deposited at the periphery. It is seen in many clients over 60 and is associated with Type II hyperlipidemia when seen in clients younger than age 40.

■ Edema of the brainstem might impair the function of cranial nerve V and cranial nerve VII and may occur after head injury or with hemorrhage or tumor.

➤**INSPECT the anterior chamber for transparency, iris surface, and chamber depth by using a penlight or ophthalmoscope.** Shine light from the side across the iris to note transparency, a flat iris, and adequate chamber depth (enough clearance between the cornea and iris) (Fig. 16-15).

■ Cloudiness or visible material or blood should be noted. The iris should not bulge toward the cornea, and the chamber should not be shallow. Also note iris or pupil shapes other than round, inconsistent iris coloration, and unequal pupil sizes. About 5% of the population normally have unequal pupils (anisocoria), but it may occur as a result of past eye surgery, trauma, or congenital anomalies.

PROCEDURES AND TECHNIQUES WITH NORMAL FINDINGS

ABNORMAL FINDINGS

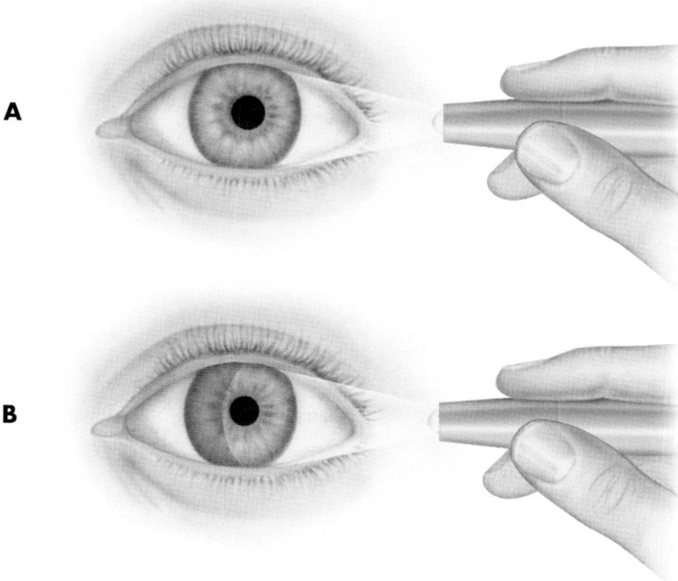

Fig. 16-15 Evaluation of depth of anterior chambers. **A,** Normal anterior chamber. **B,** Shallow anterior chamber. (From Seidel et al, 1999.)

➤**INSPECT the iris for shape and color.** It should be round with consistent coloration. Some people may have a normal variation in color in which each iris is a different color. This is due to genetic factors.

■ Clients who have had an iridectomy to correct glaucoma will have a section of the iris missing. Coloboma is a congenital defect of the iris. Blunt trauma to the eye can cause an iridodialysis, a circumferential tearing of the iris from the sclera.

➤**INSPECT the pupils for size, shape, and reaction to light.** To determine the pupil size, use a pupil gauge found at the bottom of a Rosenbaum Pocket Vision Screener (see Fig. 5-8 on p. 72). The pupil diameter is normally between 2 and 6 mm. Pupils should be round and equal in size.

Dim the room lights if possible. Ask the client to hold the eyes open and fix his or her gaze on an object across the room. Approach with a penlight beam from the side and shine it directly on the pupil. The illuminated iris should constrict (direct response) (oculomotor cranial nerve III); the other iris should constrict simultaneously (consensual response). The optic nerve (cranial nerve II) senses the light, and cranial nerve III creates the constriction of the iris, which makes the pupil appear smaller. Repeat with the other eye.

■ Failure of either one or both eyes to constrict to light in speed or magnitude indicates dysfunction of the oculomotor nerve (cranial nerve III).

■ Mydriasis is pupil size greater than 6 mm that fails to constrict; it may occur with diabetes, epilepsy, head trauma, or high blood alcohol level.

■ Miosis is constriction to less than 2 mm caused by drugs such as morphine.

➤**INSPECT pupils for accommodation** (Box 16-2). Ask the client to fix his or her gaze on a distant object across the room. The pupils should dilate when visualizing a distant object. Then ask the client to shift gaze to your finger, placed about 6 inches from the client's nose. Normally both eyes should constrict and converge (move inward toward the nose).

■ Failure of pupil to converge or constrict may occur in diabetes or syphilis.

PROCEDURES AND TECHNIQUES WITH NORMAL FINDINGS

ABNORMAL FINDINGS

Box 16-2 Acronym for Documenting Pupillary Assessment: PERRLA

Pupils are
Equal,
Round and
React to
Light and
Accommodation

INTERNAL OCULAR STRUCTURES (OPHTHALMOSCOPE EXAMINATION)

To use an ophthalmoscope, darken the room to help dilate the client's pupils. Have the client remove glasses; contact lenses may be left in. You may leave your glasses or contact lenses in place.

1. Ask the client to fixate on a distant point.
2. Turn on the ophthalmoscope light by pressing the on/off switch and turning the rheostat control clockwise. Set the diopter wheel to 0.
3. To examine the client's right eye, hold the ophthalmoscope in your right hand and use your right eye. Place your right index finger on the selection wheel so that you can change the diopter settings as needed to focus on the internal structures.
4. Direct the client to continuously gaze at a point across the room and slightly above your shoulder. Begin about 10 inches (25 mm) from client's eye at a 15° angle lateral to the client's line of vision.
5. Shine the light of the ophthalmoscope on the pupil while looking through the viewing lens.

➤**OBSERVE the red reflex.** This is a red or orange glow over the client's pupil (Fig. 16-16, *A*) created by light illuminating the retina. Keep the red reflex in sight and move closer to the eye, adjusting the lens with the diopter wheel as needed to focus; note any interruption in the red reflex. There should be none. Absence of the red reflex may be caused by movement of the light away from the pupil; correct by repositioning the light (Fig. 16-16, *B*).

■ Decreased or irregular red reflex, dark spots, and opacities should be noted.

■ Dark shadows or black dots may indicate opacities that occur with cataracts or may be due to hemorrhage in the vitreous humor.

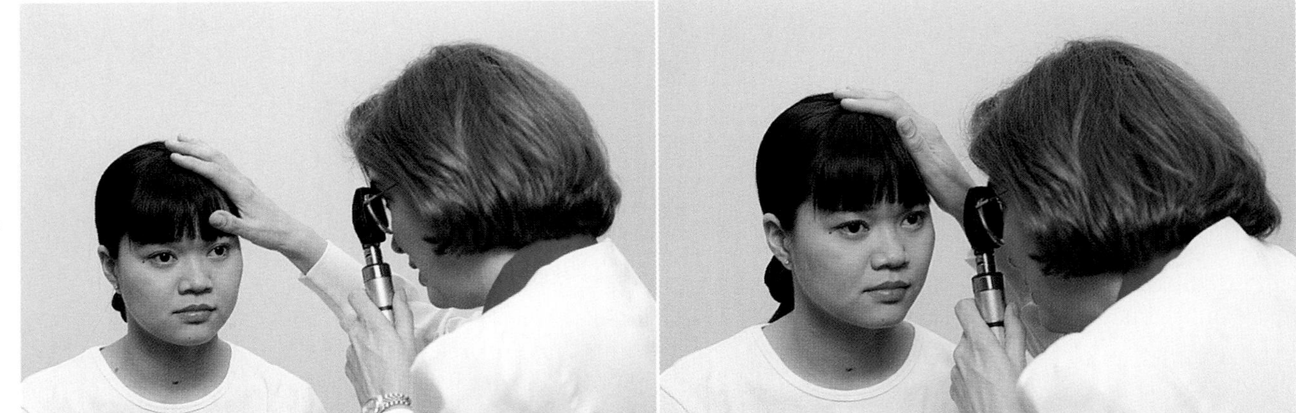

Fig. 16-16 Examining the retina. **A,** The red reflex is created by light illuminating the retina. **B,** Move close to the client until you nearly touch foreheads.

PROCEDURES AND TECHNIQUES WITH NORMAL FINDINGS

❖ ➤**INSPECT the optic disc for discrete margin, shape, size, color, and physiologic cup.** After seeing the red reflex continue to move closer until you nearly touch foreheads with the client. Placing your middle finger on the client's cheek will stabilize the ophthalmoscope.

Focusing varies depending on the refractive state of both the examiner and the client. Remember that the myopic (nearsighted) client has longer eyeballs so that light rays focus in front of the retina. To see the retina of this client, you use the minus (red) numbers by moving the diopter wheel up, or counterclockwise. By contrast, the hyperopic (farsighted) client has shorter eyeballs, so that light rays focus behind the retina. For this client, use the positive (black) numbers by moving the diopter wheel down, or clockwise. When you locate a blood vessel, follow it inward toward the nose until you see the optic disc.

The margin should be regular and have a distinct, sharp outline. Scattered or dense pigment deposits may be seen at the border. A gray crescent may appear at the temporal border.

The optic disc should be round or slightly vertically oval. Its size measures about 1.5 mm (it is magnified 15 times through the ophthalmoscope). Marked myopic refractive errors may make the disc appear larger, and hyperopic errors may make it appear smaller.

The optic disc's color should be creamy yellow to pink, lighter than the retina, possibly with tiny blood vessels visible on the surface.

The physiologic cup is a small depression just temporal to the disc center that does not extend to the border. It usually appears lighter than the rest of the disc and occupies less than one half of the disc's diameter. Vessels entering the disc may drop abruptly into the cup or appear to fade gradually.

Follow each of the four sets of retinal vessels from the disc to the periphery.

❖ ➤**INSPECT the retinal vessels for color, arteriolar light reflex, artery-to-vein (A:V) ratio, and arteriovenous crossing changes.** Arteries are on average one fourth narrower than veins; artery-to-vein width should be 2:3 to 4:5. Arteries are light red in color and may have a narrow band of light in the center. By contrast, veins are larger than arteries and have no light reflex. They are darker in color, and venous pulsations may be visible (Fig. 16-17).

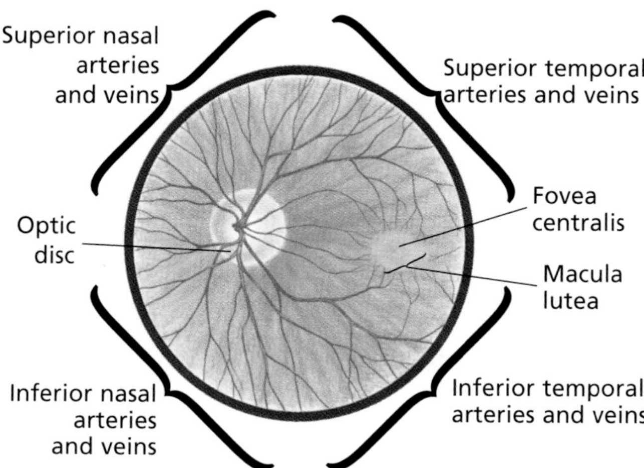

Fig. 16-17 Retinal structures of the left eye. (From Seidel et al, 1999.)

ABNORMAL FINDINGS

■ Blurred margin may indicate papilledema, which is caused by increased intracranial pressure relayed along the optic nerve.

■ Irregular disc or discs that differ in size or shape between the two eyes should be noted.

■ Note diffuse or pallor section of the disc, which always extends from the center of the disc to the border. Hyperemic discs with engorged or tortuous vessels on the surface are abnormal.

■ The depression of the physiologic cup should not extend to the border of the disc and should not occupy more than one half of the diameter of the disc. The appearance (size or placement) of the physiologic cup should not differ between eyes.

■ Extremely narrow arteries are abnormal. The width of the light reflex should not cover more than one third of the artery. They should not be pale or opaque.

■ Irregularities of caliber, either dilation or constriction, should be noted. Compact areas of tortuous, narrow vessels should be investigated. Indentations or pinched appearances where veins and arteries cross occur with hypertension and are called A-V (arteriovenous) nicking.

PROCEDURES AND TECHNIQUES WITH NORMAL FINDINGS

Overall, the caliber of both arteries and veins should be regular and uniformly decreasing in size as they branch and move toward the periphery. Artery and vein crossing should give no evidence of constricting either vessel.

ETHNIC & CULTURAL VARIATIONS

The fundi of black persons may be heavily pigmented and uniformly dark.

❖ ➤**INSPECT the retinal background for color, presence of microaneurysms, hemorrhages, and exudates.** The color is uniform throughout and may be pink, red, or orange; it varies with skin color (Fig. 16-18, *A-C*).

The retinal surface should be finely granular, with choroidal vessels possibly visible. Movable light reflections may appear on the surface, usually in young persons.

❖ ➤**INSPECT the macula for color and surface characteristics.** Ask the client to look directly into the ophthalmoscope light. The macula is about one disc diameter (DD) in size and lies about two DDs temporal to the optic disc. The macula and its center, the fovea centralis, should be slightly darker than the rest of the retina. The fovea may appear as a tiny bright light. Tiny vessels may appear on the surface. Fine pigmentation and granular appearance may be visible. The macula may be difficult to see if the client's pupil has not been chemically dilated.

Repeat the same examination of the internal eye on the other eye, holding the ophthalmoscope in the left hand and using your left eye to assess the client's left eye.

ABNORMAL FINDINGS

- Pale fundus, either in general or in localized areas, or hemorrhages (linear, flame-shaped, round, dark red, large, small) must be noted.
- Note microaneurysms, which appear as fine red dots, and any exudates, soft, hard, fuzzy, or well-defined.
- Impaired blood flow may cause the disk to appear whiter than expected.
- Drussen bodies are small, discrete spots in the retina. They are pinker than the retina, but become more yellow as the spots enlarge.

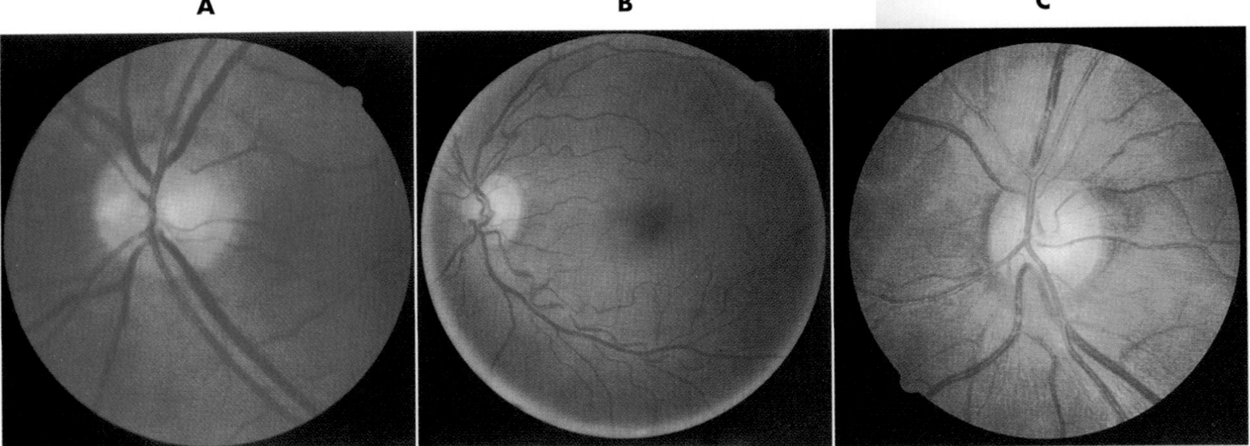

Fig. 16-18 Fundus. **A,** White client. **B,** African-American client. **C,** Asian client. (Courtesy Dr. Frances C. Gaskin.)

AGE-RELATED VARIATIONS

■ INFANTS

Anatomy and Physiology

Visual acuity at birth ranges from 20/100 to 20/400. Peripheral vision is fully developed at birth; however, central vision develops later. The 2- to 3-month-old infant begins to have voluntary control over eye muscles. At around this same time, the lacrimal ducts begin carrying tears into the nasal meatus. By 8 months the infant can distinguish colors, and by 9 months the eyes are able to perceive a single image, reflecting the eye muscles' ability to coordinate.

Health History

- Did the mother have a vaginal infection when she delivered this infant? What was the infection? How was it treated?

  Rationale Vaginal infections can cause eye infections in the neonate during the birth process.
- Have you noticed the infant looking at a toy? Does he or she reach for the toy? Can the infant follow the toy in all directions?

  Rationale These questions provide data about normal development of the eyes and vision.

Examination

Procedures and Techniques Newborns frequently have edema of the lids, either from the trauma of birth or in response to eyedrops or ointments such as prophylactic instillation of silver nitrate. The edema may delay the examination for a few days. To begin the assessment, hold or rock the infant into an upright position to elicit eye opening. An alternative strategy is to hold the infant supine with the head gently lowered.

Observe if the eyes are small or of different sizes. Inspect the eyelids for edema, epicanthal folds, and position. Note the alignment and slant of the palpebral fissures. Draw an imaginary line through the corners of the eyes (from the medial canthi to the outer canthi). Observe the space between the eyes for wide-spaced eyes (Seidel et al, 1999). Inspect the sclera for color.

Test the corneal reflex by shining a light into both eyes and noting the location of the light reflection in each eye. This tests extraocular muscles and distinguishes between pseudostrabismus and actual strabismus. Follow the corneal light reflex with the cover-uncover test to further assess for strabismus.

Test visual acuity by blinking a penlight on and off several times, then move it around slightly about 10 inches (25 cm) from the baby's face. Also test for the pupillary reaction at this time. Test red reflex by shining an ophthalmoscopic light into the pupil.

Normal and Abnormal Findings Normal findings of the eye examination of an infant reveal eyes that are usually closed; often no eyebrows are present. The eyes are symmetric, and eyelashes may be long. Eyelids may have edema. The outer canthus of the eye aligns with the pinna of the ear (Fig. 16-19). Infant sclera may have a blue tinge caused by thinness; otherwise sclera are white. Tiny black dots (pigmentation) or a slight yellow cast may appear near the limbus of dark-skinned infants. Palpebral conjunctivae are pink and intact without discharge. There are no tears until about 2 to 3 months of age.

The infant should indicate some visual recognition of light from a penlight and follow it momentarily. The blink reflex also is present in normal newborns and infants. Pupils should constrict in response to bright light and are round, about 2 to 4 mm in diameter, and equal in size. You should note a bilateral red reflex, which is a bright round, red-orange glow seen through the pupil. It may be pale in dark-skinned newborns. Presence of the red reflex rules out most serious defects of the cornea, aqueous chamber, lens, and vitreous chamber (Wong et al, 1999).

Specific age-related responses may be observed that indicate the infant's attention to visual stimuli.

- 0 to 2 weeks: Eyes do not reopen after exposure to bright light; there is increasing alertness to objects; infant capable of fixating on object.
- 1 month: Infant can fixate and follow a bright toy or light.
- 3 to 4 months: Infant can fixate, follow, and reach for a toy, since binocular vision is normally achieved at this age.
- 6 to 12 months: Infant can fixate and follow toy in all directions.

Corneal light reflex should be symmetric. Transient strabismus is common during the first few months of life due to lack of binocular vision. If it continues beyond 6 months of

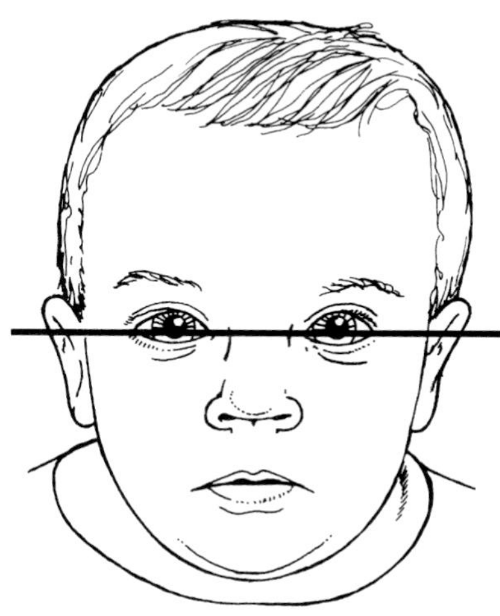

Fig. 16-19 Alignment of the outer canthus with the pinna of the ear is a normal finding.

age, however, a referral to an ophthalmologist is needed because early recognition and treatment can restore binocular vision.

Asian and Native American infants often have pseudostrabismus, the false appearance of strabismus due to the flattened nasal bridge or epicanthal fold. Pseudostrabismus disappears at about 12 months of age (Seidel et al, 1999).

Abnormal findings may include a pronounced lateral upward slant of the eyes with an inner epicanthal fold, which may indicate Down syndrome; asymmetry of eyes; wide-set eyes (hypertelorism); or those that are close together (hypotelorism). Note any discolorations of the sclera, such as dark blue sclera, or any dilated blood vessels. Hyperbilirubinemia may cause jaundiced (yellow) sclera in newborns.

Asymmetric corneal light reflex followed by malalignment of cover-uncover test indicates abnormality of eye muscles.

Excessive tearing before the third month or no tearing by the second month are deviations from normal. A purulent discharge from eyes shortly after birth is abnormal. It may indicate ophthalmia neonatorum and should be reported. Redness, lesions, nodules, discharge, or crusting of the conjunctiva is abnormal. Birth trauma may cause conjunctivitis or conjunctival hemorrhage. Birth trauma can cause eyelid capillary hemangiomas.

If the pupillary response is not present after 3 weeks, the infant may be blind. A dilated, fixed, or constricted pupil may indicate anoxia or brain damage. A white pupil may occur in retinoblastoma, a relatively rare congenital malignant tumor arising from the retina. A white pupil in conjunction with a cloudy cornea or anterior chamber may indicate congenital cataracts. Absence of the red reflex may indicate the presence of retinal hemorrhage or congenital cataracts (Wong et al, 1999).

■ CHILDREN

Anatomy and Physiology

Young children's eyes are less spherical than adults', making children's vision myopic. The globe grows gradually until the expected adult visual acuity is achieved around age 6.

HEALTH HISTORY

- Is the child's vision tested each year at school? Is the child able to see the chalk or markers on the board or overhead transparencies in the classroom without difficulty? Does the child have difficulty reading?

Rationale Participation in these preventive programs can detect visual problems early. Many times visual problems will be detected by school personnel, since the child may not be aware of the vision problem.

- What safety factors do you consider when purchasing toys? How do you protect your child's eyes from trauma? Have you taught the child how to handle and use sharp objects?

Rationale Safety is of utmost concern in the care of children's vision. Children must be taught the importance of complying with safety measures.

- Does the child rub eyes excessively? Does the child shut eyes, tilt head, or thrust head forward? Does the child blink more than usual? Does the child hold books close to his or her eyes? Sit close to television? Are the eyes inflamed or watery? Does the child develop frequent sties?

Rationale These are signs of visual problems in children and should be reported to a health care professional.

Examination

Procedures and Techniques Most of the examination of children's eyes is the same as that for adults. Vision can be assessed when performing developmental tests such as the Denver II (e.g., noting the child's ability to stack blocks or identify animals). The assessment of vision and eyes should be appropriate for the developmental stage and age of the child.

To test visual acuity use the Allen Picture Cards to screen children 2½ to 3 years of age. Show the large cards with pictures to the child up close to be sure that the child can identify them. Then present each picture at a distance of 20 feet from the child. Use Snellen's "E" chart for children 3 to 6 years of age. Have children point their fingers in the direction of the "arms" of the E. By 7 to 8 years of age, begin to use the standard Snellen's chart, as described for adults. Test each eye separately with and without glasses as is appropriate. If the child cannot cooperate for this test, wait. Be sure to screen children two separate times before referring them. Test for color vision once between the ages of 4 and 8. Use Ishihara's test, and ask the child to identify each pattern.

Perform the corneal light reflex test as described for adults, followed by the cover-uncover test if necessary (see Fig. 16-11, *A* and *B* on p. 329). Training for certification for hearing and screening in some states specifies that the child's eye be covered for 2 to 3 seconds before the hand or card is moved.

Screen for nystagmus by inspecting the movement of the eyes to the six cardinal fields of gaze. It may be necessary to stabilize the child's chin with your hand to prevent the entire head from moving.

Prepare children for the ophthalmoscope examination by showing them the light, explaining how it shines in the eye, and why the room must be darkened.

Normal and Abnormal Findings Visual acuity of 20/20 (line 7 on the chart) is achieved during toddler years, although 20/40 (line 5) is considered acceptable (Wong et al, 1999). Normally the child will be able to name three of the seven cards within three to five trials during the Allen test. A child with normal color vision will see the number or pattern embedded in Ishihara's test. A symmetric corneal light reflex is an expected finding.

Abnormal findings may include disorders of ocular muscles as well as a visual acuity greater than 20/40. A color-blind child will not be able to see the pattern against the background in Ishihara's test. Color blindness or deficiency may affect the child's school performance. If the canthus of the eye is higher or lower than the pinna, you report this as an abnormal finding.

Abnormal outcome on the corneal light reflex assessment detects exophoria and strabismus. Exophoria is the deviation of one eye outward and away from the other eye. Both eyes should exhibit coordinated parallel movements in all directions. End-point nystagmus may occur if the eye is held in extreme gaze; it is seen as mild rhythmic twitching with quick movement in the direction of gaze with slow drift in the other direction.

Screening for strabismus is important because early recognition and treatment can restore binocular vision. Diagnosis of strabismus after age 6 has a poor prognosis; it can lead to amblyopia, a type of blindness. Children who are found to have strabismus need to be referred to an ophthalmologist.

An abnormal finding when testing the six cardinal fields of gaze is involuntary, rhythmic movement of the eyes, called nystagmus. The oscillations may be horizontal, vertical, rotary or mixed and require a referral. If one or both eyes fail to follow your hand in any direction or if there are sporadic or nonpurposeful movements, a referral may be needed also.

■ ADOLESCENTS

Anatomy and Physiology

The anatomy and physiology for the adolescent is the same as for the adult.

Health History

- Can you see the chalk or markers on the board or overhead transparencies in the classroom?
  Rationale Visual problems will be detected at school when the adolescent is unaware of them or chooses not to admit them.
- Do you sit close to television or have to hold books close to your eyes?
  Rationale These actions may indicate impaired vision.
- Do you participate in sports? If yes, are your eyes at risk for injury? If so, what do you do to protect your eyes?
  Rationale Adolescents need to be aware of potential injuries that can occur with their activities so that injuries can be prevented. The American Society for Testing and Materials (ASTM) has approved eye guards for use in competitive sports (Neinstein, 1991).

Examination

Procedures and Techniques Overall the examination should be conducted in the same manner as for adults. If the client is accompanied by an adult (parent or guardian), allow the client to decide whether the adult waits in or outside the examining room during the physical examination.

Normal and Abnormal Findings The normal and abnormal findings for an adolescent's eye examination is the same as the adult. Muscle imbalances are common findings of adolescents, as well as eye strain from not wearing prescribed eyeglasses for self-esteem or image reasons.

■ OLDER ADULTS

Anatomy and Physiology

Changes in the external structure of the eye, including graying of eyebrows and eyelashes, occur, along with loss of tonus and decreased elasticity of eyelid muscles. Tearing is diminished, resulting in "dry eyes," which causes irritation and discomfort.

Corneal sensitivity often is diminished so that older adults may be unaware of infection or injury. Corneal reflexes are often diminished to absent. As the lens become more rigid, usually by the age of 45, and the ciliary muscle of the iris weakens, the near point of accommodation changes. This loss of lens elasticity is termed presbyopia. Increased density of the lens, along with degeneration of cells of the iris, cornea, and lens capsule, cause scattering of light and sensitivity to glare. Color perception is altered, with difficulty seeing blue, violet, and green (Lueckenotte, 1994).

Health History

- Do you have any trouble with vision when you are climbing stairs or driving?
  Rationale Older adults lose depth perception, which may contribute to falls or wrecks, respectively.
- Do you feel you have lost any peripheral vision? Do you have problems with night vision? Have you noticed a change in recognizing colors?
  Rationale These are common occurrences with older adults and need to be recognized and accommodated for to prevent injuries.
- Do you have cataracts? Have you had cataracts removed? Have the cataracts progressed, causing decreased vision?
  Rationale Cataracts are a frequent cause of altered vision in the older adult, but they can be surgically treated to minimize the effect on the client's quality of life.
- Do your eyes feel dry or burn? Do you have increased or decreased tearing? What do you do for these problems?
  Rationale Tears decrease in quantity, causing dry eyes, which can be treated with artificial tears.

Examination

Procedures and Techniques The eye examination should be conducted in the same manner as for younger adults.

Normal and Abnormal Findings Normal findings from expected anatomic and physiologic changes may be difficult to distinguish from the abnormal findings from pathologic conditions. Central and peripheral vision may be decreased after age 70. Acuity of 20/20 or 20/30 with corrective lenses is common. Accommodation takes longer. Color perception of blue, violet, and green may be impaired.

Eyebrows may be thin along the outer edge and the remaining brow hair may appear coarse. There may be wrinkles, or crow's-feet, in the skin around the eyes, because the elastic tissues have atrophied. Pseudoptosis, or relaxed upper eyelid, may be seen, with the lid resting on the lashes. Actual ptosis may also occur. Orbital fat may have decreased, so that the eyes appear sunken, or may herniate, causing bulging on the lower lid or inner third of the upper lid. The lacrimal apparatus may function poorly, giving the eye a lack of luster. Brown spots may appear near the limbus as a normal variation. Bulbar conjunctiva may appear dry, clear, and light pink without discharge or lesions.

The cornea is transparent, clear, often yellow; arcus senilis (a gray-white circle around the limbus) is common but not associated with any pathologic condition. Soft, raised yellow plaques (xanthelasma) may be noted on the lids at the inner canthus, but these are of no clinical significance.

Usually the retinal structures appear dull, with pale, attenuated blood vessels. The arterioles display a narrower light reflex and are straighter. More crossing defects are also seen. Benign degenerative hyaline deposits may be noted on the retinal surface (drusen); these do not interfere with vision.

Abnormal findings include ectropion, wherein the lower lid drops away from the globe, or entropion, wherein the lower lid turns inward, may be present. The difficulty or inability to visualize the internal structures of the eye may denote cataracts.

CLIENTS WITH SITUATIONAL VARIATIONS

CLIENTS WITH DECREASED OR ABSENT VISION

When performing a physical assessment on a blind person, you must remember to alert the client to all actions before you perform them.

The history questions will be revised to delete all those relating to vision and ocular problems. However, questions dealing with pain, swelling, watering, and discharge still are appropriate. Additional questions are needed concerning how the individual has adapted to the loss of sight. The physical examination includes only inspection of the external eye structures as described for the adult.

CLIENTS WITH SUSPECTED DRUG INTOXICATION

The examination should be conducted in the same manner as for adults. Include questions about recent drug use, which drugs, and what dosage.

When assessing a client whom you suspect is intoxicated, use the Rapid Eye Test in Box 16-3 to collect data to confirm or refute your suspicion. Data from Table 16-1 may help you identify from the client's eye signs which drug(s) may have been abused.

CLIENTS WITH PROSTHETIC EYE

Clients who have had an enucleation of an eye replaced by a prosthesis appear to have binocular vision. The examiner, however, must remember that the clients have no sight on the affected side and must be approached from the sighted side.

Some artificial eyes are permanently implanted. Others are removed for daily cleaning.

Box 16-3 Rapid Eye Test to Detect Current Drug Intoxication

GENERAL OBSERVATION

Look for redness of sclera, ptosis, retracted upper lid (white sclera visible above iris, causing blank stare), glazing, excessive tearing of eyes, and swelling of eyelids.

PUPIL SIZE

Dilated (>6.5 mm) or constricted (<3.0 mm).

PUPIL REACTION TO LIGHT

Slow, sluggish, or absent response.

NYSTAGMUS

Hold finger in vertical position and have the client follow finger as it is moves to the side, in a circle, and up and down. Positive test is failure to hold gaze or jerkiness of eye movements.

CONVERGENCE

Inability to hold the cross-eyed position after an examining finger is moved from 1 foot away from client's nose and held there for 5 seconds.

CORNEAL REFLEX

Decreased rate of blinking after touching cornea with cotton.

Table 16-1 Common Eye Signs Detected After Abuse of Selected Drugs

	MARIJUANA	HEROIN	ALCOHOL	COCAINE	PCP
Pupil size	Normal	Constricted	Normal	Dilated	Normal
Slow or no reaction of pupil to light	Yes		Yes	Yes	Yes
Nonconvergence	Yes				
Redness of sclera	Yes		Yes		
Glazing of cornea	Yes	Yes	Yes		
Nystagmus	Yes		Yes		Yes
Swollen eyelids	Yes	Yes			Yes
Watering eyes	Yes				
Ptosis		Yes			
Decreased corneal reflex		Yes		Yes	Yes

Data from Tennant F: Is your patient abusing drugs? *Postgrad Med 84:*108-114, 1988.
PCP, Phencyclidine.

EXAMINATION SUMMARY

Eyes and Visual System

VISION (pp. 325-328)

- Test distant vision using Snellen's chart or E chart.
- Assess near vision using Jaeger or Rosenbaum card or newspaper.
- Assess visual fields for peripheral vision using confrontation test.
- Inspect extraocular muscles for movement using six cardinal fields of gaze.
- Inspect corneal light reflex for symmetry.
  - Perform the cover-uncover test if needed.

EXTERNAL OCULAR STRUCTURES (pp. 329-333)

- Inspect eyebrows for:
  Hair distribution
  Underlying skin
  Symmetry
- Inspect eyelids and eyelashes for:
  Symmetry
  Position
  Closure
  Blinking patterns
  Discharge
  Color
- Inspect and palpate globe for:
  Position
  Indentation
- Inspect lacrimal puncta for:
  Color
  Moisture
  Discharge
  Tenderness
  Nodules
- Inspect conjunctiva for:
  Color and clarity
- Inspect sclera for:
  Color
  Clarity
- Inspect cornea for:
  Transparency
  Surface characteristics
- Inspect anterior chamber for:
  Transparency
  Iris surface
  Chamber depth
- Inspect iris for:
  Shape
  Color
- Inspect pupil for:
  Size
  Shape
  Reaction to light and accommodation

❖INTERNAL OCULAR STRUCTURES (pp. 334-336)

- Observe the red reflex.
- Inspect optic disc for:
  Margins
  Size and shape
  Color
  Physiologic cup

- Inspect retinal vessels for:
  Color
  Arteriolar light reflex
  Artery-to-vein ratio
  Arteriovenous crossing characteristics
- Inspect retinal background for:
  Color
  Presence of:
    Microaneurysms
    Hemorrhages
    Exudates
- Inspect macula and fovea centralis for:
  Color
  Surface characteristics

SUMMARY OF FINDINGS

Age Group	Normal Findings	Typical Variations	Findings Associated With Disorders
Infants and children	• *Vision:* Visual acuity 20/20 using Allen picture cards or Snellen's chart. Distinguishes colors. Symmetric corneal light reflex. • *External ocular structures:* Outer canthus of eye aligns with pinna of ear. Blink reflex present. • *Internal ocular structures:* Red reflex present bilaterally.	• *Vision:* Visual acuity 20/30 or 20/40 is acceptable. Pseudostrabismus may occur in Asian or Native American children. Transient strabismus may resolve by 6 months. • *External ocular structures:* Eyelids of newborn are edematous.	• *Vision:* Visual acuity greater than 20/40. Color-blind. • *External ocular structures:* Outer canthus of eye above or below pinna of ear. Malalignment of eyes from corneal light reflex and cover-uncover test. Purulent discharge from eyes. Absent blink and pupillary light reflexes. • *Internal ocular structures:* Absence of red reflex.
Adolescents	Same as for adult.	Same as for adult.	Same as for adult.
Older adults	• *Vision:* Color perception of blue, violet, and green impaired. • *External ocular structures:* Soft, raised yellow plaques in inner canthus. • *Globe of the eye:* Accommodation takes longer. Gray-white circle around limbus.	• *External ocular structures:* Dry bulbar conjunctiva. • *Globe of the eye:* Brown spots near limbus.	• *External ocular structures:* Lower lid moves away from the globe or moves inward toward the globe. • *Internal ocular structures:* Cloudy cornea and inability to visualize internal eye structures.
Adult	• *Vision:* Visual acuity is 20/20, peripheral visual fields are intact. Eye movement is parallel. Symmetric corneal light reflex.	• *Vision:* Corrected to 20/20 with glasses or contact lenses. Mild nystagmus at extreme lateral gaze.	• *Vision:* Visual acuity is greater than 20/20 without correction, (20/200 is legal blindness), squinting to read. Eye movement is not parallel. Corneal light reflex asymmetric.

Age Group	Normal Findings	Typical Variations	Findings Associated With Disorders
Adult—cont'd	• *External ocular structures:* Eyebrows, eyelids, and lashes symmetric. Lid margins cover part of iris. Eye globe indents slightly. Lacrimal puncta pink and intact. Conjunctivae are pink and moist. Sclerae are white, corneas and anterior chambers are transparent. • *Globe of the eye:* Pupils are equal, round, and react to light and accommodation. • *Internal ocular structures:* Red reflex is present. Optic disc is round, creamy yellow with physiologic cup occupying <1/2 disc diameter, artery-to-vein ratio is 2:3 or 4:5. Uniform pink, red, or orange color of retina. Macula 1 DD.		• *External ocular structures:* Eyelids do not cover part of iris, sclera noted above and below iris. Eyelids red, edematous. Discharge in eyes. Eye globe is firm. Lacrimal puncta are red, edematous with discharge. Conjunctivae are pale or have a discharge. Tissue growth on bulbar conjunctiva may be pterygium. Sclerae are yellow. • *Globe of the eye:* Corneas are opaque. Pupils are unequal, shape other than round, nonreactive to light and accommodation. • *Internal ocular structures:* Irregular red reflex, blurred disc margins, engorged vessels, physiologic cup > 1/2 disc diameter. Arteries narrow, A-V nicking, pale fundus or hemorrhages. Fine red dots or exudate. Fundus pale.

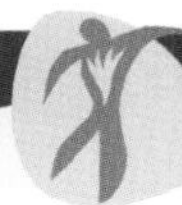

HEALTH PROMOTION

Children

Vision screening is recommended for all children before entering school, preferably at age 3 or 4 (U.S. Preventive Services Task Force, 1996). Every toddler should be screened for strabismus as part of the routine eye examination during well-child visits (Wong et al, 1999). After age 8, vision should be fully integrated. Routine vision testing is *not* recommended as a component of the periodic health examination of asymptomatic school children. Secondary visual problems may be the basis for behavioral problems.

Adolescents

Routine vision testing is *not* recommended as a component of the periodic health examination of asymptomatic clients.

Teens who participate in school shop or science laboratories or in certain sports (racquetball, squash) should wear safety lenses and safety frames approved by the American National Standards Institute. Teens with good vision in only one eye should wear safety lenses and frames to protect the unaffected eye, even if they do not otherwise need to wear glasses (USDHHS, 1994).

Adults

A comprehensive eye examination, including screening for visual acuity and glaucoma, should be performed every 2 years beginning at age 40 in African Americans and at age 60 in all other individuals. Diabetic clients, at any age, should have an annual eye examination by an ophthalmologist (U.S. Preventive Services Task Force, 1996).

Clients who work outside should protect their conjunctivae from excessive exposure to sunlight by wearing sunglasses.

Those who participate in sports need protection such as goggles or glasses when playing basketball, hockey, or football.

Older Adults

The Task Force recommends that clients over 65 years of age be tested periodically for glaucoma by an eye specialist.

COMMON PROBLEMS AND CONDITIONS

Eyes and Visual System

EXTERNAL EYE

Ectropion

An eversion of the eyelid is called ectropion. It is caused by decreased muscle tone (Fig. 16-20). The palpebral conjunctiva is exposed, increasing the risk of conjunctivitis.

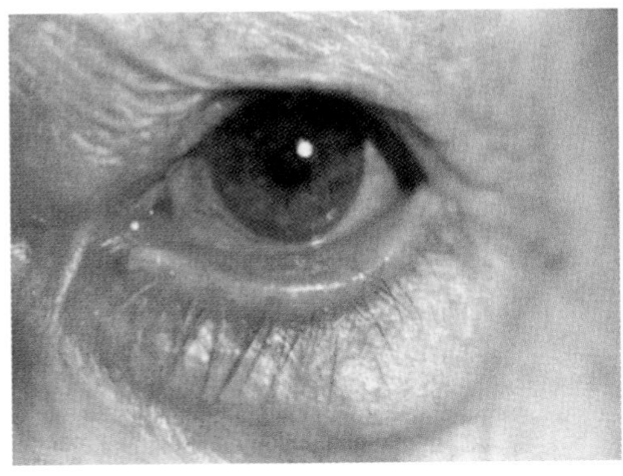

Fig. 16-20 Ectropion. (Courtesy Dr. Ira Abrahamson, Jr, Cincinnati, Ohio. From Stein HA, Slatt BJ, Stein, 1988.)

Exotropia

Outward (temporal) deviation of the eye is called *extropia* (Fig. 16-21). (See *strabismus.*)

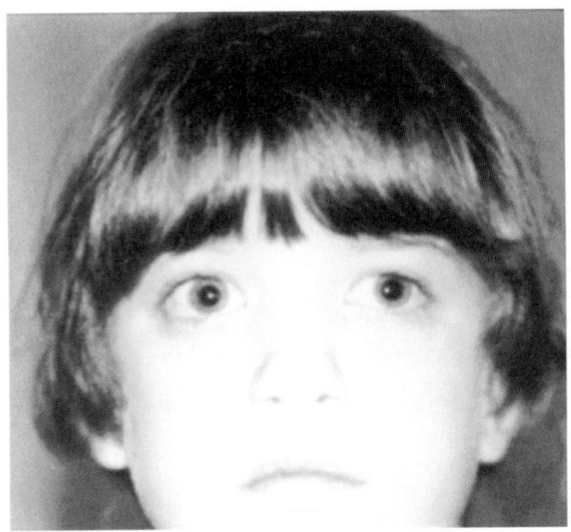

Fig. 16-21 Exotropia. Client has a 30 prism diopter exotropia at distance. (From Helveston, 1993.)

Enophthalmos

Sunken eyes are called enophthalmos. It is seen with chronic wasting illnesses such as cachexia (Fig. 16-22).

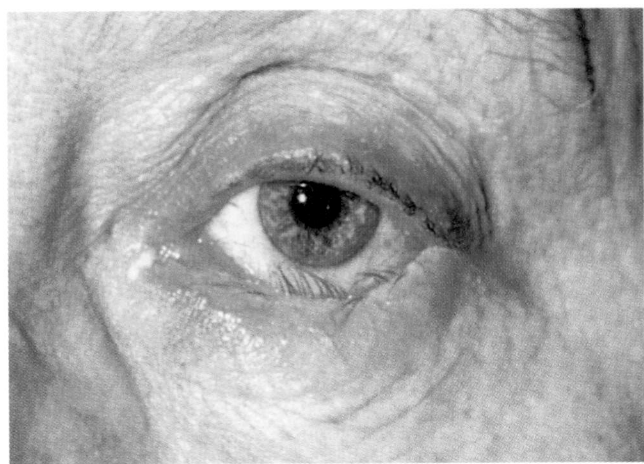

Fig. 16-22 Enophthalmos. The eyelid and lashes are rolled in. (From Bedford, 1986.)

Exophthalmos

Bulging eyes are called exophthalmos. It is associated with hyperthyroidism and caused by deposits of fat and fluid in the retro-orbital tissues, forcing the eyeballs forward (Fig. 16-23). Upper eyelids usually are retracted so that when the eye is open, the sclera above the iris is visible. Lids may not close completely.

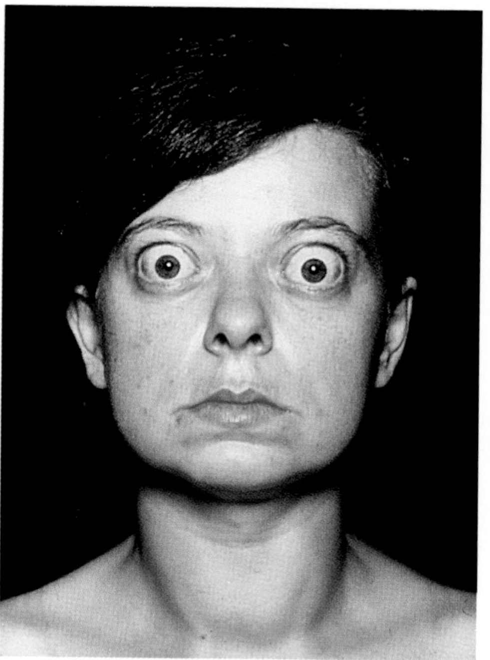

Fig. 16-23 Exophthalmos. (From Seidel et al, 1999.)

Blepharitis

Inflammation of the lash follicles and meibomian glands is known as blepharitis. It causes red, scaly, and crusted lid margins. Chronic blepharitis may be associated with seborrhea or dandruff or may be caused by bacterial infection (Fig. 16-24).

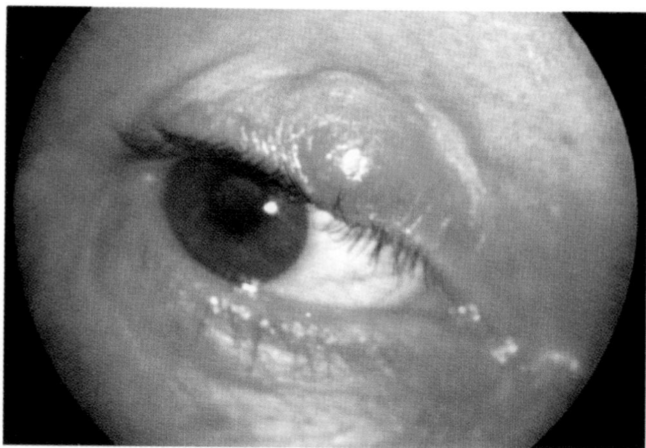

Fig. 16-24 Blepharitis. Swelling of the meibomian glands caused by eruption of sebum outside the walls of the gland. (From Bedford, 1986.)

Chalazion

A firm, nontender nodule of a meibomian gland in the eyelid is the findings of this disorder. It often follows hordeolum or chronic inflammation such as conjunctivitis, blepharitis, or meibomian cyst (Fig. 16-25).

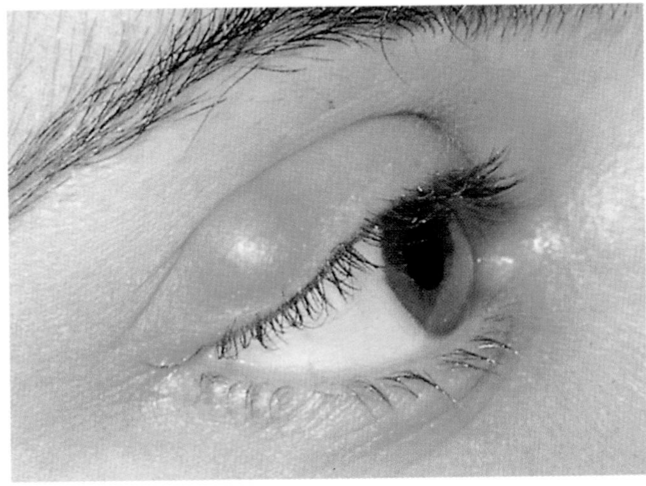

Fig. 16-25 Chalazion (right upper eyelid). (From Newell, 1992.)

Hordeolum (sty)

An acute infection of hair follicles of the eyelid is called a hordeolum. It is usually caused by *Staphylococcus aureus* (Fig. 16-26). The affected area usually is very painful, red, and edematous.

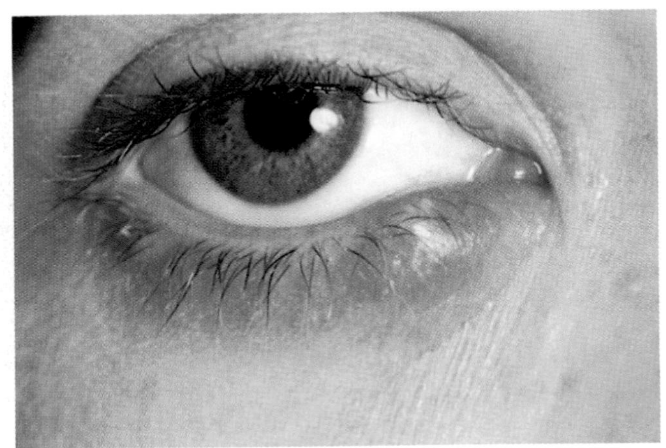

Fig. 16-26 Hordeolum (sty). (From Bedford, 1986.)

Ptosis

Drooping of the eyelid is called ptosis. It is due to paralysis of the oculomotor nerve (cranial nerve III) or systemic neuromuscular weakness such as myasthenia gravis (Fig. 16-27).

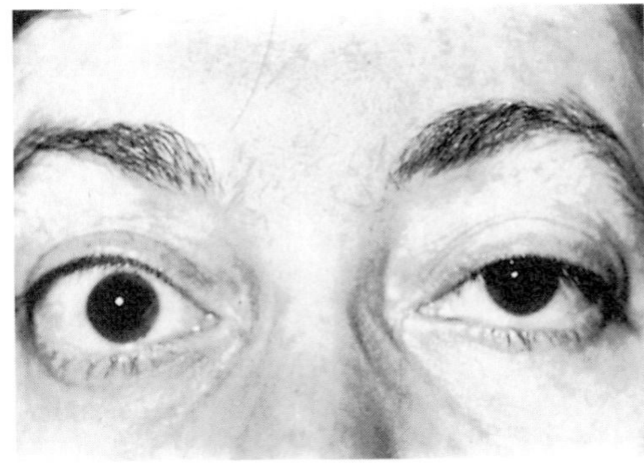

Fig. 16-27 Ptosis. Client with left ptosis and right upper lid retraction. (From Nesi et al, 1998.)

Pterygium

A growth of bulbar conjunctiva toward the center of the cornea is called pterygium. It can be caused by chronic exposure to a hot, dry, and sandy climate (Fig. 16-28). Usually it invades from the nasal side and obstructs vision as it covers the pupil.

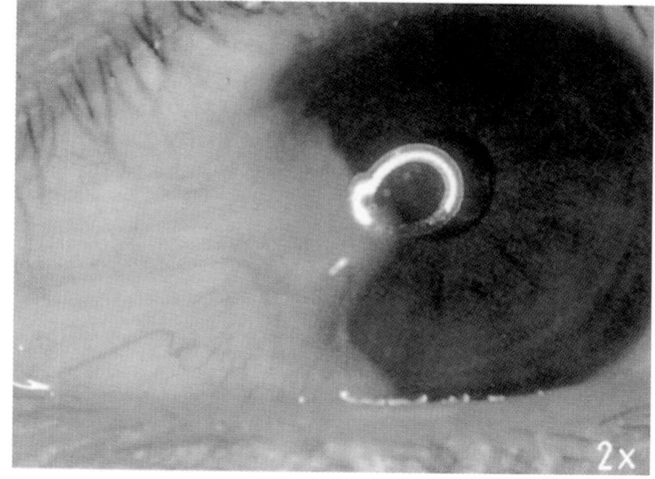

Fig. 16-28 Pterygium. (From Newell, 1996.)

Conjunctivitis

An inflammation of the palpebral or bulbar conjunctiva is known as conjunctivitis. It is caused by local infection of bacteria or virus, as well as by an allergic reaction, systemic infection, or chemical irritation (Fig. 16-29).

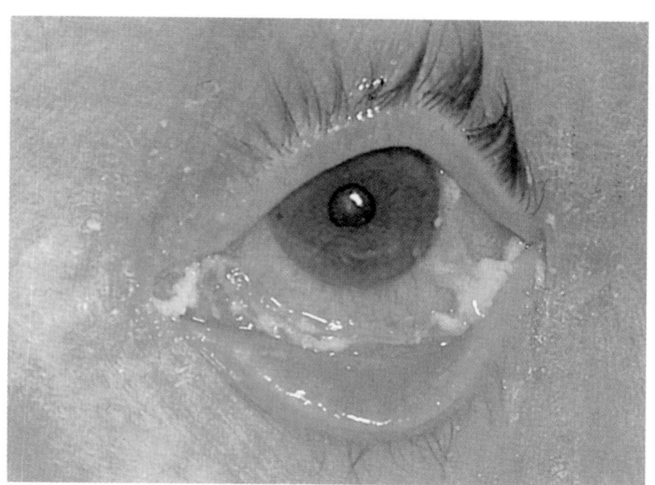

Fig. 16-29 Conjunctivitis (acute). (From Newell, 1996.)

Corneal Abrasion or Ulcer

Disruptions of the corneal epithelium and stroma create a corneal abrasion or ulcer. It is caused by fungal, viral, or bacterial infections or desiccation because of incomplete lid closure or poor lacrimal gland function (Fig. 16-30). This condition is commonly caused by scratches, foreign bodies, or contact lenses that are poorly fitted or overworn. Client feels intense pain, has a foreign body sensation, and reports photophobia. Tearing and redness are observed.

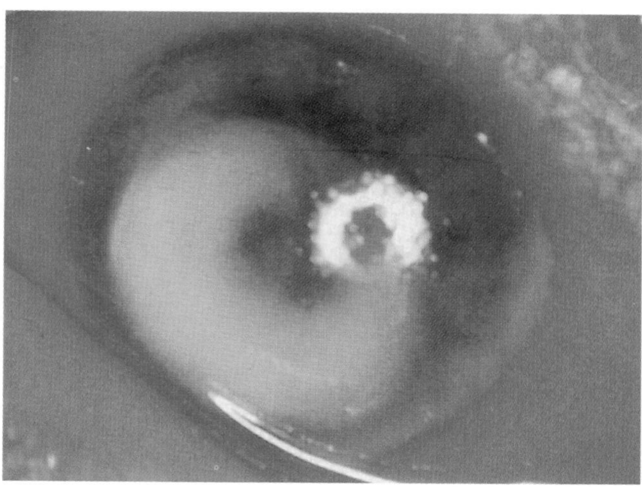

Fig. 16-30 Fungal corneal ulcer. (From Newell, 1996.)

Dacryocystitis

Inflammation of the lacrimal sac is called dacryocystitis. It is caused by an infection and blockage of the sac and duct (Fig. 16-31). Pain, warmth, redness, and swelling occur in the inner canthus. Tearing is present and may occur in newborns through older adults. Pressure on the sacs produces purulent discharge from the puncta.

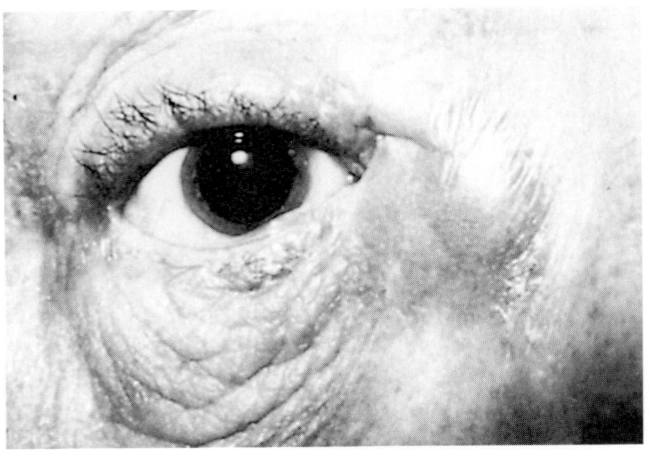

Fig. 16-31 Dacryocystitis. Acute dacryocystitis in right eye of 71-year-old man. (From Newell, 1996.)

Upward Palpebral Slant of the Eyes

This abnormal finding is seen in children with Down syndrome, along with epicanthal folds and hypertelorism (large tongue) (Fig. 16-32).

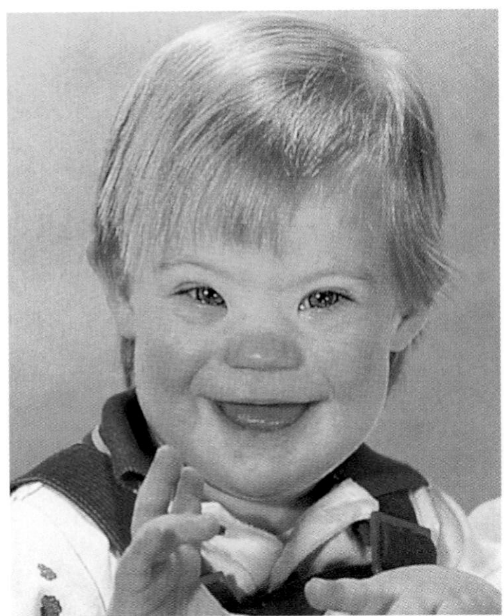

Fig. 16-32 Note upwardly slanting palpebral fissures in child with Down syndrome. (From Zitelli and Davis, 1997.)

Pupil Abnormalities (Table 16-2)

Table 16-2 Pupil Abnormalities

ABNORMALITY	CONTRIBUTING FACTORS	APPEARANCE
BILATERAL		
Miosis (pupillary constriction; usually less than 2 mm in diameter)	Iridocyclitis; miotic eyedrops (such as pilocarpine given for glaucoma)	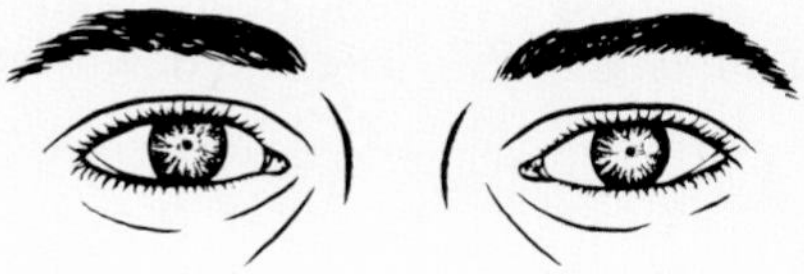
Mydriasis (pupillary dilation; usually more than 6 mm in diameter)	Iridocyclitis; mydriatic or cycloplegic drops (such as atropine); midbrain (reflex arc) lesions or hypoxia; oculomotor (CN III) damage; acute-angle glaucoma (slight dilation)	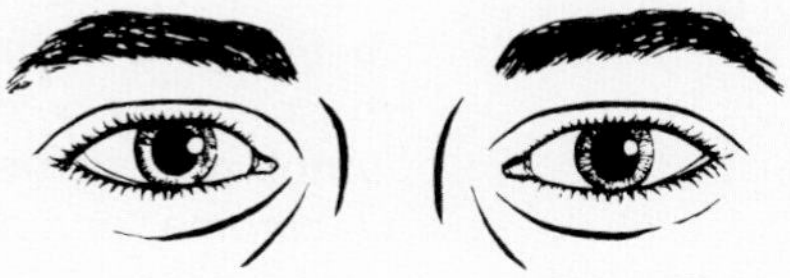
Failure to respond (constrict) with increased light stimulus	Iridocyclitis; corneal or lens opacity (light does not reach retina); retinal degeneration; optic nerve (CN II) destruction; midbrain synapses involving afferent pupillary fibers or oculomotor nerve (CN III) (consensual response is also lost); impairment of efferent fibers (parasympathetic) that innervate sphincter pupillae muscle	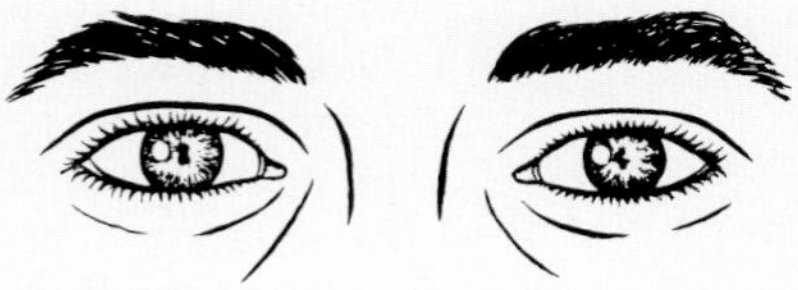
Argyll Robertson pupil	Bilateral, miotic, irregular-shaped pupils that fail to constrict with light but retain constriction with convergence; pupils may or may not be equal in size; commonly caused by neurosyphilis or lesions in midbrain where afferent pupillary fibers synapse	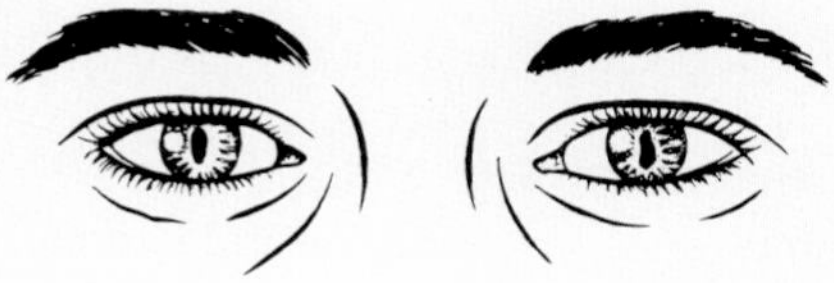
Oval pupil	Sometimes occurs with head injury or intracranial hemorrhage; transitional stage between normal pupil and dilated, fixed pupil with increased intracranial pressure (ICP); in most instances returns to normal when ICP is returned to normal	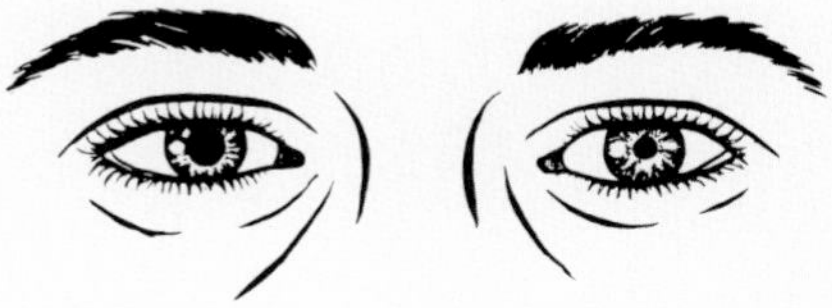
UNILATERAL		
Anisocoria (unequal size of pupils)	Congenital (approximately 20% of normal people have minor or noticeable differences in pupil size, but reflexes are normal) or caused by local eye medications (constrictors or dilators), amblyopia, or unilateral sympathetic or parasympathetic pupillary pathway destruction (NOTE: Examiner should test whether pupils react equally to light; if response is unequal, examiner should note whether larger or smaller pupil reacts more slowly [or not at all], since either pupil could be abnormal size)	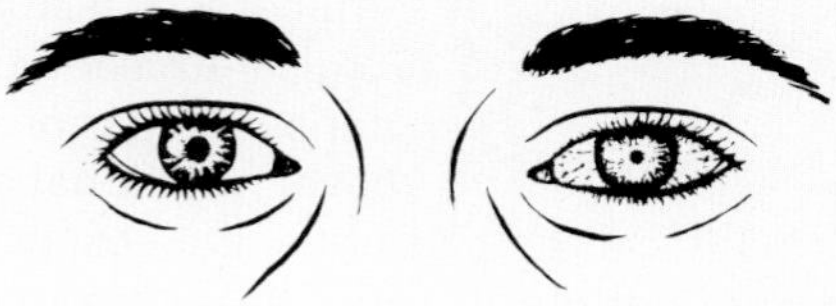
Iritis constrictive response	Acute uveitis is frequently unilateral; constriction of pupil accompanied by pain and circumcorneal flush (redness)	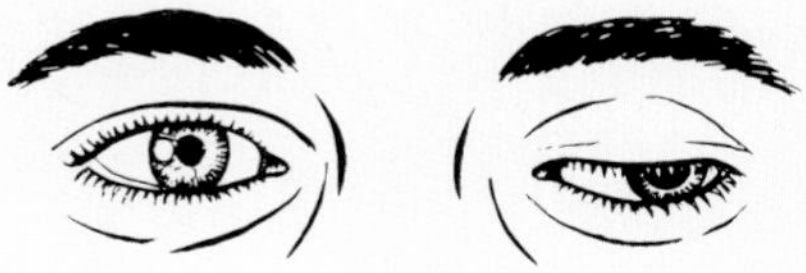

From Thompson JM et al: *Mosby's clinical nursing,* ed 4, St. Louis, 1997, Mosby.
CN, Cranial nerve.

Continued

Table 16-2 Pupil Abnormalities—cont'd

ABNORMALITY	CONTRIBUTING FACTORS	APPEARANCE
UNILATERAL—cont'd		
Oculomotor nerve (CN III) damage	Pupil dilated and fixed; eye deviated laterally and downward; ptosis	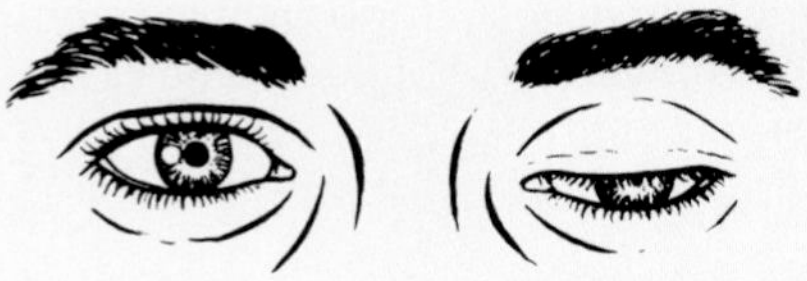
Horner's syndrome	Miotic pupil; ptosis; interruption of sympathetic nerve supply to dilator pupillae muscle; may be caused by goiter, cervical lymph enlargement, apical bronchogenic carcinoma, or surgical injury to neck	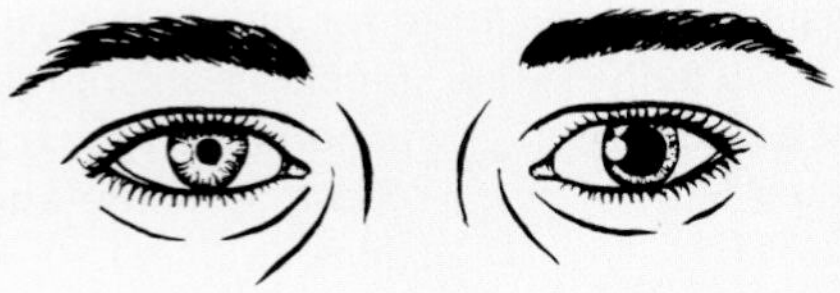
Adie's pupil (tonic pupil)	Affected pupil dilated and reacts slowly or fails to react to light; response to convergence normal; caused by impairment of postganglionic parasympathetic innervation to sphincter pupillae muscle or ciliary malfunction; often accompanied by diminished tendon reflexes (as with diabetic neuropathy or alcoholism)	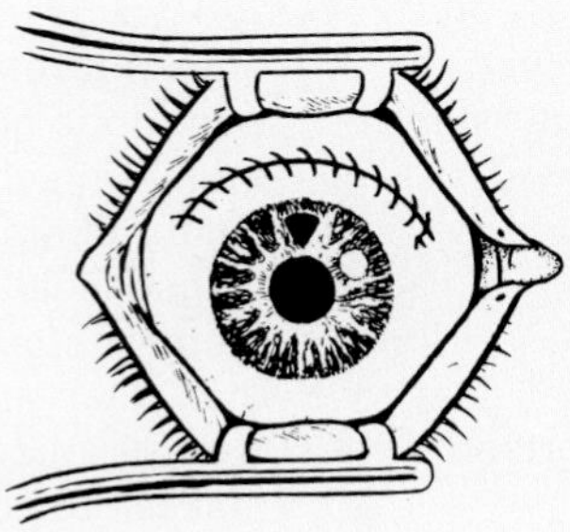
OTHER IRREGULARITIES		
Iridectomy	Sector iridectomy	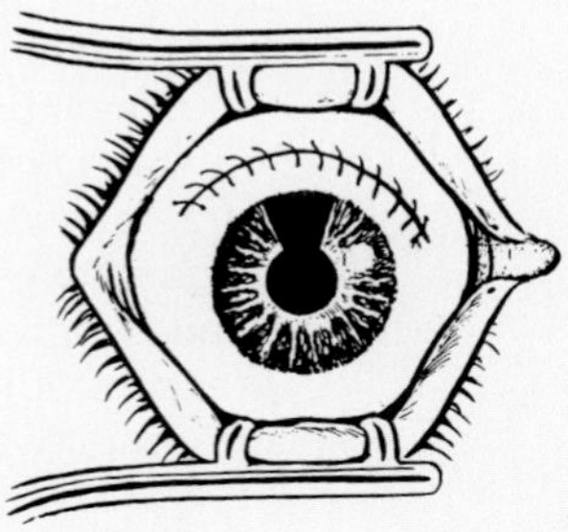
	Peripheral iridectomy Surgical excision of portion of iris usually done in superior area so upper lid will cover additional exposure	
Coloboma (localized absence of portion of iris)	Congenital absence of area of iris; remaining iris shows normal light response	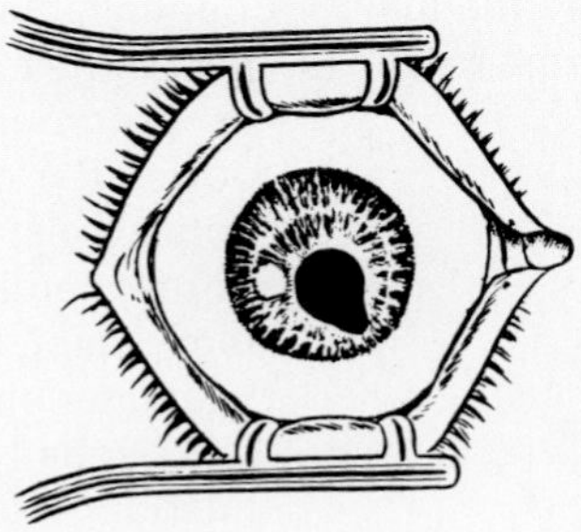
Iridodialysis (circumferential tearing of iris from scleral spur)	Blunt trauma; more than one "pupil" in eye can cause diplopia	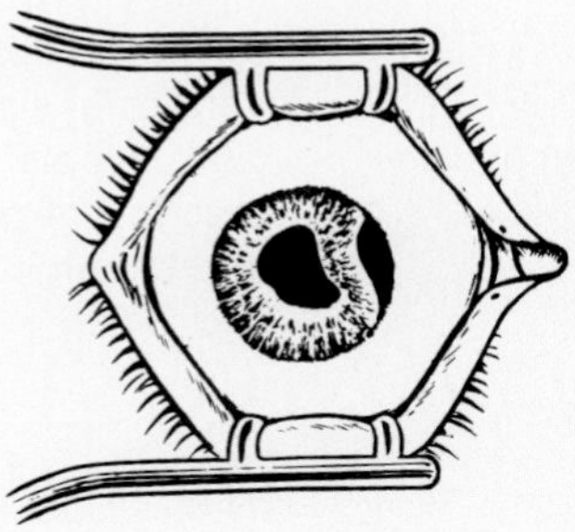

From Thompson JM et al: *Mosby's clinical nursing*, ed 4, St. Louis, 1997, Mosby.

PERIPHERAL VISUAL DEFECTS

Visual field defects can often be traced to disorders in specific anatomic locations because of the arrangement of nerve fibers (Fig. 16-33). Strokes or tumors are common causes of this type of peripheral visual defect. A left or right optic nerve lesion could cause a defect in the corresponding left or right eye. A common chiasm defect is bitemporal hemianopia, which results from a pituitary tumor.

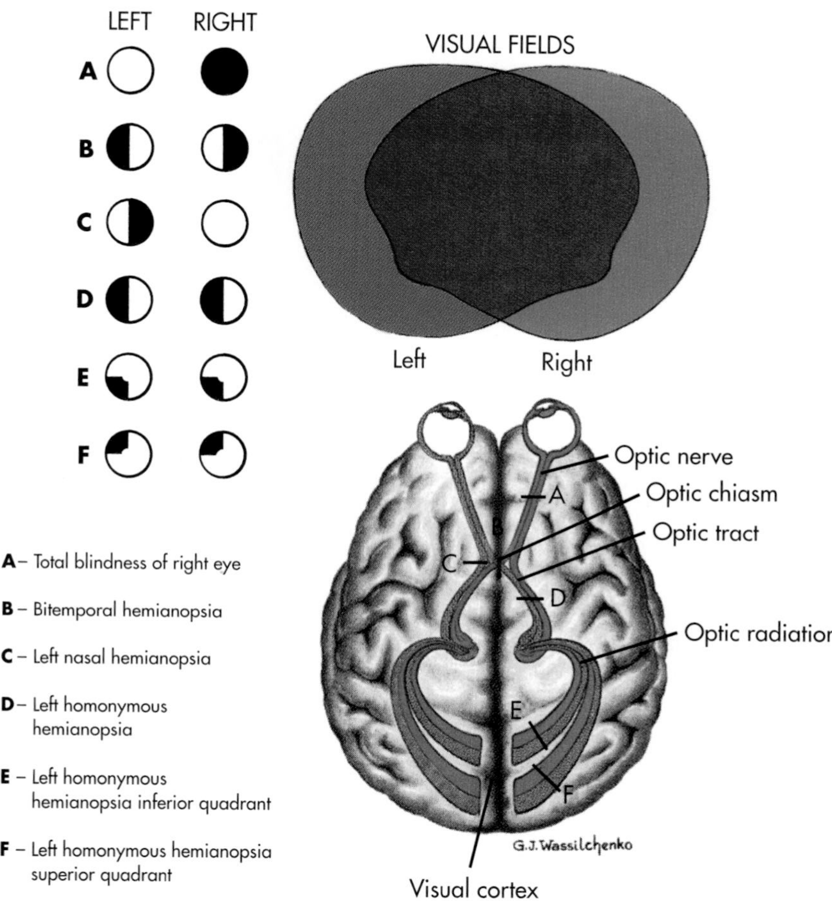

Fig. 16-33 Visual pathway defects. Fig.16-6 describes normal pathway. **A,** Lesion of the entire optic nerve to right eye. **B,** Lesion in the optic chiasm that affects only the lateral (temporal) side of the optic nerves to both eyes because those are the nerves that cross in the optic chiasm. **C,** Lesion of the medial (nasal) side of the left eye. **D,** Lesion of the optic tract on the right side distal to the optic chiasm. Since the nerve crosses at the optic chiasm, the lesion on the right affects the left side of each eye. If you follow the nerves from the lesion to the eyeball, you will see that the affected nerves are on the right side of the retina. This part of the retina provides vision for the left side of the eye. **E** and **F,** Lesions of the optic radiator that result in blindness in one quadrant of each eye as shown. (From Rudy, 1984.)

EXTRAOCULAR MUSCLES

Strabismus

An abnormal ocular alignment in which the visual axes do not meet at the desired point is called strabismus (Fig. 16-34). Nonparalytic strabismus is due to muscle weakness, focusing difficulties, unilateral refractive error, nonfusion, or anatomic differences in eyes. Paralytic strabismus is a motor imbalance caused by paresis or paralysis of an extraocular muscle. Two of the most common types of strabismus are esotropia and exotropia. Esotropia is an inward-turning eye and is the most common type of strabismus in infants. Exotropia is an outward-turning eye.

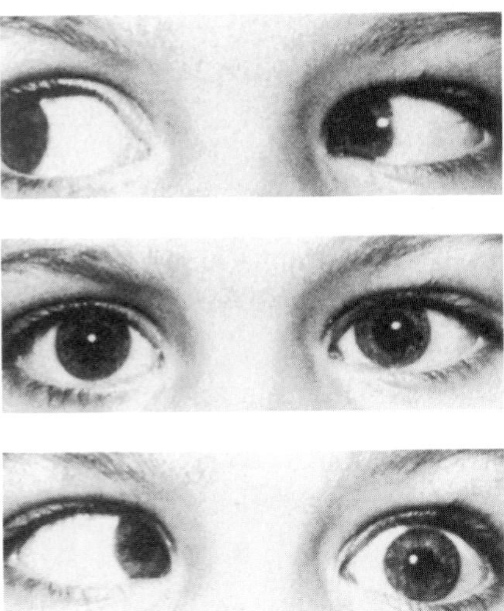

Fig. 16-34 Paralytic strabismus involving left lateral rectus muscle innervated by cranial nerve VI (abducens nerve). (From von Noorden, 1990.)

INTERNAL EYE

Cataract

An opacity of the crystalline lens is called a cataract. It most commonly occurs from denaturation of lens protein caused by aging (Fig. 16-35, *A, B*). Cataracts due to aging usually are central, but peripheral cataracts are seen in hypoparathyroidism. Congenital cataracts can result from maternal rubella or other fetal insults during the first trimester of pregnancy. Trauma to the eye can also cause cataracts.

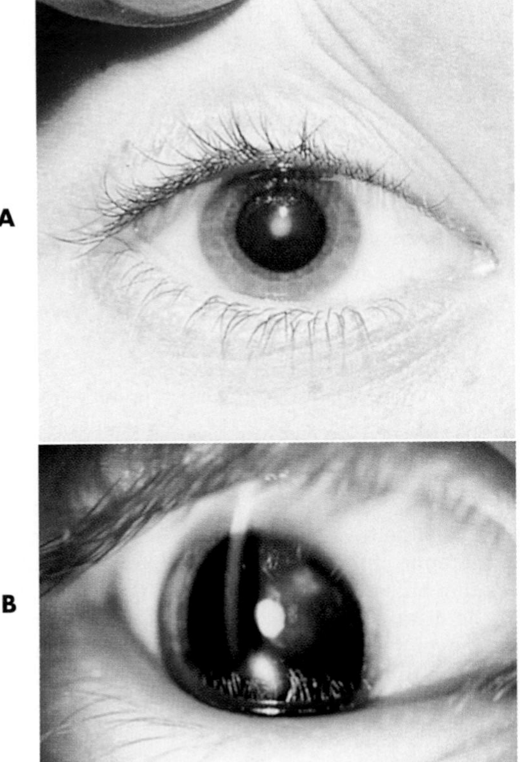

Fig. 16-35 **A,** Anterior polar cataract, a developmental abnormality, which in most cases remain stable and rarely affect vision. **B,** Cataract of galactosemia. Early lens changes in galactosemia are reversible. (From Zitelli and Davis, 1997.)

Diabetic Retinopathy

Visual alterations occurring in clients with diabetes mellitus is referred to as diabetic retinopathy. It is caused by changes in the retinal capillaries (Fig. 16-36). Diabetic retinopathy is divided into background and proliferative. Background retinopathy is marked by dot hemorrhages or microaneurysms and the presence of hard and soft exudates. Hard exudates are thought to result from lipid transudation through incompetent capillaries, have sharply defined borders, and tend to be bright yellow. Soft exudates are caused by infarctions of the nerve layer and appear as dull yellow spots with poorly defined margins.

Diabetic retinopathy (proliferative) is a form of retinopathy in which development of new vessels occurs as a result of anoxic stimulation (Fig. 16-37). New vessels lack support structures of healthy vessels and are more likely to hemorrhage. Bleeding from these vessels is a major cause of blindness in clients with diabetes.

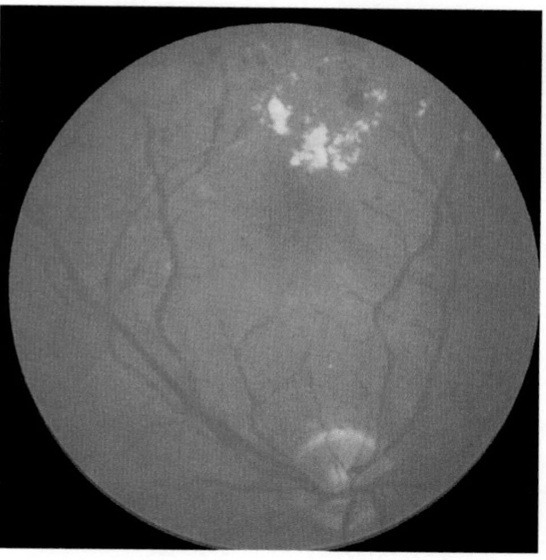

Fig. 16-36 Diabetic retinopathy. The retinal changes are predominantly at the posterior pole with microaneurysms and "dot and blot" hemorrhages, together with hard exudates in the macular area. (From Bedford, 1986.)

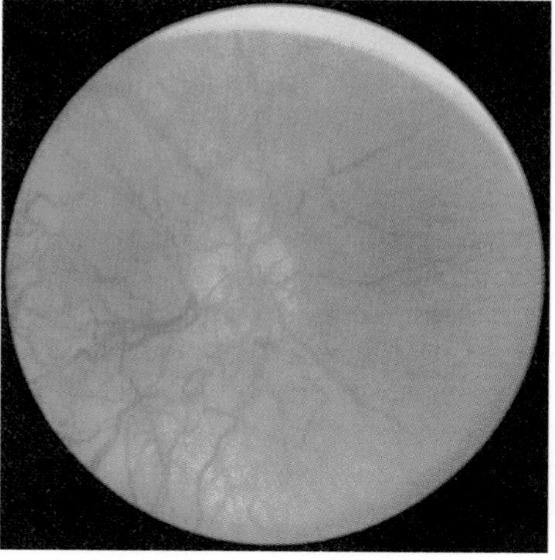

Fig. 16-37 Proliferative diabetic retinopathy. (Courtesy John W. Payne, MD, The Wilmer Ophthalmological Institute, The Johns Hopkins University and Hospital, Baltimore, Md. From Seidel et al, 1999.)

Cytomegalovirus (CMV) Infection

An increasingly common cause of blindness among clients with human immunodeficiency virus (HIV) is CMV infection of the eye (Fig. 16-38). This infection is characterized by hemorrhage, exudates, and necrosis of the retina. Cytomegalovirus infection is said to create a "pizza pie" appearance in the retina.

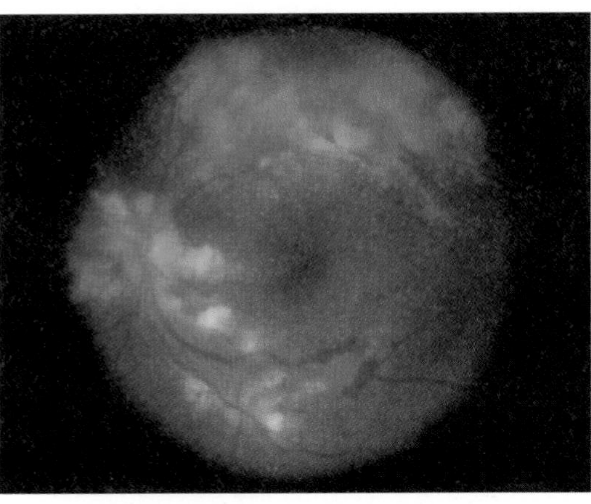

Fig. 16-38 Cytomegalovirus infection. (Courtesy Douglas A. Jabs, MD, The Wilmer Ophthalmological Institute, The Johns Hopkins University and Hospital, Baltimore. Md. From Seidel et al, 1999.)

Glaucoma

An increase in the intraocular pressure is called glaucoma. It is caused by obstruction of the outflow of aqueous humor. The increased pressure damages the retina and may cause atrophy of the optic nerve. Vision loss is gradual and painless, with loss of peripheral vision occurring first.

Hypertensive Retinopathy

Chronic hypertension can cause changes in the retina. These changes are classified using the Keith-Wagener-Barker (KWB) system, which evaluates changes in the vascular supply, the retina itself, and the optic disc. These changes occur bilaterally. The normal artery-to-vein ratio (2:3 or 4:5) decreases because of the vascular smooth muscle contraction, hyperplasia, or fibrosis (Fig. 16-39).

- Group I of the KWB classification has arterioles with an increased light reflex. There is moderate arteriolar constriction but no changes in the arteriovenous crossings.
- Group II has changes in the arteriovenous crossing. Arterioles are reduced to half the usual size, and areas of local vasoconstriction may be noted.
- Group III has shining retina and yellow areas with poorly defined margins (cotton-wool spots) that result from ischemic infarcts of the retina.
- Group IV has papilledema, edema of the optic disc (Seidel et al, 1999).

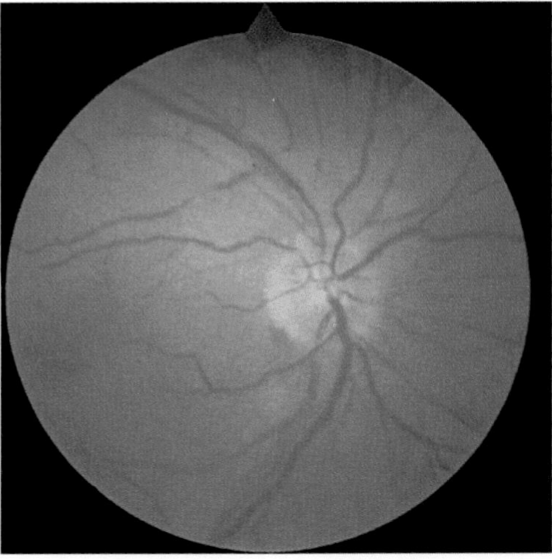

Fig. 16-39 Hypertensive retinopathy. Narrowing of the caliber of the arterioles, crossing of these arterioles over the veins, and a few hemorrhages can be seen. (From Bedford, 1986.)

CLINICAL APPLICATION and CRITICAL THINKING

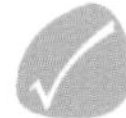

SAMPLE DOCUMENTATION

CASE 1

A 66-year-old man with blurred vision presents with a chief complaint of decreased vision.

Subjective Data

Patient states, "I can't see as well as I used to." Reports gradual changes in vision over past 6 months. Reports no eye pain, discharge, watering from eyes, excessive blinking, redness or swelling of eyes, or trauma to eyes. Last eye examination 3 years ago. Has been socially active and has volunteered at an animal shelter; has been unable to continue with activities with visual changes. Client relates he has stopped driving due to blurring vision. Is concerned vision will deteriorate to point where he will lose independence.

Objective Data

Visual acuity: O.D., 20/40; O.S., 20/40; O.U., 20/40.

Brows, lids, lashes evenly distributed; extraocular muscles intact; no lid lag; no nystagmus; visual fields equal to examiner's; no tearing; conjunctiva pink without discharge; pupils round, react to light, and accommodation. Unable to assess red reflex or perform ophthalmic examination due to opacities of lens.

Functional Health Patterns Involved

- Health perception–health management
- Cognitive–perceptual
- Self-perception–self-concept
- Role–relationship

Medical Diagnosis

Cataracts

Nursing Diagnosis and Collaborative Problems

- *Sensory/perceptual alteration* (visual) related to change in visual ability as manifested by:
  - Blurred vision
  - Decreased vision
  - Corneal opacities.
- *Altered role performance* related to change in functional status associated with reduction in vision as manifested by:
  - States inability to maintain activities due to reduced vision.
- *Anxiety* related to anticipated failing vision as manifested by:
  - Statement he lives alone
  - Concern for remaining independent.
- *Risk for social isolation* related to inability to maintain social activities.
- *Risk for injury* related to reduction in vision.

CASE 2

Erin, an 8-year-old girl, is sent to the nurse's office at school after the classroom teacher noticed her eye was red.

Subjective Data

Erin indicates her eye has been red and sore since last evening; woke this morning with large amount of dried drainage on eyelashes. Denies difficulty with vision; describes eye as a "burning pain."

Objective Data

Bilateral swelling of eyelids; mucopurulent discharge with superficial hyperemia of globes and eyelids; cornea clear; pupils round, equal, and react to light bilaterally; red reflex noted bilaterally—is sensitive to bright light; intraocular examination deferred.

Visual acuity: O.D., 20/20; O.S., 20/25; O.U., 20/25.

Functional Health Patterns Involved

- Health perception–health management
- Cognitive–perceptual

Nursing Diagnosis and Collaborative Problems

- *Sensory perceptual alteration, visual* related to inflammation of eye as manifested by:
  - Complaints of burning sensation.
  - Sensitivity to light.
- *Risk for infection* related to possible contagious pathogenic process and frequent touching of eyes.
- *PC*: Bacterial conjunctivitis.

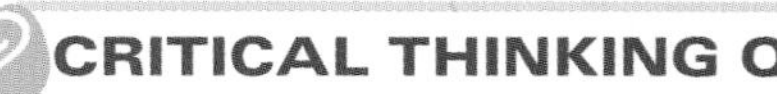

CRITICAL THINKING QUESTIONS

1. While examining the internal eye, the nurse notes retinal vessels. How are the arteries and the veins differentiated?
2. A 26-year-old white male is brought to the emergency department by ambulance after his girlfriend found him on the floor of their apartment. He is awake, but sluggish. The girlfriend tells the nurse that something is "very wrong" with him. The nurse suspects drug use. Describe a quick assessment that can help the nurse rule out drug intoxication.
3. A 5-year-old child is brought in for a routine physical examination. Describe what components of eye examination are appropriate for a child of this age without a specific eye or visual complaint.

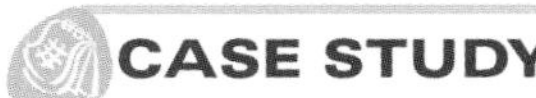

CASE STUDY

Andy Begay is a 32-year-old, single Native American man who has type 2 diabetes mellitus. Although Andy has been compliant, he has had poor control with his blood glucose levels. His reason for seeking care is a vision problem. Listed below are data collected during an interview and examination.

Interview Data

Andy presents to the clinic with complaints of significant reduction in vision over the last couple of weeks. "I can't lose my vision because I won't be able to keep my job. If I can't see, I don't know how I will take care of my diabetes or how I will maintain my income."

Examination Data

- **General survey:** Anxious, well-nourished male.
- **Eyes:** Snellen test—O.S. 20/70; O.D. 20/70 +2; O.U. 20/60 +1; reduced peripheral vision. Normal extraocular movement and corneal light reflex. Eyelids and eyelashes symmetric. Conjunctivae clear bilaterally. Sclera is white; corneas clear. Lacrimal structures without tearing. Pupils are equal and round and react to light.
- **Internal eye examination:** Retinal vessels hemorrhagic. New vessels present. Findings consistent with proliferative diabetic retinopathy.

1. What data deviate from normal findings, suggesting a need for further investigation?
2. What additional information should the nurse ask or assess for?
3. In what functional health patterns does data deviate from normal?
4. What nursing diagnosis and/or collaborative problems should be considered for this situation?

REMEMBER to check out your **companion CD-ROM**

17 Lungs and Respiratory System

www.mosby.com/MERLIN/wilson/assessment/

ANATOMY AND PHYSIOLOGY

The primary purpose of the respiratory system is to supply oxygen to the body cells and rid the cells of excess carbon dioxide. This process involves ventilation (distribution of air) and diffusion (movement of oxygen and carbon dioxide across the alveolar-capillary membrane to the blood in the pulmonary capillaries). The actual transfer of oxygen and carbon dioxide between environmental gases and the blood occurs in the alveoli. The cardiovascular system plays a role in this process by providing transportation of the oxygenated blood to the cells.

STRUCTURES WITHIN THE THORAX

There are three main structures within the chest: the mediastinum and the right and left pleural cavities (Fig. 17-1). The mediastinum is positioned in the middle section of the chest. Within it lie the heart and great vessels, the lower esophagus, and the lower part of the trachea.

The lungs are contained in the pleural cavities. The pleural cavities are lined with two types of serous membranes: the parietal and visceral pleurae. The chest wall and diaphragm are protected by the parietal pleura; the outside of the lungs is protected by the visceral pleura. A small amount of lubricating fluid coats the space between the pleurae. The lungs are not symmetric; the right lung has three lobes, and the left has two. Each lobe has a major, oblique fissure dividing the upper and lower portion; however, the right lung has a lesser horizontal fissure dividing the upper lung into upper and middle lobes (Fig. 17-2). Each lung extends anteriorly about 4 cm above the first rib into the base of the adult neck. Posteriorly, the lungs' apices rise to about the level of T1, whereas the lower borders, on deep inspiration, reach to about T12 and, on expiration, rise to about T9.

RESPIRATION

Several muscles play a role in the breathing process. The diaphragm and the intercostal muscles, however, are the primary muscles of inspiration. During inspiration, the diaphragm contracts and pushes the abdominal contents down while the intercostal muscles help to push the chest wall outward. These efforts combine to decrease intrathoracic pressure causing the lungs to fill with air. With expiration, a relatively passive action, the muscles relax, expelling the air as the intrathoracic pressure rises. Other accessory muscles that may also contribute to respiratory effort include the sternocleidomastoid, scalenus, pectoralis minor, and the rectus abdominus (Fig. 17-3, *A, B*).

During inspiration, air first enters the respiratory system through the mouth or nose, passing through the pharynx and the larynx to reach the trachea, a flexible tube approximately 10 or 11 cm long in the adult. These structures—the nose, pharynx, larynx, and intrathoracic trachea—constitute what is referred to as the upper airway (Fig. 17-4). The upper airway has three functions in respiration: to conduct air to the lower airway; to protect the lower airway from foreign matter; and to warm, filter, and humidify this inspired air.

The lower airway consists of the trachea, the mainstem and segmental bronchi, and the subsegmental and terminal bronchioles (Fig. 17-5). The trachea splits into a left and right bronchus at about the level of T4 and T5. This division occurs posteriorly and slightly below the manubriosternal junction anteriorly; the right bronchus is shorter, wider, and more upright than the left one.

The bronchi are further subdivided into increasingly smaller bronchioles. Each bronchiole opens into an alveolar duct and terminates in multiple alveoli, where the actual gas exchanges occur (Fig. 17-6). The lower airways conduct air to the alveoli and contribute to several protective mechanisms, including airway clearance, immunologic responses in the lung, and pulmonary reaction to injury.

EXTERNAL CHEST

A thoracic cage consisting of 12 thoracic vertebrae, 12 pairs of ribs, and the sternum protects the bulk of the respiratory system. All the ribs are connected to the thoracic vertebrae posteriorly. The first seven ribs are also connected to the sternum by the costal cartilages. The costal cartilages of the eighth to tenth ribs are connected immediately superior to the ribs. The eleventh and twelfth ribs are unattached anteriorly; hence their name, the "floating ribs." The tips of the eleventh ribs are located in the lateral thorax, and those of the twelfth in the posterior thorax (Fig. 17-7, *A, B*).

The adult sternum is about 17 cm long and has three components: the manubrium, the body, and the xiphoid process. The first two components articulate with the first seven ribs; the manubrium also supports the clavicle. Only the xiphoid does not articulate with any of these. The intercostal spaces (ICSs) are the spaces between the ribs. The ICS

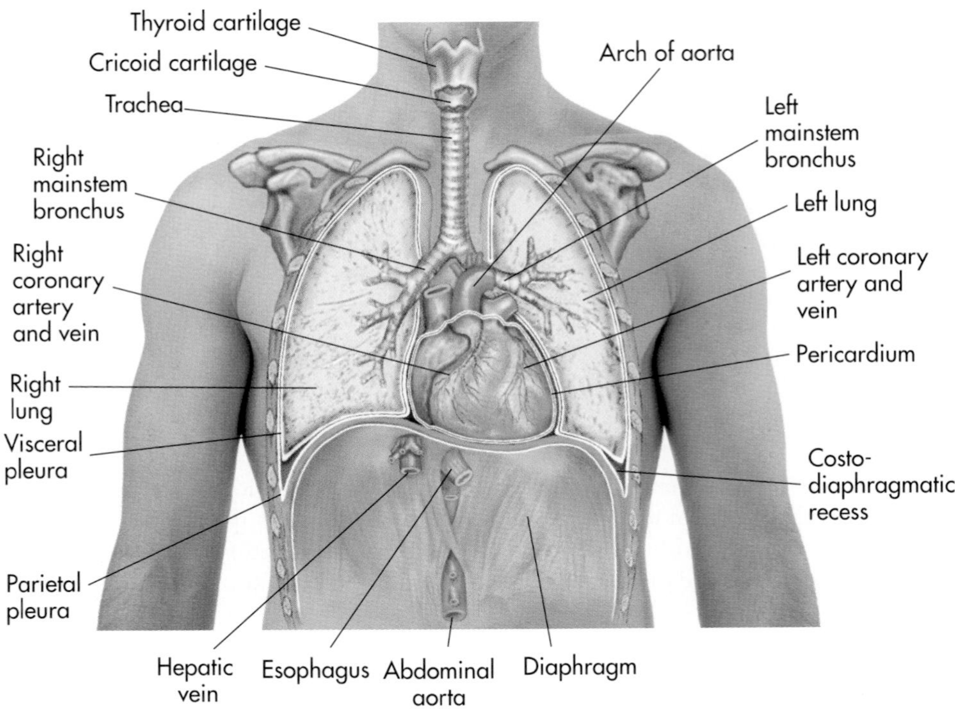

Fig. 17-1 Structures within the thoracic cavity. (From Seidel et al, 1999.)

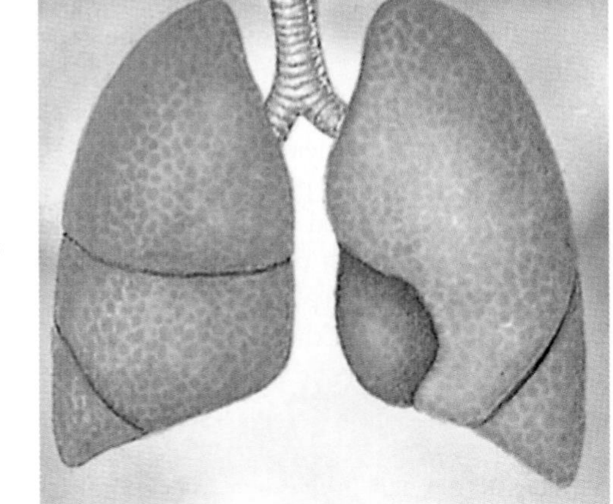

Fig. 17-2 Right and left lung. Note fissures dividing lobes of the lungs.

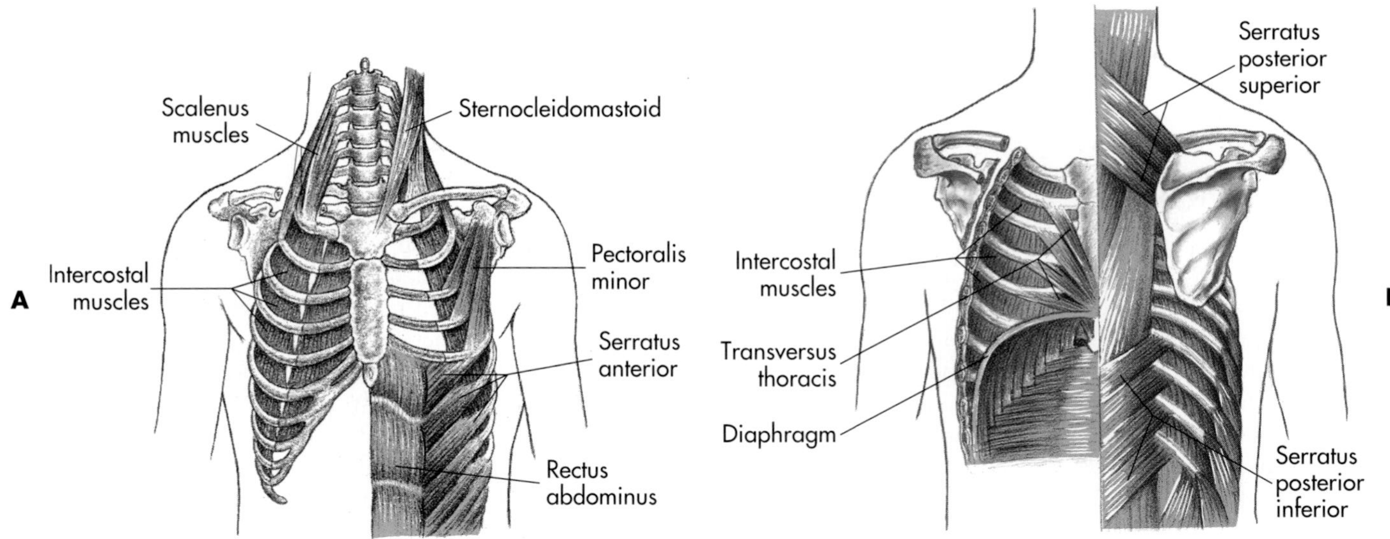

Fig. 17-3 Muscles involved in ventilation. **A,** Anterior view. **B,** Posterior view. (From Seidel et al, 1999.)

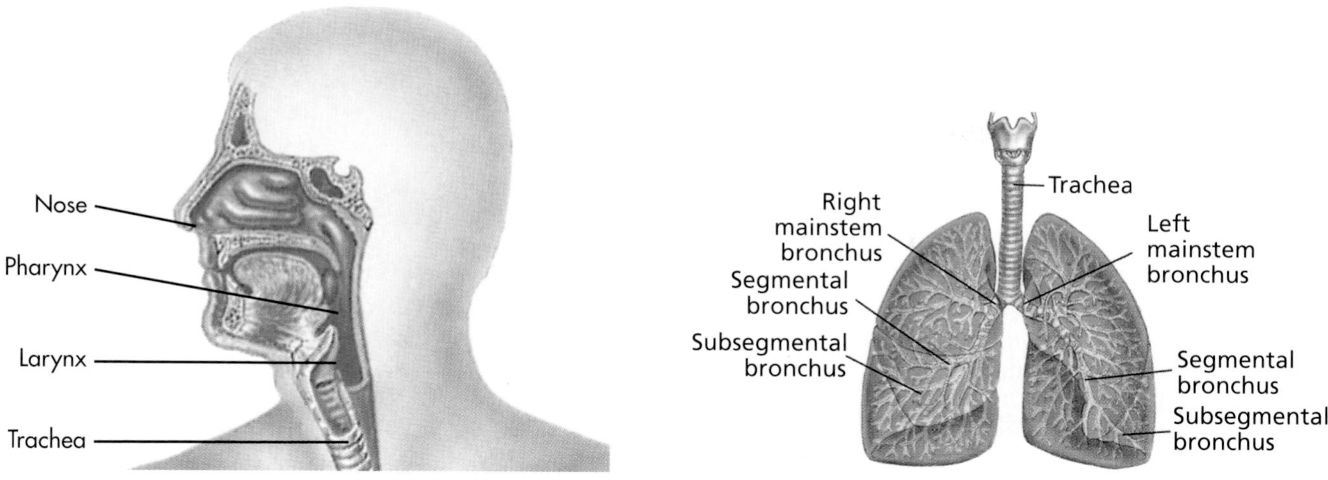

Fig. 17-4 Structures of the upper airway.

Fig. 17-5 Structures of the lower airway.

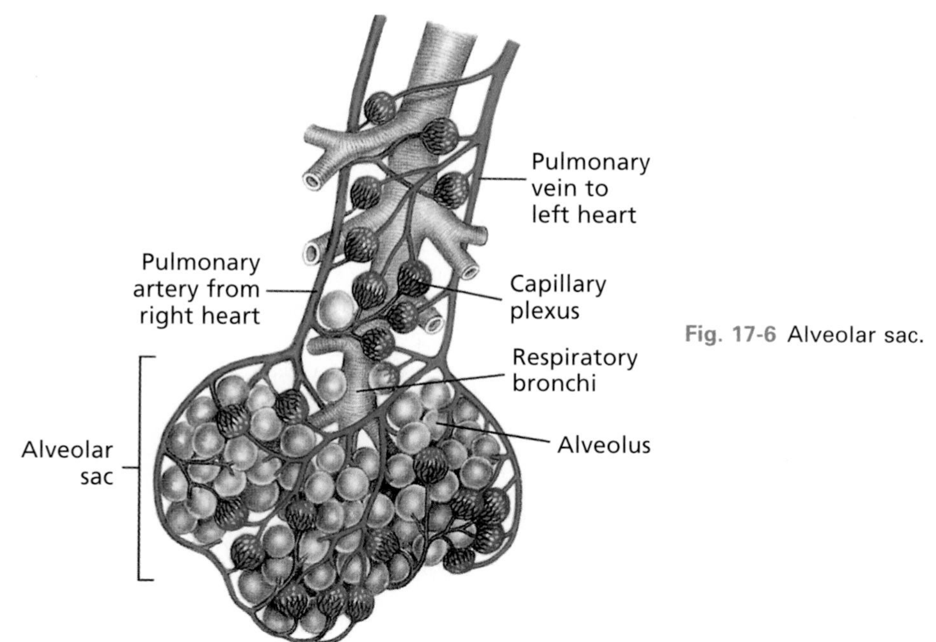

Fig. 17-6 Alveolar sac.

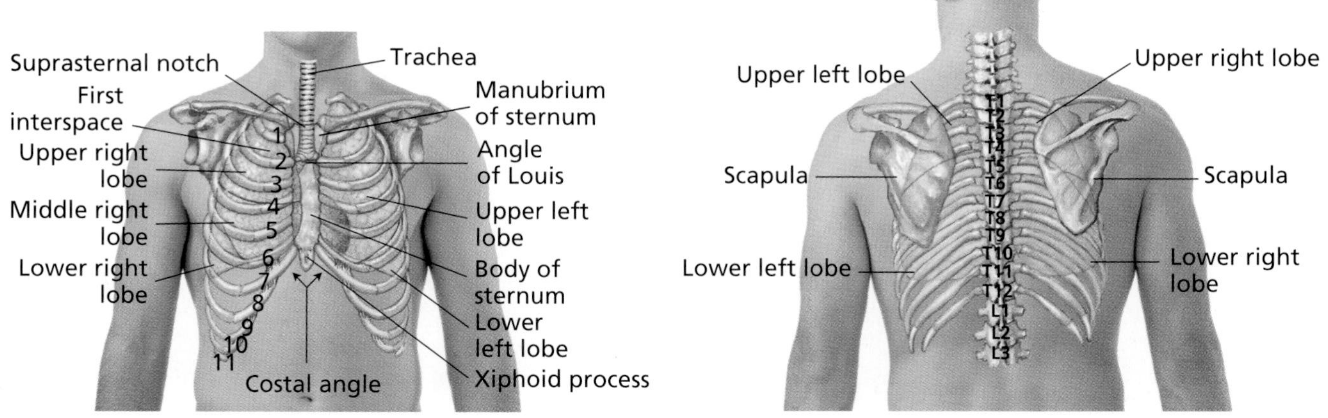

Fig. 17-7 Thorax and underlying structures.

is named according to the rib immediately superior to (above) it.

Topographic Markers

The following surface landmarks are helpful in locating underlying structures and in describing the exact location of physical findings (Fig. 17-8).

Anterior Chest Wall

- *Nipples.*
- *Manubriosternal junction (angle of Louis):* The junction between the manubrium and sternum; useful for rib identification.
- *Suprasternal notch:* The depression at the ventral aspect of the neck, just above the manubrium.
- *Costal angle:* Intersection of the costal margins, usually no more than 90°.
- *Midsternal line:* Imaginary vertical line through the middle of the sternum.
- *Clavicles:* Bones extending out both sides of the manubrium to the shoulder. They cover the first ribs.
- *Midclavicular lines:* Right and left imaginary lines through the clavicle midpoints, parallel to the midsternal line.

Lateral Chest Wall

- *Anterior axillary lines:* Left and right imaginary vertical lines from anterior axillary folds through the anterolateral chest, parallel to midsternal line.
- *Posterior axillary lines:* Left and right vertical imaginary lines from the posterior axillary folds along the posterolateral thoracic wall with abducted lateral arm.
- *Midaxillary lines:* Left and right vertical imaginary lines from axillary apices; midway between and parallel to anterior and posterior axillary lines.

Posterior Chest Wall

- *Vertebra prominens:* Spinous process of C7; visible and palpable with the head bent forward; if two palpable prominences are felt, the upper is the spinous process of C7 and the lower is that of T1.
- *Midspinal line:* Imaginary vertical line along the posterior vertebral spinous processes.
- *Scapular lines:* Left and right vertical imaginary lines, parallel to midspinal line; they pass through inferior angles of the scapulae in the upright client with arms at sides.

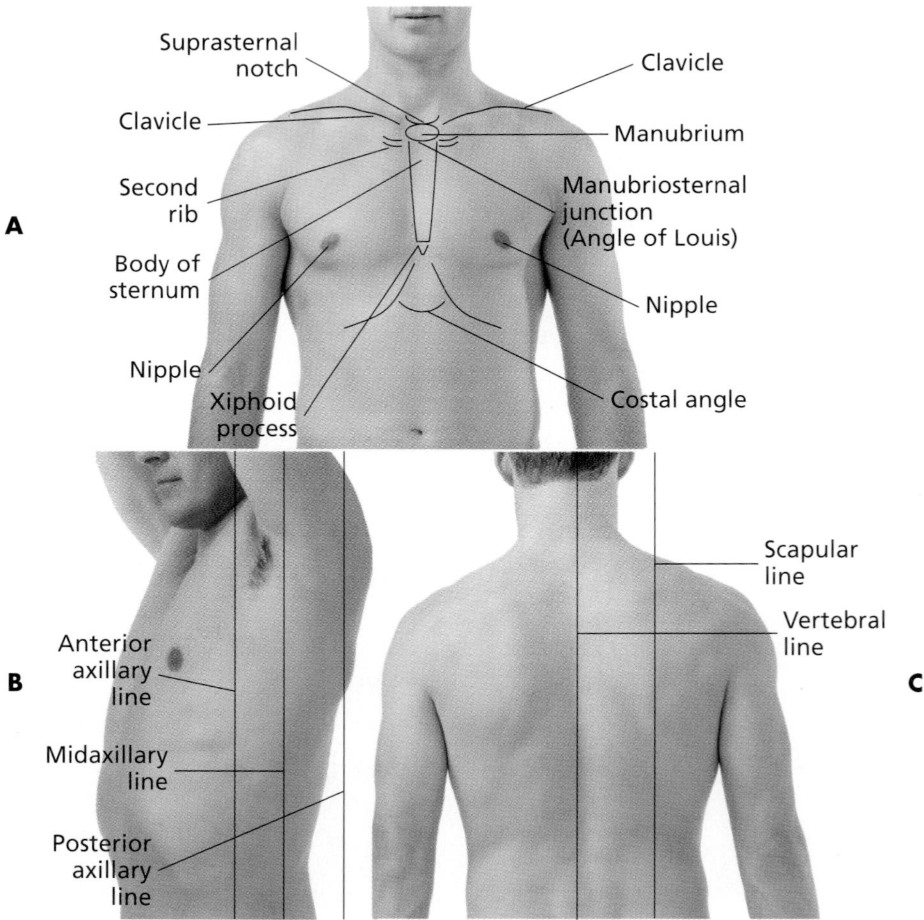

Fig. 17-8 Topographic landmarks of the thorax. **A,** Anterior. **B,** Lateral. **C,** Posterior.

HEALTH HISTORY

Lungs and Respiratory System

QUESTIONS | **RATIONALE**

PRESENT HEALTH STATUS

➤ How would you describe the condition of your lungs? What do you do, if anything, to keep healthy?

■ The client's perception of his or her health status is helpful in order to understand what the client considers a problem.

➤ Do you have any chronic illness?

■ Many chronic illnesses can cause symptoms affecting the respiratory system, including heart disease, renal disease, and diabetes mellitus.

➤ Are you currently taking any medications? If so, what are you taking, and when did you start taking the medications? Have you noticed any problems since you have been taking the medications?

■ A list of current medications being taken by the client is an important aspect of any health history. Medications can be responsible for a variety of symptoms.

➤ Do you use oxygen or an inhaler at home? If so, describe what, how much, and how often.

■ Many individuals with chronic pulmonary disease use oxygen or inhalers at home. The history must reflect current status of use.

➤ Do you have allergies? If so, what are you allergic to? Describe what your symptoms are like.

■ The severity of allergies can range from mild seasonal allergies to full anaphylactic allergic reactions. Respiratory symptoms can range from runny nose, nasal congestion and cough to wheezes and dyspnea.

➤ Do you smoke, or have you been a smoker in the past? If so, what do (did) you smoke? (cigarettes, cigar, pipe, marijuana) How long have you smoked (did you smoke)? How often do you (did you) smoke? Have you ever attempted to quit smoking? If yes, describe.

■ If the client is or has been a smoker, determine the number of pack years the client has smoked (Box 17-1).

CULTURAL NOTE

Differences in smoking habits of individuals in the United States vary by cultural group, gender, and sociologic factors. Smoking is more prevalent in African Americans, and they develop a greater number of related malignancies than do other ethnic groups (Gorin and Arnold, 1998). More men smoke than women. Smoking is prevalent among persons who experience difficulty in society and is especially high in divorced or separated men regardless of ethnicity.

Box 17-1 Recording Tobacco Use

Cigarette consumption is documented by *pack years.* A pack year is the number of years a client has smoked times the number of packs of cigarettes smoked each day. If a client tells you he or she smoked ½ pack of cigarettes a day for 40 years, it would be recorded as a 20-pack-year smoking history.

Use of pipes, cigars, marijuana, chewing tobacco, or snuff is usually recorded in the amount used daily.

QUESTIONS | RATIONALE

PAST MEDICAL HISTORY

➤ Have you ever had any problems with your lungs? If so, describe.

■ Asking the client what sort of problems he or she may have had encourages the client to describe symptoms they may be having—which may or may not have been diagnosed and treated.

➤ Have you been diagnosed as having a respiratory disease such as asthma, bronchitis, bronchiectasis, emphysema, cystic fibrosis, lung cancer, or tuberculosis? If so, please describe.

■ Background information regarding respiratory problems tells you what types of problems the client is likely to experience and clinical findings to anticipate. Other respiratory tract problems should be evaluated.

➤ Have you ever had an injury to your chest? Surgery to your chest? Lung infections? If so, describe.

■ The incidence of injury or surgery may provide additional information about a possible respiratory or lung problem.

➤ Have you ever had tests done to evaluate your lungs, such as pulmonary function tests, tuberculosis tests, or a chest x-ray examination? If so, when was it done and for what reason?

■ All of these tests provide objective measures that may be used as baseline information or used to confirm a diagnosis.

FAMILY HISTORY

➤ Is there a family history of lung disease? If so, which family member and what type of condition?

■ Family history may be used to determine risk for the client.

HOME ENVIRONMENT

➤ Are there environmental conditions that may affect your breathing at home? If so, what are they? Common things to consider include the following:

- House location (near factory, on a busy street, new construction in area, etc.)
- Possible allergens in home, such as pets
- Type of heating and/or air conditioning, including filtering system, humidification, and ventilation
- Hobbies: woodworking, plants, animals, metal work
- Exposure to the smoke of others in your home

■ There are a number of respiratory irritants found in or near the home that may cause temporary or permanent lung damage. Environmental tobacco smoke (also known as secondhand smoke) as been shown to affect nonsmokers (Gorin and Arnold, 1998).

OCCUPATIONAL ENVIRONMENT

➤ Where do you work? In a factory? Outdoors? In a mine? In a chemical plant? On a farm? In heavy traffic? Are you frequently exposed to dust? Vapors? Chemicals? Paint fumes? Irritants such as asbestos? Known allergens?

■ The client may be exposed to respiratory irritants in the workplace. The client may or may not be aware of the presence of irritants.

➤ If you are exposed to respiratory irritants, do you wear a mask or a respirator mask? Does your work area have a special ventilatory system to clear out pollutants? Do you wear a monitor to evaluate exposure? Do you have periodic health examinations, pulmonary function tests, or x-ray examinations?

■ The client may not be able to alter the presence of environmental irritants that are in the work environment. Instead, he or she must use masks, respirators, ventilation hoods, etc. to reduce the amount of exposure to respiratory irritants. Regulatory agencies such as the Occupational Safety and Health Administration (OSHA) have developed guidelines and regulations to reduce the amount of occupational exposure to respiratory irritants.

QUESTIONS

RATIONALE

RISK FACTORS

COMMON RISK FACTORS ASSOCIATED WITH Respiratory Disorders

- Smoking
- Sedentary lifestyle or recent immobility
- Extreme obesity
- Infant prematurity
- Advanced age
- Environmental exposures (work or home)
  - Chemicals
  - Vapors
  - Pesticides
  - Fertilizers
  - Paint
  - Woodworking
  - Secondhand smoke
  - Animals
- Family history of respiratory disease
- Drug use
  - Inhalants

TRAVEL

➤ Have you recently traveled to countries or areas of the United States where you may have been exposed to uncommon respiratory diseases (e.g., histoplasmosis in the Southeast and Midwest; schistosomiasis in Southwest Asia, the Caribbean, and Asia)?

■ Often, travel to areas of the country or world where the individual is exposed to unusual infections that he or she has little or no resistance to will increase that person's susceptibility to infection.

PROBLEM-BASED HISTORY

The most commonly reported problems related to the lungs are cough, shortness of breath, and chest pain. As with symptoms in all areas of health assessment, a symptom analysis is completed, which includes the location, quality, quantity, chronology, setting, associated manifestations, alleviating factors, and aggravating factors (see Box 4-2 in Chapter 4).

Cough

➤ When did you first notice the cough? Is the cough constant, or does it come and go? Has the cough changed since you first noticed it? Has it gotten worse?

■ A cough can be acute (sudden onset and usually short course lasting less than 3 weeks) or chronic (persistent for more than 3 weeks). Some conditions are characterized by a specific onset of coughing or are associated with a specific time during the day or night.

➤ What are the characteristics of your cough? Is it a dry cough? A productive cough?

■ A description of the cough may provide clues to the cause of the cough.

QUESTIONS

➤ Have you noticed any other symptoms along with the cough, such as shortness of breath, chest pain or tightness with breathing, fever, stuffy nose, noisy respiration, hoarseness, gagging, or stress? Does activity make it worse? Does the cough tire you out? Does it keep you awake at night?

RATIONALE

■ A cough may be a symptom of pulmonary problems, or it may exist in conjunction with other problems. Associated signs and symptoms are important factors to assess when trying to determine the underlying cause of the cough. For example, a cough associated with a fever, shortness of breath, and noisy breath sounds may be indicative of a lung infection, whereas tightness of the chest associated with shortness of breath and a nonproductive cough is more likely to be associated with a problem such as asthma.

➤ Have you done anything to treat the cough yourself such as medications, fluids, or a vaporizer? Have these measures been effective?

■ Determining what has been used successfully or unsuccessfully helps in understanding the problem and may guide current treatment strategies.

Sputum Production

➤ When did you first notice the phlegm or sputum? Has it changed over time? If so, how?

■ Conditions associated with sputum production may be acute and limited—or chronic and get progressively worse.

➤ How often are you coughing up sputum? (all of the time or just periodically?) How much sputum do you cough up?

■ The frequency of sputum production and the time of day most sputum is produced should be explored. Increased sputum in the morning implies an accumulation of sputum during the night and is common with bronchitis. Sputum production with a change in position is suggestive of lung abscess and bronchiectasis. The amount of sputum production can vary from a few teaspoons to a copious amount (a pint or more).

➤ What does the sputum look like? What color is it?

■ The appearance of the sputum is always important to document. Some conditions have characteristic sputum production, such as the following:
- White or clear sputum—colds, viral infections, or bronchitis
- Yellow or green material—bacterial infections
- Black–smoke or coal dust inhalation
- Rust-colored material—tuberculosis, pneumococcal pneumonia, or perhaps blood
- Bright red or dark purple—blood (hemoptysis)
- *Hemoptysis* is the expectoration of sputum containing blood. It may vary in severity from slight streaking of blood to frank bleeding.

QUESTIONS

RATIONALE

➤ What is the consistency of the sputum? (thick? thin? frothy?).

■ The consistency of sputum may be described as thin, thick, a gelatin consistency, sticky, or frothy. Pink frothy sputum with dyspnea is associated with pulmonary edema.

➤ Have you noticed if the sputum has an odor?

■ Foul-smelling (fetid) sputum is typically associated with bacterial pneumonia, lung abscess, or bronchiectasis.

➤ What do you think is causing this? Do you think you have an infection? Do you think it is related to any activity or exposure that you are aware of? If so, what?

■ Many times a client will be able to relate the cause of symptoms. Many times these perceptions are accurate and help to determine the client's understanding of conditions.

➤ What have you done to treat this condition, if anything? Has it been effective?

■ Determining what has been used successfully or unsuccessfully helps in understanding the problem and may guide current treatment strategies.

Shortness of Breath

➤ Do you experience episodes of shortness of breath? If so, how long has this been going on? Are you short of breath all the time, or does this come and go?

■ Shortness of breath, or dyspnea, occurs when breathing is difficult in an inappropriate setting such as at rest or with limited exertion. Dyspnea is the most distressing symptom of a respiratory problem (Wilkins, Krider, and Sheldon, 1995). Some conditions such as pneumonia may cause sudden onset of shortness of breath; others conditions such as chronic congestive heart failure may be associated with a longer and more gradual onset. Some clients may experience shortness of breath at intervals over a period of time.

➤ If intermittent, how often do these episodes occur? How long does an episode typically last?

■ Determine frequency and duration of symptoms.

➤ How would you describe the severity of the shortness of breath? Is it harder to inhale or exhale, or are both equally affected? Do the symptoms interfere with your activities? Do you think the shortness of breath is getting better or worse?

■ Knowing the client's perception of the severity and the extent of disablement, if any, helps you understand the problem. Inspiratory dyspnea is usually associated with obstruction of the upper airway. Expiratory dyspnea is usually associated with obstruction of smaller bronchi and bronchioles.

QUESTIONS	RATIONALE
➤ Does anything seem to trigger these episodes or make the shortness of breath worse, such as activity, exercise, or environmental factors? Do you experience shortness of breath at a certain time of day or night? If this occurs at night, what position do you sleep in? How many pillows do you use to prop behind you? Do you sleep in a recliner? Does changing your position affect the problem?	■ Causative factors should be determined. If it is brought on by activity, find out how much exercise brings on the episode (number of steps climbed, blocks walked, etc.). Dyspnea may also be brought on by positions or other conditions. *Orthopnea* is difficulty breathing when the individual is lying down. Clients may describe using several pillows to "prop" themselves up in bed so that they can sleep. The nurse should note the number of pillows needed for sleeping (Finlay, 1996). *Paroxysmal nocturnal dyspnea* is shortness of breath that awakens the individual in the middle of the night, usually in a panic with the feeling of suffocation. Comfort is usually achieved by sitting up (House-Fancher and Griego, 1996). Asthma attacks are triggered by a specific allergen. This may be external to the individual (extrinsic), such as a pet, or internal (intrinsic), such as stress or emotions.
➤ Have you noticed any other problems when you are short of breath? Cough? Chest pain? Break out in a sweat? Swelling of the feet, ankles, or legs?	■ Shortness of breath may be simply a problem of the respiratory system, or it may be a symptom associated with the cardiovascular system, such as congestive heart failure or a severe heart murmur.
➤ When these episodes of shortness of breath occur, what do you do to relieve the symptoms?	■ Assess the efficacy of treatment and any progression the client has noted. Determining what has been used successfully or unsuccessfully helps in understanding the problem and may guide current treatment strategies.
Chest Pain With Breathing	
➤ Have you had pain in your chest when you breathe? If so, when did this start? Did it start suddenly or gradually? Where do you feel the pain? Does the pain radiate to other areas, such as the neck or arms?	■ Chest pain caused by respiratory disease is usually associated with chest wall or parietal pleura. A sharp abrupt pain associated with deep breathing may be an indication of pleural lining irritation.
➤ What does the pain feel like? (viselike, tight, sharp, burning, etc.) On a scale of 1 to 10, how would you rate the intensity of the pain? Is the pain constant, or does it come and go?	■ Even though the pain is associated with breathing, it is important to evaluate the possibility of the pain being related to a cardiovascular problem.
➤ When it started, was the pain associated with an injury to your ribs or a respiratory infection? Is the pain worse with deep inspiration? Does the pain interfere with your getting enough air?	■ Injured ribs will not only cause pain when the individual breathes but also, because of the pain, the client is likely to breathe more shallowly, which may lead to respiratory congestion.
➤ Is there anything that seems to make the pain worse, such as movement or coughing?	■ Assess for aggravating factors.
➤ Have you done to anything to treat the pain, such as heat, splinting, or pain medication? Have any measures been effective?	■ Assess self-care behaviors and successful relief of pain.

EXAMINATION

Equipment

- Stethoscope to auscultate breath sounds (for infants and young children, use a stethoscope that has a small diaphragm)
- Ruler and tape measure (marked in centimeters) to measure diaphragmatic excursion
- Marking pen to mark diaphragmatic excursion

PROCEDURES AND TECHNIQUES WITH NORMAL FINDINGS

Examination of the lungs and respiratory system includes the four techniques of inspection, palpation, percussion, and auscultation. Begin with the client sitting on the edge of the examination table.

GENERAL PRESENTATION

➤INSPECT the client for general appearance, posture, and breathing effort. The client's general appearance and posture should be relaxed. The posture should be upright. Breathing should occur with no effort and at a rate that is appropriate for the client's age.

ABNORMAL FINDINGS

■ An appearance of apprehension with restlessness, possible nasal flaring, supraclavicular or intercostal retractions or bulging with expiration, or use of accessory muscles during breathing are all signs of respiratory compromise and distress.

■ *Tripod position* (leaning forward with the arms braced against the knees, against a chair or a bed) also suggests respiratory compromise. Tripod position enhances accessory muscle use (Fig. 17-9).

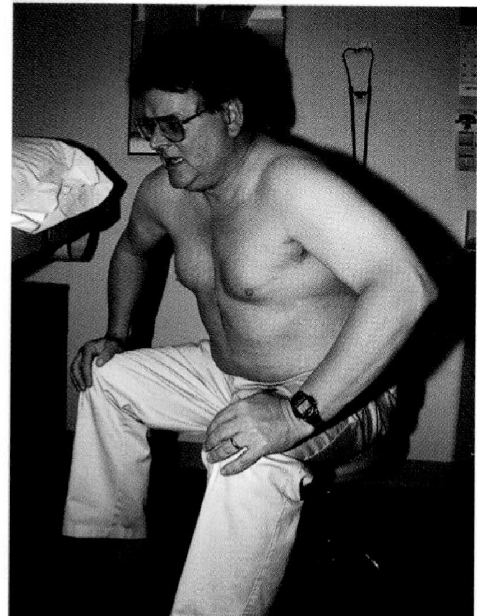

Fig. 17-9 Tripod position.

PROCEDURES AND TECHNIQUES WITH NORMAL FINDINGS

CHEST WALL CONFIGURATION

➤**INSPECT the chest for shape and symmetry, muscle development, anteroposterior (AP) diameter to transverse diameter, and costal angle.** The thorax should be symmetric. The ribs should slope down at about 45° relative to the spine. Muscle development should be equal. The spinous processes should appear in a straight line. The scapulae should be bilaterally symmetric. The AP diameter of the chest should be approximately one half the transverse diameter—or about a 1:2 ratio of AP to transverse diameter. Anteriorly the costal angle should be less than 90° (Fig. 17-10, *A, B, C*).

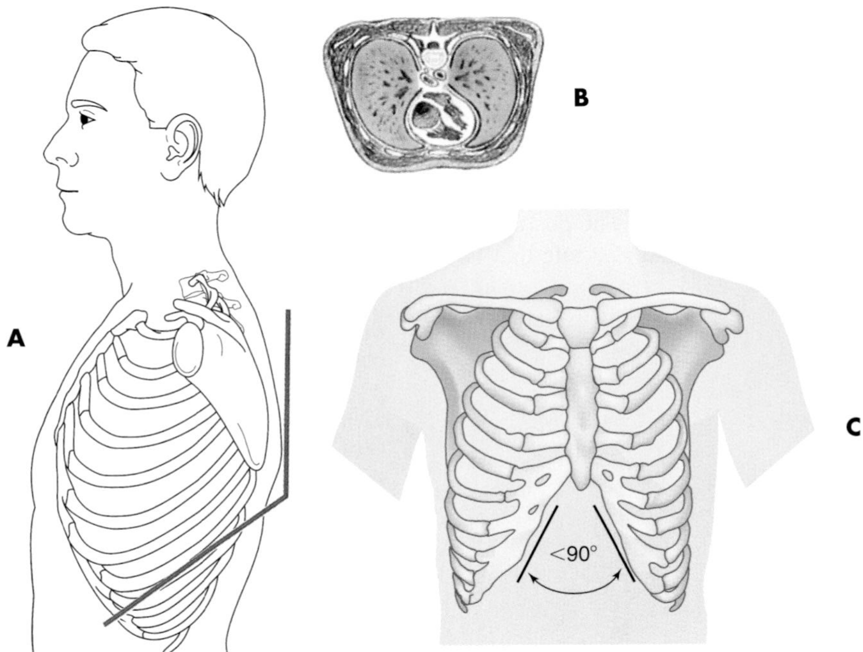

Fig. 17-10 Normal chest findings. **A,** Angulation of ribs. **B,** AP diameter is about one half the transverse diameter. **C,** Costal angle less than 90°. (**A** From Barkauskas et al, 1998.)

ABNORMAL FINDINGS

- Asymmetry or unequal muscle development is abnormal. Skeletal deformities such as scoliosis or kyphosis may limit the expansion of the chest.

PROCEDURES AND TECHNIQUES WITH NORMAL FINDINGS

ABNORMAL FINDINGS

■ In chronic lung hyperinflation conditions such as chronic emphysema, the chest wall may have a barrel-chest appearance because of an increased AP diameter. In this situation, the ribs are more horizontal, and the chest looks as if it is held in constant inspiration. The costal angle is greater than 90° (Fig. 17-11, *A, B, C*).

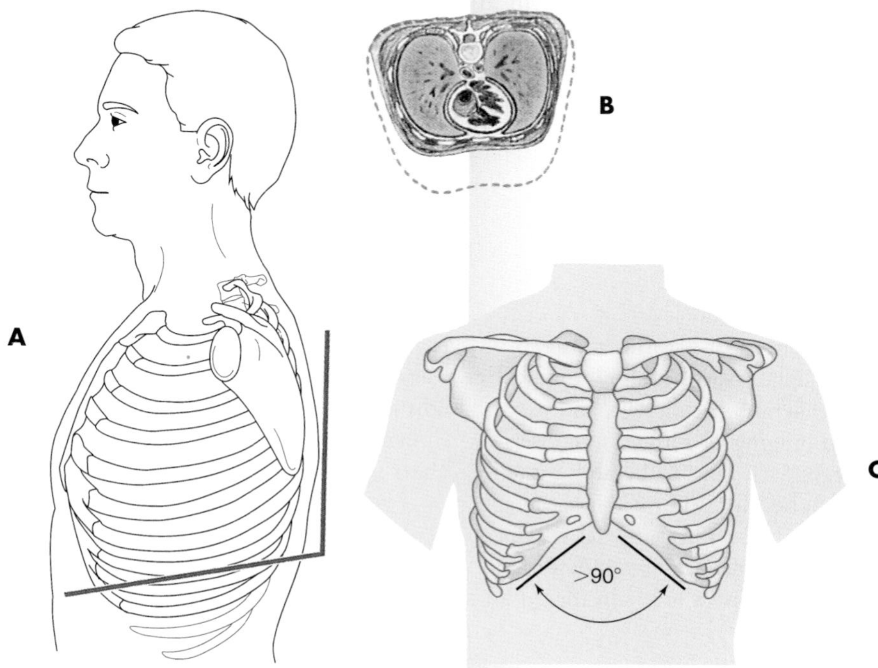

Fig. 17-11 Barrel chest. **A,** Horizontal ribs. **B,** Increased AP diameter. **C,** Costal angle greater than 90°. (**A** from Barkauskas et al, 1998.)

■ Other chest wall skeletal deformities include pectus carinatum (Fig. 17-12) and pectus excavatum (Fig. 17-13).

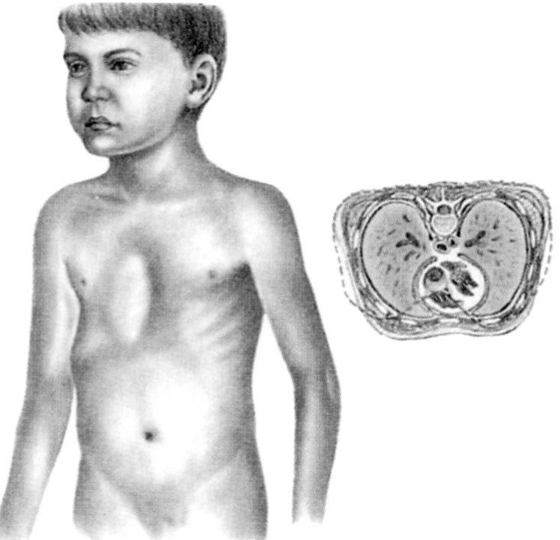

Fig. 17-13 Pectus excavatum, or funnel chest. Note sternum is indented above xiphoid.

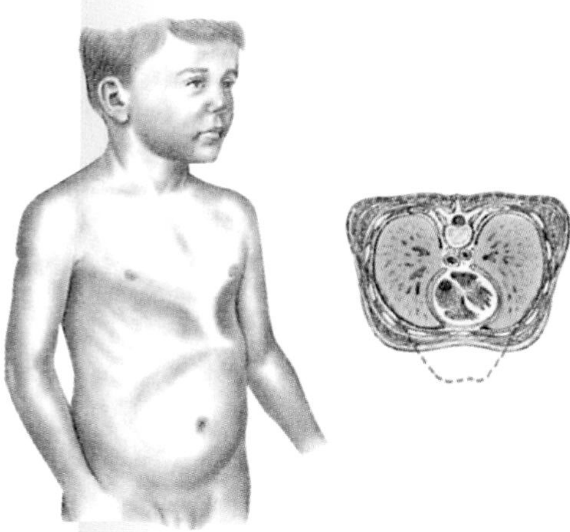

Fig. 17-12 Pectus carinatum, or pigeon chest. Note prominent sternum.

PROCEDURES AND TECHNIQUES WITH NORMAL FINDINGS

ABNORMAL FINDINGS

GENERAL OXYGENATION AND RESPIRATORY EFFORT

➤**INSPECT the client's nails, skin, and lips for color.** Skin tones vary among individuals, therefore the general color should be consistent with skin color for that individual's ethnic background. Specifically note the presence of cyanosis or pallor (see Chapters 11 and 18 for details). If there is any question about adequate oxygenation, measure the client's oxygen saturation level using pulse oximetry (see Chapter 5).

■ Cyanosis or pallor of the nails, skin, or lips may be a sign of inadequate oxygenation of tissues due to an underlying respiratory or cardiovascular condition. Clubbing of the nails is associated with chronic hypoxia.

➤**OBSERVE and EVALUATE respiration for rate and quality, breathing pattern, and chest expansion.** Note the respiratory rate. In the adult, passive breathing should occur at a rate of 12 to 20 breaths per minute (normal range respiratory rate is referred to as eupnea). The ratio of respiratory rate to pulse rate should be 1:4.

■ Abnormal breathing rates include the following:

- Bradypnea is a respiratory rate less than 12 breaths per minute. The rate and depth remains smooth and even (Fig. 17-14).
- Tachypnea is a respiratory rate greater than 20 breaths per minute. The rate and depth remains smooth and even. Tachypnea can be caused by a number of things, including fever, fear, or activity (Fig. 17-15).

➤The pattern of breathing should be even and smooth with an even respiratory depth (Fig. 17-16). It should appear easy and without effort. The chest wall should symmetrically rise and expand and then relax without effort. There should be no bulging or retractions observed. A normal variation is abdominal breathing pattern. Men tend to be abdominal breathers (or diaphragmatic) whereas women tend to be more thoracic breathers.

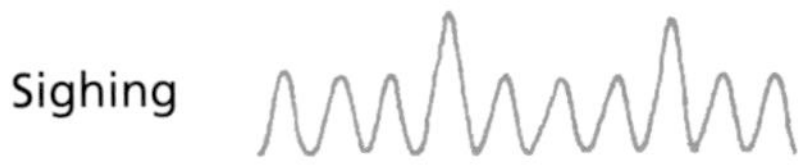

A sigh is another normal variance observed with breathing. It is an occasional interspersed deeper breath associated with a normal breathing pattern. If a sigh occurs frequently, it is considered an abnormal finding (Fig. 17-17).

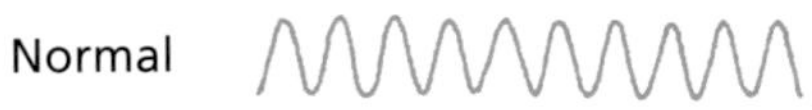

■ Abnormal breathing patterns include the following:

- *Hyperventilation* breathing is characterized by increased rate and depth of respiration. When hyperventilation occurs with ketoacidosis, it is very deep and laborious and is referred to as Kussmaul breathing (Fig. 17-18, *A, B*).

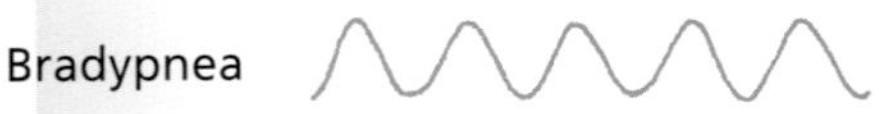

Bradypnea

Fig. 17-14 Bradypnea.

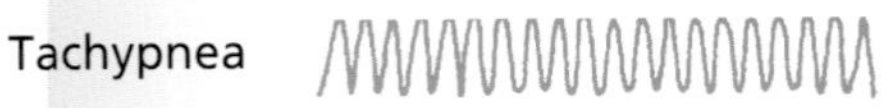

Tachypnea

Fig. 17-15 Tachypnea.

Normal

Fig. 17-16 Normal breathing pattern.

Sighing

Fig. 17-17 Sigh.

Hyperventilation (hyperpnea) **A**

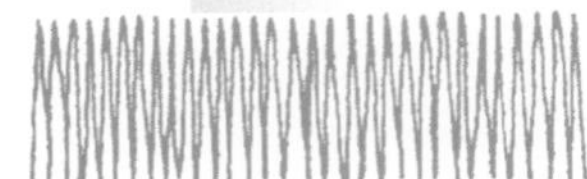

Kussmaul **B**

Fig. 17-18 **A,** Hyperventilation. **B,** Kussmaul.

PROCEDURES AND TECHNIQUES WITH NORMAL FINDINGS

ABNORMAL FINDINGS

-*Biot breathing pattern* is characterized by irregularly interspersed periods of apnea in a disorganized irregular pattern or rate and/or depth. May be associated with persistent intracranial pressure, respiratory compromise, or damage to the medulla (Fig. 17-19).

-*Cheyne-Stokes* is an abnormal pattern characterized by intervals of apnea interspersed with a deep and rapid breathing pattern. This may be seen in clients with severe illness, brain damage, or drug overdose (Fig. 17-20).

-*Air trapping* is an abnormal respiratory pattern frequently seen in clients with chronic obstructive disease (COPD). It is characterized by rapid inspirations with prolonged, forced expirations. Air is not fully exhaled; thus air becomes trapped in the lungs, which eventually overexpand (Fig. 17-21).

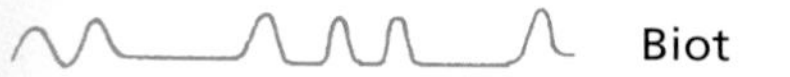

Biot

Fig. 17-19 Biot.

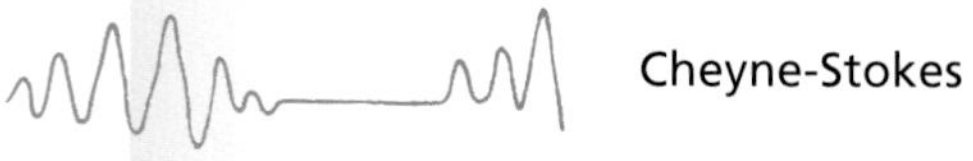

Cheyne-Stokes

Fig. 17-20 Cheyne-Stokes.

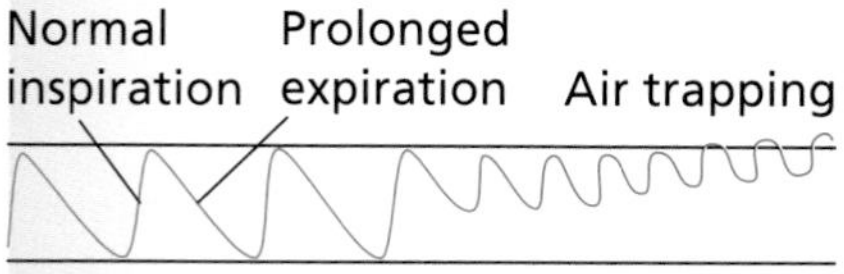

Normal inspiration
Prolonged expiration
Air trapping

Fig. 17-21 Air trapping.

PROCEDURES AND TECHNIQUES WITH NORMAL FINDINGS

ABNORMAL FINDINGS

ANTERIOR AND POSTERIOR CHEST ASSESSMENT

➤**PALPATE the trachea for position.** Stand facing the client. Using the thumbs of both hands (or your index finger and thumb of one hand), palpate the trachea on the anterior aspect of the neck by placing the thumbs on either side. It should be palpable midline and should be slightly movable (Fig. 17-22).

- If the trachea is not midline, it may be an indication of a chest mass or some degree of lung collapse.

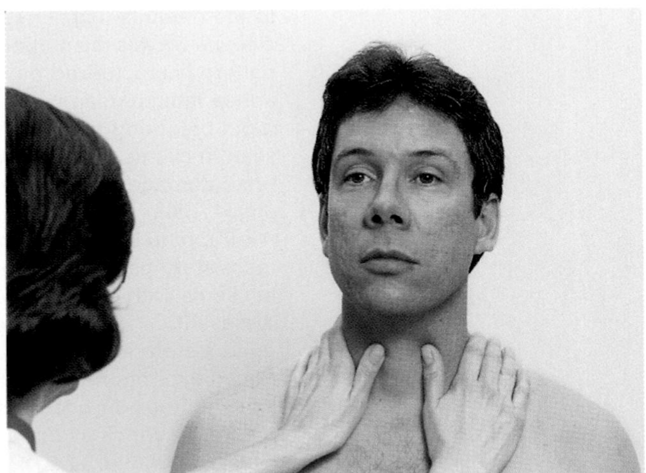

Fig. 17-22 Palpating to evaluate midline position of trachea.

➤**PALPATE the chest and thoracic muscles for tenderness, bulges, and symmetry.** With the palmar surface of your fingers, use both hands simultaneously to compare the two sides of the posterior chest wall. The skin should be smooth and warm. The spine should be straight and nontender from C7 through T12. The scapulae should be symmetric and the surrounding musculature well developed. The posterior ribs should be stable and nontender.

Repeat the palpation techniques on the anterior chest. The skin should be smooth, and the rib cage should be symmetric and firm. The sternum and xiphoid should be relatively inflexible.

- Note any crepitus, which feels like a crinkly or crackly sensation under your fingers. This abnormal finding indicates air in the subcutaneous tissue caused by an air leak from somewhere in the respiratory tree.
- Pleural friction rub may be felt as a coarse grating sensation during inspiration. It occurs secondary to inflammation of the pleural surface.
- Muscular development that is asymmetric or an unstable chest wall may indicate a thoracic disorder.

➤**PALPATE the chest wall for thoracic expansion.** Stand behind the client and place both thumbs on either side of the client's spinal processes at about the level of T-9 or T-10. While maintaining the thumb position, extend the fingers of both hands laterally (outward) over the posterior chest wall (Fig. 17-23). Instruct the client to take several deep breaths. Observe for bilateral outward movement of your thumbs during the client's inspiration. Both thumbs should move apart symmetrically with each breath.

- A unilateral or unequal movement of your thumbs suggests asymmetry of expansion—an abnormal finding. Causes of unequal chest wall expansion include pain, fractured ribs or chest wall injury, pneumonia, and atelectasis or collapsed lung. If unequal chest wall movement is noted, further evaluation is warranted.

PROCEDURES AND TECHNIQUES WITH NORMAL FINDINGS

ABNORMAL FINDINGS

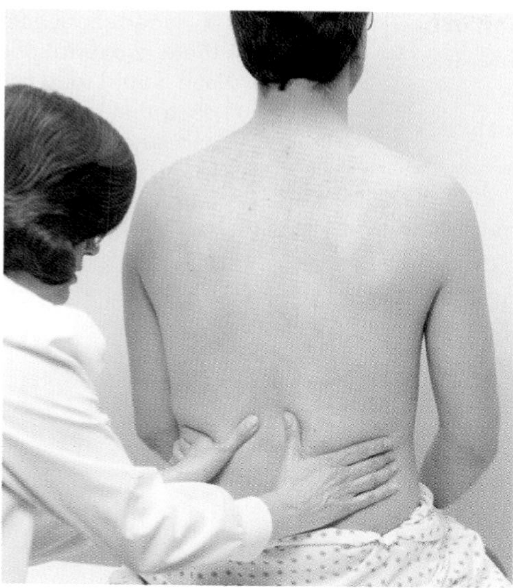

Fig. 17-23 Assessment of posterior thoracic expansion.

❖ ➤**PALPATE the chest wall for vocal (tactile) fremitus.** Vocal fremitus is a vibration resulting from speech or other verbalizations. You can feel this vibration with your hands. Place your hands on the chest over both sides of the right and left lung fields. Instruct the client to recite "One-two-three" or "ninety-nine" while you systematically palpate the chest wall (using the palmar or ulnar surface of your hands) from apices to bases (Fig. 17-24).

In a very thin client, you will probably notice increased fremitus. Conversely, in an obese or very muscular client, you will notice decreased fremitus. Although the quality of the vibrations may vary from person to person because of chest wall density and relative location of the bronchi to the chest wall, the fremitus should feel bilaterally equal.

■ Decreased or absent fremitus occurs when the vibrations are blocked. Causes include emphysema, pleural thickening or effusion, pulmonary edema, and bronchial obstruction.

■ Increased fremitus occurs when the vibrations are enhanced—sometimes described as a rougher or courser vibration. This occurs when lung tissues are congested or consolidated. Conditions commonly associated with this finding include pneumonia and a tumor.

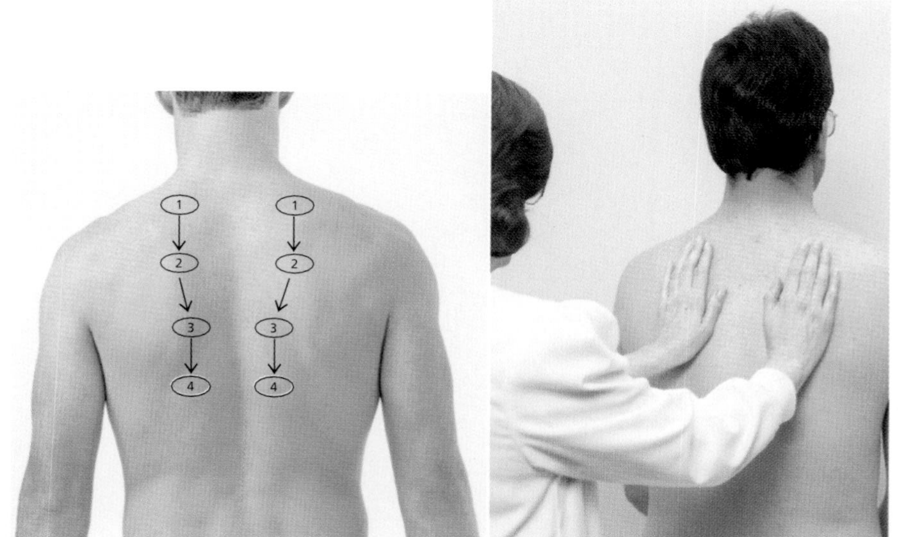

Fig. 17-24 Assessing for vocal (tactile) fremitus. **A,** Hand positions for assessment. **B,** Position hands over both lung fields.

PROCEDURES AND TECHNIQUES WITH NORMAL FINDINGS

❖ ➤**PERCUSS the thorax for tone.** Percussion is the tapping of an object to set the underlying structures in motion and thus produce a sound. If necessary, review the techniques of performing percussion in Chapter 6.

Systematically percuss first the posterior chest wall and finally the anterior and lateral chest wall. (Fig. 17-25, *A, B*).

To begin, place the client in a sitting position with arms folded in front with head bent forward to move the scapulae laterally, exposing more lung field (Seidel et al, 1999). Stand behind the client and percuss from above the scapula to the bottom of the rib area. Percuss between the ribs down the chest from side to side, comparing the two sides as you go. The sound should be resonance, which is loud in intensity, low in pitch, long in duration, and hollow in quality (Table 17-1) (Fig. 17-26). Move to the front side of the client. Ask the client to raise his or her arms over the head. Percuss down the anterior and lateral aspects of the chest, moving from side to side.

ABNORMAL FINDINGS

■ Hyperresonance is heard when there is overinflation of the lungs. It has a very loud resonance of low pitch that lasts longer than normal and seems "booming." This may be found in individuals with emphysema. Dull tones may be heard in clients with pneumonia, pleural effusion, or atelectasis.

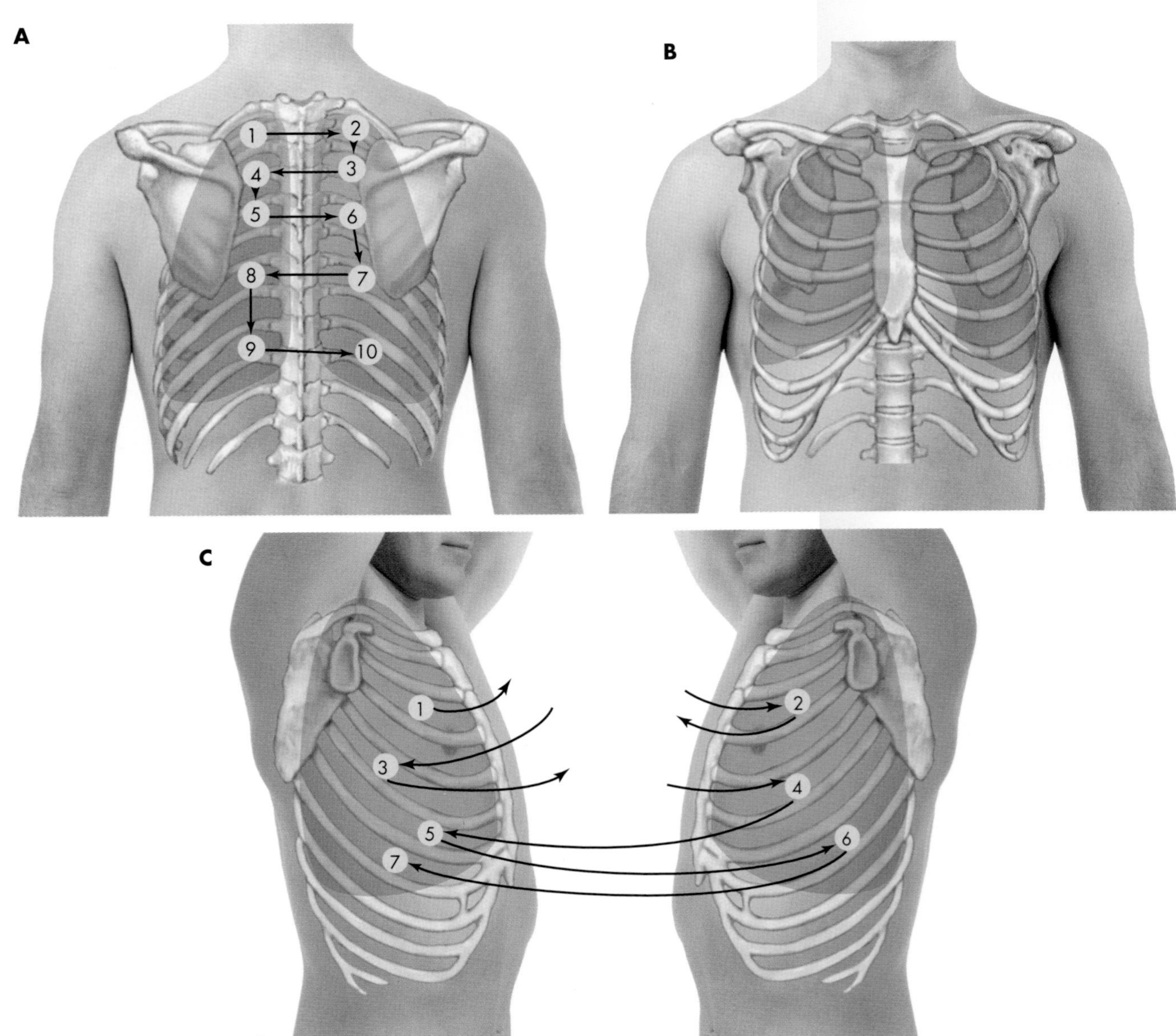

Fig. 17-25 Landmarks for chest percussion and auscultation. **A,** Posterior view. **B,** Anterior view. **C,** Lateral view. (From Seidel et al, 1999.)

Table 17-1 Percussion Tones Over the Lungs

	DESCRIPTION	ADULT PERIPHERAL LUNG	CHILD LUNG
Tone	Description of tone	Resonance	Hyperresonance
Intensity	Loudness or softness of the tone heard	Loud	Very loud
Pitch	Number of vibrations per second: Fast vibrations—high pitch Slow vibrations—low pitch	Low	Very low
Duration	Length of time a vibration note is sustained	Long	Long
Quality	Subjective assessment of characteristics of tone	Hollow	Booming

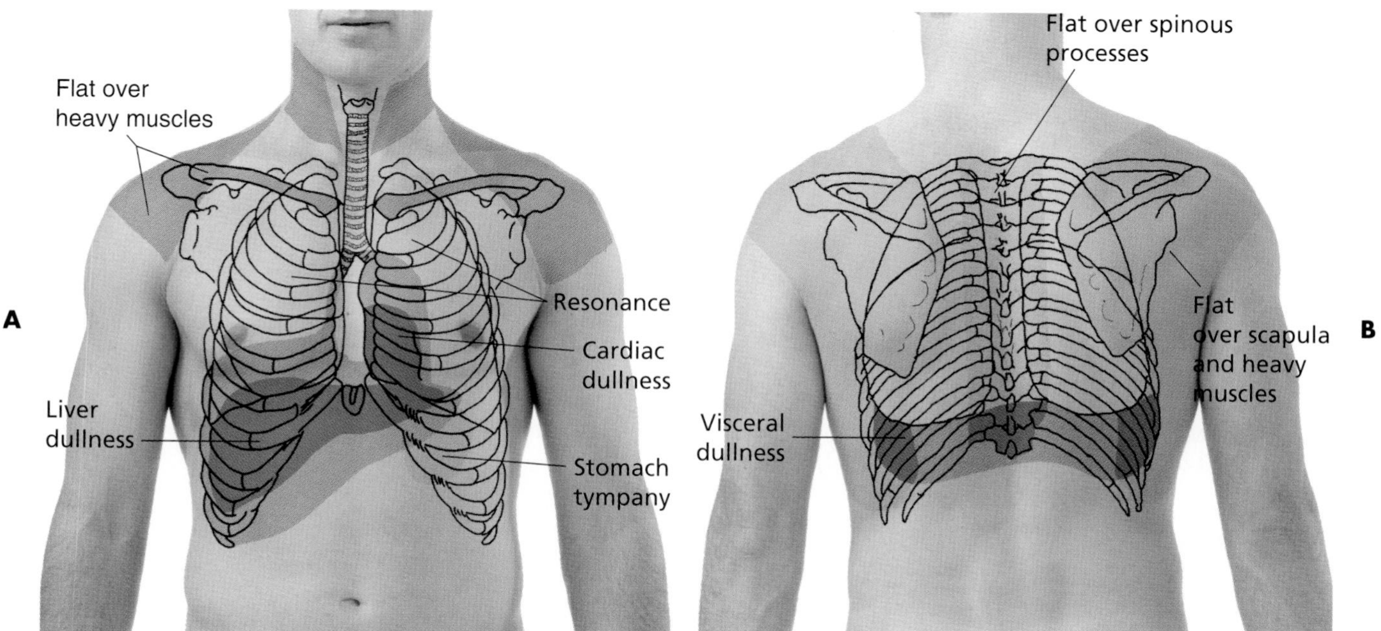

Fig. 17-26 **A,** Percussion tones of the anterior chest. **B,** Percussion tones of the posterior chest.

PROCEDURES AND TECHNIQUES WITH NORMAL FINDINGS

❖ ➤**PERCUSS the thorax for diaphragmatic (respiratory) excursion.** Diaphragmatic excursion is the upward and downward movement of the diaphragm with maximum inspiration and expiration. This allows the examiner to estimate the lower lung border during inspiration and expiration.

To measure diaphragmatic excursion, follow these steps:

1. Stand behind the client. Instruct the client to sit upright, *inhale deeply,* and hold his or her breath. *(Hold your breath at the same time so you can determine the pace of your percussion.)*
2. While the client is holding the breath, quickly percuss down the posterior chest wall along the midscapular line to determine the lower border of the lungs. (The percussion tone should change from resonant to dull.)
3. Using a marking pen, make a small line at the level where the percussion tone changed.
4. Tell the client to breathe normally. When ready, instruct the client to *exhale* as much as possible and hold.
5. Repeat the midscapular percussion down the posterior chest (same side of the chest as before), and again note and mark the point along the chest wall where the sound changes from resonant to dull at the bottom of the lungs. The difference between the two marks on each side is referred to as diaphragmatic excursion (Fig. 17-27).

Repeat the sequence on the other side of the chest. The diaphragmatic excursion should be equal bilaterally and measure at least 3 to 5 cm; in well-conditioned individuals it may measure as much as 7 to 8 cm.

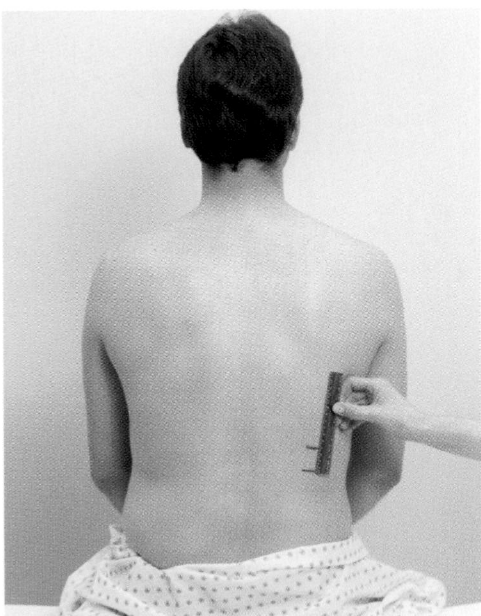

Fig. 17-27 Measuring amount of diaphragmatic excursion. Excursion usually measures 3 to 5 cm.

ABNORMAL FINDINGS

■ Any pathologic condition limiting downward lung expansion or diaphragmatic movement will result in a decreased diaphragmatic excursion. Examples include pleural effusion, emphysema, atelectasis, abdominal tumor or ascites, and severe pain with injured or fractured ribs.

PROCEDURES AND TECHNIQUES WITH NORMAL FINDINGS

ABNORMAL FINDINGS

➤**AUSCULTATE the thorax for breath sounds.** Auscultate the client's breath sounds over the posterior, anterior, and lateral chest walls. Instruct the client to sit upright and breathe deeply and slowly through the mouth. Using the diaphragm of the stethoscope, auscultate the chest from apex to base following the same pattern that was used for percussion (refer back to Fig. 17-25). When auscultating the lateral chest, ask the client to raise his or her arms for better access. Always auscultate during both inspiration and expiration, and compare one side to the other side (Table 17-2).

Table 17-2 Characteristics of Breath Sounds

	BRONCHIAL	BRONCHOVESICULAR	VESICULAR
Pitch	High	Moderate	Low
Intensity	Loud	Medium	Soft
Duration: inspiration and expiration	Insp < Exp 1:2	Insp = Exp 1:1	Insp > Exp 2.5:1
Normal location	Over trachea	First and second intercostal spaces at sternal border anteriorly; posteriorly at T4 medial to scapula	Peripheral lung fields
Abnormal location	Over peripheral lung fields	Over peripheral lung fields	Not applicable

PROCEDURES AND TECHNIQUES WITH NORMAL FINDINGS

➤Breath sounds should be clear to auscultation. Three types of breath sounds are considered normal in various parts of the chest: vesicular, bronchovesicular, and bronchial (Fig. 17-28).

Vesicular breath sounds should be heard over almost all of the posterior lung fields and all of the lateral surfaces and heard throughout the periphery of the anterior lungs fields, including the apex of the lungs above the clavicles.

Bronchovesicular breath sounds are normally heard in the posterior chest over the upper center area of the back on either side of the spine between the scapulae and over the central area of the anterior chest around the sternal border.

Bronchial breath sounds are normally heard over the trachea and the area immediately above the manubrium.

ABNORMAL FINDINGS

■ Normal breath sounds can be considered abnormal if heard in areas of the lung where they are not expected.

- Bronchial breath sounds are abnormal anywhere over the posterior or lateral chest. If heard, there is evidence of consolidation of the lung, as may be seen in clients with pneumonia. (The sound heard will be loud and high pitched. It sounds as if the air source is just under the stethoscope.)
- Bronchovesicular breath sounds should be considered abnormal when heard over the peripheral lung areas.

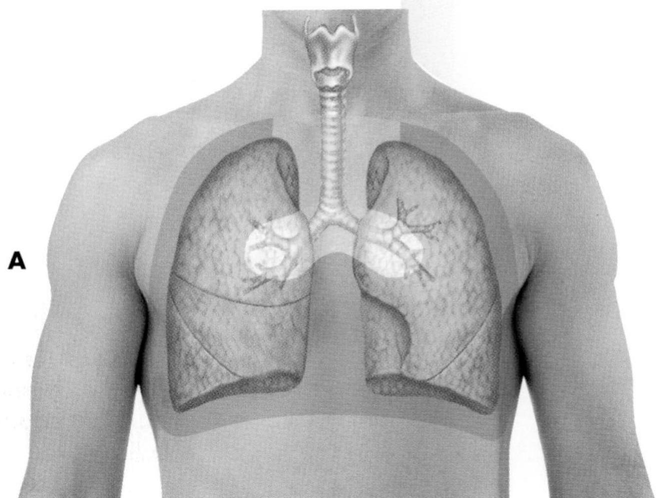

KEY:

Bronchovesicular over main bronchi

Vesicular over lesser bronchi, bronchioles, and lobes

Bronchial over trachea

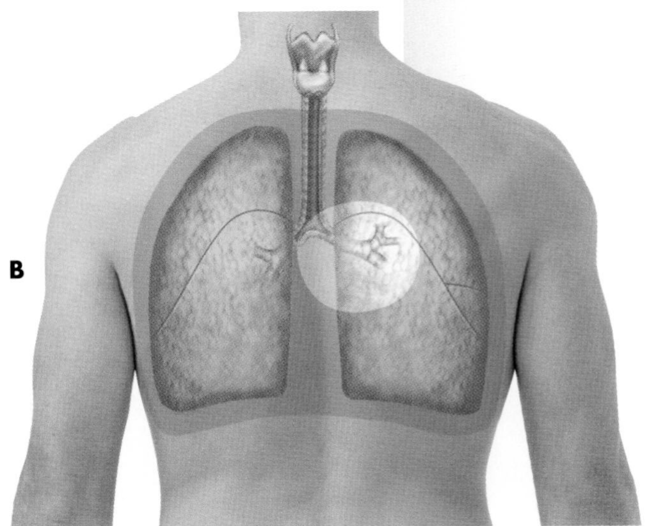

Fig. 17-28 Auscultatory sounds. **A,** Posterior chest. **B,** Anterior chest. (From Seidel et al, 1999.)

PROCEDURES AND TECHNIQUES WITH NORMAL FINDINGS

➤If an adventitious sound is heard, have the client cough; then repeat the examination to see if the sound has changed or disappeared (Box 17-2).

Box 17-2 Clinical Notes

Before you firmly decide that the client has an adventitious sound, remember that the following may also be causes of sound distortion:

- If you bump the stethoscope tubing against something or if the client touches the tubing, the sound will be distorted.
- If the client is cold and is shivering, the sound will be distorted.
- The stethoscope placed and unintentionally moved on a client's excess chest hair may give a false finding of crackles or pleural friction rub.
- Extraneous environmental noises such as the rustling of a paper gown or drape may sound like crackles or pleural friction rub.

ABNORMAL FINDINGS

■ Note the presence of adventitious breath sounds. These are extraneous sounds that are superimposed on the breath sounds. Adventitious sounds are abnormal findings (Table 17-3). If you hear adventitious sounds, identify the type of sound, the location of the sound (i.e., right lung, left lung or bilaterally; upper lobes, lower lobes; anterior and/or posterior) and the phase of breathing in which it is heard (i.e., inspiratory or expiratory). The term *respiratory stridor* is used to describe a harsh, high-pitched sound associated with breathing that is often caused by laryngeal or tracheal obstruction.

Table 17-3 Characteristics of Adventitious Sounds

ADVENTITIOUS SOUNDS	CHARACTERISTICS	CLINICAL EXAMPLES
CRACKLES (previously called rales)		
Fine crackles 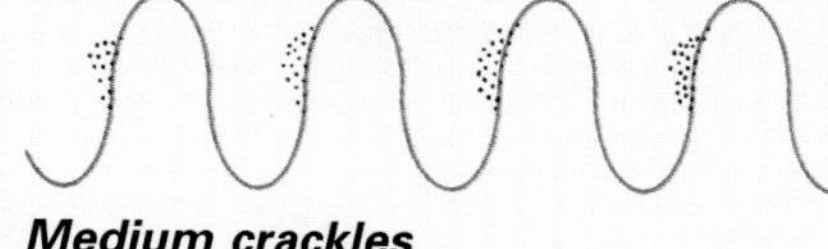	Fine, high-pitched crackling and popping noises (discontinuous sound) heard during the end of inspiration. Not cleared by cough.	May be heard in pneumonia, congestive heart failure, chronic bronchitis, asthma, and other restrictive and obstructive diseases.
Medium crackles 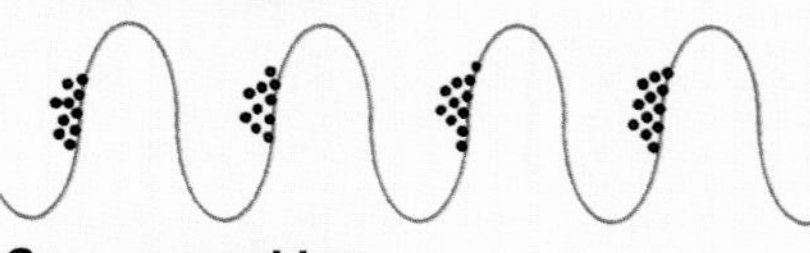	Medium-pitched, moist sound heard about halfway through inspiration. Not cleared by cough.	Same as above, but condition is worse.
Coarse crackles 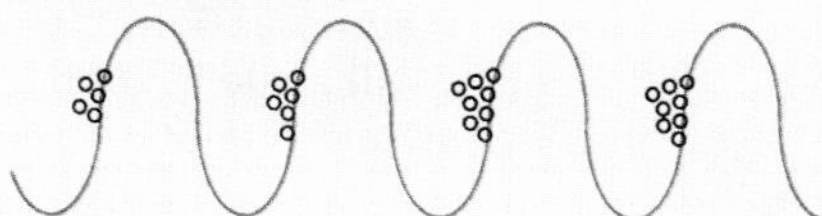	Low-pitched, bubbling or gurgling sounds that start early in inspiration and extend into the first part of expiration.	Same as above, but condition is worse or in terminally ill clients with diminished gag reflex. Also heard in pulmonary edema and pulmonary fibrosis.
WHEEZE (also called sibilant wheeze) 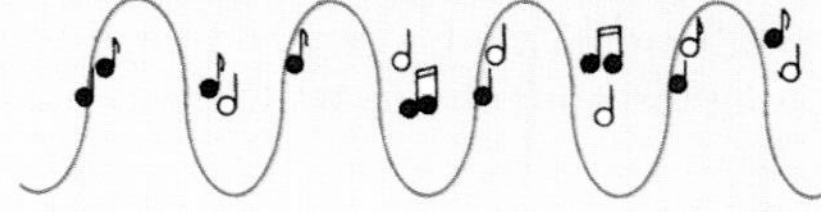	High-pitched, musical sound similar to a squeak. Heard most commonly during expiration, but may also be heard during inspiration. Occurs in small airways.	Heard in narrowed airway diseases such as asthma.

Continued

Table 17-3 Characteristics of Adventitious Sounds—cont'd

ADVENTITIOUS SOUNDS	CHARACTERISTICS	CLINICAL EXAMPLES
RHONCHI (also called sonorous wheeze)	Low-pitched, coarse, loud, low snoring or moaning tone. Actually sounds like snoring. Heard primarily during expiration, but may also be heard during inspiration. Coughing may clear.	Heard in problems causing obstruction of the trachea or bronchus, such as bronchitis.
PLEURAL FRICTION RUB	A superficial, low-pitched, coarse rubbing or grating sound. Sounds like two surfaces rubbing together. Heard throughout inspiration and expiration. Loudest over the lower anterolateral surface. Not cleared by cough.	Heard in individuals with pleurisy (inflammation of the pleural surfaces).

PROCEDURES AND TECHNIQUES WITH NORMAL FINDINGS

➤AUSCULTATE the chest for vocal sounds (vocal resonance). When there is an indication of consolidation of the lung, or if there was an abnormal finding when tactile fremitus was performed, evaluate for vocal resonance. This includes three techniques: testing for bronchophony, whispered pectoriloquy, and egophony.

The spoken voice vibrates and transmits sounds through the lung fields. These sounds are normally muffled and cannot be clearly understood. The sound is loudest medially and softer at the periphery of the lung.

First, instruct the client to repeat one of the following phrases as you auscultate the posterior chest to assess vocal resonance: "Ninety-nine," "e-e-e," or "one-two-three."

Bronchophony Using the diaphragm of the stethoscope, systematically auscultate the posterior chest. As the client repeats either "ninety-nine" or "one-two-three," listen for the response. A normal response is a muffled tone like "nin-nin" or muffled "one-two-three."

Whispered Pectoriloquy Perform when there is a positive finding of bronchophony. It is used to more clearly specify the problem and is referred to as an exaggerated bronchophony. To perform whispered pectoriloquy, ask the client to whisper "one-two-three." Again, systematically auscultate the posterior chest, listening for the quality of the whispered tones. A normal response is a muffled "one-two-three."

Egophony Egophony is the final test for vocal resonance. It evaluates the intensity of the spoken voice. Instruct the client to say "e-e-e" as you auscultate the posterior chest. If normal, the sound should be a muffled "e-e-e."

ABNORMAL FINDINGS

- It is abnormal if the sound is louder and clearer. If there is consolidation or compression of the lung, the sound will actually sound like "ninety-nine" or "one-two-three."
- An abnormal finding is increased clarity and loudness of the sounds, which may be found in consolidation or compression of the lung.
- Changes in intensity and pitch so that the sound appears to be an "a-a-a" occur if there is consolidation of the lung.

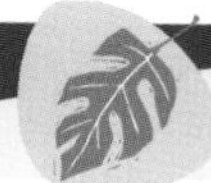

AGE-RELATED VARIATIONS

INFANTS

Anatomy and Physiology

Before birth the alveoli are collapsed, and the lungs contain no air. Throughout gestation, passive respiratory motions do not contribute to respiration; fetal gas exchange is supplied by the placenta. Instead, these passive movements prepare the lungs to respond to chemical and neurologic stimuli during and after the birth process.

Immediately following birth, rapid changes occur. Once the umbilical cord is cut, the first breath is taken, filling the lungs with air. This first breath causes blood to flow through the lungs vigorously, resulting in a decrease in pulmonary pressure. Within minutes, the foramen ovale closes, increasing oxygen tension in the arterial blood, and thus stimulates the ductus arteriosus to contract and close. These actions help both the pulmonary and systemic circulation to mature and the lungs to become fully integrated and functioning.

Newborn infants rely primarily on the diaphragm for breathing. The use of intercostal muscles occurs as they get older. The chest wall of the infant is very thin compared with that of an older child or adult.

Health History

- Was the infant premature? What was his or her birth weight? Was ventilation assistance needed? If so, for how long? Were you ever told that the baby had a breathing problem or respiratory distress syndrome?

  Rationale Low birth weight and prematurity are risk factors for respiratory difficulties. Infants placed on ventilators have increased risk for several long-term health problems.

- Is your infant congested? Has there been any obvious breathing difficulty? Have you noticed a cough? If so, how long has this been going on? Describe what it is like. What seems to make it better or worse?

  Rationale It is important to determine onset, duration, and other factors associated with the infant's current breathing difficulties. Although upper respiratory infections are common, coughing is an abnormal finding with this age group.

- Does the infant ever have spells when he or she breathes and then does not breathe for a while? Do you use an apnea monitor?

  Rationale Periods of apnea are most likely to occur if the infant is premature. Newborn apnea is usually identified while the infant is in the nursery, but if it is not, it is important to continue to assess if the infant is having apnea now. Unidentified apnea can lead to infant death.

- Have you noticed any breathing difficulty with feeding, such as increased perspiration, cyanosis, tiring quickly, or disinterest in feeding?

  Rationale Infants who tire easily or demonstrate hypoxia while feeding may have an underlying respiratory or cardiovascular disease.

- Does the baby ever have choking spells or seem to spit up a lot? Has the child had recurrent episodes of lung infections such as pneumonia?

  Rationale Recurrent choking or infection may be an indication of possible gastroesophageal reflux.

- Has anyone ever talked with you about childproofing your home? If so, what have you been told? What measures do you take to keep potentially hazardous items out of reach?

  Rationale Assess safety and emergency first-aid knowledge. Determine whether the parent protects the child by keeping small items out of reach. Suffocation is the leading cause of unintentional childhood death under the age of 1 year (Wong et al, 1999).

- Have you ever had a first-aid course about child safety? Do you know first-aid techniques? Can you demonstrate the Heimlich maneuver and rescue breathing for an infant the size of yours?

  Rationale Parents and child care providers should be taught safety and first-aid techniques so they may ensure a safe environment for the infant and implement appropriate first-aid techniques should infant choking occur.

Examination

Procedures and Techniques Assessing the respiratory status of a newborn or infant is usually straightforward and basically follows the same sequence as for an adult, although there are a few differences worth noting. The infant must be undressed at least to the diaper to perform an adequate assessment of the thorax and lungs. Be sure to provide covering for the infant when you are not performing the examination to prevent exposure and cooling. Conduct the examination while the infant is calm if at all possible; examination of a crying infant is difficult. If the infant starts to cry, take time to comfort him or her.

When inspecting the infant's chest, include a measurement of the chest circumference. To obtain a true estimate of respiratory rate, count the number of breaths for a full minute. Auscultation of the infant's breath sounds is performed in the same manner as for the older child and adult; however, the nurse should use a stethoscope with a small diaphragm. An adult-sized stethoscope diaphragm head will cover at least half of the infant's chest and is inappropriate for an accurate assessment of the infant's respiratory status. Percussion is not routinely performed during infant assessment.

Normal and Abnormal Findings Inspection of the infant's thoracic cage should show a smooth, rounded, and symmetric appearance. The "Harrison's groove" may be seen on the chest wall. This normal anatomic deviation is a horizontal groove in the rib cage at the level of the diaphragm. It extends from the sternum to the midaxillary line. Unlike the adult, the infant has a round thorax with an equal AP and transverse diameter. The average chest circumference ranges from 30 to 36 cm. This measurement should be 2 to 3 cm smaller than the child's head circumference. Room temperature may greatly affect the infant's peripheral skin color. If the infant becomes cold, mottling of the hands and feet may be noted. Once the child is warmed up, the mottling should disappear. If it remains, further evaluation is indicated.

Infants are obligate nose breathers until about age 3 months. Should their nasal passages become occluded, they may have difficulty breathing. Sneezing is a common finding for an infant and is therapeutic as it helps to clear the nose. Coughing, however, is considered abnormal and indicates a problem.

The respiratory pattern in the newborn may be irregular, having a Cheyne-Stokes type of pattern. Premature newborns may have periods of apnea for as long as 10 to 15 seconds. Stimulation by the adult caregiver can generally produce a quick breath. The respiratory rate in the newborn and infant ranges from 30 to 60 times per minute (Table 17-4). It is important to note that if the infant is ill and has a rapid respiratory rate for a prolonged period of time, he or she will tire and may subsequently become physiologically distressed.

The infant has a thin chest wall, which makes breath sounds difficult to localize with auscultation. They are commonly transmitted from one auscultatory area to another. Because of this, the predominant breath sound you will hear in the peripheral lung fields is bronchovesicular. The thin chest wall also makes the newborn's xiphoid process more prominent than that of an older child or adult.

There are several respiratory findings that indicate an infant is in respiratory distress. These include stridor, grunting, sternal or supraclavicular retractions, and nasal flaring. Any of these findings warrant immediate medical attention. Stridor is a high-pitched, piercing sound that is primarily heard in a distressed infant during inspiration. It occurs secondary to upper airway obstruction. The obstruction may cause the infant's inspiratory cycle to be 3 or 4 times longer than expiration. Respiratory grunting is a mechanism by which the infant tries to force trapped air out of the lungs while still trying to maintain adequate air in the lungs. Sternal and supraclavicular retractions and nasal flaring are indications of respiratory distress. Clinically this may be observed as "see-saw" type of breathing with alternating movements of the chest and abdomen. If any of these are observed, the infant is working very hard to try to maintain adequate breathing and should be referred to a primary care provider.

Table 17-4 Respiratory Rates in Children

AGE	RATE PER MINUTE
Newborn	30-60
Less than 1 year	30-50
1-2 years	30-40
3-5 years	20-30
6-10 years	16-20
Over 10 years	12-20

■ CHILDREN

Anatomy and Physiology

In young children, the respiratory rate is much faster than it is in adults. Children use the abdominal muscles to assist with breathing until ages 7 to 8. The chest's bony structure tends to be more prominent as well, largely due to the relatively thinner chest wall. The more cartilaginous structure is more yielding, and the xiphoid process is not only more movable but also often more prominent. By the time the child reaches 8 to 10 years of age, the respiratory rate drops to that of an adult.

Health History

- Does the child frequently eat foods such as peanuts, popcorn, hot dogs, raw carrots, and peas? If so, does he or she eat them when sitting to eat or when playing? If hot dogs are eaten, are they cut into very small pieces? Has the child ever choked on any food?

  Rationale Choking is a common problem with food substances, especially when the child is permitted to be up and playing while also eating.
- Does the child know how to swim? Do you have a swimming pool? Does the child ever play unsupervised around or near water (including the bathtub)?

  Rationale Water and swimming pools are hazardous for all unsupervised children whether they can swim or not. Drowning is the second and third leading cause of unintentional childhood death in boys and girls respectively between the ages of 1 and 14. (Wong et al, 1999).
- Does the child have recurrent respiratory infections, allergies, or breathing problems? If so, how often do the problems occur? How long does the problem usually last? What are the precipitating factors? Current medications? Effects of activities, including outdoor playing and sports?

  Rationale Children with asthma, bronchitis, or other chronic conditions such as cystic fibrosis should be questioned about the overall progress of their disease and how they are coping with it.
- Ask child: What do you understand about your breathing problem? How do you feel about having to take the treatments or medications that you have to take? How does all of this affect your ability to do what you want to do with your friends?

  Rationale Many times how the child feels about the breathing problem determines the actual sequelae of the respiratory problem.

Examination

Procedures and Techniques The techniques for examining the lungs and respiratory system of the child are generally the same as for the adult. By age 2 or 3 years, the child is usually very cooperative during the respiratory examination. Even before that age, if the examiner takes the time to develop a relationship with the child, cooperation can usually be obtained. Tricks that may help to gain cooperation include letting the child play with the stethoscope before beginning the examination, pretending that your finger is a candle and asking the child to blow it out, or having the child blow out the light of the otoscope or penlight both before and during the examination.

If performing chest palpation, the examiner should adjust the number of fingers used to palpate the chest wall to be appropriate for the size of the chest. For example, if the child is small you may use only two or three fingers. On the other hand, if the child is large, you may use three fingers or all four. Percussion is infrequently performed until the child is older, at least 10 years of age. At that time, the techniques are the same as for the adult.

Normal and Abnormal Findings Differences in findings include the following. By age 5 or 6, the rounded thorax of the child approximates the 1:2 or 5:7 ratio of AP to transverse diameter of the adult. If the child's chest proportion remains rounded, it may be an outward indication of a significant problem such as asthma or cystic fibrosis. By age 6 or 7, the child's breathing pattern should change from primarily nasal and abdominal to mostly thoracic in girls and abdominal in boys. As noted in Table 17-4, the child's respiratory rate should gradually slow as the child becomes older.

Palpation findings for the child are the same as for the adult. If percussion is performed, the examiner should note that young children will have a normal hyperresonance tone.

Auscultation findings for the child range between the findings of the infant and the findings of the adult. Depending upon the size of the child and the musculature of the chest, you may find slight variations. Findings for a small or young child with undeveloped chest musculature may include more bronchovesicular breath sounds in the peripheral lung areas, whereas if the child is larger and has started to develop more, the breath sounds will be equivalent to those of the adult (vesicular in the peripheral lung fields).

■ ADOLESCENTS

Health History

- Many young people your age smoke. Have you ever smoked a cigarette or chewed tobacco? If so, have you done it in the past week? How often and how much do you smoke or chew? How old were you when you started smoking or using tobacco? Have you tried to quit? Do you want to quit? What makes it difficult for you to quit?

Rationale Phrase question so that adolescent does not feel as threatened to answer the question truthfully. Public health authorities report that childhood and adolescent smoking is on the rise. Among high school students, cigarette use increased by 32% between 1991 and 1997 (USDHHS, 1998).

- Some young people sniff glue or spray paint to get high. Have you ever tried this? If so, what did you inhale? If so, have you done it in the past week? How often and how much do you inhale the substance? Does it make you sick? How old were you when you started inhaling? Have you tried to quit? Do you want to quit? What makes it difficult for you to quit?

Rationale The prevalence of toxic fume inhalation by school-age children and adolescents is a common, serious, and sometimes deadly problem. Inhalants are frequently the first type of drug abused by young adolescents (Espeland, 1995). One national study found that 17% of eighth graders have used inhalants; older teenagers tend to advance to other drug use (Johnston, O'Malley, and Bachman, 1993).

Examination

Procedures and Techniques Examination techniques for the adolescent are the same as for the adult. As with all clients, no matter what age, it is important to have the client disrobe to the waist. The examiner should be sensitive to the possible modesty of the adolescent and provide a drape for the breasts when the anterior chest is not being assessed.

Normal and Abnormal Findings The techniques and findings for the adolescent's lung and respiratory assessment are the same as for the adult.

■ OLDER ADULTS

Anatomy and Physiology

With aging, the individual experiences a moderate decline in lung function for several reasons. First, kyphoscoliosis, a skeletal deformity affecting the spinal curvature, is a common finding associated with aging. This can cause the thorax to shorten and the AP diameter to increase. Secondly, the chest wall may become stiffer, possibly due to calcification at rib articulation points, resulting in decreased chest wall compliance. Third, a sedentary lifestyle may contribute to diminished muscle strength of the respiratory muscles, resulting in reduced maximal inspiratory and expiratory force (Matteson et al, 1997). The lung tissue also undergoes change with aging. As the alveoli become less elastic and more fibrous, there is some loss of interalveolar folds, decreasing the amount of alveolar surface area available for gas exchange. As a result, breathing on exertion becomes more difficult; exceeding a tolerant level of exertion may result in dyspnea. Also, with age, mucous membranes become drier and less able to clear retained mucus; this predisposes the older adult to bacterial growth and respiratory infection.

Health History

- Do you get a flu shot every year? Do you get a shot to prevent you from getting pneumonia?

Rationale Assess the client's level of preventive care, as well as his or her exposure to respiratory pathogens.

- Have you noticed any fatigue or shortness of breath while following your daily routine? Does it seem to be harder to breathe than it used to be? Do you feel that you cannot breathe as deeply as you used to? Have you experienced a decrease in energy or ability to complete your activities?

Rationale Older adults may have a reduced ability to exercise because pulmonary function tends to decrease with age. Specific changes that may occur are addressed in the previous section.

- Have you gained or lost weight over the last few months? If so, how much?

Rationale Changes in weight may be clues to problems, particularly with specific respiratory complaints. Weight gain can be associated with pulmonary edema; complaints of weight loss could be associated with infection, disease, or general shortness of breath.

- Have you noticed sweating at night? Have you had a low-grade fever periodically? Do you feel any sensations in the chest other than pain—perhaps a feeling of heaviness?

Rationale The incidence of chronic respiratory disease is higher in older adults, and these questions make note of symptoms of respiratory disorders.

Examination

Procedures and Techniques The procedure and techniques are the same as for the younger adult. It is important to correlate the client's history with the physical findings. For example, if the client has been a 35-year smoker and now has adventitious sounds present on auscultation, it may have a different meaning and significance than it would for a client who has never smoked and now has shortness of breath and presence of adventitious sounds.

Normal and Abnormal Findings The findings of the assessment of the lungs and respiration in the older person are basically the same as for the adult, but several structural and functional differences may be seen. Posterior thoracic stooping or bending or kyphosis may alter the chest wall configuration and make adequate lung expansion more difficult. This in turn may result in decreased tidal volume and thus more shallow breathing. The older adult may also have decreased expansion of the lungs secondary to a sedentary lifestyle or general physical health disability or weakness.

CLIENTS WITH SITUATIONAL VARIATIONS

CLIENTS WITH CHRONIC OBSTRUCTIVE PULMONARY DISEASES (COPD)

Health History

- Do you use oxygen at home? If so, when is it used—or how many hours a day is it used? How many liters of oxygen do you use? Does it seem to meet your oxygen needs? Do you have any limitations in your activity because of the oxygen use?

Rationale Clients with severe disease may require continuous oxygen therapy. If the client being examined is using oxygen, it is important to inquire about the number of hours per day that oxygen is required, the oxygen concentration required, and the limitation of activity because of either the disease or the oxygen use.

- Have you had recent weight loss or weight gain? If so, how much? Does your shortness of breath give you difficulties eating and drinking enough fluids? Do you use nutritional supplementation?

Rationale Clients who have chronic shortness of breath tend to have poor appetites. Maintaining adequate nutrition and hydration becomes a challenge for these individuals. It is imperative that the nurse continually monitor nutritional status.

- What medications do you take every day? Do you remember to take them regularly? How do you keep track of what you need to take and when?

Rationale Because these clients are also usually on multiple medications, obtaining a careful medication history is important. It is also important to determine if the medications are taken correctly. Many clients use medication organizers or some specific system to keep track of all the medications.

Examination

Procedures and Techniques There are no differences in examination procedure and techniques from the adult.

Normal and Abnormal Findings It is difficult to generalize the degree of findings of an individual with an obstructive lung disease because findings are dependent upon the severity of the condition. If the disease is in early stages, the client may have only symptoms that are exacerbated by illness or stress, but no obvious physical changes.

Clients with advanced disease may have an increased AP diameter or have a "barrel-shaped" chest. Percussion of the chest may indicate hyperresonance secondary to chronic hyperinflation of the lungs. Pursed-lip breathing may be observed.

A client who develops an acute exacerbation of COPD may have significant respiratory compromise. If the client is in distress, he or she may have forward posturing of the upper trunk or may sit in a tripod position with arms forward and supported on knees or on an overbed table. This is known as "the position of air hunger." The nurse may first note dyspnea, cough, and an audible expiratory wheeze. Auscultation of breath sounds may indicate prolonged expiration and diminished breath sounds over the affected area.

EXAMINATION SUMMARY

Lungs and Respiratory System

PROCEDURE

General Presentation

- Inspect the client for:
  General appearance
  Posture
  Breathing effort

Chest Wall Configuration

- Inspect the chest for:
  Shape and symmetry
  Muscle development
  Anteroposterior (AP) diameter
  Costal angle

General Oxygenation

- Inspect skin, nails, and lips for:
  Color

Respiratory Rate

- Observe and evaluate respiration for:
  Rate and quality
  Breathing pattern
  Chest expansion

Anterior and Posterior Chest Assessment

- Palpate the trachea for:
  Position
- Palpate chest and thoracic muscles for:
  Tenderness
  Bulges
  Symmetry
- Palpate the chest wall for:
  Thoracic expansion
- ❖ Palpate the chest wall for:
  Vocal (tactile) fremitus
- ❖ Percuss the thorax for:
  Tone
- ❖ Percuss the thorax for:
  Diaphragmatic (respiratory) excursion
- Auscultate the thorax for:
  Vesicular breath sounds
  Bronchovesicular breath sounds
  Bronchial breath sounds
- ❖ Auscultate the chest for vocal sounds (vocal resonance)

SUMMARY OF FINDINGS

Age Group	Normal Findings	Typical Variations	Findings Associated With Disorder
Infants and children	• Prominent xiphoid and sharp tip. • Harrison groove seen on chest wall. • AP to transverse diameter 1:1 for infants and 1:2 by age 6. • Respiratory rate of infants 30-40/min; gradually slows during childhood; reaches adult rate/min range by age 10. • Infants are obligatory nose breathers.	• Crackles and rhonchi are common. • Transient tachypnea. • Preterm infants may have irregular respiratory rate or apneic periods. • Hyperresonance is a common finding.	• Chest roundness (increased AP diameter) after age 2 suggests chronic obstruction. • Indictors of respiratory distress include flared nostrils; intercostal, sternal, or supraclavicular retractions. • Clubbing of nail indicates chronic heart or lung disease. • Dry, hoarse, barking cough suggests croup. • Stridor indicates high respiratory obstruction in infants and children.

Age Group	Normal Findings	Typical Variations	Findings Associated With Disorder
Adolescents older adults	Same as for adult. • Loss of muscle strength of thorax and diaphragm, thus a decreased lung resiliency. • Alveoli are less elastic and more fibrous.	Same as for adult. • Older adults have less chest expansion, marked bony prominences, and larger AP diameter. • Aging is associated with kyphosis, use of accessory muscles, and hyperresonance.	Same as for adult. • Shortness of breath and fatigue may indicate lung disease. • Chest pain could indicate cardiac or respiratory problem.
Adults	• AP diameter half size of transverse diameter. • Respiratory rate 12-20/min. • Rate of respiration to heart rate is 1:4. • Bilateral equal chest expansion. • Bronchial and vesicular and bronchovesicular breath sounds auscultated.	• Pectus carinatum and pectus excavatum normal findings in absence of disease.	• Shallow respiration associated with injured rib, pleurisy, liver enlargement, or abdominal ascites. • Change in respiratory rate may indicate neurologic, metabolic imbalance, infection, or pleurisy, respiratory distress, or anxiety imbalance or neurologic disorder. • Tripod position, flared nostrils, pursed-lip breathing associated with dyspnea. • Barrel chest with kyphosis, prominent sternal angle associated with COPD. • Asymmetry, unequal expansion may be extrapleural air, fluid, or mass. • Decreased tactile or vocal fremitus is associated with emphysema. • Hyperresonance indicates hyperinflation of the lungs. • Dullness indicates lung consolidation.

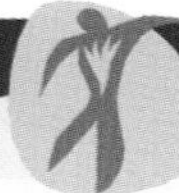

HEALTH PROMOTION

SMOKING

Cigarette smoking is the most important single and preventable cause of death in society. In fact, it is one of the most potent known human carcinogens, causing more cancer deaths than any other known agent (Gorin and Arnold, 1998). To compound the problem further, the number of young people who are smoking in the United States is increasing (Wechsler et al, 1998).

The American Cancer Society and most large health care facilities have a variety of "stop-smoking" programs that use a variety of strategies. Successful smoking cessation has been shown to enhance the client's commitment to health and change the client's conceptualization of smoking from positive to negative (Puskar, 1995).

Factors that seem to contribute to the success of a stop-smoking program are client readiness and finding a program that works for that individual client. The clinician can be effective with a brief, unambiguous, informative message regarding the need to stop using tobacco. Reinforcement by the clinician and self-help materials enhance success (U.S. Preventive Services Task Force, 1996). Giving the client only written materials about the hazards of smoking and ways to quit smoking is thought to have minimal impact on the client's success in actually quitting smoking. The use of nicotine patches or gum may be useful to gradually wean the client's dependence.

SMOKELESS TOBACCO

Tobacco chewing and the use of smokeless tobacco have many of the same harmful effects on the body as does smoking cigarettes. In addition, persons with this behavior are at increased risk for mouth cancer and leukoplakia. The same strategies apply to stopping smokeless tobacco as for smoking. The American Cancer Society has programs and related materials.

INHALANTS

Inhalants such as gasoline, glue, hair spray, deodorant sprays, correction fluid, and liquid cement are used, primarily by young persons, to "get high." These are often the first mood-altering substances used by children. Inhalants may be attractive to the child and adolescent because of their rapid onset of action, low cost, and easy availability. They are typically used by inhaling from a plastic bag containing the substance or by inhaling a cloth saturated with the substance. The initial effect is usually stimulation and excitation, but use of inhalants may lead to death or cause permanent lung, liver, kidney, or brain damage. It is vitally important to determine if the client is now using or has ever used an inhaled agent—even on a single occasion. If you assess that the client is either at risk for using inhalants or is currently a user of inhalants, the client should be clearly informed of the risks associated with their continued use and ultimately referred to a clinical resource that can provide adequate counseling. Your local public health office or teen clinic will most likely have materials and resources that may be helpful.

OCCUPATIONAL OR HOME EXPOSURE TO IRRITANTS AND CARCINOGENS

All individuals who work in areas where there are fumes are at risk for lung damage and subsequent respiratory problems. The exposure could be to a known harmful agent such as asbestos, or it could be to less obvious toxins such as hair spray, paint fumes, pesticides, herbicides, coal dust, secondary cigarette smoke, wood-burning fireplace fumes, or even dust. Exposure to environmental tobacco smoke has been shown to increase the frequency of middle ear effusions and lower respiratory infection in children (U.S. Preventive Services Task Force, 1996).

Regardless of the toxin or irritant, individuals should be cautioned either to avoid areas where the toxins are present or to wear a filtering mask or respirator to keep from inhaling the fumes. An ounce of prevention is worth a pound of cure.

PREVENTING RESPIRATORY INFECTIONS

Respiratory infections are most serious for the older adult and any person with chronic lung disease. The following guidelines may be helpful for those clients at high risk for infection:

- Follow all guidelines from health care providers, such as taking prescribed medications or using supplemental oxygen if ordered.
- Take care of yourself: Drink at least 6 glasses of water each day (unless advised otherwise), eat nutritious meals, get adequate sleep each night (7 to 8 hours), take several short rest periods during the day, learn to conserve your energy so as not to get too tired.
- Stay away from people who have colds and the flu. If this is not possible, wear a disposable mask when around ill people.
- Avoid air pollution, including tobacco smoke, wood or oil smoke, car exhaust, and industrial fumes.
- If you are older or in a group at high risk for infection, consult your health care provider about receiving a pneumococcal vaccine every 5 years and a flu vaccine every fall.
- Take special precautions with personal hygiene, and always wash your hands.
- If you should become ill, seek medical attention.

COMMON PROBLEMS AND CONDITIONS

Lungs and Respiratory System

INFECTIONS AND INFLAMMATORY CONDITIONS

Acute Bronchitis

Acute bronchitis is an inflammation of the mucous membranes of the bronchial tree caused by pulmonary infection. Most cases of acute bronchitis are viral, but some may be bacterial in origin. Bronchitis most commonly occurs in clients with COPD; however, it can occur in other clients with pulmonary infection as well. Clinical findings include fever, cough, tachypnea, and purulent sputum production (Mitchell, 1996). Some clients complain of a pleuritic chest pain as well. Rhonchi and crackles are frequently heard with auscultation (Fig. 17-29).

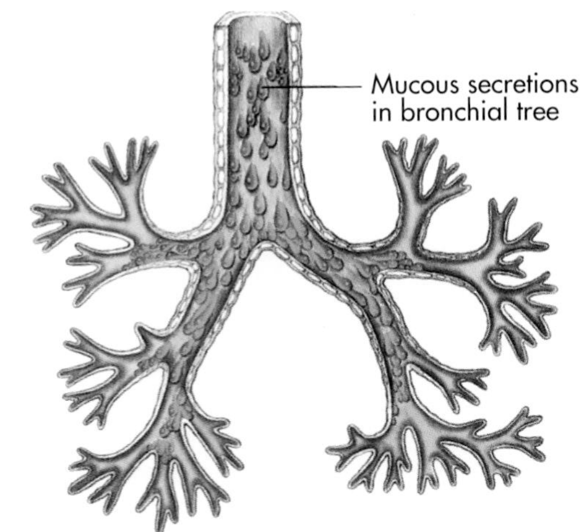

Fig. 17-29 Bronchitis. Irritation of the bronchi causes inflammation.

Pneumonia

Pneumonia is an infection of the lung tissue. Pneumonia can be bacterial, fungal, or viral. The infectious process causes an inflammatory process within the bronchioles and alveolar spaces and a consolidation of inflammatory fluid (Fig. 17-30). Clinical findings associated with pneumonia include fever, tachypnea, labored breathing, productive cough, and restlessness. Sputum production may be copious or minimal, and the sputum may appear white, green, yellow, pink, or rusty (Mitchell, 1996). Increased fremitus and dull tone to percussion may be noted over the area of consolidation. Crackles and wheezes may be heard with auscultation of the lungs. An increase in clarity and volume may be noted with egophony, bronchophony, and whispered pectoriloquy.

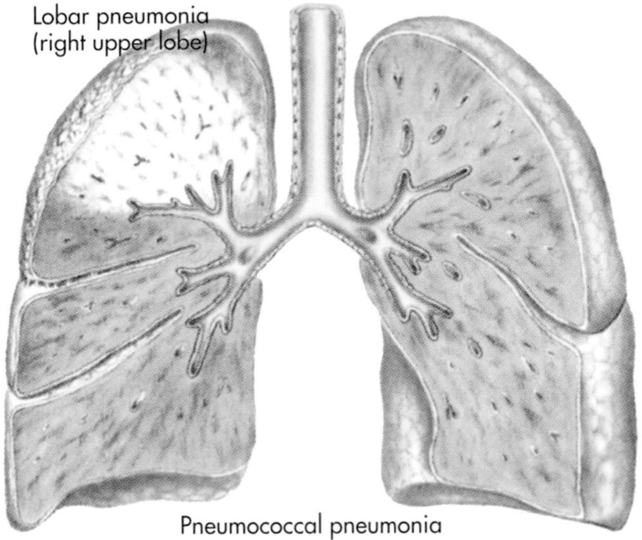

Fig. 17-30 Right upper lobe pneumonia.

Bronchiectasis

Repeated respiratory infections may cause a chronic dilation of the bronchi or bronchioles known as bronchiectasis (Fig. 17-31). This condition most commonly affects the older adult, although it can also be seen in younger individuals with cystic fibrosis. Common clinical findings include respiratory distress, tachypnea, and possibly a barrel or rounded chest wall. The client frequently has crackles and wheezing noted upon auscultation; however, these may clear after coughing (Mitchell, 1996).

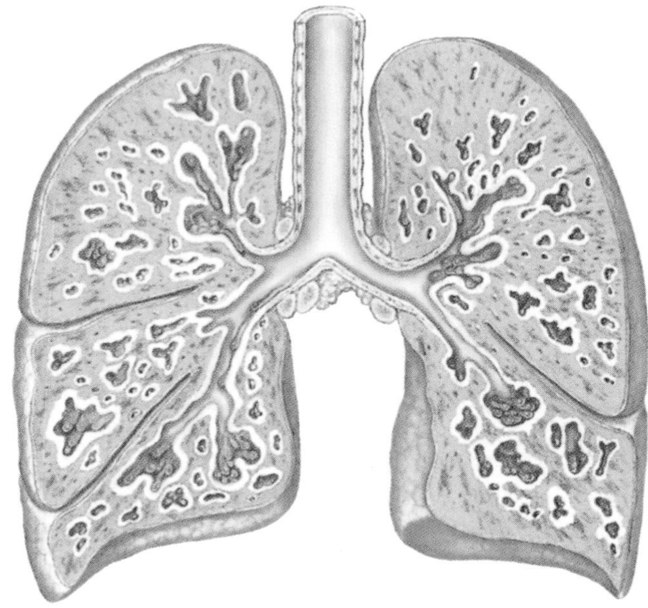

Fig. 17-31 Bronchiectasis.

Pleural Effusion

A pleural effusion is an accumulation of nonpurulent fluid in the pleural space between the visceral and parietal pleurae (Fig. 17-32). Normally, less than 10 ml of fluid is in pleural space. The accumulation of the excess fluid usually occurs secondary to another problem, such as infection, cancer, or injury. The degree of clinical symptoms depends greatly on the amount of fluid accumulation and the position of the client. Fluid tends to accumulate to the most dependent position in the lung.

If the effusion has occurred rapidly and if it is large, there may be dyspnea, intercostal bulging, or decreased chest wall movement. Fremitus ranges from normal to absent, depending on the amount of fluid that has accumulated. If present, it will be decreased over the affected area. Percussion tones over the affected area will be dull to flat. The tone may change as the client changes position. Breath sounds are diminished or "muted" over the affected area as well.

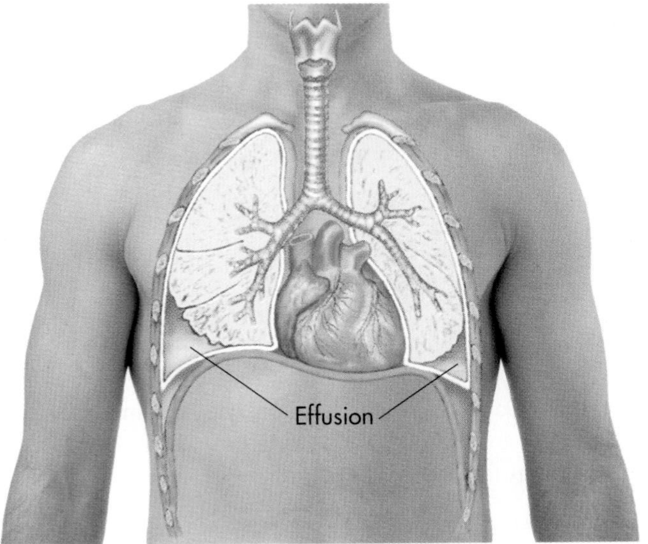

Fig. 17-32 Pleural effusion.

Empyema

An accumulation of purulent exudate in the pleural space is called empyema (Fig. 17-33). The purulent exudate commonly arises from adjacent infected or traumatized tissue within the lung. The client with empyema often has a fever and an increased respiratory rate (if severe, may have respiratory distress). With empyema, fremitus may range from normal to absent (depending on the amount of fluid that has accumulated), and a dull area with percussion over the affected area may be noted. Breath sounds are distant to absent over affected area as well.

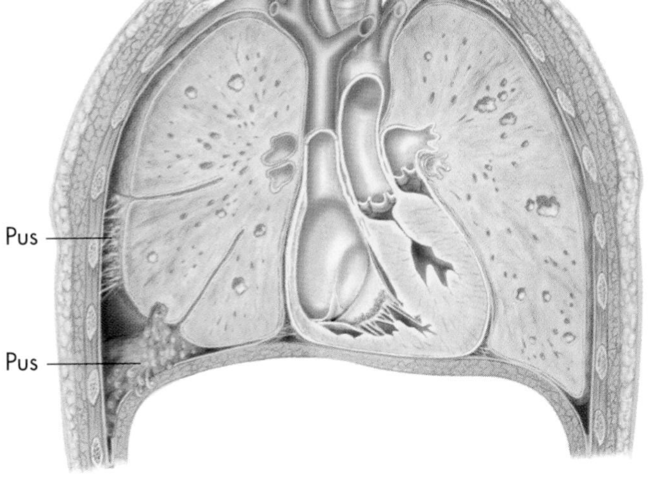

Fig. 17-33 Empyema. (Modified from Wilson and Thompson, 1990. From Seidel et al, 1999.)

Tuberculosis

Tuberculosis (TB) is a bacterial infectious disease caused by *Mycobacterium tuberculosis.* It causes infection primarily to the lungs, but kidney, bone, lymph node and meninges can also be involved (Fig. 17-34). The client is usually asymptomatic during the early stages of the disease. The initial clinical manifestations may consist of fatigue, anorexia, weight loss, night sweats, and fever. The characteristic pulmonary finding is a cough that becomes increasingly frequent, producing a mucopurulent sputum. Chest pain may also be present. Blood-streaked sputum is not a common initial finding and is usually associated with more advanced infection (Mitchell, 1996). Screening for TB is done by tuberculin skin test or chest x-ray examination.

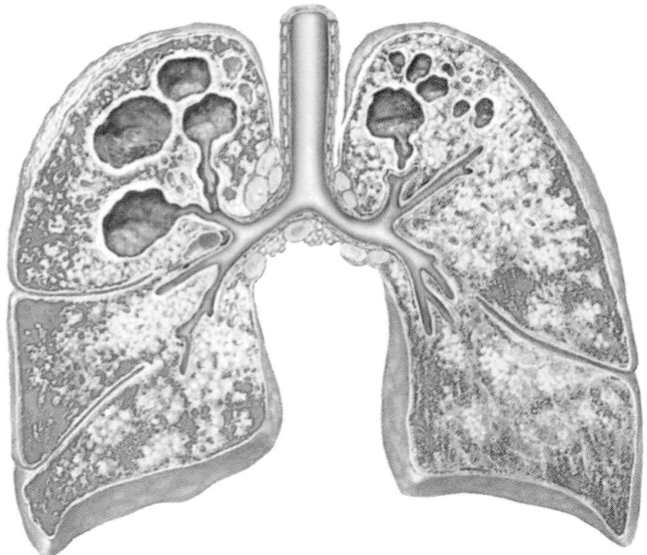

Fig. 17-34 Tuberculosis.

Croup

Croup is a syndrome that usually results from a viral infection. It is seen almost exclusively in young children under the age of 3 years. The child suffering from croup usually appears anxious with labored breathing and a fever. A classic "bark" type of cough is a common finding, sometimes accompanied by inspiratory stridor. The examiner may hear crackles or inspiratory stridor with auscultation, but it not uncommon for the breath sounds to be clear.

CHRONIC OBSTRUCTIVE PULMONARY DISEASE

Chronic obstructive pulmonary disease is a descriptive term given to a cluster of respiratory diseases characterized by increased resistance to airflow due to airway narrowing or obstruction.

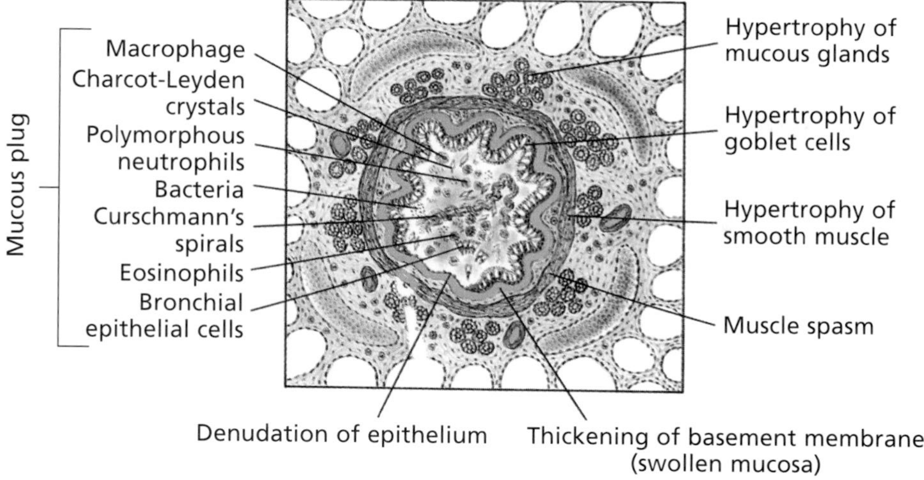

Fig. 17-35 Asthma.

Asthma

Asthma (sometimes referred to as reactive airway disease) is a common lung disease characterized by airway obstruction and inflammation. In this condition, there is an increased responsiveness of the airways to various stimuli, resulting in widespread narrowing of the airways and bronchospasm with increased mucous secretions (Fig. 17-35). The stimuli triggering an acute asthmatic condition may be allergens or irritants such as dust, pollen, smoke, mold, food, medications, and respiratory infections (Cronin, 1997).

Clinical findings include increased respiratory rate with prolonged expiration, audible wheeze, shortness of breath, tachycardia, anxious appearance, possible use of accessory muscles, and cough. Prolonged expiration, expiratory and occasionally inspiratory wheeze, and diminished breath sounds are common findings with auscultation. Decreased tactile fremitus, possibly hyperresonance, and a decreased diaphragmatic excursion may be noted.

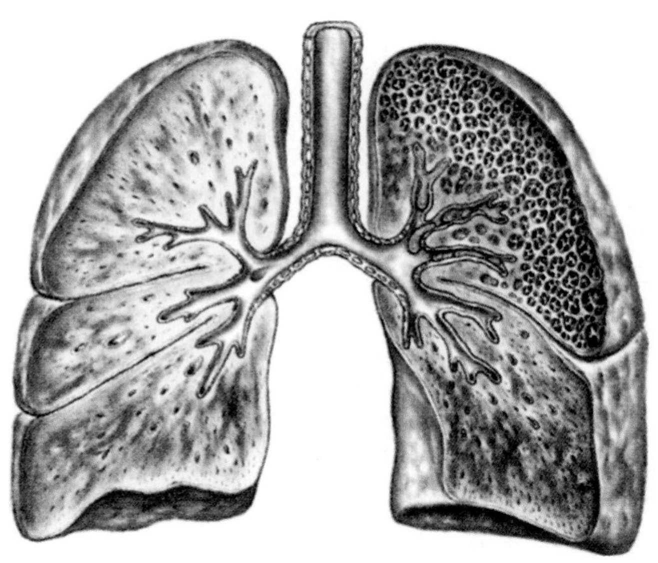

Fig. 17-36 Emphysema in upper left lobe.

Emphysema

Emphysema is a disease in which there is an anatomic alteration of the air spaces distal to the conducting airways (Fig. 17-36). There is a permanent abnormal enlargement of the air spaces. This results in destruction of the alveolar walls and, finally, increased airway resistance.

The classic general appearance of a client with advanced emphysema is a thin, underweight individual with a barrel chest. Although these individuals are not always short of breath when their disease is well managed, they easily become short of breath with minimal exertion and are susceptible to respiratory failure with acute exacerbation of their disease or with an acute pulmonary infection. When the client is short of breath, pursed-lip breathing and tripod position are frequently observed. Other clinical findings typically reveal diminished breath and voice sounds, possible wheezing or crackles to auscultation, a diminished fremitus to palpation, hyperresonance and decreased diaphragmatic excursion to percussion.

Cystic Fibrosis

Cystic fibrosis (CF) is an autosomal recessive genetic disorder of the exocrine glands. It is a multisystem disease affecting almost all body systems but especially the lungs, pancreas, and sweat glands. It causes respiratory system dysfunction because of heavy, thick mucus production from the mucous glands (Fig. 17-37). The abnormally thick mucus production leads to a chronic, diffuse obstructive pulmonary disease in almost all clients (Weilitz and Sciver, 1996).

Clinical findings consistent with CF include cough and congestion with thick mucous secretions, tachypnea, retractions, decreased chest movement, dyspnea, and barrel chest. Moist breath sounds with crackles and wheezes are noted with auscultation; breath sounds may be unequal or decreased. Decreased fremitus is noted with palpation; tympanic percussion tones are noted over consolidation or areas of atelectasis.

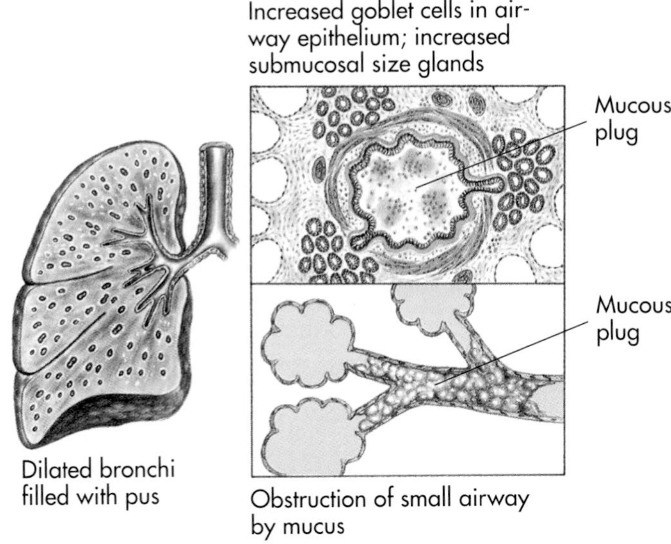

Fig. 17-37 Cystic fibrosis.

ACUTE OR TRAUMATIC CONDITIONS

Pneumothorax

When air enters the pleural space, pneumothorax results. Three types of pneumothorax exist: (1) closed, which may be spontaneous, traumatic, or iatrogenic; (2) open, which occurs following penetration of the chest by either injury or surgical procedure; and (3) tension, which develops when air leaks into the pleura and cannot escape (Fig. 17-38). While all types cause respiratory compromise, the tension pneumothorax is life-threatening and requires immediate intervention.

The clinical signs vary depending on the amount of lung collapse. If there is very minor collapse, the client may be slightly short of breath, anxious, and have chest pain. If there is a large amount of lung collapse, the client will be in severe respiratory distress, including dyspnea, tachypnea, and cyanosis. Distant and hyperresonant breath sounds over the affected area are noted to auscultation. Decreased chest wall movement on the affected side may be noted; the client may also have paradoxical chest wall movement. If severe, there may be tracheal displacement toward the unaffected side with a mediastinal shift. A "booming" quality percussion tone over the affected area may be noted.

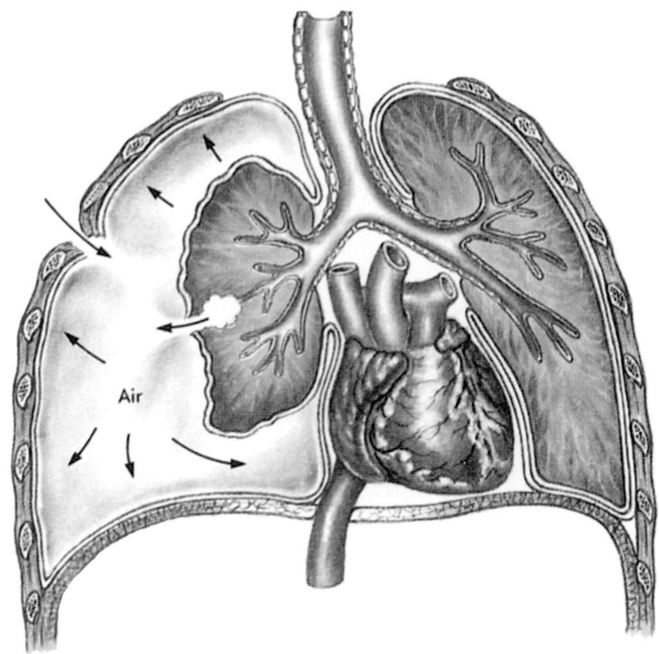

Fig. 17-38 Tension pneumothorax.

Hemothorax

A hemothorax is caused by the presence of blood in the pleural space (Fig. 17-39). It occurs most frequently following either blunt or penetrating injury to the chest wall but may also be a complication after thoracic surgery. Clinical findings are similar to those described in pneumothorax, although it is common to note distant muffled breath sounds and dullness with percussion over affected area.

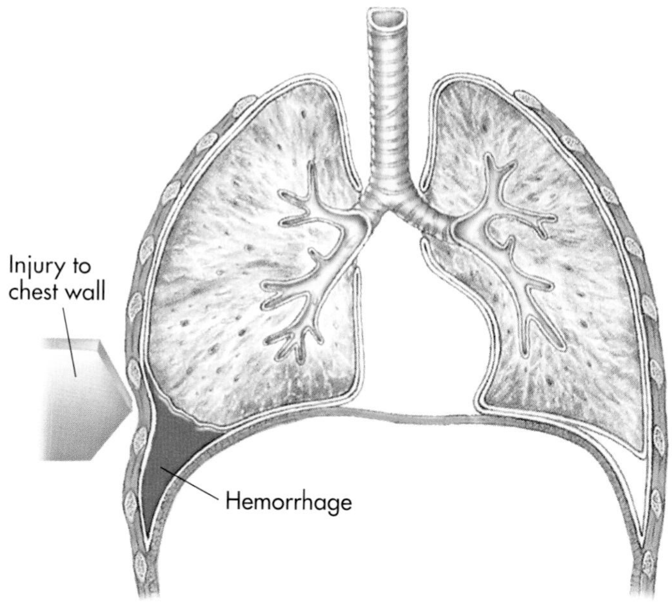

Fig. 17-39 Hemothorax.

OTHER PULMONARY CONDITIONS

Atelectasis

Atelectasis refers to an airless state of alveoli (Fig. 17-40). Alveoli may become airless due to an accumulation of secretions. This may be the collapse of a previously expanded lung or an acquired condition secondary to a disease process or immobility. Clients who develop atelectasis frequently have a cough, tachypnea, tachycardia, decreased chest wall movement on the affected side, and possible tracheal deviation if a large portion of the lung is involved.

The affected lung lobe will have diminished or absent breath sounds; areas above the affected area may have increased volume and clarity with egophony and whispered pectoriloquy. The examiner may note diminished fremitus to palpation and dull percussion tones over the affected area.

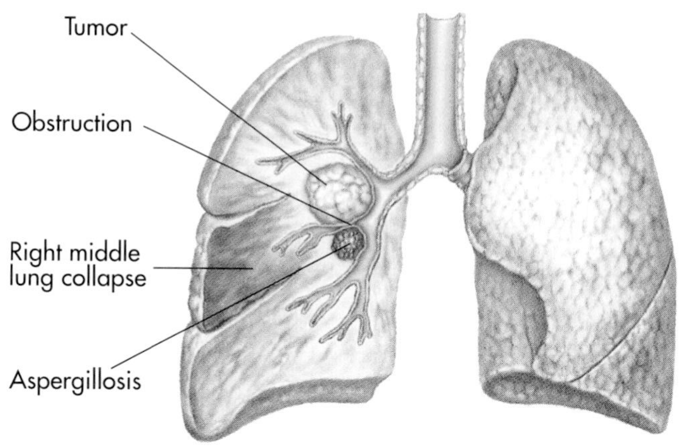

Fig. 17-40 Atelectasis.

Lung Cancer

Lung cancer is caused by an uncontrolled growth of anaplastic cells in the lung (Fig. 17-41). Etiologic factors include such agents as tobacco smoke, asbestos, ionizing radiation, and other noxious inhalants. Cancer develops when the genes responsible for sequential cell division, called proto-oncogenes, change to cells called oncogenes. Adenocarcinoma appears to be increasing in frequency and is probably the most common type, accounting for 40% of all cases. Adenocarcinoma arises in peripheral lung tissue or in areas scarred from pulmonary infarction, infection, or idiopathic fibrosis. Squamous cell carcinoma accounts for about 30% of all lung cancers.

Depending on stage, client may appear healthy, or client may have weight loss, cough, congestion, wheezing, hemoptysis, labored breathing, or dyspnea. Lung sounds may be normal or diminished over the affected area; if there is a partial obstruction of airways from the tumor, wheezes may be heard. Percussion tones may be normal or may be dull over the tumor, particularly if the cancer is large or the client has associated atelectasis.

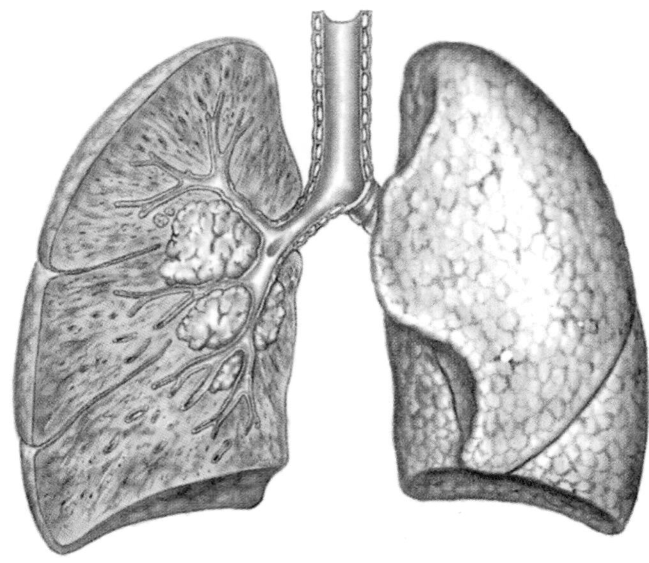

Fig. 17-41 Lung cancer.

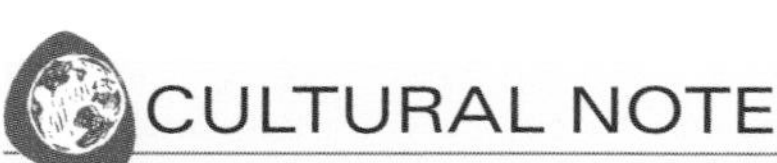

African Americans have the highest incidence rates of cancer and are at greater risk of dying from cancer than any other racial or cultural group. Among men, African Americans have the highest incidence of lung cancer (Landis et al, 1999).

CLINICAL APPLICATION and CRITICAL THINKING

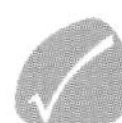

Sample Documentation

CASE 1

K.B., a 9-year-old boy comes to the emergency department with a 2-hour history of wheezing.

Subjective Data

Child states he has asthma. Mother indicates he woke this morning with a "cold" and coughing with mucus production. Earlier today was playing soccer until he couldn't breathe; then got scared. Mother present; appears frightened and frustrated. Reports history of asthma since 5 years old. Medications: albuterol and cromolyn sodium by nebulizer BID; uses Proventil inhaler PRN. Usually responds well to Proventil inhaler. Had two puffs just before coming to clinic, approximately 30 minutes ago—no noted relief. No previous hospitalizations for asthma. States no other health problems.

Objective Data

9-year-old boy appears anxious, sitting in tripod position, leaning forward, attempting to breathe with mouth open; coughing up mucus.

Vital signs: Pulse, 132 beats/min; Respiratory rate, 48; Oxygen saturation on room air, 91%; Temperature, 100.3° F (37.9° C).

Inspection: Chest wall smooth and normal configuration; no retractions or bulges noted.

Palpation: Deferred because of client's anxious state.

Percussion: Deferred because of client's anxious state.

Auscultation: Noted expiratory wheezes bilaterally; prolonged expiration; diminished breath sounds throughout.

Functional Health Patterns Involved

- Health perception–health management
- Activity–exercise
- Self-perception–self-concept

Medical Diagnosis

Asthma

Nursing Diagnosis and Collaborative Problems

- *Ineffective airway clearance* related to increased mucus production and bronchospasm as manifested by:
  - Difficulty breathing.
  - Coughing mucus.
  - Expiratory wheezes.
  - Diminished breath sounds.
  - Inhaler reported as "ineffective".
- *Anxiety* related to difficulty breathing as manifested by:
  Client and mother report feeling scared.
  Client and mother appear anxious.
- *Risk for ineffective management of therapeutic regimen* related to lack of knowledge of symptoms that could trigger episode.
- *PC*: Hypoxemia.

CASE 2

M.V. is a 61-year-old white woman with weight loss and a dry, hacking cough.

Subjective Data

States "dry hacking cough" for the past 3 months, won't go away. Reports decreased appetite and 12-pound weight loss during same period; denies other symptoms or other problems. Reports 41-year history of cigarette smoking. Amount has decreased during past 6 months from 1½ packs of nonfiltered cigarettes to ½ pack per day. Reports that cough is worse in the morning when she awakens. On two unrelated occasions during the past week she has coughed up "small amount of bright red blood." Reports dyspnea on exertion especially when going up and down stairs. Toward end of interview client started crying and stated fear of having cancer. Current medications: Coumadin 2.5 mg PO qd.

Objective Data

Height, 5′3″ (160 cm); Weight, 104 lb (47.2 kg); Temperature, 98.6° F (37.0° C); Pulse, 96 beats/min; Respiratory rate, 22.

Inspection: Small-framed, pale, and very thin appearing white woman sitting erect on examination table; no noted respiratory distress; multiple areas of ecchymosis noted all over body—client states she "bruises easily"; AP chest diameter without noted enlargement; slight kyphosis noted; thoracic expansion symmetric; respirations even and without noted distress.

Palpation: No friction rubs or rib tenderness noted; tactile fremitus increased over most of posterior left lung.

Percussion: Resonance over right lung fields; dullness over most of left lung.

Auscultation: Breath sounds present bilaterally; (R) vesicular breath sounds heard throughout; without adventitious sounds; (L) combination of bronchovesicular and vesicular breath sounds heard; slightly diminished breath sounds on (L) when compared to (R); egophony and whispered pectoriloquy present on (L).

Functional Health Patterns Involved

- Health perception–health maintenance
- Nutritional–metabolic
- Activity–exercise
- Self-perception–self-concept

Medical Diagnosis

Left lung mass, rule out malignancy

Nursing Diagnosis and Collaborative Problems

- *Impaired gas exchange* related to left lung consolidation as manifested by:
  - Dyspnea on exertion
  - Smoking history
  - Left lung dull to percussion
  - Diminished breath sounds on left
  - Egophony and whispered pectoriloquy on left.
- *Activity intolerance* related to inadequate oxygenation for activity as manifested by:
  - Dyspnea on exertion
- *Altered nutrition: less than body requirements* related to decreased appetite, decreased food intake, and possible increase in metabolic demands as manifested by:
  - Weight loss of 12 pounds in 3 months
  - Reports decreased appetite and food intake
- *Fear* related to possible lung malignancy as manifested by:
  Statement of fear of cancer
  - Crying
- *Altered health maintenance* related to unhealthy lifestyle as manifested by 41-year history of smoking
- *PC*: Hypoxemia related to consolidation of lung
- *PC*: Anticoagulant therapy adverse effects

CRITICAL THINKING QUESTIONS

1. Mrs. Cantrell has brought her 14-month-old daughter to the clinic. She tells the nurse that she has had a fever and cough. The child cries when her mother sets her down on the examination table. What could you do to gain cooperation from the child as you auscultate her lungs?
2. Mrs. Chaves tells you all three of her young children have had problems with coughing and some trouble breathing ever since they moved into a new apartment 2 months ago. She also tells you they have not had fevers with these symptoms. What type of interview questions should be asked to further explore these symptoms?
3. Mr. Stein is a 78-year-old man with mild emphysema. You are preparing to teach him how to

reduce his risk for respiratory infection. What specific guidelines could you share with him?

4. Mr. Pena is a 42-year-old migrant worker from Mexico who comes to the clinic where you work. Through an interpreter, you learn he has had a fever with night sweats, fatigue, frequent coughing with reddish sputum, and weight loss. What significance do these symptoms have?
5. Mr. Louis Jackson is a 73-year-old man who is seen in the clinic for a routine examination. During the interview, Mr. Jackson tells the interviewer that he smokes. When questioned further, he indicates he has been smoking "roughly 60 years." He states, "I started smoking cigarettes when I was about 14 years old. Until I was about 25, I smoked a pack—maybe every 3 days or so. Then I started smoking about ½ pack a day until the age of 40. Since that time, I've smoked about a pack a day." Mr. Jackson adds, "I knew I should quit, but I never really wanted to very much. I decided that when I got up to a pack a day, I would never smoke more than that."
   a. Based on the information given, calculate Mr. Jackson's pack-year history.

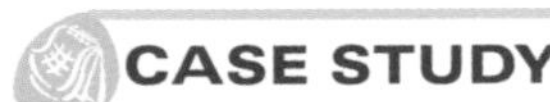

CASE STUDY

Sharon Martin is a 66-year-old woman complaining of shortness of breath. Listed below are the initial data collected.

Interview Data

Sharon says she's had breathing problems "for years" but is getting worse. She tells the examiner that she gets short of breath with activity, adding that she can do things around the house only for a few minutes before she has to sit down to rest and catch her breath. She says she can sleep only a couple hours at a time. She sleeps best with two pillows at night, but on some nights she just sits in a chair. Sharon does not currently use oxygen, but she thinks oxygen would help. She admits to smoking 1 ½ packs of cigarettes a day. She has never quit because she says she just can't do it.

Examination Data

- **General survey**: Alert and slightly anxious female, sitting slightly forward, with moderately labored breathing. Skin is pale with slight cyanosis around the lips and in nail beds. Appears extremely thin.
- **Chest wall configuration**: Chest is round shaped and symmetrical with increased AP diameter and costal angle greater than 90°. Small muscle mass noted over chest: ribs protrude.
- **Breathing effort**: Respiratory rate 24 and labored.
- **Chest assessment**: Chest wall expansion with respirations is reduced but symmetrical. Chest wall tactile fremitus diminished. Sibilant wheeze are auscultated throughout lung field. Lung sounds are diminished in lung bases bilaterally.
- **Vocal sound auscultation**: Muffled tones auscultated.

1. What data deviate from normal findings, suggesting a need for further investigation?
2. What additional information should the nurse ask or assess for?
3. In what functional health patterns does data deviate from normal?
4. What nursing diagnosis and/or collaborative problems should be considered for this situation?

REMEMBER to check out your **companion CD-ROM**

18 Heart and Peripheral Vascular System

www.mosby.com/MERLIN/wilson/assessment/

ANATOMY AND PHYSIOLOGY

The cardiovascular system transports oxygen, nutrients, and other substances to all the body's tissues and carries metabolic waste products to the kidneys and lungs. The heart and blood vessels provide this transportation. The heart is about the size of a fist and beats 60 to 100 times a minute without rest, responding to both external and internal demands such as exercise, temperature changes, and stress. Many of these stimuli are communicated to the cardiovascular system through the endocrine and nervous systems. In turn, the cardiovascular system adjusts to these stimuli by constricting or dilating blood vessels, altering the cardiac output, and redistributing blood flow.

THE HEART AND GREAT VESSELS

The heart is a pump divided into right and left sides. Each side of the heart has two chambers, an atrium and a ventricle. The right side receives blood from the superior and inferior venae cavae and pumps it through the pulmonary arteries to the pulmonary circulation; the left side receives blood from the pulmonary veins and pumps it through the aorta into the systemic circulation.

The upper part of the heart is the base, and the lower left ventricle is called the apex. The heart lies behind the sternum and above the diaphragm in the mediastinum at an angle so that the right ventricle makes up most of the anterior surface and the left ventricle lies to the left and posteriorly. The right atrium forms the right border of the heart, and the left atrium lies posteriorly. The aorta curves upward out of the left ventricle and bends posteriorly and downward just above the sternal angle. The pulmonary arteries emerge from the superior aspect of the right ventricle near the third intercostal space (Fig. 18-1).

PERICARDIUM AND CARDIAC MUSCLE

The heart wall has three layers: pericardium, myocardium, and endocardium (Fig. 18-2). The heart is encased in the pericardium, a double-walled fibrous sac of elastic connective tissue that shields the heart from trauma and infection. The outer wall, the parietal pericardium, is fibrous pericardium. The inner wall, the visceral pericardium, is also called the epicardium. It covers the heart surface and extends to the great vessels. A small amount of pericardial fluid between the visceral and parietal pericardium reduces friction as the heart beats. The middle layer, or myocardium, is thick muscular tissue that controls the pumping action. The endocardium lines the inner chambers and valves (McCance and Huether, 1998).

BLOOD FLOW THROUGH THE HEART: THE CARDIAC CYCLE

Four valves govern blood flow through the four chambers of the heart. The tricuspid valve on the right and mitral valve on the left are called the atrioventricular (AV) valves because they separate the atria from the ventricles. The aortic valve emerges from the left ventricle into the aorta, and the pulmonic valve opens from the right ventricle into the pulmonary artery (Fig. 18-3). The aortic and pulmonic valves are called semilunar valves because of their half-moon shape.

Diastole

Blood flows into the atria from the systemic and pulmonic circulation and creates positive pressure. When the pressure in the atria is higher than the pressure in the ventricles, the AV valves passively open, and the ventricles fill with blood. About 80% of the blood from the atria flows into relaxed ventricles. Then a contraction of the atria forces the remaining 20% of the blood into the ventricles. This added atrial thrust is referred to as the "atrial kick." This phase in the cardiac cycle when the ventricles are relaxed and filling with blood is called diastole.

Systole

When the pressure of blood in the ventricles becomes higher than the pressure in the atria, the AV valves close, preventing the backflow or regurgitation of blood into the atria. When the pressure in the ventricles exceeds the pressure in the great vessels, the semilunar valves open, and blood flows into the pulmonary artery and aorta (Fig. 18-4). The ejection of blood out of the ventricles lowers the pressure in the ventricles, causing the semilunar valves to close. This phase in the cardiac cycle when the ventricles are contracting is called systole.

ELECTRIC CONDUCTION

The heart is stimulated by an electric impulse that originates in the sinoatrial (SA) node in the superior aspect of

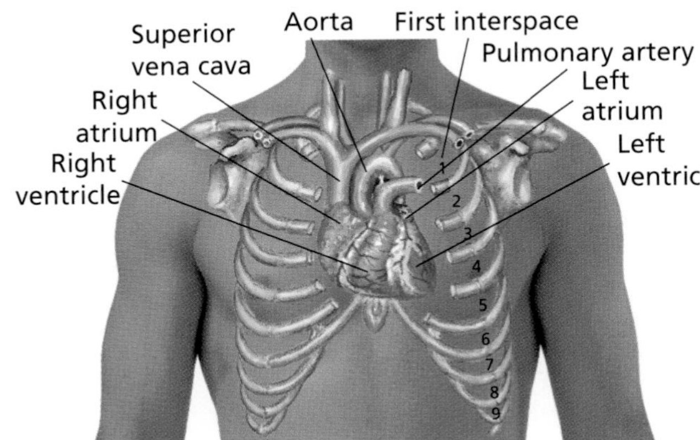

Fig. 18-1 Position of the heart chambers and great vessels. Intercostal spaces 1 to 9 are numbered.

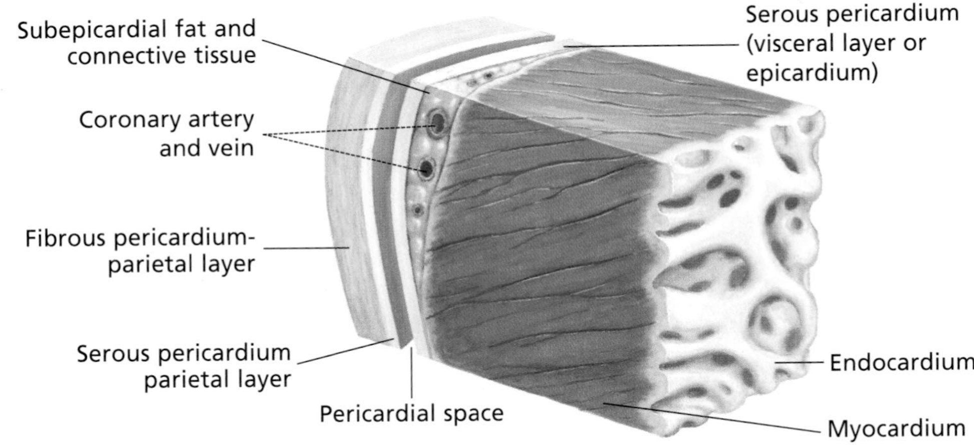

Fig. 18-2 Cross section of cardiac muscle. (From Canobbio, 1990.)

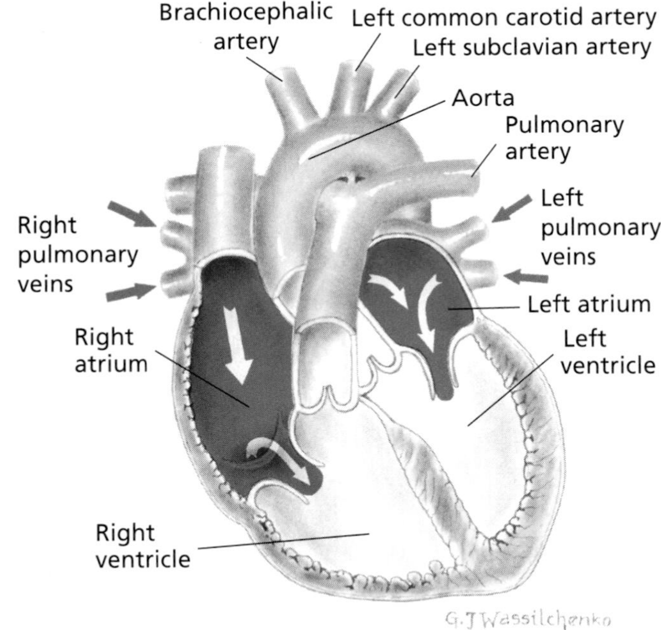

Fig. 18-3 Blood flow during diastole. (From Canobbio, 1990.)

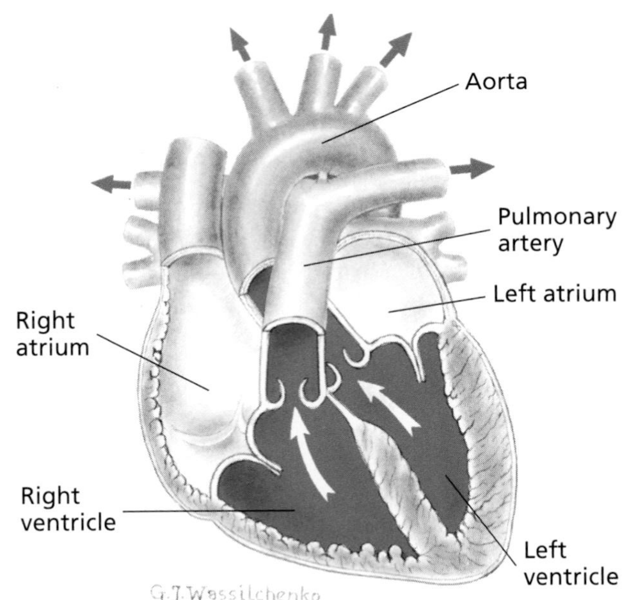

Fig. 18-4 Blood flow during systole. (From Canobbio, 1990.)

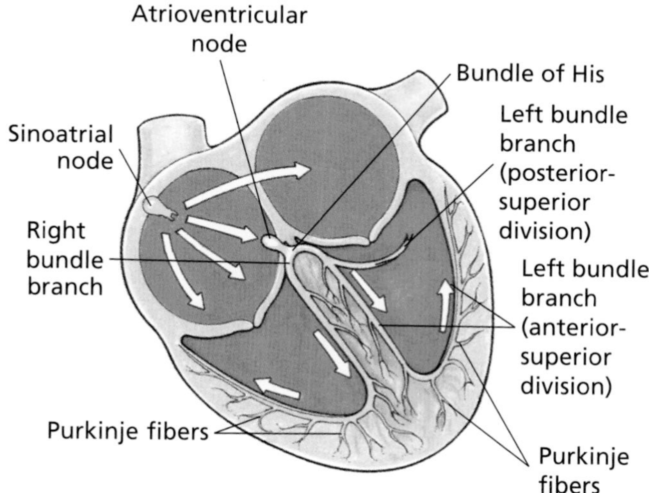

Fig. 18-5 Cardiac conduction. (From Canobbio, 1990.)

the right atrium. The node, called the cardiac pacemaker, discharges about 60 to 100 impulses per minute. The electric impulse stimulates contraction of both atria and then flows to the AV node in the inferior aspect of the right atrium. The impulses are then transmitted through a series of branches (bundle of His) and Purkinje fibers in the myocardium, which results in ventricular contraction (Fig. 18-5). The AV node prevents excessive atrial impulses from reaching the ventricles. If the SA node fails, the remaining electrical system can generate ventricular contraction at a slower rate, 40 to 60 impulses per minute. If both SA and AV nodes are ineffective, the bundle branches may take over contraction, but at a very slow rate of 20 to 40 impulses per minute.

BLOOD CIRCULATION

The circulatory system is composed of arteries, capillaries, and veins. The tough and tensile arteries and their smaller branches, the arterioles, are subjected to remarkable pressures (Fig. 18-6, *A*). They maintain blood pressure by constricting or dilating in response to stimuli from parasympathetic and sympathetic nervous system, aldosterone, and body temperature. The more passive veins (Fig. 18-6, *B*) and their smaller branches, the venules, are less sturdy but more expansible, enabling them to act as a reservoir for extra blood, if needed, to decrease the workload on the heart. Pressure within the veins is low, compared with arterial circulation. The valves in each vein keep blood flowing in a forward direction toward the heart.

Blood leaving the heart in the aorta is oxygen-rich. It flows from the aorta to arteries to arterioles and into capillaries. Capillaries deliver oxygen and nutrients to cells and collect waste products. The capillary blood flows into the venules, through the veins, and delivers the deoxygenated blood to the right side of the heart. The blood is then pumped into the pulmonary circulation, where the carbon dioxide diffuses across the alveolocapillary membranes to be exhaled. Oxygen diffuses in the opposite direction, from alveoli into pulmonary capillaries. Other waste products are eliminated as the blood flows through the glomeruli of the kidneys.

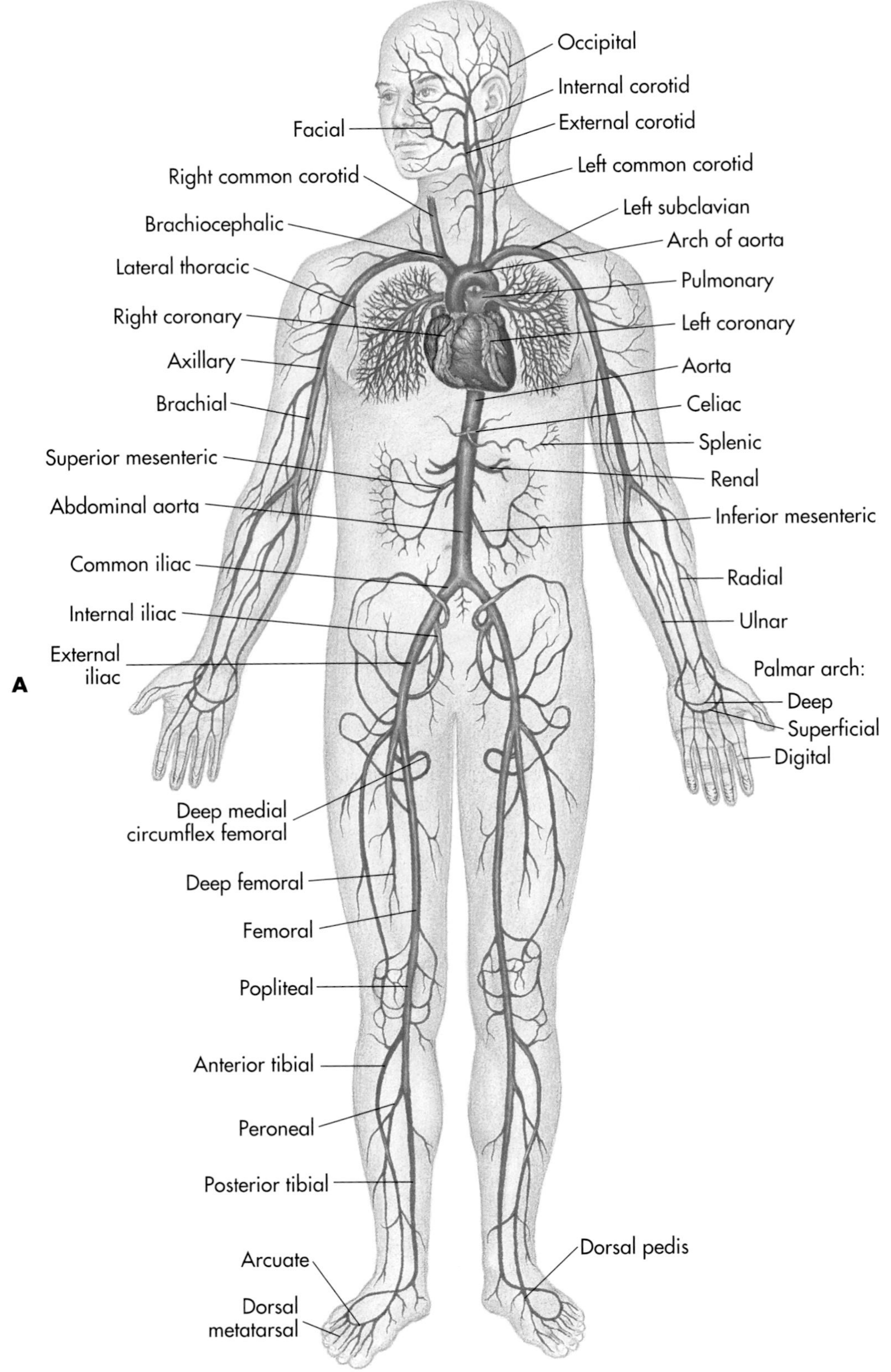

Fig. 18-6 **A,** Arteries. (From Seidel et al, 1999.)

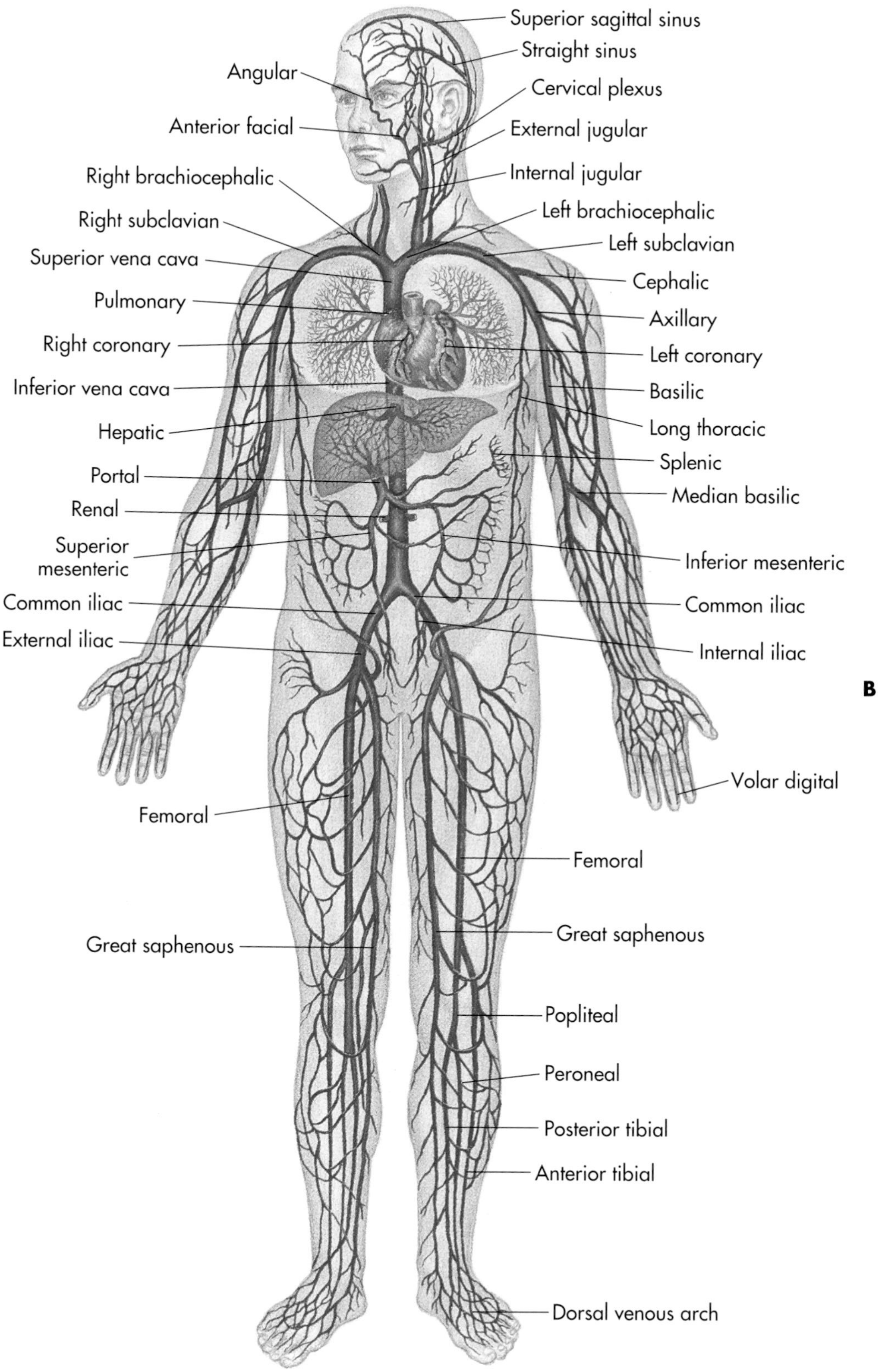

Fig. 18-6, cont'd B, Veins.

HEALTH HISTORY

Heart and Peripheral Vascular System

QUESTIONS | **RATIONALE**

PRESENT HEALTH STATUS

➤ How healthy are your heart and blood vessels?

■ The client's perception of his or her cardiovascular health is helpful in order to understand what the client considers a problem and to understand what is important to him or her.

➤ Do you have any chronic illnesses, such as diabetes mellitus, renal failure, chronic hypoxia, or hypertension? If yes, describe.

■ Chronic illnesses can cause symptoms affecting the cardiovascular system when they increase the workload of the heart by narrowing the vessels (diabetes, hypertension), increase the fluid volume to be pumped (renal failure), or increase the heart rate (hypoxia).

➤ Are you taking any medications? If yes, what are you taking, and when did you start taking the medications? Have you had any side effects from these medications? Do you take them as prescribed?

■ Medications may be to taken treat a cardiovascular problem or may cause side effects affecting the cardiovascular system. For example, tricyclic antidepressants, phenothiazines, or lithium can cause dysrhythmias; hormonal contraceptives can cause thrombophlebitis; corticosteroids can cause sodium and fluid retention; and theophylline and recreational drugs can cause tachycardia and dysrhythmias.

➤ What over-the-counter drugs do you take? Do you take an aspirin on a regular basis to help thin your blood? Do you use cocaine? Other street drugs? How often do you use these drugs?

■ These nonprescription drugs may affect the cardiovascular system. For example, aspirin prevents platelet aggregation to reduce clot formation. Decongestants containing pseudoephedrine may aggravate hypertension. Cocaine use has been associated with myocardial infarction and stroke.

➤ Do you exercise? If yes, what kind of exercise? How often do you exercise? How much time do you spend exercising?

■ Physical activity for at least 30 minutes 5 times weekly increases energy and improves self-esteem, as well as preventing coronary artery disease, hypertension, and obesity.

➤ If no, have you ever exercised? If yes, what exercises have you tried in the past? What motivated you to start in the past? What influenced you to stop your exercising?

■ Clients who no longer exercise must be encouraged to resume an exercise program. Exploring reasons for stopping can begin the problem-solving process to determine what can motivate them to start again.

QUESTIONS	RATIONALE
➤ How would you describe your personality type? Are you intense? Often angry? How do you deal with stress?	■ Stress and persistent intensity are risk factors for heart disease. (Observe the client as he or she responds, and throughout the examination, to detect stress or intensity.)
➤ Do you work in an area where there are factors that may affect your heart or blood vessels? For example, are there extensive physical demands? Emotional stress?	■ Physical exertion may increase the workload on the heart if the client has a history of cardiovascular disease. ■ Stress is a risk factor for heart disease. In a psychologically stressful environment, the client should be encouraged to use several strategies to relieve stress and to change his or her perception of the situations so that they are perceived as less stressful.
➤ How often do you take time to relax? What do you do to relax? Hobbies? Sports? Meditation? Yoga? Music?	■ Ask about ways to relax so that you can suggest ways the client may use on a regular basis. Physical relaxation can reduce blood pressure.
➤ Describe your usual eating habits. How often do you eat red meat? How much red meat do you eat at a meal? Do you monitor your fat and salt intake? Do you eat whole grains each day?	■ Selecting foods consistent with the food pyramid provides balanced nutrition. Calories from fat should be limited to 20% of daily calories with 10% limited to saturated fat. Frequent consumption of large servings of red meat is associated with high cholesterol. A serving of red meat is 4 oz and should be limited to 3 times weekly. Whole grains (e.g., cereals) have been found to reduce heart disease.
➤ Do you drink alcoholic beverages? What type of alcohol do you drink? How much? How often?	■ Excessive alcohol intake has been associated with hypertension. Research suggests that moderate consumption of alcohol may increase high-density lipoproteins (HDL) and prevent blood clot formation (Gaziano et al, 1993; Ridker et al, 1994). Moderate alcohol intake is defined as two drinks per day for men and one drink per day for women and those over 65 years of age. One drink is defined as 12 oz of beer, 5 oz of wine, or 1.5 oz of 80-proof distilled spirits (Camargo et al, 1997).
➤ Do you consume caffeine? In coffee? Chocolate? How much caffeine do you consume? How often?	■ Excessive caffeine intake can cause tachycardia, which can increase the workload of the heart.

QUESTIONS

➤ Do you smoke or have you been a smoker in the past? If yes, what forms of tobacco do (did) you use? (cigarettes, cigars, pipe, marijuana, smokeless or chewing tobacco) How long have you used (did you use) tobacco? How often do you use tobacco? Have you ever quit smoking? If yes, how did you accomplish it and for what length of time? Are you interested in quitting smoking? Do you know how smoking affects the cardiovascular system?

RATIONALE

■ Nicotine in tobacco causes vasoconstriction, which may decrease blood flow to extremities and increase blood pressure, both of which increase the workload on the heart.

■ Clients who previously have successfully stopped their tobacco use may be more easily convinced to repeat their success. Clients must be interested in stopping tobacco use; otherwise, there is little motivation to change behavior. Perhaps educating them about the negative effects of nicotine on the cardiovascular system will provide some motivation.

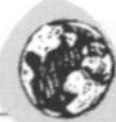

ETHNIC & CULTURAL VARIATIONS

White men are heavier smokers than other ethnic groups, but more African-American and Hispanic men smoke than whites. Black men often have increased high-density lipoproteins (HDLs) than other groups. Mexican Americans and Puerto Ricans have higher cholesterol levels than whites.

PAST MEDICAL HISTORY

➤ As a child did you have congenital heart disease or heart defect?

■ Data from past medical history gives information about clinical findings to anticipate.

➤ During childhood did you have "growing pains," unexplained joint pains? Recurrent tonsillitis? Rheumatic fever? Heart murmur?

■ These questions relate to diagnosis of rheumatic fever caused by autoimmune reaction to group A beta-hemolytic streptococcal pharyngitis that may have contributed to rheumatoid arthritis or rheumatic heart disease.

➤ Have you been told that you have high levels of cholesterol or elevated triglycerides?

■ Hyperlipidemia is a risk factor for coronary artery disease since the fat lines the arteries, which decreases the blood flow to tissues and increases workload on the heart.

➤ Have you ever had coronary artery disease? How was it treated? What lifestyle changes did you make after your recovery?

■ Having coronary heart disease increases the risk for a myocardial infarction. If the client has made changes in his or her life (e.g., exercising, stopping smoking, losing weight), then the risk is not as great.

➤ Have you ever had surgery on your heart? On your blood vessels? If so, what procedure was done? When was it done? How successful was the surgery?

■ Knowledge of past surgical procedures may provide additional information about a possible cardiovascular problem. These data also explain the presence of scars you will observe on examination.

➤ Have you ever had any tests on your heart? Electrocardiogram (ECG), stress ECG, or other heart test? When were the tests? What did the tests reveal? What, if any, treatment did you receive?

■ These tests provide objective measures that provide baseline data on the health of the client's cardiovascular system.

FAMILY HISTORY

➤ In your family, is there a history of diabetes, heart disease, hyperlipidemia, hypertension, or sudden death syndrome, especially among young and middle-aged relatives?

■ These conditions are risk factors for heart disease and have familial tendencies.

QUESTIONS

RATIONALE

RISK FACTORS

COMMON RISK FACTORS ASSOCIATED WITH Cardiovascular Disease

NONMODIFIABLE RISK FACTORS

Gender: Men develop more coronary heart disease and at an earlier age than women; postmenopausal women have a risk equal to men because they lose the protective effect of estrogen
Family history of cardiovascular disease, diabetes, hyperlipidemia, and hypertension
Ethnicity: Black Americans have a higher incidence of hypertension
Increasing age: Due to increase in peripheral vascular resistance

MODIFIABLE RISK FACTORS

Hypertension: Systolic pressure >140 mm Hg; diastolic pressure >90 mm Hg
Smoking
Elevated serum cholesterol level (>200 mg/dl) and lowered high-density lipoprotein (HDL) (<35 mg/dl); elevated low-density lipoproteins (>130 mg/dl); total cholesterol-to-HDL ratio >7.5
Diabetes mellitus
Physical inactivity
Long-term use of oral contraceptives
Environmental stress

PROBLEM-BASED HISTORY

The focus of the history includes descriptions of chest pain, shortness of breath, nocturia, cough, fatigue, syncope, dependent edema, and leg pain. As with symptoms in all areas of health assessment, a symptom analysis is completed that includes the location, quality, quantity, chronology, setting, associated manifestations, and alleviating and aggravating factors. (See Box 4-2 in Chapter 4.)

Chest Pain

➤ Are you having chest pain? If yes, where are you feeling the pain? Does the pain radiate to any location? How severe is the pain on a scale of 1 to 10? What does the pain feel like? Is it crushing? Stabbing? Burning? Viselike? (Note: Allow the client to describe the pain in his or her own words before suggesting any of these descriptors.) (Table 18-1)

■ Angina is an important symptom of coronary artery disease. It indicates that the heart cannot supply the body's demand for oxygen. Pain frequently is felt behind the sternum and may radiate down the left or both arms, toward the neck or jaws, and toward the scapula area. The origin of chest pain may be cardiac, pulmonary, musculoskeletal, or gastrointestinal. If the client uses a clenched fist placed on the sternum (Levine's sign) to describe the pain, angina is extremely likely.

➤ When did the pain start? Is the pain intermittent or constant? If intermittent, how long does it last?

■ These questions help distinguish angina from other causes of chest pain.

➤ What symptoms have you noticed along with the pain? Sweating? Turning pale or gray? Heart skipping beats or racing? Shortness of breath? Nausea or vomiting? Dizziness? Anxiety?

■ These associated symptoms frequently accompany a myocardial infarction (O'Hanlon-Nichols, 1997).

Table 18-1 Differentiation of Chest Pain

CAUSE	LOCATION	QUALITY OF PAIN	QUANTITY OF PAIN	CHRONOLOGY	ASSOCIATED MANIFESTATIONS	AGGRAVATING FACTORS	ALLEVIATING FACTORS
Stable angina	Precordial or retrosternal, radiates to L > R arm, jaw, interscapular or epigastrium not above C3 or below T10	Pressure, burning, dull, or sharp	Variable, usually worse with activity	>1 min or < 1 hr	Dyspnea, diaphoresis, palpitations, nausea, weakness	Physical exertion, emotional stress, cold	Rest, nitroglycerin, beta-blocker, calcium channel blocker
Unstable angina/ myocardial infarction	Precordial or retrosternal, radiates to L > R arm, jaw, interscapular or epigastrium not above C3 or below T10	Pressure, squeezing, crushing; burning, dull, or sharp	10 of 10 on pain scale	Sudden onset or progressing <30-40 min for unstable angina, >1 hr to 2-3 days MI	Dyspnea, diaphoresis, palpitations, nausea, weakness	Chest pain during exercise or at rest	Beta-blocker, aspirin, heparin, oxygen
Cocaine-induced chest pain	Similar to myocardial infarction	Sharp, pressure-like, squeezing	Severe 8 to 10 of 10 on pain scale	Gradual onset over minutes lasting minutes to hours	Tachycardia, tachypnea, hypertension	During and shortly after cocaine use	Nitroglycerin or calcium channel blockers
Mitral valve prolapse	Anywhere in chest, localized or diffuse; does not radiate	Variable, often sharp or "kick"	Variable within same client	Sudden, current onset. Lasts seconds or persists for days	Often asymptomatic; palpitations when lying on left side, dyspnea, dizziness	Usually nonexertional, occasionally positional	Position change, nitroglycerin, analgesics
Acute pericarditis	Precordial, posterior neck, trapezius muscle	Boring, oppressive, pleuretic, or positional	Moderate, 4 to 6 of 10 on pain scale	Onset hours to days, lasts hours to weeks	Fever, dyspnea, orthopnea, friction rub	Reclining	Leaning forward
Panic disorder	Localized retrosternally, abdomen	Tightness, vague, diffuse; unrelated to exertion	May be described as disabling	Lasts 30 min or more	Hyperventilation, fatigue, anorexia, emotional strain	Emotional strain	Variable by client
Peptic ulcer disease	Epigastric radiating to lower bilateral chest (T6 to T10)	Burning, gnawing	Moderate, 4 to 6 of 10 on pain scale	Gradual, recurrent onset, lasts hours	Nausea, abdominal tenderness	Empty stomach	Food, antacids, histamine$_2$ (H_2) blocker
Esophageal reflux	Midepigastric to xiphoid area ,C7 to T12, radiates to neck, ear, or jaw	Burning, pressure-like, sqeezing	Moderate to severe	Spontaneous onset, lasts min to days	Dysphagia	Spicy or acidic meal, alcohol, lying supine	Oral fluids, belching, antacids, nitroglycerin, H_2 blocker
Costo-chronditis (inflammation of rib or cartilage)	2nd to 4th costochondral junction, xiphoid, radiates to precordium, arms, shoulders	Variable	Variable	Gradual onset, constant pain lasts for days	None	Coughing, deep breathing, laughing, sneezing	Localized heat, analgesics, anti-inflammatories

Adapted with permission from B Hill and SA Geraci, MD: A diagnostic approach to chest pain based on history and ancillary evaluation, *The Nurse Practitioner* 23(4):20-45, © Springhouse Corporation/www.springnet.com.

QUESTIONS | **RATIONALE**

➤ What factors seem to precede the pain? Exercise? Rest? Highly emotional situations? Eating? Sexual intercourse? Cold?

■ Chest pain that begins during exertion such as exercise and then diminishes after exertion is stopped may be caused by myocardial ischemia. Factors in the other questions can occur prior to a myocardial infarction.

➤ What makes it worse? Moving the arms or neck? Deep breathing? Lying flat? Exercise?

■ The chest pain from pericarditis is aggravated by deep breathing, coughing, or lying supine.

➤ What relieves the pain? Rest? Nitroglycerin? How many nitroglycerin tablets does it take to relieve chest pain?

■ These questions assess for alleviating factors. Chest pain that is relieved by nitroglycerin may be caused by myocardial ischemia, whereas chest pain that is not relieved by 4 or more nitroglycerin tablets taken 5 minutes apart may be caused by myocardial infarction.

Shortness of Breath (Dyspnea, Orthopnea)

➤ Do you have episodes of shortness of breath or times when it is hard to breathe? If yes, how long has this been going on?

■ Dyspnea may be caused by a respiratory or cardiac problem. A gradual onset may be caused by heart failure that develops slowly from backup of fluid from the heart into the alveoli.

➤ When does the shortness of breath happen? How often does it occur? How long does it last?

■ These questions determine the frequency and duration of dyspnea.

➤ Does the shortness of breath interfere with your daily activities? How many level blocks can you walk before you become short of breath? How many blocks could you walk 6 months ago?

■ Dyspnea that interferes with activities of daily living (ADL) may require the client to use supplemental oxygen. If the ability to walk is shortened, it is a sign the dyspnea is getting worse. As the client is talking, note how many words he or she can say without taking a breath. Normally a person can say 8 to 12 words before the next breath. As dyspnea becomes worse, the client is able to say fewer words in between breaths. If the client can say 3 words before taking a breath, this can be documented as "3-word dyspnea."

➤ Do you have any other symptoms with the shortness of breath such as cough? Is the cough productive? If yes, what color is the sputum? Clear? Frothy? White? Do your feet swell during the day when you are up?

■ White, frothy sputum may be a sign of pulmonary edema that occurs with left-sided heart failure. Dependent edema seen in the ankles and/or feet develops because of right-sided heart failure.

QUESTIONS	RATIONALE
➤ What makes the shortness of breath worse? Walking upstairs? Lying down? How many pillows do you require when you lie down to sleep? Do you sleep in a recliner?	■ Walking up stairs increases the workload of the heart. When dyspnea becomes worse upon lying down, the term orthopnea is used. Orthopnea occurs when a person must sit up or stand to breathe easily. The number of pillows that are necessary to relieve the orthopnea is documented (e.g., two-pillow orthopnea means the client must elevate his or her chest with two pillow to breathe easily). Some clients sleep in a recliner for elevation rather than using pillows.
➤ When these episodes of shortness of breath occur, what do you do to breathe more easily?	■ Determine the effectiveness of the action(s) to relieve dyspnea. This information may be helpful in planning future treatment strategies.
Nocturia	
➤ Have you been awakened at night with an urgent need to urinate? How long has this been happening? How many times a night do you get up to urinate?	■ Nocturia occurs with heart failure in persons who are ambulatory during the day. Lying down at night creates a fluid shift by gravity that promotes the reabsorption of fluid and its excretion.
➤ What have you done to prevent this from happening? How successful have your efforts been?	■ This information may guide future teaching and treatment strategies.
Cough	
➤ Do you have a cough? If yes, when did it start? How often do you cough? Do you cough up anything? What does it look like? Is there blood mixed with the mucus?	■ Coughing up blood (hemoptysis) is a symptom of mitral stenosis, as well as of pulmonary disorders. Coughing up frothy sputum may occur in heart failure.
➤ Is your cough associated with position (more coughing when lying down), with anxiety, or with talking or activity? What makes it worse? What actions do you take to relieve the cough?	■ Coughing more when lying down may indicate heart failure. Knowing how the client relieves the cough may help identify treatment strategies.
Fatigue	
➤ Have you noticed any unusual or persistent fatigue? Is the fatigue worse in the morning or evening? Is it worse at work or home? Do you have trouble keeping up with your friends? Are you too tired to take part in normal activities? Does rest reduce the fatigue? Do you go to bed earlier because you are too tired to stay awake?	■ When cardiac output is decreased, fatigue results. It is generally worse in the evening. Fatigue due to other causes, for example, psychogenic (depression or anxiety) occurs all day or is worse in the morning and varies by location. Fatigue from anemia lasts all day.
➤ When did you first notice the fatigue? Was the onset sudden or gradual?	■ This question determines chronology. Fatigue from anemia and heart disease occurs gradually, while fatigue from acute blood loss occurs more rapidly.
➤ Do you take vitamin or iron pills? Do you eat foods with iron, such as green leafy vegetables and liver? For women: Do you have a heavy menstrual flow?	■ These questions relate to iron deficiency anemia. Iron pills and nutrition can prevent or treat this anemia. Women may have iron deficiency from monthly blood loss.

QUESTIONS

RATIONALE

➤ Have you been short of breath? Are there any other symptoms associated with the fatigue, such as rapid heart rate, headache, pale skin, sore tongue or lips, or changes in your nails?

■ Fatigue and exertional dyspnea are manifestations of mild anemia. Additional signs of tachycardia, headache, pallor, brittle, spoon-shaped nails, glossitis (inflammation of the tongue), and cheilitis (inflammation of the lips) occur with moderate to severe anemia (Marantides and Lottman, 1999).

➤ Have you noticed any unusual feelings in your feet and hands, muscle weakness, or trouble thinking?

■ Neurologic symptoms in addition to those described above may indicate anemia from vitamin B_{12} deficiency.

Syncope

➤ What were you doing just before you fainted? Did you feel dizzy? Did you lose consciousness?

■ Syncope is a brief lapse of consciousness. When syncope occurs with activity or position changes and causes dizziness, it may be due to hypotension.

➤ Has this happened to you before? How often has this occurred?

■ These questions determine frequency of syncope.

➤ Was fainting preceded by any other symptoms? Nausea? Chest pain? Headache? Sweating? Rapid heart rate? Confusion? Numbness? Hunger? Ringing in your ears?

■ These questions attempt to determine whether the cause of fainting is a cardiovascular, neurologic, or ear problem. It may be due to small emboli in the cerebral circulation. Emboli may be the result of atrial fibrillation, valvular disease, or cardiac dysrhythmias. Cerebral emboli may cause a stroke resulting in reports of headache, confusion, and numbness. Ask about tinnitus to rule out Ménière's disease.

Dependent Leg Edema

➤ When did you first notice the swelling in your legs? Are both legs affected equally?

■ Localized edema of one leg may be caused by venous insufficiency from varicosities or thrombophlebitis. Edema of both legs may be caused by systemic disease (e.g., heart failure, renal failure, or liver disease).

➤ What makes the swelling go away? Does elevating your feet reduce the swelling? Does the swelling disappear after a night's sleep? Do you wear support stockings?

■ Edema that increases during day and decreases at night or with elevation may be related to venous stasis (e.g., heart failure). Support stockings may help relieve edema.

➤ Are there any associated symptoms that occur with the swelling? Shortness of breath? Swelling in your abdomen? Yellowing of your eyes? Weight gain?

■ Dyspnea may be due to heart failure or ascites caused by liver disease. Jaundice suggests liver disease. Weight gain occurs anytime there is fluid retention regardless of cause.

➤ Do you have pain in your legs? Do you have sores on your legs?

■ Edema of legs can cause pain on palpation. Venous insufficiency can produce ulcers.

QUESTIONS | **RATIONALE**

➤ For women: Are you taking hormonal contraceptives? Is the swelling associated with your menstrual period?

■ Hormonal contraceptives may be associated with thrombophlebitis, which may cause unilateral leg edema. Changes in estrogen and progesterone blood levels can contribute to fluid retention, resulting in dependent edema.

Leg Cramps or Pain

➤ Are you having leg cramps or leg pain? Do your legs feel heavier than usual? If yes, when did it start?

■ Determine the chronology of the pain. Arterial insufficiency produces pain that may make legs feel heavier.

➤ Describe the pain location. Calf? Feet? Thighs? Buttocks? How severe is the pain on a scale of 1 to 10?

■ Pain from arterial insufficiency is most commonly felt in the calf but may occur in other locations mentioned. Determine quantity or severity of pain.

➤ What makes the pain worse? Activity? Rest? What relieves the pain? Elevating your feet? Lowering your feet?

■ Arterial insufficiency produces pain that worsens with activity, especially prolonged walking. Leg pain is worse when legs are elevated, improved when legs are lowered. The pain is usually relieved quickly (within 2 minutes) when movement ceases. Determine exactly how much activity brings on the pain. By contrast, pain due to venous insufficiency intensifies with prolonged standing or sitting in one position. Pain is worse when legs are lowered, relieved when legs are elevated. Discomfort increases throughout the day, being worse at the end of the day.

➤ Have you noticed any changes in the skin of your legs, such as coldness, pallor, hair loss, sores, redness or warmth over the veins, or visible veins?

■ These signs may indicate arterial insufficiency of the legs.

EXAMINATION

Equipment

- Stethoscope, with a bell and diaphragm to auscultate heart sounds and detect vascular bruits
- Sphygmomanometer with appropriately sized cuff to measure blood pressure
- Tape measure (paper or cloth) for measuring circumference of limbs when edema occurs
- ❖ Marking pen or pencil and centimeter ruler (optional; used if cardiac percussion performed)
- Penlight to illuminate jugular veins and inspect chest
- ❖ Tongue blade and ruler to measure jugular venous pressure.

PROCEDURES AND TECHNIQUES WITH NORMAL FINDINGS

➤**EVALUATE the client's general condition.** Observe the client while he or she is lying supine or at an elevation of 30° to 45°. The client should have a relaxed, comfortable posture with deep, even respirations.

ABNORMAL FINDINGS

■ Abnormal findings include the sensation of chest or leg pain, coughing, choking, or smothering, with an inability to lie flat for an extended period of time; uneven, shallow, or gasping respirations with inadequate exchange of gases; cyanosis or gray pallor to the skin; mottling; or abnormal color around the lips, neck, or upper chest.

ARTERIAL ASSESSMENT: BLOOD PRESSURE

➤**PALPATE, then AUSCULTATE the brachial artery to evaluate arterial blood pressure in both arms.** (See Chapter 6 for procedure.) Blood pressure will vary with sex, body weight, and time of day, but the upper limits for adults are 140 mm Hg systolic, 90 mm Hg diastolic, and 30 to 40 mm Hg pulse pressure. The pressure should not vary more than 5 to 10 mm Hg systolic between the two arms (Fig. 18-7).

■ Note elevated systolic or diastolic pressures (hypertension) and lowered systolic or diastolic pressures (hypotension). Also note significant discrepancies in measurements between the two arms.

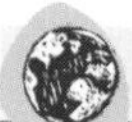

ETHNIC & CULTURAL VARIATIONS

African Americans have generally higher blood pressure readings than whites. These higher readings are thought to be related to differences in renin activity and the regulation of angiotensin II, which acts as a vasoconstrictor. African Americans also retain sodium and chloride better in heat-related situations than do whites.

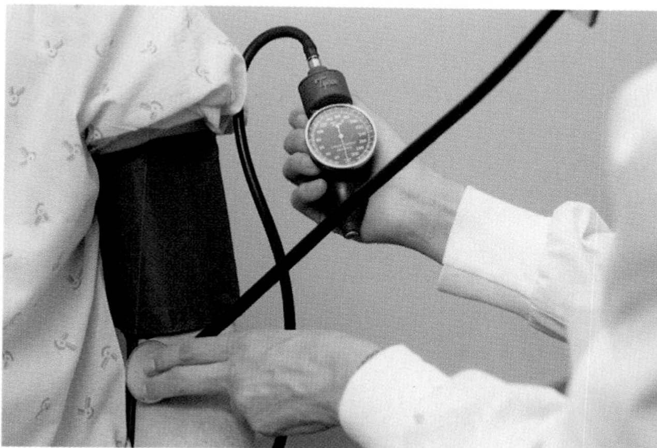

Fig. 18-7 Assessing blood pressure.

➤If the client offers a history of syncope or dizziness or is taking antihypertensive medications, measure the client's blood pressure and heart rate while he or she is sitting, standing, and lying. On standing, pressure may drop 10 to 15 mm Hg systolic and 5 mm Hg diastolic.

■ A decrease in systolic blood pressure greater than 20 mm Hg and symptoms such as dizziness indicate orthostatic (postural) hypotension. Diastolic pressure may decrease also. This may be due to a fluid volume deficit, drugs (e.g., antihypertensives), or prolonged bed rest.

PROCEDURES AND TECHNIQUES WITH NORMAL FINDINGS

ABNORMAL FINDINGS

ARTERIAL ASSESSMENT: PERIPHERAL PERFUSION

➤**PALPATE arterial pulses for rate, rhythm, amplitude, and contour.** Palpate arteries using the finger pads of the first two fingers. Comparing pulses on both sides of the body is customary. All pulses are assessed for amplitude and contour. The pulses palpated for assessment of rate and rhythm typically are the apical, brachial, and radial. The remaining six pulses usually are assessed to determine perfusion

Rate 60 to 100 beats/min (athletes may be as low as 50 beats/min). Pulse rates in women tend to be 5 to 10 beats/min faster than men.

■ Rates above 100 beats/min (tachycardia) or below 60 beats/min (bradycardia) are abnormal, although recent exertion, smoking, or anxiety will elevate the rate.

Rhythm Regular, that is, equal spacing between beats.

■ Irregular rhythms without any pattern should be noted. Coupled beats (two beats that occur close together) are abnormal also.

Amplitude Easily palpable, smooth upstroke. Compare the strength of upper extremity pulses with lower extremity and the left with the right (Box 18-1).

■ Note any exaggerated or bounding upstroke or, conversely, pulses that are weak, small, or thready, or where the peak is prolonged. Upstrokes should not vary (seen in pulsus alternans). The force of the beat should not be reduced during inspiration (known as paradoxical pulse).

Box 18-1 Pulse Amplitude Ratings

0+	Absent
1+	Diminished, barely palpable
2+	Normal
3+	Full volume
4+	Full volume, bounding hyperkinetic

Contour (Outline of the Pulse That Is Felt) Smooth and rounded, a series of unvaried, symmetric pulse strokes. (Note: There may be a slight transient increase in rate during inspiration, especially in clients younger than 40.)

■ Note any asymmetry in force or pulse contour, as well as any increased resistance to compression.

Temporal. Palpate over the temporal bone on each side of the head lateral to each eyebrow (Fig. 18-8).

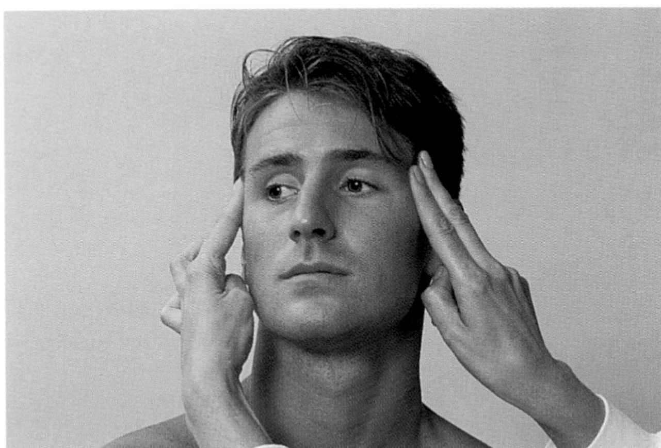

Fig. 18-8 Palpating temporal pulse lateral to each eyebrow.

PROCEDURES AND TECHNIQUES WITH NORMAL FINDINGS

ABNORMAL FINDINGS

Carotid. Palpate along medial edge of sternocleidomastoid muscle in lower third of the neck. Palpate one carotid pulse at a time to avoid reducing blood flow to the brain (Fig. 18-9).

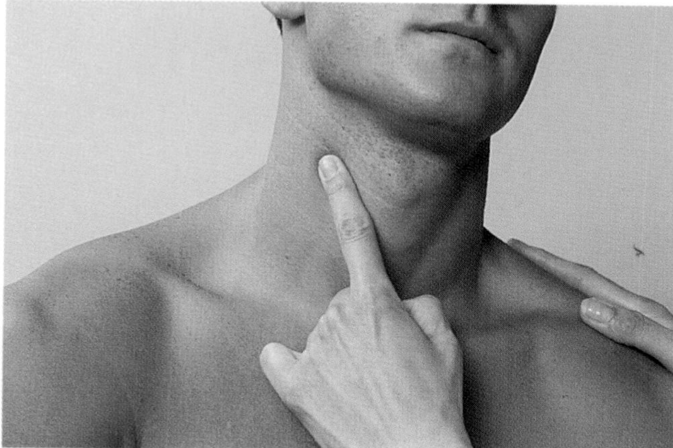

Fig. 18-9 Palpating carotid pulse in the lower third of the neck.

Apical. Palpate over the apex of the heart at the fourth or fifth intercostal space, left midclavicular line (Fig. 18-10). The apical pulse can be assessed as part of the palpation of the heart.

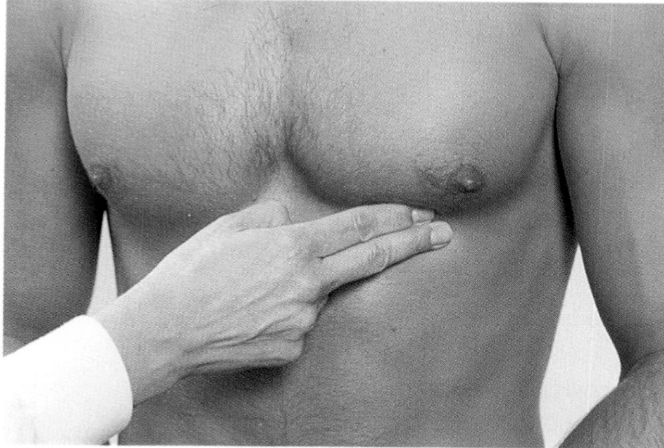

Fig. 18-10 Palpating apical pulse at the fourth or fifth intercostal space, left midclavicular line.

Brachial. Palpate in the groove between the biceps and triceps muscle just medial to the biceps tendon at the antecubital fossa (in the bend of the elbow) (Fig. 18-11).

PROCEDURES AND TECHNIQUES WITH NORMAL FINDINGS

ABNORMAL FINDINGS

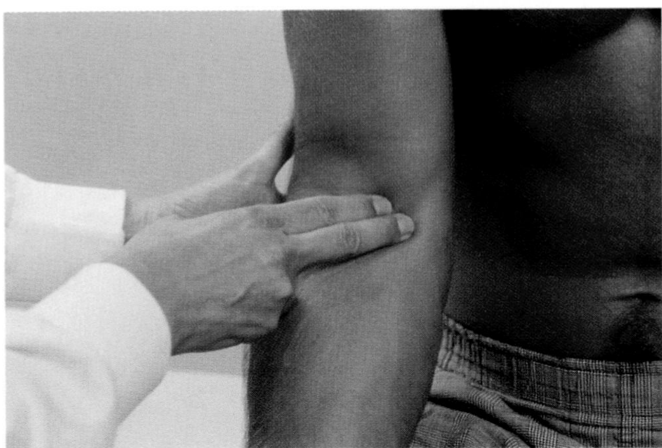

Fig. 18-11 Palpating brachial pulse at the antecubital fossa.

Radial. Palpate at the radial or thumb side of the forearm at the wrist (Fig. 18-12).

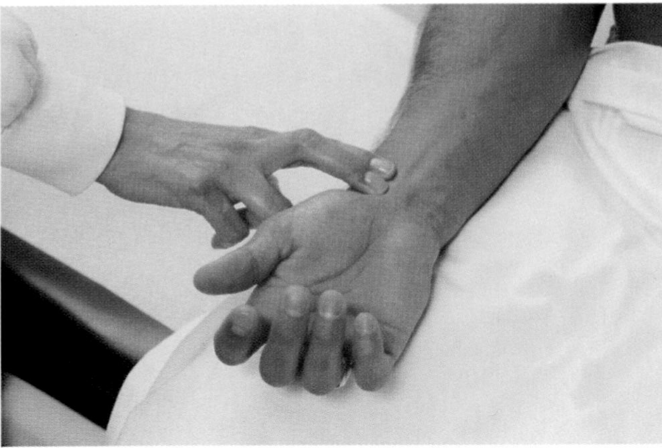

Fig. 18-12 Palpating radial pulse on the thumb side of the forearm at the wrist.

Femoral. Palpate below the inguinal ligament, midway between the symphysis pubis and anterior superior iliac. To find the femoral pulse move inward toward the genitalia. You can locate the anatomy using the mnemomic NAVEL: **N**, nerve; **A**, artery; **V**, vein; **E**, empty space; **L**, lymph. Firm compression may be needed for obese clients (Fig. 18-14).

PROCEDURES AND TECHNIQUES WITH NORMAL FINDINGS

ABNORMAL FINDINGS

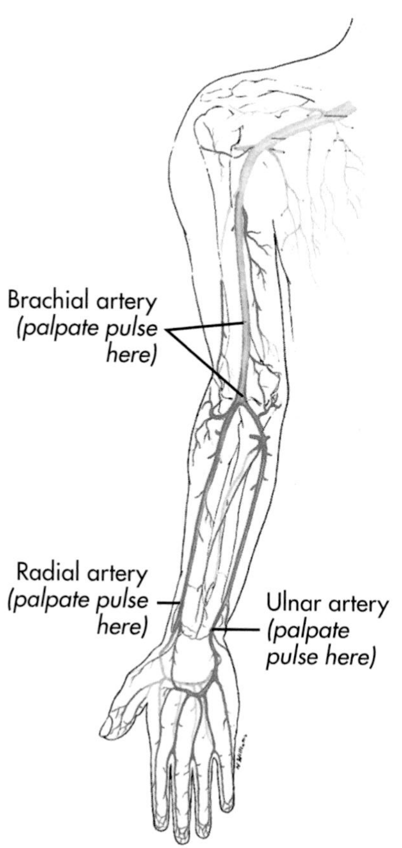

Fig. 18-13 Arteries of the upper extremity that are palpated. (Modified from Francis and Martin, 1975.)

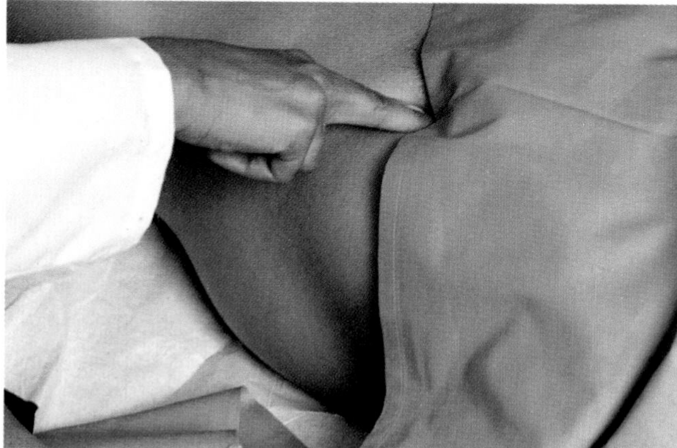

Fig. 18-14 Palpating femoral pulse between the symphysis pubis and anterior superior iliac. (From Canobbio, 1990.)

PROCEDURES AND TECHNIQUES WITH NORMAL FINDINGS

ABNORMAL FINDINGS

Popliteal. Palpate behind the knee in the popliteal fossa (Fig. 18-15). This pulse may be difficult to find. Having the client in the prone position may help in finding this pulse.

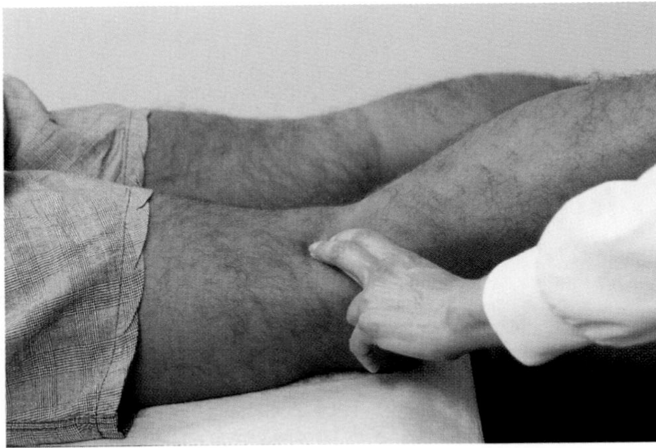

Fig. 18-15 Palpating popliteal pulse behind the knee.

Posterior tibial. Palpate on the inner aspect of the ankle below and slightly behind the medial malleolus (ankle bone) (Fig. 18-16).

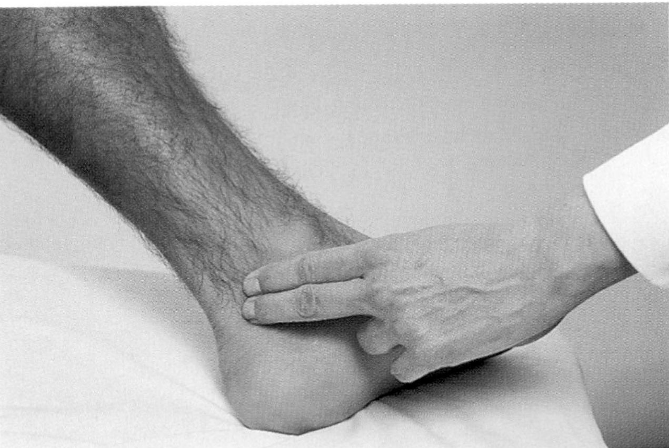

Fig. 18-16 Palpating posterior tibial pulse on the inner aspect of the ankle.

Dorsalis pedis. Palpate lightly over the dorsum of the foot between the extension tendons of the first and second toe (Fig. 18-17). (This pulse may be difficult to find or absent in normal persons.)

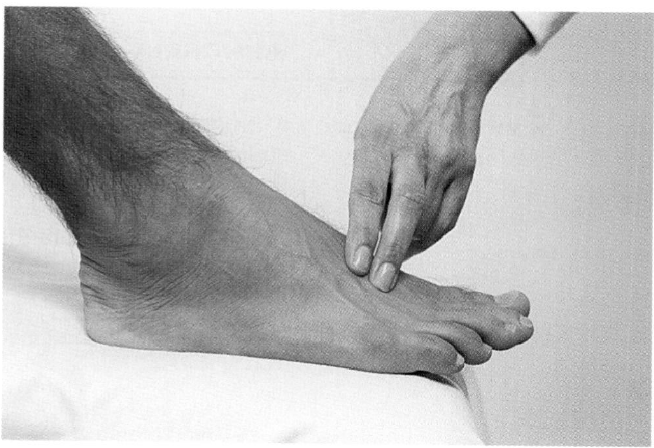

Fig. 18-17 Palpating dorsalis pedis pulse on top of the foot between first and second toe.

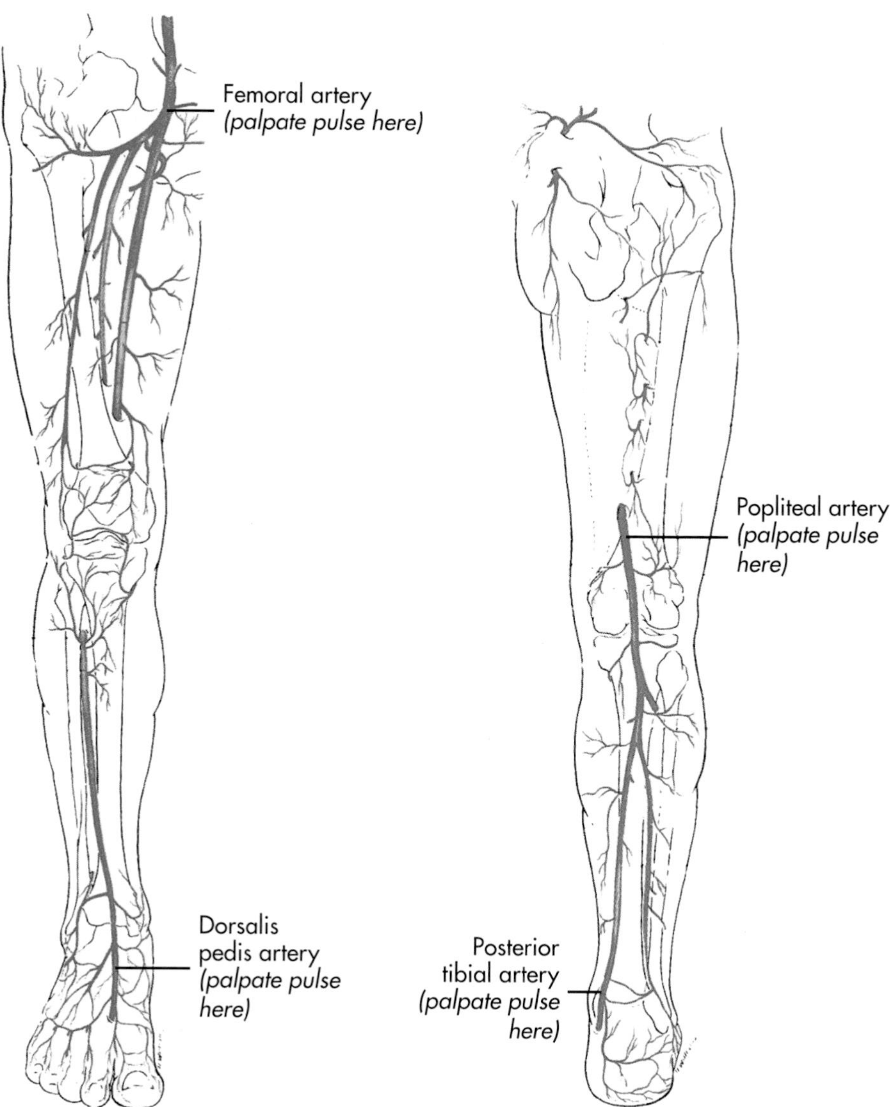

Fig. 18-18 Arteries of the leg that are palpated. (From Francis and Martin, 1975.)

PROCEDURES AND TECHNIQUES WITH NORMAL FINDINGS	ABNORMAL FINDINGS

➤**AUSCULTATE the carotid artery for bruits using the bell of the stethoscope.** Ask the client to hold breath while you listen. Normally you hear no sound over these arteries (Fig. 18-19).

■ Bruits are low-pitched blowing sounds usually heard during systole that indicate a narrowing of the vessel by arteriosclerosis. Other arteries to listen to are the temporal, abdominal aortic, renal, and femoral arteries.

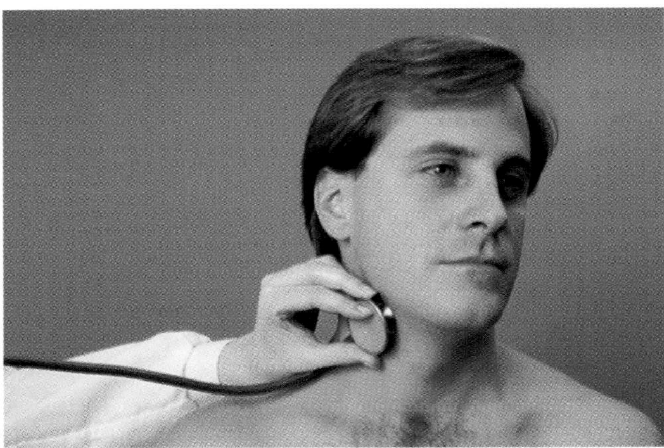

Fig. 18-19 Auscultating carotid pulse. (From Canobbio, 1990.)

➤**INSPECT and PALPATE the extremities for appearance, color, temperature, hair distribution, and capillary refill.** There may normally be no hair over the digits or dorsum of the hands and feet. Hair on men's legs is expected but is less abundant in Asian men. Some women shave leg hair, but others do not. The skin should be pink or brown (as appropriate) and warm with no evidence of edema. Gently squeeze pads of fingers and toes until they blanche. Release pressure and observe capillary refill, that is, how many seconds it takes for the original color to appear; it should be 2 seconds or less.

■ Arterial insufficiency may cause a decrease in or lack of hair peripherally or skin that appears thin, shiny, and taut. Cold extremities in a warm environment and mild edema are also abnormal. Note marked pallor or mottling when the extremity is elevated or any ulcerated digit tips. There should not be tenderness on palpation or the sensation of "stocking anesthesia," wherein the legs feel numb in a pattern resembling the area covered by a sock. A capillary refill time greater than 2 seconds indicates poor perfusion.

➤Nails should be pink, with an angle of 160° at the nail bed.

■ Clubbing of fingers (angle of nail disappears, becoming greater than 160°) indicates chronic hypoxia (Fig. 18-20).

Clubbing—early

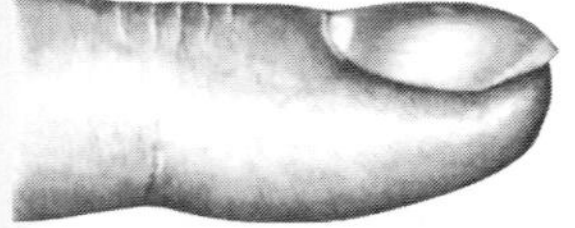

Clubbing—middle

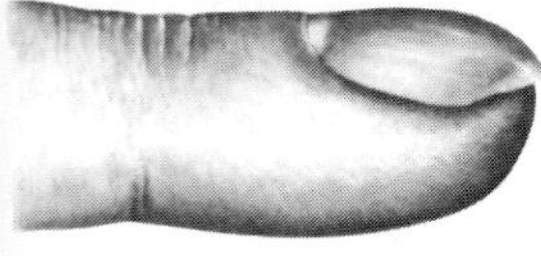

Clubbing—severe

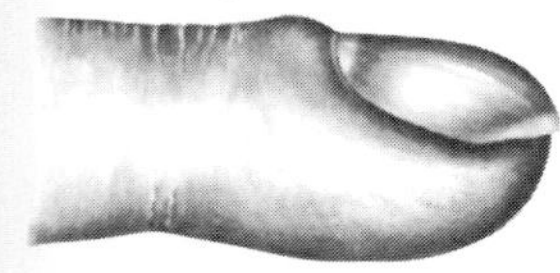

Fig. 18-20 Clubbing of fingers. (From Canobbio, 1990.)

PROCEDURES AND TECHNIQUES WITH NORMAL FINDINGS

ABNORMAL FINDINGS

➤If arterial insufficiency is suspected, have the client lie down. Elevate his or her legs 12 inches (30 cm) above the level of the heart. Then ask the client to flex and dorsiflex the feet for 60 seconds. The feet should exhibit mild pallor. Next have the client sit up and dangle the legs. Original color should return in about 10 seconds, with the foot veins filling up in about 15 seconds. (Note: This can also be done with the arms and hands.)

■ Note any marked pallor in one or both feet, any delayed return of color or mottled appearance, delay in filling of the veins, or marked redness in the dependent foot (or hand).

VENOUS ASSESSMENT

➤**INSPECT jugular vein for pulsations.** Elevate the head of the bed until venous pulsation in the internal jugular vein is seen. The angle may be 30° to 45° or as high as 90° if venous pressure is elevated. Inspect both sides of the client's neck for venous pressure as he or she lies at a angle. Elevate the client's chin slightly and tilt the head away from the side being examined. Illuminate the jugular veins for pulsations with a tangential light source, such as a penlight (Fig. 18-21).

■ Note any fluttering or oscillating of the pulsations. Note irregular rhythms or unusually prominent waves. These may indicate right-sided heart failure.

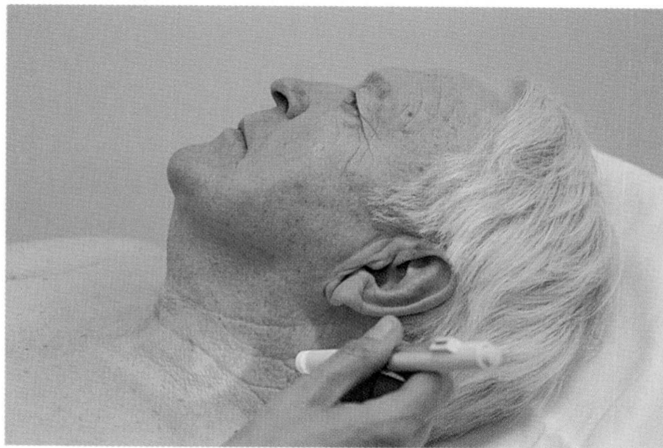

Fig. 18-21 Tangential light to view jugular veins and pulsations.

➤Pulsations should be regular, soft, and of a wavelike quality. The level of pulsation decreases with inspiration, and the pulsation increases in recumbent position.

■ Note any fluttering or oscillating of the pulsation. Note irregular rhythms or unusually prominent waves.

PROCEDURES AND TECHNIQUES WITH NORMAL FINDINGS

❖ ➤**ESTIMATE jugular venous pressure.** With the client's head elevated at the same angle, identify the highest level that jugular vein pulsations are visible, then identify the manubriosternal joint (angle of Louis). Use a tongue blade to create an imaginary line from the highest venous pulsation to the manubriosternal angle. Measure the vertical distance between the tongue blade and the manubriosternal angle to estimate jugular venous pressure in centimeters (Fig. 18-22). This pressure should not rise more than 1 inch (2.5 cm) above the sternal angle. (Note: If you cannot find the jugular vein, have the client lie down flat for a few minutes so that it will distend.)

ABNORMAL FINDINGS

■ Note if the jugular venous pressure exceeds 1 inch (2.5 cm) above the level of the manubrium. (Note: If venous pressure is elevated, meaning that the vein is distended up to the neck, the client's head is raised until the highest jugular pulsation can be detected. The distance in inches above the sternal angle and the angle at which the client is reclining should be recorded.) Also note if other veins in the neck, shoulder, or upper chest are distended.

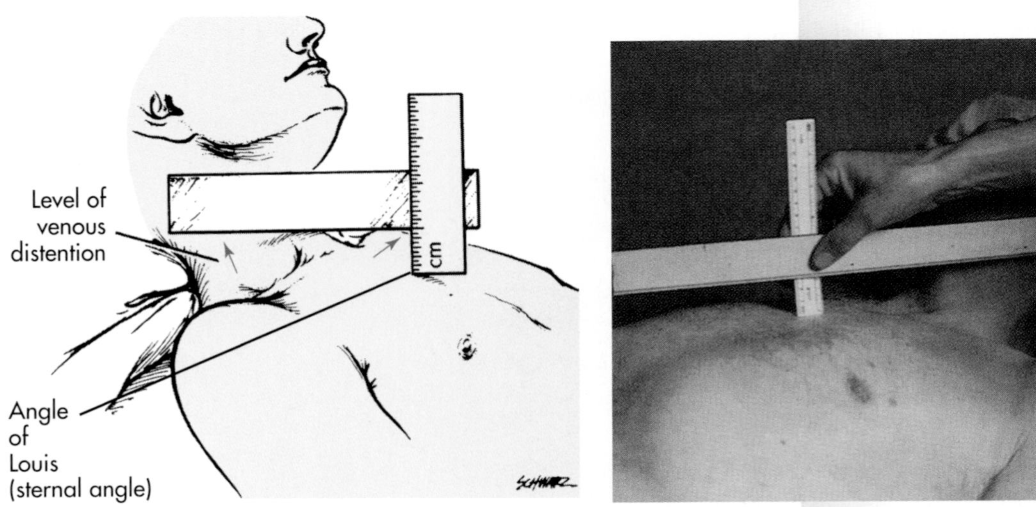

Fig. 18-22 Measuring jugular venous pressure. (From Barkauskas et al, 1998.)

PROCEDURES AND TECHNIQUES WITH NORMAL FINDINGS

ABNORMAL FINDINGS

➤**INSPECT and palpate the legs for the presence or appearance of superficial veins.** There should be distention in the dependent position, and the venous valves may appear as nodular bulges. The veins collapse with elevation of the limbs.

■ Note if there are distended veins in the anteromedial aspect of the thigh and lower leg or on the posterolateral aspect of the calf from the knee to the ankle.

➤**INSPECT and palpate the thigh and calf for surface characteristics.** The legs should be symmetric, nontender, and without excess warmth or coolness.

■ Note any swelling of one or both legs (especially if one calf appears larger than the other), tenderness on palpation, warmth, or redness (Table 18-2). Measure any apparent swelling of the thighs and calves with a tape measure to determine progress toward resolving. Measure at the widest point; measure the other leg in the same location. Clients who are immobile with reduced sensation, such as client with spinal cord injury, may manifest an increase in thigh circumference as the first sign of deep vein thrombosis.

Table 18-2 Pitting Edema Scale

SCALE	DESCRIPTION	"MEASUREMENT"*
1+	A barely perceptible pit	2 mm (3/32 in)
2+	A deeper pit, rebounds in a few seconds	4 mm (5/32 in)
3+	A deep pit, rebounds in 10-20 seconds	6 mm (1/4 in)
4+	A deeper pit, rebounds in > 30 seconds	8 mm (5/16 in)

*"Measurement" is in quotation marks because depth of edema is rarely actually measured but is included as a frame of reference.

Descriptions column data from Kirton C: Assessing edema, *Nursing 96* 26(7):54, 1996. Illustrations from Canobbio MM: *Cardiovascular disorders*, St. Louis, 1990, Mosby.

➤Sharply dorsiflex the client's foot (with the knee slightly flexed) to assess the calf pain response. No pain should be reported.

■ If pain results, this is known as Homan's sign and may indicate thrombophlebitis, but it is not a reliable indicator.

PROCEDURES AND TECHNIQUES WITH NORMAL FINDINGS

ABNORMAL FINDINGS

Box 18-2 Definitions of Lift, Heave, Thrill, and Retraction

A *lift* feels like a more sustained thrust than an expected apical pulse and is felt during systole. A *heave* is more prominent thrust of the heart against the chest wall during systole. Lifts and heaves may occur from left ventricular hypertrophy due to increased workload. A *thrill* is a palpable vibration over the precordium or artery; it feels like fine, palpable, rushing vibration. A thrill is associated with aortic valve stenosis. *Retraction* of the chest is a visible sinking in of tissues between and around the ribs. Retraction begins in the intercostal spaces. It occurs with increased respiratory effort. If additional effort is needed to fill the lungs, supraclavicular and infraclavicular retraction may be seen.

➤**INSPECT and PALPATE the extremities for skin turgor, color, and skin integrity.** Pinch an area of the skin between your finger and thumb and then release the skin. It should immediately fall back into place, indicating elasticity. Skin turgor should be elastic without tenting or edema (see Fig. 11-8). Color is as appropriate for race. Skin integrity is intact without lesions.

■ Peripheral cyanosis, edema (bilaterally or unilaterally; see Table 18-2 for interpretation), pigmentation around the ankles, thickening skin, and ulceration, especially around the ankles, are abnormal findings. Varicose veins appear as dilated, often tortuous, veins when legs are in a dependent position.

➤**PERFORM Trendelenburg's test to evaluate competence of venous valves in clients who have varicose veins.** With client in supine position, lift one leg above the level of the heart to allow veins to empty, then assist the client to stand. If veins are competent, veins fill slowly. Repeat the test on the other leg.

■ If the veins fill rapidly, the valves may incompetent, and varicose veins may be present.

CARDIAC ASSESSMENT

➤**INSPECT the anterior chest wall for contour, pulsations, lifts, heaves, or retractions.** Provide modesty and privacy while inspecting the female client's unclothed chest. Movement may be subtle. Use tangential light to inspect client's chest at eye level. Chest should be rounded and symmetric. Slight retraction medial to the left midclavicular line at the fourth or fifth intercostal space is normal; this is the apical pulse (Box 18-2).

■ Note any kyphosis, sternal depression, or asymmetry. A retraction is noted when some of the tissue is pulled into the chest on the precordium. Marked retraction of apical space may indicate pericardial disease or right ventricular hypertrophy.

➤The apical pulse may be visible only when the client sits up and leans forward, bringing the heart closer to the anterior chest. It may be obscured by obesity, large breasts, and muscularity.

■ Apical pulsation may be observed after exertion, in hyperthyroidism, or in left ventricular hypertrophy. Pulsations may be displaced left, right, or downward due to cardiac anomalies or change in heart size.

➤**PALPATE the precordium for pulsations, thrills, lifts, and heaves using the palmar surface of the hand and finger pads.** Supine is the preferred position for cardiac palpation; however, the sitting position may be necessary to feel impulses. Use a gentle touch, allowing the movements of the chest to lift the hands.

Palpate systematically from the base to the apex or from apex to base.

■ Observe whether the entire chest seems to lift or heave with the heartbeat. A lift or heave may indicate left ventricular enlargement.

➤Palpate the base of the heart (Fig. 18-23, *A*).

■ Pulsations may indicate an aortic aneurysm. A thrill may be associated with a murmur from some disorder of the aortic or pulmonic valve.

➤Palpate the LSB (Fig. 18-23, *B*) with the heel of the hand between the third, fourth, and fifth left ICS (Box 18-3).

■ Sustained lifts or palpations may indicate right ventricular hypertrophy; pulsations may indicate pulmonary hypertension. A thrill is associated with pulmonic valve stenosis.

Box 18-3 Abbreviations for Topographic Landmarks

ICS	intercostal space
RICS	right intercostal space
LICS	left intercostal space
SB	sternal border
RSB	right sternal border
LSB	left sternal border
MCL	midclavicular line
RMCL	right midclavicular line
LMCL	left midclavicular line

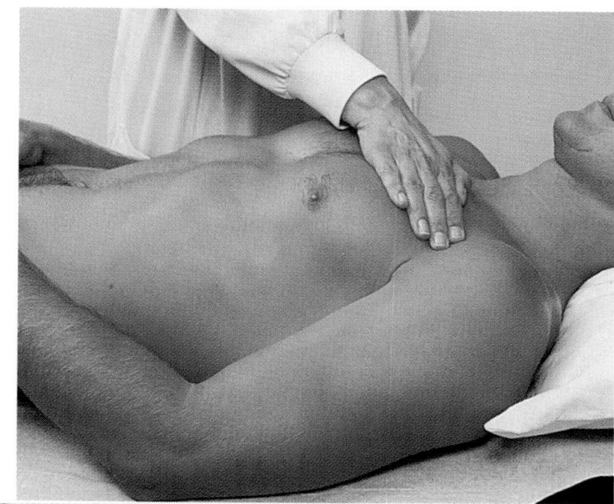

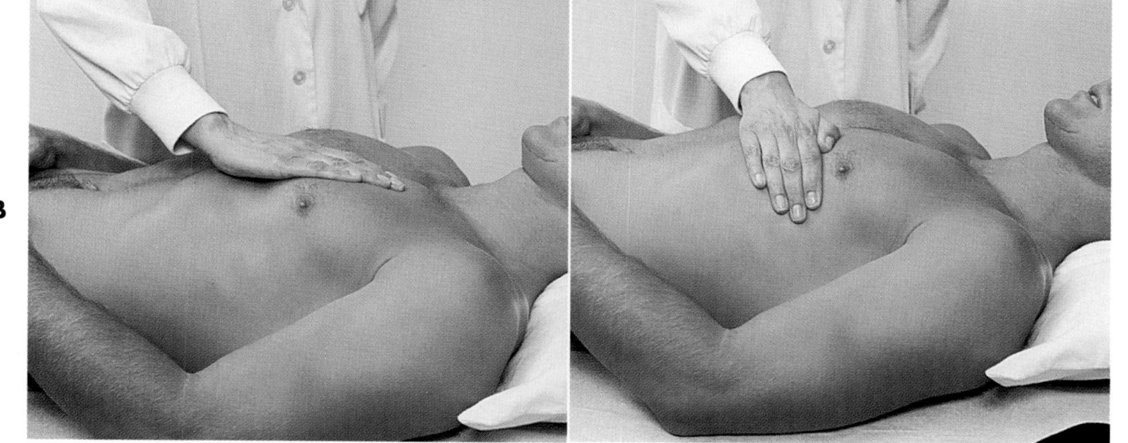

Fig. 18-23 Palpation of precordium. **A,** Palpating base. **B,** Palpating left sternal border. **C,** Palpating apex.

PROCEDURES AND TECHNIQUES WITH NORMAL FINDINGS

➤Palpate the apex of the heart at the fifth ICS midclavicular line (Fig. 18-23, *C*). This is the point of maximum impulse (PMI). Apical pulse has small amplitude, brief duration, and is no larger than 2 to 3 cm in diameter.

➤Palpate the epigastric area for pulsations. There should be an aortic pulsation.

ABNORMAL FINDINGS

■ Forceful pulsation, displaced laterally or downward, is associated with increased cardiac output or left ventricular hypertrophy. Presence of a thrill may indicate a murmur.

■ Bounding pulsations may indicate abdominal aortic aneurysm or aortic valve regurgitation.

PROCEDURES AND TECHNIQUES WITH NORMAL FINDINGS

❖ ➤**PERCUSS the heart borders for the heart size.** (This is an optional assessment technique because chest x-ray examination provides more precise information.) Percussion is performed at the third, fourth, and fifth ICS from the left anterior axillary line to the right anterior axillary line. The expected finding is a change from resonance to dullness about 6 cm lateral to the left of the sternum. The areas of dullness are marked with a pencil and the distance from the sternum measured with a ruler. Percussion of the heart may be difficult with obese or large-breasted clients.

ABNORMAL FINDINGS

■ Deviation of the left border further to the left is associated with dilated left ventricle, right pneumothorax, or pericardial effusion. Deviation of the left border to the right is associated with dextrocardia or left pneumothorax.

AUSCULTATION

➤**AUSCULTATE S_1 and S_2 heart sounds for rate, rhythm, pitch, and splitting** (Box 18-4). All five areas should be auscultated, first with the diaphragm using firm pressure and then with the bell using light pressure. The sounds are generated by valve closure and are best heard where blood flows away from the valve instead of directly over the valve area (Fig. 18-24). Heart sounds are low pitched, making them difficult to hear (Box 18-5). When first learning heart sounds, you may want to close your eyes to concentrate on each specific sound (i.e., selective listening). Begin with the client sitting upright. A systematic approach is used to listen in the five auscultatory areas, with the client breathing normally and then holding the breath in expiration. This allows you to hear the heart sounds better. Using the diaphragm, begin with the aortic valve area (second ICS, RSB) (Fig. 18-25, *A*), then the pulmonic valve area (second ICS, LSB) (Fig. 18-25, *B*), then Erb's point (third ICS, LSB) (Fig. 18-25, *C*), tricuspid valve area (fourth ICS, LSB) (Fig. 18-25, *D*), and finally the mitral valve area/apical pulse (fifth ICS, left MCL) (Fig. 18-25, *E*).

Repeat the auscultation of the five areas using the bell of the stethoscope.

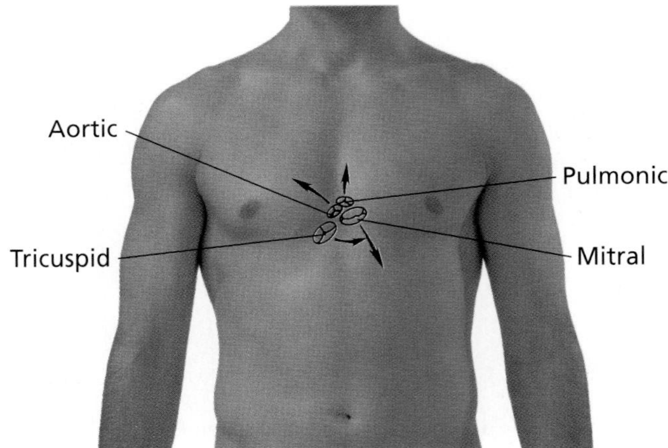

Fig. 18-24 Transmission of closure sounds from the heart values.

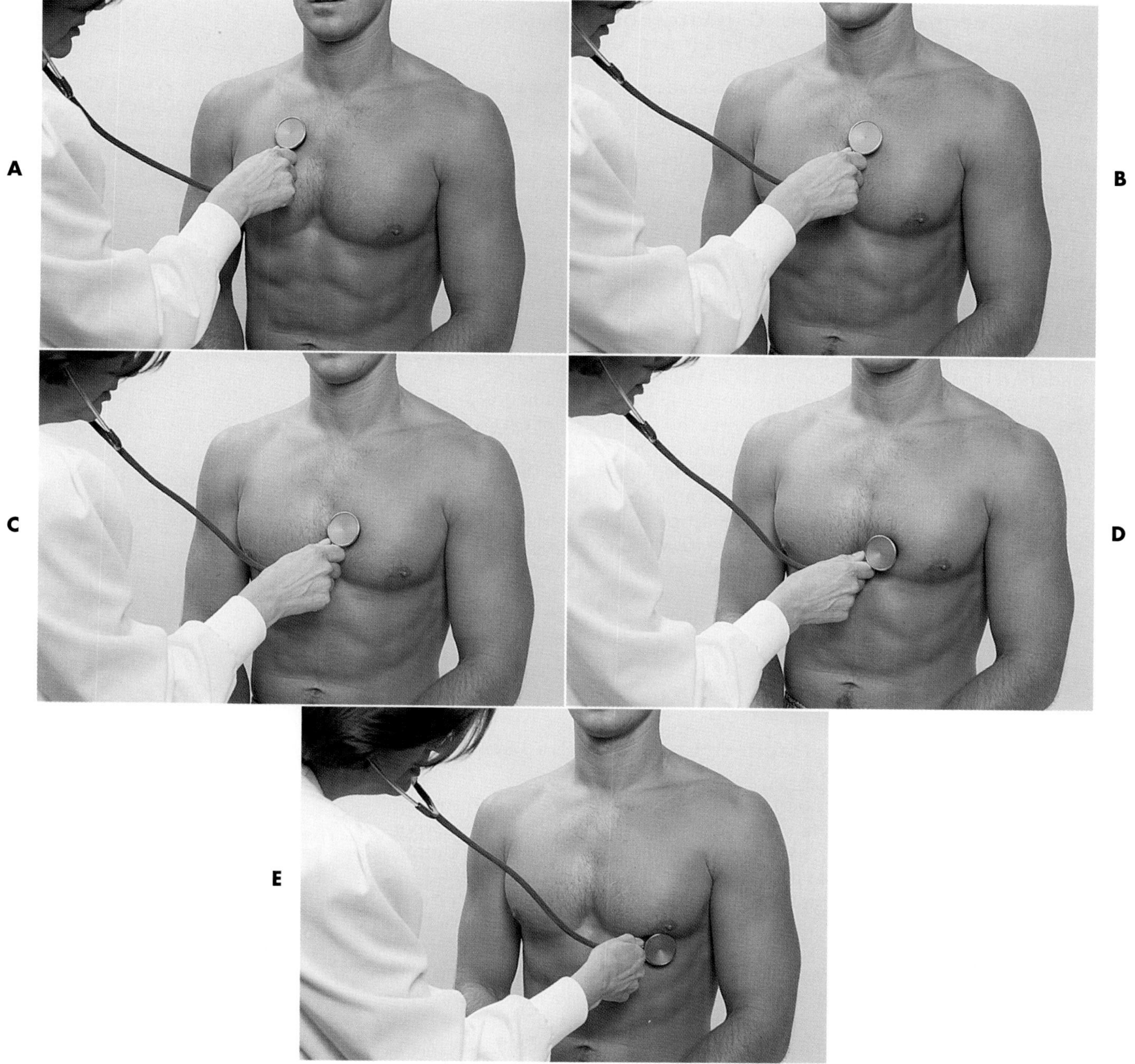

Fig. 18-25 Position for cardiac auscultation. **A,** Aortic area. **B,** Pulmonic area. **C,** Erb's point. **D,** Tricuspid area. **E,** Mitral area.

Box 18-4 Technique for Locating Intercostal Spaces for Auscultation of the Heart

A systematic approach is needed for this assessment. Some examiners begin at the apex and proceed upward toward the base of the heart, whereas others begin at the base and proceed downward toward the apex. The sequence is irrelevant as long as the assessment is systematic. Listen first with the diaphragm to hear high-pitched sounds, then with the bell to hear low-pitched sounds.

- When auscultating from base to apex, begin at the second intercostal space (ICS). Locate this ICS by palpating the right sternoclavicular joint (where the right clavicle joins the sternum).
- Palpate the first rib and then move down to palpate the space between the first and second ribs; this is the first ICS.
- Continue palpating downward to the space between the second and third ribs. This is the second ICS at the right sternal border (RSB), the auscultatory site for the aortic valve area. This is not the anatomic site of the aortic valve, but the site on the chest wall where sounds produced by the valve are heard best.
- Moving to the left side of the sternum at the second ICS, the area for auscultating the pulmonic valve area is found.
- Remaining at the LSB, move the stethoscope down to the third ICS, which is called Erb's point, an area to which pulmonic or aortic sounds frequently radiate. The fourth ICS, LSB is over the tricuspid valve area.
- At the fifth ICS, move the stethoscope laterally to the left midclavicular line, where the mitral valve area is located.

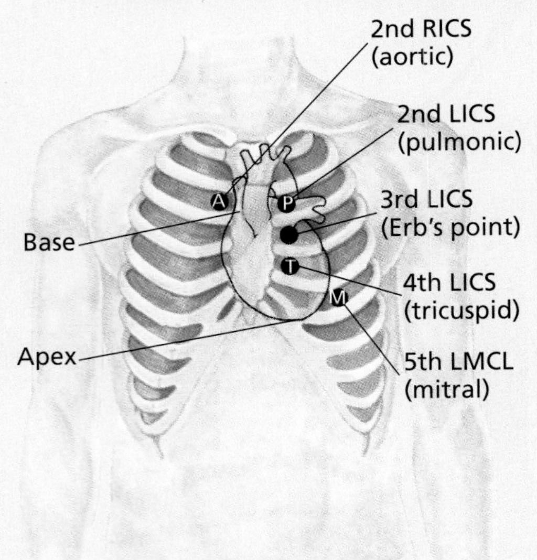

Box 18-5 Low- and High-Pitched Sounds of the Heart

In chapter 6 you read that the heart had low-pitched (low-frequency) sounds best heard with the bell of the stethoscope and that breath sounds were high pitched (high frequency), best heard with the diaphragm of the stethoscope. In this chapter you read that S_1 is lower in pitch than S_2 or that S_2 is higher in pitch than S_1 and that bruits are low pitched. How can both statements be true? The pitch of the sounds is relative, depending on which sounds you are comparing. When comparing breath sounds with heart sounds, heart sounds are low pitched. However, when comparing the sounds of S_1 with S_2, the pitch of S_1 is lower than S_2. Now, if you compared the pitch of breath sounds to the pitch of S_2, you would find S_2 is low pitched. These sounds could be put on a continuum from high to low pitch. Breath sounds would be high pitched, S_2 would be a lower pitch than breath sounds but higher than S_1, and S_1 would be the lowest pitch of all three sounds.

PROCEDURES AND TECHNIQUES WITH NORMAL FINDINGS

Rate Count the apical heart rate. Normal range is 60 to 100 beats/min; conditioned athletes or joggers may have slower rates normally.

ABNORMAL FINDINGS

■ Note rates that are over 100 or under 60 beats/min.

Tip to Remember

To help you remember which valve you are listening to (aortic, pulmonic, tricuspid, or mitral), use the mnemonic **Apartment M** or **APT M:**
Aortic
Pulmonic
Tricuspid

Mitral

or

APE TO MAN
Aortic
Pulmonic
Erb's point
To tricuspid
Mitral

Rhythm Normally the heart rate is regular, that is, an equal space between beats.

■ Irregular, nonpatterned rhythm or sporadic extra beats or pauses between beats should be noted.

Pitch The first and second heart sounds have low and high pitches, respectively (Box 18-5). Pitch is the quality of the sound dependent on the relative speed of the vibrations by which it is produced.

➤First heart sound (S_1) is made by the closing of the mitral (M_1) and tricuspid (T_1) valves. (When the heart sounds are described as *lubb-dubb,* the *lubb* represents S_1.) This heart sound should be heard at all sites; often louder at the apex; usually lower in pitch than the second heart sound; almost synchronous with the carotid pulse.

Splitting When the mitral and tricuspid valves do not close at the same time, S_1sounds as if it were split into two sounds instead of one. Splitting is heard occasionally in the tricuspid area with deep inspiration and varies from beat to beat, occasionally heard as a narrow split.

■ Note if the first heart sound appears accented, diminished or muffled, or varying in intensity with different beats. Note whether the frequency (pitch) becomes higher with accented intensity. Note that the fourth heart sound is sometimes mistaken for the splitting of the first heart sound.

➤Second heart sound (S_2) is made by the closing of the aortic (A_2) and pulmonic (P_2) valves. (S_2 is the *dubb* of the *lubb-dubb* heart sound.) This heart sound is usually heard at all sites; often louder at the base where the aortic and pulmonic sites are auscultated; usually higher in pitch than the first heart sound; duration shorter than with the first heart sound; splitting (physiologic splitting) is commonly heard in the pulmonic area on inspiration in young adults and usually disappears on expiration.

■ Note any increased intensity, especially in the aortic or pulmonary areas, or any decreased intensity. Wide, fixed, or paradoxic splitting are abnormal.

■ One form of pathologic splitting is paradoxic or reversed splitting that appears on expiration and disappears on inspiration. The most common cause is a left bundle branch block.

➤Palpation and auscultation may be repeated with the client lying in the left decubitus position and sitting.

■ Box 18-6 discusses abnormal heart sounds.

Box 18-6 Abnormal Heart Sounds

Abnormal heart sounds and murmurs are described by where they occur in the cardiac cycle. The normal sequence of events in the cardiac cycle can be diagrammed as shown below:

$S_1 \rightarrow$ systole $\rightarrow S_2 \rightarrow$ diastole $\rightarrow S_1 \rightarrow$ *etc.*

To determine if an abnormal sound occurs in systole or diastole, determine if the sound occurs after S_1 or after S_2.

- During diastole, when 80% of the blood in the atria rapidly fills the ventricles, a third heart sound may be heard (S_3). It is often heard at the apex. An S_3 occurs just after the S_2 and lasts about the same time as it takes to say "me too." The "me" is the S_2 and the "too" is the S_3. An S_3 is normal in children and young adults. However, when an S_3 is heard in adults over 30 years of age, it signifies fluid volume overload to the ventricle that may be due to heart failure or mitral or tricuspid regurgitation (Swartz, 1994).
- At the end of diastole, when atrial contraction completes the filling of the ventricle, a fourth heart sound may be heard (S_4). An S_4 occurs just before the S_1 and lasts about the same time as it takes to say "middle." The "mi" is the S_4 and the "ddle" the S_1. An S_4 is normal in children and young adults. However, when an S_4 is heard in adults over 30 years of age, it signifies a noncompliant or "stiff" ventricle. Hypertrophy of the ventricle precedes a noncompliant ventricle. Also, coronary artery disease is a major cause of a stiff ventricle (Swartz, 1994). Useful mnemonics for remembering the cadence and pathophysiology of the third and fourth heart sounds (Swartz, 1994) are as follows.

SLOSH′-ing-in	SLOSH′-ing-in	SLOSH′-ing-in
S_1 S_2 S_3	S_1 S_2 S_3	S_1 S_2 S_3
a-STIFF′-wall	a-STIFF′-wall	a-STIFF′-wall
S_4 S_1 S_2	S_4 S_1 S_2	S_4 S_1 S_2

Another way to remember the cadence of the S_3 and S_4 heart sounds is using the words "Kentucky" and "Tennessee."

Ken-tuck-y	Ken-tuck-y	Ken-tuck-y
S_1 S_2 S_3	S_1 S_2 S_3	S_1 S_2 S_3
Ten-ness-ee	Ten-ness-ee	Ten-ness-ee
S_4 S_1 S_2	S_4 S_1 S_2	S_4 S_1 S_2

Thus the third and fourth heart sounds can be abnormal when they occur in adults over 30. Both sounds occur in diastole.

The opening *snap* caused by the opening of the mitral or tricuspid valves is another abnormal sound heard in diastole when either valve is thickened, stenotic, or deformed. The sounds are high-pitched and occur early in diastole.

- In systole, *ejection clicks* may be heard if either the aortic or pulmonic valve is stenotic or deformed. The aortic valve ejection click is heard at either apex or base of the heart and does not change with respiration. The less common pulmonic valve ejection click is heard over the second or third left ICS. It increases with expiration and decreases with inspiration.
- *Pericardial friction rubs* are caused by inflammation of the layers of the pericardial sac. A rubbing sound is usually present in both diastole and systole and is best heard over the apical area.

ABNORMAL FINDINGS

Table 18-3 Characterization of Heart Murmurs

	CLASSIFICATION	DESCRIPTION
Timing and duration*	Early systolic	Begins with S_1, decrescendoes, ends well before S_2
	Midsystolic (ejection)	Begins after S_1, ends before S_2; crescendo-decrescendo quality sometimes difficult to discern
	Late systolic	Begins mid to late systole, crescendoes, ends at S_2; often introduced by mid to late systolic clicks
	Early diastolic	Begins with S_2
	Middiastolic	Begins at clear interval after S_2
	Late diastolic (presystolic)	Begins immediately before S_1
	Holosystolic (pansystolic)	Begins with S_1, occupies all of systole, ends at S_2
	Holodiastolic (pandiastolic)	Begins with S_2, occupies all of diastole, ends at S_1
	Continuous	Starts in systole, continues without interruption through S_2, into all or part of diastole; does not necessarily persist throughout entire cardiac cycle
Pitch	High, medium, low	Depends on pressure and rate of blood flow; low pitch is best heard with bell
Intensity†	Grade I	Barely audible in quiet room
	Grade II	Quiet but clearly audible
	Grade III	Moderately loud
	Grade IV	Loud, associated with thrill
	Grade V	Very loud, thrill easily palpable
	Grade VI	Very loud, audible even with stethoscope not on chest, thrill palpable and visible
Pattern	Crescendo	Increasing intensity caused by increased blood velocity
	Decrescendo	Decreasing intensity caused by decreased blood velocity
Quality	Harsh, raspy, machine-like, vibratory, musical, blowing	Quality depends on several factors, including degree of valve compromise, force of contractions, blood volume
Location	Anatomic landmarks (e.g., second left intercostal space on sternal border)	Area of greatest intensity, usually area to which valve sounds are normally transmitted
Radiation	Anatomic landmarks (e.g., to axilla)	Site farthest from location of greatest intensity at which sound is still heard; sound usually transmitted in direction of blood flow
Respiratory phase variations	Intensity, quality, and timing may vary	Venous return increases on inspiration and decreases on expiration

*Systolic murmurs are best described according to time of onset and termination; diastolic murmurs are best classified according to time of onset only.

†Discrimination among the six grades is more difficult for the diastolic murmur than for the systolic.

From Seidel HM et al: *Mosby's guide to physical examination,* ed 4, St. Louis, 1999, Mosby.

Murmur

■ A series of prolonged heart sounds heard either during systole or diastole is called a murmur. These abnormal heart sounds are produced by vibrations created when blood flow is altered. Murmurs are heard when there are structural abnormalities in the aortic or pulmonary arteries or defects in the heart itself or the valves. Murmurs are best heard over the auscultatory areas, rather than over the actual heart defect. Table 18-3 shows the characterization of heart murmurs.

Systolic Murmur A murmur occurring during the ventricular ejection phase of the cardiac cycle is called a systolic murmur. Most systolic murmurs are caused by obstruction of the outflow of the semilunar valves or by incompetent AV valves. The vibration is heard during all or part of systole. Other causes of systolic murmurs are structural deformities of the aorta or pulmonary arteries and anemia and thyrotoxicosis (hyperthyroidism). A ventricular septal defect results in a murmur classified as pansystolic or holosystolic because it occupies all of systole.

Diastolic Murmur A murmur occurring in the filling phase of the cardiac cycle is called a diastolic murmur. Incompetent semilunar valves or stenotic AV valves create diastolic murmurs. These murmurs almost always indicate heart disease. Early diastolic murmurs usually result from insufficiency of a semilunar valve or dilation of the valvular ring. Mid- and late-diastolic murmurs are generally caused by stenosed mitral and tricuspid valves that obstruct blood flow.

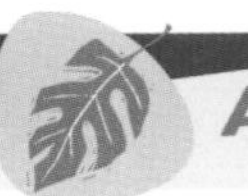

AGE-RELATED VARIATIONS

NEWBORNS AND INFANTS

Anatomy and Physiology

The newborn's heart is developmentally similar to the adult's, even before birth, with one notable exception: oxygenation occurs through the placenta to compensate for the nonfunctional fetal lungs. Arterial blood is returned via the umbilicus to the right side of the heart. The foramen ovale is an opening between the left and right atria that allows blood to flow into the left side of the heart, where about two thirds is pumped into the aorta. The remaining third is pumped from the right ventricle directly into the aorta through the patent ductus arteriosus. After birth, as the pressure in the left atrium rises, the foramen ovale closes, usually within the first hour. The ductus arteriosus usually closes within 10 to 15 hours (Wong et al, 1999).

Health History

- What was the mother's health status during pregnancy? Did she have rubella during the first trimester? Unexplained fever? Any infections? Did she use drugs (over-the-counter, prescribed, or illicit)?

  Rationale Congenital rubella, fever, and drug use may cause congenital heart defects (e.g., patent ductus arteriosus).
- Have you noticed any breathing changes in the infant? Does the infant breathe more heavily or rapidly than expected while feeding or having a bowel movement? Does the infant seem to tire easily while eating? Does the infant take breaks from feeding to catch his or her breath? Does the infant turn blue around his or her mouth while feeding? Does the infant's skin tone turn blue at other times such as when crying? Is the infant gaining weight as expected? Is the infant growing like other infants?

  Rationale An infant with heart failure takes only a few ounces during each feeding, becomes short of breath during sucking, may be diaphoretic or cyanotic, falls asleep as if exhausted, and then awakens a short time later, hungry again.
- Does the infant tire easily while playing? How many naps does the infant take each day? How long does a nap last?

  Rationale Infants with cardiovascular problems have poor sleeping patterns and tend to sleep more than expected (Wong et al, 1999).

Examination

Procedures and Techniques Blood pressure measurement is difficult to obtain for newborns and young infants. The electronic sphygmomanometer with a Doppler technique is relatively sensitive and useful for this age group. The apical pulse of the newborn normally is felt in the fourth or fifth ICS just medial to the midclavicular line. Examine the heart within the first 24 hours of birth and again at 2 to 3 days to assess changes from fetal to systemic and pulmonic circulation. Auscultation of the heart must be done when the client is quiet. Thus it may be performed out of sequence when you can take advantage of a quiet infant. The stethoscope used must have a small diaphragm and bell to detect specific cardiac sounds of the newborn or infant. If the infant is having dyspnea, estimate size and position of heart.

Normal and Abnormal Findings Normally the heart rate of infants is faster when they are awake and slower when they are asleep. Sinus dysrhythmia is an expected finding when the heart rate increases during inspiration and decreases during expiration. Splitting of heart sounds is common in infants until about 48 hours after birth due to the transition from fetal circulation to systemic and pulmonic circulation. Innocent murmurs, grade I or II, accompanied by no other signs or symptoms frequently disappear within 2 to 3 days. Capillary refill in infants is very rapid—less than 1 second.

Acrocyanosis (cyanosis of hands and feet) without central cyanosis is of little concern and usually disappears within hours to days of birth.

Abnormal findings include changes in the skin and cardiovascular system. Central cyanosis may indicate congenital heart defects. Note if cyanosis increases with crying or sucking. Severe cyanosis that appears shortly after birth may indicate transposition of great vessels, tetralogy of Fallot, a severe septal defect, or severe pulmonic stenosis. Cyanosis that appears after the first month of life suggests pulmonic stenosis, tetralogy of Fallot, or large septal defects.

Murmurs that persist after 3 days or radiate must be referred for further evaluation. Pushing on the infant's liver increases pressure to the right atria. Murmur with a left-to-right shunt through a septal opening or patent ductus will disappear briefly with pressure to the liver, whereas murmurs of right-to-left shunt will increase. A pneumothorax shifts the apical impulse away from the area of the chest where the pneumothorax is located. The infant's heart may be shifted to the right by a diaphragmatic hernia commonly found on the left. Dextrocardia causes the apical impulse to be on the right.

Weak or thin pulses may be due to decreased cardiac output or peripheral vasoconstriction. Bounding pulses may indicate a patent ductus arteriosus creating a left-to-right shunt. Coarctation of the heart is suspected when the femoral pulses are absent or there is a difference in pulse amplitude between upper extremities or between femoral and radial pulses. Prolonged refill times (more than 2 seconds) may indicate dehydration or hypovolemic shock.

CHILDREN

Anatomy and Physiology

The anatomy and physiology for the child is the same as for the adult.

Health History

- Is the child developing like other children in your family or other children his or her age? Has the child gained weight and height as expected?
  Rationale These questions are asked to determine if the parents perceive the child has met developmental milestones.
- Does he or she tire easily during play? What activities are tiring? Can he or she keep up with other children? Is he or she reluctant to go out to play because of an inability to keep up? Does the child turn "blue" or become short of breath during activities? Does the child take longer-than-usual (for his or her age) naps? Does the child squat instead of sit while at play or watching television? Does the child complain of leg pains during exercise?
  Rationale A positive response to these questions may indicate congenital heart disease. Squatting relieves dyspnea.
- Has the child had any unexplained fever? Does the child have frequent respiratory infections? How many per year? How are these treated? Have any been streptococcal infections? Unexplained joint pain?
  Rationale These questions help to rule out rheumatic fever caused by group A beta-hemolytic streptococcal pharyngitis.
- Is there a brother or sister in the family with a heart defect? Does anyone in the family have Down syndrome?
  Rationale These are disorders caused by chromosomal anomalies that may be present in this child if they are present in other family members.

Examination

Procedures and Techniques Auscultation can be difficult and requires a quiet, extremely cooperative child. Although the child's chest is auscultated in the same areas as the adult's, it may take a considerably longer time to be sure of the sounds, which may be upsetting to the parents. Explanations should be given in advance. All of the techniques used require that the child wear only underwear and sit on the table or the caregiver's lap. Cooperative children may recline at a 45° angle. If this is not possible, the child may lie supine to allow you to hear more cardiovascular sounds.

If an irregular rhythm is noted, have the child hold his or her breath so that only heart sounds are heard. Auscultate with the bell of the stethoscope over the right supraclavicular space at the medial end of the clavicle along the anterior border of the sternocleidomastoid muscle (Fig. 18-26) for a venous hum. It is a vibration heard over the jugular vein caused by turbulent blood flow and has a continuous, low-pitched sound that is louder during diastole. A venous hum may be stopped by gentle pressure between the trachea and the sternocleidomastoid muscle at the level of the thyroid cartilage. Note differences between pulses, particularly the radial and femoral.

Normal and Abnormal Findings A child's pulse may normally increase on inspiration and decrease on expiration. Sinus dysrhythmia may be an expected finding during childhood. Changes in heart rates in children are listed in Table 6-3. An expected finding in children is a venous hum in the jugular vein.

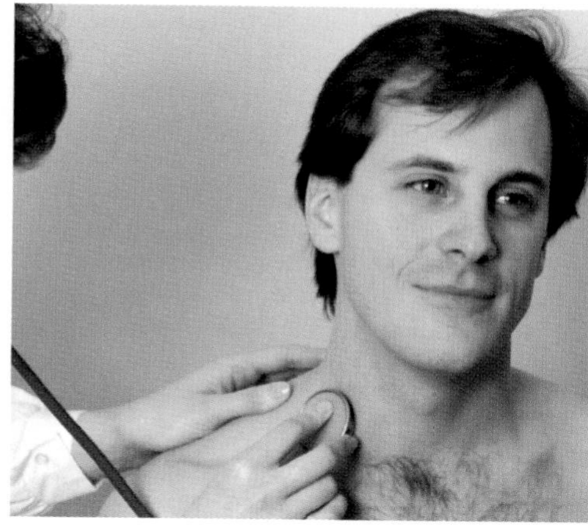

Fig. 18-26 Auscultation for venous hum. (From Canobbio, 1990.)

It is important to record the abnormal findings observed during the child's activities. Note any poor weight gain or cyanosis. Squatting may be a compensatory position for a child with a heart defect. Cyanosis or pallor may indicate poor perfusion due to congenital heart defects. Note if there is more cyanosis with crying and if there is facial or ankle edema. Note signs of poor feeding (e.g., low weight) and reports of caregiver that child stops eating to get his or her breath, which may indicate a heart problem. Labored respirations could indicate a cardiovascular problem. Weak or absent femoral pulses may indicate coarctation of the aorta.

■ OLDER ADULTS

Anatomy and Physiology

The aging heart functions well under normal conditions but may be unable to compensate for extremes of stress, blood loss, tachycardia, unusual exertion, or fever. With increased age the heart size tends to decrease. The cardiac output declines 30% to 40% because of decreased heart rate and myocardial contractility. Response to stress or increased oxygen demand is less efficient, and the return to baseline heart rate takes longer. Physiologic changes, such as thickening of the endocardium and decreased elasticity of the myocardium, contribute to delayed recovery from myocardial contractility and irritability. Artrial walls and some superficial vessels become less efficient in complying with changing needs as they become more dilated, prominent, tortuous, and calcified. Increased blood pressure, both systolic and diastolic, occurs in response to increased peripheral vascular resistance. In addition, the older adult's cardiac function is affected by fibrosis and sclerosis of the SA node and mitral and aortic valves.

Health History

- Have you experienced any confusion, dizziness, blackouts, or fainting? Have you noticed any palpitations?
  Rationale Decreased cerebral perfusion can cause confusion, dizziness, or fainting.

- Have you been short of breath or nauseated, or have you vomited or had any weakness?

Rationale When older adults have a myocardial infarction (MI) they may not experience the typical chest pain, referred to as a "silent MI." The most common symptom reported in the silent MI is dyspnea, and it may be the only presenting symptom. Other symptoms that may be reported are gastrointestinal complaints of nausea and vomiting and neurologic complaints of weakness, vertigo, confusion, or impaired consciousness (Matteson, McConnnell, and Linton, 1997).

Examination

Procedures and Techniques The examination for the older adult is the same as for the younger adult.

Normal and Abnormal Findings Older adults may have variations in heart rate normally. It may be slower due to increased vagal tone or more rapid, with a range from the low 50s to greater than 100 beats/min. Clients with these extreme ranges would require future assessment to determine if the heart rates were significant. Occasional ectopic beats are common and may or may not be significant. The S_4 heart sound is common in older adults and may be associated with decreased left ventricular compliance.

Systemic blood pressure increases with age due to stiffness of the aorta. Check the pressure in both arms when the client is lying down and when standing up. A maximum of 160 mm Hg systolic may be within normal limits if it remains stable over time and the client has no symptoms or evidence of end-organ damage. Pressures in both arms should not vary more than 5 to 10 mm Hg systolic. Soft, early systolic murmurs may be "functional," or nonsignificant. They are often found and represent the effects of aortic lengthening, tortuosity, and sclerotic changes.

Abnormal findings include postural or orthostatic hypotension identified by a systolic pressure that drops more than 20 mm Hg with a change in posture from sitting to lying. Note loud aortic (ejection) murmurs that radiate into the neck, which can indicate obstructive aortic disease. Systolic murmurs heard at the apex may indicate mitral calcification.

EXAMINATION SUMMARY

Heart and Peripheral Vascular System

PROCEDURE

- Evaluate client's general condition.

Arterial Assessment (pp. 411-419)

Blood Pressure

- Palpate, then auscultate arterial blood pressure in both arms.

Peripheral Perfusion

- Palpate each pulse for:
  Rate
  Rhythm
  Amplitude
  Contour
- Auscultate carotid artery for:
  Bruits
- Inspect and palpate extremities for:
  Appearance
  Color
  Temperature
  Hair distribution
  Capillary refill

Venous Assessment (pp. 419-421)

- Inspect jugular veins for:
  Pulsations
- ❖ Estimate jugular venous pressure
- Inspect and palpate lower extremities for:
  Superficial veins
  Surface characteristics
  Skin turgor
  Color
  Skin integrity

Cardiac Assessment (pp. 421-427)

- Inspect anterior chest for:
  Contour
  Pulsations
  Lifts
  Heaves
  Retractions
- Palpate precordium for:
  Pulsations
  Thrills
  Lifts
  Heaves
- ❖ Percuss heart borders for heart size (optional).
- Auscultate heart sounds over aortic area, pulmonic area, tricuspid area, mitral area, and apical areas for:
  Rate
  Rhythm
  Pitch
  Splitting
  Murmurs
  Extra sounds

SUMMARY OF FINDINGS

Age Group	Normal Findings	Typical Variations	Findings Associated With Disorders
Infants and children	Same as for adults. • Stethoscope with a smaller diaphragm is used. Capillary refill is <1 sec. Important to palpate for femoral pulse.	• Grade I or II murmur with no other signs disappears first 2 or 3 days. • *Sinus dysrhythmia:* An expected variation when heart rate increases during inspiration and decreases during expiration for infants and children. • *Splitting heart sounds:* Common in infants. • Children may have a venous hum in a jugular vein.	• *Central cyanosis and dyspnea:* May indicate congenital heart defects. • *Murmurs:* If persist after 3 days, should be evaluated further. • *Pulses:* Weak thin pulses may be due to deceased cardiac output or peripheral vasoconstriction. Bounding pulse may indicate patent ductus arteriosus creating a left-to-right shunt. Coarctation of the heart is suspected when femoral pulses are absent. • *Weight loss and cyanosis:* In a child with report of squatting, may indicate heart disease.
Adolescents Adults	Same as for adults. • *Blood pressure:* Upper limit is 140/90 mm Hg. • *Heart rate:* Between 60 and 100 beats/min. Nine pulses are regular, easily palpable, smooth, and rounded. • *Extremities:* Have color appropriate for race, warm, expected hair distribution for race, with capillary refill <2 sec. • *Nails:* Pink with 160° angle. • *Jugular vein pulsations:* Regular, soft and wavelike and do not rise more than 1 inch (2.5 cm). • *Chest:* Rounded and symmetric. • *S_1 and S_2:* Present and regular.	Same as for adults. • *Athletes:* May have a heart rate as low as 50 beats/min. • *Pulses:* Are not palpable but can be assessed by Doppler.	Same as for adults. • *Blood pressure drops:* > 15 mm Hg systolic and 5 mm Hg diastolic when standing, sitting, and lying. • *Tachycardia:* Pulse rate >100 beats/min; bradycardia is a pulse rate <60 beats/min. Irregular pulse rates may occur in dysrhythmias. • *Faint-to-absent peripheral pulses:* Occur with peripheral vascular disease. • *Carotid artery for bruits:* Found in arteriosclerosis. • *Arterial insufficiency:* Lack of hair with shiny, taut skin may occur, as well as color not returning to feet for >10 sec after they are elevated above the heart. Capillary refill >2 sec. • *Jugular vein distention:* >1 inch (2.5 cm). • *Positive Homan's sign:* May indicate thrombophlebitis. • *Trendelenberg's test:* Reveals varicose veins. • *Heave and lift:* If observed and palpated, may indicate ventricular hypertrophy.

Age Group	Normal Findings	Typical Variations	Findings Associated With Disorders
Older adults	• Same as for adults with the following exceptions in vital signs: Heart rate may range from 50 to over 100 beats/min. Systemic blood pressure may be elevated due to stiffness of aorta. A maximum of 160 mm Hg systolic may be within normal limits.	• Occasional ectopic beats are common. • *S_4 heart sound:* Common due to decreased left ventricular compliance. • *Soft early systolic murmurs:* May be functional.	• *Orthostatic hypotension:* When the systolic pressure drops >20 mm Hg when changing from sitting to lying. • *Loud aortic ejection murmur:* May radiate to the neck. • *Systolic murmurs heard at the apex:* May indicate mitral calcification. • *Dyspnea:* May be a common symptom of a myocardial infarction, called a "silent MI." Other symptoms of the MI may be nausea, vomiting, and neurologic symptoms such as vertigo, confusion, and impaired consciousness.

HEALTH PROMOTION

SMOKING

The nicotine in tobacco vasoconstricts blood vessels, which increases the workload on the heart, increases blood pressure, and decreases peripheral perfusion. Smokers have more than twice as many heart attacks as nonsmokers. Peripheral vascular disease is almost exclusively a disease of smokers. When people stop smoking, their risk of heart disease drops rapidly, and 10 years after quitting their risk of death from heart disease is about the same as for people who never smoked. Stop-smoking programs are available through the American Lung Association, American Cancer Society, and American Heart Association.

HYPERTENSION

Elevated blood pressure—over 140 systolic or 90 mm Hg diastolic on more than one measurement—indicates hypertension. The Joint National Committee (JNC) VI lifestyle recommendations to reduce hypertension are as follows:

- Stop smoking for overall cardiovascular health.
- Reduce intake of dietary fat and cholesterol.
- Lose weight if overweight.
- Increase aerobic activity to 30 to 45 minutes most days of the week.
- Reduce sodium intake to not more than 100 mmol per day.
- Maintain potassium intake of 90 mmol per day.
- Maintain adequate intakes of calcium and magnesium for general health.
- Limit alcohol intake.

(The National High Blood Pressure Education Program, 1999).

Blood pressure screening is recommended every 2 years for clients with a diastolic pressure below 85 mm Hg and systolic below 140 mm Hg. Screening is recommended annually for clients with a diastolic between 85 and 89. Persons with higher blood pressures require more frequent measurements (U.S. Preventive Services Task Force, 1996).

OBESITY AND HYPERCHOLESTEREMIA

Cholesterol levels between 200 and 240 mg/dl increase the risk of heart disease. Obesity increases the workload on the heart, and excessive lipids, cholesterol, and triglycerides increase the fatty plaque that forms on blood vessels, making them narrow. Exercise and a low-fat diet are recommended to maintain an ideal body weight and a cholesterol level under 200 mg/dl. A progressive walking program, beginning with 5 minutes of brisk walking and progressing to 30 minutes on most days, is recommended. A low-fat diet can be accomplished by eating more chicken, turkey, fresh fruits and vegetables, and less beef and yellow cheese. Preparing food by baking or broiling is preferred over frying.

STRESS

Psychologic stress increases the heart rate and can increase the workload on the heart. Relaxation techniques are useful in reducing stress. Techniques such as relaxation, yoga, music therapy, and mental imagery are some of the techniques proven to reduce stress.

COMMON PROBLEMS AND CONDITIONS

Heart and Peripheral Vascular System

CARDIAC DISORDERS

Valvular Heart Disease (VHD)

An acquired or congenital disorder of the cardiac valve is known as valvular heart disease. It is characterized by stenosis of a heart valve, causing obstruction of blood flow, or by valvular degeneration, causing regurgitation of blood. A stenotic valve is one that does not open completely so that blood flow through the valve is reduced and a backflow is created. Conversely, valvular degeneration causes an incompetent or insufficient valve that does not close completely, causing regurgitation of blood. For example, some of the blood that normally would be pumped from the left ventricle through the aortic valve will flow back into the left atrium through the incompetent mitral valve. Rheumatic fever and endocarditis account for most cases of acquired VHD (Table 18-4).

Left Ventricular Hypertrophy

An increase in the size of the myocardial cells of the left ventricle caused by chronic overwork is called left ventricular hypertrophy. Aortic stenosis or hypertension increases the resistance that the left ventricle must work against to maintain adequate cardiac output. The hypertrophy creates a lift palpable during systole and displaces the apical pulse laterally.

Right Ventricular Hypertrophy

An increase in the size of the myocardial cells of the right ventricle caused by chronic overwork is called right ventricular hypertrophy. Idiopathic pulmonary hypertension increases the resistance that the right ventricle must pump against to maintain adequate blood flow to the lungs. Pulmonary hypertension can also be caused by chronic hypoxia. Pulmonary capillaries compensate for chronic hypoxia by constricting, which increases the workload of the right ventricle. Chronic obstructive pulmonary disease and cystic fibrosis are causes of chronic hypoxia. Right ventricular hypertrophy can cause a lift along the left sternal border in the third and fourth left intercostal spaces.

Angina Pectoris

Chest pain due to ischemia of the myocardium as a result of atherosclerosis of the coronary arteries is called angina pectoris. Angina can occur during activity, stress, or exposure to intense cold because of an increased demand on the heart, or it can occur during rest as a result of spasms of the coronary arteries. Clients describe the pain as squeezing, suffocating, or constricting. Angina is a steady pain, lasting less than 5 minutes, and it is relieved by rest or vasodilating drugs (e.g., nitroglycerin).

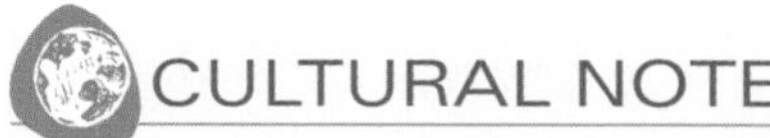

Heart disease and stroke are major killers of individuals in the United States, and minority cultural groups have disproportionately high losses. American Indians and Alaskan natives have a cardiac disease mortality rate twice the rate of the general population. African Americans have a higher morbidity and mortality rate from coronary artery disease and stroke than the general population.

Myocardial Infarction

When myocardial ischemia is severe, myocardial cells are destroyed, causing necrosis of the muscle, which is called a heart attack or myocardial infarction. The left ventricle is more commonly affected, but the right ventricle may be affected. Description of pain given is that this pain is the worst chest pain ever experienced, a pain that lasts longer than 5 minutes; it may radiate to the left shoulder, jaw, arm, or other areas of the chest; and is not relieved by rest or nitroglycerin. Dysrhythmias are common. Heart sounds may be distant with a thready pulse.

Heart Failure

When either ventricle fails to pump blood efficiently into the aorta or pulmonary arteries, the condition is called heart failure.

Left Ventricular Failure Left ventricular failure is caused by (1) increased resistance that occurs with aortic stenosis or hypertension when the ventricle can no longer compensate effectively for the increased workload or (2) weakening of the left ventrical contraction that occurs after a myocardial infarction when myocardial cells are necrosed, rendering the ventricle ineffective. Since the left ventricle cannot pump sufficient blood forward, some of the blood backs up into the left atria and eventually into the pulmonary capillaries, causing pulmonary edema. Assessment finds precordial movement, displaced apical pulse and palpable thrill, S_3, and systolic murmur at apex. In the acute phase the client usually has crackles bilaterally from pulmonary edema.

Right Ventricular Failure Right ventricular failure is caused by hypertrophy from pulmonary hypertension or from necrosis from a myocardial infarction. The failure of the right ventricle to pump blood into the pulmonary arteries causes a backflow of blood into the inferior and superior venae cavae. Assessment findings are precordial movement at xiphoid or left sternal border, elevated jugular venous pressure, S_3 at lower left sternal border, and systolic murmur.

Table 18-4 Murmurs due to Valvular Defects

SYSTOLIC EJECTION MURMUR

Systole Diastole

Systolic ejection murmur

S_1 S_2 S_1 S_2 S_1 S_2

TYPE		DETECTION	QUALITY/PITCH	VARIABLES
Aortic stenosis	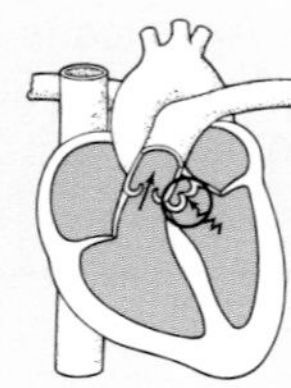	Heard over aortic valve area; ejection sound at second right intercostal border. Radiates to neck, down left sternal border.	Medium pitch, coarse, with crescendo-decrescendo pattern. Pitch low.	May radiate as far as apex and to carotid with thrill; S_1 may be followed by ejection click; S_2 soft or absent; S_4 palpable.
Pulmonic stenosis	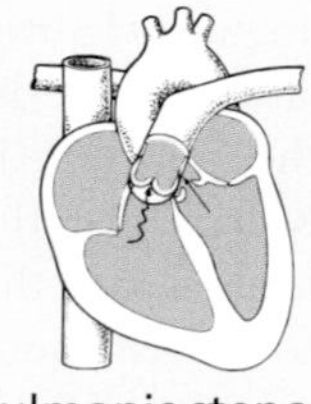 Pulmonic stenosis	Heard over pulmonic valve; radiates left to neck; thrill at second and third left intercostal spaces.	Same as for aortic stenosis. Pitch medium.	S_1 usually followed by quick ejection click; S_2 often diminished with wide split; P_2 may be soft or absent; S_4 common if right ventricular hypertrophy present.

DIASTOLIC REGURGITANT MURMUR

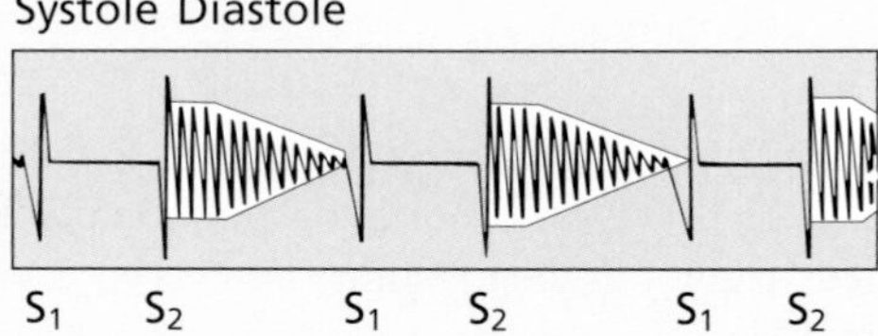

TYPE		DETECTION	QUALITY/PITCH	VARIABLES
Aortic regurgitation	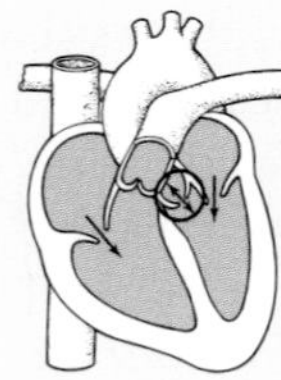	Diaphragm, client sitting and leaning forward. Second right intercostal space radiates to left sternal border.	Blowing in early diastole. Pitch high.	Decrescendo midsystolic murmur common; early ejection click may be present; S_1 soft; S_2 split may have drum-like quality; summation gallop common. Wide pulse pressure; bisferial pulse common in carotid, brachial, and femoral arteries.
Pulmonic regurgitation	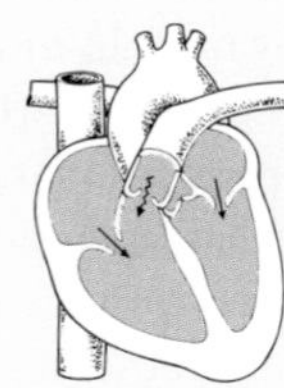 Pulmonic Regurgitation	Diaphragm, client sitting or leaning forward. Third and fourth left intercostal spaces.	Blowing. Pitch high or low.	Difficult to distinguish from aortic regurgitation on physical examination.

Table 18-4 Murmurs due to Valvular Defects—cont'd

TYPE	DETECTION	QUALITY/PITCH	VARIABLES
DIASTOLIC MURMUR 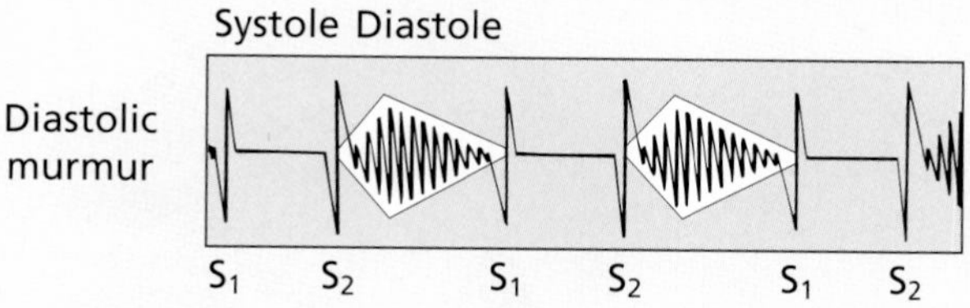			
Mitral stenosis	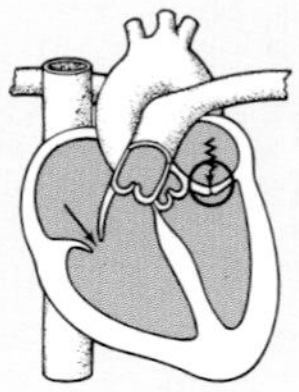 Bell at apex with patient in left lateral decubitus position.	Low rumble more intense in early and late diastole. Pitch low.	Thrill at apex in late diastole common; S_1 increased and often palpable at left sternal border; accentuated P_2 common, followed closely by opening snap. Decreased arterial pulse amplitude.
Tricuspid stenosis	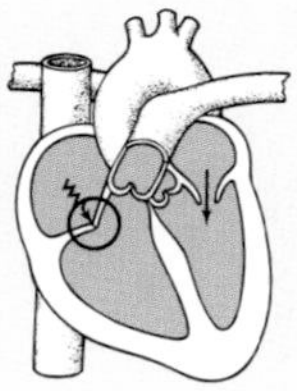 Bell over tricuspid area.	Similar to mitral stenosis but louder on inspiration. Pitch low.	Thrill over right ventricle; S_2 may split during inspiration. Decreased arterial pulse amplitude. Jugular pulse prominent.
HOLOSYSTOLIC MURMUR 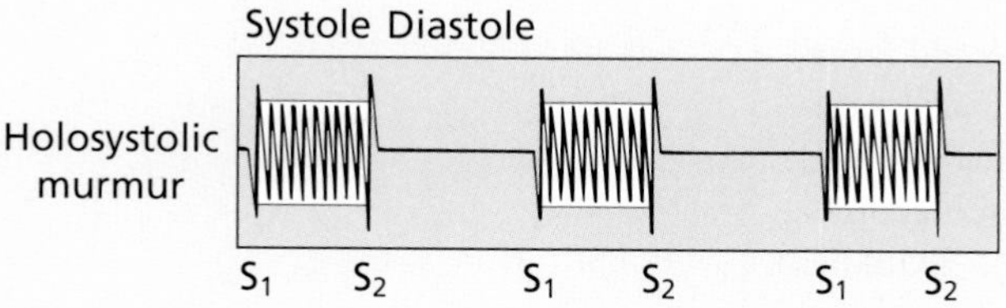			
Mitral regurgitation	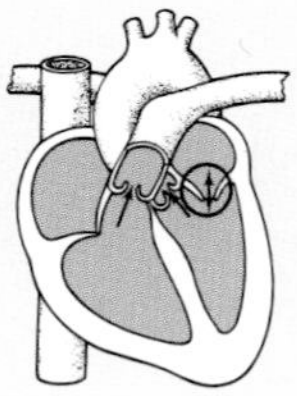 Diaphragm at apex, radiates to left axilla or base.	Harsh blowing quality. Pitch high.	Thrill may be palpable at base; S_1 decreased; S_2 increased, with P_2 often accentuated; S_3 often present. If mild, late systolic crescendo present; if severe, early systolic decrescendo and summation gallop present.
Tricuspid regurgitation	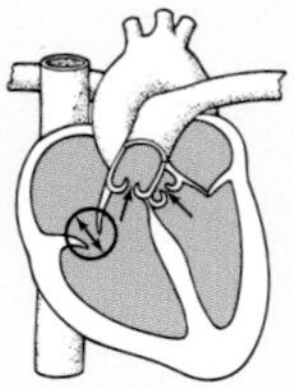 Fifth intercostal space, left lower sternal border.	Blowing. Pitch high.	Murmur increases during inspiration, decreases during expiration.

Diastolic murmur: Systole Diastole; S_1 S_2 S_1 S_2 S_1 S_2

Holosystolic murmur: Systole Diastole; S_1 S_2 S_1 S_2 S_1 S_2

Cor Pulmonale Cor pulmonale is the term used when right-sided heart failure is caused by pulmonary disease such as chronic obstructive disease or cystic fibrosis. The mechanism of altered blood flow is the same as that in right-sided heart failure, but the cause is different. The pulmonary capillaries compensate for chronic hypoxia by constricting, which increases the workload on the right ventricle. After continual stress on the right ventricle, it fails to pump blood effectively. A backflow of blood occurs into the superior and inferior venae cavae.

Infective Endocarditis

An infection of the endothelial layer of the heart, including the cardiac valves, is called infective endocarditis. This infection develops when the endocardial surface is damaged by turbulent blood flow as a result of valvular heart disease, congenital lesions, or direct injury from intravenous lines or injections, cardiac catheterization, or artificial valves. Circulating bacteria, viruses, fungi, or rickettsiae may be introduced from respiratory or skin infections (Fig. 18-27). Microorganisms attach to the endothelial membrane and form an infective vegetation. A thrombus forms where endocardial tissue is damaged. The thrombus can break apart and become emboli, producing infarctions or abscesses in heart, lungs, brain, kidneys, spleen, or extremities. Heart sounds are normal during the early infection. In late infection, a murmur is heard if valve damage occurs (DeJong, 1998).

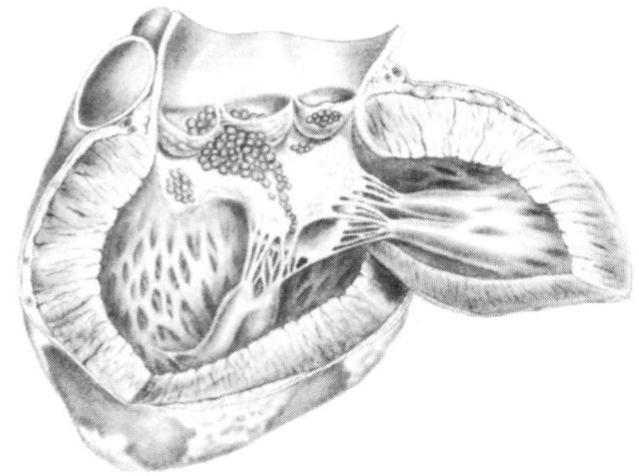

Fig. 18-27 Bacterial endocarditis. (From Cannobio, 1990.)

Pericarditis

An inflammatory process of the parietal and visceral layers of the pericardium and outer myocardium is called pericarditis (Fig. 18-28). It may be idiopathic or the result of myocardial infarction, uremia, cancer, trauma, infections, cardiac surgery, or an autoimmune reaction. Exudates formed may be serous, fibrinous, or purulent. Two classic clinical findings are pericardial friction rub and chest pain. A pericardial friction rub develops as the inflamed layers of pericardium move against each other. The friction rub is best heard with client leaning forward so that the heart is closer to the chest wall. Listen in the second, third, or fourth intercostal spaces at the left sternal border or at the apex; it is louder during inspiration. Chest pain experienced is described as a sharp pleuretic pain that is aggravated by deep breathing, lying supine, or coughing (Dugan, 1998).

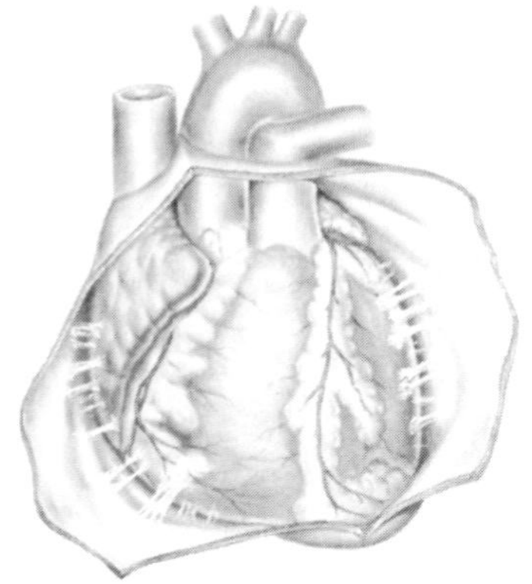

Fig. 18-28 Pericarditis. (From Canobbio, 1990.)

CONGENITAL HEART DEFECTS

Patent Ductus Arteriosus (PDA)

Patent ductus arteriosus is a vascular connection that, during fetal life, permits blood to flow from the pulmonary artery to the aorta, bypassing the lungs (Fig. 18-29). Functional closure usually occurs shortly after birth. If the ductus remains open, or patent, blood is shunted from the high systemic pressure in the aorta through the ductus to the pulmonary artery, raising the pressure in the pulmonary circulation and increasing the workload of the right ventricle. Children's growth and development are normal. Blood pressure has wide pulse pressure and bounding pulses. Thrill may be palpable at left upper sternal border. Continuous murmur heard in systole and diastole is called a machinery murmur.

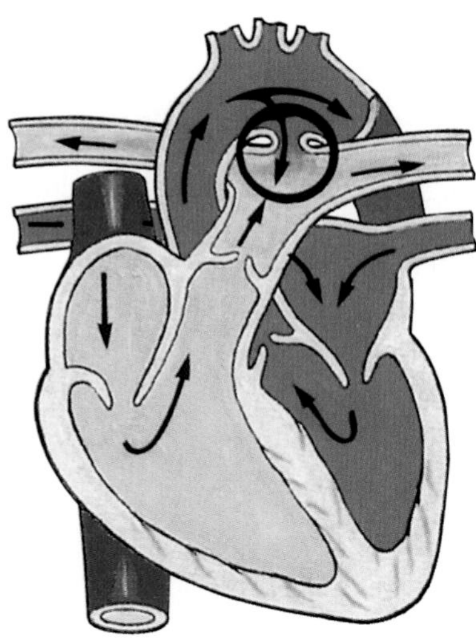

Fig. 18-29 Patent ductus arteriosus. (From Wong et al, 1999.)

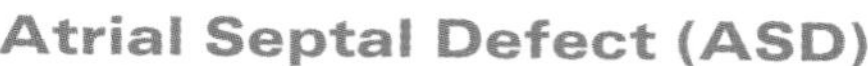

Atrial Septal Defect (ASD)

A defect in the septum that allows blood flow between the left and right atria is called an atrial septal defect (Fig. 18-30). With increasing age this defect increases pressure on the right ventricle, causing fatigue and dyspnea in children or young adults. The S_2 sound splits, with P_2 often being louder than A_2. The murmur is due to increased blood flow through the pulmonic valve. It is heard at the base in the second left intercostal space and is called a systolic ejection murmur of medium pitch.

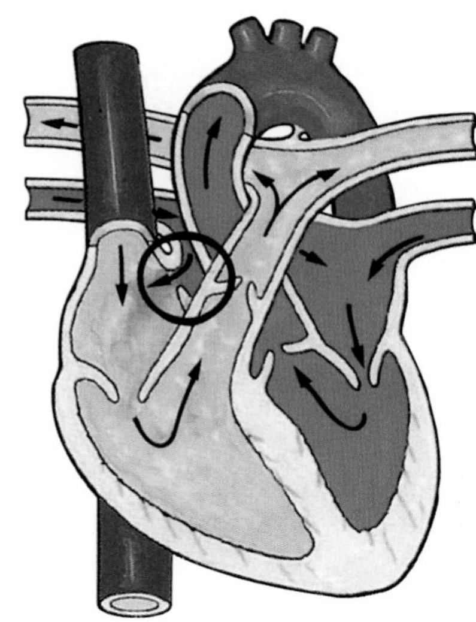

Fig. 18-30 Atrial septal defect. (From Wong et al, 1999.)

Ventricular Septal Defect (VSD)

A defect in the septum between the ventricles is called a ventricular septal defect (Fig. 18-31). The side of the defect determines the extent of the shunting of blood and clinical findings. Infants with large defects have slow weight gain, dyspnea, and feeding problems. A loud, harsh, holosystolic murmur is best heard at the left lower sternal border and may be accompanied by a thrill.

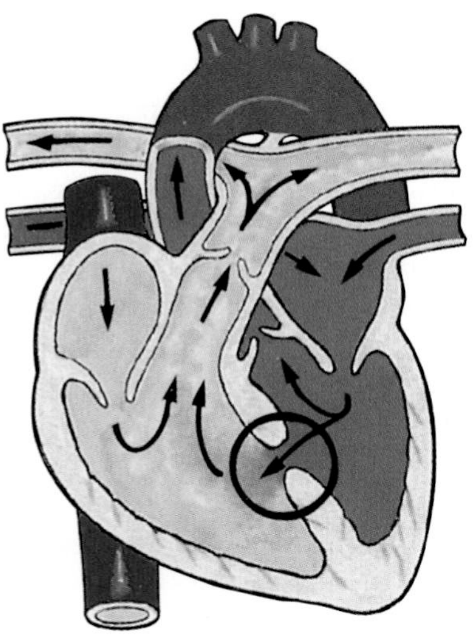

Fig. 18-31 Ventricular septal defect. (From Wong et al, 1999.)

Tetralogy of Fallot

Tetralogy of Fallot involves four cardiac defects, comprising ventricular septal defect, pulmonic stenosis, dextroposition of the aorta (aorta overrides ventricular septum), and right ventricular hypertrophy (Fig. 18-32). The right ventricular outflow is obstructed, resulting in right ventricular hypertrophy and shunting of venous blood directly into the aorta away from the pulmonary artery, preventing blood from being oxygenated. Infants have severe cyanosis as they grow, and the pulmonic stenosis becomes worse. Infants have dyspnea and use squatting position when walking begins. Assessment reveals palpable thrill at the left sternal border, normal S_1, a loud A_2 and diminished P_2, and a loud, pansystolic systolic murmur.

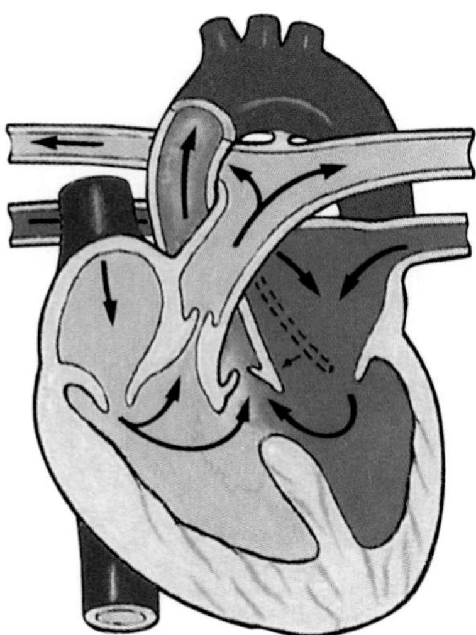

Fig. 18-32 Tetralogy of Fallot. (From Wong et al, 1999.)

Coarctation of the Aorta

A narrowing or partial obstruction of a section of the aorta is called coarctation of the aorta (Fig. 18-33). The narrowing increases pressure in the proximal aorta and diminishes output distal to the narrowing, which decreases blood flow to the kidneys. The increased pressure in the aorta increases the workload on the left ventricle. Symptoms are usually not present in childhood. Blood pressure in the arms may be 10 to 15 mm Hg higher than the legs. Most important finding is absent-to-diminished femoral pulses.

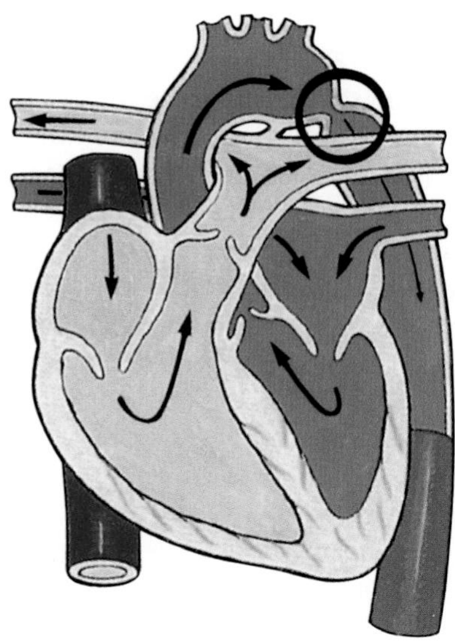

Fig. 18-33 Coarctation of the aorta. (From Wong et al, 1999.)

VESSEL DISORDERS

Hypertension

Sustained elevation in systolic blood pressure on two or more occasions above 140 mm Hg or diastolic blood pressure above 90 mm Hg is called hypertension (Sixth Report, 1997). The elevated blood pressure results from an increase in peripheral resistance due to vasoconstriction of arterial vessels or excess fluid volume in the vascular space. The exact cause of hypertension is unknown. There are no specific symptoms of hypertension, which is why periodic screening is important (Box 18-7). Hypertension increases the workload of the heart by increasing the resistance against which the left ventricle must pump to maintain cardiac output. Some factors that contribute to hypertension are obesity; high fat, cholesterol, and salt intake; race; and genetic factors (Tobin, 1999).

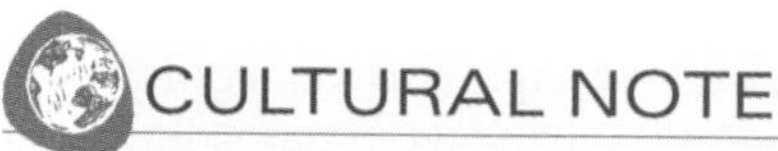

CULTURAL NOTE

Hypertension is generally more prevalent in minority cultural groups in the United States than in whites. Higher incidences have been reported in African Americans, Hispanics, and Pacific Islanders. Asian Americans and American Indians and Alaskan natives have lower prevalence of hypertension than the general population.

Box 18-7 Classification of Blood Pressure for Adults Age 18 and Older*

Category	Systolic (mm Hg)		Diastolic (mm Hg)
Optimal†	<120	or	<80
Normal	<130	or	<85
High normal	130-139	or	85-89
Hypertension‡			
Stage 1	140-159	or	90-99
Stage 2	160-179	or	100-109
Stage 3	>180	or	>110

*Not taking antihypertensive drugs and not acutely ill. When systolic and diastolic blood pressures fall into different categories, the higher category should be selected to classify the individual's blood pressure.
†Optimal blood pressure with respect to cardiovascular risk is below 120/80 mm Hg. However, unusually low readings should be evaluated for clinical significance.
‡Based on an average of two or more readings taken at each of two or more visits after an initial screening.
Modified from National Heart, Lung, and Blood Institute: *The Sixth Report of the Joint Commission on Prevention, Detection, Evaluation and Treatment of High Blood Pressure (JNC VI)*, Pub No 98-4080, Bethesda, Md, 1997, National Institutes of Health.

Venous Thrombosis/ Thrombophlebitis

Venous thrombosis is an abnormal condition in which a thrombus (clot) develops within a vein. In contrast, thrombophlebitis is inflammation of a vein that may or may not be accompanied by a clot. The triad of stasis, damage to the inner layer of veins, and hypercoagulability usually is responsible for both venous thrombosis and thrombophlebitis. Either may occur in the lower extremity (Fig. 18-34), usually in deep veins, and are sometimes recognized by calf pain and tenderness when the foot is dorsiflexed (Homan's sign, described under venous assessment), dilated superficial veins, edema of the involved extremity, and increased circumference of the involved leg. In the upper extremity, either may occur in superficial veins and are recognized by redness, warmth, and tenderness over the affected area. Veins may be visible and palpable.

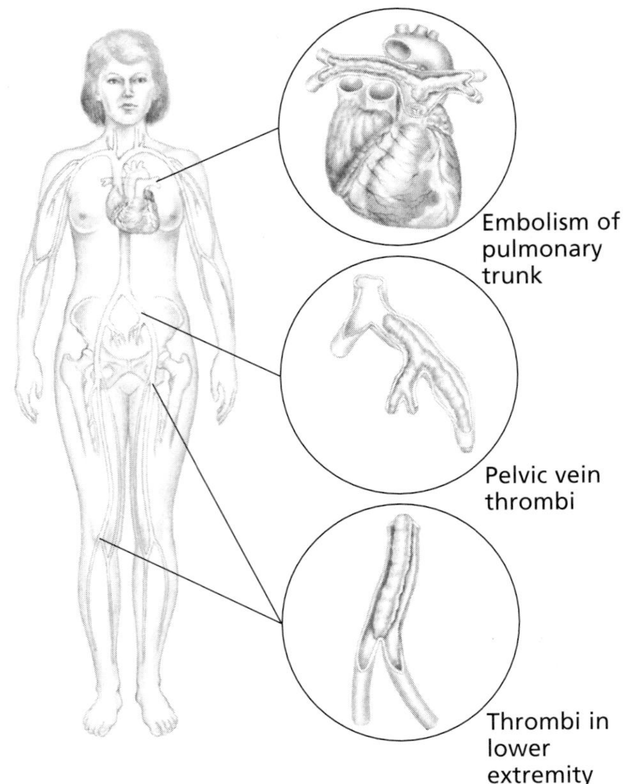

Fig. 18-34 Sites of venous thrombosis. (From Canobbio, 1990.)

Peripheral Atherosclerosis Disease (Arteriosclerosis Obliterans)

Chronic arterial insufficiency that occurs when atherosclerotic plaques occlude the blood supply to the legs is called arteriosclerosis obliterans. A primary symptom is intermittent claudication, which produces leg pain, cramping, and aching during exercise that is relieved by a brief rest period. Progressive occlusion results in severe ischemia, in which the leg or foot becomes cold and numb and skin appears dry and scaly with poor hair and nail growth.

Raynaud's Phenomenon and Disease

An idiopathic intermittent spasm of arterioles of the digits, nose, and ears is known as Raynaud's phenomenon or disease. Vasospasms may last minutes to hours and may occur bilaterally. They are secondary to connective tissue diseases such as scleroderma, rheumatoid arthritis, and systemic lupus erythematosis, and to drug intoxication, myxedema, and primary pulmonary hypertension. Signs and symptoms include blanching of the extremities followed by cyanosis, then redness along with numbness, tingling, burning, and pain. Ulcers may form on the tips of the digits. The diagnosis of Raynaud's disease is applied when there is a history of symptoms for at least 2 years with no progression of symptoms and no evidence of underlying cause.

Arterial Aneurysm

Localized dilation of an artery caused by weakness in the arterial wall is called an arterial aneurysm (Fig. 18-35). Aneurysms occur anywhere along the aorta and iliac vessels; abdominal aortic aneurysm is most common. A thrill or bruit may be noted over the aneurysm.

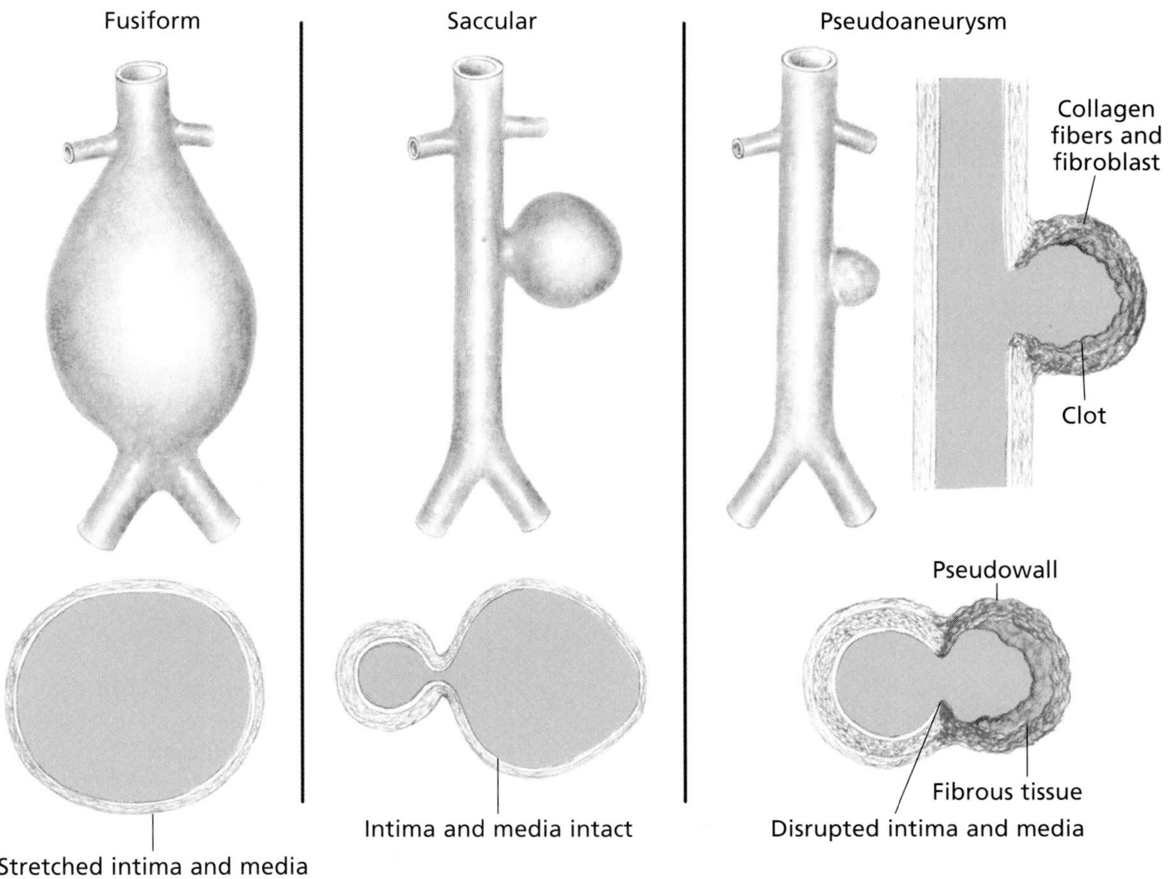

Fig. 18-35 Arterial aneurysm. (From Canobbio, 1990.)

CLINICAL APPLICATION and CRITICAL THINKING

SAMPLE DOCUMENTATION

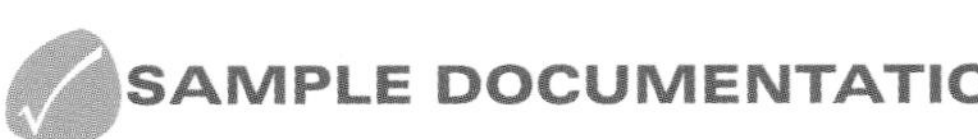

CASE 1

R.D is a 45-year-old male who is here for an annual physical examination as required by his employer.

Subjective Data

Has no presenting complaint. Had appendectomy at age 15 and vasectomy at age 44. Does not remember last medical examination; last dental examination was 2 years ago. Father had myocardial infarction at age 47; died from second MI at age 54. Paternal grandfather died of heart attack at age 65; paternal grandmother died of breast cancer at age 50. "Heart attacks just run in my family." Married with two teenage sons, employed full time as engineer. Worked for this company for 1 year, likes job; becomes stressed with deadlines every 2 to 3 months. Rarely exercises, currently smokes ½ pack of cigarettes per day; 10-pack-year history. Interested in stopping smoking since there are "so few places I can smoke anymore." No medications; no alcohol use, no use of street drugs.

Objective Data

Alert, cooperative, healthy-appearing man.

Height, 6′1″ (185 cm); weight, 190 lb (86 kg); Temperature, 98.5° F (36.9° C); Pulse, 88; Respiratory rate, 16.

Blood pressure, 150/95 mm Hg, right arm—sitting; 148/97 mm Hg, left arm—sitting.

Serum cholesterol, 230 mg/dl.

Heart: No lifts, heaves, or pulsations on inspection or palpation. PMI palpable at fifth ICS, MCL, S_1 loudest at apex, and S_2 loudest at base; regular rate and rhythm without murmur or S_3 or S_4.

Pulses: Temporal, carotid, brachial, radial, femoral, posterior tibial, dorsalis pedis 2+, symmetric. No carotid bruits.

Extremities: Warm, dry without pallor, cyanosis, or edema; elastic skin turgor, usual male hair distribution.

Functional Health Patterns Involved

- Health perception–health maintenance
- Cognitive–perceptual

Nursing Diagnosis and Collaborative Problems

- *Altered health maintenance* related to inadequate information about exercise, healthy diet, stress reduction, and lowering blood pressure as manifested by:
  - Rarely exercises
  - Eats whatever he desires
  - Smokes ½ pack per day
  - Family history of heart disease
  - Stressful job
  - Cholesterol 230 mg/dl
  - Blood pressure 150/95 mm Hg
- *Knowledge deficit* related to stopping smoking as manifested by:
  - Smokes ½ pack per day; 10-pack-year history
  - Desires to stop smoking

CASE 2

J.J. is a 79-year-old African-American man with complaints of cold feet and hair loss on legs.

Subjective Data

Reports changes in his feet over the last 6 months. Has pain in calf when walking; pain subsides with rest. Toes with burning sensation; increased pain in feet when he elevates his feet when sitting in recliner. Reports no other problems or illnesses. Lives with wife in apartment with small garden, which he cares for; volunteers at the church. Smokes 1½ packs of cigarettes per day; has 52-pack-year history.

Objective Data

Alert, cooperative man with a slow gait.

Temperature, 97.8° F (36.5° C); Pulse, 88 beats/min; Respiratory rate, 20; Blood pressure, 140/88 mm Hg.

Lower extremities: Glossy, cool, smooth skin; pallor that increases with elevation of extremity; hair loss of lower leg bilaterally.

Ulceration: (1 cm) over lateral malleolus with clear exudate. Numbness in tips of toes bilaterally.

Pulses, pressure: Temporal, carotid, brachial, radial strong and symmetric. Femoral, posterior tibial and dorsalis pedis palpable by Doppler. Capillary refill >2 sec. Bruits over abdominal and femoral arteries.

Functional Health Patterns Involved

- Nutrition–metabolic
- Activity–exercise
- Cognitive–perceptual

Medical Diagnosis

Peripheral arterial vascular disease.

Nursing Diagnosis and Collaborative Problems

- *Pain* related to reduced oxygenation to peripheral tissue as manifested by:
  - Pain in legs with activity
  - Pain in legs when elevated
  - Complaint of burning sensation in toes.
- *Altered peripheral tissue perfusion* related to arterial insufficiency as manifested by:
  - Glossy, cool, smooth skin
  - Pallor that increases with elevation of extremity
  - Hair loss of lower leg bilaterally
  - Bruits over abdominal and femoral pulses, increased capillary refill
- *Impaired skin integrity* related to inadequate circulation as manifested by:
  - Ulceration over lateral malleolus (1 cm) with clear exudate
  - Decreased capillary refill
- *Risk for impaired physical mobility* related to insufficient perfusion of lower extremities
- *PC*: Peripheral vascular insufficiency

CRITICAL THINKING QUESTIONS

1. A 10-year-old girl is brought to the clinic by her mother. The mother tells the examiner that the girl has been very tired and short of breath and has been running a low grade fever. These symptoms have been getting progressively worse over the last few weeks. The only significant health history is treatment for strep throat last month. What specifically should the examiner focus on to aid in the diagnosis?
2. Mr. Yazzie is a 42-year-old American Indian with type 1, or immune-mediated, diabetes mellitus. He is seen in the clinic for an ulcer on his right foot that does not heal. In taking the pulses of his lower right leg, you can palpate the femoral and popliteal pulses. What additional assessment do you need to perform?
3. Mr. Dexter tells you he is awakened at night, needing to urinate. He has not had this problem in the past. What relevance does this symptom have to cardiac functioning? What additional questions should be asked of Mr. Dexter?
4. Mrs. Murphy has brought her 3-month-old male infant to the clinic. She says he doesn't eat well and has been losing weight. Upon further questioning, you learn that the infant takes only 1 ½ oz with each feeding and that Mrs. Murphy is feeding him every couple of hours or so. What significance do these symptoms have?

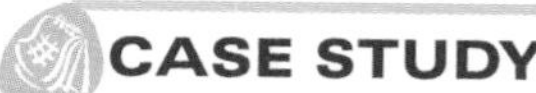

CASE STUDY

Howard is a 76-year-old man complaining of difficulty breathing. Listed below are the initial data collected.

Interview Data

Howard doesn't know exactly when his breathing difficulty started, but it has gotten noticeably worse the last couple of days. He volunteers at the church library three mornings a week and plays golf twice a week. However, he tells the examiner that this last week he has "just felt too tired to do anything." Howard says that he has not been able to sleep very well at night because of his breathing difficulty. He adds, "I keep coughing out this bubbly-looking phlegm." Howard denies taking any medications. He says that he doesn't smoke or drink alcoholic beverages.

Examination Data

- **General survey:** Alert, anxious, cooperative, well-groomed male. Appears stated age. Breathing is labored.
- **Vital signs:** Temperature, 98.8° F (37.1° C); Pulse, 120 beats/min; Respiration, 26: Blood pressure, 142/112 mm Hg, right arm, 144/110 mm Hg, left arm.
- **Pulses:** All pulses palpable 2+. No carotid bruits bilaterally.
- **Neck:** Jugular distension and pulsation noted with client in supine position.
- **Lower extremities:** Skin warm and dry, without cyanosis. Even hair distribution. 2+ pitting edema noted bilaterally; no lesions present.

1. What data deviate from normal findings, suggesting a need for further investigation?
2. What additional information should the nurse ask or assess for?
3. In what functional health patterns does data deviate from normal?
4. What nursing diagnosis and/or collaborative problems should be considered for this situation?

REMEMBER to check out your **companion CD-ROM**

19 Breasts and Axillae

www.mosby.com/MERLIN/wilson/assessment/

ANATOMY AND PHYSIOLOGY

The breasts are paired mammary glands located on the ventral surface of the thorax, within the superficial fascia of the anterior chest wall. Breasts are a feature of all mammals, evolving as milk-producing organs to provide nourishment for offspring. During embryologic development these paired glands develop along paired "milk lines," an embryonic ridge that extends between the limb buds of what will become the axillae and the inguinal regions. Normally, only one gland develops on each side in the pectoral region. After birth, the glands undergo little additional development in the male. In the female, however, the breasts undergo considerable development during adolescence, under the influence of estrogen and progesterone.

FEMALE BREAST

The breast of the mature female has a distinctive shape; however, there is a tremendous variation in "normal" breast size and volume. The breasts extend vertically from the second or third rib to the sixth or seventh intercostal space and laterally from the sternal margin to the midaxillary line. The breast is divided into four quadrants by an imaginary vertical and horizontal line intersecting at the nipple (Fig. 19-1).

The female breast is composed of three types of tissue: glandular tissue, fibrous tissue, and subcutaneous and retromammary fat tissue (Fig. 19-2). The glandular tissue is arranged into 15 to 20 lobes per breast, radiating around the nipple in a circular, spokelike pattern. Each lobe is composed of 20 to 40 lobules, or alveoli, containing the milk-producing acini cells. During lactation, milk produced by acini cells empties into the lactiferous ducts. A lactiferous duct drains milk from the lobes to the surface of the nipple. The largest amount of glandular tissue lies in the upper outer quadrant of each breast. From this quadrant, the breast tissue extends into the axilla, forming the axillary tail of Spence. The breast is supported by a layer of subcutaneous fibrous tissue and by multiple fibrous bands called Cooper's ligaments. These sensory ligaments extend from the connective tissue layer and run through the breast, attaching to the underlying muscle fascia. Subcutaneous and retromammary fat surrounds the glandular tissue and composes most of the bulk of the breast.

Centrally located on the breast, the nipple is surrounded by the pigmented areola. The nipples are composed of epithelium intertwined with circular and longitudinal smooth muscle fibers. These muscles contract in response to sensory, tactile, or autonomic stimuli, producing erection of the nipple and causing the lactiferous ducts to empty. A number of sebaceous glands, called Montgomery's glands, are located within the areolar surface, aiding in lubrication of the nipple during lactation.

Throughout the reproductive years, the breasts undergo a cyclical pattern of size change, nodularity, and tenderness during the menstrual cycle. The breasts are smallest during days 4 through 7 of the menstrual cycle. Three to four days before the onset of menses, many women experience breast tenseness, fullness, tenderness, and pain because of hormonal changes and fluid retention.

The breasts undergo a dramatic change during pregnancy and lactation in response to luteal and placental hormones. These changes include an increase in the number of lactiferous ducts and an increase in the size and number of alveoli. Refer to Chapter 26 for further information.

Lymphatic Network

Each breast contains an extensive lymphatic network, which drains into lymph nodes in several areas. More than 75% of lymph drainage from the breast flows outward toward the axillary lymph node groups and then upward to the subclavicular and supraclavicular nodes (Romrell and Bland, 1998). Other routes for lymph drainage include flow through the interpectoral nodes (above the breast), internal mammary nodes (in the thorax), subdiaphragmatic nodes (toward the abdomen), and through cross-mammary pathways to the opposite breast (Fig. 19-3). Palpation of lymph nodes in the axilla and supraclavicular areas are included with breast examination because they are accessible and may provide clues regarding the presence of inflammation or lesions.

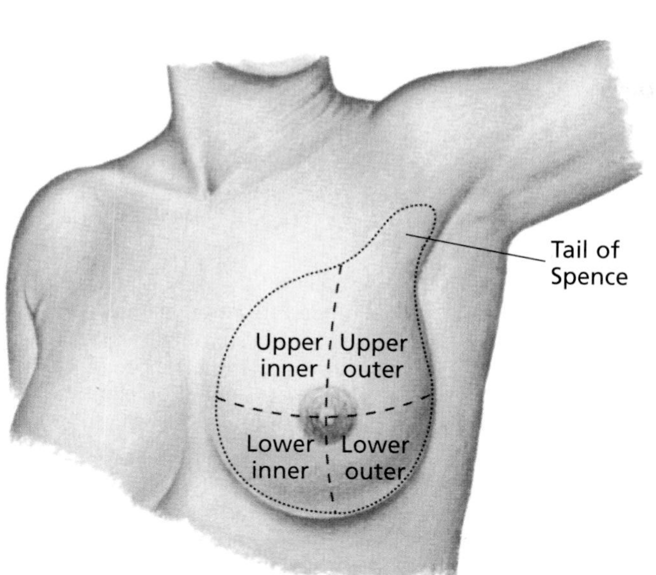

Fig. 19-1 Quadrants of the left breast and axillary tail of Spence. (From Seidel et al, 1999.)

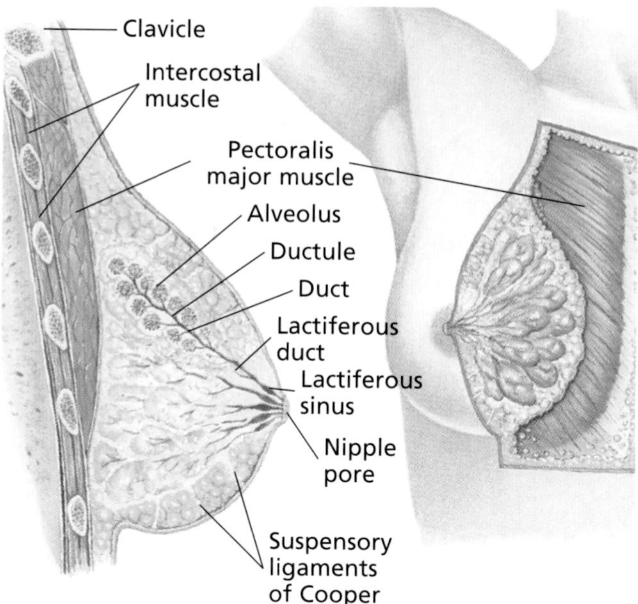

Fig. 19-2 Anatomy of the breast, showing position and major structures. (From Seidel et al, 1999.)

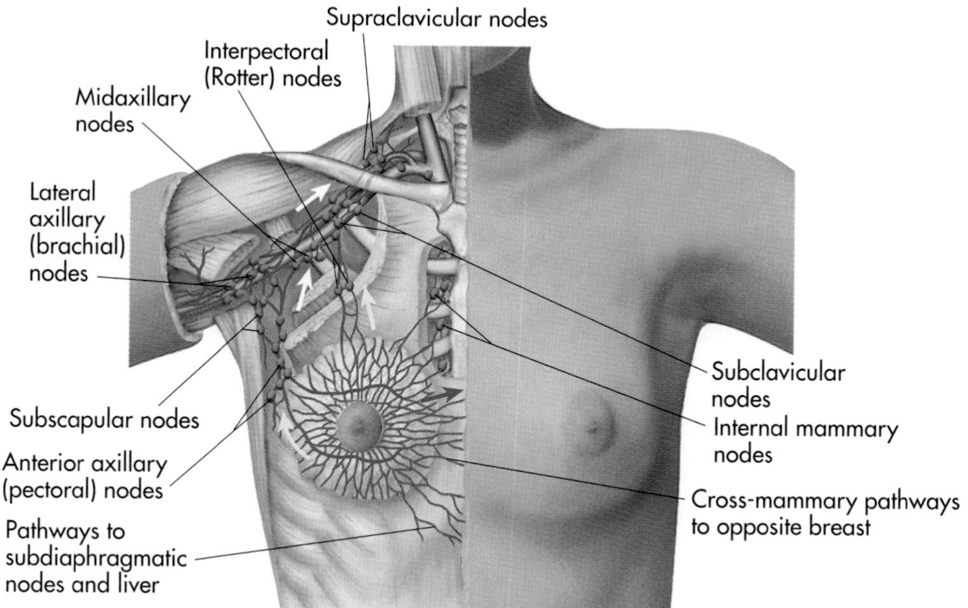

Fig. 19-3 Lymphatic drainage of the breast. (From Seidel et al, 1999.)

MALE BREAST

The male breast undergoes very little additional development after birth, and the gland remains rudimentary. It consists of a thin layer of undeveloped tissue beneath the nipple. The areola of the nipple is small when compared with the female counterpart. During puberty, the male breast may become slightly enlarged, producing a temporary condition called gynecomastia. Although gynecomastia is usually unilateral, it may occur bilaterally. The older male may also have gynecomastia secondary to a decrease in testosterone.

HEALTH HISTORY

Breasts and Axillae

QUESTIONS

RATIONALE

PRESENT HEALTH STATUS

Self-Care Pattern

➤ Do you perform breast self-examination? If so, how often? When do you do this?

■ Evaluating self-care behaviors will help guide further education and encouragement of health-enhancing behaviors. It is important to determine not only if the client performs self-breast examination, but also if it is done routinely and correctly.

➤ Have you ever had a mammogram? If so, when was your last mammogram? How frequently do you have a mammogram?

■ It is important to note if and when a baseline mammogram was done. It is recommended that a baseline be done by the time a woman is 40 (American Cancer Society, 1998). Routine mammograms are done based on age, risk factors, and clinical findings.

➤ What medications do you currently take?

■ Some medications such as oral contraceptives can cause cyclic breast discomfort or nipple discharge.

➤ How much chocolate and caffeine do you consume each day or each week?

■ A diet high in methylxanthines (found in foods containing caffeine) may cause benign breast disease such as fibrocystic changes to the breast.

➤ Do you take any vitamin supplements? If so, which vitamins?

■ Some individuals take vitamin supplementation to reduce symptoms of breast swelling and tenderness.

PAST MEDICAL HISTORY

➤ Have you ever had breast problems such as fibrocystic breast changes, fibroadenomas, or breast cancer? If so, describe. When? How was it diagnosed? How was it treated?

■ A history of breast cancer increases the risk of recurrences. Fibrocystic breast complicates the evaluation of the breasts because the general lumpiness of the breast makes it difficult to detect new lumps.

➤ Have you ever had surgery on a breast? If so, when was it, and what was it for? Was it a biopsy? Mastectomy? Lumpectomy? Mammoplasty, either to reduce or augment your breast(s)?

■ This is helpful background information; it may impact findings noted with examination.

➤ How old were you at menarche and/or menopause?

■ Menarche before age 12 or menopause after age 55 increases the risk for breast cancer.

➤ Have you ever been pregnant? If so, at what age did you have your children?

■ Nulliparous or first child born after age 30 is a risk factor for breast cancer.

QUESTIONS

RATIONALE

FAMILY HISTORY

➤ Is there a history of breast cancer or breast disease in your family? If so, in whom? At what age did this relative have breast cancer or disease? How was the cancer treated? What were the results?

■ If first-degree relatives have breast cancer, it is helpful to know if it affected one or both breasts and if the onset was premenopausal or postmenopausal. A family history of breast cancer occurring before menopause increases the risk for a woman having cancer (Ziegfeld, 1998).

RISK FACTORS

COMMON RISK FACTORS ASSOCIATED WITH Breast Cancer

Female gender
Age (incidence increases dramatically with age after 40)
Personal history of cancer
First-degree relatives with breast cancer
Menarche before age 12
Menopause after age 55
Nulliparous or first child after 30 years of age

PROBLEM-BASED HISTORY (FEMALE)

The most commonly reported problems related to the breasts are pain or tenderness, breast lump, nipple discharge, and pain or lumps in the axillae. As with symptoms in all areas of health assessment, a symptom analysis is completed, which includes the location, quality, quantity, chronology, setting, associated manifestations, alleviating factors, and aggravating factors. (See Box 4-2 in Chapter 4.)

Breast Pain or Tenderness

➤ Do you ever have pain or tenderness in your breasts? If so, when did you first become aware of it?

■ Establish the onset of the breast pain. Determine if this is a new pain, or if this has been occurring for some time.

➤ Describe the pain. Is it like an ache? Sharp pain? Gnawing pain? Rate the severity of the pain on a scale from 1 (not very painful) to 10 (very painful). Does the pain or tenderness prevent you from carrying out routine activities?

■ Determine the characteristics of the pain. Cystic disease of the breast and breast cancer may not have any associated pain. On the other hand, some women with breast cancer report a burning or pulling sensation in addition to a vague pain. Rapidly growing cysts may be very painful. Limitations in activity may also help the examiner understand how the pain affects the client.

➤ Where does it hurt? Is it in one breast or both? Is there a specific location, or is the pain general? Can you point to the area that hurts? Is the area tender to the touch?

■ Determine the location of the pain. Pain occurring bilaterally is more likely attributed to hormonal effects; pain in one breast could suggest a pathologic condition.

QUESTIONS

➤ Is the pain constant, or does it come and go? When have you noticed the pain occurs? Does the pain come and go in relation to your menstrual cycle?

RATIONALE: ■ Determine the duration of the pain. Discomfort that is associated with the menstrual cycle is a common finding caused by hormonal fluctuations.

➤ Have you noticed any specific activities that bring on the pain? For example, do you experience pain during sexual activity? When you exercise? When wearing a certain bra, or when not wearing a bra?

RATIONALE: ■ Determine any aggravating factors for the pain. Strenuous activity can bring on pain, as can the other specific causes noted.

➤ Have you noted any recent changes in your breasts, such as changes in size, shape, skin characteristics, or tenderness? Is the breast pain associated with a breast lump? Nipple discharge? Nipple retraction?

RATIONALE: ■ Question the client for associated symptoms with the breast pain such as fullness, discharge, and nausea.

➤ Is the breast tenderness associated with a swollen feeling to the breasts? If yes, when do you notice the swelling? Is the swelling related to your menstrual cycle? Has the swelling been significant enough to increase your bra size?

RATIONALE: ■ Cyclic bilateral breast swelling or fullness is a normal occurrence caused by hormonal fluctuations associated with the menstrual cycle. Significant swelling should be further evaluated, especially if it is unilateral, has other associated findings, or influences the woman's ability to participate in normal activities.

Breast Lump

➤ Have you noticed a lump in your breast? If so, where is this lump? How long have you had it?

RATIONALE: ■ Establish the onset and location of all breast lumps. Some lumps may be present over a period of several years. If such lumps do not undergo change, they may be insignificant but still should be carefully examined. Any new lumps or changes in a previously identified lump should be of particular concern.

➤ Is the lump tender to the touch? If yes, does the severity of the tenderness change related to menstruation?

RATIONALE: ■ Determine the characteristics of the lump. Some lumps are tender—others painless. The degree of pain or tenderness may be affected by hormonal fluctuations.

➤ Is the lump always present, or does it seem to come and go? If always present, does it seem to change in size related to your menstrual cycle? If it comes and goes, does the lump appear related to your menstrual cycle?

RATIONALE: ■ Lumps that change in size in relation to the menstrual cycle may be influenced by hormonal fluctuations.

➤ Have you recently suffered any trauma to the breasts? If yes, did the lump develop after the injury?

RATIONALE: ■ Lumps resulting from an injury may be associated with a hematoma. Typically these will resolve in a short period of time.

➤ Have you noticed any other symptoms such as redness, swelling, or dimpling associated with this lump?

RATIONALE: ■ Determine associated changes to the breast—redness, localized heat, rash, and dimpling are all symptoms requiring further evaluation.

Nipple Discharge

➤ Have you noticed any discharge from either nipple? If so, how long has this been going on? Have you ever noticed this before?

RATIONALE: ■ Determine onset and duration of nipple discharge.

➤ Describe the discharge. Color? Is it thick or thin? Is there an odor associated with the discharge? Does the discharge occur at specific times, such as always before your menstrual period or with breast manipulation?

RATIONALE: ■ Nipple discharge may indicate a pathologic condition. A bloody or blood-tinged discharge is an alarming finding and must be investigated.

QUESTIONS | **RATIONALE**

➤ Is the discharge from one or both breasts?

■ Unilateral nipple discharge is a concerning finding because it is more commonly associated with a pathologic condition than is bilateral nipple discharge (Morrison, 1998).

➤ Does the discharge occur spontaneously, or does it only occur when expressed?

■ If the discharge is spontaneous, it is helpful to know if this occurs intermittently or constantly. Spontaneous discharge is considered an abnormal finding. Discharge that is not spontaneous may result from medications or from endocrinologic causes (Morrison, 1998).

➤ Have you noticed other symptoms such as breast pain or a breast lump? Have you been having headaches or changes in your vision?

■ Determine if there are any other associated breast symptoms or onset of other symptoms. Headaches or changes in vision along with nipple discharge may suggest a pituitary tumor or mass (Morrison, 1998).

➤ Are you taking any medications, such as oral contraceptives, phenothiazines, digitalis, diuretics, or steroids?

■ Several medications can cause clear nipple discharge, such as those listed on the left.

Breast Skin Characteristics

➤ Have you had any changes to the skin on your breasts such as a rash? If so, when did you first become aware of it? Where did you first notice the rash? Has it spread? If so, describe. Is the rash found on one or both of your breasts? Is the rash just on your breasts, or is it elsewhere on your body?

■ Note the onset, location, and duration of the rash. A rash on the breast could be caused by dermatitis, breast-feeding, or Paget's disease of the breast. A rash found on both breasts and skin elsewhere on the body is likely to be dermatitis, whereas a unilateral breast rash suggests another pathologic condition.

➤ Have you noticed any other symptoms such as itching or bleeding?

■ Associated symptoms may provide important clues to the cause of the rash.

➤ Have you recently changed detergents, soaps, perfumes, lotions, etc?

■ Sometimes a rash on the breasts or axilla can be traced back to an irritation by a substance applied by the client or to irritation from detergent used to clean clothes.

➤ What have you done to treat the rash, if anything?

■ Explore self-care practices; this may be helpful to guide future treatment strategies.

Axilla Characteristics

➤ Have you noticed any pain or tenderness in the area under your arms? Any lumps? If so, when did this begin?

■ Since the tail of Spence extends up into the axilla, and since most lymphatic drainage flows toward the axillary nodes, a symptom analysis for lumps and/or tenderness is in order. Determine the onset of symptoms.

➤ Where is the lump or tenderness located? Under one arm or both arms? Does this come and go, or is it always present? Has the tenderness or lumps gotten worse?

■ Determine the location and characteristics of the lump or tenderness.

QUESTIONS

RATIONALE

➤ Do you shave your underarms? If so, how often? Do you notice a relationship to shaving your arms and the tenderness? Do you use deodorant or antiperspirant under your arms?

■ Shaving and/or use of deodorants and antiperspirants can cause discomfort and a mild inflammation to the axilla.

➤ What have you done to treat this, if anything?

■ Explore self-care practices; this may be helpful to guide future treatment strategies.

PROBLEM-BASED HISTORY (MALE)

➤ Have you noticed any enlargement or swelling in either of your breasts? If so, what is the change, and when did it occur? Has the swelling been on one or both sides?

■ Gynecomastia is the enlargement of one or both breasts in the male. Although it may occur at any time, it is most prevalent during puberty and in the older adult man.

➤ Do you have any masses in either breast? If so, what are their locations? Are they tender or nontender?

■ Breast cancer in men is very uncommon. However, the most common presenting symptom is a breast mass.

➤ Have you noticed any discharge from either one or both of your nipples?

■ Nipple discharge is an uncommon associated symptom of breast cancer in the male, but when it occurs, it is usually bloody or serosanguineous (Morrison, 1998).

EXAMINATION

Equipment

- Small pillow or towel (to place under the client's shoulder)
- Ruler marked in centimeters (to measure lesions or masses)
- Examination gloves (if there is suspicion of nipple discharge or tissue lesions)
- Glass slide and cytologic fixative (if nipple discharge is present)

PROCEDURES AND TECHNIQUES WITH NORMAL FINDINGS

ABNORMAL FINDINGS

FEMALE

Always explain the procedure to the client before you begin. Let her know you will be touching her breasts, and be sure to obtain her permission before you begin the examination. Initially, position the client so she is sitting on the examination table facing you. She should be sitting erect with her gown dropped to the waist (Fig. 19-4). Following the breast inspection, assist the client into a supine position so the breasts and nipples may be palpated.

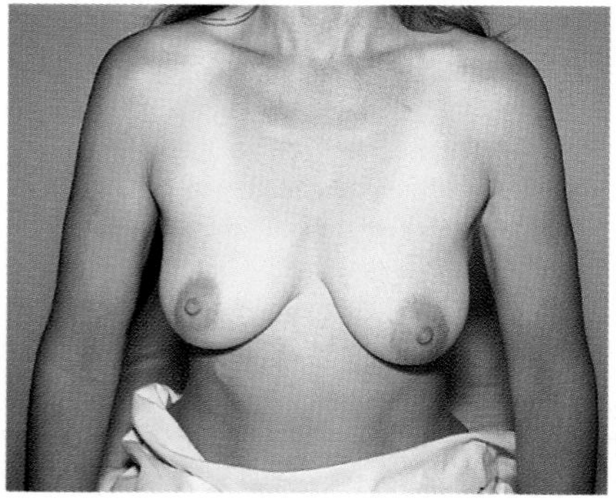

Fig. 19-4 Client should be seated, arms at sides, with gown dropped to the waist.

PROCEDURES AND TECHNIQUES WITH NORMAL FINDINGS

➤**INSPECT both breasts, noting size, shape, and symmetry.** It is common for the breasts to be slightly unequal in size. Breast size may vary significantly, but symmetry or only slight asymmetry should be considered normal. The breast contour should be smooth, convex, and even.

Gently lift each breast with your fingers and inspect the lower and outer aspects of each breast for dimpling or different characteristics.

➤**INSPECT the skin of the breasts for appearance, color, pigmentation, vascularity, surface characteristics and lesions.** The skin of the breast should appear smooth and evenly pigmented. The venous patterns should be bilaterally similar. The venous pattern may be pronounced in obese or pregnant females.

ABNORMAL FINDINGS

■ Note evidence of marked asymmetry of size and/or shape of the breasts. Significant and rapid changes in the size of one breast could indicate an inflammatory process or a growth.

■ Note any localized or generalized areas of discoloration or change in surface characteristics such as dimpling, retraction, or bulging. Inflammation, cellulitis, or breast abscess in the breast tissue may cause surface erythema and heat (Fig. 19-5). Unilateral hyperpigmentation is also considered an abnormal finding.

■ Unilateral venous patterns on the breast may occur secondary to dilated superficial veins from a increased blood flow to a malignancy.

■ Note any roughened, tough skin, lesions, or thickening. Edema may give the skin a peau d'orange texture, like an orange (Fig. 19-6).

■ Note any lesions or newly developed moles or those that have changed or are tender.

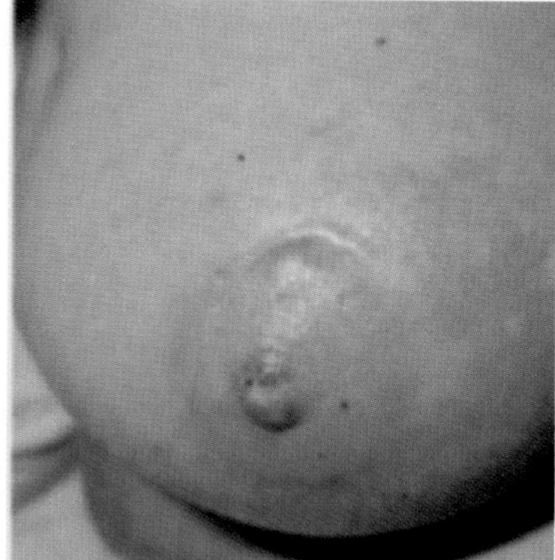

Fig. 19-5 Erythema of the breast. (From Swartz, 1994.)

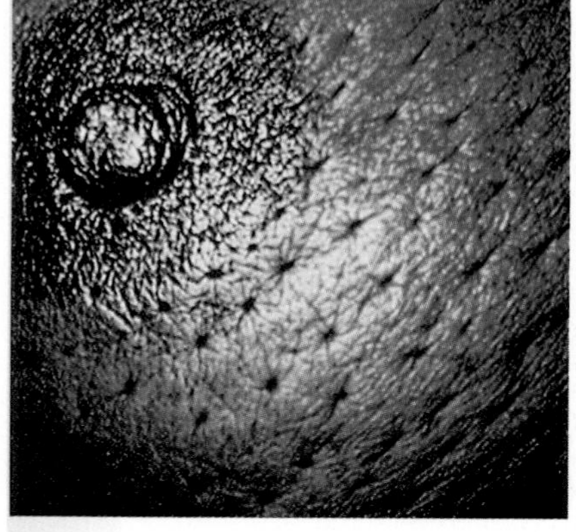

Fig. 19-6 Peau d'orange appearance caused by edema. (From Gallager et al, 1978.)

PROCEDURES AND TECHNIQUES WITH NORMAL FINDINGS

➤**INSPECT the areolae for color and surface characteristics.** The color of the areolae may vary depending on the client's skin color. Figure 19-7 shows the variations of areola color, ranging from pink to black. The areolae should be round or oval and should appear bilaterally similar. Montgomery's tubercles (Fig. 19-7, *B*) may appear as slightly raised bumps on the areola tissue. Hairs on the nipple may also be seen. These are all normal variations.

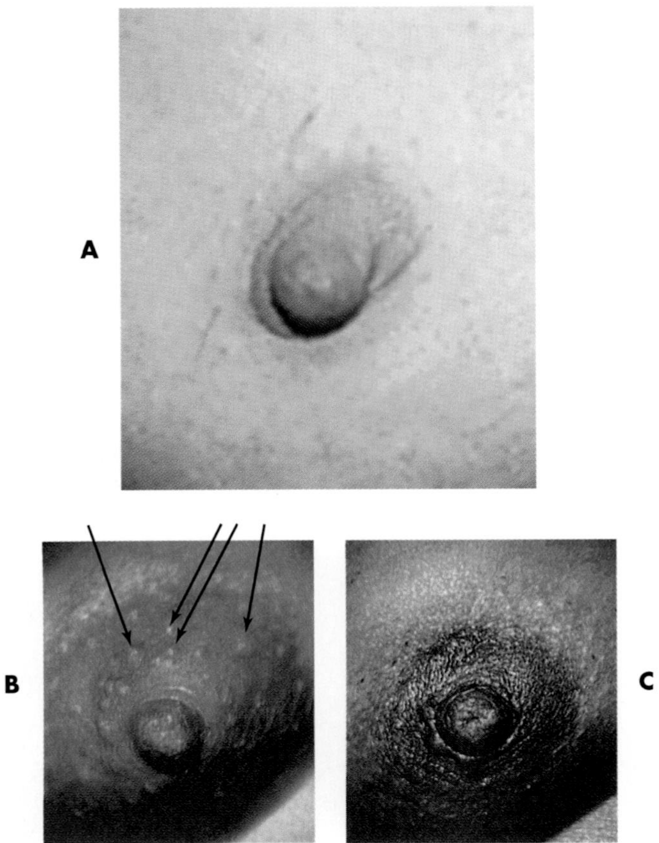

Fig. 19-7 Variations in color of areola. **A,** Pink. **B,** Brown. **C,** Black. Note presence of Montgomery's tubercles in **B.** (**B** and **C** from Seidel et al, 1999.)

ABNORMAL FINDINGS

- Areolae that are unequal bilaterally, other than round or oval, with obvious masses or lesions and with pigment changes, either bilaterally or unilaterally, are abnormal.

PROCEDURES AND TECHNIQUES WITH NORMAL FINDINGS

➤INSPECT the nipples for position and symmetry. Most women's nipples protrude, although some may appear to be flat or actually inverted. All should be considered normal if they have remained unchanged throughout adult life. Normal nipple inversion may be unilateral or bilateral and can usually be everted with manipulation (Fig. 19-8).

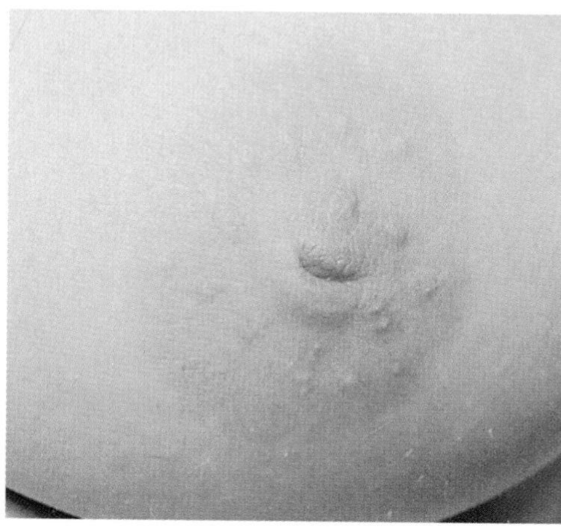

Fig. 19-8 Nipple inversion. (From Mansel and Bundred, 1995.)

ABNORMAL FINDINGS

- Nipples that point in different directions, or those that are not symmetric should be considered abnormal.
- Recent change in the nipple such as inversion or retraction is suggestive of malignancy, and the client should be referred for further evaluation (Fig. 19-9).

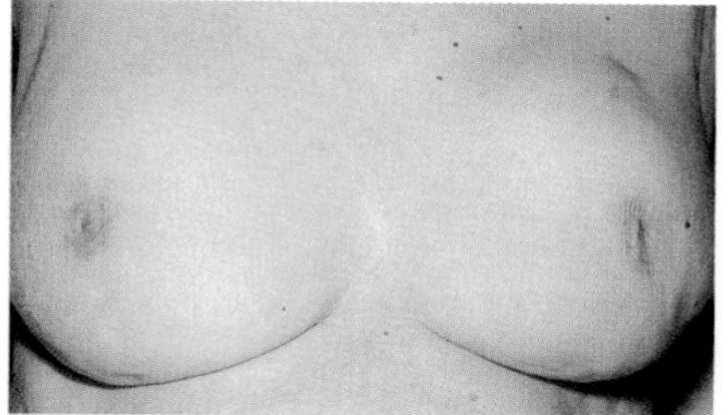

Fig. 19-9 Nipple retraction. (From Mansel and Bundred, 1995.)

PROCEDURES AND TECHNIQUES WITH NORMAL FINDINGS

➤INSPECT the nipples for intactness, scaling, lesions, bleeding, or discharge. Nipples are normally smooth and intact without evidence of crusting, bleeding or discharge. If the nipple appears to have drainage or a lesion, put on gloves before actually touching the nipple.

Note presence of supernumerary nipples. Supernumerary nipples are considered a normal variation, although they are fairly uncommon. These nipples look similar to pink or brown moles and generally appear along the embryonic "milk line" (Figs. 19-10 and 19-11).

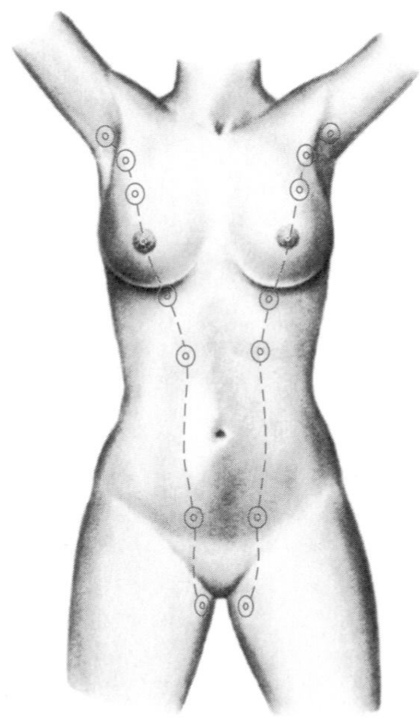

Fig. 19-10 Supernumerary nipples and tissue may arise along the "milk line," an embryonic ridge. (From Thompson et al, 1997.)

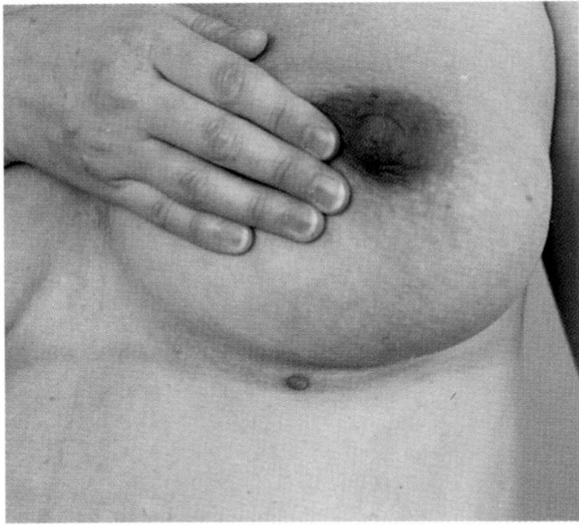

Fig. 19-11 Supernumerary nipple without glandular tissue. (From Seidel et al, 1999.)

ABNORMAL FINDINGS

■ Deviations from normal include nipple edema, redness, pigment changes, ulceration or crusting, erosion or scaling, and wrinkling or cracking. Recent development of nipple discharge should be considered abnormal until further evaluation. Any discharge should be saved for cytologic examination. (See Box 19-1.)

■ A red, scaly nipple with discharge and crusting that lasts more than a few weeks could indicate a rare type of breast cancer called Paget's disease of the breast.

Box 19-1 Preparation of Nipple Discharge for Cytologic Evaluation

EQUIPMENT
- Examination gloves
- Cotton-tipped applicator
- Clear microscopic slide
- Cytologic fixative

STEPS
1. Wearing gloves, gently squeeze the nipple to express a small amount of discharge.
2. Use a cotton-tipped applicator to collect a small sample of the discharge.
3. Using a rolling technique, smear the specimen on the slide and spray with the cytologic fixative.
4. Label the specimen with the client's name, date, and source—right or left breast. On the requisition, describe the characteristics of the discharge and other relevant clinical information, such as duration of discharge.

PROCEDURES AND TECHNIQUES WITH NORMAL FINDINGS

❖ ➤**COLLECT nipple discharge specimen for cytologic examination.** This is done only if nipple discharge is present (Box 19-1). Note the color, consistency, and odor of the nipple

ABNORMAL FINDINGS

■ There are several types of nipple discharge (Table 19-1).discharge.

Table 19-1 Nipple Discharge

COLOR OF DISCHARGE	POSSIBLE CAUSE
Serous (yellow)	Usually normal
Serosanguineous (straw colored)	Carcinoma Ductal ectasia
Sanguineous (bloody)	Carcinoma Intraductal papilloma Ductal ectasia Prepartum women from vascular engorgement
Clear (watery)	Pharmacologic causes Carcinoma
Milky	Pituitary adenoma Pharmacologic causes Galactorrhea
Purulent	Infectious process Ductal ectasia
Multicolored (green, gray, brown)	Fibrocystic changes Carcinoma Infectious process Ductal ectasia

PROCEDURES AND TECHNIQUES WITH NORMAL FINDINGS

➤**INSPECT the breasts in various postures for bilateral pull, symmetry, and contour.** Ask the client to remain seated and raise her arms over her head (Fig. 19-12, *A*). This position adds tension to the suspensory ligaments and will accentuate dimpling or retractions. Observe and compare all of the areas already mentioned. Then evaluate for any bilateral pull on the suspensory ligaments. It should be equal on both sides, so that the breasts are bilaterally symmetric.

With her arms still raised, have the client lean forward (Fig. 19-12, *B*). It may be helpful for the nurse to hold onto the client's hands to provide balance.

Inspect the breasts for symmetry and bilateral pull, as previously described. The breasts should hang equally with a smooth contour, and pull should be symmetric. This is an especially useful technique if the client has large and pendulous breasts, because the breasts will fall away from the chest wall and will hang freely.

Next, inspect the breasts while the seated client pushes her hands onto her hips or pushes her palms together, thus contracting the pectoral muscles (Fig. 19-12, *C*). There should be no deviations in contour and symmetry.

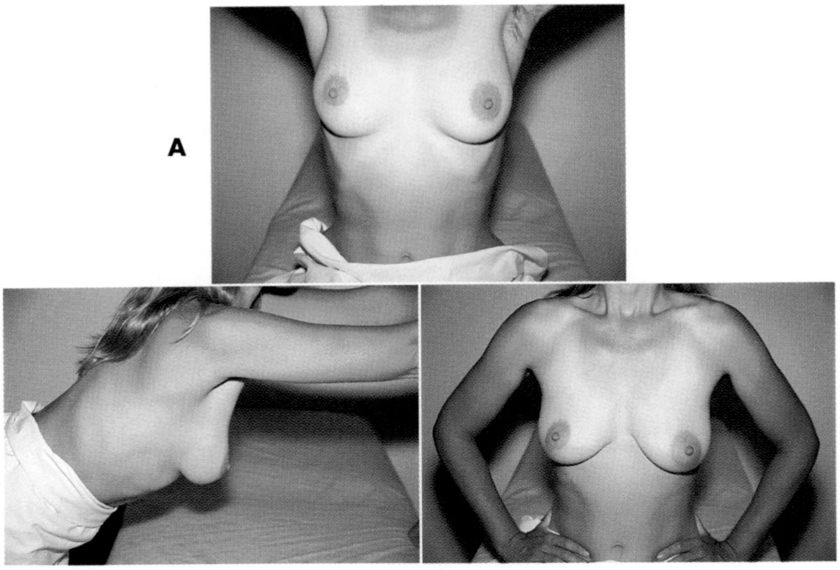

A

B

C

Fig. 19-12 **A,** Client with arms extended overhead. **B,** Client with arms raised and leaning forward. **C,** Client sitting and pressing her hands on hips.

ABNORMAL FINDINGS

- Note any asymmetry or appearance of attachment (fixation) of either breast.
- Note asymmetry or any bulging retraction. Note fixation as described previously.

PROCEDURES AND TECHNIQUES WITH NORMAL FINDINGS

➤INSPECT and PALPATE the axillae for evidence of rash, lesions, or masses. While the client is still in the sitting position, instruct the client to lift each arm. Next, instruct the client to relax both arms at her sides. Using your hand (generally your left if you are right-handed), lift one of the client's arms and support it so that her muscles are loose and relaxed (Fig. 19-13). While in this position, use your other hand (right if you are right-handed) to palpate each axilla.

Reach your fingers deep into the axilla, and slowly and firmly slide your fingers along the client's chest wall, first down the middle of the axilla, then again along the anterior border of the axilla, and finally along the posterior border. Then turn your hand over and examine the inner aspect of the client's upper arm. (CAUTION: You must have short fingernails to adequately perform this maneuver.) During all maneuvers, position the client's arm with your other hand to maximize the examining area. In all positions, palpate for areas of enlargement, masses, lymph nodes, or isolated areas of tenderness. Repeat with the client's other arm.

If the client has a rash or lesion in the axilla, be sure to wear examining gloves during the palpation.

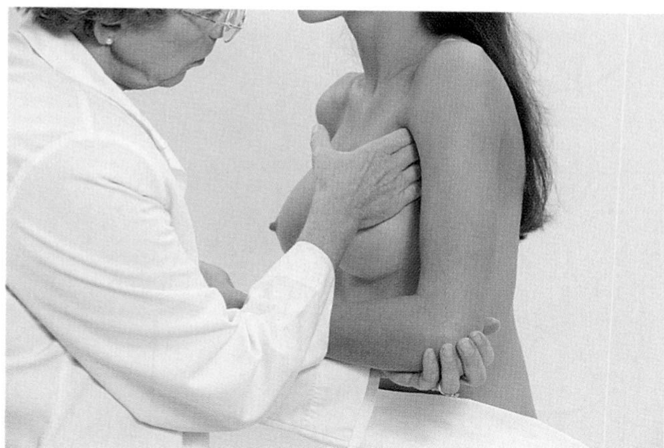

Fig. 19-13 Raise and support client's arm while palpating axilla.

➤PALPATE the breast for tissue characteristics. Assist the client into a supine position and place a small pillow or towel under the shoulder of the breast to be examined. Instruct the client to place her arm over her head. The combination of the slight shoulder elevation and the arm positioning flattens the breast tissue evenly over the chest wall. Other position options are provided in Box 19-2.

ABNORMAL FINDINGS

■ Infections in the breast, arms, and even the hand may have lymphatic drainage into the axillary area. Enlargement and tenderness of lymph nodes in the axilla may indicate such an infection. Hard, fixed nodules or masses may suggest metastatic carcinoma or lymphoma.

■ Breasts that are engorged (very full and hard) are an abnormal finding in clients who are not pregnant or premenstrual.

PROCEDURES AND TECHNIQUES WITH NORMAL FINDINGS

ABNORMAL FINDINGS

Using the finger pads of the first two or three fingers of your examining hand, gently, firmly, and systematically palpate all four quadrants of the breast and the tail of Spence (see Fig. 19-2). Use a systematic approach to breast palpation that begins and ends at a designated point. This will ensure that all areas of the breast are examined. There are several motions that may be used for breast palpation (Table 19-2).

The breast should feel firm, smooth, and elastic. After pregnancy or menopause, the breast tissue may feel softer and looser. During the premenstrual period, the client's breasts may be engorged, slightly tender, and have generalized nodularity.

Table 19-2 Methods for Breast Palpation

CIRCULAR METHOD

This is the most common palpation technique. Place the finger pads of your middle three fingers against the outer edge of the breast. Press gently in small circles around the breast until you reach the nipple. Try not to lift your fingers off the breast as you move from one point to another.

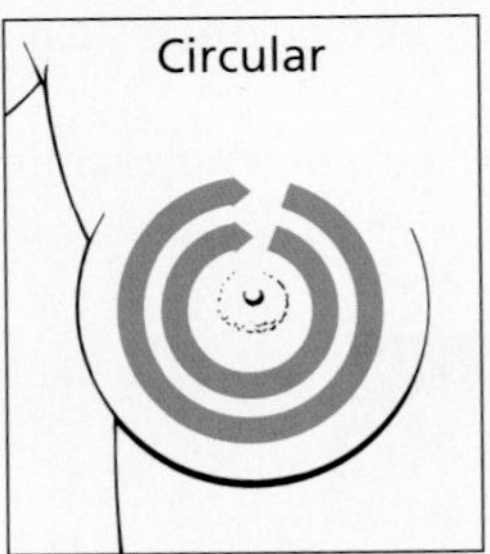

WEDGE METHOD

Place the finger pads of your middle three fingers on the areola, and palpate from the center of the breast outward. Return your fingers to the areola and again palpate from center outward covering another section of the breast (in a spokelike fashion). Repeat this until the entire breast has been covered.

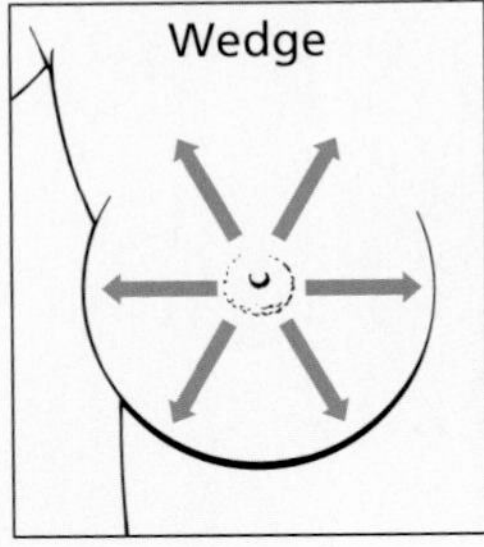

VERTICAL STRIP METHOD

Place the finger pads of your middle three fingers against the top outer edge of the breast. Palpate downward, then upward working your way across the entire breast.

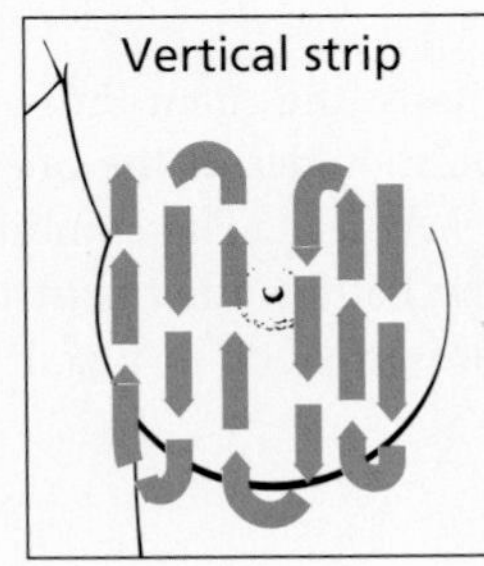

PROCEDURES AND TECHNIQUES WITH NORMAL FINDINGS

➤**PALPATE the breast for masses, nodules, or tenderness.** Press firmly enough to get a good sense of the underlying tissue, but not so firmly that the tissue is compressed against the rib cage. Do not lift your fingers from the chest wall during the palpation. This will break the continuity of the palpation. Instead, gently slide your fingers over the breast tissue, moving along the designated pattern of palpation (Fig. 19-14).

Most women have a firm transverse ridge along the lower edge of the breast called the inframammary ridge. This firm ridge is normal and should not be mistaken for a breast mass.

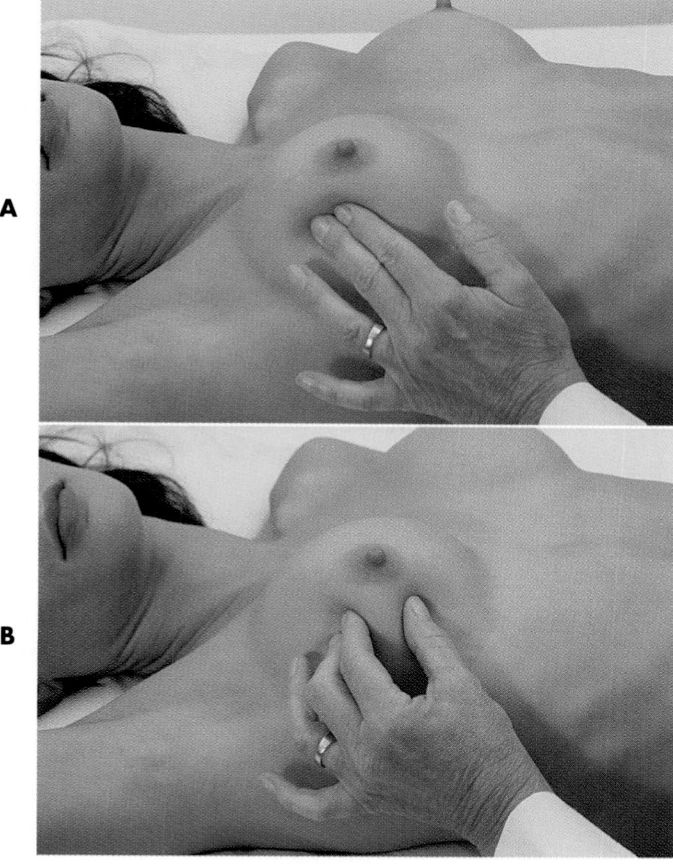

Fig. 19-14 **A,** Palpating for consistency of breast lesion. **B,** Palpating for delineation of borders and mobility of breast mass.

ABNORMAL FINDINGS

■ Abnormal findings during the breast palpation include masses or isolated areas of tenderness or pain. If a mass is identified, note its specific location, size, shape, consistency, tenderness, mobility, delineation of borders, and retraction (Box 19-3). Transillumination may be used to confirm the presence of fluid in superficial masses.

Box 19-3 Breast Mass Characteristics

Note and record the following:

- *Location:* Which breast; which quadrant (may describe as position on the clock or draw on chart to show location).
- *Size:* Measure the width, length, and thickness in centimeters.
- *Shape:* Is the mass oval, round, lobed, irregularly shaped, or indistinct?
- *Consistency:* Is the mass hard, soft, or firm, or rubbery?
- *Tenderness:* Is the mass tender during palpation?
- *Mobility:* Does the lump move during palpation or is it fixed to the overlying skin or the underlying chest wall?
- *Borders:* Are the edges of the mass discrete or poorly defined?
- *Retractions:* Is there any dimpling of the tissue around the mass?

Modified from Seidel HM et al: *Mosby's guide to physical examination,* ed 4, St. Louis, 1999, Mosby.

PROCEDURES AND TECHNIQUES WITH NORMAL FINDINGS

ABNORMAL FINDINGS

Box 19-2 Positioning Options for Breast Palpation

Although the supine position is usually the preferred position for breast palpation, alternative positions may be indicated. A sitting position may be used if the client has difficulty lying down, if the client is young and has very small breasts, or if the client has very large breasts making it difficult to palpate her breasts while in a supine position.

If the sitting position is used for a woman with large breasts, assist her to a sitting position and instruct her to lean slightly forward. Take the breast between your hands and, while supporting the inferior side of the breast with one hand, use the other hand to palpate the breast (Fig. 19-15). Start at the top of the breast and slowly and purposefully feel the underlying breast tissue while sliding the top examining hand's fingerpads down the breast. Repeat the technique until all breast tissue is examined. As with the previously described techniques, do not lift your fingers during the palpation. Be sure to include the tail of Spence in the palpation.

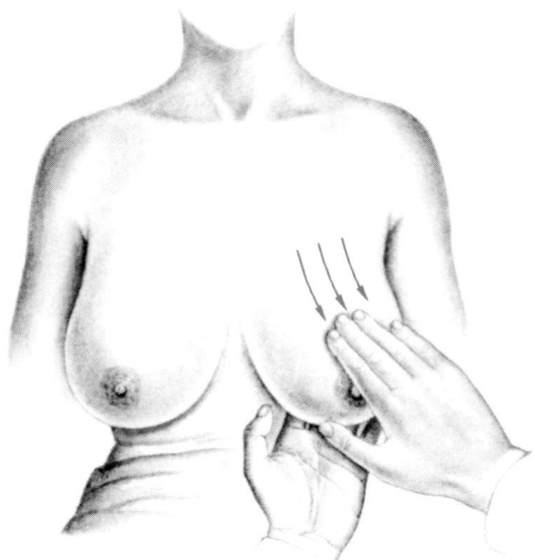

Fig. 19-15 Manual palpation of large breasts. (From Seidel et al, 1999.)

PROCEDURES AND TECHNIQUES WITH NORMAL FINDINGS

➤PALPATE the nipples for surface characteristics and discharge. With the client in the supine position, palpate the nipples. To do this, gently compress the nipple between your index finger and thumb (Fig. 19-16). Inspect the nipple for discharge. If a discharge is present, note the color, consistency, and odor. Gently palpate the area around the nipple to determine if the origin of the discharge can be ascertained. It is advisable to wear gloves during the nipple palpation to protect the examiner from possible discharge contamination.

When the palpation of the first breast is completed, place the towel or pillow under the other shoulder, instruct the client to lift her arm above her head, and repeat the entire procedure.

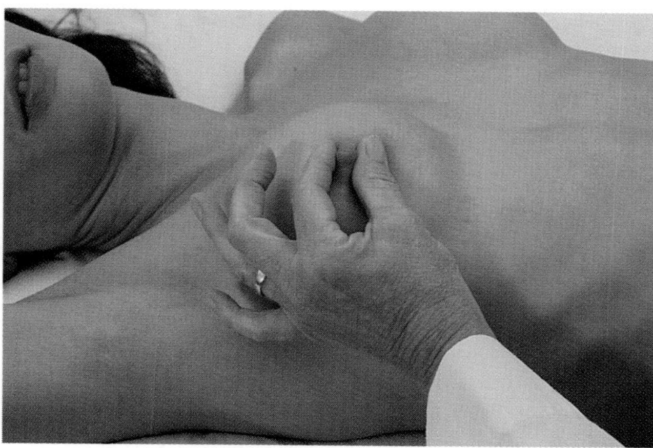

Fig. 19-16 Palpating the nipple.

➤TEACH breast self-examination (BSE). Use the opportunity of breast examination to teach the woman breast self-examination. If she states that she already does this, have her briefly show you what she does and explain how often she does it and what she looks or feels for during the self-assessment. Be sure to explain that this should be performed at the same time each month. (Box 19-4 provides a full discussion of the breast self-examination procedures.)

ABNORMAL FINDINGS

■ Nipple discharge may occur secondary to fluid retention of the ducts, infection, hormonal flux, or carcinoma. If a nipple discharge is present, a specimen should be sent for cytologic evaluation. (The directions for preparing a smear are discussed in Box 19-1.)

■ BSE is a simple method that is thought to be helpful in the identification of breast mass.

PROCEDURES AND TECHNIQUES WITH NORMAL FINDINGS

ABNORMAL FINDINGS

Box 19-4 Teaching Breast Self-Examination

Teach the client to do breast self-examination by instructing the following:

1. Undress and stand in front of a mirror with your arms at your sides. Look for any changes in the shape or size of your breasts or anything unusual, such as discharge from the nipples or puckering or dimpling of the skin.
2. Raise your arms above and behind your head, and press your hands together. Look for the same things as in Step 1.
3. Place the palms of your hands firmly on your hips; look again for any changes.
4. Raise your left arm over your head. Examine your left breast by firmly pressing the fingers of your right hand down and around in a circular motion until you have examined every part of your breast. You may use the wedge section, circular, or vertical strip examination method *(instruct the client in one of these three techniques; see Table 19-2 for directions).* Be sure to include the area between your breast and armpit and the nipple itself. You are feeling for any lump or mass under the skin. If you find a lump, notify your health care provider.
5. Apply gentle pressure with both hands on the breast and stroke toward the nipple. Look for any discharge. If there is any, notify your health care provider.
6. Repeat Steps 4 and 5 on your right breast. (You may also perform Steps 4 and 5 in the shower.)
7. Now, lie down on your back with a pillow under your right shoulder. Put your right arm over your head. This position flattens the breast and makes it easier to examine. Examine your right breast just as you did in Steps 4 and 5. Repeat the examination on your left breast.

From *Mosby's patient teaching guides,* St. Louis, 1995, Mosby.

MALE

As part of a comprehensive examination, it is essential to examine the male client's breasts. Inspect the male breast while the client is seated with his arms at his sides.

➤**INSPECT the breasts and nipples.** With the client in a seated position, inspect both breasts, looking for breast symmetry, color, skin lesions, and enlargement. The breasts should be flat and without rashes or lesions. Men who are overweight often have a thicker fatty layer of tissue on the chest, giving the appearance of breast enlargement. If this is noted, it is important to assess the client's situation with a careful history of weight gain. If the client reports that his breasts became full as he gained weight, the condition is most likely within normal limits.

The nipple and areolar areas should be intact, smooth, and of equal color, size, and shape bilaterally.

■ Note any asymmetry or distinct differences between the two sides. Note any ulcerations, masses, or swelling. If the client reports a sudden bilateral or unilateral breast enlargement with associated tenderness, the examiner should consider the situation possibly abnormal and should send the client for further evaluation.

PROCEDURES AND TECHNIQUES WITH NORMAL FINDINGS	ABNORMAL FINDINGS
➤**PALPATE the breasts and nipples.** With the client in the same position, palpate the breasts and areolar areas. The tissue should feel smooth, intact, and nontender. Note evidence of tenderness, unilateral enlargement, or masses. Gently compress the nipples of both breasts to assess for nipple discharge.	■ Unilateral or bilateral breast enlargement in men may be gynecomastia, which may occur secondary to a hormonal imbalance, liver failure, or certain medications. (See Common Problems and Conditions later in this chapter for a more detailed discussion.) ■ Breast cancer can occur in men. It most commonly presents as a hard, painless, irregular nodule often fixed to the area under the nipple or in the upper outer quadrant of the breast. Breast cancer affected approximately 1,400 men in the United States in 1997 (Parker et al, 1997).
➤**PALPATE the axilla.** If not already done as part of the lymphatic assessment, palpate the client's axillary area for tenderness or lymphatic enlargement.	■ Palpation of the axilla of a male client provides information about the lymphatic system. Lymph nodes should not be palpable, or should be small, soft and nontender.

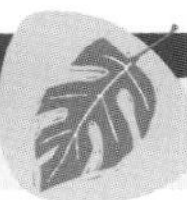

AGE-RELATED VARIATIONS

■ INFANTS AND YOUNG CHILDREN

Anatomy and Physiology

The function and structure of the breast changes throughout life. Breast development is latent during infancy and childhood, with only minimal branching of primary ducts occurring. Before age 10 little difference exists in the appearance of male and female breasts. The nipples are small and slightly elevated. No palpable glandular tissue or areolar pigmentation exists.

Health History

Generally, there are no questions for infants or young children. Newborns may have hypertrophic breast tissue with full raised areola buds. This is a normal phenomenon that lasts 1 to 2 months. Should a parent report that the infant or young child has any breast symptoms such as breast redness or swelling or increased pigmentation around the areola, then further questioning about hormonal or systemic problems is necessary.

Examination

Procedures and Techniques The examination of the newborn's breasts may be done quickly and easily. The infant should be lying supine and be undressed to the waist. Young children should also be disrobed for the breast and chest examination. With a little encouragement, most children will generally readily remove their tops, exposing the chest and breast area.

Normal and Abnormal Findings Newborns of both genders may have full, slightly enlarged breasts secondary to the mother's estrogen level before the infant was born (Fig. 19-17). The newborn may have a small amount of watery or milky nipple discharge, also secondary to maternal hormones. This discharge is commonly referred to as "witch's milk." Both the discharge and breast swelling are normal findings and should last only a few days to a few weeks.

■ SCHOOL-AGE CHILDREN

Anatomy and Physiology

Before the onset of puberty, the breasts remain small and only slightly elevated. However, breast development begins during the preadolescent phase, usually preceding the onset of menarche by approximately 2 years. Tanner (1962) has described the five stages of breast development in the female (Fig. 19-18). Stage 1 is the preadolescent phase that begins for most girls during the late grade school or early middle school years. During this stage, the nipple is only slightly raised above the level of the breast and still appears as in younger children.

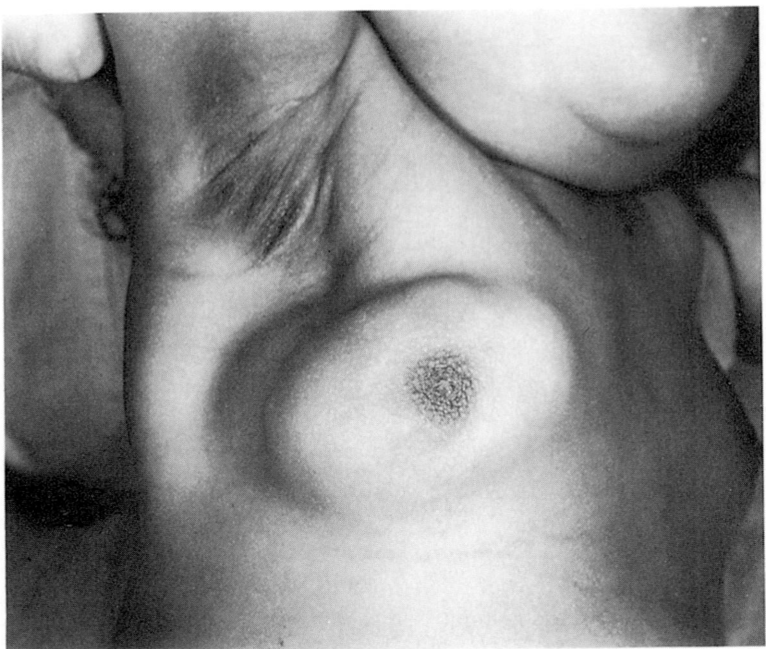

Fig. 19-17 Marked enlargement of breast bud in neonate. This is an exaggerated response to maternal hormones. (From Gallager et al, 1978.)

Health History

Girls

- Have you noticed your breasts changing? If so, when did this start? Have you noted other changes in your body that come with growing up? What changes have you noticed?
  Rationale Breast development is the most obvious sign of puberty, and girls focus a great deal of attention on this development. It occurs about the same time as the growth spurt and before the onset of pubic hair development and menarche.
- How do you feel about these changes?
  Rationale Evaluate the adolescent's perception of the changes she is undergoing, and provide teaching and guidance as needed.

Boys

- Have you noticed any tenderness, redness, lumps, or inflammation in the breast area? If so, is it on one side or both sides?
  Rationale Hypertrophy may be normal for stocky or heavy boys, but the symptoms noted should be evaluated for possible gynecomastia secondary to hormonal changes or systemic disease.

Examination

Procedures and Techniques School-age girls may show increasing modesty as they get older. The nurse should be sensitive to this but should also provide a gown for the girl and then use a matter-of-fact approach to expose the girl's entire chest area for a complete breast examination.

School-age boys will usually expose their chest without embarrassment. If the boy is obese and has slightly enlarged breast tissue, he may be self-conscious.

Normal and Abnormal Findings Although the breast should be examined at each well-child evaluation, no significant findings are generally noted until puberty. As noted above, obese children may have slightly full bilateral breast tissue. Any unilateral breast enlargement or changes may be abnormal and should be further evaluated.

As the girl reaches prepubertal age, sometimes as young as age 8, her breasts will show prepubertal budding (see Fig. 19-18). At this time the breasts change from flat to slightly convex. Although both breasts may not appear exactly alike, they should both show maturational development. If only one breast shows development, other causes for the enlargement such as a cyst or hormonal imbalance must be evaluated.

■ ADOLESCENTS

Anatomy and Physiology

Thelarche (breast development) represents an early sign of puberty in adolescent females. At this time the estrogen hormones stimulate breast changes. Between the ages of 10 and 14, the mammary tissue beneath the areola begins to grow. The diameter of the areola increases, and a "mammary bud" is formed. The nipple and breast protrude as a single mound. Eventually the nipple begins to separate from the areola as the breasts become further elevated. The full development of the breast from Tanner stages 2 through 5 (see Fig. 19-18) takes an average of 3 years (range 1½ to 6 years). Menarche begins when the breasts reach stages 3 or 4, usually just after the peak of the adolescent growth spurt, which is about age 12 (Fig. 19-19). Tanner developed the stages from studies conducted on British white females. Because of

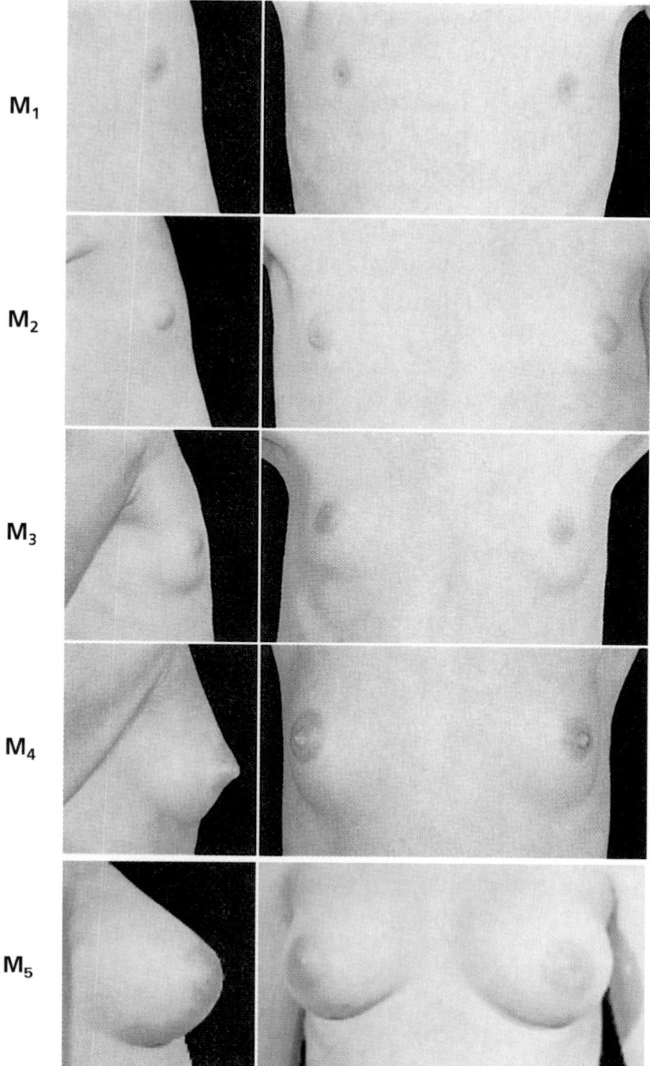

Fig. 19-18 Tanner's five stages of breast development in females. M_1—Only the nipple is raised above the level of the breast, as in the child. M_2—Budding stage: bud-shaped elevation of the areola. On palpation, a fairly hard "button" can be felt, disk- or cherry- shaped. Areola increased in diameter and surrounding area slightly elevated. M_3—Further elevation of the mamma. Diameter of areola increases further. Shape of mammary tissue now visibly feminine. M_4—Increasing fat deposits. The areola forms a secondary elevation above that of the breast. This secondary mound apparently occurs in roughly half of all young females and in some cases persists in adulthood. M_5—Adult stage. The areola (usually) subsides to the level of the breast and is strongly pigmented. (From Van Wieringen et al, 1971. Reprinted by permission of Kluwer Academic Publishers.)

this, the nurse is cautioned about generalizing the stages to other cultural groups. For example, Harlan (1980) found that African-American girls developed secondary sex characteristics earlier than white girls of the same age.

By age 14, most females have developed breasts that resemble those of the adult female. The continuing breast development, including size and form, is affected by heredity, nutrition, and individual sensitivity to hormones.

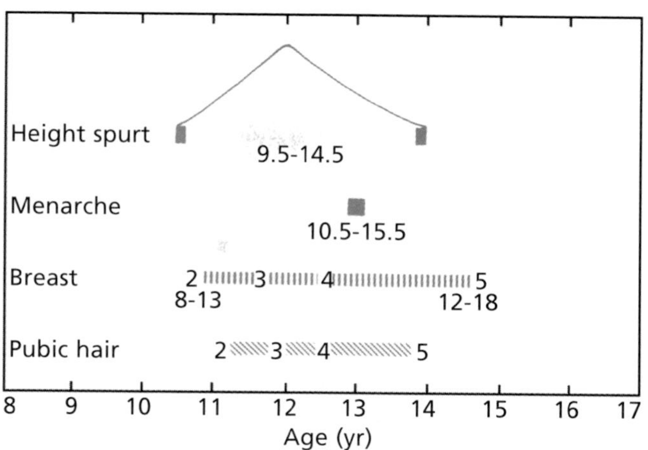

Fig. 19-19 Summary of maturational development of girls. See Fig. 19-18 for explanation of numbers 2 through 5. Number ranges in graph (e.g., 9.5-14.5) indicate average or common range of age for development of characteristic. (From Marshall WA, Tanner JM: Variations in pattern of pubertal changes in girls, *Arch Dis Child* 44:291-303, 1969.)

Health History

Females

- Are your breasts developing? Are your breasts the same size, or is one larger than the other?

  Rationale It is common for the adolescent's breasts to develop at different rates. Usually the breast size equalizes by the end of adolescence. Occasionally the asymmetry remains after puberty and must be surgically corrected.
- Have you started your menstrual period yet? If yes, at what age did you begin?

  Rationale Information about the onset of menarche will provide general information about the adolescent's maturational development.
- Do you have any tenderness or pain in your breasts? Have you ever noticed any lumps or unusual areas of discoloration?

  Rationale Any report of a lump or localized area of tenderness requires further evaluation. If a mass is identified, it is most generally a benign tumor such as a fibroadenoma.
- Do you have any discharge or drainage from either or both of your nipples? If so, how often does it occur, and what does it look like? Do you use hormonal contraceptives?

  Rationale Hormonal contraceptives or breast manipulation may be a contributory factor to nipple discharge.

Males

- Have you noticed any tenderness, redness, or lumps in the breast or nipple area? If so, is the area tender or painful? Is it on one side or both sides?

Rationale Hypertrophy may be normal for stocky or heavy boys, but the symptoms noted should be evaluated for possible gynecomastia secondary to hormonal changes or systemic disease.

Examination

Procedures and Techniques The adolescent female may be sensitive to having her breasts exposed. The nurse should take time to reassure the client that although her privacy is important, it is also important to adequately expose the chest for a complete breast examination. The breast examination should include all of the components as presented in the discussion of the adult female. Note the developmental stage of the client. Adolescence is also the time to teach breast self-examination techniques and to stress the importance of regular self-examination.

Male adolescents should be taught that breast examination is also important for them and that, although infrequent, they may also develop diseases of the breast such as gynecomastia and breast cancer.

Normal and Abnormal Findings The right and left breasts may develop at different rates. It is important to reassure the client that this is very common and, in time, the development may equalize. The breast tissue in the adolescent female should feel firm and elastic throughout both breasts. Refer to the anatomy section of this chapter for a review of the developmental stages of the female breast to ensure that the client is adequately developing.

Male adolescents, especially obese males, may have transient unilateral or bilateral subareolar masses (Fig. 19-20). These firm and sometimes tender masses may be of great concern. Reassure the teen that these are generally transient and should disappear within a year or so. Gynecomastia, on the other hand, is an unexpected enlargement of one or both breasts in the male that may occur secondary to a hormonal imbalance, testicular or pituitary tumors, or illicit or prescription medications.

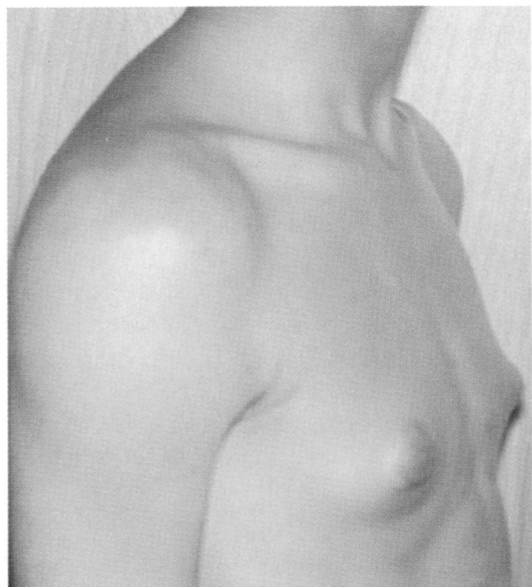

Fig. 19-20 Prepubertal gynecomastia. (Courtesy Wellington Hung, MD, Children's National Medical Center, Washington, DC. From Seidel et al, 1999.)

■ OLDER ADULTS

Anatomy and Physiology

By age 40, the breast begins atrophic changes. Before menopause, a moderate decrease in glandular tissue occurs. After menopause, the glandular tissue in the breast continues to atrophy and is replaced by fat and connective tissue. As the release of ovarian hormones diminishes, the acini cells of the alveoli degenerate and disappear, although some of the ducts remain. These changes to the breast tissue, and the relaxation of the suspensory ligaments, result in a tendency for the breast to hang more loosely from the chest wall, giving it a flattened appearance.

Health History

Women

- At what age did you reach menopause? Since that time, have you taken hormone therapy? If so, what is the name and dosage of the medication? Do you take it every day or just at certain times of the month?

  Rationale It is currently thought that a small association exists between hormone therapy and breast cancer. Although hormone therapy is not thought to cause breast cancer, it may increase the growth of an estrogen cancer should it occur.
- Do you have any irritation or rash under your breasts? If so, what do you do to treat it?

  Rationale It is common, especially during warm weather, for pendulous breasts to cause skin-to-skin contact irritation.

Examination

Procedures and Techniques Postmenopausal women should continue to have regular breast examinations. The techniques for examining the breasts in older women are the same as for younger women. Because the women are no longer subject to hormonal changes and menstruation, it may be difficult for the woman to remember to perform breast self-examination. The woman should be taught to pick one day each month (such as the day of her birth date) to perform the examination. Likewise, she should be encouraged to receive regular clinical breast examination (CBE) and mammograms.

Older males should also have a systematic breast examination. The techniques for examining the older adult man's breasts are the same as for the younger man.

Normal and Abnormal Findings The breasts in postmenopausal women may appear flattened and elongated or pendulous secondary to a relaxation of the suspensory ligaments.

Palpation findings that may be normal variations in the older adult include a granular feeling of the glandular tissue of the breast. If the woman had cystic disease earlier in life, her breasts are now more likely to feel smoother and less cystic. The inframammary ridge thickness may now be more prominent, and the nipples may be smaller and flatter.

CLIENTS WITH SITUATIONAL VARIATIONS

CLIENTS WITH A MASTECTOMY

Health History

Be sure to question the client about self-examination practices as well as other routine screening. The client should be encouraged to routinely perform monthly breast self-examination on the remaining breast and have regular screening (yearly clinical breast examination and mammography). Also explore with the client the impact the mastectomy has had on her. Many women experience anxiety and/or fear as they worry about the recurrence of cancer or metastasis. Some women may also have personal issues regarding self-concept and body image. Interview questions should be directed toward assessing these potential issues.

Examination

Women who have had a mastectomy require the same careful breast assessment as all other women. The woman may feel self-conscious about removing her brassiere and prosthesis, if she wears one. The examiner should be sensitive to this but should also reassure the client that it is necessary to perform a comprehensive examination. In addition to examining the remaining breast in the usual manner, careful assessment should be made of the mastectomy site, including the area of the scar (Fig. 19-21, *A*). If a malignancy recurs, it may be at the scar site. The mastectomy site and axilla should be inspected for color changes, redness, rash, irritation, and visible signs of swelling, thickening, or lumps. Note areas that may have had muscle resection. Also note any signs of proximal or distal lymphedema.

Using the finger pads of your examining hand, carefully palpate the side with the mastectomy, especially around the area of the scar. Use a small circular motion assessing for thickening, lumps, swelling, or tenderness, then use a sweeping motion to palpate the entire chest area on the affected side to ensure that nothing has been missed. Finally, palpate the axillary and supraclavicular areas for lymph nodes.

If the client has had breast reconstruction or augmentation, perform the breast examination in the usual manner. Pay particular attention to any scars and new tissue (Fig. 19-21, *B*).

Breast cancer is a major health problem for women and is the number one killer of women age 35 to 54 years. In-

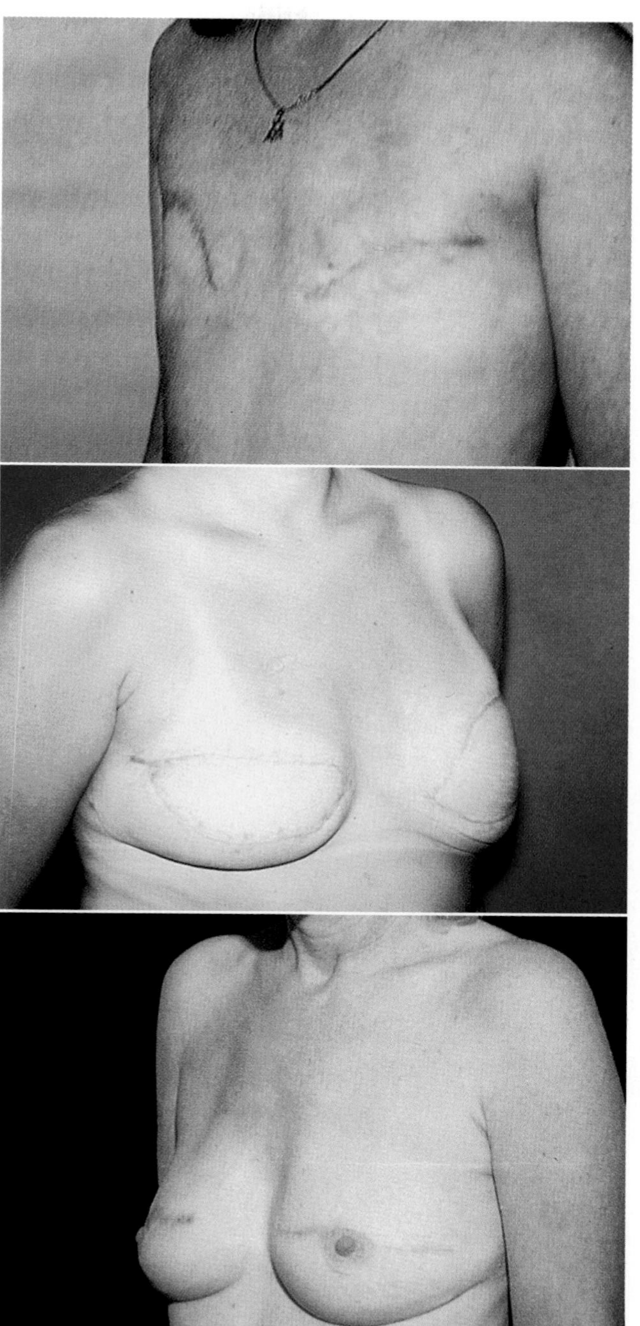

Fig. 19-21 **A,** Appearance of chest following bilateral mastectomy. Postoperative breast reconstruction before, **B,** and after, **C,** nipple-areolar reconstruction. (Courtesy Brian W. Davies. From Fortunato and McCullough, 1998.)

ETHNIC & CULTURAL VARIATIONS

Breast size, shape, and symmetry vary widely with individual women. Asian women tend to have smaller breasts than white women (Algaratnam and Wong, 1985). African-American women have a higher prevalence of supernumerary nipples (Christianson et al, 1981), but other racial differences in breasts are not well documented. African-American adolescents develop secondary sex characteristics, most notably breasts and axillary hair, at an early age. The onset of puberty in adolescent females continues to occur at a young age across all racial groups in the United States.

cidence of breast cancer varies widely across cultural lines for reasons that are not well understood. White women are more likely to develop breast cancer than women of any other racial or ethnic group; however, African-American women are more likely to die of breast cancer than women in other cultural or racial groups (Landis et al, 1999). Hispanic and Asian women are in the midrange of breast cancer incidence compared with other cultural and racial groups, whereas American Indian and Alaskan native women have the lowest incidence. There is a possible association of fat intake and incidence of breast cancer (Knobf, 1996).

EXAMINATION SUMMARY

PROCEDURE

Female

- Inspect the breasts for:
  Size
  Shape
  Symmetry
- Inspect the skin of the breasts for:
  Appearance
  Color
  Pigmentation
  Vascularity
  Surface characteristics
  Lesions
- Inspect the areolae for:
  Color
  Surface characteristics
- Inspect the nipples for:
  Position and symmetry
  Intactness
  Evidence of scaling, lesions, bleeding, or discharge
- Inspect the breasts in various positions for:
  Bilateral pull
  Symmetry
  Contour
- Inspect and palpate the axillae for:
  Evidence of rash, lesions, or masses
- Palpate the breasts and axillae for:
  Tissue characteristics
  Masses, nodules, tenderness
- Palpate the nipples for:
  Surface characteristics
  Discharge
- Teach breast self-examination

Male

- Inspect the breasts and nipples
- Palpate the breasts and nipples
- Palpate the axillae

SUMMARY OF FINDINGS

Age Group	Normal Findings	Typical Variations	Findings Associated With Disorders
Infants and young children	• At birth, breasts may be enlarged from maternal estrogen. • Newborns may also have milky nipple discharge.	• Supernumerary nipples may be present and may appear as moles.	
School-age children	• Breasts remain flat and unchanged until late childhood. Nipple budding is first indication of breast development.		• Female prepubertal breast enlargement (premature menarche).

Age Group	Normal Findings	Typical Variations	Findings Associated With Disorders
Adolescents	• Breasts of female adolescents in process of development. • Tanner's stages are useful to assess breast development. • Boys' breasts may be slightly enlarged (gynecomastia).	• Breasts develop at different rates that can cause increased temporary asymmetry. • During menstrual cycle there may be increased nodularity and tenderness.	
Adults	• Breasts are nearly equal in size and bilaterally convex. • Breasts have equal smoothness, contour, and pigmentation. • Slight venous markings are bilateral, and nipples and areolae are bilaterally equal.	• Breast size varies tremendously among women. Slight asymmetry of breasts common. Striae may be visible on breast. • Fibrocystic cysts, which are soft, mobile masses, are common. During menstrual cycle there may be increased nodularity and tenderness. • Both nipples may be bilaterally inverted.	• Breast mass, especially if unilateral, hard, fixed, stonelike mass. • Red scaling, crust patch on nipples; retractions or dimpling; thickened skin; unilateral breast drainage; unilateral venous patterns.
Older adults	• There is a gradual decrease in glandular, alveolar, and lobular tissue. • After menopause, glandular tissue atrophies and is replaced by fat; relaxation of suspensory ligaments also occurs, causing breast to hang more loosely from chest wall. • Men's breasts may be slightly enlarged (gynecomastia).	• Breasts of postmenopausal women may be flatter, and longer. • Breast tissue of older women becomes fine and soft.	• Blocked subareolar ducts of menopausal women (mammary duct ectasia); firm discolored irregular mass.

HEALTH PROMOTION

BREAST CANCER PREVENTION AND SCREENING RECOMMENDATIONS

Breast cancer is the leading cause of cancer involving females in the United States. It is estimated that 175,000 new cases of breast cancer are expected to occur among women during 1999 (American Cancer Society, 1998). Because of this, much attention has been directed at prevention and screening. Massive public education has had only marginal success in improving cancer detection (Nichols, 1996). It has been suggested that the perception of a client's cancer risk may differ from the biomedical risk factors preached by health care providers, which may partly explain the marginal success (Lawson, 1998).

Most authorities agree that a combination of screening methods is an important and necessary aspect of breast cancer detection and health promotion; however, there is a variety of opinion regarding frequency of examinations.

BREAST SELF-EXAMINATION

Breast self-examination has been recommended for over 40 years. The value of BSE comes under question primarily because only 15% to 40% of women reportedly perform this on a regular basis (Knobf, 1996). Nevertheless, all women should be taught to perform breast self-examination. The breasts should be examined at the same time each month—ideally between the fourth and fourteenth day of the menstrual cycle, when the breasts are least congested (see Box 19-4).

CLINICAL BREAST EXAMINATION

The CBE is a professional clinical examination of the breast. For women under the age of 40, it is suggested this be done every 1 to 3 years; for women over age 40 it should be done annually. This examination ideally should occur near the same time as a mammogram.

MAMMOGRAM

A baseline mammogram is recommended for women between ages 35 and 40. Depending on personal risk factors, mammograms are done every 1 to 2 years for women between the ages of 40 and 50. From age 50 and up, most recommend a mammogram every year, although some authorities suggest every other year is sufficient for those individuals with low-risk factors (U.S. Preventive Services Task Force, 1996). The American Cancer Society (1998), however, now recommends that all women over the age of 40 have annual mammograms.

COMMON PROBLEMS AND CONDITIONS

Breasts and Axillae

FEMALES

Fibrocystic Breast Condition

Fibrocystic breast condition is a benign mass of the breast caused by ductal enlargement and cyst formation (Fig. 19-22). The cysts are filled with fluid, which may be aspirated for diagnostic purposes. Typically, a fibrocystic condition will present bilaterally as well delineated, slightly mobile and tender lumps and occur in multiples. Premenstrually the breasts may be tender and have heavy dull pain. The disease is most prevalent in women ages 30 to 55 and will decrease after menopause (Table 19-3).

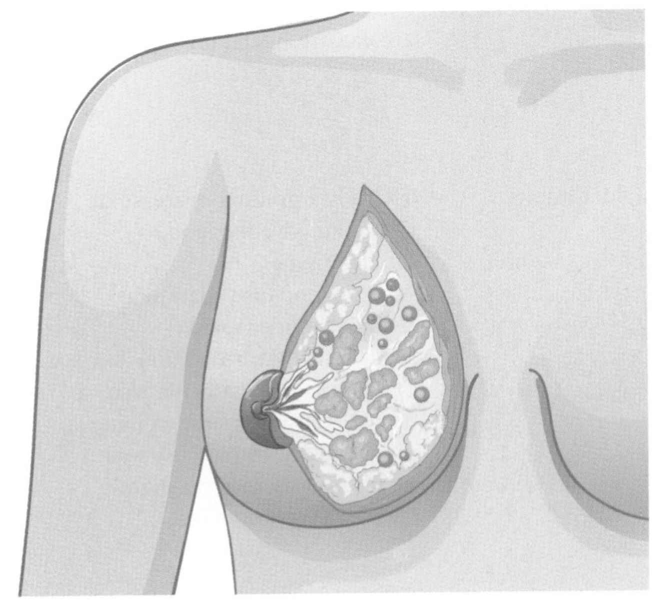

Fig. 19-22 Fibrocystic breast.

Table 19-3 Differentiation of Breast Masses

	FIBROCYSTIC BREAST CONDITION	FIBROADENOMA	CANCER
Age range	20-49	15-55	30-80
Occurrence	Usually bilateral	Usually bilateral	Usually unilateral
Location	Upper outer quadrant	No specific location	48% occur in the upper outer quadrant, but may occur in any part of the breast or axillary tail
Nipple discharge	No	No	If present, may be bloody or clear
Pain	Yes	No	Usually none
Number	Multiple or single	Single; may be multiple	Single
Shape	Rounded	Rounded or discoid	Irregular or stellate
Consistency	Soft to firm; tense	Firm, rubbery	Hard, stonelike
Mobility	Mobile	Mobile	Fixed
Retraction signs	Absent	Absent	Often present
Tenderness	Usually tender	Usually nontender	Usually nontender
Borders	Well delineated	Well delineated	Poorly delineated; irregular
Variations with menses	Yes	No	No

Modified from Seidel HM, et al: *Mosby's guide to physical examination,* ed 4, St. Louis, 1999, Mosby; and Fogel CI, Woods NF: *Health care of women: a nursing perspective.* St. Louis, 1981, Mosby.

Fibroadenoma

This is a common benign breast tumor that occurs most frequently in young women (Fig. 19-23). The tumor, which consists of glandular and fibrous tissue, usually presents unilaterally as a solitary, firm, rubbery, nontender lump (Houlihan, 1996). It is generally mobile and well-delineated. This tumor does not change premenstrually. Surgical excision or biopsy is generally performed to rule out cancer. The lesion is most prevalent in young women less than 25 years of age but may be seen until menopause (see Table 19-3).

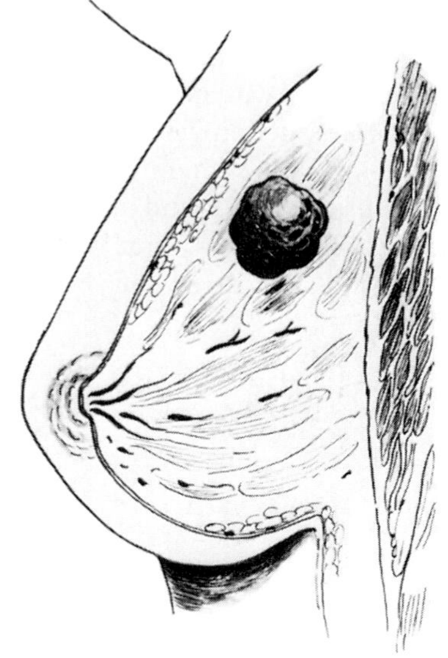

Fig. 19-23 Fibroadenoma. (From Gallager et al, 1978.)

Malignant Breast Tumor

A malignancy of the breast usually presents as a solitary, unilateral, nontender lump, thickening, or mass (Fig. 19-24). As the mass grows, there may be breast asymmetry, discoloration (erythema or ecchymosis), unilateral vein prominence, peau d'orange, ulceration, dimpling, puckering, or retraction of the skin. The lesion is sometimes fixed to underlying tissue. Its borders are irregular and poorly delineated. The nipple may be inverted or diverted to one side. A bloody or clear nipple discharge may be present. There may be crusting around the nipple or erosion of the nipple or areola. Lymph nodes may be palpable in the axilla. Breast cancer is most prevalent in women ages 40 to 60 years (see Table 19-3).

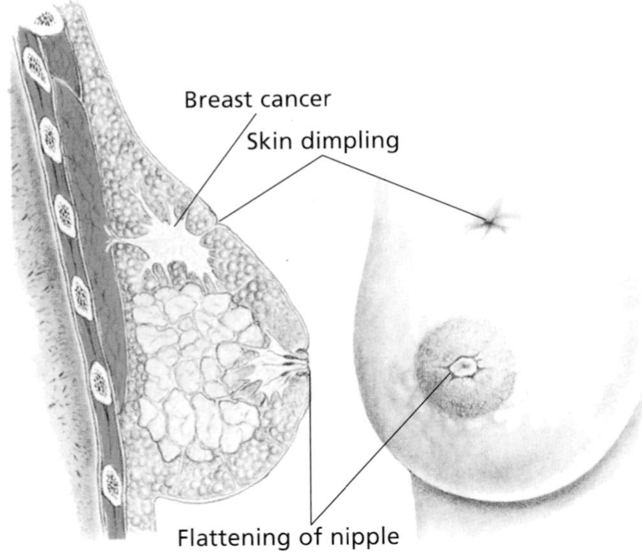

Fig. 19-24 Clinical signs of breast cancer: nipple retraction and dimpling of skin. (From Seidel et al, 1999.)

Intraductal Papilloma

An intraductal papilloma is a small 2- to 3-cm tumor of the subareolar duct. It may consist of single or multiple tumors. Clinically, no mass is usually palpable, but there is serous or bloody discharge from the nipple. About 75% of the time, this occurs directly beneath the areola, making it difficult to palpate. The tumors should be removed surgically and cytologically examined for malignancy.

Paget's Disease of the Breast

This condition manifests on the nipple and areolar area of an underlying intraductal carcinoma of the breast (Fig. 19-25). In the early stages, the nipple and areola becomes friable, dry, and scaling. As the condition worsens, the nipple becomes reddened, excoriated, and finally ulcerated. The condition may be differentiated from more common dermatologic conditions such as eczema because it appears unilaterally.

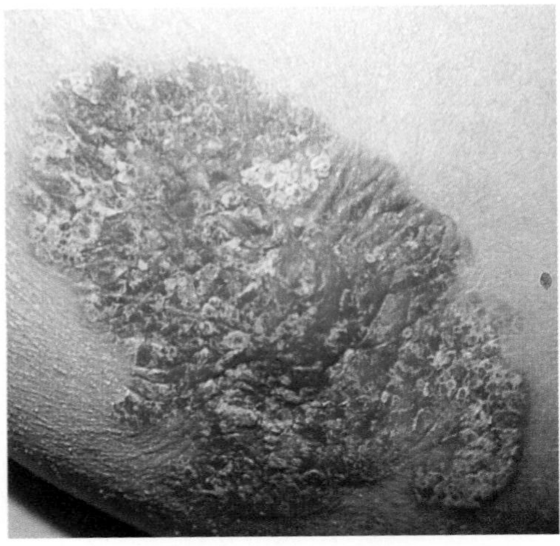

Fig. 19-25 Paget's disease. (From Habif, 1996.)

Mastitis

This is an inflammatory condition of the breast usually caused by a bacterial infection. The infection generally occurs in one area of the breast, which appears as red, swollen, tender, warm to the touch, and hard. The client will usually have associated fever and chills. The condition occurs most frequently in lactating women secondary to milk stasis or a plugged duct (Fig. 19-26).

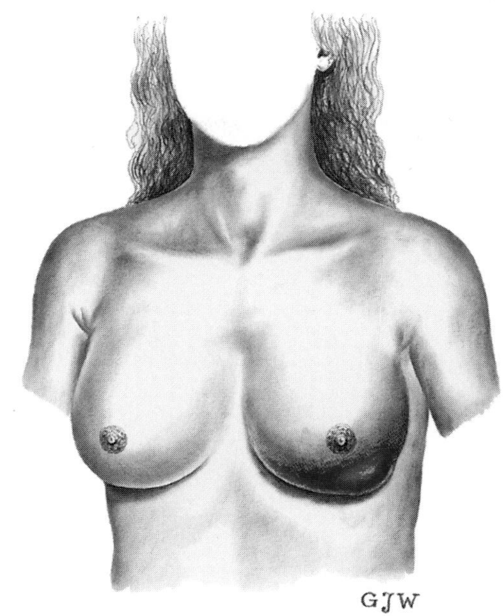

Fig. 19-26 Mastitis. (From Lowdermilk, Perry, and Bobak, 1999.)

Ductal Ectasia

Ductal ectasia is a benign breast disease involving one or multiple subareolar ducts. The only initial symptom is a multicolored and sticky nipple discharge. As the disease progresses inflammatory signs occur. The woman may experience burning or itching of the nipple and swelling in the areolar area. The discharge may become purulent and or bloody. A complication that can occur is a breast abscess.

Galactorrhea

This condition is manifested by lactation not associated with childbearing. It occurs most frequently in women taking medications such as phenothiazines, tricyclic antidepressants, estrogens, and select antihypertensive agents. It may also occur secondary to breast manipulation and diseases such as hypothyroidism, Cushing's syndrome, and hypoglycemia and in prolactin-secreting tumors (Fig. 19-27).

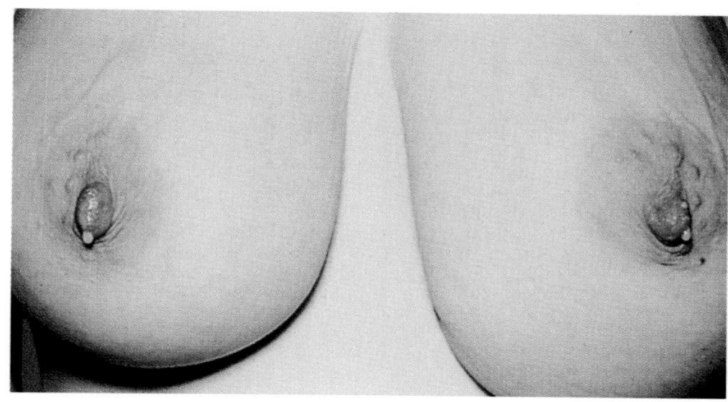

Fig. 19-27 Galactorrhea produced by a prolactin-secreting pituitary tumor. (From Mansel and Bundred, 1995.)

MALES

Gynecomastia

This is a noninflammatory enlargement of one or both male breasts (Fig. 19-28). It is most commonly seen in the neonate, adolescent, and older adult. At puberty the condition is idiopathic and transient. Common causes in adult men include adrenal or testicular tumors, liver disease, renal disease, and hyperthyroidism. This can also be a side effect of certain medications, especially hormone therapy, cimetidine, digitoxin, and spironolactone (Braunstein, 1996).

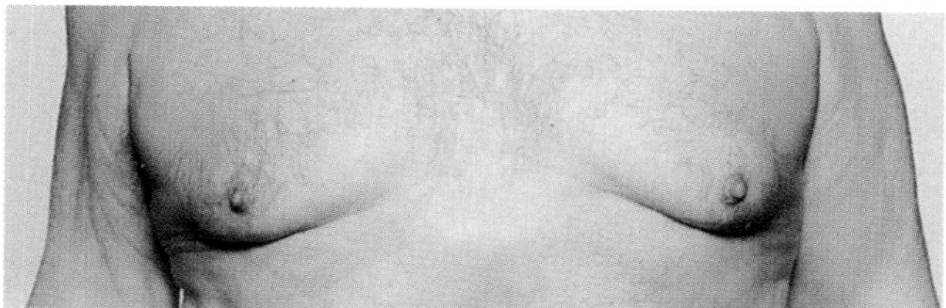

Fig. 19-28 Gynecomastia in older adult. (From Mansel and Bundred, 1995.)

Cancer of the Breast

Cancer of the breast is uncommon in men but accounts for 1% to 2% of all breast cancers (Fig. 19-29). The lesion occurs most frequently around the nipple as a hard, irregular, and nontender mass.

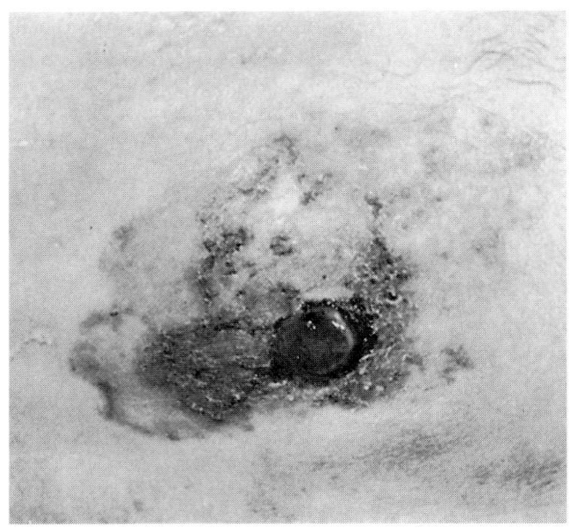

Fig. 19-29 Carcinoma of breast has infiltrated overlying skin, producing ulceration of nipple and areola.
(From Crichlow, Kaplan, and Kearney, 1972.)

CLINICAL APPLICATION and CRITICAL THINKING

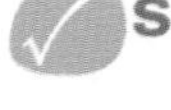

SAMPLE DOCUMENTATION

CASE 1

K.M. is a 23-year-old female with complaint of a tender breast.

Subjective Data

K.M. is 10 days post-partum. Reports 2 days ago she noticed tenderness in left breast and is getting progressively worse. States the breast is swollen, hot, and painful. Pain constant; affecting only left breast area and is "8" on a 1 to 10 pain scale. K.M. has been breast-feeding but has stopped using the left breast due to intolerable pain; right nipple has become sore. Concerned about the baby's health and nutritional status. Feels tired and sick; has had her own mother taking care of baby. Feels "horrible" about not being able to meet baby's needs. Taking no medications; reports no allergies.

Objective Data

Temperature, 101.6° F (38.7° C); Pulse, 116 beats/min; Respirations, 28; Blood pressure, 114/76 mm Hg.

Left breast swollen; erythema around nipple; skin warm to touch; no exudate observed. Client extremely sensitive to pain with even slight manipulation and palpation to breast.

Lymph nodes in left axilla slightly enlarged, tender. Right nipple red and cracked, no inflammation noted.

Functional Health Patterns Involved

- Nutrition–metabolic
- Self-perception–self-concept
- Cognitive–perceptual

Medical Diagnosis

Mastitis

Nursing Diagnosis and Collaborative Problems

- *Pain* related to inflammation of breast tissue as manifested by:
  - Rating of pain at 8 on 1 to 10 pain scale.
  - Pain too great to continue breastfeeding.
- *Self-esteem disturbance* related to inability to care for infant as verbalized by:
  - Feeling bad can't breast-feed.
  - Feeling too sick to care for baby.
  - Concern regarding how her illness may affect infant.
- *Risk for ineffective breast-feeding* related to maternal discomfort and illness.
- *PC*: Breast abscess

CASE 2

R.R. is a 12-year-old male with complaint of a big breast.

Subjective Data

Client reports that 1 month ago he noticed that his left breast was "getting big"; verbalizes concern that he may be "growing boobs." Denies any previous episodes of breast enlargement or health problems. Client denies any use of medications or illicit drugs. Denies any nipple discharge or breast tenderness. States boys in PE class laugh at him. Reports poor diet that lacks intake of fruits and vegetables.

Objective Data

Height, 4′11″ (1.5 m); Weight, 160 lb (72.7 kg)
Obese male who appears to be stated age.
Chest/breast: Appearance provides evidence of an enlarged left breast area. The right breast shows only slight fullness congruent with body weight.
Palpation of the left breast: Feels smooth and slightly firm. There is no evidence of a mass or nodularity. There is no tenderness with palpation and no nipple discharge.

Functional Health Patterns Involved

- Nutrition–metabolic
- Self-perception–self-concept

Medical Diagnosis

Idiopathic, unilateral gynecomastia, left breast

Nursing Diagnosis and Collaborative Problems

- *Body image disturbance* related to disfigurement of body as manifested by:
  - Left breast is "getting big"
  - Client being teased at school
- *Altered nutrition: more than body requirements* related to excessive intake in relation to metabolic need as manifested by:
  - Lack of exercise
  - Diet deficit of fruits and vegetables
  - Height, 4′11″; weight, 160 lb

CRITICAL THINKING QUESTIONS

1. A 43-year-old woman tells you her mother died of breast cancer, and her 50-year-old sister currently has breast cancer. She is worried about developing breast cancer as well. Her gynecologic history includes menarche at age 11. She has one child, a 7-year-old son. She has no history of other pregnancies. She has no history of illness. List her current risk factors. Would you consider her to be at high risk for breast cancer?
2. A 72-year-old client presents with a complaint of nipple discharge. She informs the nurse that the discharge is "reddish yellow" in appearance. What additional questions should be asked, and what specifically should be examined?
3. A 23-year-old woman requests information on how to perform breast self-examination. Describe essential elements you would want to include in a teaching plan.

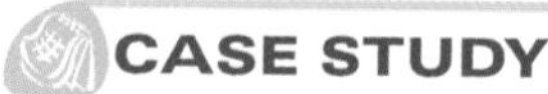

CASE STUDY

Julie Fisher is a 46-year-old woman who came to the clinic because she had discovered a lump in her left breast. Listed below are data collected during an interview and examination.

Interview Data

Julie tells the examiner that she first noticed the lump about 9 months ago. Because it seemed small and did not hurt, she did not feel that it was much to worry about. Recently, Julie began noticing that the lump felt bigger and decided she better have someone look at it. Julie tells the examiner, "I just know it is not cancer because I am much too young and healthy. And if it is, I am not about to let some doctor mutilate me with a knife. I'd rather die than have my breast cut off." The examiner asks her if she has noticed any redness or dimpling of the breast. Julie tells the nurse, "No, not really, but I don't pay attention to those sorts of things." Julie tells the examiner that she started having regular menstrual cycles at the age of 11 and still has not reached menopause. She has never been married and has no children.

Examination Data

- **General survey:** Very nervous, well-nourished female. Is hesitant to expose her breast for examination.
- **Breast examination:** Inspection reveals breasts of typical size with right and left breast symmetry. The skin of both breasts is smooth, with even pigmentation. The nipples protrude slightly with no drainage noted. The left nipple is slightly retracted. Significant dimpling noted on left breast in upper outer quadrant when arms are raised over her head. Right breast appears normal. Palpation of the left breast reveals a large hard lump in the upper outer quadrant. No lumps or masses noted in right breast. The left nipple produces a clear bloody-type discharge when squeezed; the right nipple is unremarkable.

1. What data deviate from normal findings, suggesting a need for further investigation?
2. What additional information should the nurse ask or assess for?
3. In what functional health patterns does data deviate from normal?
4. What nursing diagnosis and/or collaborative problems should be considered for this situation?

REMEMBER to check out your **companion CD-ROM**

20 Abdomen and Gastrointestinal System

www.mosby.com/MERLIN/wilson/assessment/

ANATOMY AND PHYSIOLOGY

The abdominal cavity, the largest cavity in the human body, contains vital organs, including the stomach, small and large intestines, liver, gallbladder, pancreas, spleen, kidneys, adrenal glands, and in women the uterus and ovaries, as well as major vessels. Lying outside the abdominal cavity, but a vital part of the gastrointestinal (GI) system, is the esophagus (Fig. 20-1). Protection is provided by a muscular structure and peritoneum.

PERITONEUM, MUSCULATURE, AND CONNECTIVE TISSUE

The abdominal lining, the peritoneum, is a serous membrane forming a protective cover. It is divided in two layers, the parietal and the visceral peritoneum. The parietal peritoneum lines the abdominal wall, whereas the visceral peritoneum covers organs. The space between the parietal and visceral peritoneum is the peritoneal cavity. It usually contains a small amount of serous fluid to reduce friction between abdominal organs and their membranes.

The rectus abdominis muscles form the anterior border of the abdomen, whereas the vertebral column and lumbar muscles form the posterior border. Lateral support is provided by the internal and external oblique muscles. A tendinous band, the linea alba, protects the midline of the abdomen between the rectus abdominis muscles. This band extends from the xiphoid process to the symphysis pubis. The abdomen is bordered superiorly by the diaphragm and inferiorly by the superior aperture of the lesser pelvis (Fig. 20-2).

ALIMENTARY TRACT

The digestive system can be thought of as one long tube, the alimentary tract. From the mouth to the anus, the adult alimentary tract extends 27 feet (8.2 m) and includes the esophagus, stomach, small intestine, large intestine, rectum, and anal canal (Fig. 20-3). One of its main functions is to ingest and digest food, absorbing nutrients, electrolytes, and water. Its other main function is to excrete resultant waste products. Products of digestion are moved along the digestive tract by peristalsis, under the control of the autonomic nervous system. The esophagus is a tube about 10 inches (25.4 cm) long connecting the pharynx to the stomach, extending just posterior to the trachea, through the mediastinal cavity and diaphragm.

Stomach

The stomach is located directly below the diaphragm in the left upper quadrant. It is a hollow, flask-shaped, muscular organ that secretes digestive juices and mixes food with the digestive enzymes and hydrochloric acid (Fig. 20-4). Gastric acid continues the breakdown of carbohydrates that was begun in the mouth. Pepsin breaks down proteins, converting them to peptones and amino acids, whereas gastric lipase acts on emulsified fats to convert triglycerides to fatty acids and glycerol. The stomach also liquifies food into chyme and propels it into the duodenum of the small intestine.

Two sphincters control the flow of contents into and out of the stomach. The lower esophageal sphincter controls the flow of food from the esophagus into the stomach, and the pyloric sphincter regulates the outflow of chyme into the duodenum. The gastric mucosa contains parietal cells that absorb vitamin B_{12}, necessary for erythrocyte production.

Small Intestine

The longest section of the alimentary tract, the small intestine, is about 21 feet (6.4 m) long, beginning at the pyloric orifice and joining the large intestine at the ileocecal valve. In the small intestine, ingested food is mixed, digested, and absorbed. The small intestine is divided into three segments: the duodenum, jejunum, and ileum. The duodenum occupies the first foot (30 cm) of the small intestine and forms a C-shaped curve around the head of the pancreas. Absorption then takes place through the walls of the duodenum, jejunum (8 feet [2.4 m] long) and ileum (12 feet [3.6 m] long). The ileocecal valve between the ileum and the large intestine prevents backward flow of fecal material (see Fig. 20-3).

Large Intestine (Colon) and Rectum

The large intestine begins at the cecum, a small blind pouch, and ends at the anus. It is about 5 feet (1.5 m) long, consisting of cecum, appendix, colon, rectum, and anal canal. The ileal contents empty into the cecum through the ileocecal valve; the appendix extends from the base of the cecum. The colon is divided into three parts: the ascending, transverse, and descending colon. The end of the descending colon turns medially and inferiorly to form the S-shaped sigmoid colon. The rectum extends from the sigmoid colon to the pelvic floor, where it continues as the anal canal, terminating at the anus. The large intestine absorbs water and elec-

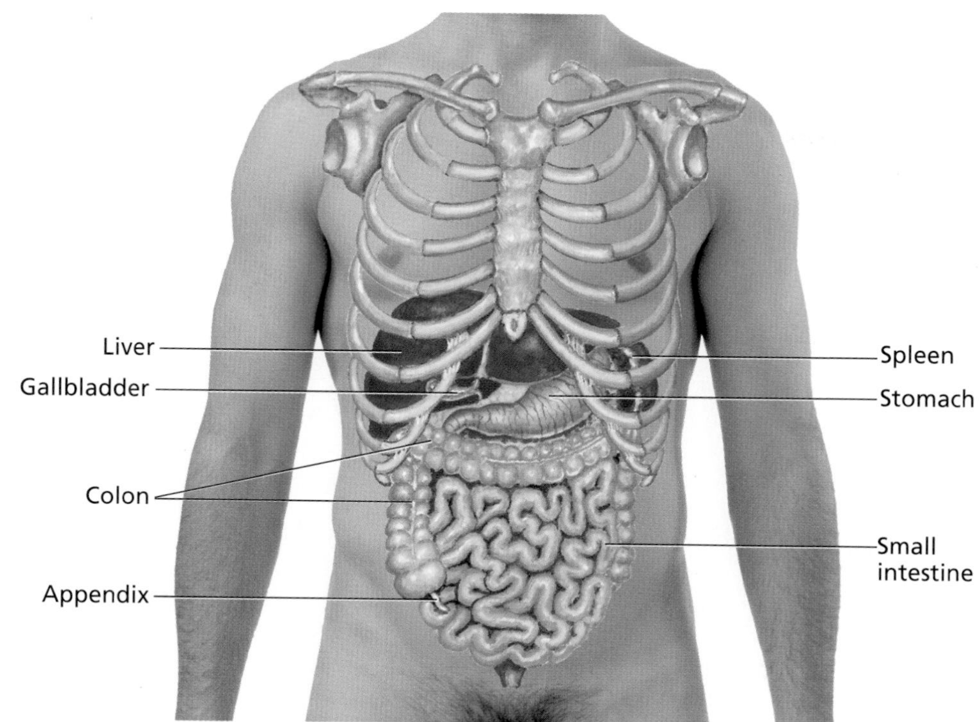

Fig. 20-1 Major structures of abdominal cavity.

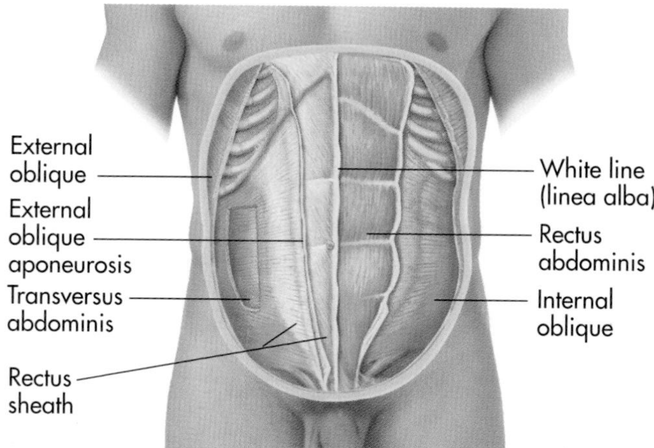

Fig. 20-2 Muscles of the abdomen. (Seidel et al, 1999.)

trolytes. Feces are formed in the large intestine and held until defecation (see Fig. 20-3).

Liver

The largest organ in the body, weighing about 3.5 lb (1.6 kg), the liver lies under the right diaphragm, spanning the upper quadrant of the abdomen from the fifth intercostal space to slightly below the costal margin (Fig. 20-5). The rib cage covers a substantial portion of the liver; only the lower margin is exposed beneath it. The liver is divided into right and left lobes.

This complex organ has a variety of functions, including the following:

- Bile production and secretion, to emulsify fat
- Transfer of bilirubin from the blood (conjugated or direct) to the duodenum (unconjugated or indirect)
- Protein, carbohydrate, and fat metabolism
- Glucose storage in the form of glycogen
- Production of clotting factors and fibrinogen for coagulation
- Synthesis of most plasma proteins (albumin and globulin)
- Detoxification of a variety of substances, including drugs and alcohol
- Storage of certain minerals (iron and copper) and vitamins (A, B_{12}, and other B-complex vitamins).

Gallbladder

The gallbladder is a pear-shaped sac, 3 inches (7.6 cm) long, attached to the inferior surface of the liver (see Fig. 20-5). It concentrates and stores bile produced in the liver. The cystic duct combines with the hepatic duct to form the common bile duct, which drains bile into the duodenum. The presence of bile in the feces is evident by the brown color.

Pancreas

The pancreas lies in the upper left abdominal cavity, immediately under the left lobe of the liver, behind the stomach (see Fig. 20-5). It has both endocrine and exocrine functions. First, it produces endocrine enzymes such as insulin, glucagon, and gastrin for carbohydrate metabolism. Its exo-

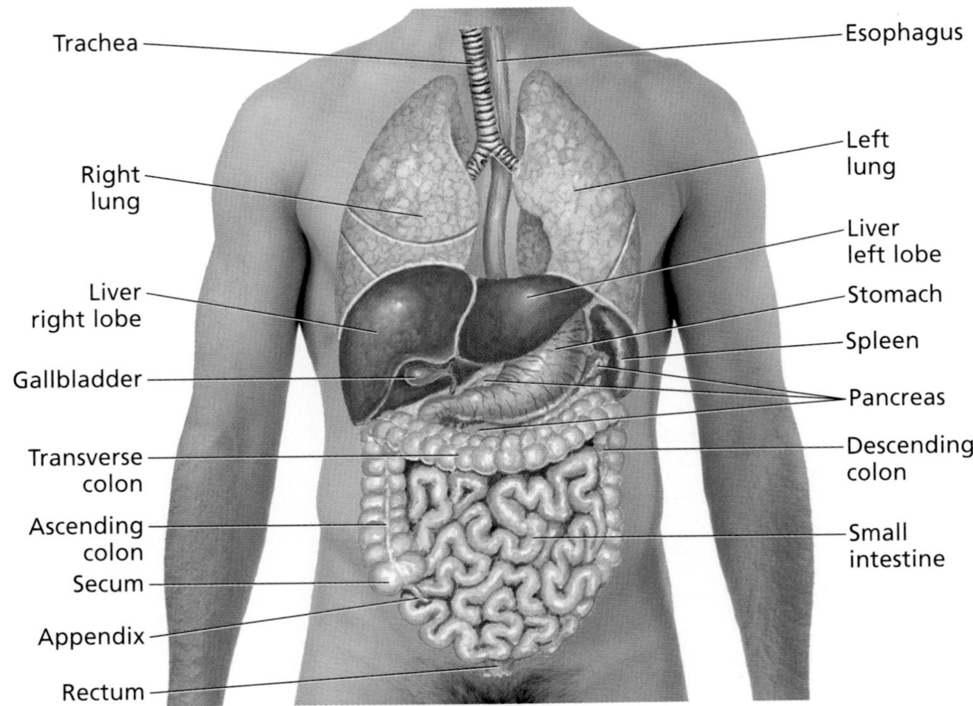

Fig. 20-3 Anatomy of the gastrointestinal system.

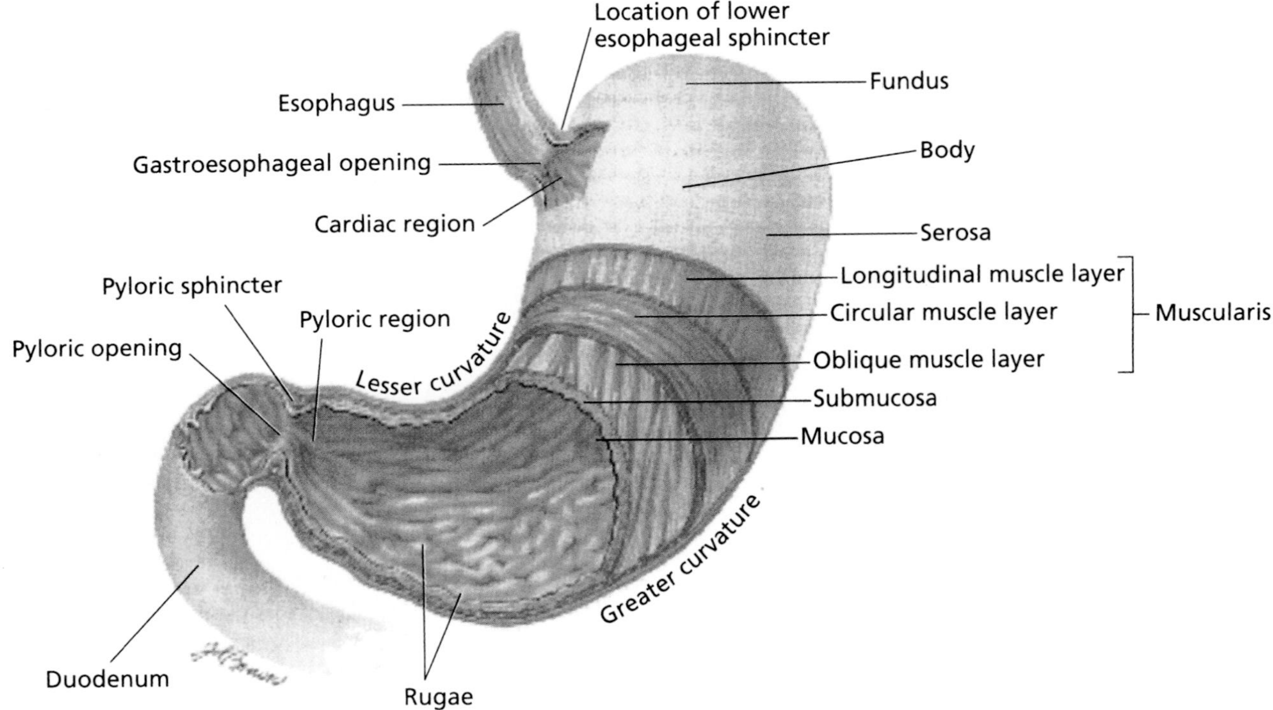

Fig. 20-4 Gross anatomy of the stomach. Cutaway section reveals muscular layers and internal anatomy. (From Seeley, Stephens, and Tate, 1995.)

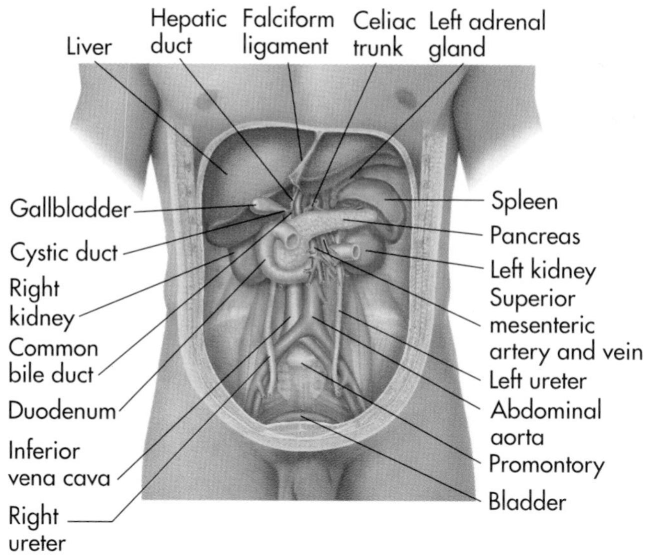

Fig. 20-5 Anatomy of liver, gallbladder, pancreas, spleen, kidney, and major vessels of abdominal cavity. (From Seidel et al, 1999.)

crine secretions contain bicarbonate and pancreatic enzymes that flow into the duodenum to break down proteins, fats, and carbohydrates for absorption.

Spleen

The concave, encapsulated spleen is a small organ about the size of a fist. It is located in the upper left abdominal cavity, posterior to the greater curvature of the stomach, in front of the first and second lumbar vertebrae (see Fig. 20-5). Its main functions include the following:

- Storage of 1% to 2% of erythrocytes and platelets
- Removal of old or agglutinated erythrocytes and platelets by macrophages
- Activation of B and T lymphocytes
- Production of erythrocytes during bone marrow depression

URINARY TRACT

The urinary tract includes the kidneys, ureters, urinary bladder, and urethra. Together, they remove water-soluble waste materials.

Kidneys

The kidneys are located in the posterior abdominal cavity on either side at the spinal levels of T12 through L3, where they are covered by the peritoneum and attached to the posterior abdominal wall (see Fig. 20-5). Each kidney is approximately 4 inches × 2 inches × 1 inch (10 × 5 × 2.5 cm) and partially protected by the ribs and a cushion of fat and fascia. The right kidney is slightly lower than the left, due to displacement by the liver. Additional kidney functions include the following: (1) secretion of erythropoietin to stimulate red blood cell production, (2) secretion of renin to constrict blood vessels influencing blood pressure, and (3) production of a biologically active form of vitamin D. The nephron regulates fluid and electrolyte balance through an elaborate microscopic filter and pressure system that eventually produces urine.

Ureters

The urine formed in the nephrons flows from the distal tubes and collecting ducts into the ureters and on into the bladder through peristaltic waves. Each ureter is composed of long, intertwining muscle bundles that extend for approximately 12 inches (30 cm) to insertion points at the base of the bladder (see Fig. 20-5).

Bladder

The bladder, a sac of smooth muscle fibers, is located behind the symphysis pubis in the anterior half of the pelvis (see Fig. 20-5). The bladder contains an internal sphincter, which relaxes in response to a full bladder. Generally, when the bladder's urine volume reaches about 300 ml, moderate distention is felt; a level of 450 ml causes discomfort. On voiding, the urine exits through the urethra, which extends out of the base of the bladder to the external meatus.

Vasculature of the Abdomen

In the abdomen, the descending aorta travels from the diaphragm just to the left of midline until it branches into the two common iliac arteries at about the level of the umbilicus.

HEALTH HISTORY

Abdomen and Gastrointestinal System

Questions regarding nutrition and eating habits are asked in the general evaluation of the client (see Chapter 10).

QUESTIONS

RATIONALE

PRESENT HEALTH STATUS

➤ How would you describe the health of your digestive system? How about the health of your urinary system?

■ It is important to obtain the client's perception of his or her health of these body systems.

➤ Do you have any chronic diseases? If yes, describe.

■ Some chronic diseases may affect the GI or urinary systems such as diabetes mellitus. Diseases such as chronic hepatitis or cirrhosis may impair the liver's ability to metabolize nutrients and drugs.

➤ Do you take any medications? If yes, what do you take and how often? Are you taking the medications as they were prescribed?

■ Both prescription and over-the-counter medications should be documented. Many medications, such as analgesics, cause GI side effects. Drugs are not metabolized well in clients with chronic liver disease.

➤ Do you drink alcohol? How much? How often? When was your last drink (of alcohol)?

■ Alcohol is a risk factor for peptic ulcer disease, stomach cancer, and cirrhosis.

➤ Do you smoke? How much? Have you considered stopping or cutting down?

■ Cigarette smoking is a risk factor for peptic ulcer disease.

➤ How often do you have a bowel movement? When was your last bowel movement? What are the color and consistency of the stool?

■ Frequency of bowel movement is documented in the client's history along with color and consistency of stool as baseline data. This question also gives the client an opportunity to describe disorders of the colon such as diarrhea, constipation, dark or lights stools, or blood in stool.

PAST MEDICAL HISTORY

➤ Have you had problems with your digestive system in the past? Esophagus? Stomach? Intestines? Liver? Gallbladder? Pancreas? Spleen? If yes, describe.

■ History of gastrointestinal disorders tells what types of disorders the client has experienced and may provide insight into findings to anticipate at this visit.

➤ Have you had problems with your urinary tract in the past? Kidneys? Uterers? Bladder? If yes, describe.

■ History of urinary disorders tells you what types of disorders the client has experienced and may provide insight into findings to anticipate at this visit.

➤ Have you had injury to or surgery on your digestive system or urinary tract? If yes, describe.

■ The incidence of injury or surgery may provide additional information about a possible GI or urinary problem.

FAMILY HISTORY

➤ In your family, is there a history of diseases of the GI system such as gastroesophageal reflux disease (GERD)? Peptic ulcer disease? Stomach cancer? Colon cancer?

■ Family history may be used to determine client's risk factors for gastrointestinal disorders.

➤ In your family, is there a history of diseases of the urinary tract such as kidney stones, cancer? Kidney cancer? Bladder cancer?

■ Family history may be used to determine client's risk factors for urinary disorders.

QUESTIONS

RATIONALE

PROBLEM-BASED HISTORY

Specific areas to be covered in the assessment of the abdomen and gastrointestinal system include abdominal pain, nausea and vomiting, indigestion, abdominal distention, change in bowel habits, jaundice, and urination. As with symptoms in all areas of health assessment, a symptom analysis is completed, which includes the location, quality, quantity, chronology, setting, associated manifestations, alleviating factors and aggravating factors (see Box 4-2 in Chapter 4).

Abdominal Pain

➤ Do you have abdominal pain? How long have you had this pain? Where is it located? When did you first feel the pain? What activity were you doing at that time?

■ Time, location, and activity when pain occurs are important to diagnosis. Sudden, severe pain that awakens the client may be associated with acute perforation, inflammation, or torsion of an abdominal organ.

➤ Describe the pain. It is dull or sharp? Burning? Cramping? Colicky? Is it constant, or does it come and go? Have you had episodes of this pain before? Did the pain start suddenly? Have you ever had gallstones or kidney stones? Table 20-1 provides a differentiation of abdominal pain.

■ Pain description is important to diagnosis. Intense pain may be caused by a stone in the biliary tract or ureter, rupture of a fallopian tube from an ectopic pregnancy, perforation of a gastric ulcer, peritonitis, or acute appendicitis. Diffuse, deep, and dull pain is visceral in origin, due to localized distention, inflammation, or ischemia. Sharp, localized pain is parietal or peritoneal, due to generalized inflammation.

➤ Has the pain changed its location since it started? Do you feel the pain in any other parts of your body?

■ Pain radiation patterns are shown in Table 20-1. Pain from acute appendicitis starts around the umbilicus and radiates to the right lower quadrant. Pain from an abdominal aneurysm may start in the chest and travel to the abdomen. Back pain is associated with abdominal aneurysms. Pain from gallbladder disease may be felt in the right shoulder.

➤ Is the pain worse when your stomach is empty? Is it affected by eating? Is the pain worse at night or during the day?

■ Patterns of GI pain may help identify the cause. For example, the pain of peptic ulcer disease is worse when the stomach is empty because food acts as a buffer from the acid, whereas pain in gastroenteritis and irritable bowel disease is worse in the presence of food because peristalsis is stimulated, which causes pain.

➤ What relieves the pain? Is there any particular position that relieves the pain? What have you done to relieve the pain?

■ A particular position may relieve abdominal pain. Pancreatitis pain is relieved in the knee-chest position. Colicky (sharp visceral) pain (gallbladder or kidney stone) is relieved with restless movement. The pain of appendicitis is relieved by lying very still.

Table 20-1 Differentiation of Abdominal Pain

CAUSE	CLIENT CHARACTERISTICS	QUALITY	LOCATION*
Gastroesophageal reflux	Any age	Gnawing, burning	Midepigastric; may radiate to jaw
Gastroenteritis	Any age	Crampy	Diffuse
Gastritis	Alcoholism	Constant, burning	Epigastric
Peptic ulcer	30-50 years; more males than females	Gnawing, burning	Epigastric radiating to sides, back, right shoulder
Pancreatitis	Alcoholism, cholelithiasis	Steady, severe to mild, knifelike, sudden onset	LUQ and epigastric; radiates to back
Appendicitis	Any age; peak 10-20 yr	Colicky, progressing to constant	Umbilicus, moving to RLQ
Cholecystitis or cholelithiasis	Adults; more females than males	Colicky, progressing to constant	RUQ radiates to right scapula
Ectopic pregnancy	History of menstrual irregularity	Sudden onset, persistent pain	Lower quadrant
Diverticular disease	Older adults	Intermittent cramping	LLQ
Irritable bowel disease	Young women	Crampy, recurrent, sharp, burning	LLQ
Intestinal obstruction	Older adults; those with prior abdominal surgery	Colicky, sudden onset	May be localized or generalized

**LUQ*, left upper quadrant; *LLQ*, left lower quadrant; *RUQ*, right upper quadrant; *RLQ*, right lower quadrant.

QUESTIONS

➤ Is pain associated with other factors, such as stress, fatigue, nausea and vomiting, gas, eating certain foods, fever, chills, constipation, diarrhea, rectal bleeding, frequent urination, or vaginal or penile discharge?

➤ Is the pain associated with your menstrual period? When was your last menstrual period?

Nausea and Vomiting

➤ Have you been experiencing nausea or vomiting.? How often? For how long? How much do you vomit?

➤ What does the vomitus look like? Does it contain blood? Does it have an odor?

RATIONALE

■ Identifying symptoms associated with pain may assist in determining the cause.

■ Dysmenorrhea (pain associated with menstruation) may cause lower abdominal pain and vomiting due to the increase in prostaglandin.

■ Vomiting may be caused by severe irritation of the peritoneum caused by (1) obstruction of the intestine, bile duct, or ureter, (2) toxins, or (3) perforation of an abdominal organ (Sellers, 1996).

■ The characteristics of the vomitus may help to determine its cause. Acute gastritis leads to vomiting of stomach contents, whereas obstruction of the bile duct results in greenish-yellow vomitus, and an intestinal obstruction may have a fecal odor to the vomitus. Vomiting stomach contents is associated with acute gastritis. Stomach or duodenal ulcers or esophageal varices may cause blood in vomitus (hematemesis).

ASSOCIATED SYMPTOMS	AGGRAVATED BY	ALLEVIATED BY	FINDINGS
Weight loss	Recumbency, bending, stooping	Antacids, sitting up	
Nausea and vomiting, fever, diarrhea	Food	Some relief with vomiting, diarrhea	Hyperactive bowel sounds
Hemorrhage, nausea and vomiting, diarrhea, fever	Alcohol, food, salicylates	Antacids	
	Empty stomach, stress, alcohol, recumbency	Food, antacids	Epigastric tenderness to palpation or percussion
Nausea and vomiting, diaphoresis	Lying supine	Leaning forward	Abdominal distention, $\downarrow$ bowel sounds, diffuse rebound
Vomiting, constipation, fever	Worse with moving, coughing	Lying still	Rebound tenderness RLQ, positive obturator, positive iliopsoas
Nausea and vomiting, dark urine, light stools, jaundice	Fatty foods, drugs		Tender to palpation or percussion of RUQ
Tender adnexal mass, vaginal bleeding			Palpable mass on affected side
Constipation, diarrhea	Eating	Bowel movement, passing flatus	Palpable mass LLQ
Mucus in stools		May be relieved by defecation	Colon tender to palpation
Vomiting, constipation			Hyperactive bowel sounds in small obstruction

QUESTIONS

➤ Could you be pregnant?

➤ Do you have nausea without vomiting?

➤ Did the symptoms begin over the last 24 hours? What foods did you eat over this period? Where did you eat? How long after you ate did you vomit? Has anyone else who ate with you had these symptoms over the same time period?

➤ Do you have other symptoms with the nausea or vomiting? Pain? Constipation? Diarrhea? Change in color of stools? Change in color of urine? Fever or chills?

Indigestion

➤ Do you have indigestion or heartburn? Where do you feel the discomfort? In your stomach? Chest? How long has this been happening? How often does this occur?

RATIONALE

■ Pregnancy should be ruled out as a cause of nausea and vomiting. Pregnant women have high serum levels of chorionic gonadotrophin, which stimulates vomiting. As with any disorder, treatment may be altered for the pregnant client.

■ Nausea without vomiting is a common symptom of pregnant clients or those with metastatic disease.

■ These questions are asked to detect food poisoning or stomach influenza.

■ Knowing associated symptoms may help determine the cause of nausea and vomiting. For example, liver disease may change stool color from brown to clay colored. Infection such as hepatitis may cause fever and chills.

■ Heartburn felt in the chest, over the esophagus, or in the stomach that occurs after eating may indicate GERD.

QUESTIONS | **RATIONALE**

➤ What makes the symptoms worse? Does a change in position, such as lying down, affect your indigestion?

■ Heartburn caused by GERD is often worse when the client lies down because the gastric aids move by gravity toward the esophagus.

➤ What relieves these symptoms? Do you take antacids or acid blockers?

■ When antacids relieve pain, then excessive acid can be assumed to part of the cause of the indigestion.

➤ Are there any other symptoms associated with the heartburn? Radiating pain? Sweating? Light-headedness?

■ Knowing associated symptoms may help determine the cause of indigestion. Angina or myocardial infarction may be the cause of the "indigestion-like" symptoms. Radiating pain to the arms or jaw, along with other questions, are asked with these cardiovascular disorders in mind.

Abdominal Distension

➤ How long has your abdomen been distended? Does it come and go? Is it related to eating? What relieves the distension? Passing gas? Burping?

■ Distention associated with eating is intermittent and relieved by passing gas. Constipation contributes to distention and develops slowly but is not relieved without bowel movement. Distention caused by ascites is a progressive process and increases abdominal girth.

➤ Are there other symptoms associated with it? Vomiting? Loss of appetite? Weight loss? Change in bowel habits? Shortness of breath? Pain?

■ Vomiting may indicate intestinal obstruction as a cause of distension. Loss of appetite is associated with cirrhosis and malignancy. Shortness of breath and ascites are associated with heart failure or chronic liver disease.

Change in Bowel Function

➤ Describe the change in your bowel movements. Change in frequency? Change in consistency of feces? When did you first notice the change? How long has this been happening? Have you changed your diet? Have you changed your activity level?

■ Changes in bowel function can be related to a number of factors, including changes in diet, activity, stress, and medications. A change in bowel habits is one of the seven signs of cancer.

➤ Are there other associated symptoms such as increased gas, pain, fever, nausea, vomiting, abdominal cramping, diarrhea?

■ Knowing associated symptoms may help determine the cause of the change in bowel function. Some foods cause increased gas, fever suggests inflammation or infection, and abdominal cramping with diarrhea may indicate gastroenteritis.

Jaundice (Icterus)

➤ When did you first notice the yellow discoloration of your skin or eyes? Has it become more noticeable?

■ Jaundice indicates elevated serum bilirubin that can be caused by liver disease or obstruction of bile flow from gallstones.

➤ Is the yellow discoloration of your skin or eyes associated with abdominal pain? Loss of appetite? Nausea? Vomiting? Fever?

■ Fever, nausea, vomiting, and loss of appetite are also symptoms of hepatitis.

QUESTIONS	RATIONALE
➤ In the last year, have you had a blood transfusion or tattoos? Are you using any intravenous drugs? Do you eat raw shellfish, for example, oysters? Have you traveled abroad in the last year? Where? Did you drink unclean water?	■ These are possible sources of transmission of the hepatitis virus.
➤ Has your urine or stools changed in color?	■ Urine changing from amber to brown and stools changing from brown to clay colored suggest high serum bilirubin.

Urination

QUESTIONS	RATIONALE
➤ Have you felt any pain or burning when urinating? Urinating frequently in small amounts, feeling you cannot wait to urinate? If yes, when did this begin?	■ Pain, burning, or frequency may indicate a bladder infection. For women, frequent bubble baths or wearing a wet swimsuit for a prolonged period increases the risk of cystitis.
➤ Have you had associated symptoms? Have you had fever, chills, and back pain?	■ These symptoms may indicate a kidney disorder such as pyelonephritis.
➤ Describe the color of the urine. Is there blood in the urine?	■ Dark amber urine is associated with kidney or liver disease. Blood in the urine is associated with menstrual periods in women or with kidney disease.
➤ Have you had an unexpected weight gain? Have you noticed swelling in your ankles at the end of the day or shortness of breath? Are you urinating less?	■ These signs and symptoms may indicate renal failure, when kidneys fail to produce urine and fluid normally excreted is retained.

EXAMINATION

Equipment

- Stethoscope to auscultate the abdomen
- Tape measure to measure abdominal girth
- Penlight or other light source to inspect the abdomen
- ❖ Small ruler to measure liver borders on inhalation and exhalation
- ❖ Marking pencil or pen to mark liver borders

PROCEDURES AND TECHNIQUES WITH NORMAL FINDINGS	ABNORMAL FINDINGS
➤**OBSERVE client's general behavior and position.** The client should appear relaxed, sitting or lying quietly with slow, even respirations.	■ Note abnormal findings such as emaciation, obesity, marked restlessness, marked immobility or a rigid posture, the knees drawn up, facial grimacing, and rapid, uneven, or grunting respirations. Clients with pancreatitis prefer knee-chest position; those with peritonitis or appendicitis will lie very still; those with colicky gallstones or ureteral stones may rock.

PROCEDURES AND TECHNIQUES WITH NORMAL FINDINGS

ABNORMAL FINDINGS

ABDOMEN

➤**INSPECT the abdomen for skin color, surface characteristics, contour, and surface movements.** Direct a light source at a right angle to the client's long axis.

➤Skin color may be paler than other parts of the skin, due to lack of exposure.

■ Jaundice indicates elevated serum bilirubin, erythema may indicate inflammation, bruises indicate trauma, cyanosis indicates hypoxia, and pink, purple, or red striae may indicate abdominal distension.

➤Surface characteristics should be smooth. There may be silver-white striae, scars, and a very faint, fine vascular network present. The umbilicus should be centrally located (Fig. 20-6).

■ Note prominent venous patterns or engorgement of the veins around the umbilicus. Glistening or taut appearance is associated with ascites. The umbilicus should not be displaced upward, downward, or laterally, nor should a hernia be visible around or slightly above the umbilicus. Note if the umbilicus is inflamed or has drainage.

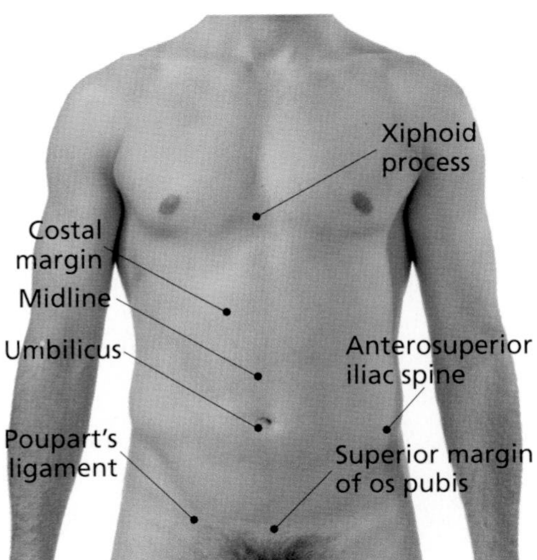

Fig. 20-6 Landmarks of the abdomen.

➤Contour is usually sunken, although it may protrude slightly, and should be smooth. Adjusting the light source to form shadows may highlight small changes in the contour. Evaluate symmetry of features by viewing the abdomen at eye level from the side, as well as from behind the client's head. Ask the client to take a deep breath and hold it. The contour of the abdomen should remain smooth and symmetric.

■ Check for marked concavity, which is associated with general wasting signs or anteroposterior rib expansion. When abdominal distention is noted, place a measuring tape around the abdomen at the level of the superior iliac crests to measure the abdominal girth (circumference). This provides an objective measure to assess the increase or decease in abdominal distention. Abdominal distention may result from the 7 *F* s—fat (obesity), fetus (pregnancy), fluid (ascites), flatulence (gas), feces (constipation), fibroid tumor, or fatal tumor. Note any bulges or masses, particularly of the liver or spleen. Abdominal or incisional hernias can also create bulges of the abdomen.

PROCEDURES AND TECHNIQUES WITH NORMAL FINDINGS

➤Inspect the surface for movements. Peristalsis is usually not visible, but there may be an upper midline pulsation visible in thin individuals. Generally, the abdomen should move smoothly and evenly with respirations. Generally females exhibit thoracic movements during inhalation, whereas males exhibit abdominal movements. Ask the client to raise his or her head without using the arms for support. The rectus abdominis muscles become prominent, and a midline bulge may appear. Areas of bulges considered normal variations are pregnancy or marked obesity.

➤**AUSCULTATE the abdomen for bowel sounds.** Be sure to auscultate *before* palpating and percussing the abdomen so that the presence or absence of bowel sounds or pain is not altered. A quiet environment may be necessary. Box 20-1 lists the anatomic correlates of the quarters of the abdomen (Fig. 20-7). Box 20-2 shows an alternate way to section the abdomen for examination using nine regions (Fig. 20-8).

ABNORMAL FINDINGS

■ Note visible peristalsis or marked pulsations. Grunting or labored movements or restricted abdominal movements with respirations should be recorded.

■ Report any absence of sound after listening for several minutes in each quadrant. Decreased or absent bowel sounds occur with mechanical obstruction or paralytic ileus. Decreased bowel sounds are associated with peritonitis and bowel obstruction. Increased bowel sounds, also called borborygmus, are high-pitched "tinkles" associated with increased peristalsis from diarrhea, use of a laxative, gastroenteritis, or an area anterior to an early intestinal obstruction.

Box 20-1 Anatomic Correlates of the Quadrants of the Abdomen

RIGHT UPPER QUADRANT	LEFT UPPER QUADRANT
Liver and gallbladder Pylorus Duodenum Head of pancreas Right adrenal gland Portion of right kidney Portions of ascending and transverse colon	Left lobe of liver Spleen Stomach Body of pancreas Left adrenal gland Portion of left kidney Portions of transverse and descending colon
RIGHT LOWER QUADRANT	**LEFT LOWER QUADRANT**
Lower pole of right kidney Cecum and appendix Portion of ascending colon Bladder (if distended) Ovary and salpinx Uterus (if enlarged) Right spermatic cord Right ureter	Lower pole of left kidney Sigmoid colon Portion of descending colon Bladder (if distended) Ovary and salpinx Uterus (if distended) Left spermatic cord Left ureter

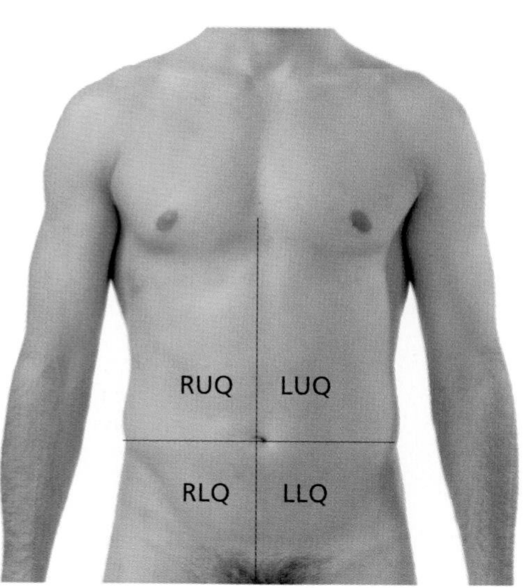

Fig. 20-7 Quadrants of the abdomen.

Box 20-2 Anatomic Correlates of the Nine Regions of the Abdomen

RIGHT HYPOCHONDRIAC	EPIGASTRIC	LEFT HYPOCHONDRIAC
Right lobe of liver Portion of gallbladder Portion of duodenum Portion of right kidney Right adrenal gland	Pyloric end of stomach Duodenum Pancreas Portion of liver Portion of gallbladder	Stomach Spleen Tail of pancreas Upper pole of left kidney Left adrenal gland
RIGHT LUMBAR	**UMBILICAL**	**LEFT LUMBAR**
Ascending colon Lower half of right kidney Portion of duodenum and jejunum	Lower duodenum Jejunum and ileum	Descending colon Lower half of left kidney Portions of jejunum and ileum
RIGHT INGUINAL	**HYPOGASTRIC**	**LEFT INGUINAL**
Cecum Appendix Ileum (lower end) Right ureter Right spermatic cord Right ovary	Ileum Bladder Uterus (in pregnancy)	Sigmoid colon Left ureter Left spermatic cord Left ovary

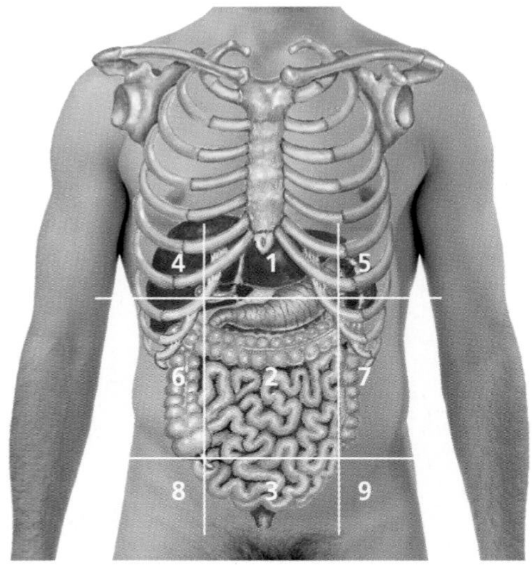

Fig. 20-8 Nine regions of the abdomen.

PROCEDURES AND TECHNIQUES WITH NORMAL FINDINGS

ABNORMAL FINDINGS

Use the diaphragm of the stethoscope and press lightly. Listen in a systematic progression, such as from right upper quadrant (RUQ) to left upper quadrant (LUQ) to left lower quadrant (LLQ) and finally to right lower quadrant (RLQ). Bowel sounds should be noted every 5 to 15 seconds. The duration of a single bowel sound may range from 1 to several seconds. The sounds are high-pitched gurgles or clicks, although this varies greatly.

➤**AUSCULTATE the abdomen for arterial and venous vascular sounds.** Listen with the bell of the stethoscope. Listen over aorta and renal, iliac, and femoral arteries for bruits that make "swishing" sounds, occur during systole, and are continuous regardless of the client's position (Fig. 20-9). Normally vascular sounds are not heard.

■ Bruits indicate a turbulent blood flow caused by narrowing of a blood vessel. Bruits over the aorta suggest an aneurysm. Two sound patterns may indicate renal arterial stenosis: soft, medium-to low-pitched murmurs heard over the upper midline or toward the flank or epigastric bruits that radiate laterally.

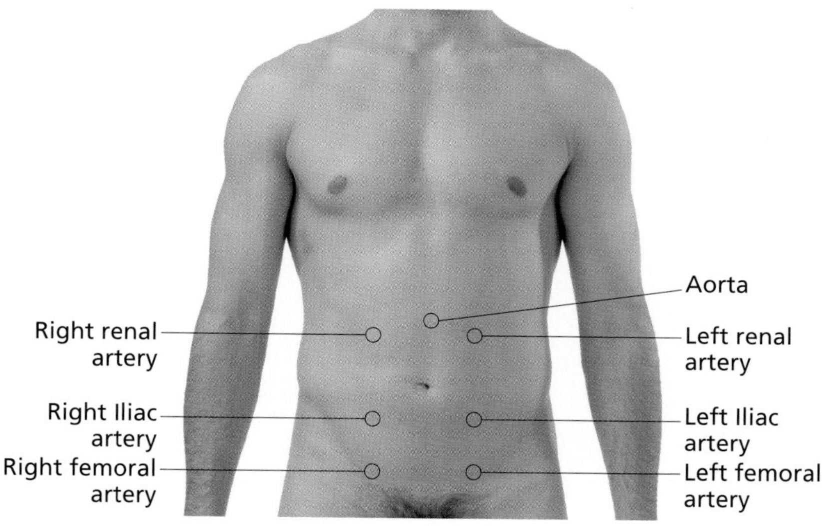

Fig. 20-9 Sites to auscultate for bruits: renal arteries, iliac arteries, aorta, and femoral arteries.

PROCEDURES AND TECHNIQUES WITH NORMAL FINDINGS

ABNORMAL FINDINGS

➤Also listen with the bell over the epigastric region and around the umbilicus for a venous hum, a soft, low-pitched, and continuous sound.

■ Venous hums are rare but associated with portal hypertension and cirrhosis.

❖ ➤**PERCUSS the abdomen for tones.** Percuss all quadrants for tones, using indirect percussion to assess density of abdominal contents. (Develop a system or routine for the percussion process to ensure that all areas are covered.) (Fig. 20-10.) Percuss in each quadrant for tympany and dullness. Tympany is the most common percussion tone heard due to the presence of gas. The suprapubic area may be dull when the urinary bladder is distended. See Chapter 6 for the procedures for percussion.

■ Note any marked dullness in a localized area that may indicate an abdominal mass.

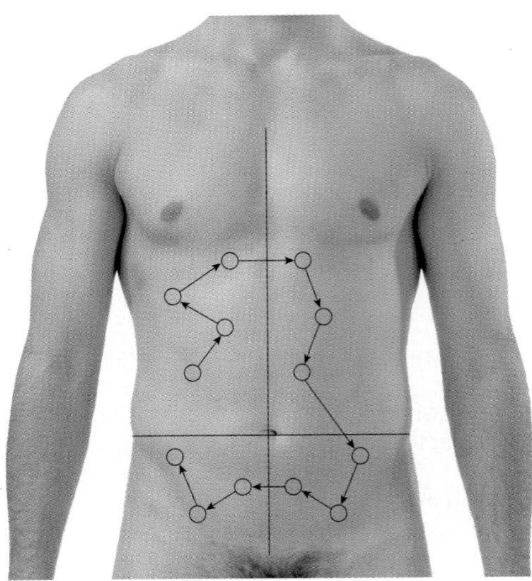

Fig. 20-10 Systematic route for abdominal percussion.

❖ ➤**PERCUSS the liver to determine span.**

1. Beginning below the level of the umbilicus at the right midclavicular line (RMCL); percuss upward over the tympanic area until dull percussion tone indicates the liver border. Mark the border with the marking pencil or pen. The lower border is usually at the costal margin or slightly below it (see Figs. 20-6 and 20-11, *A*).

■ Note when the lower border of the liver exceeds ¾ to 1 ³⁄₁₆ inches (2 to 3 cm) below the costal margin. This indicates an enlarged liver (hepatomegaly), which is associated with cirrhosis and hepatitis.

2. Beginning over the lung in the RMCL, percuss the intercostal spaces downward until tone changes from resonant to dull, indicating the upper liver border. Mark the location with the pencil or pen. The upper border usually begins in the fifth to seventh intercostal space (Fig. 20-11, *B*).

■ Note when dullness extends above the fifth intercostal space, indicating hepatomegaly.

3. Measure the span between the two lines to estimate the midclavicular liver span. Normally it is 2.5 to 4.5 inches (6 to 11 cm) (Fig. 20-11, *C*). Liver span correlates with body size and gender; large people and men tend to have larger spans (O'Hanlon-Nichols, 1998).

■ Note any span exceeding 4 ¾ inches (12 cm). Hepatomegaly is associated with cirrhosis. Also, clients with chronic obstructive pulmonary disease may have a flat diaphragm, which makes percussion of the upper border of the liver difficult. Obesity can make percussion difficult.

4. Ask the client to take a deep breath and hold; then percuss upward in the RMCL again to estimate the liver descent. The lower border of the liver should descend inferiorly ¾ to 1 ³⁄₁₆ inches (2 to 3 cm.)

■ Note if the liver fails to move with inspiration or if movement is less than ¾ inch (2 cm).

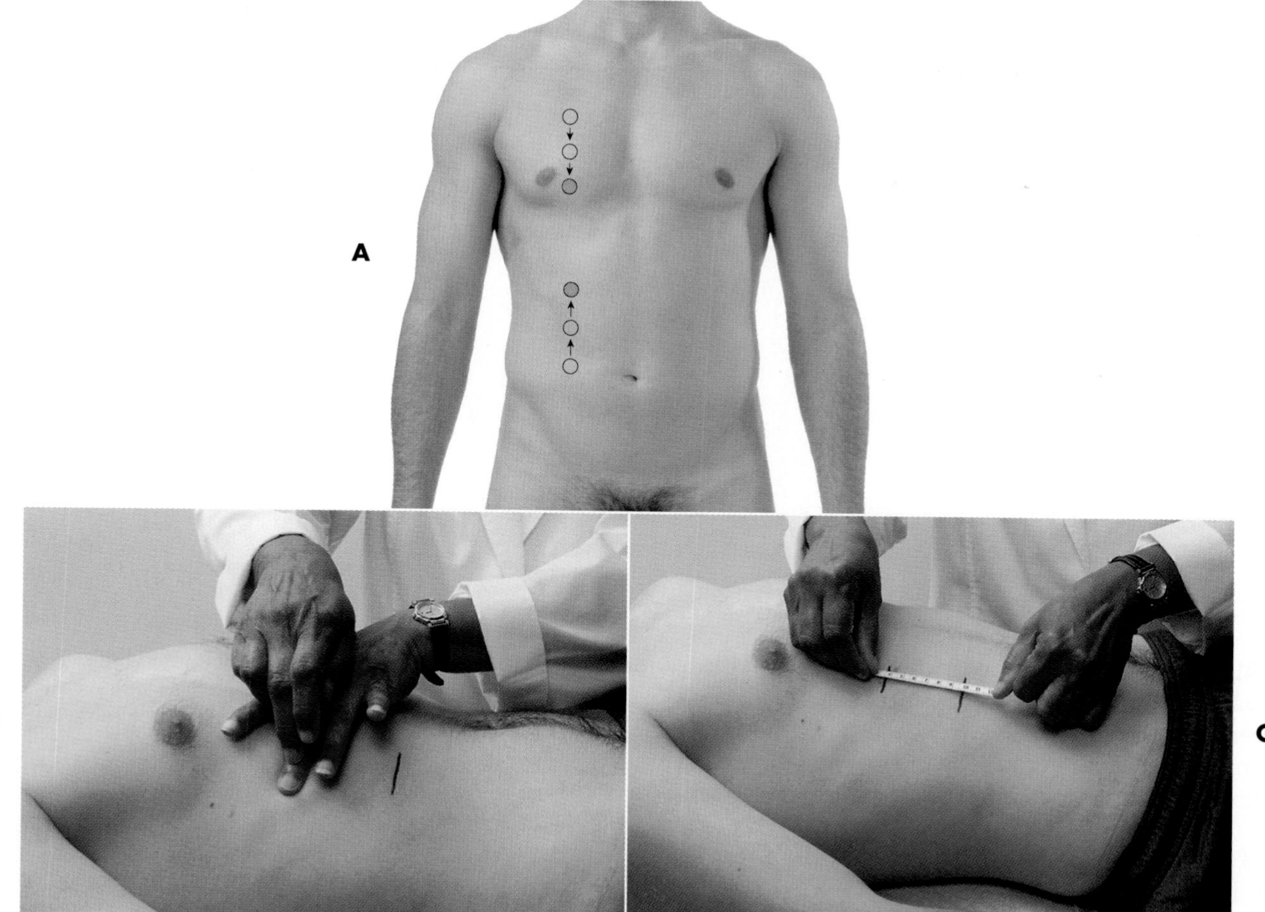

Fig. 20-11 **A,** Liver percussion route. **B,** Percussion method of estimating size of liver in the midclavicular line. **C,** Distance between the two marks measured in estimating the liver span in midclavicular line is usually 2 ⅜ to 4 ¾ inches (6 to 12 cm).

PROCEDURES AND TECHNIQUES WITH NORMAL FINDINGS

❖ ➤**PERCUSS the spleen for size.** Begin with the resonance of the lung and percuss from the seventh to tenth intercostal spaces at about the left midaxillary line (LMAL) (Fig. 20-12). Try to outline the spleen by percussing in several directions from dullness to resonance or tympany. Normally the spleen cannot be percussed, or you may hear a small area of splenic dullness at the sixth to the tenth intercostal spaces. A full stomach and feces in the transverse or descending colon may mimic dullness of splenic enlargement.

➤Percuss the lowest intercostal space in the left anterior axillary line before and after the client takes a deep breath. The area is usually tympanic.

ABNORMAL FINDINGS

■ Splenic enlargement may indicate infection, trauma, or chronic liver disease.

■ Note whether the tympany changes to dullness on inspiration. An enlarged spleen is brought forward on inspiration to produce a dull percussion note. Caution: A full stomach or feces-filled intestine may create dullness in this area also.

PROCEDURES AND TECHNIQUES WITH NORMAL FINDINGS

ABNORMAL FINDINGS

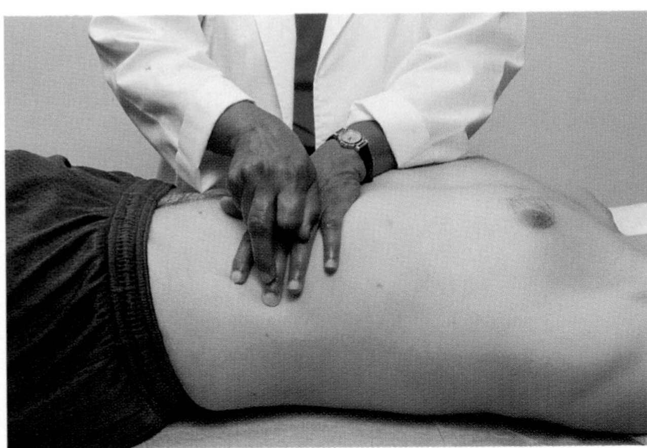

Fig. 20-12 Percussion of the spleen.

➤**PALPATE the abdomen lightly for tenderness, muscle tone, and surface characteristics.** Palpate all quadrants of the abdomen. Use the pads of the fingertips to depress the abdomen ⅜ to ¾ inches (1 to 2 cm) (Fig. 20-13). Some examiners reduce ticklishness by maintaining contact with the client's skin by sliding their hands into each palpation position. No tenderness should be present, and the abdominal muscles should be relaxed, although anxious clients may have some muscle resistance on palpation. Note consistent tension as you move across the smooth surface.

■ Note any cutaneous tenderness or hypersensitivity, as well as any involuntary resistance that cannot be relaxed on command. Note superficial masses or localized areas of rigidity or increased tension. Rigidity is associated with peritoneal irritation and may be diffuse or localized.

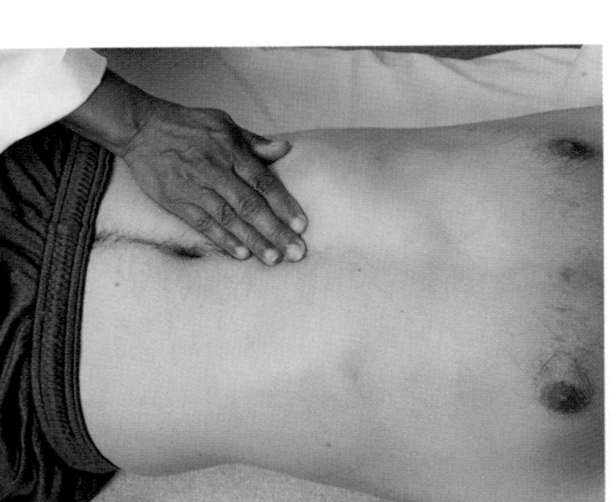

Fig. 20-13 Light palpation of the abdomen.

PROCEDURES AND TECHNIQUES WITH NORMAL FINDINGS

➤PALPATE the abdomen deeply for tenderness, masses, and aortic pulsation. Palpate all quadrants. Use either the distal flat portions of the finger pads (Fig. 20-14) and press gradually and deeply 1 ⅝ to 2 ⅜ inches (4 to 6 cm) into the palpation area, or use a bimanual technique, with the lower hand resting lightly on the surface and the upper hand exerting pressure for deep palpation (Fig. 20-15). Observe for facial grimaces during palpation that may indicate areas of tenderness. Ask the client to breathe slowly through the mouth to facilitate muscle relaxation.

The aorta is often palpable at the epigastrium, as well as above and slightly to the left of the umbilicus (Fig. 20-16). The borders of the rectus abdominis muscles can be felt, as can the sacral promontory and feces in the ascending or descending colon (see Fig. 20-5).

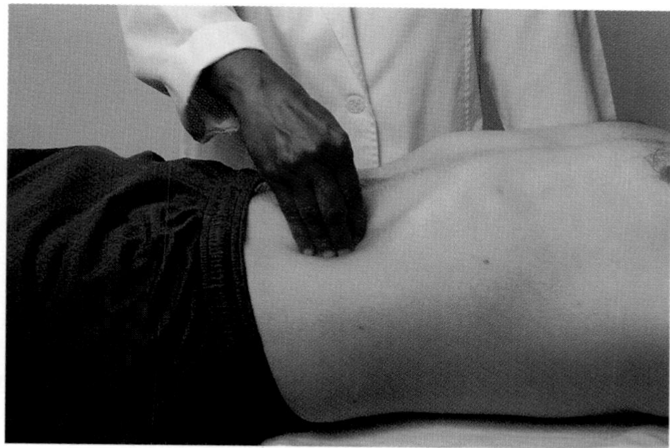

Fig. 20-14 Deep palpation of the abdomen.

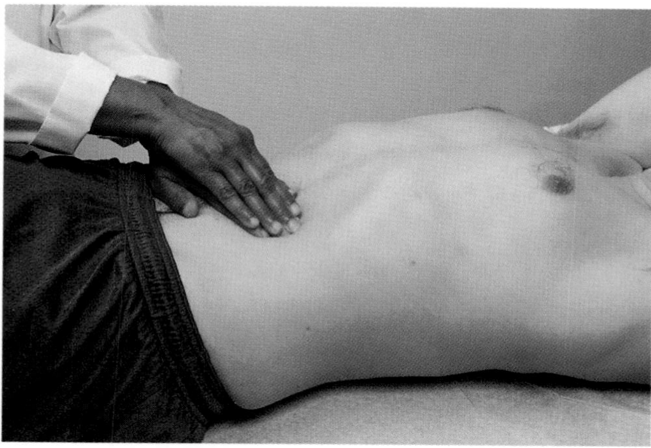

Fig. 20-15 Deep bimanual palpation.

ABNORMAL FINDINGS

- Note any pain that is present in local or generalized areas. The client may respond to pain by using muscle guarding, facial grimaces, or pulling away from the examiner.
- Abnormal findings include masses that descend during inspiration, lateral pulsatile masses (abdominal aortic aneurysm), laterally mobile masses, and fixed masses.

PROCEDURES AND TECHNIQUES WITH NORMAL FINDINGS

ABNORMAL FINDINGS

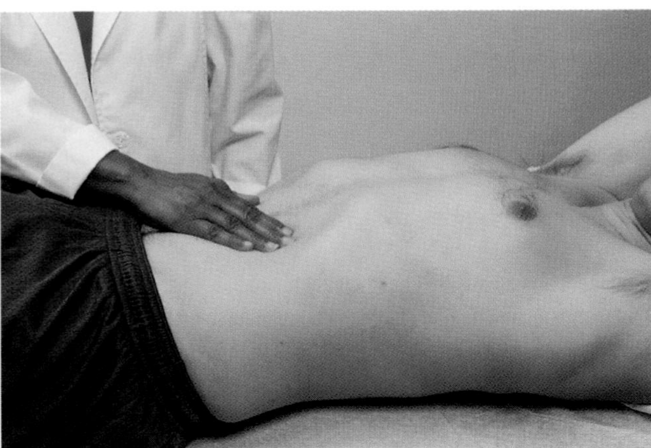

Fig. 20-16 Palpating the aorta.

➤**PALPATE around the umbilicus for bulges, nodules, and the umbilical ring.** The ring should be round with no irregularities or bulges. The umbilicus itself may be inverted or slightly everted.

■ Note if the umbilical ring is incomplete or soft in the center.

❖ ➤**PALPATE the liver for lower border and tenderness.** There are two different techniques for this assessment. Be sure your fingernails are short for this procedure.

1. Place the left hand under the eleventh and twelfth ribs to lift the liver closer to the abdominal wall, while the right hand is parallel to the right costal margin (Fig. 20-17, *A, B*). Press your right hand down and under the costal margin (see Fig. 20-6). Ask the client to take some deep breaths. The border and contour of the liver is often not palpable. It may "bump" against the fingers during inspiration, especially in thin clients.
2. To use the "hooking" technique, stand on the client's right side facing the feet. Place your hands side by side at the right costal margin and curve your fingers to "hook" them under the right costal margin (Fig. 20-17, *C*). Ask the client to take a deep breath, and you may feel the liver bump against your fingers during inspiration. The border of the liver should feel smooth. No tenderness should be present.

■ A very enlarged liver may lie under the examiner's hand as it extends downward into the abdominal cavity.

■ Note any irregular surfaces or edges as well as any tenderness. With pain, the client may abruptly stop inspiration.

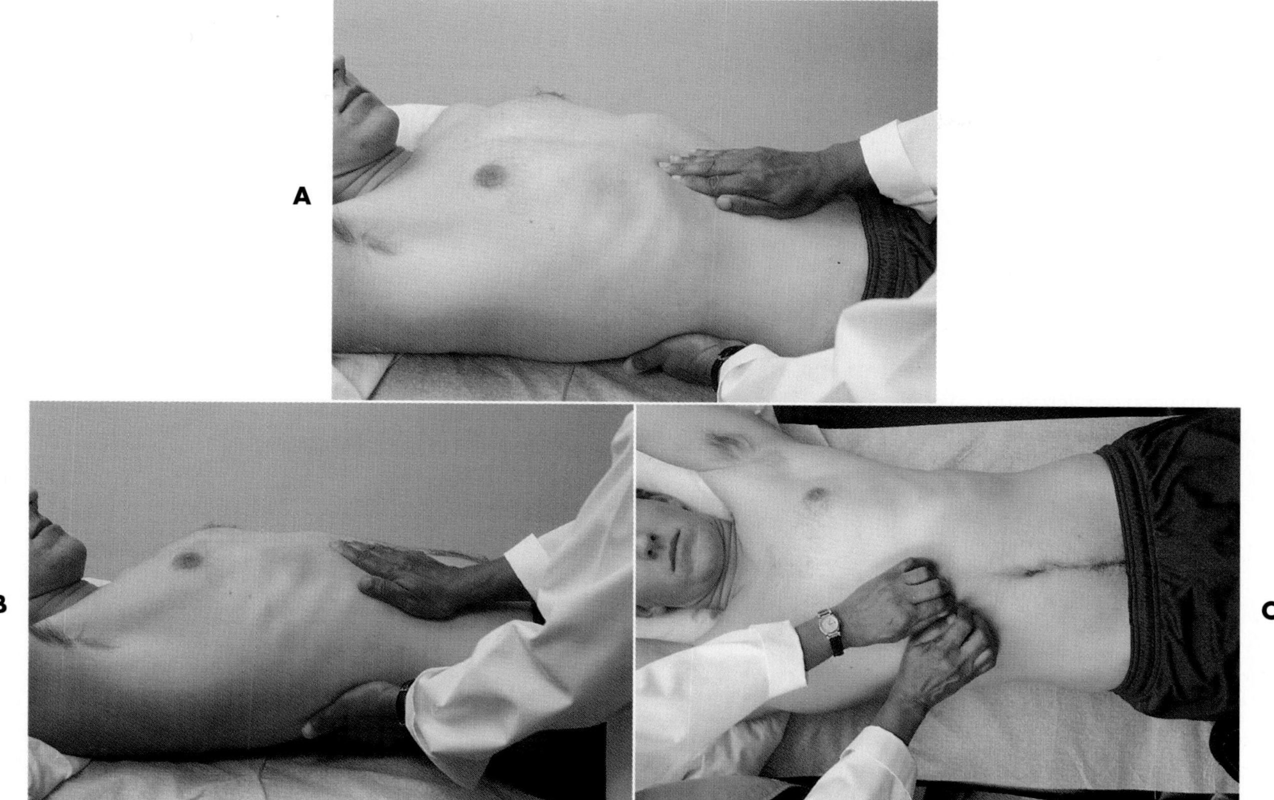

Fig. 20-17 Methods of palpating the liver. **A,** Fingers are extended, with tips on right midclavicular line below the level of liver tenderness and pointing toward the head. **B,** Fingers parallel to the costal margin. **C,** Fingers hooked over the costal margin.

PROCEDURES AND TECHNIQUES WITH NORMAL FINDINGS

❖ ➤**PALPATE the gallbladder for tenderness.** Palpate below the liver margin at the lateral border of the rectus abdominis muscle for the gallbladder. A healthy gallbladder is not palpable.

ABNORMAL FINDINGS

■ A palpable, tender gallbladder may indicate cholecystitis. Test for cholecystitis by asking the client to take in a deep breath during deep palpation. Cholecystitis is suspected if the client experiences pain and abruptly stops inhaling during palpation. This is called Murphy's sign. A nontender, enlarged gallbladder suggests common bile duct obstruction.

PROCEDURES AND TECHNIQUES WITH NORMAL FINDINGS

ABNORMAL FINDINGS

❖ ➤**PALPATE the spleen for border and tenderness.** Standing at the client's right side, place the left hand under the client's left flank at the costovertebral angle and exert pressure upward to move the spleen anteriorly. Press the right hand gently under the left anterior costal margin (Fig. 20-18).

Ask the client to take a deep breath and then exhale. With the exhalation, follow the tissue contour under the border of the ribs to try to palpate the spleen; normally it is not palpable.

An alternate strategy for spleen palpation is to perform the procedure with the client lying on the right side with the legs and knees flexed. Stand on the client's right and place your left hand over the client's left costovertebral angle while pressing your right hand under the left anterior costal margin.

■ A palpable spleen will feel like a firm mass that bumps against examiner's fingers. Spleen tenderness may indicate infection or trauma.

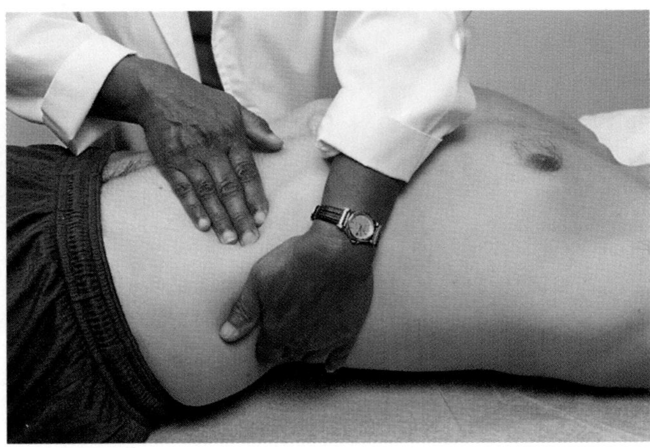

Fig. 20-18 Palpation of the spleen.

❖ ➤**PALPATE the kidneys for presence, contour, and tenderness.** Normally the kidney is not palpable and is excluded for the routine health assessment unless data from the history indicates a need.

Left Kidney Stand to the client's right side with the client in a supine position. Place the left hand at the left posterior costal angle (left flank) and the right hand at the client's left anterior costal margin (see Fig. 20-6). Ask the client to take a deep breath and elevate the client's left flank with your left hand and palpate deeply with your right hand (Fig. 20-19). Occasionally the lower pole of the kidney can be felt during inhalation in thin clients, but rarely in the average client. The contour should be smooth with no tenderness.

■ Tenderness is associated with kidney trauma or infection, for example, pyelonephritis.

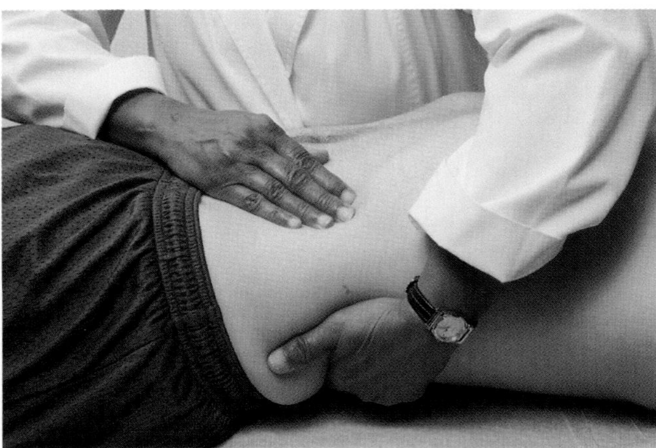

Fig. 20-19 Palpation of left kidney.

PROCEDURES AND TECHNIQUES WITH NORMAL FINDINGS

ABNORMAL FINDINGS

Right Kidney Repeat the same maneuver on the right side, which is easier to palpate since it lies lower than the left kidney (Fig. 20-20). The lower pole of the right kidney may be palpated during inspiration as smooth, firm, and nontender.

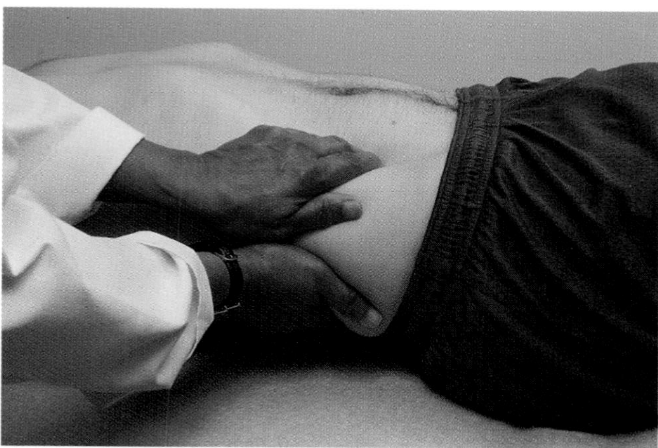

Fig. 20-20 Palpation of right kidney.

❖ **➤ELICIT abdominal reflexes for presence.** Elicit the abdominal reflexes by stroking each quadrant with the end of a reflex hammer or tongue blade (Fig. 20-21). For upper abdominal reflexes, stroke upward and away from the umbilicus; for lower abdominal reflexes, stroke downward and away from the umbilicus. The expected response to each stroke is contraction of the rectus abdominis muscle and movement of the umbilicus toward the side stroked.

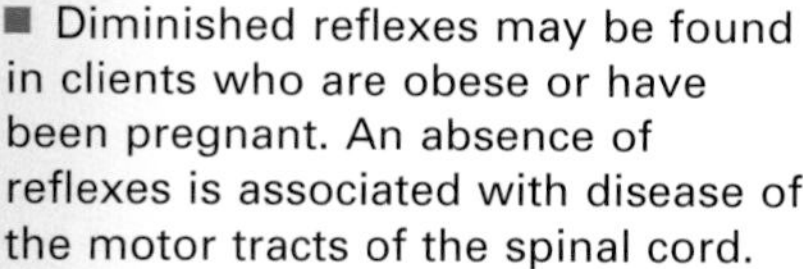

■ Diminished reflexes may be found in clients who are obese or have been pregnant. An absence of reflexes is associated with disease of the motor tracts of the spinal cord.

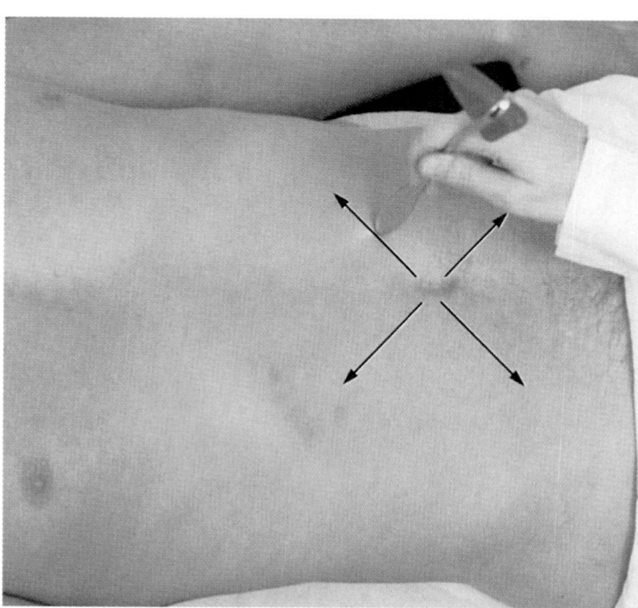

Fig. 20-21 Eliciting superficial abdominal reflexes. Stroke the upper abdominal area upward, away from the umbilicus, and the lower umbilicus area downward, away from the umbilicus. (From Seidel et al, 1999.)

PROCEDURES AND TECHNIQUES WITH NORMAL FINDINGS

ABNORMAL FINDINGS

❖ ADDITIONAL ASSESSMENT TECHNIQUES FOR SPECIAL CASES

➤**PERCUSS the kidneys for costovertebral angle (CVA) tenderness.** Approach the client from behind as he or she is seated. Use direct percussion to tap each CVA with the ulnar surface of the dominant fist (Fig. 20-22, *A*). An alternative method is to use indirect percussion. Place the palmar surface of the nondominant hand over the CVA, and tap the dorsum of that hand with the dominant fist (Fig. 20-22, *B*). The client should perceive a thud.

■ Costovertebral angle tenderness or severe pain may indicate pyelonephritis.

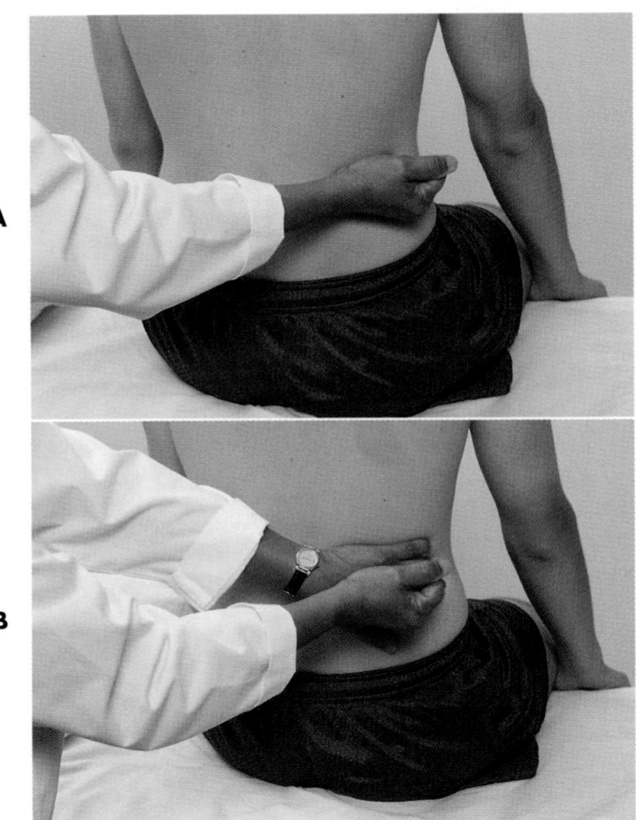

Fig. 20-22 Fist percussion of costovertebral angle for kidney tenderness. **A,** Direct percussion. **B,** Indirect percussion.

PROCEDURES AND TECHNIQUES WITH NORMAL FINDINGS

➤ASSESS the abdomen for fluid. If fluid is suspected within the abdomen, perform the following tests:

- *Shifting dullness.* Ask the client to lie supine so that any fluid will pool in the lateral (flank) area. Percuss the abdomen. Draw lines on the abdomen to indicate the midline tympany (the expected tone) in contrast to lateral dullness (tone created by fluid). Then have the client turn to the right side and repeat percussion. Listen as the tympanic tone shifts to the upper (left) side and the area of dullness rises toward the midline (Fig. 20-23). Finally, have the client turn to the left lateral position and percuss. Listen as the dullness rises toward the midline.
- *Fluid wave.* Another examiner's or the client's hand is placed sideways in the middle of the client's abdomen to stop the transmission of a tap across the skin (Fig. 20-24). Tap one flank while palpating the other side. You will feel the fluid with the other hand on the opposite side of the abdomen.

ABNORMAL FINDINGS

■ Movement of dullness as the client shifts position reflects the shift of fluid in the peritoneal cavity (ascites).

■ If ascites is present, the tap will cause a fluid wave through the abdomen.

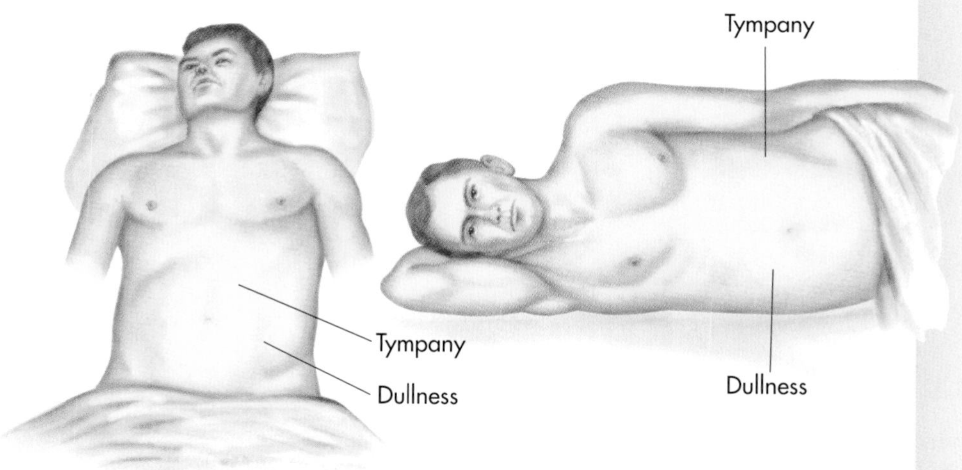

Fig. 20-23 Testing for shifting dullness. Dullness shifts to the dependent side. (From Seidel et al, 1999.)

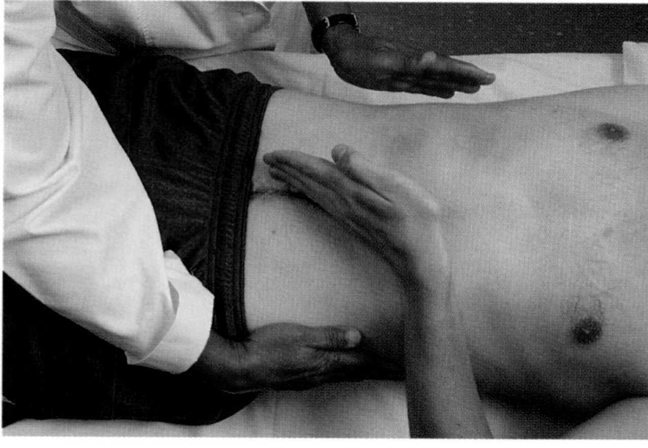

Fig. 20-24 Testing for fluid wave. Strike one side of the abdomen sharply with the fingertips. Feel for the impulse of a fluid wave with the other hand.

PROCEDURES AND TECHNIQUES WITH NORMAL FINDINGS

➤**ASSESS the abdomen for pain (see Table 20-1).** If the client has abdominal pain, test for rebound tenderness as follows: Press down firmly at a 90° angle to the abdomen in an area away from the point of pain. Press inward deeply (Fig. 20-25), then release your hand quickly.

➤Testing for McBurney's sign is a test for appendicitis. Palpate McBurney's point, which is located halfway between the umbilicus and the right anterior iliac crest. Press firmly into the abdomen, and release pressure quickly. Absence of pain is a negative McBurney's sign.

➤Perform the iliopsoas muscle test when acute appendicitis is suspected. With the client supine, place your hand over the lower right thigh. Ask the client to raise the right leg, flexing at the hip. Push down to resist the raising of the leg (Fig. 20-26). When the client reports no pain from the pressure on the iliopsoas muscle, the test is negative.

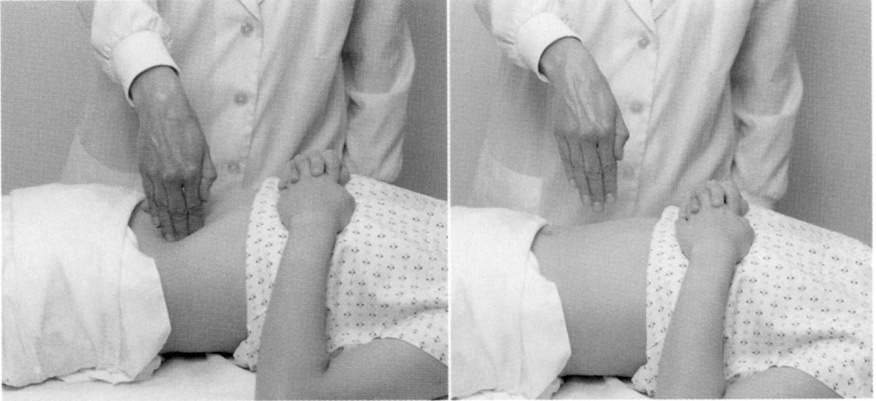

Fig. 20-25 Testing for rebound tenderness. **A,** Press deeply and gently into the abdomen; then **B,** rapidly withdraw the hands and fingers.

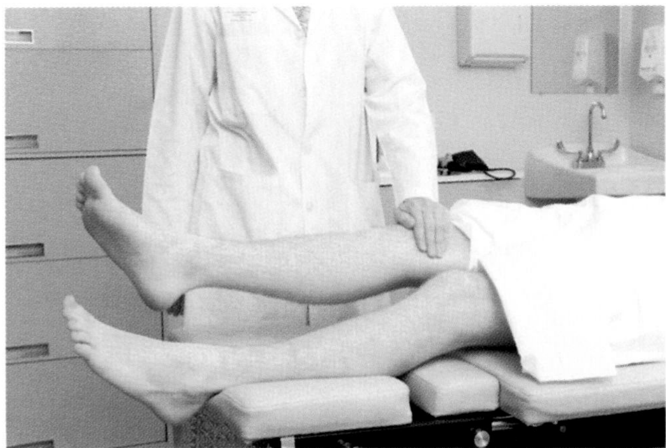

Fig. 20-26 Iliopsoas muscle test. (From Doughty and Jackson, 1993.)

ABNORMAL FINDINGS

■ Rebound tenderness is present if the client experiences more pain when pressure is released than when pressure exerted and indicates peritoneal inflammation.

■ Positive rebound tenderness over McBurney's point indicates appendicitis.

■ An inflamed appendix may irritate the lateral iliopsoas muscle. When the client reports LLQ pain to pressure against the raised leg, the iliopsoas muscle test is positive.

PROCEDURES AND TECHNIQUES WITH NORMAL FINDINGS

➤Perform the obturator muscle test when a ruptured appendix or pelvic abscess is suspected. The client lies supine and flexes the right hip and knee to 90°. The examiner, holding the leg just above the knee and at the ankle, rotates the leg medially and laterally (Fig. 20-27). If the client has no pain, the test is negative.

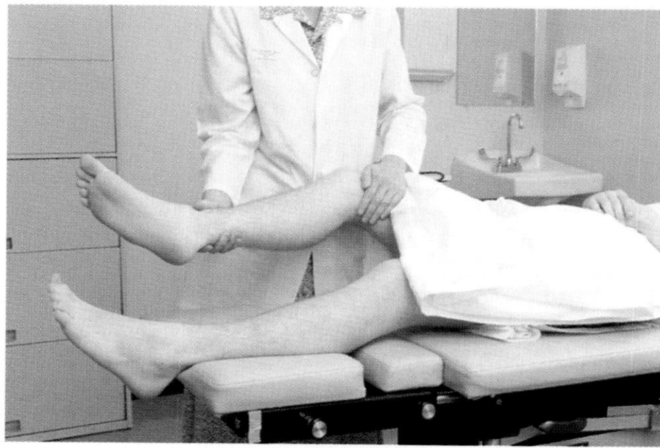

Fig. 20-27 Obturator muscle test. (From Doughty and Jackson, 1993.)

➤**ASSESS abdomen for floating mass.** Ballottement is a palpation technique used to determine a floating mass. Ballottement can be performed with one or two hands.

Place one hand perpendicular to the abdomen and push in toward the mass with fingertips (Fig. 20-28, *A*). A freely movable mass will float upward and touch the fingertips as fluids and other structures are displaced.

When using the bimanual method, place one hand on the anterior abdomen to push down. The other hand is placed against the flank to push up and palpate the mass to determine presence and size (Fig. 20-28, *B*).

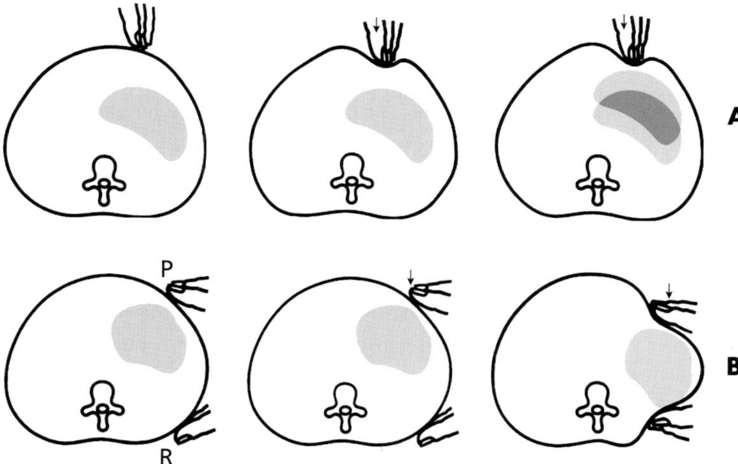

Fig. 20-28 Ballottement technique. **A,** Single-handed ballottement. Push inward at a 90° angle; if the object is freely movable, it will float upward to touch the fingertips. **B,** Bimanual ballottement. *P,* Pushing hand; *R,* receiving hand. (From *GI Series,* 1981, Whitehall-Robins Healthcare.)

ABNORMAL FINDINGS

■ Pain in the hypogastric region is a positive sign indicating irritation of the obturator muscle, which may be caused by a ruptured appendix or pelvic abscess.

■ A floating mass may be an abnormal growth or a fetal head.

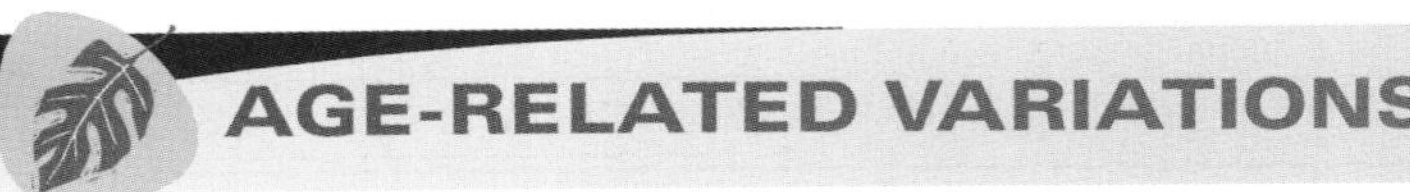

AGE-RELATED VARIATIONS

Refer to Chapter 10 for additional questions about nutrition.

INFANTS

Anatomy and Physiology

Anatomy and physiology for the infant are the same as for the adult.

Health History

- Has the infant had a distended abdomen? Vomited?
  Rationale These signs may suggest intestinal obstruction.
- Has your infant been spitting up, crying more than usual, been irritable, arching the back and had trouble sleeping? Have you noticed him or her coughing or wheezing?
  Rationale These symptoms are consistent with GERD in the infant (Ault and Schmidt, 1998).

Examination

Procedures and Techniques The abdominal examination is straightforward, with the infant lying supine on an examining table. Follow the same procedures for examining the abdomen as for adults.

Normal and Abnormal Findings Inspecting the abdomen of a healthy infant finds a symmetric, soft, and round abdomen with a slight protrusion, and no masses are present. There is synchronous abdominal and chest movement with breathing. Diastasis swelling and a gap between the rectus muscles may be noted during crying. Inspect the umbilicus in the newborn. Immediately after the umbilical cord is cut, two arteries and one vein should be noted. After the cord is clamped, it will change from white to black as it dries; it should be dry in 5 days and fall off spontaneously in 7 to 14 days. Visible pulsations in the epigastric areas are common.

Abnormal findings include discharge, odor, or redness around the umbilicus; a protrusion or nodular appearance of the umbilicus; thick Wharton's jelly; and a thin or green cord. Note any distention, masses, and concave, sunken, or flat appearance. A scaphoid, turnip-shaped abdomen suggests diaphragmatic hernia. Respiratory signs such as cough, wheeze, pneumonia, and stridor may indicate GERD (Ault and Schmidt, 1998).

The edge of the infant's liver should be ⅜ to ¾ inch (1 to 2 cm) below the right rib cage (costal margin). The spleen is generally not palpable, although the tip may be felt in the left upper quadrant (far left costal margin). The left kidney is noted with deep palpation; both should be ⅜ to ¾ inch (1 to 2 cm) above the umbilicus. Dull tones are noted on percussion over the bladder above the symphysis pubis. Abnormal findings include an enlarged liver 1 ¼ inch (3 cm) or more below the margin, palpable spleen, masses near the kidneys, and enlarged kidneys.

CHILDREN

Anatomy and Physiology

Anatomy and physiology for the children is the same as for the adult.

Health History

- Has your child complained about heartburn, abdominal pain, or difficulty swallowing? Have you noticed a chronic cough, wheezing at night, or vomiting?
  Rationale These are symptoms of GERD in children (Ault and Schmidt, 1998).
- Is the child toilet trained? Has toilet training been successful? If not, describe.
  Rationale Most parents begin to toilet train children by age 2 or 2 ½. By this age the child has enough muscle development to exert some control over elimination.
- Does the child ever wet the bed at night? If so, does it occur frequently or on rare occasions? What have you done about this? How does the child feel about wetting the bed? How do you, as a parent, feel about it?
  Rationale Almost all children wet the bed at some time. Assess if the bed-wetting occurs frequently, whether it occurs because of physiologic or psychosocial dysfunction or a full bladder before the child goes to bed. Parents should be encouraged not to scold the child for bed-wetting and to seek help from a primary care practitioner on how to deal with frequent bed-wetting.

Examination

Procedures and Techniques Children may resist abdominal palpation because they are ticklish. Assessment of children is generally the same as for adults, with the exception of the areas noted below.

Normal and Abnormal Findings Inspect the contour of the abdomen. It is normally rounded (a potbelly) in toddlers both while standing and while lying down. School-age children may show this roundedness until about 13 years of age when standing; when lying, the abdomen should be scaphoid. Inspect and palpate for any umbilical hernia. This type of hernia is common in African-American children until 7 years of age and in white children under 2 years of age (Wong et al, 1999). Note movement of the abdomen on respiration. Until about age 7, children are abdominal breathers; after age 7, boys exhibit chiefly abdominal movement whereas girls exhibit chiefly thoracic movement. Note any grunting or labored breathing accompanied by restricted abdominal movement. Check the tenseness of the abdominal muscles. The condition of diastasis recti abdominis (two rectus muscles fail to approximate one another) is common in African-American children but should disappear during the preschool years (Wong et al, 1999).

Abnormal findings include scaphoid abdomen in toddlers and any generalized distention. Note any hernia still present after age 7 years in African-American children and age 2 years in white children (Wong et al, 1999). Abdominal pain is a symptom in a number of childhood illnesses, including upper respiratory infection, pharyngitis, right lower lobe pneumonia, pyelonephritis, constipation, appendicitis, and gastroenteritis.

❖ Percuss the liver for tone and span. Averages vary by age as follows: 5 years of age, 2 ¾ inches (7 cm); 12 years of age, 3 ½ inches (9 cm). Percuss for spleen tone and span. In young children the area of dullness may extend to ⅜ to ¾ inches (1 to 2 cm) below the costal margin.

❖ Palpate the liver to locate the border. The lower edge of the liver may be palpable in young children as a superficial mass ⅜ to ¾ inch (1 to 2 cm) below the right costal margin. Normally the liver descends during inspiration. The liver may not be palpable in older children (Wong et al, 1999).

■ ADOLESCENTS

Anatomy and Physiology

Anatomy and physiology for the adolescent are the same as for the adult.

Health History

Health history is the same as for the adult.

Examination

Procedures and Techniques Procedures and techniques, as well as normal and abnormal findings, are the same for the adolescent as for the adult.

■ OLDER ADULTS

Anatomy and Physiology

Changes in the structure and function of the gastrointestinal system occur with aging. Motility of the esophagus is reduced due to a decreased number of cells, causing dilation of the lower end of the esophagus. As aging occurs, less gastric acid is secreted; however, sufficient enzymes are available for digestion. Decreased motor activity delays the emptying of the stomach into the duodenum. With degeneration of the gastric mucosa, there is a reduction in parietal cells, which normally secrete intrinsic factor needed for vitamin B_{12} absorption.

The small intestine contains fewer absorbing cells, but this usually does not affect function. A decrease in lipase production may contribute to an intolerance of fatty foods. In the large intestine, weakened muscle and decreased peristalsis contribute to constipation. Bacterial flora in the intestines become less biologically active, contributing to food intolerance and impaired digestion. For example, older adults may have faulty absorption of vitamins B_1, B_{12}, calcium, and iron.

The liver decreases in size after age 50, reducing its storage capacity and ability to synthesize proteins. A decrease in cardiac output reduces the blood flow to the liver. As a result, the liver metabolism of drugs, hormones, and alcohol is less efficient (Matteson, McConnell, and Linton, 1997).

Health History

- Have you had any abdominal pains recently that you have not felt before?

  Rationale Degenerative vascular disease of local arteries may contribute to the development of gastric pain in older adults. These clients frequently do not complain of epigastric pain until hemorrhage or perforation occurs (Yamada, 1998).

- Do you have difficulty with constipation? How do you define constipation? How much liquid do you drink a day? How much bulk or fiber do you eat? Do you take any laxatives for constipation? How often?

  Rationale Definitions of constipation vary by individual. Constipation is a common problem of older adults that they may not mention to the health care provider. These questions help identify the problem and what the client usually does to prevent constipation.

- Have you had urinary incontinence? When does it occur? Suddenly or only when you laugh or sneeze? What do you do to stay dry?

  Rationale Clients may be reluctant to initiate a discussion about incontinence. Urinary incontinence is reported by 15% to 30% of older adults living at home and almost 50% for those in nursing homes. Urge incontinence occurs suddenly and is caused by detrusor overactivity, whereas stress incontinence is more common in women and caused by relaxation of the pelvic muscles (Matteson, McConnell, and Linton, 1997).

Examination

Techniques and Procedures Techniques and procedures for assessing the GI and renal systems for the older adult are the same as for the younger adult.

Normal and Abnormal Findings Older adults may have increased fat deposits over the abdominal area even with decreased subcutaneous fat over the extremities. The abdomen may feel soft due to loss of abdominal muscle tone, making palpation of organs easier (Lueckenotte, 1994). Note any marked distention or concavity associated with general wasting signs or anteroposterior rib expansion.

CLIENTS WITH SITUATIONAL VARIATIONS

CLIENTS WITH ILEOSTOMY OR COLOSTOMY

Clients who have had either an ileostomy or colostomy have had to deal with many issues ranging from altered body functioning to body image changes to concern about "accidents and odors" to possibly dealing with a serious disease such as cancer (Box 20-3). Because the client is usually skilled in caring for the ostomy, the examiner should encourage the client to be a participant in the examination by having him or her remove the external pouch bag (if present) and have the client describe how the ostomy appears.

Health History

- How long have you had the ostomy?
  Rationale Clients who have a new ostomy may need more teaching and referrals for support than clients who have had more time to adjust.
- How have you changed your diet because of the ostomy?
  Rationale Clients are encouraged to eliminate foods that cause gas such as raw vegetables. Clients who have an ileostomy need to replace fluids lost through the stoma.
- What is your daily routine for caring for the ostomy?
  Rationale The client may need a referral for education and/or support if he or she is having difficulty adjusting to the ostomy and skin care required.
- How well do you think you have been able to cope with having the ostomy? Are there activities that you have been unable to do because of the ostomy? If yes, describe.
  Rationale Assess client's perception of how well he or she has adjusted so that referrals can be made.

Examination

Procedures and Techniques Observe the skin characteristics around the stoma, as well as inspecting the stoma itself. Observe the characteristics of the stool from the stoma.

Box 20-3 Types of Ostomies

COLOSTOMY

A surgical procedure that creates an opening, or stoma, between the colon and the abdominal wall. A colostomy is performed when a portion of the large bowel, including the colon, rectum, or anus, is diseased and must be bypassed or removed. The most common reasons for a colostomy are diverticulitis, tumors, injury, or birth injury.

ILEOSTOMY

A surgical procedure in which an opening, or stoma, is created by bringing the ileum of the small intestine through the abdominal wall.

Normal and Abnormal Findings The stoma of either the ileostomy or the colostomy should appear red and moist. Because the stoma is actually inverted bowel, it has no sensory nerve endings. The area where the ostomy attaches to the skin should appear well-healed and without lesions, irritation, or areas of excoriation. If skin irritation is noted, inquire about cleaning techniques and use of preparations that will help prevent skin breakdown.

The stool characteristics of an individual with an ostomy will depend upon the level of the ostomy. Clients with an ileostomy (small-bowel area) will have uncontrollable drainage of stool that is of a thick liquid consistency. If the client has had a transverse (upper colon) level colostomy, the stool will be mushy and uncontrollable. If the client's colostomy is in the area of the descending or sigmoid (lower) colon, the stool will be more solid and may actually become controllable, so that some clients may elect to not wear a pouch.

EXAMINATION SUMMARY

Abdomen and Gastrointestinal System

PROCEDURE

- Observe client for:
  General behavior
  Position

Abdomen (pp. 488-499)

- Inspect the abdomen for:
  Skin color
  Surface characteristics
  Contour
  Surface movements
- Auscultate the abdomen with diaphragm of stethoscope for:
  Bowel sounds
- Auscultate abdomen with bell of stethoscope for:
  Arterial (aorta, renal, iliac, femoral) bruits
  Venous hum

❖ • Percuss abdomen for:
Tones (tympany) in all quadrants

❖ • Percuss liver for:
Span

❖ • Percuss spleen for:
Size

• Palpate abdomen lightly in all quadrants for:
Tenderness
Muscle tone
Surface characteristics

• Palpate abdomen deeply for:
Tenderness
Masses
Aortic pulsation

• Palpate around the umbilicus for:
Bulges
Nodules
Umbilical ring

❖ • Palpate the liver for:
Lower border and tenderness

❖ • Palpate gallbladder for:
Tenderness

❖ • Palpate spleen for:
Border
Tenderness

❖ • Palpate kidneys for:
Presence
Contour
Tenderness

❖ • Elicit abdominal reflexes for:
Presence

❖ Additional Assessment Techniques for Special Cases (pp. 500-503)

• Percuss kidneys for costovertebral angle tenderness

• Assess abdomen for fluid:
Shifting dullness
Fluid wave

• Assess abdomen for pain:
Rebound tenderness
McBurney's sign
Iliopsoas test
Obturator test

• Assess abdomen for floating mass:
Ballottement

SUMMARY OF FINDINGS

Age Group	Normal Findings	Typical Variations	Findings Associated With Disorders
Infants and children	• Height and weight are within expected normal range for age and gender. • Infants have synchronous abdominal and chest movement with breathing. Superficial veins are seen in infants. • Pulsations in epigastric area are common. • Liver palpated 1-3 cm below right costal margin. • Left kidney may be palpable. • Abdomen appears rounded or convex and protrudes in toddlers.		• Height and weight less than expected indicate a growth problem. • Height and weight greater than expected may indicate overnutrition or hormonal imbalance.
Adolescents	Same as for adult.	Same as for adult.	Same as for adult.
Older adults	Same as for adult.		• Left lower quadrant pain may suggest diverticulitis. • The incidence of colon cancer is increased. • Constipation and urinary incontinence are common problems.

Age Group	Normal Findings	Typical Variations	Findings Associated With Disorders
Adults	• Skin of abdomen is pale in color, smooth, with flat or rounded contour. • Bowel sounds are present in all quadrants with no vascular sounds heard. • Percussion tones are tympany except for dull tones over liver and bladder. Liver span is 2.5 to 4.5 inches. No percussion tones over spleen. • No pain to palpation. • No masses, tenderness, or aortic pulsations on deep palpation. • No bulges around umbilicus. • Liver, spleen, and kidneys not palpable. • Abdominal reflexes intact.	• Bulges may appear due to pregnancy or marked obesity. Pulsations may be visible in thin persons. • Tones over spleen may be dull. • The umbilicus may be inverted or may protrude. • Liver span is larger in men and tall persons. • Decreased reflexes may be found in pregnancy or in obese people.	• Jaundiced skin indicates high serum bilirubin. • Erythema may indicate trauma, rash, or other inflammation. • Engorged veins and taut skin occurs in ascites. • Bulges over the liver or spleen may indicate masses. • Pain on palpation. Masses, tenderness, or aortic pulsations on deep palpation. • Decreased to absent bowel sounds occur with mechanical obstruction or paralytic ileus. • Bruits over the aorta suggest an aneurysm. • Dull percussion tone in areas other than over the bladder and liver would suggest fluid or masses. • An enlarged liver suggests cirrhosis or hepatitis and may occur with jaundice. • Enlarged spleen that feels firm occurs during a systemic infection or after abdominal trauma. • The umbilical ring is incomplete or soft. • CVA tenderness suggests pyelonephritis. • Diminished reflexes suggest a neurologic disorder.

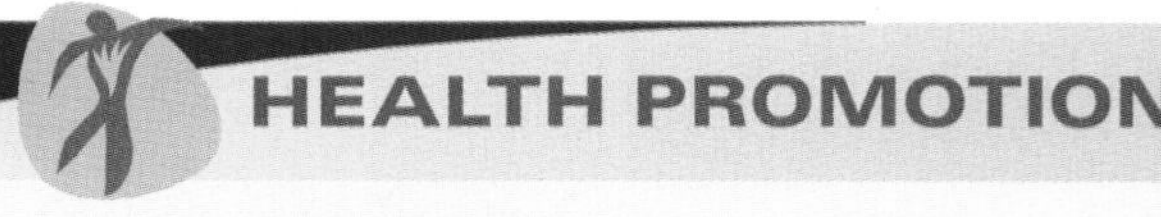

HEALTH PROMOTION

IMMUNIZATIONS

Parents need education about the importance of immunizing their children. Hepatitis B vaccine is started at birth or by 2 months of age. The second injection is due 1 month after the first, and the third and final injection is due 6 months after the first.

FOOD POISONING

Prevent food poisoning by refrigerating foods containing eggs and milk products and cooking meat and fish thoroughly before eating.

LEAD POISONING

Childhood lead poisoning has declined in the United States because of the limits of lead in gasoline, paint, food cans, and other products. Lead poisoning is still a significant health problem affecting an estimated 890,000 preschoolers. The Centers for Disease Control estimates that 4.4% of children age 1 to 5 have too much lead in their bodies.

Although lead poisoning crosses all socioeconomic, geographic, and racial boundaries, the majority of cases are from low-income families and children of color. African-American children are 5 times more likely to be poisoned than white children.

Text continued on p. 510

RISK FACTORS

COMMON RISK FACTORS ASSOCIATED WITH Cancers Affecting the Abdomen and Gastrointestinal System

	Age (yr)	Gender	Race	Tobacco Use	Alcohol Use	Diet	Other
Esophagus	45-70	Men 3 times greater than women	African Americans 3 times greater than whites	Increases risk	Long-term use increases risk	Deficient in fruits and vegetables; vitamins A, C, riboflavin	Barrett's esophagus (long-term gastroesophageal reflux) Lye ingestion Achalasia (lower esophageal stricture)
Stomach	50-70	Men 2 times greater than women	Φ	Increases risk	Increases risk	Large amounts smoked foods, salted fish and meat, pickled foods; low fiber	*Helicobacter pylori* infection, previous stomach surgery, pernicious anemia, blood group A, family history of stomach cancer, stomach polyps
Colon	>50	Φ*	Φ	Φ	Φ	Red meat, high-fat, low-fiber diet	Rectal polyps, family history, chronic inflammatory bowel disease, e.g., Crohn's ulcerative disease or ulcerative colitis, physical inactivity
Liver	Φ	Φ	Φ	Increases risk	Φ	Φ	Hepatitis B or C, cirrhosis, anabolic steroids
Pancreas	50-80	Men 3 times greater than women	African Americans greater than whites or Asians	Increases risk	Φ	High meat and fat	Diabetes mellitus, chronic pancreatitis, stomach surgery, occupational exposure to insecticides, family history
Kidney	50-70	Men 2 times greater than women	Φ	Increases risk	Φ	High fat	Obesity, family history, exposure to asbestos, inherited and acquired gene mutation, long term kidney failure

*Φ, No risk factors for this type cancer.

Data from *www.cancer.org* Prevention and risk factors, American Cancer Society, December 1998 to April 1999.

Table 20-2 Prevention of Some Common Cancers of the Abdomen and Gastrointestinal System

	HEALTHY BEHAVIORS TO START/CONTINUE			UNHEALTHY BEHAVIORS TO MODIFY
	DIET	ALCOHOL	ADDITIONAL BEHAVIORS	SMOKING
Esophagus	Eat fruits and vegetables.	Limit intake from 0 to 2 drinks per day.		Smoking cessation.
Stomach	Eat fresh fruits and vegetables, bread, cereals, pasta, rice, and beans.		Treat *Heliocobacter pylori* infection, which causes peptic ulcer disease (see discussion of common problems).	Smoking cessation.
Colon	Eat 5 servings of fresh fruits and vegetables, 6 servings from other plant sources (e.g., whole grains in bread and cereal, rice, pasta, beans), low-fat dairy products.		Physical activity 30 minutes most days.	
Liver		Limit intake from 0 to 2 drinks daily.	Prevent infection of hepatitis B and C (e.g., Hepatitis B vaccine, protected sexual intercourse). Stop using intravenous drugs or if that is impossible, use sterile needles.	Smoking cessation. Stop intravenous drug use or if that is not possible, use sterile needles.
Pancreas	Eat diet low in fat, high in fiber. Eat 5 servings of fresh fruits and vegetables, 6 servings from other plant sources (e.g., whole grains in bread and cereal, rice, pasta, beans), low-fat dairy products.			Smoking cessation.
Kidney			Reduce exposure to asbestos.	Smoking cessation.

Data from *www.cancer.org* Prevention and risk factors, American Cancer Society, December 1998 to April 1999.

Lead is most harmful to children under age 6 because it is easily absorbed. Children are poisoned by chronic low-level lead exposure. Lead interferes with brain development, causing reduced intelligence, reduced attention span, hyperactivity, hearing loss, and disabilities in reading and learning. In addition, physical growth is impaired. Since the lead exposure occurs over time, there may not be symptoms to alert parents of the poison. A blood test is the only way to determine if the child is poisoned. Except for severely poisoned children, there is no medical treatment for this disease.

The only way to prevent this poisoning is to remove the source of exposure. The most common source is lead-based paint found in older homes. Children are exposed by normal hand-to-mouth activity after getting lead dust on their hands and toys. Soil also can be contaminated from flaking exterior paint or previous deposits of leaded gasoline. Drinking water can contain lead from pipes or solder. Parents who work in lead-related industries can bring lead home on their clothes (Alliance to End Childhood Lead Poisoning, *www.aeclp.org*, July 15, 1999).

COMMON PROBLEMS AND CONDITIONS

Abdomen and Gastrointestinal System

ALIMENTARY TRACT

Gastroesophageal Reflux Disease

Flow of gastric secretions up into the esophagus is called gastroesophageal reflux disease. It is due to weakened lower esophageal pressure or increased intraabdominal pressure. Clients complain of epigastric pain and heartburn, aggravated by lying down and relieved by sitting up, antacids, and eating.

Hiatal Hernia

A protrusion of the stomach through the esophageal hiatus of the diaphragm into the mediastinal cavity is called a hiatal hernia (Fig. 20-29). Muscle weakness is a primary factor in developing this type of hernia. It is associated with pregnancy, obesity, and ascites and occurs more frequently in women and older adults.

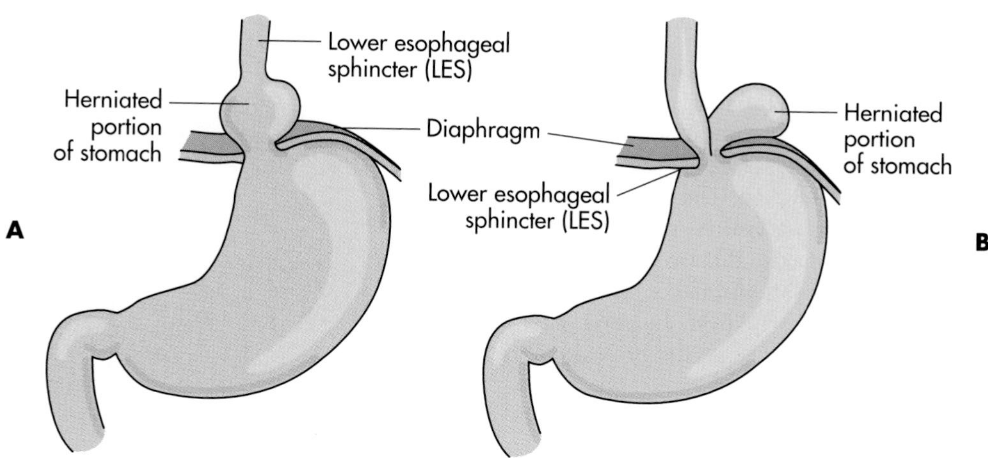

Fig. 20-29 Hiatal hernia. **A,** Sliding hernia. **B,** Paraesophageal. (From Phipps, Sands, and Marek, 1999.)

Peptic Ulcer Disease

An ulcer occurring in the lower end of the esophagus, in the stomach, or the duodenum is known as a peptic ulcer. Duodenal ulcer is the most common form, caused by a break in the duodenal mucosa that scars with healing (Fig. 20-30). Ulcers may result from infection with *Helicobacter pylori* and cause increased gastric secretion. Clients complain of localized epigastric pain when the stomach is empty, which is relieved by food or antacids. Gastric bleeding may occur as a result of the ulcer, causing signs of hematemesis, melena, dizziness, hypotension, or tachycardia. Perforation of a duodenal ulcer may be life threatening. Ulcers on the anterior walls are more likely to perforate, whereas ulcers on the posterior wall are more likely to bleed.

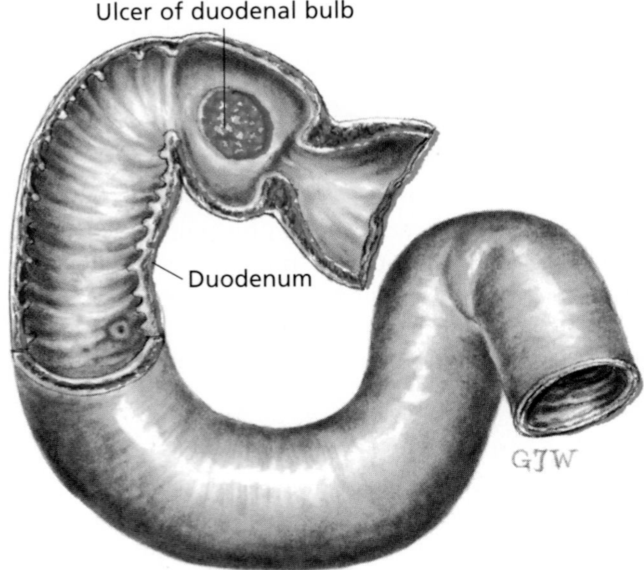

Fig. 20-30 Duodenal peptic ulcer. (From Doughty and Jackson, 1993.)

Crohn's Disease

A chronic inflammatory bowel disease of unknown origin is called Crohn's disease (Fig. 20-31). Inflammation may occur from mouth to anus, but it most commonly affects the terminal ileum and colon. Diseased sections of bowel become thicker, which narrows the lumen. The mucosa is ulcerated, with formations of fistulas, fissures, and abscesses. Normal bowel segments may separate diseased sections of bowel. Clients complain of severe abdominal pain, cramping, diarrhea, nausea, fever, chills, weakness, anorexia, and weight loss. It is also called regional enteritis or regional ileitis.

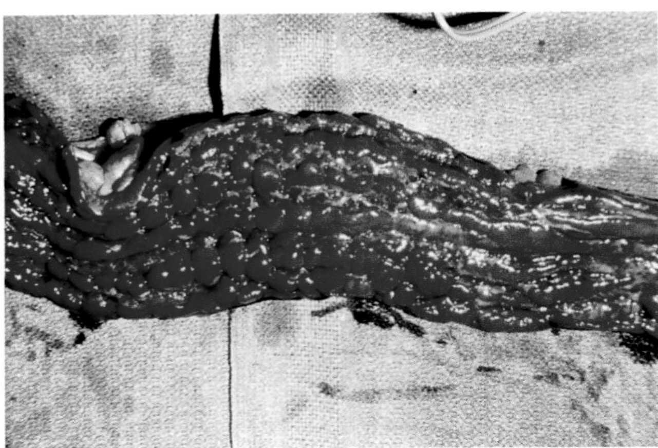

Fig. 20-31 Crohn's disease showing deep ulcers and fissures, creating "cobblestone" effect. (From Doughty and Jackson, 1993.)

Ulcerative Colitis

A chronic, episodic inflammatory disease that starts in the rectum and progresses through the large intestine is called ulcerative colitis (Fig. 20-32). The submucosa becomes engorged, and mucosa becomes ulcerated and denuded with granulation tissue. Ulcerative colitis is characterized by profuse watery diarrhea of blood, mucus, and pus and may progress to colon cancer. Clients complain of severe abdominal pain, fever, chills, anemia, and weight loss.

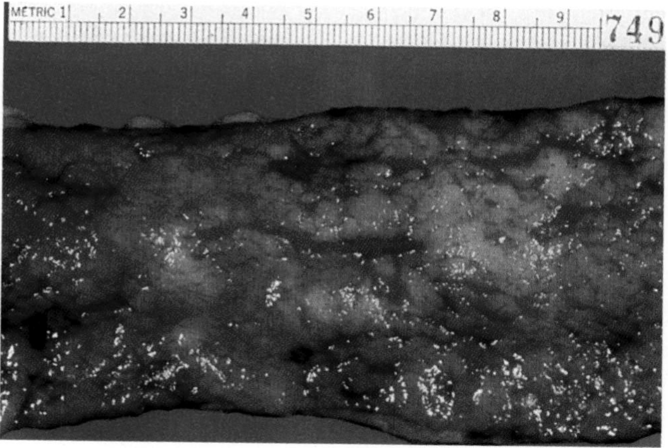

Fig. 20-32 Ulcerative colitis showing severe mucosal edema and inflammation with ulcerations and bleeding. (From Doughty and Jackson, 1993.)

Diverticulitis

Inflammation of diverticula is termed diverticulitis. Diverticula are pouch type of herniations through the muscular wall in the colon (Fig. 20-33). Presence of fecal material through the thin-walled diverticula causes inflammation and abscesses. It is probably secondary to a diet low in fiber. Clients complain of cramping pain in the LLQ, nausea, vomiting, and altered bowel habits, usually constipation. The abdomen may be distended and tympanic, with decreased bowel sounds and localized tenderness.

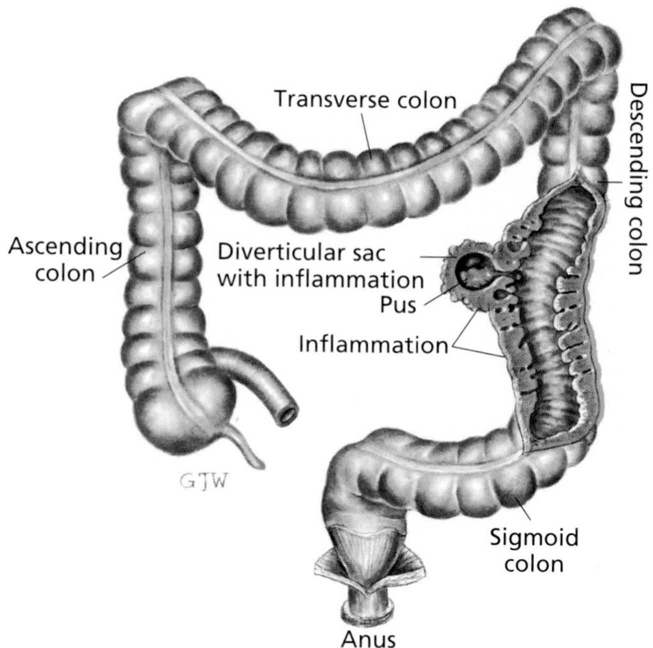

Fig. 20-33 Diverticulosis (diverticulitis). (From Doughty and Jackson, 1993.)

Table 20-3 Comparison of Hepatitis A, B, C, D, E, and G

	HEPATITIS A	HEPATITIS B	HEPATITIS C	HEPATITIS D	HEPATITIS E	HEPATITIS G
Mode of transmission	Fecal-oral	Blood borne/ sexual/ perinatal	Blood borne/ sexual/ perinatal	Blood borne* sexual	Fecal-oral†	Blood borne Frequent coinfection with hepatitis C
Incubation period	2-6 wk	4-24 wk	2-23 wk	4-24 wk	2-8 wk	
Chronicity	None	6%-10%	>85%	70%-80%	None	
Vaccine	Yes	Yes	No	No	No	No

*Hepatitis D is acquired as a coinfection with hepatitis B or as a superinfection with chronic hepatitis B.

†All cases of acute hepatitis E in the United States have been reported among travelers returning from high hepatitis E areas outside the country.

From *http://www.cdc.gov/ncidod/diseases/hepatitis*

HEPATOBILIARY SYSTEM

Viral Hepatitis

Viral hepatitis is the name given to an inflammation of the liver resulting from different viruses. Table 20-3 shows modes of transmission and incubation periods for all known types of hepatitis. Pathologic changes in the liver are similar regardless of the causative virus. Edema and cell infiltration in parenchyma and portal ducts, hepatic cell necrosis, proliferation of Kupffer's cells, and accumulation of necrotic debris produce changes in the lobules and ducts that ultimately disturb bilirubin excretion. Common symptoms are anorexia, vague abdominal pain, nausea, vomiting, malaise, fever, and jaundice. An enlarged liver and spleen are classic findings. The liver inflammation may alter the bilirubin conjugation so that the stools appear clay colored and urine is dark amber.

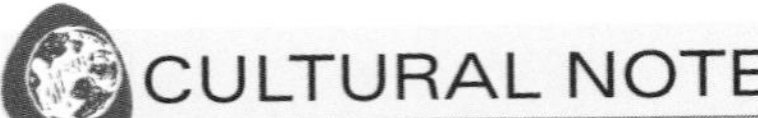

CULTURAL NOTE

Cirrhosis of the liver and other liver diseases are the fifth leading cause of mortality among American Indians and Alaskan natives (U.S. Department of Health and Human Services, 1995).

Cirrhosis

Cirrhosis is a chronic degenerative disease of the liver in which diffuse destruction and regeneration of hepatic parenchymal cells occur (Fig. 20-34). Lobes of the liver become fibrotic and infiltrated with fat. A diffuse increase in connective tissue results in disorganization of the lobular and vascular structure. Causes of cirrhosis include viral hepatitis, biliary obstruction, and alcohol abuse. The liver becomes palpable, hard, and nontender. The proliferation of connective tissue spreads throughout the liver, changing the normal lobular structure. Associated signs include ascites, jaundice, cutaneous spider angiomas, dark urine, clay-colored stools, and spleen enlargement. End-stage cirrhosis is characterized by hepatic encephalopathy and coma.

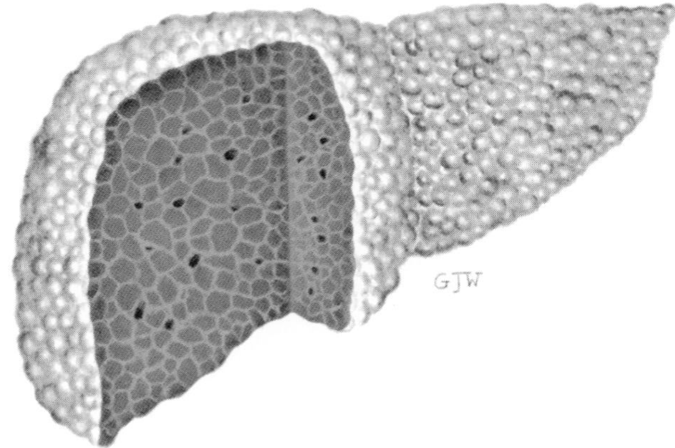

Fig. 20-34 Cirrhosis of the liver. (From Doughty and Jackson, 1993.)

Cholecystitis With Cholelithiasis

Acute or chronic inflammation of the gallbladder with stone formation is called cholecystitis (inflammation of the gallbladder) with cholelithiasis (gallstones) (Fig. 20-35). The bile duct becomes obstructed either by edema from inflammation of the gallbladder wall or by gallstones. The primary symptom is RUQ colicky pain that may radiate to midtorso or right scapula. Other indications include indigestion and mild transient jaundice.

PANCREAS

Pancreatitis

Pancreatitis is acute or chronic inflammation of the pancreas resulting from autodigestion of the organ. The flow of pancreatic digestive enzymes into the duodenum is obstructed, so that the digestive enzymes act on the pancreas itself. Clients complain of pain, described as steady, boring, dull, or sharp, that radiates from the epigastrium to the back. Clients prefer the fetal position with knees to the chest. Other manifestations include nausea and vomiting, weight loss, steatorrhea, and glucose intolerance.

URINARY SYSTEM

Urinary Tract Infection

Infections of the lower urinary tract may involve the urinary bladder (cystitis), the urethra (urethritis), or the prostate (prostatitis) (see Chapter 23). Upper urinary tract infections (UTIs) may involve the kidney and renal pelvis (pyelonephritis). Most UTIs result from gram-negative organisms such as *Escherichia coli, Klebsiella, Proteus,* or *Pseudomonas* that originate from the client's own intestinal tract and ascend through the urethra to the bladder. Urinary tract infections are more common in women due to the short urethra. Also rectal bacteria tend to colonize the perineum and vaginal vestibule. Sexual intercourse has been shown to be a major precipitating factor for UTIs. Symptoms for urethritis include frequency, urgency, and dysuria. For cystitis the symptoms are the same as urethritis plus signs of bacteriuria and perhaps fever. Clients with pyelonephritis complain of flank pain, dysuria, nocturia, and frequency. Costovertebral angle tenderness, bacteriuria, and pyuria may be found (Marantides, Marek, and Morgan, 1999).

Glomerulonephritis

Inflammation of the renal glomeruli caused an autoimmune process is called glomerulonephritis. Clients complain of fever, chills, nausea, malaise, and arthralgia. Costovertebral angle tenderness is present.

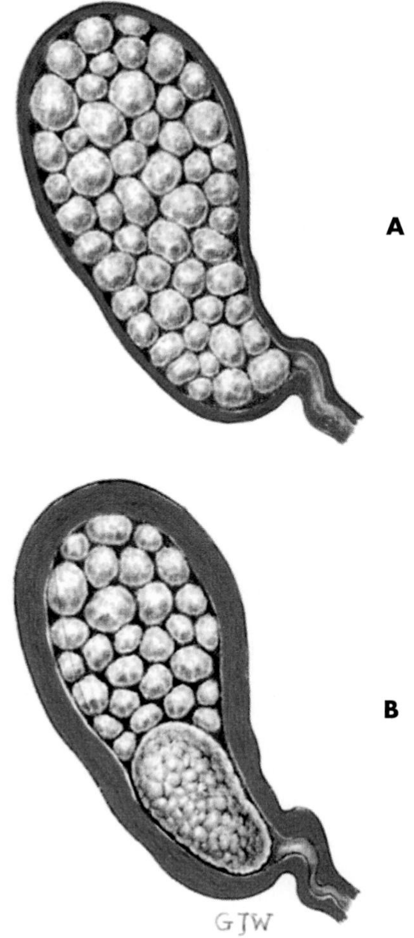

Fig. 20-35 Cholelithiasis. **A,** Multiple-faceted stones. **B,** Large and numerous small stones in chronic cholecystitis. (From Doughty and Jackson, 1993.)

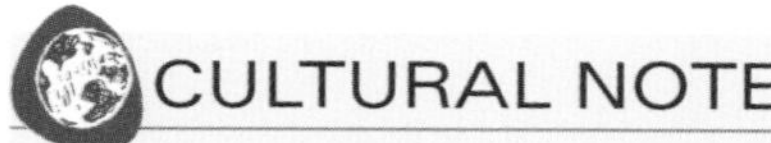

CULTURAL NOTE

American Indians and Alaskan natives have a higher incidenc of liver and gallbladder disease than other ethnic and culture groups (Chandrasome a and Taylor, 1998).

Nephrolithiasis, or Renal Calculi

The condition in which stones form in the kidney pelvis is called nephrolithiasis. Formation of stones is associated with obstruction and urinary tract infections (Fig. 20-36). These stones or calculi are made of calcium salts, uric acid, cystine, or struvite. Alkaline urine facilitates formation of stones made of calcium phosphate, whereas acid urine facilitates stones formed of cystine. Men develop renal calculi more often than women. Signs and symptoms include fever, hematuria, and flank pain that may radiate to the groin and genitals.

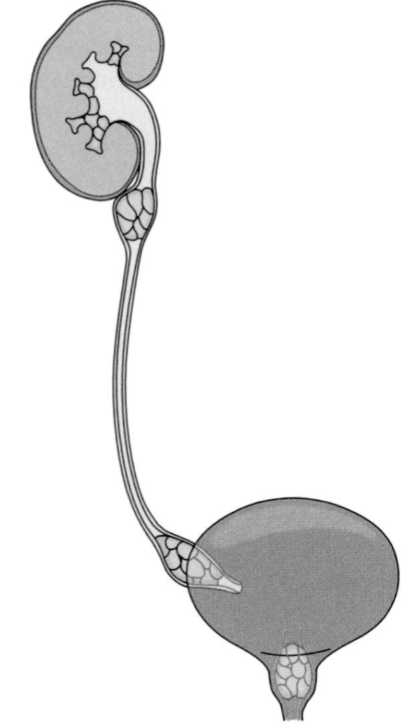

Fig. 20-36 Most common locations of renal calculi formation. (From Phipps, Sands, and Marek, 1999.)

Acute Renal Failure

Acute renal failure is the name given to a sudden, severe impairment of renal function, causing an acute uremia episode. Impairment may be due to changes in the prerenal phase (e.g., reduced cardiac output), intrarenal phase (e.g., acute pyelonephritis, acute tubular necrosis, acute glomerulonephritis, and nephrotoxic agents, including drugs), or postrenal phase (e.g., acute urinary tract obstruction). Urine output may be normal, decreased, or absent.

Chronic Renal Failure

Slow, insidious, and irreversible impairment of renal function is called chronic renal failure. Uremia usually develops gradually. Major causes include diabetic nephropathy, glomerulonephritis, and polycystic kidney disease. The client complains of oliguria or anuria and has signs of fluid volume overload (dependent edema, weight gain, and pulmonary edema).

INFANTS

Intussusception

Intussusception is diagnosed when there is prolapse of one segment of the intestine into another, causing intestinal obstruction. It occurs in infants aged 3 to 12 months. The cause is unknown. Manifestations include abdominal distention, intermittent abdominal pain, vomiting, and stools that are mixed with blood and mucus with a currant-jelly appearance. A mass is found on palpation of the upper quadrants, whereas the lower quadrants feel empty (Fig. 20-37).

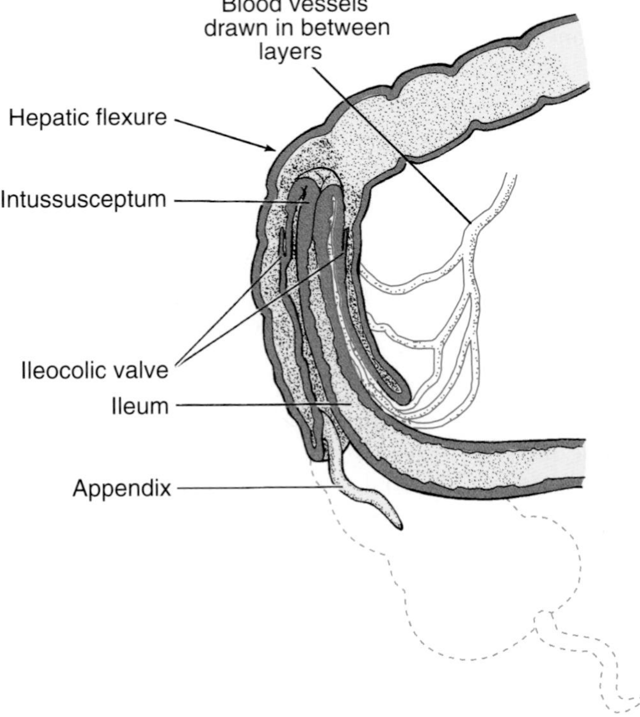

Fig. 20-37 Ileocolic intussusception. (From Wong et al, 1999.)

Hypertrophic Pyloric Stenosis

Pyloric stenosis occurs when the pyloric sphincter is obliterated by hypertrophied circular muscle (Fig. 20-38). It occurs during the first month after birth. Signs and symptoms include regurgitation progressing to projectile vomiting and failure to gain weight with signs of dehydration.

Meconium Ileus

Meconium ileus occurs when there is an obstruction of the lower intestine, caused by thickening and hardening of meconium. It is characterized by failure of the newborn to pass a meconium stool in the first 24 hours after birth and abdominal distention.

Biliary Atresia

Congenital obstruction or absence of some or all of the bile duct system is called biliary atresia. Signs include jaundice, hepatomegaly, abdominal distention, and failure to gain weight. Urine is a dark color, while stools are clay colored.

Meckel's Diverticulum

Outpouching of the ileum proximal to the ileocecal valve is known as Meckel's diverticulum. It is the most common congenital anomaly of the GI tract. Signs and symptoms, if present, resemble intestinal obstruction, diverticulitis, or appendicitis. There may be bright or dark bleeding with little abdominal pain.

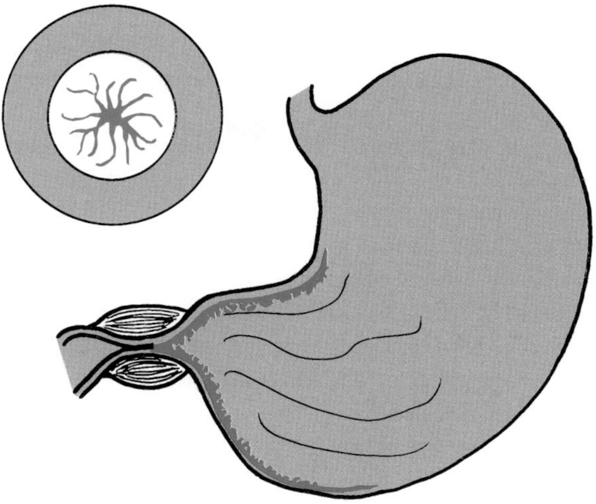

Fig. 20-38 Hypertrophic pyloric stenosis. (From Wong et al, 1999.)

CLINICAL APPLICATION and CRITICAL THINKING

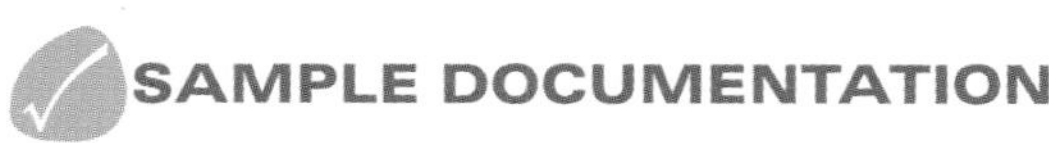

SAMPLE DOCUMENTATION

CASE 1

B.Y. is a 55-year-old man with epigastric pain.

Subjective Data

Alert, cooperative man with hand on stomach. Reports 2-week episode of gnawing epigastric pain that does not radiate. Pain worse before meals and relieved somewhat after meals. Denies nausea and vomiting. Stools described as regular but "much darker than usual—almost black." Has taken antacids with some relief. Reports fatigue and shortness of breath with activity since pain onset. Current medications: nonsteroidal inflammatory drugs daily for arthritis. Smoker—has smoked 1 pack of cigarettes/day for 40 years; drinks a fifth of whiskey per week. Employed full-time at an insurance company; married with two children. Reports occasional stress at work, minimal stress at home.

Objective Data

Blood pressure, 140/80 mm Hg; Pulse, 88 beats/min; Respirations, 18; Temperature, 98.8° F (37.1° C).

Height, 6′3″ (190 cm); Weight, 180 lb (82 kg).

Abdomen: Scaphoid, soft, no scars; aorta midline with bruit; no bruit in iliac, renal, or femoral arteries; bowel sounds heard in all quadrants, epigastrium tender to deep palpation; liver span 9 cm (3.5 inches) RMCL; liver palpable 2 cm (¾ inches), nontender; spleen and kidneys nonpalpable; superficial reflexes intact; no CVA tenderness. Stool is guaiac positive.

Functional Health Patterns Involved

- Health perception–health management
- Activity–exercise
- Cognitive–perceptual

Medical Diagnosis

Peptic ulcer disease and anemia

Nursing Diagnosis and Collaborative Problems

- *Pain* related to gastric hypersecretion as manifested by:
  - Two-week episode of gnawing epigastric pain that does not radiate
  - Pain is worse before meals and relieved somewhat after meals
  - Epigastrium tender to light and deep palpation. History of smoking, alcohol intake
  - Self-medication with nonsteroidal antiinflammatory drugs (NSAIDs) for arthritic pain
- *Altered health maintenance* related to inadequate information about effect of smoking and alcohol on abdominal pain as manifested by:
  - Gastric hypersecretion
  - Smokes
  - Drinks alcohol
- *Activity intolerance* related to compromised oxygen transport as manifested by:
  - Complaints of shortness of breath with activity
  - Complaints of fatigue with activity
- *PC*: Hemorrhage.

CASE 2

M.T. is a 54-year-old woman with complaints of abdominal pain.

Subjective Data

States pain "off and on" for a few months; increasingly worse over time. Pain intermittent gassy or crampy pain; the intensity of pain increases and decreases as it comes and goes. Pain radiates to right shoulder blade area. Associated symptoms: nausea and indigestion; symptoms are worse after eating. Diet "healthy."

Objective Data

Height, 5′1″ (155 cm); Weight, 172 lb (78 kg).

General appearance: Obese female in no acute distress; slight jaundice noted in sclera of eyes. Bowel sounds positive in all quadrants. Abdomen is soft, no tenderness, no masses with palpation; unable to palpate liver. Liver span, 7 inches; no CVA tenderness.

Functional Health Patterns Involved

- Health perception–health management
- Nutrition–metabolic
- Cognitive–perceptual

Medical Diagnosis

Cholecystitis and cholelithiasis

Nursing Diagnosis and Collaborative Problems

- *Pain* related to inflammatory process as manifested by:
  - Complaints of pain
  - Radiation of pain to shoulder
  - Pain becoming increasingly worse
- *Altered health maintenance* related to intake in excess of metabolic requirements as evidenced by:
  - Height 5′1″ with weight of 172 lb

CRITICAL THINKING QUESTIONS

1. As you auscultate the abdomen, you should listen not only for bowel sounds, but vascular sounds and a friction rub as well. List specifically what you are listening to and what abnormal findings may indicate.
2. Ms. Quintana is in the clinic with her newborn infant. You ask her if anyone has talked with her about immunizations. Ms. Quintana says to you, "My friend told me about a liver disease shot that my baby should have. What is it? Should my baby get it?" What education should you provide regarding her question?
3. Two clients come to the health care facility. Mr. Nguyen, age 45 years, complains of crampy abdominal pain that is aggravated by food. Ms. Martinez, age 23 years, complains of sharp crampy abdominal pain that is aggravated by food. What questions do you ask to distinguish the causes of the abdominal pain of these two clients? What do you expect to find on abdominal examination?

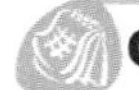

CASE STUDY

Katie is an 18-year-old woman complaining of abdominal pain. Listed below are data collected by the examiner during an interview and examination.

Interview Data

Katie tells the examiner the pain started yesterday evening and has gotten progressively worse. She describes the pain as "really bad." The pain is constant and located in her right lower abdomen, toward her umbilicus. She says that her pain feels a little better if she stays curled up and does not move. She tells the examiner that she is in good health and that she has never had a problem with her stomach. Katie indicates that normally she has a good appetite and can eat anything—except for now. She says she ate breakfast and lunch yesterday, but by dinner time she was nauseated and had no appetite. She has not eaten anything since. She has had no recent weight changes, but she would like to weigh about 5 lb less than she currently does. Katie does not smoke or drink alcoholic beverages, and she takes no medication. She denies discomfort or problems with urination, describing her urine as "usual looking."

Examination Data

- **General survey:** Alert and anxious female in moderate distress lying in a fetal position on the examination table, with her eyes closed. Appears well nourished. Her skin is hot.
- **Abdominal inspection:** Abdomen is flat and symmetric. No lesions or scars noted. No surface movements are seen except for breathing.
- **Abdominal auscultation:** Bowel sounds absent.
- **Abdominal percussion:** Tympany noted over most of abdominal surface; dullness over liver. Midclavicular liver span is 4 inches.
- **Light abdominal palpation:** Demonstrates pain and guarding in right lower quadrant. Unable to palpate deep structures because of excessive abdominal discomfort. Demonstrates positive rebound tenderness in right lower quadrant.

1. What data deviate from normal findings, suggesting a need for further investigation?
2. What additional information should the nurse ask or assess for?
3. In what functional health patterns does data deviate from normal?
4. What nursing diagnosis and/or collaborative problems should be considered for this situation?

REMEMBER to check out your companion CD-ROM

21 Female Genitalia and Reproductive System

www.mosby.com/MERLIN/wilson/assessment/

ANATOMY AND PHYSIOLOGY

EXTERNAL GENITALIA

The external female genitalia are collectively referred to as the vulva. The vulva includes the mons pubis, prepuce, clitoris, labia majora, labia minora, vaginal vestibule, ducts of the Skene's and Bartholin's glands, vaginal orifice, urethral meatus, and perineum (Fig. 21-1).

The mons pubis is a layer of adipose tissue that lies over the symphysis pubis. After puberty this surface is covered with coarse hair that extends down over the outer labia to the perineal and anal areas. The labia majora are folds of tissue that extend downward from the mons pubis, surround the vestibule, and meet at the perineum. The outer surfaces are covered with hair, whereas the inner surfaces are hairless and smooth.

Lying inside the labia majora are darker, hairless folds called the labia minora. In some women, the labia minora are completely enclosed within the labia majora, whereas in others the labia minora protrude between the labia majora. Each of the labia minora divides into a medial and lateral aspect. The medial aspects join superior to the clitoris to form the clitoral hood (prepuce), and the lateral aspects join inferior to the clitoris to form the frenulum. The clitoris is a small, cylindrical bud of erectile tissue, homologous to the male penis and a primary center of sexual excitement. It is approximately ¾ inch (2 cm) in length and 3⁄16 inch (0.5 cm) in diameter.

The vestibule is the area that lies between the labia minora and contains the urethral (urinary) meatus, the vaginal orifice (introitus), hymenal tissue, and Bartholin's and Skene's glands. The urethral meatus is located about ¾ inch (2 cm) below the clitoris and appears as an irregularly shaped slit. The vaginal orifice lies immediately below the urethral meatus and varies in size and shape. The hymen is a fold of mucous membrane at the vaginal opening. The hymen usually ruptures during the perinatal period and remains as a fold of mucous membrane around the vaginal opening. These edges may appear as small, fleshy tags of skin (sometimes referred to as hymenal remnants) or completely disappear. Failure of the membrane to rupture results in imperforate hymen—a rare occurrence.

The ducts of Skene's glands and Bartholin's glands open within the vestibule. Skene's glands are numerous, tiny organs located in the paraurethral area. During sexual intercourse, they secrete a lubricating fluid. The ducts are not usually visible. Bartholin's glands are small and round, located on either side of the introitus, at approximately the 5 and 7 o'clock positions. The ducts of the Bartholin's glands open onto the sides of the vestibule in the space between the hymen and the labia minora. The ductal openings are usually not visible. During sexual excitement, Bartholin's glands secrete a mucoid material into the vaginal orifice for lubrication.

The perineal surface is the triangular-shaped area between the vaginal opening and the anus. The pelvic floor consists of a group of muscles that form a suspended sling supporting the pelvic contents. These muscles attach to various points on the bony pelvis and form functional sphincters for the vagina, rectum, and urethra.

INTERNAL GENITALIA

The internal genitalia include the vagina, uterus, fallopian tubes, and ovaries (Fig. 21-2). They are supported by four pairs of ligaments: cardinal, uterosacral, round, and broad ligaments.

Vagina

The vagina is a musculomembranous canal extending posteriorly from the vestibule to the uterus. It inclines posteriorly at an angle of approximately 45° to the vertical plane of the body. Its posterior length is approximately 3½ to 4 inches (9 to 10 cm), and its anterior length is 2⅜ to 3⅛ inches (6 to 8 cm). The canal is transversely rugated in the reproductive years, lined with a moist mucous membrane. The uterine cervix enters superiorly and anteriorly into the vaginal cavity to form a recess, or fornix, around the cervix. This pocket is divided into anterior, posterior, and lateral fornices, through which the internal pelvic walls can be palpated. The vagina carries menstrual flow from the uterus and is the receptive organ for the penis during sexual intercourse. During birth, the vagina becomes the terminal portion of the birth canal.

Uterus

The uterus is a hollow, thick, pear-shaped, muscular organ. It is approximately 2⅛ to 3⅛ inches (5.5 to 8 cm) long, 1 ⅜ to 1 ¾ inches (3.5 to 4 cm) wide, and ¾ to 1 inch (2 to 2.5 cm) thick. The uterus is suspended and stabilized in the pelvic cavity by four sets of ligaments. It is fairly mobile, usu-

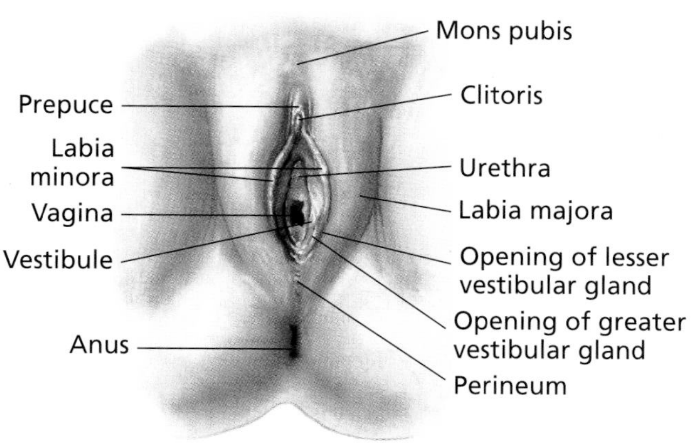

Fig. 21-1 Female external genitalia. (From Lowdermilk, Perry, and Bobak, 1999.)

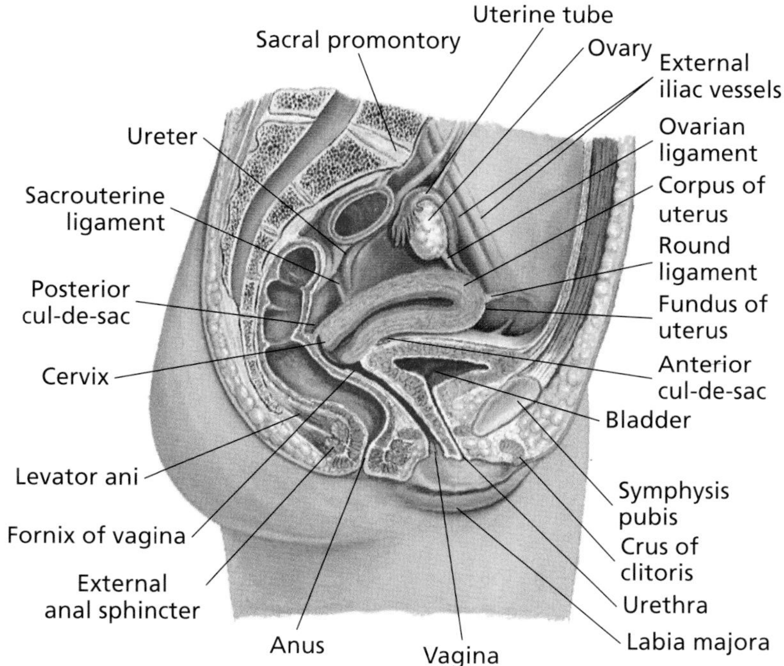

Fig. 21-2 Midsagittal view of female pelvic organs. (From Seidel et al, 1999.)

ally loosely suspended in position between the bladder and rectum; the exact positions of the organ may normally vary in individuals. The uterus is inclined forward at an angle of about 45°. The angle of the uterus can be found in any of the following positions: anteverted, anteflexed, retroverted, or retroflexed.

The two main parts of the uterus are the cervix and the corpus. The cervix is a mucus-producing gland that is the lowest portion of the uterus. It is visible and palpable in the upper vagina. The cervical opening, or the os, is visible on the surface of the cervix. It appears as a small round opening in a nulliparous woman or as an irregular slit in parous women. The outer surface of the cervix (known as the ectocervix) is layered with squamous cells whereas the cervical canal is layered with columnar cells. The juncture of these two types of cells (the squamocolumnar junction) can be observed as a circumscribed red circle around the os in some women—especially in the adolescent and in clients who take oral contraceptives (Fig. 21-3).

The portion of the uterus above the cervix is known as the corpus. The corpus is composed of three sections: the isthmus (the narrow neck from which the cervix extends into the vagina), the main body of the uterus, and the fundus, which is the bulbous top portion of the uterus (Fig. 21-4). The fundus maintains its anterior position by the attached round ligaments, which are occasionally palpable on either side of the uterus.

Fallopian (Uterine) Tubes

The fallopian tubes insert into the fundus and extend laterally from 3⅛ to 5½ inches (8 to 14 cm) to the ovaries. The fimbriated ends of the fallopian tubes partially project

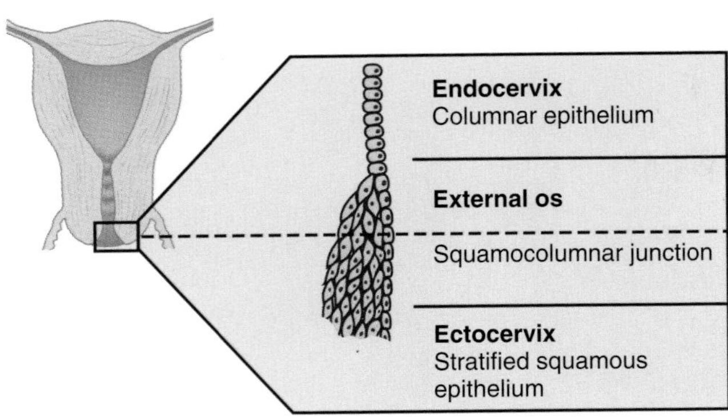

Fig. 21-3 Types of cervical cells: endocervical, external os, and ectocervix. (Used with permission from Mashburn J and Scharbo-DeHaan M: "A clinician's guide to pap smear interpretation," *The Nurse Practitioner* 22(4):115-143, © Springhouse Corporation/www.springnet.com.)

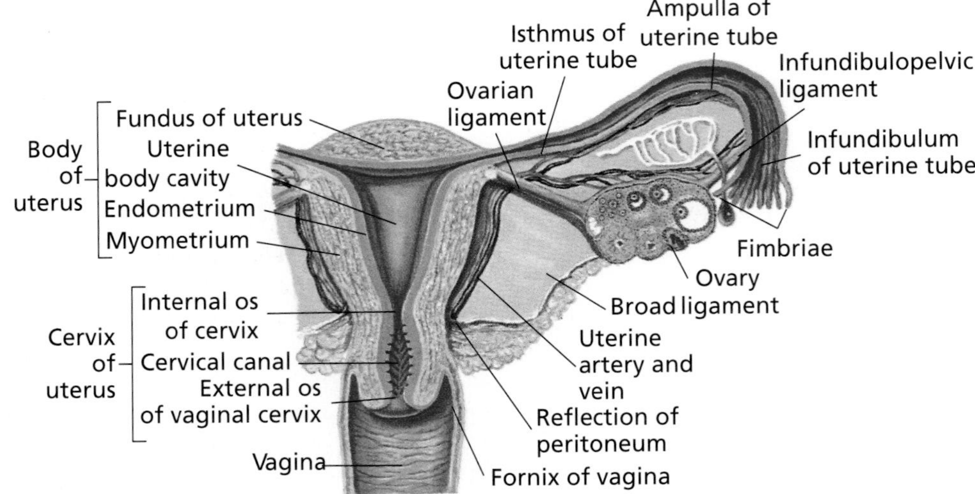

Fig. 21-4 Cross-sectional view of internal female genitalia and pelvic contents. (From Seidel et al, 1999.)

around the ovary to capture and draw ova into the tube for fertilization. The ova are transported to the uterus by rhythmic contractions of the tubal musculature. The inner tube is lined with cilia that further assist in transport of the ova.

Ovaries

The ovaries, a pair of almond-shaped organs on the lateral pelvic wall, are connected to the uterine body by the ovarian ligaments. They secrete estrogen and progesterone, which have several functions, including control of the menstrual cycle and pregnancy support. They are usually located at the level of the anterosuperior iliac spine. The ovaries are approximately 1⅛ inches (3 cm) in length, ¾ inch (2 cm) wide, and ⅜ inch (1 cm) thick during the reproductive years.

MENSTRUAL CYCLE

The hypothalamus and pituitary in the brain and the ovaries in the pelvis are the main sites of regulation of the menstrual cycle. The cycle moves predictably through a 28-day cycle. Table 21-1 and Fig. 21-5 detail the stages.

BONY PELVIS

The bony pelvis is structured to accommodate both fetal growth and the birth process. It is composed of four bones: two innominate (each consisting of ilium, ischium, and pubis); the sacrum; and the coccyx. The pelvis contains four joints of very limited movement: the symphysis pubis, the sacrococcygeal, and two sacroiliac joints. The pelvis is divided into two parts: the false pelvis (the shallow upper section) and the true pelvis (the lower curved bony canal, including the inlet, cavity, and outlet) (Fig. 21-6). The fetus will pass through this lower canal during birth. The lower border of the outlet is bounded by the pubic arch and the ischial tuberosities. The upper border of the outlet is at the level of the ischial spines. These project into the pelvic cavity and are important landmarks during labor.

Table 21-1 The Menstrual Cycle

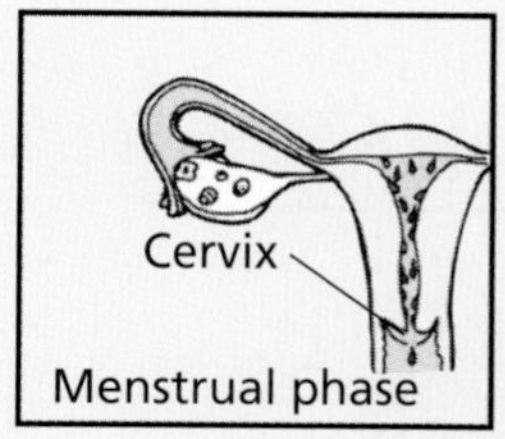

MENSTRUAL PHASE: DAYS 1 TO 4

Ovary	Estrogen levels begin to rise, preparing follicle and egg for next cycle.
Uterus	Progesterone stimulates endometrial prostaglandins that cause vasoconstriction; upper layers of endometrium shed.
Breast	Cellular activity in the alveoli decreases; breast ducts shrink.
Central nervous system (CNS) hormones	FSH and LH levels decrease.
Symptom	Menstrual bleeding may vary, depending on hormones and prostaglandins.

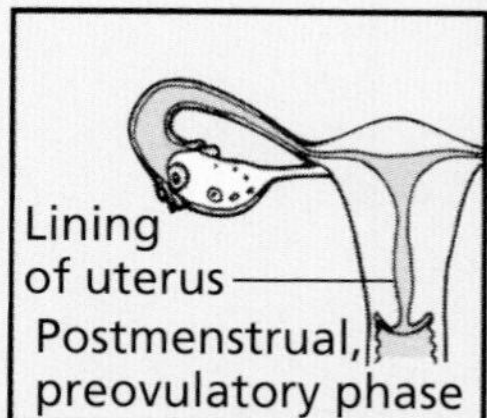

POSTMENSTRUAL, PREOVULATORY PHASE: DAYS 5 TO 12

Ovary	Ovary and maturing follicle produce estrogen. *Follicular phase*—egg develops within follicle.
Uterus	*Proliferative phase*—uterine lining thickens.
Breast	Parenchymal and proliferation (increased cellular activity) or breast ducts occurs.
CNS hormone	FSH stimulates ovarian follicular growth.

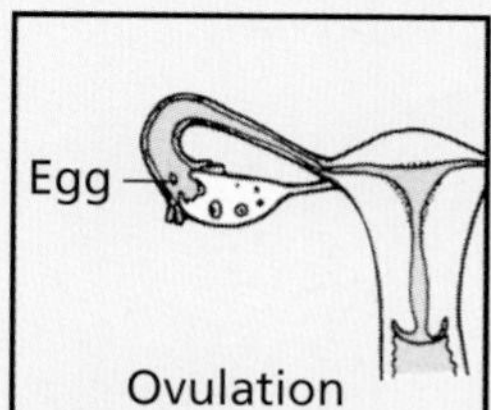

OVULATION: DAY 13 OR 14

Ovary	Egg is expelled from follicle into abdominal cavity and is drawn into the uterine (fallopian) tube by fimbriae and cilia; follicle closes and begins to form corpus luteum. Fertilization of egg may occur in the outer one third of tube if sperm are unimpeded.
Uterus	End of proliferative phase; progesterone causes further thickening of the uterine wall.
CNS hormones	LH and estrogen levels increase rapidly; LH surge stimulates release of egg.
Symptom	Mittelschmerz (pain) may occur with ovulation; cervical mucus is increased and is stringy and elastic (spinnbarkeit).

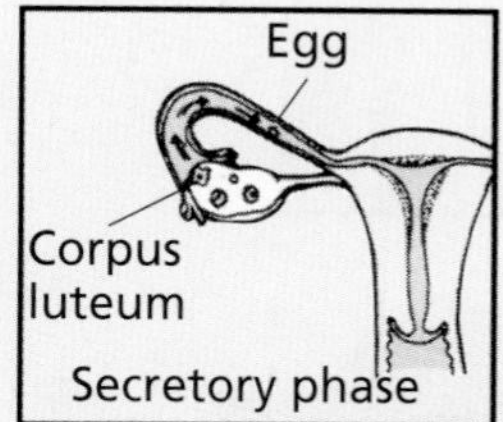

SECRETORY PHASE: DAYS 15 TO 20

Ovary	Egg (ovum) is moved by cilia into the uterus.
Uterus	After the egg is released, the follicle becomes a corpus luteum; secretion of progesterone increases and predominates.
CNS hormones	LH and FSH decrease.

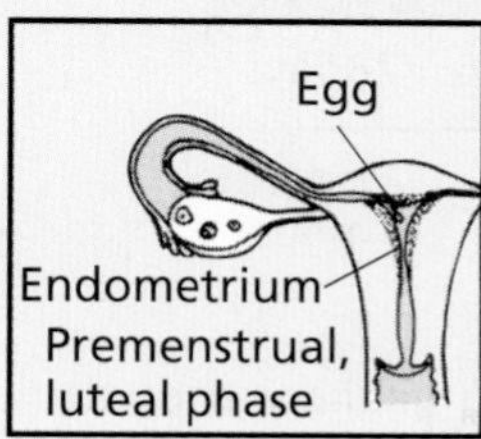

PREMENSTURAL, LUTEAL PHASE: DAYS 21 TO 28

Ovary	If implantation does not occur, the corpus luteum degenerates. Progesterone production decreases, and estrogen production drops and then begins to rise as a new follicle develops.
Uterus	Menstruation starts around day 28, which begins *day 1* of the menstrual cycle.
Breast	Alveolar breast cells differentiate into secretory cells.
CNS hormones	Increased levels of GnRH cause increased secretion of FSH.
Symptoms	Vascular engorgement and water retention may occur.

Modified from Edge V, Miller M: *Women's health care,* St. Louis, 1994, Mosby.

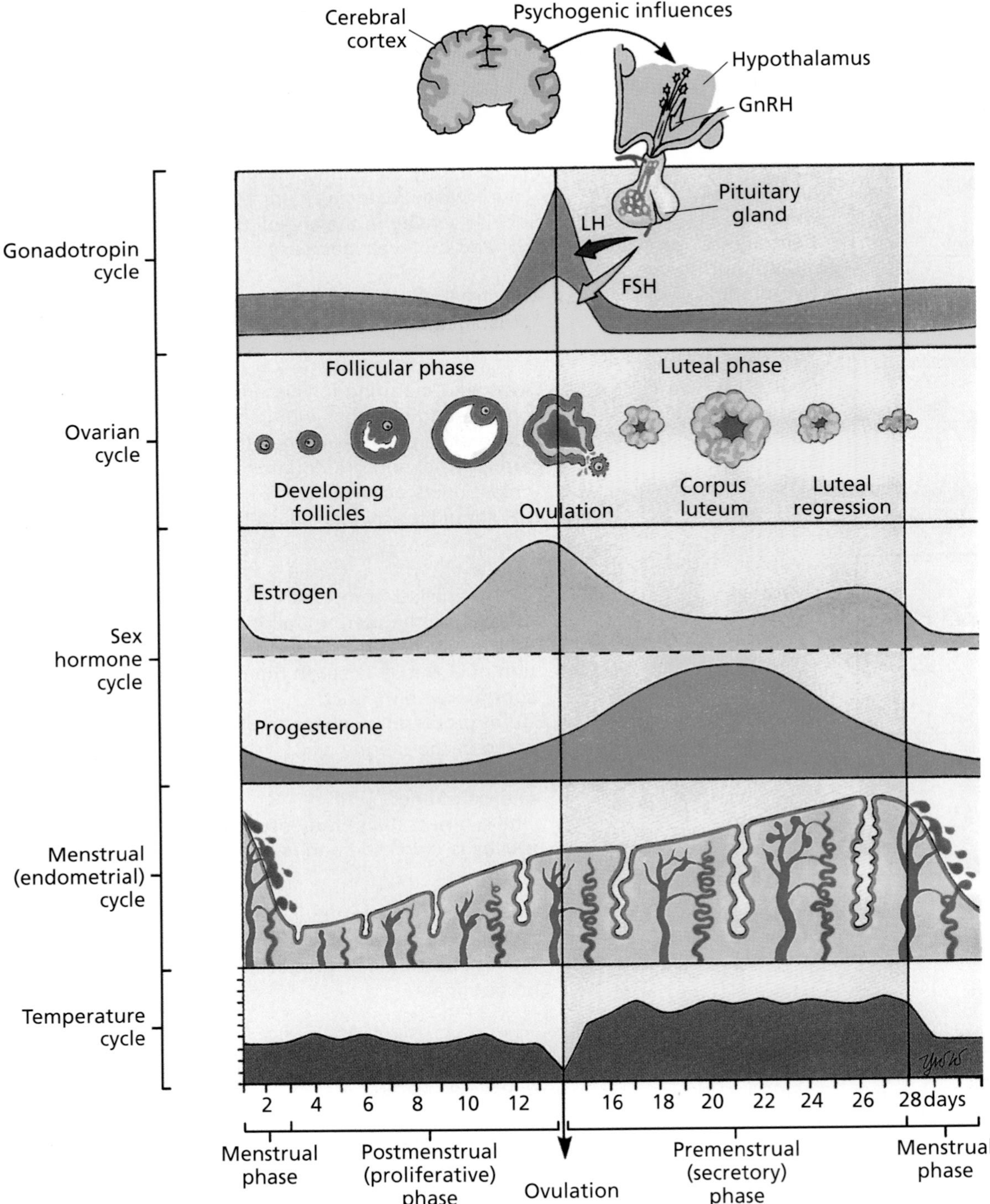

Fig. 21-5 Female menstrual cycle. Diagram shows the interrelationship of the cerebral, hypothalamic, pituitary, and uterine functions throughout a standard 28-day menstrual cycle. The variations in basal body temperature are also shown. (From Thibodeau and Patton, 1999.)

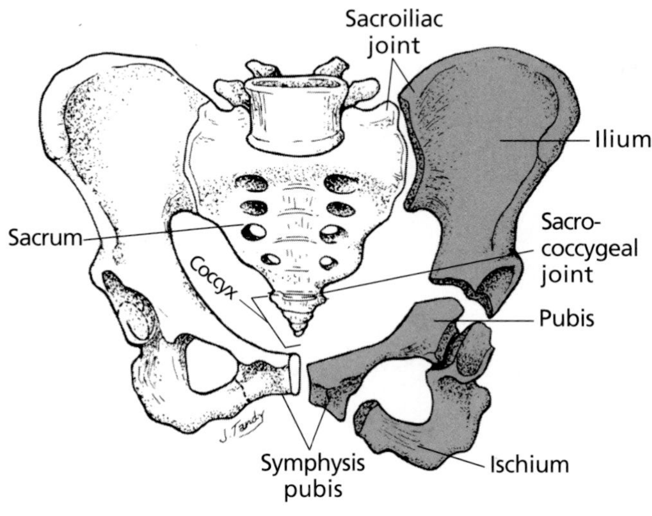

Fig. 21-6 Adult female pelvis. Note the pelvis joints. (From Lowdermilk, Perry, and Bobak, 1999.)

HEALTH HISTORY

Female Genitalia and Reproductive System

QUESTIONS	RATIONALE
PRESENT HEALTH STATUS	
➤ Do you have any chronic illness? If so, describe.	■ Some chronic illness such as diabetes or other endocrine disorders may affect the female reproductive system or make the client more susceptible to problems with the female reproductive system.
➤ Do you take any medications? If so, what do you take, and how often?	■ Both prescription and over-the-counter medications should be noted. Assess if they are taking medications as prescribed. Medications, particularly hormones, can affect reproductive system functioning.
➤ How often do you have a pelvic examination? When was your last Papanicolaou (Pap) smear? What were the results?	■ Assess self-care behaviors. Ideally, women should have examination and Pap smear done on a regular basis.
➤ Do you ever examine your genitalia? Do you feel comfortable looking at your female parts?	■ Although many women perform breast self-examination, many do not perform genitalia examination. This information may help direct client teaching.
PAST MEDICAL HISTORY	
➤ Have you had problems with your uterus or ovaries in the past? If so, describe.	■ Identify previous problems with reproductive system as this information may be helpful when documenting current problems.
➤ Have you ever had surgery on the uterus, vagina, or ovaries. If so, when? Why? How did you feel about having the surgery? How has it affected you?	■ Past surgical procedures should be noted. Removal of ovaries may affect hormonal balance.

QUESTIONS

RATIONALE

FAMILY HISTORY

➤ Has any woman in your family ever had cancer of the cervix, ovary, uterus, breast, or colon? If so, who? When? How was it treated?

■ A family history of these cancers increases cancer risk in the client.

RISK FACTORS

COMMON RISK FACTORS ASSOCIATED WITH Female Reproductive System Cancer

CERVICAL CANCER

Sexual intercourse at early age
Lifetime history of multiple sex partners
Infection with human papilloma virus (HPV)
Age between 40 and 50 years
Cigarette smoking
Lower socioeconomic status

OVARIAN CANCER

Age 50 or older
Early menarche and late menopause (increased number of ovulatory cycles)
Nulliparity or few pregnancies
History of infertility
Family history of ovarian, breast, colorectal, or endometrial cancer
White race

ENDOMETRIAL CANCER

Nulliparity
Infertility
Menstrual irregularities
Late onset of menopause
Dysfunctional uterine bleeding during menopause
History of diabetes or hypertension
Family history of endometrial, breast, colon, or ovarian cancer

MENSTRUATION

➤ What was the date of the first day of your last menstrual period? How often do you have periods? How long do they usually last?

■ A menstrual history consists of the last menstrual period (LMP), usual menstrual interval, and the duration of menses.

➤ How would you describe your usual amount of flow—light, moderate, heavy? How many pads or tampons do you use over the course of a day? An hour?

■ Normal flow is difficult to determine, but any change from what is "normal" for the client should be noted.

➤ Have you noted any change in your periods recently?

■ Change in menstruation could reflect hormonal imbalance.

➤ How old were you when you started having periods?

■ Normal onset of menarche is between ages 12 and 14 years, although the range spans ages 8 to 16. Onset between ages 16 and 17 suggests an endocrine problem.

QUESTIONS

RATIONALE

SEXUAL ACTIVITY

➤ Are you currently in a relationship that involves sexual intercourse? If yes, do you have one or multiple partners? How frequently do you engage in sexual activities? Are you and your partner(s) satisfied with the sexual relationship? Do you communicate comfortably about sex?

■ It is important to determine the type of sexual activity the individual has, as well as the client's satisfaction regarding that activity. The rationale for asking about client satisfaction is to determine if the client is satisfied with her sexuality and the sexual practices in which she engages.

➤ How many sexual partners have you had in the past 6 months? Do you prefer relationships with men, women, or both? (If client is a lesbian, inquire if she is in a significant relationship and has a partner.)

■ The rationale for this type of questioning is to determine the numbers and types of sexual encounters. This information may be used to determine the client's risk for sexually transmitted disease. Lesbians need to feel acceptance to discuss their health concerns. If the examiner seems genuinely interested and concerned, the client may appreciate the opportunity to discuss sexuality issues or problems.

➤ What are you doing to protect yourself from sexually transmitted infection (STI)? If protection is used, what type? Do you use protection every time you have intercourse?

■ Assess client's level of understanding and risk for sexually transmitted infection.

➤ How old were you when you first had intercourse? Was it by choice? Have you ever been in a relationship with anyone who hurt you? Have you ever been forced into sexual acts as a child or an adult? Is sexual activity associated with drug or alcohol use?

■ Inquire about possible past sexual abuse. Many times this causes ongoing sexual difficulties. There is a high incidence of sexual activity associated with substance abuse such as alcohol or marijuana. Assess for pattern of behavior. Several studies indicate that as many as 15% to 30% of women have been sexually abused as children. Some of these women may feel relieved to discuss this—others may choose to not disclose this information. (Roberts, 1996).

BIRTH CONTROL

➤ Are you currently using any birth control measures? If so, what type? How long have you been using this product? How effective do you feel this has been? Do you have any difficulty using it (problems with inserting it, remembering it, retaining it)?

➤ Has it affected your general physical or mental health?

➤ Do you use birth control measures every time you have intercourse?

■ All women who have the potential to become pregnant in heterosexual relationships should be questioned about contraceptive practices. Information should be gathered about appropriate use of the contraception, length of use, and satisfaction with the product.

OBSTETRIC HISTORY

➤ Have you ever been pregnant? If so, how many times? How many babies have you had? Have you had any miscarriages, abortions, or babies that died before they were born? If so, how many? (Box 21-1)

■ This forms the obstetric history. Gravida refers to the number of pregnancies; para refers to the number of births; abortion refers to any interrupted pregnancies—both spontaneous miscarriages and elective abortions. See Chapter 26 for more information regarding documentation of obstetric history.

Box 21-1 Documentation Tip

Gravida
Para
Term
Abortions
Living

QUESTIONS | RATIONALE

➤ Do you think you may be pregnant now? What symptoms have you noticed?

■ Symptoms may include missed or abnormal periods, history of sexual activity, nausea or vomiting, breast changes or tenderness, and fatigue.

➤ Have you ever had difficulty becoming pregnant? If so, have you seen a health care practitioner? What have you tried to do to become pregnant? How do you feel about not being able to become pregnant?

■ It is as important to inquire about difficulty becoming pregnant as it is to inquire about actual pregnancy. It is often quite distressing for the couple trying unsuccessfully to become pregnant.

PROBLEM-BASED HISTORY

The most commonly reported problems related to the female reproductive system are problems or changes with menstruation, pelvic pain, and vaginal discharge. As with symptoms in all areas of health assessment, a symptom analysis is completed, which includes the location, quality, quantity, chronology, setting, associated manifestations, alleviating factors, and aggravating factors. (See Box 4-2 in Chapter 4.)

Problems With Menstruation

➤ Have you noted any clotted blood during your periods? If so, when did this begin? Is it becoming worse over time? Have you talked with a health care provider about this?

■ *Menorrhagia* is a term for heavy menses. Clotting of blood indicates a heavy flow or vaginal pooling.

➤ Do you have cramps or other pains associated with your period? Does this occur each month? What relieves the discomfort? Do the cramps or pains interfere with your normal activities?

■ *Dysmenorrhea* is a term for painful or difficult menses. It is often associated with hormonal imbalance.

➤ Do you ever have spotting between periods?

■ Spotting between periods may indicate hormonal imbalance or a need for dose adjustment if the client is taking hormonal contraceptives or hormonal replacement.

➤ Do you have any other problems or symptoms prior to menses, such as headaches, bloated feeling, weight gain, breast tenderness, irritability, or moodiness? Does this seem to be associated with all of your periods or just occasionally? Does it interfere with your routine activities? What do you do to treat the problem? Does the treatment work?

■ Hormonal fluctuation associated with the menstrual cycle may cause the client to have symptoms that are frequently referred to as premenstrual syndrome (PMS). Asking how routine activities are affected by symptoms helps the nurse gain a better understanding of the significance of the symptoms.

QUESTIONS	RATIONALE
Lower Abdominal or Pelvic Pain	
➤ Do you ever experience pain either associated with your periods or between your periods? If so, when did you first become aware of this?	■ Lower abdominal pain or discomfort may be caused by many problems. It may include problems with the gastrointestinal tract, the urinary tract, or the reproductive system. If the client is having discomfort, it is important to try to determine the cause of the pain. Common problems may be associated with the uterus, the ovaries, or the vagina. Determine the onset of the pain.
➤ Describe the characteristics of the pain. Sharp? Aching? Nagging? Dull? On a scale of 1 to 10, how would you rate the intensity of the pain?	■ Note the characteristics of the pain and the intensity of the pain. This information may provide important clues to the cause of the problem.
➤ Is the pain affected by any other activity or function, such as menstruation, sexual activities, having a bowel movement, urinating, exercise, or walking?	■ Determine if there are any aggravating factors contributing to the pelvic pain.
➤ Do you have associated symptoms such as vaginal discharge or bleeding, gastrointestinal symptoms, abdominal distention or tenderness, or pelvic fullness? Are you able to put your finger on the place where the pain is, or is the discomfort more generalized?	■ Determine if there are any associated symptoms with the pelvic pain, as well as location.
➤ What have you done, if anything, to treat the pain?	■ Knowledge of previous self-treatment measures may be helpful in identifying appropriate treatment strategies.
Vaginal Discharge	
➤ Do you have any unusual vaginal discharge? If so, when did it begin? Has the onset of the vaginal discharge been sudden or gradual?	■ Identify onset and pattern of symptom.
➤ What color is it? What does it look like? Describe its odor, consistency, changes in characteristics.	■ Normal discharge is clear or cloudy, with minimal odor. A change may suggest a vaginal infection. Specific appearance or odor of the discharge may help to identify the causative organism.
➤ Do you feel that there is more discharge than usual? Have you noted any connection with vaginal itching, rash, pelvic pain, or pain with intercourse?	■ These are associated symptoms. Irritation from the discharge can cause itching, rash, or pain on intercourse. Pelvic or abdominal pain associated with new discharge suggests infection.

QUESTIONS

RATIONALE

➤ Do you use a vaginal douche? How often? Do you use feminine hygiene products? If yes, describe. Taking medications? What kind of underwear or pantyhose do you wear?

■ All of these factors can affect the discharge by increasing glycogen content, altering pH, or producing local irritation or contact dermatitis. Tight-fitting nylon underwear and hose can contribute to yeast infections. Medications that can cause problems include oral contraceptives, which increase the glycogen content of the vaginal epithelium and provide a fertile ground for organisms, and broad-spectrum antibiotics, which alter the balance of the normal vaginal flora.

➤ If sexually active, does your partner have a discharge?

■ If the client has developed discharge and the partner is known to have discharge, this could suggest STI.

Changes in Urination

➤ Do you have pain or burning with urination? If yes, when did this first begin?

■ Symptoms such as burning with urination suggest urinary tract infection (UTI). Note the onset of the problem.

➤ Do you have any other symptoms such as frequent urination in small amounts? Feeling that you cannot wait to urinate? Is there ever any blood in your urine? Is it dark, cloudy, or foul smelling?

■ These are common associated symptoms with UTI.

➤ Do you have difficulty controlling your bladder, wetting yourself? Do you urinate when you laugh, sneeze, bear down, cough, or pick up a heavy load? If yes, how long has this been going on?

■ Urinary tract problems such as urinary incontinence are common problems for many women, especially as they get older. Women at highest risk for problems with urinary incontinence are those who have had children, who are overweight, and who have weak musculature of the pelvic floor.

Menopause

➤ Have your menstrual periods slowed down or stopped? Do you have any of the following symptoms: hot flashes, numbness or tingling, back pain, palpitations, headaches, painful intercourse, changes in sexual desire, excessive sweating, mood swings, or vaginal dryness or itching?

■ Amenorrhea means absent menses. The perimenopausal period occurs from ages 40 to 55 years. These are common symptoms experienced during menopause.

➤ Are you being treated for any symptoms associated with menopause? Are you taking hormonal replacement? If so, what are you taking and how much? Is this helping? Have you noted any side effects?

■ The side effects of estrogen replacement therapy include fluid retention, breast pain or enlargement, and vaginal bleeding.

➤ How do you feel about going through menopause?

■ Although this is a normal life stage, psychologic reactions range from a sense of loss to positive acceptance.

QUESTIONS | **RATIONALE**

Sexually Transmitted Infection: Lesions and Discharges

➤ Do you have any other problems in the genital area, such as sores or lesions? If so, when did you first become aware of the problem?

■ Sexually transmitted infections frequently manifests as a lesion or a sore. Establish when the lesion was first noticed as this may be important in identifying the problem. Common problems include herpes, genital warts, molluscum contagiosum, gonorrhea, syphilis, chlamydia, monilial vaginitis, and trichomoniasis (see the Common Problems and Conditions section at the end of this chapter).

➤ Do you have any other symptoms, such as tender, inflamed, or bleeding external tissues; vaginal discharge; rash; burning pain with urination; pelvic fullness? Do you have any abdominal pain?

■ These are common symptoms associated with STI.

➤ Have you had a sexual relationship with someone who has a sexually transmitted infection, such as gonorrhea, herpes, acquired immunodeficiency syndrome (AIDS), chlamydia infection, venereal warts, or syphilis? If so, when? Have you ever been treated for any of these problems? If so, was the treatment successful? Were there any complications?

■ Sexual contact with a partner with untreated STI increases a person's risk for STI.

EXAMINATION

Equipment

- Disposable gloves for barrier protection
- ❖ Vaginal speculum of appropriate size to inspect the vagina and cervix
- Mirror to allow client to aid in client teaching (if desired)
- Sterile cotton swabs or large cotton-tipped applicators (Fox swabs) to manage secretions
- ❖ Materials for cytologic study (these vary):
  Glass slides
  Sterile cotton-tipped applicator
  Endocervical swab
  Endocervical spatula
  Ayre's spatula
  Cytologic fixative spray
  Small bottle of normal saline solution
  Small bottle of potassium hydroxide (KOH)
  Bottle of acetic acid (white vinegar)
- Water-soluble lubricant to lubricate hands prior to palpation
- Examination lamp (goosenecked, with a strong light) to visualize vagina and cervix

PROCEDURES AND TECHNIQUES WITH NORMAL FINDINGS | **ABNORMAL FINDINGS**

Before you begin this procedure, prepare the room. Assemble the equipment, obtain a sheet and gown, and be sure the room temperature is warm. If necessary, arrange for an assistant.

Prior to bringing the woman to the examination room, ask her to empty her bladder. Next, ask the woman to undress and put on a gown. Some woman may be more comfortable with their socks on. Allow for privacy while she prepares.

PROCEDURES AND TECHNIQUES WITH NORMAL FINDINGS

ABNORMAL FINDINGS

Box 21-2 Clinical Note

It may be uncomfortable for both the client and the examiner if they are of the opposite sex. If there is no objection by the client, proceed in a professional manner. Also remember that it may be helpful to have an escort in the examination room during the assessment.

Once the woman is ready for the examination, help her into the lithotomy position, with body supine, feet in the stirrups, and knees apart. Provide adequate draping with a sheet. Position the client with her buttocks at the edge of the examination table. Ask the woman to place her arms at her sides or across her chest, but not over her head (this tightens the abdominal muscles). Position the drape completely over the client's lower abdomen and upper legs, exposing only the vulva for your examination. Push the drape down so that you can see the woman's face as you proceed. Sit on a stool at the end of the table between the client's legs.

Help the woman to relax. The lithotomy position may make the woman feel embarrassed and vulnerable. If the client seems uncomfortable or embarrassed, you may ask her if she would like her head elevated so that she can see you better. Also it may help to readjust the stirrups either outward or inward to reduce the stress on the pelvis and legs. In addition, make sure that the client is adequately draped and that you are in a private location where others may not walk in during the examination.

As you start the examination reassure her that you will tell her everything that you are going to do before you actually do it. Assure her that if she becomes too uncomfortable, you will stop what you are doing and reassess what is happening. Always remember to touch the inner aspect of her thigh before you actually touch the external genitalia. (Don't be tentative with your touch—once you make physical contact, maintain it throughout the procedure.) Be sure to talk to the woman throughout the examination to tell her what you are doing, what you are seeing or feeling, and how long it will be until you are finished.

PROCEDURES AND TECHNIQUES WITH NORMAL FINDINGS

EXTERNAL GENITALIA

➤**INSPECT the pubic hair for distribution.** Hair distribution varies but usually covers an inverse triangle with the base over the mons pubis; some hair may extend up midline toward the umbilicus (Fig. 21-7).

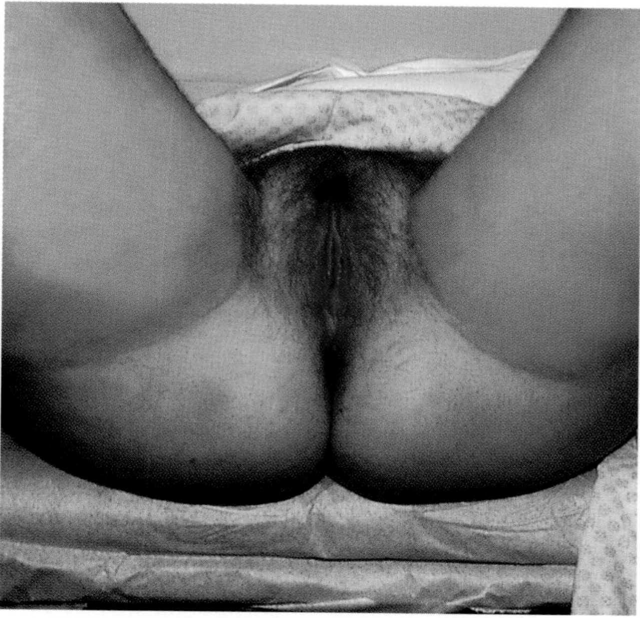

Fig. 21-7 Inspection of the external genitalia.

➤**INSPECT the skin over the mons pubis and inguinal area for surface characteristics.** The skin should be smooth and clear (Fig. 21-7).

➤**INSPECT and PALPATE the labia majora for pigmentation and surface characteristics.** Pigmentation should be darker than the client's general skin tone, and the tissues should appear shriveled or full, gaping or closed, usually symmetric, with a smooth skin surface and a dry or moist texture.

Begin palpation by gently touching the client on the inner thigh. Tell her that you are going to touch her external genitalia and that you are going to spread the labia apart.

Spread the labia majora with the fingers of one hand to view the inner surface of the labia majora and the labia minora and the surface of the vestibule (Fig. 21-8). Pigmentation should be dark pink. The area should appear moist, and the tissue should appear symmetric and without lesions or sores.

ABNORMAL FINDINGS

- Note any male hair distribution (diamond-shaped pattern), patchy loss of hair, or absence of hair in any client over 16 years of age.
- Observe for presence of skin lesions or infestations of skin or pubic hair.
- Observe for signs of inflammation, swelling, excoriation, leukoplakia (white patches), ulceration, lesions, nodules, or marked asymmetry.

PROCEDURES AND TECHNIQUES WITH NORMAL FINDINGS

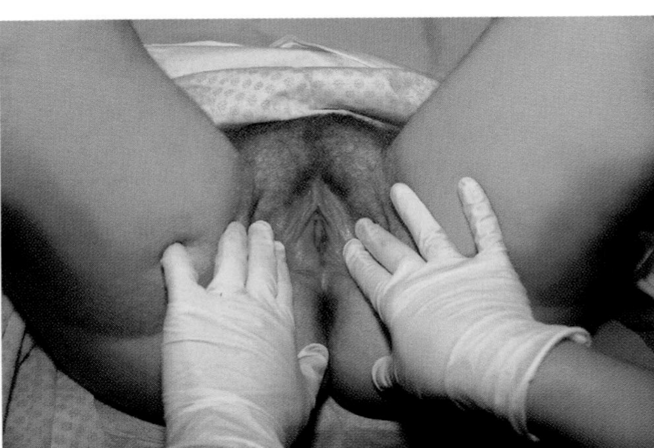

Fig. 21-8 Inspection of the labia.

➤**INSPECT and PALPATE the labia minora for pigmentation and surface characteristics.** Palpate the labia minora between your thumb and second fingers of your other hand. The tissue should feel smooth and soft, without nodules, masses or statements of discomfort from the client.

➤**INSPECT the clitoris for size and length.** The typical size of the clitoris should be approximately 2 cm (3/4 inch) or less in length (visible length) and 3/16 inch (0.5 cm) in diameter.

➤**INSPECT the urethral meatus, vaginal introitus, and perineum for positioning and surface characteristics.** Inspect the urethral meatus and the tissues immediately surrounding it. There should be a midline location of an irregular opening or slit close to or slightly within the vaginal introitus.

Inspect the vaginal introitus and the tissues immediately surrounding it. The introitus may appear as a thin vertical slit or a large orifice with irregular edges from the hymenal remnants; the tissues should appear moist.

Inspect the posterior skin surface of the perineum between the vaginal introitus and the anus. The skin should appear smooth and without lesions or discoloration. If the client has had an episiotomy, a scar (midline or mediolateral) may be visible.

➤**INSPECT the anus for color and surface characteristics.** The anus should exhibit increased pigmentation and coarse skin; no lesions should be present. Hemorrhoids may be seen in the adult; differentiate hemorrhoids from other lesions.

ABNORMAL FINDINGS

■ Look for areas of inflammation, irritation, excoriation, or vaginal discharge. Discoloration or tenderness may be the result of traumatic bruising.

■ Note any enlargement, atrophy, or inflammation.

■ Note any discharge from the surrounding (Skene's) glands or the urethral opening, polyps, inflammation, or a lateral position of the meatus. Note any surrounding inflammation, discolored or foul-smelling vaginal discharge, bleeding or blood clots, swelling, skin discoloration indicative of tissue bruising, or lesions. Note scars, skin tags, lesions, inflammation, fissures, lumps, or excoriation. Imperforate hymen is a very uncommon finding in young women; it is usually congenital or could be associated with past sexual abuse.

■ Note lesions or fissures around the anus. Lesions associated with sexually transmitted infections frequently appear on or around the anus.

PROCEDURES AND TECHNIQUES WITH NORMAL FINDINGS

➤**PALPATE the Skene's and Bartholin's glands for surface characteristics, discharge, and pain or discomfort.** With the labia still spread apart, insert the index finger of your other hand (palm surface up) into the vagina as far as possible. Exert upward pressure on the anterior vaginal wall surface and milk the Skene's glands by moving your finger outward toward the vaginal opening (Fig. 21-9). The glands area should be nontender and without discharge.

Next, palpate the lateral tissue of the vagina bilaterally. Use your thumb and index finger to palpate the entire area, paying attention to the posterolateral portion of the labia majora where the Bartholin's glands are located (Fig. 21-10). The surface should be homogeneous, nontender, and without discharge.

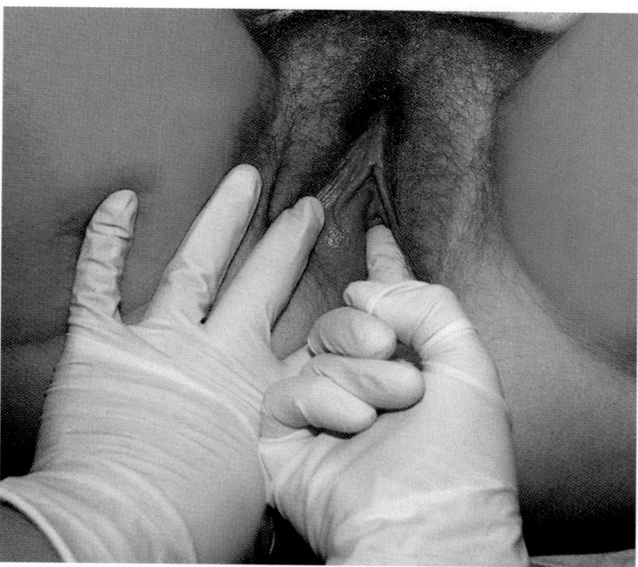

Fig. 21-9 Palpation of Skene's gland.

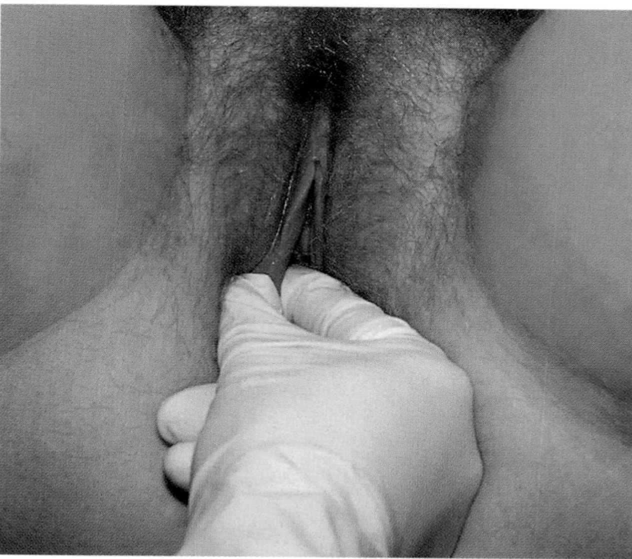

Fig. 21-10 Palpation of Bartholin's gland.

ABNORMAL FINDINGS

■ Note any tenderness or discharge; prepare a culture of any discharge that is present. Discharge from the Skene's and Bartholin's glands is usually indicative of an infection. Swelling in the area of the Bartholin's glands that is painful and "hot to the touch" may indicate an abscess of the Bartholin's gland. The abscess is generally pus filled and is gonococcal or staphylococcal in origin. A nontender mass, which is the result of chronic inflammation of the gland, is usually indicative of a Bartholin's cyst.

PROCEDURES AND TECHNIQUES WITH NORMAL FINDINGS

➤**INSPECT and PALPATE muscle tone for vaginal wall tone, rectal muscle tone, and urinary incontinence.** With your examining finger still in the vagina, instruct the client to squeeze the vaginal orifice around your finger. The nulliparous client (has had no children), usually squeezes tightly, so that you will feel the vaginal wall tissue firmly around your examining finger (Fig. 21-11). If the woman is parous (has had a baby), she may not squeeze as tightly.

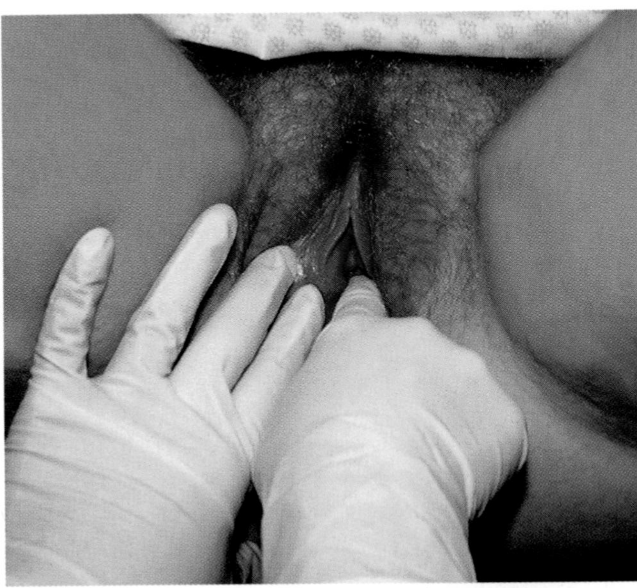

Fig. 21-11 Assessing vaginal tone.

➤Remove your finger from the vagina. Next, ask the client to bear down as you watch for vaginal wall bulging and urinary incontinence. Ask the client to cough and again inspect for bulging and incontinence.

ABNORMAL FINDINGS

- Note inability of client to constrict the vaginal orifice around your finger.

- Bulging of the anterior wall may indicate a cystocele.
- Bulging of the posterior vaginal wall may indicate a rectocele.
- If the cervix is visible at the opening of the vagina, it may indicate signs of a uterine prolapse.
- The presence of urine during either bearing down or coughing may be indicative of stress incontinence.

PROCEDURES AND TECHNIQUES WITH NORMAL FINDINGS

ABNORMAL FINDINGS

❖ INTERNAL GENITALIA: SPECULUM EXAMINATION

Tell the client that you will now use a speculum to do the internal examination (Box 21-3).

Box 21-3 Clinical Notes

- Make sure that you know how to use the speculum before you start. Especially know how to lock the blades open in place, and know how to release the lock.
- Make sure that the speculum is warm (especially if it is metal). If necessary, run it under warm water to warm it up. The speculum may also be kept warm by wrapping it in a heating pad or placing it under a warming light.
- Pick the correct size speculum of the client. Do not assume that a wide-blade Graves' speculum will be comfortable for all women. If the client is not sexually active, she will most likely need a narrower-blade speculum.
- Lubricate the speculum with warm water. Do not use lubricant. This will interfere with cytologic analysis.
- Make sure that you have all of the necessary supplies within handy reach before you start (e.g., slides, applicators, test tubes with KOH and saline).

Using a speculum of appropriate size, follow these steps:

- Locate the cervix using the middle finger on the nondominant hand; visualize the location in your "mind's eye"—this will help to locate the cervix with the speculum.
- Place the index and middle fingers of the nondominant hand inside the vaginal introitus and spread it apart about 2.5 cm (1 inch). Exert downward pressure against the posterior wall; wait for the vaginal wall muscles to relax (Fig. 21-12).

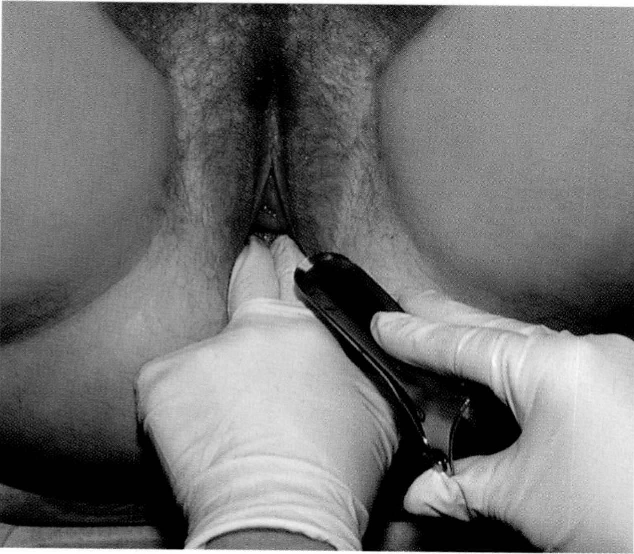

Fig. 21-12 Apply downward pressure on vagina before inserting the speculum.

PROCEDURES AND TECHNIQUES WITH NORMAL FINDINGS

ABNORMAL FINDINGS

- As downward pressure is exerted, simultaneously insert the closed speculum, holding the blades closed using one of two techniques:
  -Insert the speculum over your spread fingers, holding the speculum in a horizontal position (Fig. 21-13, *A*). (The opening made with the fingers should be wider than the width of the speculum.) Many practitioners prefer this technique because it prevents discomfort to the highly sensitive urethra adjacent to the anterior vaginal wall and avoids pubic hair being pulled with speculum placement. (Wheeler, 1995; Secor, 1999).

  OR

  -Insert the speculum over your fingers, holding the speculum at an oblique angle (Fig. 21-13, *B*). After the blades pass over the fingers, the speculum must be rotated to a horizontal position as it is inserted.
- After the blades have passed the introitus, remove the fingers while exerting downward pressure. Maintain downward and posterior pressure on the blades directed at a 45° angle until the speculum is completely inserted (Fig. 21-14).
- With speculum fully inserted and blades horizontal, open the blades of the speculum and look for the cervix. Reposition the speculum if unable to visualize the cervix. Once the cervix is visualized, lock the blades in the open position (Fig. 21-15).

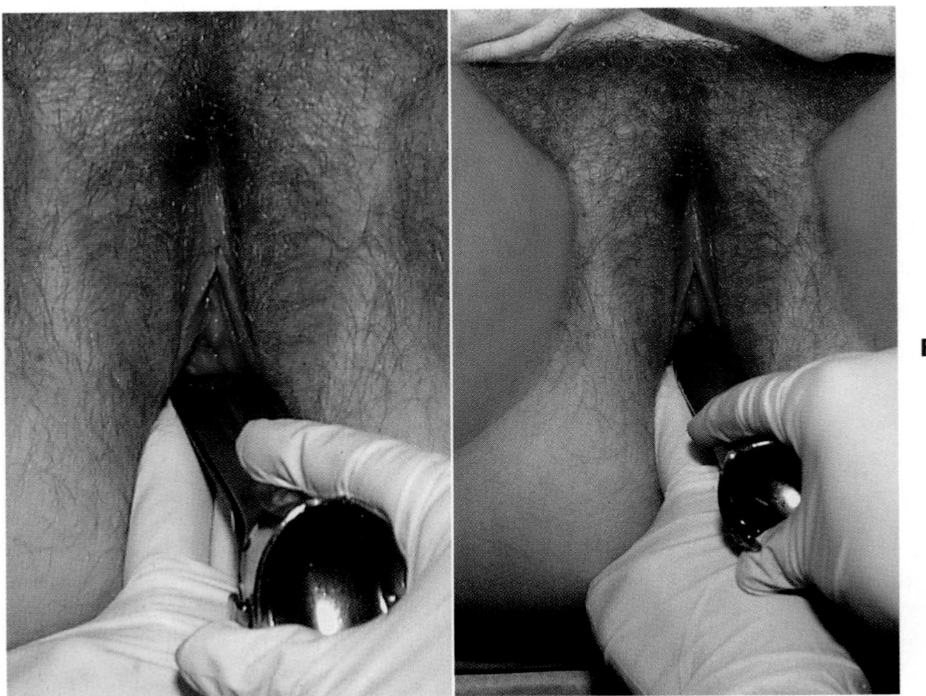

Fig. 21-13 **A,** Insertion of closed speculum blades in horizontal position. **B,** Insertion of closed speculum blades with oblique angle.

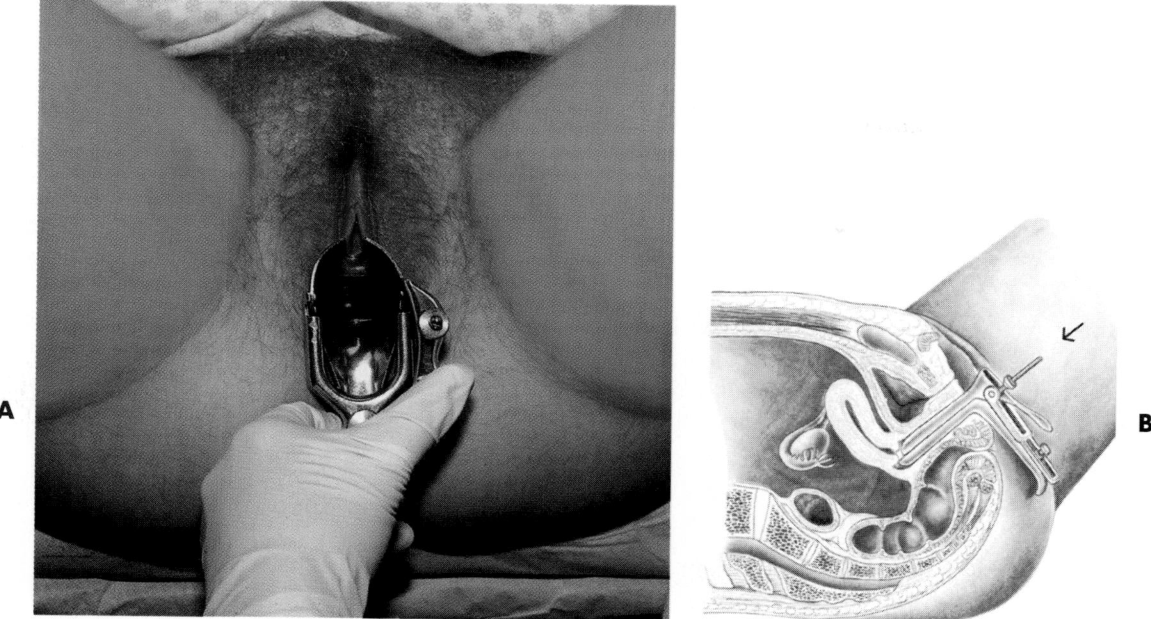

Fig. 21-14 **A,** Direct the speculum downward at 45° angle. **B,** Cross-sectional view. (**B** From Seidel et al, 1999.)

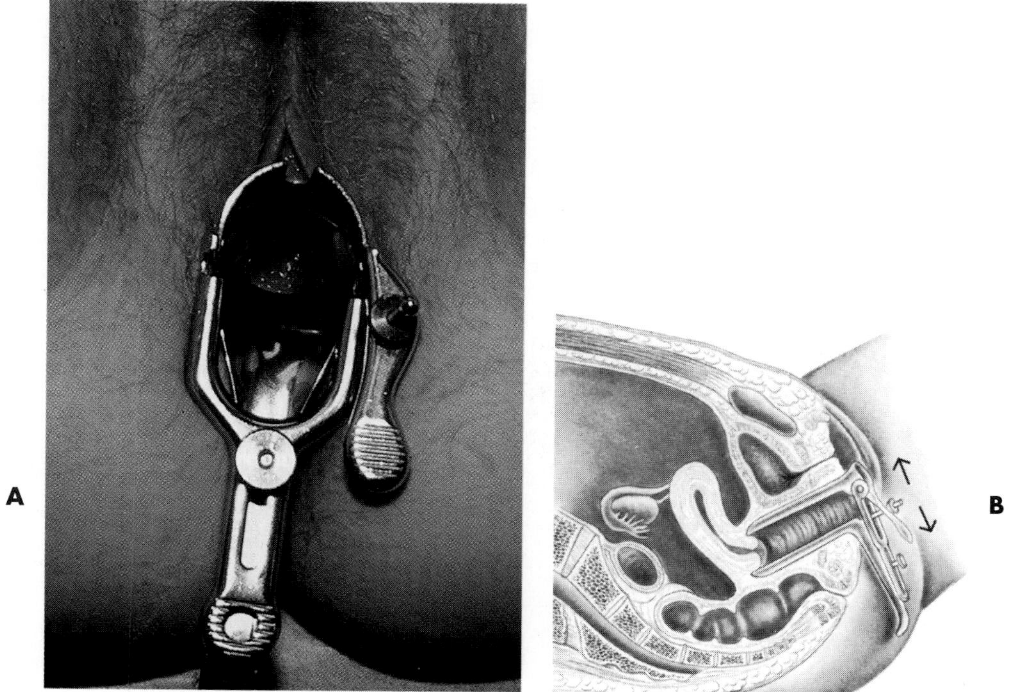

Fig. 21-15 **A,** Open speculum blades. **B,** Cross-sectional view. (**B** From Seidel et al, 1999.)

PROCEDURES AND TECHNIQUES WITH NORMAL FINDINGS

❖ ➤**INSPECT the cervix for color.** The cervix should be an evenly distributed pink color or, in pregnancy, a blue color secondary to increased vascularity. A symmetric, circumscribed erythema surrounding the os (the opening) may indicate the normal condition of exposed columnar epithelium—known as squamocolumnar junction.

❖ ➤**INSPECT the cervix for surface characteristics.** Inspect the surface of the cervix. It should appear smooth, with an occasional squamocolumnar junction (symmetric reddened circle around the os) visible. You may see nabothian cysts, which appear as smooth, round, small, yellow raised areas (Fig. 21-16).

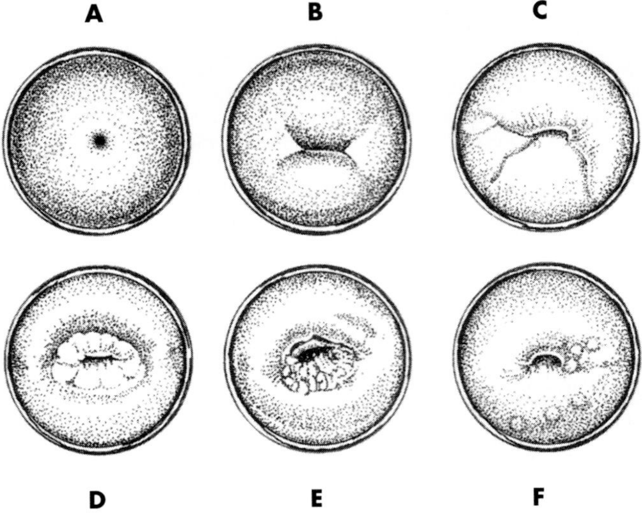

Fig. 21-16 Common appearances of the cervix. **A,** Nulliparous cervix. Note rounded os. **B,** Parous cervix. Note slit appearance of os. **C,** Multigravidous, lacerated. **D,** Everted. **E,** Eroded. **F,** Nabothian cysts. (From Seidel et al, 1999.)

ABNORMAL FINDINGS

- Note any reddened granular area around the os (especially if asymmetric), friable tissue, red patches or lesions, strawberry spots, or white patches. A pale-appearing cervix may be associated with menopause or anemia.
- Reddened, irregular color or patchy appearance with irregular borders can be an abnormal finding and requires further investigation.

PROCEDURES AND TECHNIQUES WITH NORMAL FINDINGS

❖ ➤**INSPECT the cervix for position.** It should be midline and point in a direction that is related to the position of the uterus. An anterior-pointing cervix indicates a retroverted uterus. A posterior-pointing cervix indicates an anteverted uterus. A cervix in the midline indicates a midposition uterus. The cervix should project into the vagina ⅜ to 1⅛ inches (1 to 3 cm), causing ⅖- to 1$\frac{1}{10}$-inch (1- to 3-cm) fornices surrounding the cervix.

❖ ➤**INSPECT the cervix for size and shape.** The cervix is usually about 2.5 cm (1 inch) in diameter. The os of a nulliparous client is small, round, and oval. The os of a parous client is generally slit shaped and may be irregular. A lacerated cervix has a torn slit appearance. An everted cervix (a normal variant) is manifested by a circular raised erythematous area around the os (see Fig. 21-16).

❖ ➤**INSPECT the cervical os for discharge.** First, if a discharge is present, determine whether it is coming from the cervix itself or whether it is from the vagina and has only pooled near the cervix. A mucous plug may be present at the os of the cervix. If a discharge is present, it should be odorless, creamy or clear, thin, thick, or stringy. At the middle of the menstrual cycle or immediately after menstruation, the discharge may be heavier.

❖ ➤**OBTAIN vaginal smears and cultures.** Often during the speculum examination, a culture or smear is indicated. These specimens should be collected while the speculum is still in place, but after the cervix and surrounding tissue have been inspected. It is important that specimens are not collected while the client is menstruating, or if the client took a bath, used a vaginal douche, or inserted topical vaginal inserts or lubrications within the last 48 hours. Also, do not use lubrication jelly on the speculum if specimens are to be collected. These will affect the quality of samples taken and could result in false negative results.

ABNORMAL FINDINGS

■ Report if the cervix is situated laterally. A cervix deviating to either the right or left from a midline position may indicate a pelvic mass, uterine adhesions, or pregnancy. Report if there is a projection of more than 1⅛ inches (3 cm) into the vaginal canal. If the cervix projects into the vagina more than this, it may indicate a pelvic or uterine mass.

■ Note if the cervix is over 1¾ inches (4 cm) in diameter. Injury secondary to childbirth, abortion, or removal of an intrauterine device may cause a change in the shape of the cervical os.

■ A discharge with an odor or a discharge that is colored, such as yellow, green, or gray, most probably indicates a bacterial or fungal infection.

PROCEDURES AND TECHNIQUES WITH NORMAL FINDINGS

Papanicolaou (Pap) Smear The Pap smear should always be the first specimen collected. It is used as a screening test to detect cervical and endometrial dysplasia and cancer. The Pap smear is recommended as a routine part of the annual pelvic examination in women once they become sexually active, or between 18 and 21 years of age, whichever comes first. In clients whose mothers received diethylstilbestrol (DES) while pregnant with the client, annual screening should begin at age 14 or the onset of menses. Annual screening can be stopped at the age of 65 if previous smears have been negative. False negative results may be as high as 20%; most are attributed to laboratory error and poor specimen collection (U.S. Preventive Services Task Force, 1996). Follow the guidelines in Table 21-2 for specimen collection. Be sure to inform the client that she may experience spotting or a slight amount of bleeding following this procedure.

ABNORMAL FINDINGS

■ Results of Pap smears are now reported describing squamous intraepithelial lesions (SIL) (Mashburn and Scharbo-DeHaan, 1997). Abnormal labels from least to most severe include:
-Atypical squamous cells of undetermined significance (ASCU)
-Low-grade squamous intraepithelial lesions (LSIL) (lesions equivalent to changes associated with human papillomavirus [HPV])
-High-grade squamous intraepithelial lesions (HSIL)
-Invasive cancer

Table 21-2 ❖Procedure for Collecting Pap Smear Specimen

	PROCEDURE	RATIONALE	
Ectocervical specimen	Insert vertical projection of spatula into os until lateral projection is against cervix. Rotate 360°, maintaining contact with cervix, scraping the entire cervical surface. Remove and spread the material from both sides of the spatula thinly on a glass slide; immediately spray slide with cytologic fixative; label slide "ectocervical specimen."	Avoid applying a thick sample on the slide—this will make it difficult to visualize cells.	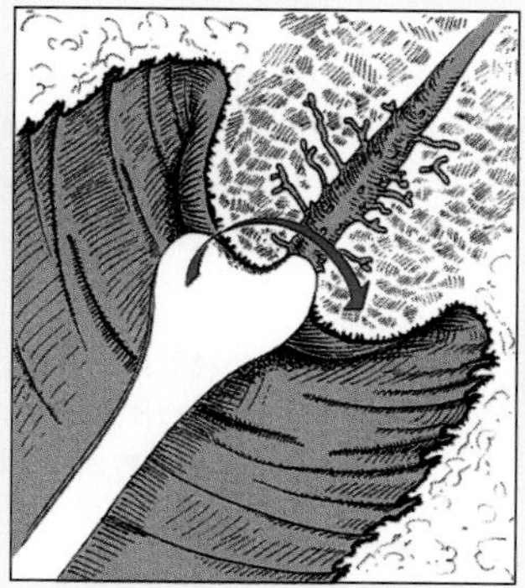 (From Barkauskas et al, 1998.)
Endocervical specimen	Insert a cytobrush into cervical os. Rotate 360°. Remove and place sample on slide using a rolling or twisting motion on the slide. Immediately spray slide with cytologic fixative; label slide "endocervical specimen."	Use of brush as opposed to cotton-tipped applicator has improved the quality of the sample of endocervical cells.	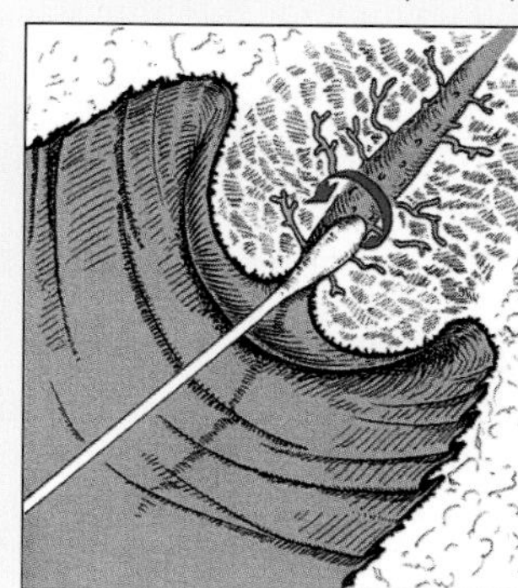 (From Barkauskas et al, 1998.)
Another type of device frequently used for Pap smear is a Cervex-brush. It collects both ectocervical and endocervical specimens at the same time.			
Ectocervical/ endocervical specimen	Use a Cervex-brush. Insert the central long bristles into the os until the lateral bristles bend against the ectocervix. Apply gentle pressure and rotate the brush 3 to 5 times to the left and right. Withdraw brush and paint the glass slide with two single stokes in the same place on the slide applying the first stroke with one side to the brush, the second stroke with the other side of the brush. Apply a fixative and label "ectocervical and endocervical specimen."	Use of a cervex-brush reportedly causes less spotting after the examination, yet provides a quality sample of ectocervical and endocervical cells.	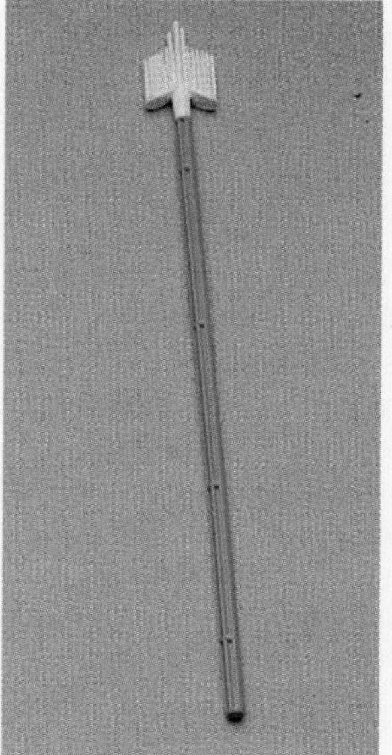 (Courtesy Cooper Surgical, Shelton, Conn.)

PROCEDURES AND TECHNIQUES WITH NORMAL FINDINGS

ABNORMAL FINDINGS

Other Specimens for Screening, Culture, or Microscopic Evaluation There are a variety of additional screening tests or cultures that will be taken based on risk factors, the history, or clinical findings (Box 21-4). Individuals with these risk factors should be screened. Follow the guidelines in Table 21-3 for specimen collection. It is important to get a detailed history regarding sexual activity.

Box 21-4 High-Risk Population Requiring Routine Screening for Various Sexually Transmitted Infections (STIs).

CHLAMYDIA

- All sexually active adolescent females
- All sexually active females under age of 25 with other following risk factors:
  - New or multiple sex partners
  - Inconsistent use of barrier contraceptives
  - Cervical ectopy
  - History of previous STI

GONORRHEA

- Commercial sex workers (prostitutes)
- Individuals with a history of gonorrhea infection
- Individuals under 25 who have had 2 or more sex partners in last year
- Pregnant females in high risk group

SYPHILIS

- All pregnant women
- Commercial sex workers (prostitutes)
- Individuals who trade sex for drugs
- Persons who have had sex with partner infected with syphilis
- Individuals who have other STIs or Human Immunodeficiency virus (HIV)

From U.S. Preventive Services Task Force, 1996.

❖ ➤**INSPECT the vaginal walls for color and surface characteristics.** Following the specimen collection, carefully unlock the speculum and, while the blades are still partially open, gently begin to remove the speculum from the vagina. The blades of the speculum tend to close by themselves. As the speculum is being removed, slowly rotate the blades of the speculum and inspect the walls of the vagina. Apply posterior, downward pressure to avoid causing discomfort to the sensitive urethra with blade removal.

➤The walls should be pink, with transverse rugae (which diminish after vaginal deliveries), moist and smooth, and homogeneous in consistency.

■ Note if the wall is reddened or pale; if there are lesions, leukoplakia, cracks, a dried surface, or bleeding; or if it appears nodular or swollen.

➤Inspect any vaginal secretions. They should be thin, clear or cloudy, odorless, and minimal to moderate in amount.

■ Report any secretions that are thick, curdy, frothy, gray, green, yellow, foul smelling, or profuse.

Table 21-3 Collection of Samples for Screening, Culture, or Microscopic Evaluation

	PROCEDURE	RATIONALE
CHLAMYDIA AND GONORRHEA SCREENING OR CULTURE		
Screening	Specimen taken from cervical os. Insert dacron swab into os, leave in place for 30 seconds to allow adequate absorption. Remove swab from os—be careful not to touch walls of vagina as this will contaminate specimen. Place in container provided and follow instructions. (Newer tests are using vaginal secretions and urine samples for screening.)	DNA probes and enzyme immunoassays are the most widely used nonculture diagnostic tests. Both are rapid and have high sensitivity and specificity—particularly the DNA probe. Since products used for screening vary, the examiner must follow instructions on the label of the specimen collection kits for accurate results.
Culture*	Culture for both chlamydia and gonorrhea requires endocervical specimen. If using Thayer-Martin culture plate for gonococcal culture, use a cotton-tipped swab, leave in cervical os for 30 seconds, remove, and apply in Z pattern.	Culture is most specific test for asymptomatic persons—not used as widely as screening because of several limitations, including expense, special handling of specimen, and results not available for 3-7 days.
***CANDIDIA, TRICHOMONAS,* AND BACTERIAL VAGINOSIS MICROSCOPIC EXAMINATION**		
Wet mount	Use cotton-tipped swab to obtain sample of vaginal secretion. Remove swab, apply specimen to slide. Apply one drop of saline to slide, cover with glass cover slip. Label slide appropriately.	Wet mount is used to diagnose bacterial vaginosis and *Trichomonas.*
KOH preparation	Use cotton-tipped swab to obtain sample of vaginal secretions. Remove swab, apply specimen to slide. Apply one drop of potassium hydroxide (KOH) to slide, cover with glass cover slip. Label slide appropriately.	KOH dissolves epithelial cells, and debris KOH is used to diagnosis *Candida* by allowing visualization of budding filaments and spores. A fishy odor is indicative of *Gardnerella,* a common organism causing bacterial vaginosis.

*Many products test for both chlamydia and gonorrhea. Follow instruction provided with the culture kit.

PROCEDURES AND TECHNIQUES WITH NORMAL FINDINGS | **ABNORMAL FINDINGS**

INTERNAL GENITALIA: BIMANUAL EXAMINATION

It is important to first tell the client that you are going to perform an internal examination with your fingers and hand. Next, move to a standing position at the end of the examination table between the client's legs. If your gloves have become soiled or contaminated, put on a clean pair of gloves. Lubricate the index and middle fingers of the hand that will be placed internally. Gently insert the middle and index fingers into the vaginal opening. Insert downward pressure on the posterior vaginal wall. Wait for a moment for the vaginal opening to relax. Then gradually insert your fingers their full length into the vagina.

❖ ➤**PALPATE the vagina for surface characteristics and discomfort.** Palpate the vaginal wall as you insert your fingers. The wall should feel smooth and should be nontender. Once your fingers are fully extended into the vaginal wall, position your thumb (which is outside the vagina and near but not on the urethra and clitoris) out of the way so that it is not uncomfortable for the client.

■ Abnormalities of the vaginal wall include nodules, cysts, discomfort, or unusual tissue growths.

PROCEDURES AND TECHNIQUES WITH NORMAL FINDINGS

❖ ➤**PALPATE the cervix for position, size, surface characteristics, mobility, and discomfort.** Locate the cervix with the fingers of your internal hand. Place the palmar surface of the fingers of your other hand on the lower abdomen midway between the umbilicus and the pubis (Fig. 21-17). The hand on the abdomen should be used to gently hold the uterus downward against the internal examination hand so that the cervix can be evaluated. Palpate the cervix and vaginal fornices with the palmar surfaces of the fingers of your internal hand. The cervix should measure 1 to 1¾ inches (2.5 to 4 cm), be evenly rounded or slightly ovoid, feel firm (like the tip of a nose) and smooth, and move ⅕ to ⅘ inches (1 to 2 cm) in each direction without causing the woman discomfort. It should be located in the midline position; the fornices (pockets surrounding the cervical protrusion) should be pliable and smooth, and there should be no tenderness.

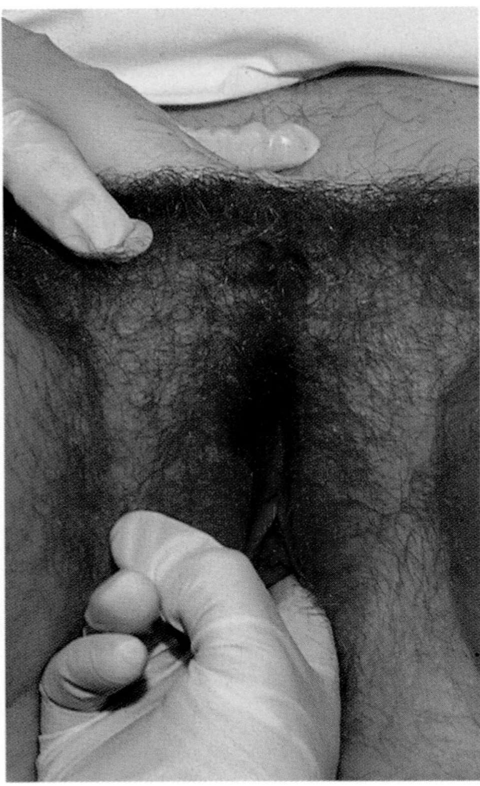

Fig. 21-17 Bimanual palpation of the uterus.

ABNORMAL FINDINGS

■ Note if the cervix is enlarged, irregular, soft or nodular, hard, immobile or associated with discomfort as it moves, and laterally displaced (not in the midline). Painful cervical movement suggests a pelvic inflammatory process such as acute pelvic inflammatory disease (PID) or a ruptured tubal pregnancy.

PROCEDURES AND TECHNIQUES WITH NORMAL FINDINGS

❖ ➤**PALPATE the uterus for size and position.** Move the fingers from the cervical os into the anterior fornix of the vagina. Slowly slide the hand that is on the abdomen toward the pubis with the palmar surface of your fingers pressing downward to push the pelvic organs closer for your internal fingers to palpate. It may be helpful to visualize the hands working together to "trap" the uterus between the two hands. The non-pregnant uterus is small and usually lies under the symphysis pubis in the pelvis. Normally, it is not palpable abdominally by the external hand, rather it is assessed with the internal fingers. In a parous client, the uterus may feel larger.

- *Anteverted:* The uterus is palpated at the level of the pubis between the abdominal and internal hands; the uterus points anteriorly, the cervix will be aimed posteriorly. Most women have an anteverted uterus (Fig. 21-18).

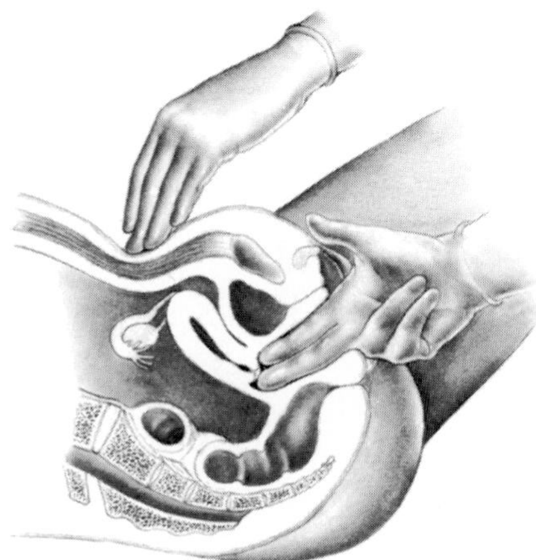

Fig. 21-18 Anteverted uterus. (From Seidel et al, 1999.)

- *Anteflexed:* The uterus is palpable at the level of the pubis between the abdominal and the internal hands; the uterus points anteriorly, the cervix points along the axis of the vaginal canal (Fig. 21-19).

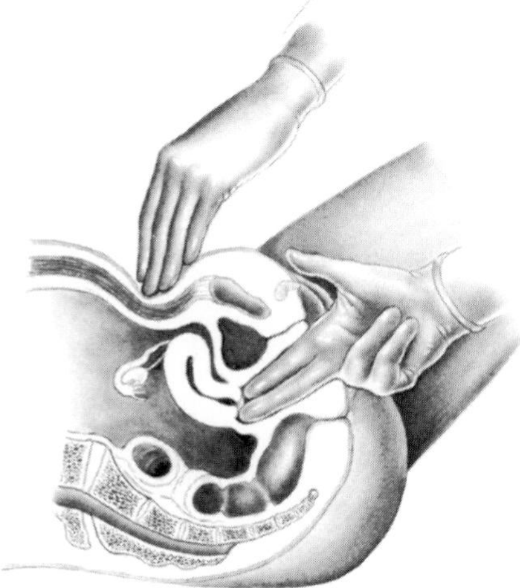

Fig. 21-19 Anteflexed uterus. (From Seidel et al, 1999.)

ABNORMAL FINDINGS

■ An enlarged uterus in a nonpregnant woman is abnormal and requires further evaluation. An enlarged uterus may be caused by fibroid tumor, adenomyosis, or carcinoma.

PROCEDURES AND TECHNIQUES WITH NORMAL FINDINGS

ABNORMAL FINDINGS

- *Midposition:* The uterus may not be palpable between the external and internal hands; the uterus points upward, the cervix is pointed along the axis of the vaginal canal (Fig. 21-20).

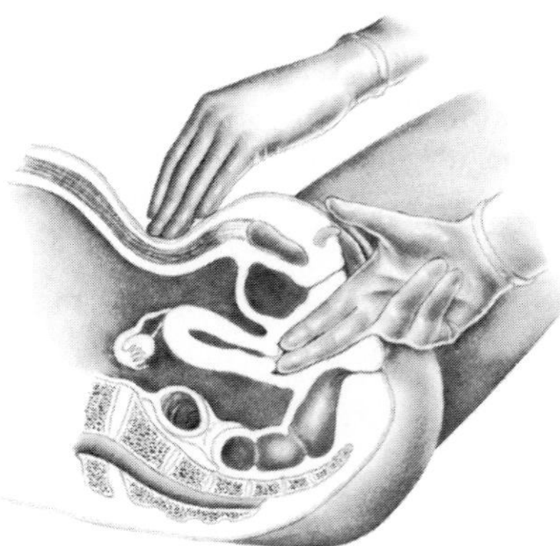

Fig. 21-20 Uterus at midposition. (From Seidel et al, 1999.)

- *Retroverted:* The uterus is positioned posteriorly and is not palpable between the external and internal hands. The cervix is pointed anteriorly (Fig. 21-21).

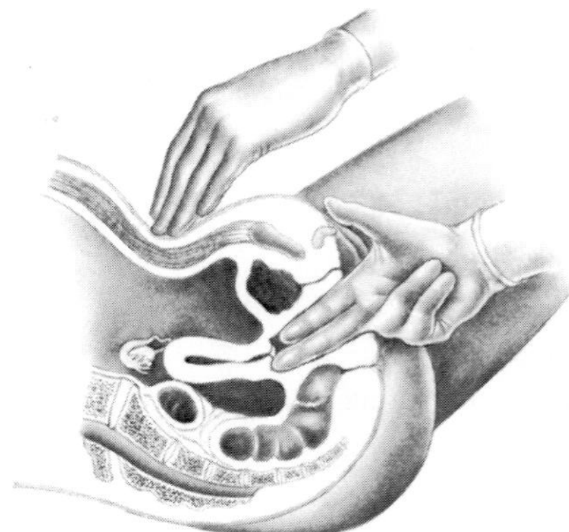

Fig. 21-21 Retroverted uterus. (From Seidel et al, 1999.)

PROCEDURES AND TECHNIQUES WITH NORMAL FINDINGS

- *Retroflexed:* The uterus is positioned posteriorly and is not palpable between the external and internal hands. The cervix is directed along the axis of the vaginal canal (Fig. 21-22).

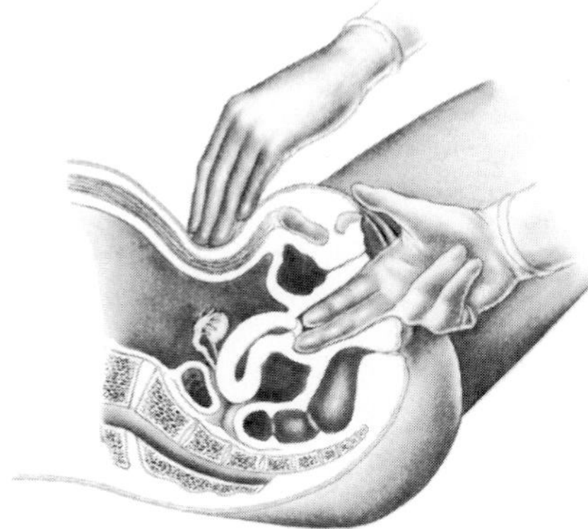

Fig. 21-22 Retroflexed uterus. (From Seidel et al, 1999.)

❖ ➤**PALPATE the uterus for surface characteristics, mobility, and discomfort.** Palpate the uterine wall with the internal fingers in the vaginal fornices. Normally, it feels smooth and firm. Gently move the uterus between your external hand and internal fingers. It should move freely and be nontender.

❖ ➤**PALPATE the adnexa and ovaries for size, shape, and tenderness.** Place the abdominal hand on the left lower abdominal quadrant and the intravaginal hand in the left fornix of the vagina. Lift the internal fingers upward as the external fingers press down and inward to "trap" the ovary between the hands. You will know if you have located the ovary when you reach a slight bulging area in the lower quadrant and when the client complains of a "twinge" sensation of slight tenderness. The ovary may not always be palpable, but if it is, it should feel smooth, firm, and ovoid. The ovaries are approximately walnut-sized (about 1¾ inches [4 cm]) and should be mobile. Fallopian tubes have a very small diameter and normally are not palpable or sensitive. In thin women, the only other structure that may be palpable is the round ligament. Reverse the position of the hands to the right side and use the same techniques to evaluate the right ovary and adnexa (Fig. 21-23).

ABNORMAL FINDINGS

■ Report any irregular contour, soft, nodular consistency, or masses. A uterus that feels irregular or nonsmooth is abnormal and requires further evaluation. A soft uterus is usually associated with pregnancy; an irregular surface suggests fibroids. Note if the uterus is fixed or tender during this maneuver. A fixed uterus may indicate adhesions. Tenderness may indicate pelvic inflammation or a ruptured tubal pregnancy.

■ An ovary over 5 cm (2 inches) is considered abnormal and requires further evaluation. If any masses are noted in the adnexa, evaluate their characteristics: size, shape, location, tenderness, and consistency.

PROCEDURES AND TECHNIQUES WITH NORMAL FINDINGS

ABNORMAL FINDINGS

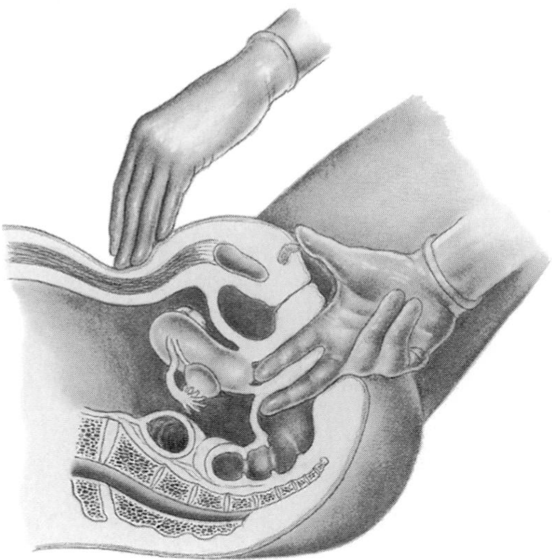

Fig. 21-23 Bimanual palpation of the adnexa. (From Seidel et al, 1999.)

RECTOVAGINAL EXAMINATION

To prepare for rectovaginal examination, change the intravaginal glove. (This prevents transfer of organisms from the vagina to the rectum.) Tell the client what you will be doing and that the procedure will be uncomfortable; she may feel the urgency of a bowel movement. Lubricate the first two fingers of the newly gloved hand. Place your middle finger, palm side up, over the anus. Ask the client to bear down; while she is doing so, gently insert your middle finger into the rectum. Insert your index finger into the vagina and locate the cervix.

❖ ➤**PALPATE the rectal wall for surface characteristics.** With the index and middle fingers inserted as far as possible, instruct the client to bear down. This will bring more rectal wall into the range of palpation. Gently rotate the finger in the rectum (middle finger) to evaluate the characteristics of the rectal wall. The wall should feel smooth and be without any areas of masses, fistulas, fissures, or tenderness. The septum between the vagina and the rectum should be thin, smooth, and intact.

■ Note any areas of masses, polyps, nodules, irregularities, and tenderness.

❖ ➤**PALPATE the uterus and ovaries for surface characteristics.** Place the external hand on the lower abdomen and apply downward pressure. Repeat the steps as described in the bimanual examination. Keep the index finger of the internal hand under the cervix as a landmark. The rectovaginal examination allows for a more complete evaluation of the posterior side of the uterus. The findings should be the same as previously described in the bimanual examination procedure section (Fig. 21-24).

■ Note marked tenderness, nodularity, enlargement, and masses that seem immobile. All of these findings should be considered abnormal. If a mass is detected in the adnexa, evaluate its characteristics including size, shape, location, tenderness, and consistency.

PROCEDURES AND TECHNIQUES WITH NORMAL FINDINGS

ABNORMAL FINDINGS

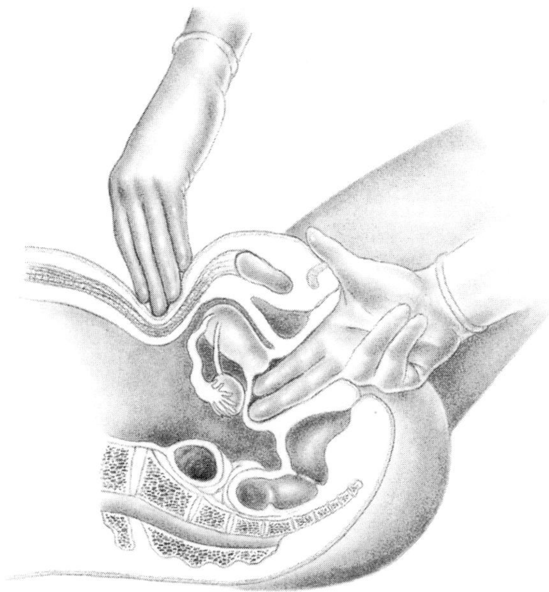

Fig. 21-24 Rectovaginal examination. (From Seidel et al, 1999.)

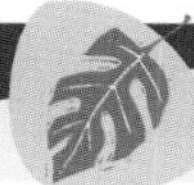

➤PALPATE the anal sphincter for tone. Withdraw your fingers slowly and evaluate the characteristics of the anal tone with the middle finger. The anus should tighten evenly around the examination finger. Examine the characteristics of the stool on the examination finger. For techniques and findings of the anus and stool characteristics, see Chapter 23.

Following the examination, assist the client in scooting back on the examination table. Offer her a tissue or cloth to clean her perineum. Provide her with privacy so that she may clean herself and get dressed.

■ Note the presence of rectal stricture.

AGE-RELATED VARIATIONS

■ INFANTS

Anatomy and Physiology

The female infant possesses functionally immature ovaries, and the cervix constitutes about two thirds of the entire uterus. The vagina is simply a small narrow canal with few epithelial folds. The nonprominent labia majora have a smooth, dry appearance. The thin, avascular labia minora are much more prominent and lighter in color in the infant than in the adolescent and adult. It is not unusual for the infant to have an irregular urethral opening. The clitoris is very small. The hymen, a thin membranous tissue just inside the introitus, may or may not be across the vaginal opening. It may appear as a crescent-shaped opening in the midline.

Health History

- When the child was born, did anyone tell you that there was anything wrong with the infant's genitalia? Does the infant have any congenital problems?
  Rationale This information provides baseline data.

Examination

Procedures and Techniques During infancy and childhood the examination is limited to an evaluation of the external genitalia to determine if the structures are intact, the vagina is present, and the hymen is patent. The infant is placed on the examination table in frog-leg position (hips flexed with the soles of the feet together and up to the buttocks). Using gloved hands, place both thumbs on either side of the labia major and gently push the tissue laterally while pushing the perineum down. This should permit visualization of the perineal area, the urethra, the clitoris, the hymen, and possibly the vaginal opening.

Normal and Abnormal Findings Secondary to maternal hormones, the newborn's genitalia appear somewhat engorged, with swollen labia majora and prominent and protruding labia minora. The clitoris also looks relatively enlarged and the hymen may appear thick. It may be difficult to see the vaginal opening. A mucoid, whitish vaginal discharge may be observed during the early period following birth. This should disappear by 1 month. Vaginal discharges noted after the child is a month old may occur secondary to diaper or powder irritation.

■ CHILDREN

Anatomy and Physiology

The anatomy and physiology is similar to that previously described for the infant.

Health History

- Does the child have any sores, rashes, or complaints of itching on the genitalia? Does she ever cry when she urinates? Do you ever put bubble bath in the bathtub when the child is bathing?

  Rationale Vaginal discharge, itching, and rash may be caused by poor hygiene or the presence of a foreign body. If any of these symptoms are present, ask about similar problems or past urinary tract infections or the use of bubble bath. Bubble bath frequently is an irritant for girls.
- Does the child frequently play with her own genitalia? Does her playing with herself bother you? Has the child ever placed foreign objects into her vagina?

  Rationale Exploration of the genitalia is a normal developmental phenomenon. It does not arouse sexual feelings equivalent to those in the adult. It is important to assess how the parent feels about this and how the parent interacts with the child regarding the self-play.
- To preschool or young children: Has anyone ever asked you to touch them? Have you ever been touched on your vagina or between your legs by someone when you did not want them to? If so, when did this happen? Who did it? Did you tell anyone? If the answer is no, ask child, Would you tell me if they did? (Box 21-5)

  Rationale Screen for sexual abuse.

Examination

Procedures and Techniques The extent of the genitalia examination in children depends on their age and the presence of problems. An inspection of a young girl's external genitalia should be included with each routine examination. If this examination is performed consistently, the child will experience less anxiety and embarrassment in later years when internal examination become necessary (Hairston, 1997). Internal examination is not routinely performed because the internal female genitalia is underdeveloped in the prepubertal girl.

Box 21-5 Talking With Children Who Reveal Abuse

- Provide a private time and place to talk.
- Do not promise not to tell; tell the child that you are required to report the abuse.
- Do not express shock or criticize the family.
- Use the child's vocabulary to discuss the body part.
- Avoid using any leading statements that can distort the child's story.
- Reassure the child that he or she has done the right thing by telling.
- Tell the child that the touching or abuse is not his or her fault; he or she is not bad or to blame.
- Determine the child's immediate need for safety.
- Let the child know when you report the situation.

(From Wong DL et al: *Whaley & Wong's Nursing care of infants and children,* ed 6, St. Louis, 1999, Mosby.

There are, however, occasional situations that warrant a more complete examination. The decision to do this is usually based on external examination findings or the history. For example, if the child has a history of urinary tract problems, vaginal discharge or irritation, or complaints of itching, rash, or pain, then a more complete examination is necessary. A complete examination is also necessary if there is any indication of sexual abuse or mishandling of the child.

Regardless of what level of examination is necessary, the nurse must take the time to gain the cooperation and understanding of the child; how this is done is largely dependent on the age of the child and previous experiences. By the time a child is 4 to 6 years of age, you will need to spend considerable time reassuring the child that the procedure involves looking at her genitalia and touching her on the outside only. It is often quite difficult to get the child to understand that it is okay for you to perform a genitalia examination but that if someone else touches her in a way that she should not be touched, that it is not okay. It is often important to include the parent in the discussion of the necessity for the examination and to actually be with the child and help to position the child during the examination.

In all cases, ensure privacy for the child. School-age girls will dislike the examination even more than younger children. It is best to approach the child in a matter-of-fact manner and to tell her what you are going to do. If you take your time and tell the child that you need her cooperation, the examination will usually occur without incident. The child should participate in the decision about whether the parent is present in the room or not during the examination. Some girls may want a parent present, and some may not. Confer with the child before the examination and, if appropriate, ask the parent to wait outside.

Occasionally a girl will refuse to be examined. This may be due to a previous bad experience from an examination or possibly from prior sexual abuse. If you are unable to obtain the cooperation from the girl, the genitalia examination should be discontinued and scheduled at another time. Forcible restraint and examination of the girl is never indicated. Not only will the quality of the examination be affected (due to poor relaxation of the perineal area), but this will also convey to the girl that adults with power have control over what is done to her body.

Position the child on her back and place her legs in a frog-leg position (hips flexed with the soles of the feet together and up to her buttocks), with the head slightly elevated so she can observe the examiner. The older girl may have difficulty obtaining adequate relaxation of the knees with the feet together and thus it may be necessary to assume the lithotomy position with feet in stirrups (Hairston, 1997). The techniques of the external genitalia examination are the same as for the infant. Using gloved hands, gently spread the labia so that the genitalia may be inspected. If internal inspection of the vagina and cervix is necessary, a pediatric Pederson speculum may be used for an older girl. For young girls, a nasal speculum with an attached light source is a useful instrument, as the Pederson speculum is too large (Hairston, 1997). A rectal examination is necessary if there is any expected history of fondling, abuse, or the possibility of a foreign body in the rectum.

Normal and Abnormal Findings Until approximately age 7, the labia majora are flat, the labia minora are thin, and the clitoris is relatively small. Usually the hymen membrane has a visible opening, although there are a number of normal variations in the appearance of the hymen. Following that time, the mons pubis thickens, the labia majora thicken, and the labia minora become slightly rounded. By the time the child reaches pubescence (usually between the ages of 8 and 11), pubic hair will begin to develop. (See the anatomy and physiology section for adolescent development.) There should be no vaginal discharge, vaginal odor, or evidence of bruising. Just before menarche, there is a physiologic increase in the amount of vaginal secretions.

■ PREADOLESCENTS AND ADOLESCENTS

Anatomy and Physiology

The onset of puberty (pubescence) usually occurs over a 3- to 5-year span. Pubertal development begins with a growth spurt, followed by budding of the nipples (thelarche), followed by adrenarche, or the development of axillary and pubic hair (Table 21-4). Menarche (the onset of menstruation) usually begins between ages 8 and 14, at the time when the breast and pubic hair development is in Tanner's developmental stages 3 or 4. The age of menarche has decreased over the past three or four decades, for reasons not fully understood. Most white females reach menarche at a mean age of 12.88; for African-American girls, the mean is 12.16 (Herman-Giddens et al, 1997). At the time of puberty, the external genitalia become larger, gaining adult proportions and adult functional maturation. In particular, the labia majora and mons pubis become prominent and develop pubic hair, while the labia minora darken and recede. These phenomena tend to occur simultaneously with breast development. During this time, the vagina also lengthens with a thickening of its epithelial layers; if the hymen is intact, the vaginal opening will be about 1 cm (⅖ inch) in diameter.

The internal reproductive organs also grow larger. The main reason for the darkening pigmentation evidenced in the labia minora is the increased vascular supply, especially to the uterus. In preparation for the onset of menstruation, the endometrial lining thickens. For 2 to 3 years before the onset of menstruation, a watery discharge will be present; within 1 year after onset, the discharge will become the same as that observed in the adult. Vaginal secretions become acidic under the influence of estrogen.

Health History

In addition to the questions asked of adults, ask the following of girls showing sexual maturity, such as signs of breast and pubic hair development. Use the following guidelines when asking questions: (1) Ask questions appropriate for the girl's age but be aware that "normal" varies widely; it is better to ask too many questions than to omit anything. (2) Ask questions that are direct and professional; avoid judgmental phrases. Begin by establishing that it is normal to feel or think a certain thing, for example, "Girls your age often feel. . . ." (3) Ask questions that assume rather than ask for an admission. You may say, "When you . . ." rather than "Do you . . . ." This implies that the individual is normal.

In addition, the interviewer should explore with an adolescent girl her perceptions and feelings regarding her history and should be prepared to address concerns.

- What changes have you noticed in your body over the last 2 years? What do you like about the changes? What don't you like?

  Rationale Note the adolescent's attitude toward changes taking place.

- Have you started having periods? How did you feel about this? Were you ready, or was it a surprise?

  Rationale This establishes menarche, as well as the adolescent's feelings about the event. Her level of information is also noted.

- Who do you usually talk to about body changes and sex information? Are you comfortable in these talks? Do you think you get enough information? Have you taken sex education classes in school? Is there someone outside of the family, maybe at school or church, with whom you can discuss these issues?

  Rationale It is important to assess where and how the client gets her information. In addition, it is important to assess how accurate and complete the information is.

- Often girls your age have questions about sexual activity. Do you? Have you ever had sex? Are you dating someone now? Do you and your partner have sex? If you do, do you use some type of protection? If so, what method of birth control are you using? Do you always use this method of

Table 21-4 Tanner's Sex Maturity Development

STAGE	PUBIC HAIR DEVELOPMENT
Stage 1	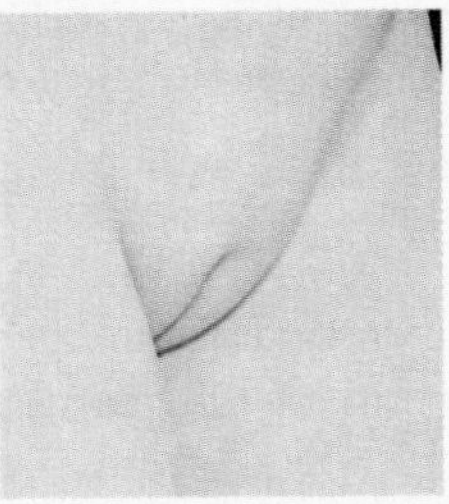 No growth of pubic hair.
Stage 2	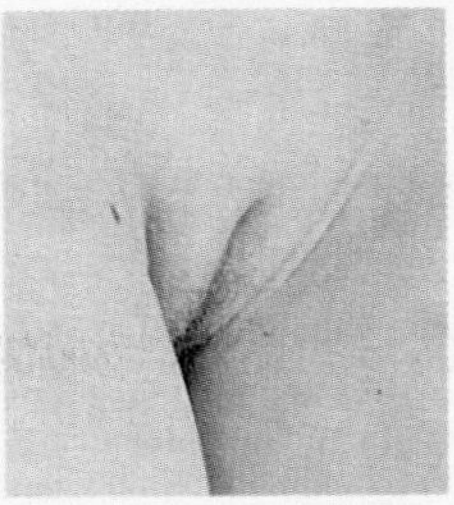 Initial, scarcely long, straight, downy and slightly pigmented hair, especially along the labia
Stage 3	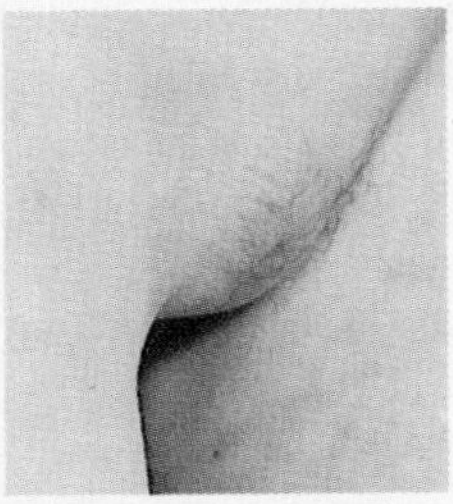 The hair is darker, coarser, and curly, and spread sparsely over the entire pubis in the typical female triangle
Stage 4	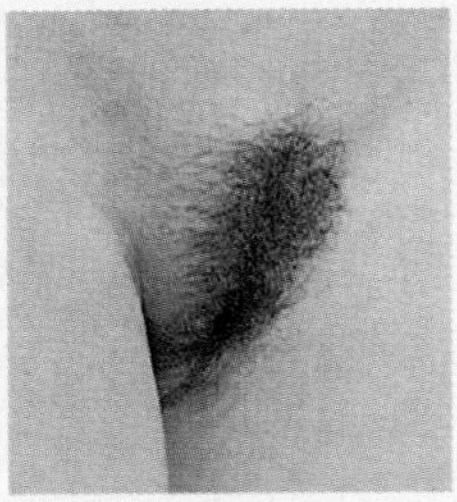 Pubic hair is denser, curled, and in an adult distribution, but less abundant and restricted to the pubic area
Stage 5	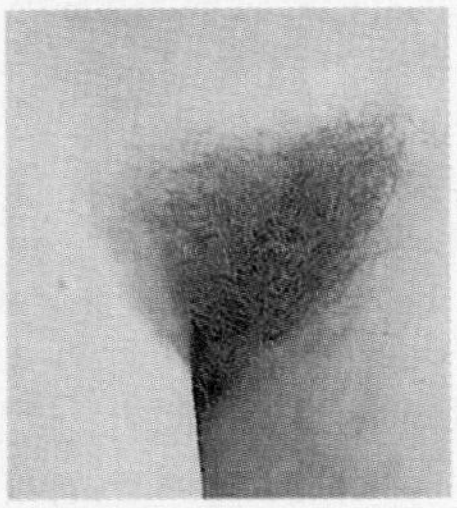 The pubic hair is adult in quantity, type, and pattern, with lateral spreading to the inner aspect of the thighs
Stage 6	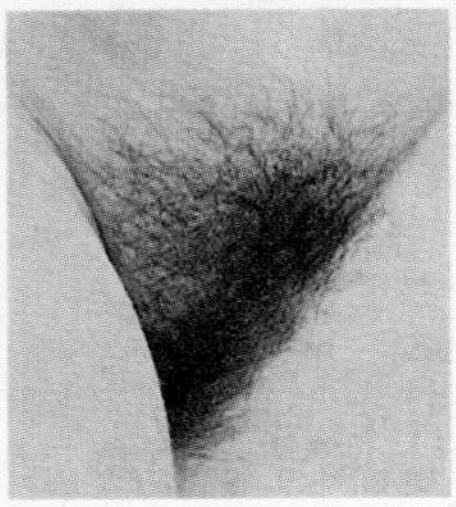 Further extension laterally, upward, or over the upper thighs (this stage may not occur in all women)

Photographs from Van Wieringen JC: *Growth diagrams 1965 Netherlands, second national survey on 0-24-year-olds,* Groningen, Netherlands, 1971, Wolters-Noordhoff. Reprinted by permission of Kluwer Academic Publishers.

protection every time you have sex or just once in a while? What questions do you have about sex?

Rationale It is important to establish a history of sexual activity, as well as to assess methods of contraception used. Adolescent girls are very sensitive to questions regarding number of sexual partners; thus the client may not be truthful during an interview (Rosenthal et al, 1996).

- Have you ever had an infection on your genitalia? If so, what kind? How was it treated? If not, has anyone ever discussed information about sexually transmitted infection or how you get AIDS or other infections? Tell me about what you know about how these infections or diseases are spread. Do you know what you can do to keep from getting these diseases?

Rationale It is important to establish a baseline about knowledge that the adolescent either has or does not have, as well as to assess the accuracy of that information. This will provide the platform for health promotion education. Adolescent girls are very sensitive to questions regarding history of STI; thus they may not be truthful during an interview (Rosenthal et al, 1996).

- Sometimes someone touches a girl in a way she does not want to be touched or sometimes has sex with her when the girl does not want to. Has this happened to you? If that happens, remember that it is not your fault and you need to tell an adult about it immediately.

Rationale A screening assessment should always be made for child abuse, sexual assault, or incest.

Examination

Procedures and Techniques The adolescent should be given a choice to be examined alone, and she should be assured of privacy and confidentiality. Discuss with her the normal growth and development process, including any questions and health concerns she may have. Assess her growth, menstrual history, and sexual maturity development using Tanner's stages (referred to in the anatomy and physiology and history sections of this chapter). Reassure the client of the normal aspects of the changes her body is undergoing. The adolescent's first pelvic examination is probably the most important of her entire life. Time and care should be taken to explain the procedures, show the equipment, and tell the client exactly what she may expect. Because many are becoming very interested in their own bodies and the changes that may be taking place, they may want to actually take part in the examination. This may be a perfect opportunity to teach the child about her own anatomy and the changes that she will experience. A mirror may be used during the examination for instruction.

The size and type of vaginal speculum used is based on the size of the client and the sexual history. The speculum most commonly used to reduce discomfort is a pediatric speculum with blades that are 1.0 to 1.5 cm wide. If the client is sexually active, a larger speculum may be used.

The positioning and techniques for examination of the external genitalia and possibly pelvic examination are the same as for the adult. A pelvic examination should be performed if the adolescent desires contraception, if she is sexually active and has sexual intercourse, or if she is 18 years of age or older. Additionally, a pelvic examination is warranted any time the client has any signs of genital or vaginal irritation, infection, or related problems. This will include periodic Pap tests when intercourse begins. The procedures to be followed are the same as for an adult woman, but additional time must be allowed for the counseling and support needed with an adolescent client.

Normal and Abnormal Findings All findings for the genitalia examination of the adolescent are the same as for the adult.

■ OLDER ADULTS

Anatomy and Physiology

Women undergo a period of changing hormonal function starting between the ages of 35 and 40. This period is known as the climacteric or transitional period. The climacteric is a long transition phase extending many years. It includes endocrine, somatic, and psychologic changes involving a complex relationship between the ovarian and hypothalamic-pituitary factors. During this period, the woman undergoes a series of changes associated with aging and estrogen depletion (Matteson et al, 1997). Menopause is just one phase of the climacteric. Menopause is defined as the permanent cessation of menses and is considered complete after the woman has experienced an entire year with no menses. Ovulation usually ceases 1 to 2 years before menopause. Menopause typically occurs around the age of 50, although the age may range from 35 to 60 years.

During menopause, the labia and clitoris become smaller and paler in color, and the epithelial layers become thinner and flatter, losing their subcutaneous fat as a result of decreased estrogen levels. Pubic hair grays and thins. The vaginal introitus may diminish in size, with a shortening and narrowing of the vagina; a thinning and drying of the mucosa may result in dyspareunia (painful intercourse). The cervix becomes smaller and paler. The uterus and ovaries also decrease in size, with the ovarian follicles gradually disappearing.

Finally, in some women, the ligaments and connective tissue of the pelvis may lose their muscle tone and elasticity, resulting in less structural support for the pelvic contents, including the vaginal walls.

Health History

Because we remain sexual beings throughout our lifetime, the older adult woman should be asked all of the questions for adults, especially the questions related to menopause and urinary incontinence. Additional questions dealing with issues specific to her age include the following:

- Do you have any problems with urination or vaginal itching or dryness?

Rationale Physiologic changes may cause a decrease in vaginal fluids, which may lead to vaginal itching and dryness. In addition, a relaxation of the pelvic floor and decreased sphincter tone may lead to urinary incontinence or a feeling of urgency.

- Have you had any vaginal bleeding since menopause?

  Rationale Postmenopausal bleeding may result from numerous causes, from friable vaginal tissue to cancer of the uterus. If the client has postmenopausal bleeding, she should be referred to a health care practitioner for further evaluation.

- Are you in a relationship in which you have sexual intercourse? If so, is it satisfying to you? Does it ever hurt when you have intercourse? If so, what have you done to decrease the discomfort? Do you have difficulty with urinary frequency or urgency during sexual stimulation?

  Rationale Sexual activity is normal at any adult age. As the client becomes older, it is most important to assess if the client is satisfied with her sexual activity and if it occurs in a manner that feels satisfying to her. If the client has vaginal dryness secondary to hormonal changes, intercourse may be painful for her. It is important to assess if this is the case and, if so, determine what she is doing to treat the problem.

- Do you have other physical problems that interfere with sexual behavior (for example, painful joints, fatigue, dyspnea, or fear of injuring yourself or causing illness)?

  Rationale Sexual activity for the older adult should be pleasurable. If the client has physical difficulties that interfere, it is important to assess what these are, how much they interfere, and what the client or her partner has done about them.

Examination

Procedures and Techniques The examination procedures for the older adult are the same as for the younger adult. Often there is a temptation to defer the routine pelvic examination of the older woman because it may be difficult for her to be positioned in stirrups, she is postmenopausal, or she is no longer sexually active. None of these are reasons to defer the examination. Instead, older women have different problems, such as urinary incontinence, pelvic relaxation, vaginal irritation, dryness, or rectal problems that warrant evaluation. What is important to remember when examining an older adult is that she may need assistance to help hold her legs if she is unable to tolerate positioning in the stirrups. In addition, she may need more assistance in assuming a modified lithotomy position and may not be able to stay in the position as long as a younger woman. If the client is no longer sexually active, a smaller speculum with narrower blades may be necessary to prevent discomfort from the introital constriction. Also, because of the decrease in the amount of natural lubrication in the vagina, it becomes necessary to lubricate the speculum and the fingers of the examining hand adequately to avoid causing discomfort during the examination.

Normal and Abnormal Findings The labia of the older woman become flatter and smaller. The skin may appear dry and have a shiny appearance. The pubic hair often appears sparse and fine. There may be patchy loss of pubic hair or, in some cases, total absence. The clitoris also becomes smaller. During the bimanual examination the examiner may find that the client's introitus is smaller and may admit only one finger, or, in parous women, the introitus may be gaping, with vaginal walls rolling toward the opening. Either should be noted and evaluated accordingly.

The examiner may also find that the client's vagina is narrower and shorter and that there is an absence of rugation of the vaginal wall. Likewise, the cervix may appear smaller and paler, and the fornices may be smaller or absent. Following menopause, the uterus also diminishes in size and may actually not be palpable upon examination. If the uterus is palpable, it should be smooth, firm, freely movable, and nontender. Any uterine enlargement; nodular, irregular, hardened, or indurated areas; areas that are tender on palpation; and fixed, nonmobile areas in the pelvis should be further evaluated. Ovaries atrophy with age and are rarely palpable in aging women.

During the rectovaginal examination, you will most likely feel the rectovaginal septum to be thin, smooth, and pliable. The anal sphincter tone may be somewhat diminished, and because of pelvic musculature relaxation, the client may have stress incontinence and prolapse of the vaginal walls or uterus.

CLIENTS WITH SITUATIONAL VARIATIONS

CLIENTS WHO HAVE HAD A HYSTERECTOMY

Examination

Procedures and Techniques Performing a pelvic examination on a client who has had a hysterectomy is essentially no different than examining any other client. Before the examination, it is important to assess if the client had the hysterectomy by the abdominal or vaginal approach and to determine if she has had a total (fallopian tubes and ovaries removed) or a partial (tubes and ovaries not removed) hysterectomy. In addition, it is important to find out why she had the hysterectomy, when it was performed, if she had any accompanying bowel or bladder repairs, and what problems or concerns she has had since the surgery.

A thorough vaginal examination should be performed. In women who have undergone a hysterectomy in which the cervix was removed, Pap testing is not required unless the hysterectomy was performed because of cervical cancer or its precursors (U.S. Preventive Services Task Force, 1996). If a routine Pap smear is indicated, the sample should be collected from along the suture line, using the blunt end of a spatula. Label the specimen as vaginal cells taken from the suture line.

Normal and Abnormal Findings Probably the most obvious finding during the assessment will be the absence of a cervix and uterus. If the client has had her ovaries removed, many findings are consistent with findings that are present in older, postmenopausal women.

EXAMINATION SUMMARY

Female Genitalia and Reproductive System

PROCEDURE

External Genitalia

- Inspect the pubic hair for:
  Distribution
- Inspect the skin of the mons pubis and inguinal area for:
  Surface characteristics
- Inspect and palpate the labia majora for:
  Pigmentation
  Surface characteristics
- Inspect and palpate the labia minora for:
  Pigmentation
  Surface characteristics
- Inspect the clitoris for:
  Size and length
- Inspect the urethral meatus, vaginal introitus, and perineum for:
  Positioning
  Surface characteristics
- Inspect the anus for color and surface characteristics.
- Palpate the Skene's and Bartholin's glands for:
  Surface characteristics
  Discharge
  Pain or discomfort
- Inspect and palpate muscle tone for:
  Vaginal wall tone
  Rectal muscle tone
  Urinary incontinence

❖ Internal Genitalia: Speculum Examination

- Inspect the cervix for:
  Color
  Surface characteristics
  Position
  Size and shape
- Inspect the cervical os for:
  Discharge
- Obtain all cervical and vaginal cultures and smears
- Inspect the vaginal walls for:
  Color
  Surface characteristics

❖ Internal Genitalia: Bimanual Examination

- Palpate the vagina for:
  Surface characteristics and discomfort
- Palpate the cervix for:
  Position
  Size
  Surface characteristics
  Mobility
  Discomfort
- Palpate the uterus for:
  Size
  Position
- Palpate the uterus for:
  Surface characteristics
  Mobility
  Discomfort
- Palpate the adnexa and ovaries for:
  Size
  Shape
  Tenderness

❖ Rectovaginal Examination

- Palpate the rectal wall for:
  Surface characteristics
- Palpate the uterus and adnexa for:
  Surface characteristics
  Tenderness
- Palpate the anal sphincter for:
  Tone

SUMMARY OF FINDINGS

Age Group	Normal Findings	Typical Variations	Findings Associated With Disorders
Infants and children	• In newborns, labia majora are separate, and clitoris is prominent up to 36 weeks' gestation. • Newborn's genitalia may be swollen, with prominent minora. Hymen often protrudes and central opening is about 0.5 cm in diameter. • Mucoid whitish vaginal discharge may be seen from birth to 1 month of age due to hormonal transfer in utero. • In children, Bartholin's and Skene's glands and ovaries are not usually palpable.	• Vaginal discharge problems should be assessed for relationship to diapers, use of powders or lotions.	• Swelling of vulvar tissues with bruising suggests sexual abuse. • Enlarged clitoris in newborn suggests adrenal hyperplasia. • In children, vaginal discharge may cause redness and excoriation. • Perineal irritation may be related to infection or irritation.
Adolescents	• In adolescents, vaginal secretions increase before menarche. • By menarche, vaginal opening should be at least 1 cm wide.	• Menstrual cycle characteristics may include dysmenorrhea, breast tenderness or headaches.	
Adults	• Skin is smooth. • Hair is in triangular pattern. • Majora are symmetric, soft, and homogenous. • Minora are moist and dark pink. • Clitoris is 2 cm in length and 0.5 cm in diameter. • No swelling, mass, or pain present.	• After hymen tears, hymenal tags may be visible. • Uterus is usually flattened and anteroposterior at 45° angle, but it may also be anteverted, anteflexed, retroverted, or retroflexed. • Episiotomy scar may be evident. • Perineum is thinner and more rigid in multiparous women and more thick and smooth in nulliparous women. • Squamocolumnar epithelium on cervical canal may be visible. • Nabothian cysts may be seen around cervix. • Os of nulliparous women may be small, round, or oval, and os of multiparous women may be more horizontal, irregular, or stellate.	• External labia swelling, pain, warmth, and redness may mean Bartholin's gland abscess. • Vaginal discharge (yellow, green, or gray) with odor suggests infection. • Labia minora irritation may be caused by vaginal infection. • Ulcers or vesicles may be from sexually transmitted disease. • Urethral inflammation or dilation suggests repeated urinary tract infections. • Discharge from Skene's glands suggests infection. • Pale cervix suggests anemia.

Age Group	Normal Findings	Typical Variations	Findings Associated With Disorders
Older adults	• In older women, the labia are flatter and smaller. The clitoris is smaller, and the vagina becomes narrower and has decreased rugation. • With age, the cervix becomes smaller, paler, and less mobile. • The cervical os may be smaller, and uterus diminishes in size and may not be palpable.	• Feelings about menopause, self-image, sexual desires should be explored.	• Bulging of anterior vaginal wall with urinary incontinence indicates cystocele. • Bulging of posterior wall indicates rectocele. • Protrusion of cervix or uterus through vaginal introitus indicates uterine prolapse.

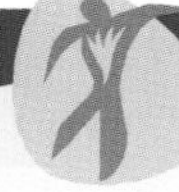

HEALTH PROMOTION

SAFE SEX—REDUCING RISK OF SEXUALLY TRANSMITTED INFECTION

The only way to prevent transmission of STIs is to abstain from sexual intercourse with an infected partner. Since many individuals with STIs are asymptomatic, it is nearly impossible to know for sure who might carry an infection. Reduce the risk of STIs by taking the following safe-sex measures:

- Abstain from sexual intercourse and oral sex.
- Maintain a mutually faithful, monogamous relationship with a partner known to be uninfected.
- Consistently and correctly use barrier protection.
- Avoid sexual contact with casual partners.
- Avoid sexual contact with high-risk individuals (those who have multiple partners).
- Maintain an awareness that drug and alcohol use lead to high-risk sexual behaviors.

Latex Condom (Fig. 21-25, *A*)

The best barrier protection is a latex condom. (These have shown to be effective in preventing transmission of STIs and HIV if used consistently and correctly.) Condom breakage is estimated at 2% if used correctly (CDC, 1998). Most condom failure results from incorrect use. Correct use includes the following principles:

- Handle condom carefully—be sure not to break before application.
- Use a new condom with each act of intercourse.
- Ensure adequate lubrication during intercourse with water-based lubrication. Avoid petroleum jelly, mineral oil, hand lotion, baby oil, massage oil, etc. because these oil-based products damage the condom.
- After sex, hold the condom against the base of the penis while withdrawing the penis—this should be done while the penis is still erect.

Female Condom (Fig. 21-25, *B*)

If the male partner does not wear a condom, the best protection option is a female condom. It is considered an effective mechanical barrier to viruses, including HIV, and will reduce risk of transmission. It is not as effective, however, as the male condom.

Spermacides, Diaphragm, Cervical Cap (Fig. 21-25, *C, D*)

These methods may reduce the risk of gonorrhea and chlamydia transmission, but they have not been shown to be effective against HIV or other STIs. These methods are not as effective as the male condom and should not be used alone as barrier protection.

VULVAR SELF-EXAMINATION

A vulvar self-examination includes inspection of all of the external genital organs, including the pubic mound, clitoris, urinary opening, vaginal opening, and anus (Fig. 21-26, *A*).

To perform a self-examination, use a flashlight and a hand mirror and follow these steps:

1. Sit on the edge of a toilet seat, your bed, or the bathtub. Sit with your legs spread apart and inspect the entire vulvar region (Fig. 21-26, *B*).
2. Examine both sides of the labia and see if they are similar. With your fingers, separate the inner lips of the vulva, and check the clitoris, the urinary opening, the vagina, and the skin between the vagina and the anus (Fig. 21-26, *C*).
3. Press down on all areas of the vulva, feeling for any lumps or masses (Fig. 21-26, *D*).
4. Gently squeeze the vaginal opening between your thumb and forefinger. It should feel soft and moist (Fig. 21-26, *E*).
5. If you notice any lumps, masses, growths, or changes in skin color, see your health care professional.

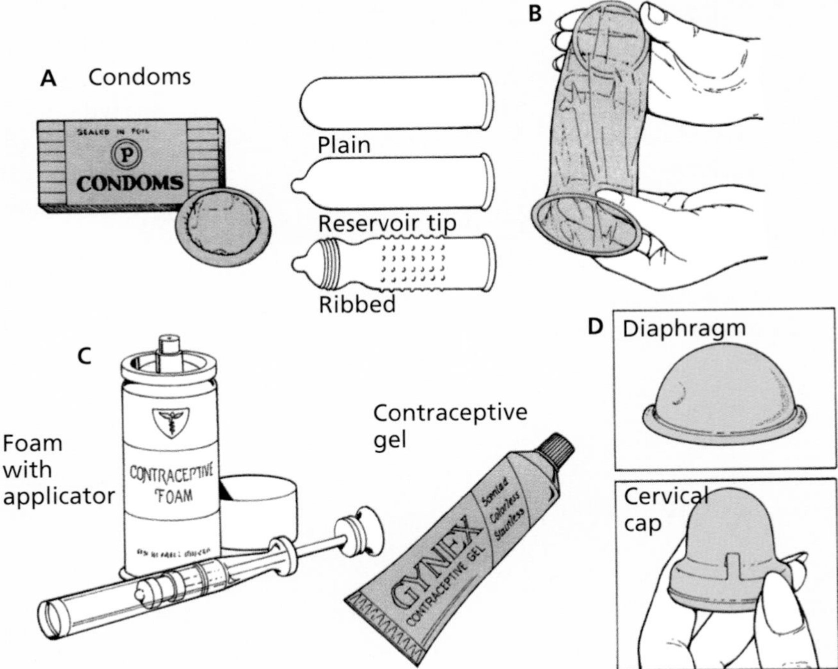

Fig. 21-25 **A,** Latex condom. **B,** Female condom. **C,** Vaginal spermicides. **D,** Diaphragm and cervical cap. (From Edge and Miller, 1994.)

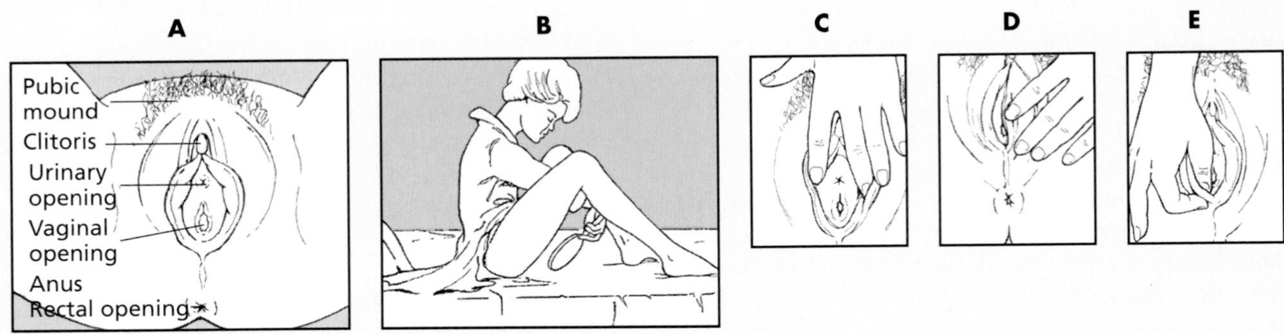

Fig. 21-26 Vulvar self-examination (see text for details). (From Edge and Miller, 1994.)

PELVIC MUSCLE EXERCISES

Kegel exercises are perineal exercises that help to decrease stress incontinence by strengthening the perineal floor muscles. To be effective, Kegel exercises should be performed at least 4 times each day. To perform the exercises, do the following:

1. During urination, tighten the muscles and stop the flow of urine in midstream. You should feel a sensation of pulling upward into the vagina, and the buttocks will be squeezed together.
2. Repeat the procedure by stopping and starting the urine flow. Stop urination for 3 to 5 seconds, then relax and start the flow again.
3. Repeat this sequence 12 to 24 times during urination.

PREMENSTRUAL SYNDROME (PMS)

Because PMS is a progesterone-deficiency illness, taking synthetic progesterone, or a natural progesterone such as wild yams, may help, but by itself this will not control PMS. Treatment involves relieving the symptoms and, when possible, correcting the cause. Things that you can do to control your body's response include:

1. Reduce your salt intake to reduce bloating and fluid retention.
2. Do some form of moderate, enjoyable exercise at least 4 times each week.
3. Reduce your intake of caffeine and sugar.

COMMON PROBLEMS AND CONDITIONS

Female Genitalia and Reproductive System

MENSTRUATION

Premenstrual Syndrome (PMS)

This is a combination of affective (emotional) and somatic (physical) symptoms that begins shortly after ovulation (about 14 to 16 days) and diminishes after menstruation begins. Premenstrual syndrome is most prevalent in women over 30 years of age. It has been estimated that 50% of all women will experience PMS at some time during their lives.

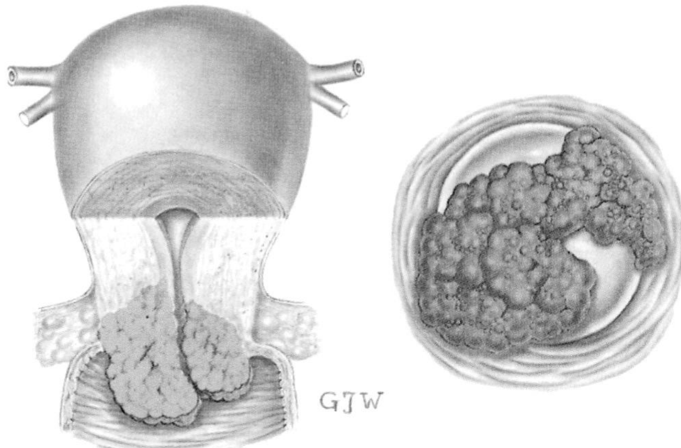

Fig. 21-27 Advanced cervical cancer. (From Belcher, 1992.)

CERVIX

Cervical Cancer

Cancer of the cervix begins as a neoplastic change at or near the cervical os. The lesion usually has a hard granular surface that bleeds easily and has irregular borders. There is a strong link between development of cervical cancer and HPV infection; an estimated 90% of cervical cancers are caused by HPV infection; however, infection alone does not lead to cervical cancer (Verdon, 1997) (Fig. 21-27).

Infected Nabothian Cyst

A nabothian cyst is considered a normal finding; however, if infected it will become an enlarged fluid-filled cyst. It may occur singly or in multiples and may vary in size. The presence of a cyst may distort the shape of the cervix.

UTERUS

Endometriosis

Endometriosis is an inflammatory process characterized by the development of stroma (connective tissue) and endometrial glands (identical to uterine tissue) outside the uterus (Fig. 21-28). It has been estimated that as many as 20% to 25% of all women have some degree of endometriosis during their lives. The most common sites of endometriosis are the uterosacral ligaments, round ligaments, sigmoid colon, rectovaginal septum, pelvic peritoneum, ovaries, cul-de-sac, and urinary bladder. Common symptoms include pelvic pain, dysmenorrhea, and heavy or prolonged menstrual flow. Examination findings include small, firm, nodular-like masses palpable along the uterosacral ligaments. The uterus may be tender with movement.

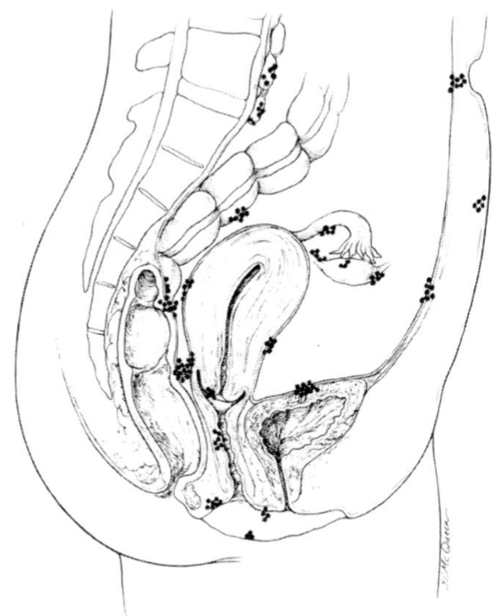

Fig. 21-28 Common sites of endometriosis. (From Droegemueller, 1987.)

Fibroids (Myomas)

Fibroids are common, benign uterine tumors that are firm and irregular in shape (Fig. 21-29). They may vary in size and may occur as a single tumor or in multiples. The prevalence in women over the age of 35 is 20% to 25%.

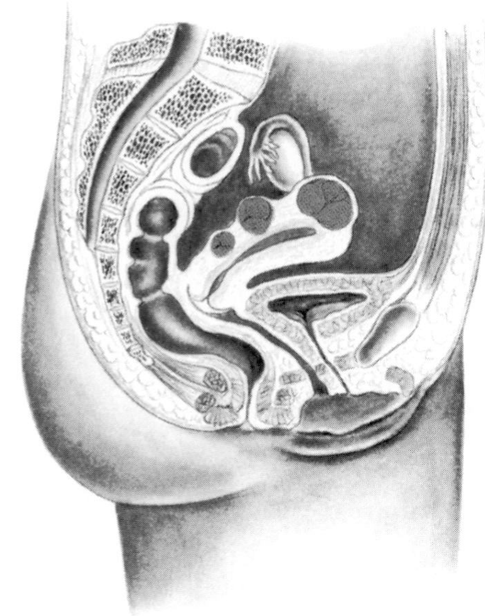

Fig. 21-29 Myomas of the uterus (fibroids). (From Seidel et al, 1999.)

Uterine Prolapse

When the supporting structures of the pelvic floor weaken, the uterus, bladder, and rectum may prolapse. When there is a prolapse, the uterus becomes progressively retroverted and descends into the vagina. In first-degree prolapse the cervix remains within the vagina (Fig. 21-30, *A*). In second-degree prolapse the cervix is in the introitus (Fig. 21-30, *B*). In third-degree prolapse the cervix and vagina drop outside the introitus (Fig. 21-30, *C*).

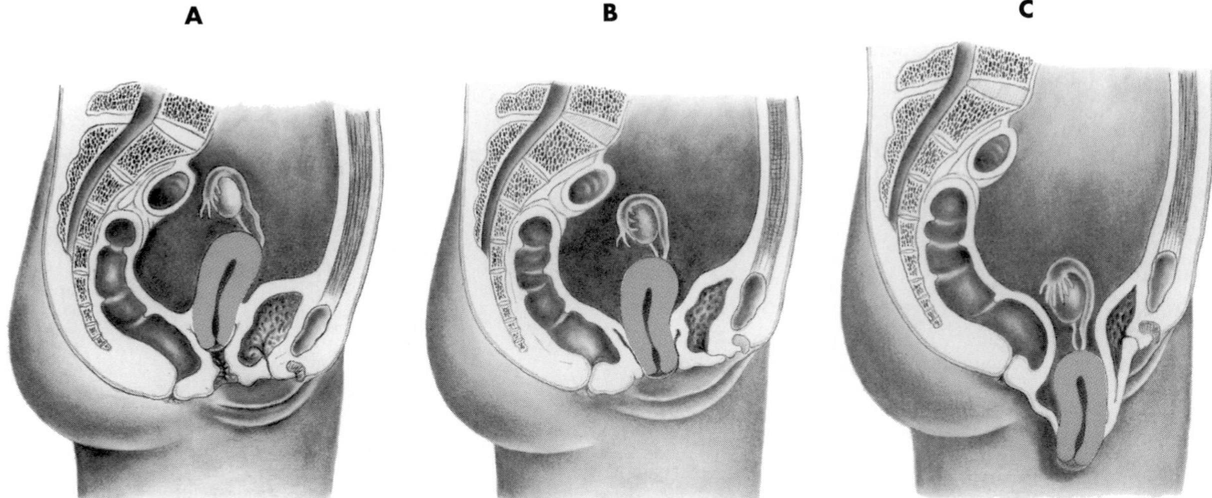

Fig. 21-30 Uterine prolapse. **A,** First-degree prolapse of the uterus. **B,** Second-degree prolapse of the uterus. **C,** Third-degree prolapse of the uterus. (From Seidel et al, 1999.)

Endometrial Cancer

Endometrial cancer is the most common gynecologic malignancy (Fig. 21-31). It occurs most often in postmenopausal women, especially those women taking estrogen. The cardinal symptom is uterine bleeding, although a watery vaginal discharge is frequently noted several weeks to months prior to the bleeding.

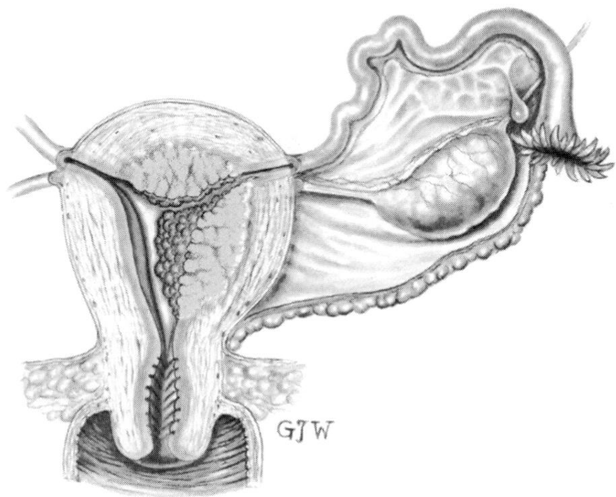

Fig. 21-31 Endometrial cancer. (From Belcher, 1992.)

OVARIES

Ovarian Cyst

This is a cystic growth within the ovary. It can occur unilaterally or bilaterally. Examination findings for an ovarian cyst include a nontender, fluctuant, mobile, and smooth mass on the ovary (Fig. 21-32).

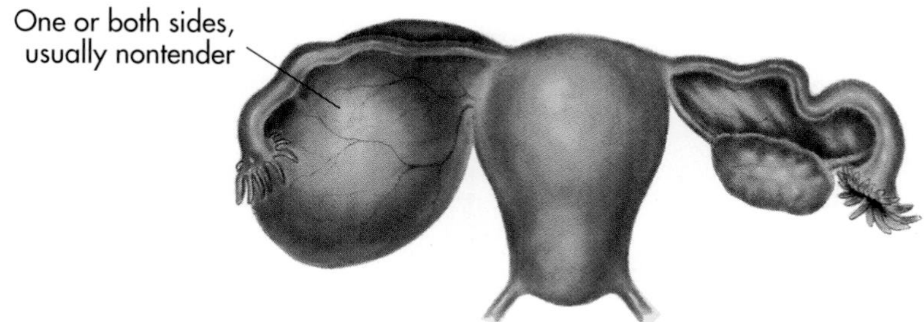

Fig. 21-32 Ovarian cyst. (From Seidel et al, 1999.)

Ovarian Cancer

The incidence of ovarian cancer is rising and is highest among western, industrialized, white women over the age of 50 (Fig. 21-33). It is the fourth leading cause of cancer-related deaths in women and has the highest mortality of the gynecologic cancers (Parker et al, 1997). An ovarian tumor will feel more solid and nodular compared with an ovarian cyst. Any enlarged ovary should raise suspicion. It is very difficult to detect, however, because by the time ovarian malignancies are palpable, the disease is usually advanced. In addition, there are frequently no symptoms until advanced stages. Research has found that 94% of women diagnosed with ovarian cancer had at least one symptom prior to diagnosis. Gastrointestinal symptoms and menstrual cycle changes were most frequently reported (Igo, 1997). A screening test for early detection of ovarian cancer is CA-125, a tumor antigen. Unfortunately, CA-125 lacks specificity and sensitivity in early-stage disease and is not recommended as an annual routine screening test at this time (Thompson et al, 1997).

Pelvic Inflammatory Disease (PID)

Pelvic inflammatory disease is an inflammatory process affecting the adnexal areas that is most commonly caused by untreated gonococcal and chlamydia infections. Acute PID is associated with very tender adnexal areas (ovaries and fallopian tubes). Typically, the pain is so severe that the client is unable to tolerate bimanual examination. Chronic PID is associated with tender, irregular, and fixed adnexal areas (Fig. 21-34).

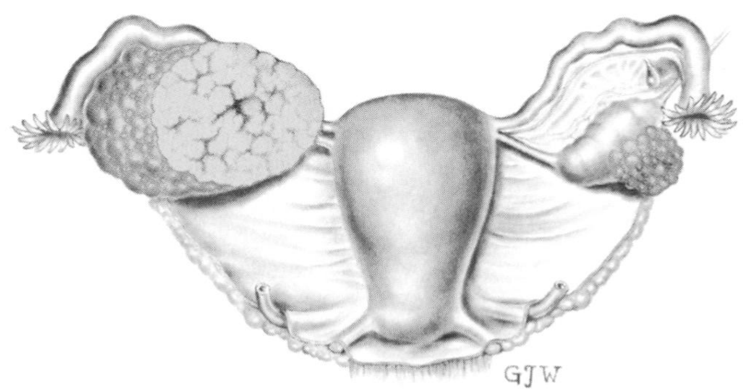

Fig. 21-33 Cancer of the ovaries. (From Belcher, 1992.)

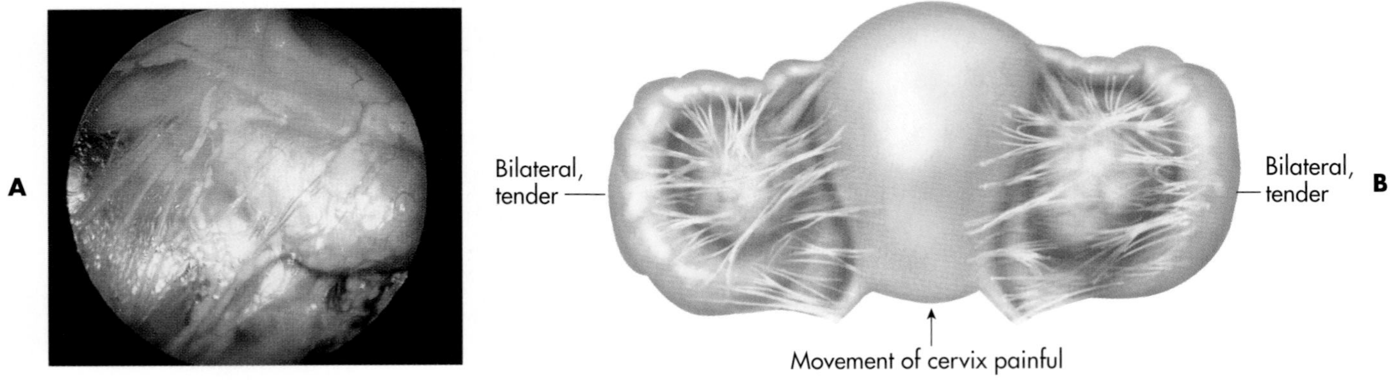

Fig. 21-34 Pelvic inflammatory disease. (Drawing from Seidel et al, 1999. Photograph from Symonds and MacPherson, 1994.)

VULVA AND VAGINA

Monilia Vaginitis (Candidiasis)

Candidiasis is a fungal or yeast infection caused by *Candida albicans.* It has been estimated that 75% of all women have a yeast infection sometime during their lifetime. Some women are prone to many infections (see Risk Factors box below). Yeast infections are more prevalent in women in tropical climates and occur most frequently before menstruation and during pregnancy. Some women are asymptomatic, whereas others may have a thick, cheesy, white vaginal discharge that may cause mild to moderate discomfort.

Inflamed Bartholin's Glands

An acute inflammation of the Bartholin's gland causes swelling of the gland, which is very painful. The mucosa at the duct opening appears very red; the examiner may be able to express a purulent discharge (Fig. 21-35). Nonacute or chronic inflammation causes a nontender cyst on the labia. This condition is commonly (but not always) caused by gonococcal infection.

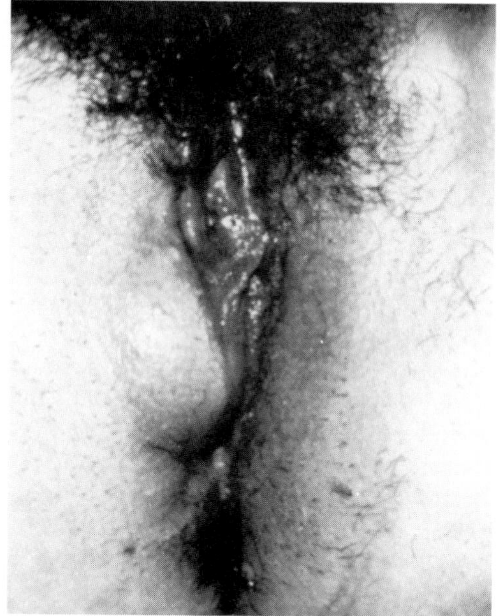

Fig. 21-35 Inflammation of Bartholin's glands. (From Kaufman et al, 1994.)

Cystocele

This is a hernia type of protrusion of the urinary bladder through the anterior wall of the vagina (Fig. 21-36). The bulging is usually seen and felt as the woman bears down. If the cystocele is severe, it may be accompanied by stress incontinence.

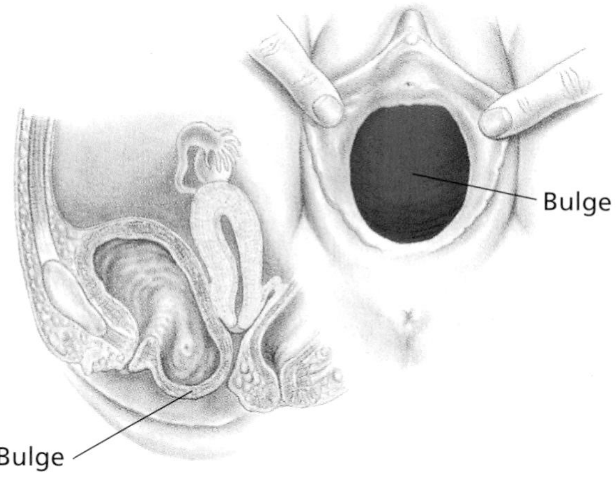

Fig. 21-36 Cystocele. (From Seidel et al, 1999.)

RISK FACTORS

COMMON RISK FACTORS ASSOCIATED WITH
Asymptomatic Vaginal Candidiasis

- Pregnancy
- Uncontrolled diabetes mellitus
- Tight-fitting synthetic underclothing
- Corticosteroid therapy
- Antimicrobial therapy
- Estrogen therapy
- Contraceptives
- Frequent sexual intercourse

Box 21-6 Clinical Note

Sexually transmitted infection can occur on the genitalia, rectum, and in the oral cavity. Furthermore, an STI can concurrently occur in more than one location. Therefore, if an STI is suspected, examination in the other areas is also warranted.

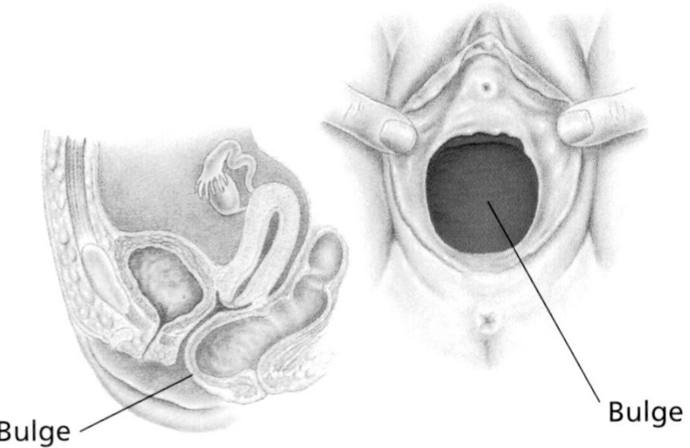

Fig. 21-37 Rectocele. (From Seidel et al, 1999.)

Rectocele

This is a hernia type of protrusion of the rectum through the posterior wall of the vagina (Fig. 21-37). Bulging of the posterior vaginal wall may be seen as the woman bears down.

SEXUALLY TRANSMITTED INFECTION

There are well over 50 different STIs. Listed below are those the examiner may observe in conjunction with examination of genitalia. Many other STIs do not have symptoms that manifest with examination of the genitalia (Table 21-5).

Bacterial Sexually Transmitted Infections

Chlamydia Trachomatis This is the *most common* sexually transmitted infection in the United States. The infection usually does not cause enough inflammation to produce symptoms. It is estimated that 75% of women infected with chlamydia are asymptomatic, making this a very difficult infection to diagnose (Weinstock, Dean, and Bolan, 1994). If untreated, chlamydia can cause pelvic inflammatory disease. If symptoms occur, the most common are urinary symptoms (such as dysuria, frequency, or urgency) and vaginal symptoms (such as spotting or bleeding after sex or purulent cervical discharge). The most important examination finding in a chlamydia infection is a purulent or mucopurulent cervical discharge. Cervical bleeding on introduction of a cotton swab (friability) may also be observed (Fogel, 1995). It is recommended to screen all sexually active adolescents and women age 20 to 24 (particularly those who have new or multiple sex partners and who do not routinely use barrier contraceptives) during routine annual examinations—even if asymptomatic (CDC, 1998). Although culture is considered the "gold standard" for diagnosis, it is very expensive, not uniformly available, and takes from 3 to 7 days to get results. Many clinics are now using new screening techniques using urine or vaginal swab specimens. These newer screening techniques are both rapid and sensitive (U.S. Preventive Services Task Force, 1996).

Gonorrhea This STI is caused by the aerobic, gram-negative diplococcus *Neisseria gonorrhoeae.* It is currently the most *frequently reported* sexually transmitted disease in the United States. If left untreated, gonorrhea may lead to pelvic inflammatory disease. It is transmitted from genital-genital, oral-genital, and rectal-genital contact. Some individuals are asymptomatic; however, in many individuals

Table 21-5 Sexually Transmitted Infections

NAME	CAUSE	SYMPTOMS/CLINICAL FINDINGS	SEQUELAE IF UNTREATED	DIAGNOSIS	TREATMENT
Genital herpes simplex	HSV2	Painful vesicles and ulcers on genitalia or mouth	• Spread of infection • Discomfort	• Clinical findings	• Antivirals—no cure
Hepatitis	Hepatitis B virus	Frequently asymptomatic until advanced liver disease	• Liver failure	• Serology • Hepatitis surface antigen	• Preventable with vaccination • Immune globulin
Human immunodeficiency virus	HIV1 HIV2	Asymptomatic for years—symptoms develop after immune system weakens	• AIDS	• Enzyme immunoassay • Antibody test	• Antivirals—no cure
Human papillomavirus	HPV (over 20 types)	Asymptomatic or may have warty lesions on vulva or cervix	• Spread of infection • Possible cervical cancer	• Clinical findings • Abnormal Pap smear	• Podophyllin • Cryotherapy • Surgical removal
Molluscum contagiosum	MCV	Asymptomatic. Genital lesion differentiated from wart by umbilicated center	• Spread of virus to other sexual contacts	• Clinical findings	• None
Chlamydia	Bacterial: *Chlamydia trachomatis*	75% Asymptomatic Pelvic discomfort; friability of cervix	• Spread of infection • PID • Infertility • Ectopic pregnancy	• DNA probe • Immunoassay • Culture	• Antibiotic
Gonorrhea	Bacterial: *Neisseria gonorrhoeae*	Pelvic discomfort; vaginal, vulvar itching; dysuria; yellowish green vaginal discharge	• Spread of infection • PID • Infertility	• DNA probe • Immunoassay • Culture	• Antibiotic
Syphilis	Bacterial: *Treponema pallidum*	Primary lesion—single painless ulcer on genitalia or mouth; Secondary lesion—skin rash; flat oval or round grayish lesions	• Spread of infection • Tertiary illness neurosyphilis	• Serology	• Antibiotic
Bacterial vaginitis	Bacterial: *Gardnerella vaginalis; Prevotella, Mobiluncus, Mycoplasma hominis.*	Malodorous whitish vaginal discharge; no inflammation	• Spread of infection • Discomfort	• Clinical findings • Whiff test • Microscopic examination of "wet prep"	• Antibiotic
Trichomonas	Protozoan: *Trichomonas vaginalis*	Green-gray, foul-smelling vaginal discharge—may have vaginal bleeding as well	• Spread of infection • Discomfort	• Clinical findings • Microscopic examination of "wet prep"	Metronidazole
Lice/crabs	Ectoparasite: *Pediculosis pubis*	Vaginal itching; visualization of lice and nits	• Spread of infection • Discomfort	Microscopy—visualization of lice and nits	• Permethrin or Lindane

gonorrhea causes a yellow or green vaginal discharge, dysuria, pelvic or abdominal pain, and abnormal menses. The vaginal itching and burning may be severe. Examination findings are nonspecific, thus diagnosis is not made by symptoms and clinical findings alone. It is recommended that symptomatic clients or high-risk individuals be screened for gonorrhea. DNA probes and enzyme immunoassays are the most widely used nonculture diagnostic tests—these provide rapid, accurate results. The culture is considered the "gold standard" for diagnosis of gonorrhea; however, since results take a couple of days, many clinics are now using the non-culture screening tests (U.S. Preventive Services Task Force, 1996).

Syphilis Syphilis is a chronic systemic disease caused by *Treponema pallidum* that is transmitted congenitally or by sexual contact. Syphilis lesions may be during the primary or secondary phase. Primary syphilis produces a single, firm, painless open sore or chancre at the site of entry on the genitals or mouth (Fig. 21-38). Secondary syphilis occurs 6 to 12 weeks after the initial lesion. It is characterized by round or oval, flat grayish lesions known as condyloma latum (Fig. 21-39). Diagnosis during these stages may be made based on clinical findings and by direct fluorescent antibody tests of lesion exudate or by serologic tests for syphilis. If left untreated, clients may develop tertiary syphilis, which causes neurologic complications—confusion and insanity may result. Routine serologic screening for syphilis is recommended for all pregnant women and for high-risk individuals (CDC, 1998).

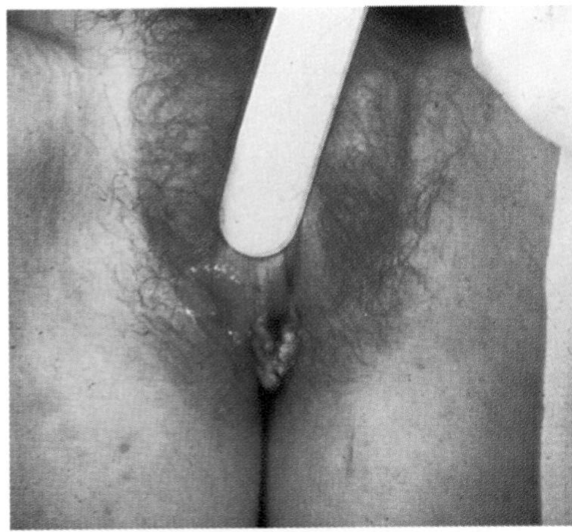

Fig. 21-38 Primary syphilis of the vulva with condyloma at bottom of labia near rectum. (From Edge and Miller, 1994.)

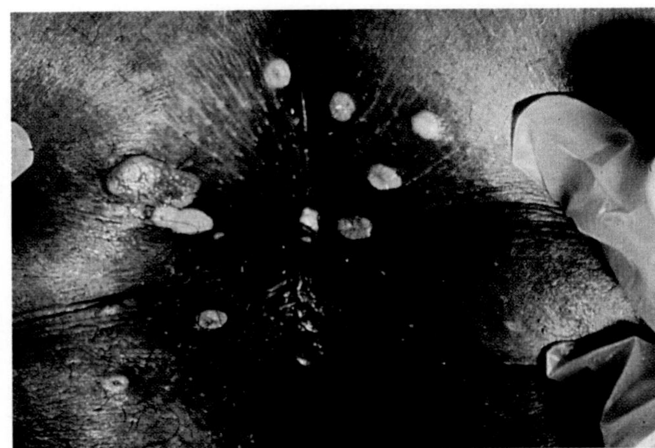

Fig. 21-39 Secondary syphilis lesions (condyloma latum). (Courtesy Antoinette Hood, University of Indiana School of Medicine, Indianapolis. From Seidel et al, 1999.)

Trichomoniasis This is a vaginal infection caused by the protozoan *Trichomonas vaginalis.* Trichomoniasis produces a frothy or bubbly, heavy greenish-gray malodorous discharge with vulvar redness and irritation. The walls of the vagina and the cervix may have petechial "strawberry patches." Some women may be asymptomatic. Diagnosis is made by microscopic inspection of vaginal secretions; the examiner would prepare a wet mount specimen (see Table 21-3 and Fig. 21-40).

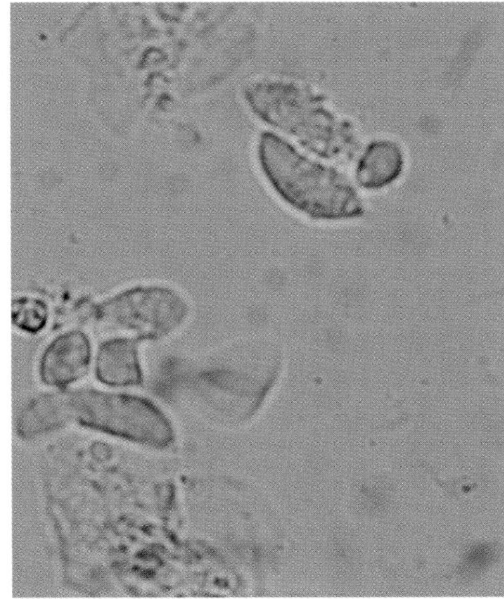

Fig. 21-40 Trichomoniasis as it appears under microscope. (From Zitelli and Davis, 1997.)

Bacterial Vaginosis (BV) Bacterial vaginosis is a clinical syndrome characterized by malodorous vaginal discharge or vulvar itching and irritation. It is caused by an alteration of the normal vaginal flora with other bacteria; there are a number of bacteria that can cause BV including *Gardnerella vaginalis, Mobiluncus,* and *Mycoplasma hominis.* The cause of the alteration in vaginal flora remains unclear; however, it presents in women with multiple sex partners, but rarely in women who are not sexually active. Diagnosis is made based on clinical findings (white, malodorous, noninflammatory discharge that smoothly coats the vaginal walls), by microscopic examination including Gram's stain, a pH vaginal discharge greater than 4.5, and presence of "clue cells" (Fig. 21-41).

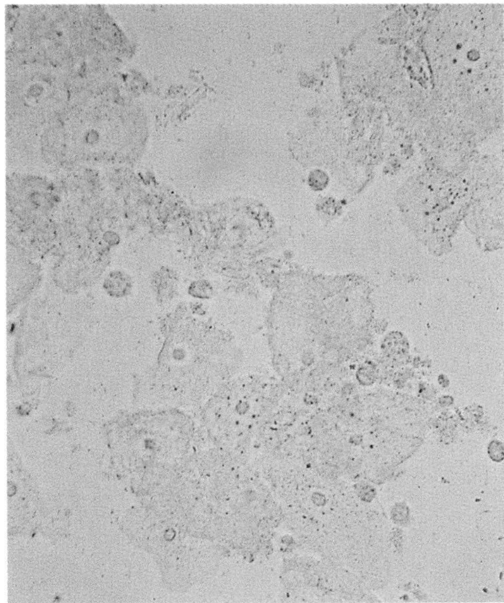

Fig. 21-41 Bacterial vaginosis "clue cells" under the microscope. (From Zitelli and Davis, 1997.)

Viral Sexually Transmitted Infections

Herpes Genitalis Herpes is a sexually transmitted viral infection caused by the herpes simplex virus. Herpes simplex virus type 1 (HSV1) and herpes simplex virus type 2 (HSV2) are two different antigen subtypes of the herpes simplex virus. HSV1 is more commonly associated with gingivostomatitis and oral ulcers (fever blisters) whereas HSV2 is usually associated with genital lesions. However, both types can be transmitted to both sites through genital-oral contact. Typical early symptoms include burning or pain with urination, pain in the genital area, and fever. Examination findings reveal single or multiple vesicles that can be found on the genital area or the inner thigh. After vesicles rupture, small painful ulcers are observed (Fig. 21-42). The initial infection may involve several areas and usually lasts 7 to 10 days. Subsequent infections tend to be less severe, are usually localized to one area, and usually last 3 to 10 days. Women contract herpes genitalis far more often than men and typically have a more severe clinical course than men (Fogel, 1995).

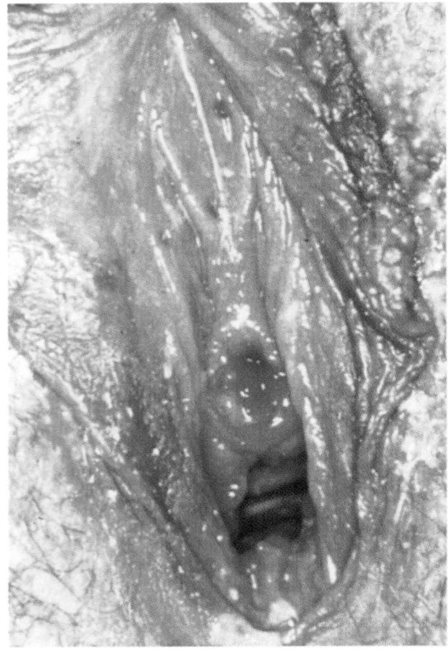

Fig. 21-42 Herpes infection of the labia. (From Edge and Miller, 1994.)

Human Papillomavirus (HPV) (Genital Warts, Condylomata) Human papillomavirus is one of the most common sexually transmitted infections because it is highly contagious. Infection with HPV can cause wartlike growths that are referred to as condylomata acuminata (Fig. 21-43). The warts typically appear as soft, papillary, pink to brown, elongated lesions that may occur singularly or in clusters on the internal genital, external genitalia, and anal-rectal region. When in clusters they take on a cauliflower-like resemblance. The incubation period for HPV is 1 to 6 months. Although it previously was considered benign, HPV has been linked to cervical neoplasms. Positive diagnosis of HPV is made based on clinical findings and Pap smear.

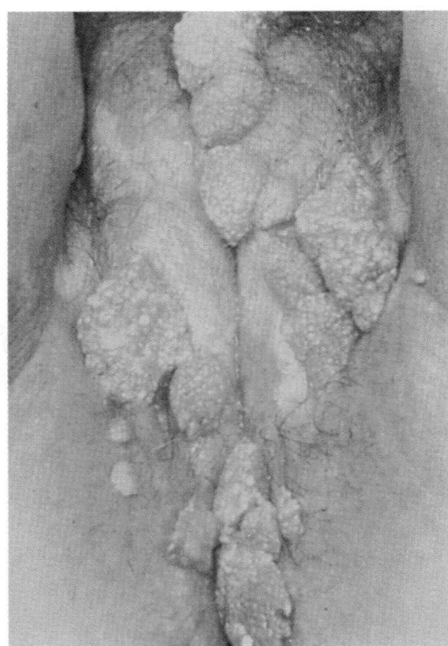

Fig. 21-43 Condyloma acuminatum. (From Grimes, 1991.)

Molluscum Contagiosum This is a benign condition caused by the molluscum contagiosum virus (MCV). It affects the mucous membranes and skin, producing genital lesions or papules. It is differentiated from HPV warts by an umbilicated center from which a thick creamy white core can be expressed (Fig. 21-44). This virus is transmitted by sexual contact and is most frequently seen in girls and young women ages 10 to 16.

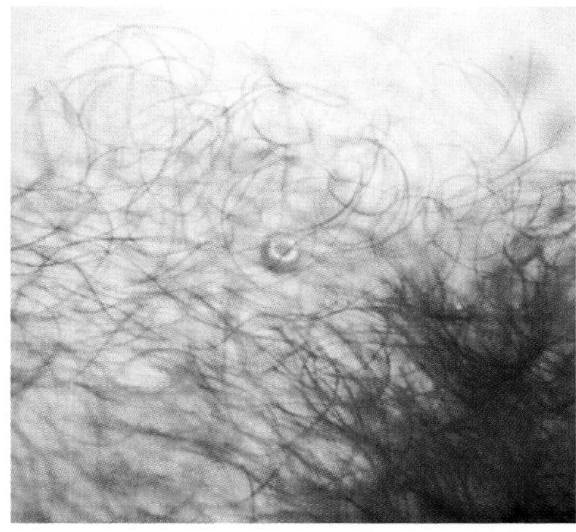

Fig. 21-44 Papule caused by molluscum contagiosum virus. (From Edge and Miller, 1994.)

Ectoparasitic Sexually Transmitted Infections

Pediculosis Pubis (Crabs, Pubic Lice) Pediculosis pubis is a parasitic infection transmitted by close physical contact. Infection is characterized by complaints of severe pruritus in the perineal area. Clients may also notice the lice and/or nits (eggs) in the pubic hair. Examination findings include excoriation and an area of erythema; on close inspection the lice and nits can be seen—they will appear as small dark spots.

CLINICAL APPLICATION and CRITICAL THINKING

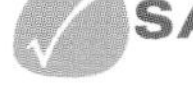

SAMPLE DOCUMENTATION

Case 1

L.T. is a 48-year-old woman with complaints of "hot flashes."

Subjective Data

Client thinks she is "going through the change"; states periods have become very irregular, sometimes lasting only 1 day; time between periods is 3 to 7 weeks. Last period was 4½ weeks ago; awakens frequently during the night "in a sweat" with increased perspiration. Has not slept well for several weeks. Sexually active and wants to know if she can still get pregnant now that she is entering menopause. Concerned about the effect of "the change" on the way she looks and on her sexuality. Last Pap smear was 10 months ago during routine examination.

Objective Data

Inguinal nodes: Nonpalpable, nontender.

External genitalia: Unremarkable; no lesions or discoloration.

Vagina: Rugated, scant amount of clear, odorless discharge; small cystocele noted; no rectocele. No lesions noted.

Cervix: Pink, midline, parous, without lesions; vaginal discharge clear, odorless, and scant.

Uterus: Anteverted, small, firm, mobile, nontender, no masses.

Adenexa: Ovaries palpated bilaterally; smooth, 1 ½ cm × 3 cm mild tenderness with deep palpation; no masses.

Rectovaginal examination: No tenderness; no masses, fissures, or fistulas.

Functional Health Patterns Involved

- Cognitive–perceptual
- Self-perception–self-concept
- Sleep–rest
- Sexuality–reproductive

Nursing Diagnosis and Collaborative Problems

- *Knowledge deficit* related to lack of information about self-care management as manifested by:
  - Hot flashes.
  - Irregular periods.
- *Body image disturbance* related to body change as manifested by:
  - Concerned about appearance and sexuality associated with menopause.
- *Risk for sleep pattern disturbance* related to discomfort while sleeping.
- *Risk for altered sexual patterns* related to verbalized concern about sexuality.

CASE 2

M.M. is a 77-year-old woman complaining of pressure in pelvic area.

Subjective Data

Client states she was having a bowel movement and felt part of her insides slip—as though part of her insides are coming out of her vagina. States that this condition is uncomfortable. M.M. also states she is worried she will be unable to have sex and worried that she may have to have an operation. She states she has been in good health.

Objective Data

External genitalia: No lesions noted.
Vagina: Cervix appears at the introitus with straining.
Cervix: Pink without lesions or bleeding.
Bimanual examination: Deferred.

Functional Health Patterns Involved

- Cognitive–perceptual
- Self-perception–self-concept
- Sexuality–reproductive

Medical Diagnosis

Second-degree uterine prolapse

Nursing Diagnosis and Collaborative Problems

- *Altered comfort* related to pressure in pelvic region as manifested by:
  - Client states she is uncomfortable
- *Fear* related to unknown prognosis and concern about surgery as manifested by:
  - Client states she is scared.
  - Client states she is worried about possible surgery.
- *Risk for altered sexual patterns* related to change in body image.

CRITICAL THINKING QUESTIONS

1. A 51-year-old woman tells the nurse that she experiences urinary dribbling with activity. She wants to know what she can do about this problem. What should the nurse discuss with her?
2. An imperforate hymen is a rare finding in a young women. Signs and symptoms may first occur when the young women reaches menarche. What does the onset of menses have to do with recognition of this condition? What kind of symptoms might you expect?
3. Acacia is a 16-year-old girl who is in the clinic for a routine physical examination. How should her health history and the examination of her genitalia differ from that of an adult?
4. During a pelvic examination, the examiner determines the need to screen the client for chlamydia and gonorrhea, prepare a slide for wet mount and KOH preparation, and do a routine Pap smear. In which order should the specimens be taken?

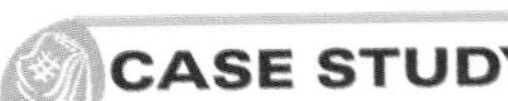

CASE STUDY

Melinda Robertson is a 33-year-old woman who presents to the urgent care center. Listed below are data collected by the nurse.

Interview Data

Melinda tells the examiner, "I have a really bad pain in front of my butt. It hurts so much that I can't even wipe with a tissue after I go to the bathroom. There is no way I could have a stool right now." Melinda indicates the pain started 2 days ago and is "much worse now." When asked about her sexual activity she says, "I'm with a guy, but it's not exclusive or anything. We see other people and try not to be real serious."

Examination Data

- **External examination:** Typical hair distribution, urethral meatus intact, no redness or discharge. Perineum intact. Extreme pain response to palpation of vaginal opening; swelling, redness, and mass detected on right side. Foul-smelling discharge noted.
- **Internal examination:** Deferred due to extreme pain associated with inflammation.

1. What data deviate from normal findings, suggesting a need for further investigation?
2. What additional information should the nurse ask or assess for?
3. In what functional health patterns does data deviate from normal?
4. What nursing diagnosis and/or collaborative problems should be considered for this situation?

REMEMBER to check out your **companion CD-ROM**

22 Male Genitalia

www.mosby.com/MERLIN/wilson/assessment/

ANATOMY AND PHYSIOLOGY

THE GENITALIA

The male genitalia consist of the penis, urethra, scrotum, testicles, epididymides, vas deferens, seminal vesicles, and prostate gland (Fig. 22-1).

Penis

The penis serves two functions: it is the final excretory organ in urination, and during intercourse it introduces sperm into the vagina. The body of the penis contains three layers; the two outer layers of spongy tissue, the corpora cavernosa and the corpus spongiosum, encase the urethra (see Fig. 22-1). This smooth, semifirm, spongy tissue becomes firm when engorged with blood, forming an erection. The corpus spongiosum expands at its distal end to form the glans penis.

The glans penis is lighter pink in color than the rest of the penis. It is exposed when the prepuce (the foreskin) is either pulled back or surgically removed (circumcision). The corona is the ridge that separates the glans from the shaft of the penis. The skin covering the penis is thin, hairless, and a little darker than the rest of the body; it adheres loosely to the shaft to allow for expansion with erection.

Erection is a neurovascular reflex that occurs when the two corpora cavernosa become engorged with blood, caused by increased arterial dilation and decreased venous outflow. This reflex can be induced by psychogenic and local reflex mechanisms, both under the control of the autonomic nervous system. The psychogenic erection can be initiated by any type of sensory input—auditory, visual, tactile, or imaginative—whereas the local reflex mechanisms are initiated by tactile stimuli. Cortical input can also suppress erection. Ejaculation—the emission of semen from the vas deferens, epididymides, prostate, and seminal vesicles—is followed by constriction of the vessels supplying blood to the corpora cavernosa and gradual return of the penis to its relaxed, flaccid state.

Urethra

The innermost tube of the penis, the urethra, is usually about 7 to 8 inches (18 to 20 cm) from bladder to meatus. It extends out of the base of the bladder, traveling through the prostate gland into the pelvic floor and through the penile shaft (see Fig. 22-1). The urethral orifice is a small slit at the tip of the glans.

Scrotum

The scrotum is a pouch covered with thin, darkly pigmented, rugous (wrinkled) skin. A septum divides the scrotum into two pendulous compartments, or sacs. Each sac contains a testis and an epididymis, which is suspended by the spermatic cord—a network of nerves, blood vessels, and the vas deferens (Fig. 22-2). Because sperm production requires a temperature slightly below body temperature, the testes are suspended outside the body cavity; its temperature is controlled by a layer of muscle under the scrotal skin that contracts when the outside temperature is cold and retracts the pouch and its contents upward toward the body. Conversely, when body heat rises, the sac allows it to relax, expand, and drop downward. The left side of the scrotum is usually slightly lower than the right side due to the spermatic cord.

Testicles and Epididymides

The testicles each contain a series of coiled ducts (seminiferous tubules), where sperm production (spermatogenesis) occurs. Each testicle is approximately 1½ × 1 × ¾ inches (4 × 2.5 × 2 cm), ovoid, rubbery in texture, and smooth on the surface (see Fig. 22-2). On production, the sperm move toward the center of the testis, traveling into the efferent tubules adjacent to the comma-shaped epididymis on the posterolateral surface of each testis. The epididymis is about 2 inches (5 cm) long. The sperm receive nutrients and mature in an elaborate, coiled duct within the epididymis. They are stored in the ductus epididymis and eventually travel through the vas deferens into the penis.

Vas Deferens

The vas deferens begins at the tail of the epididymis. It ascends from the scrotum through the external inguinal ring to the posterior aspect of the bladder. It unites with the seminal vesicle, forming the ejaculatory duct.

Seminal Vesicles

The seminal vesicles, small pouches lying between the rectum and the posterior bladder wall, join the ejaculatory duct at the base of the prostate (see Fig. 22-1). These vesicles, along with the vas deferens, the prostate, and the bulbourethral glands, produce all secretions and nutrients needed within the semen to maximize the health, life span, and motility of the sperm.

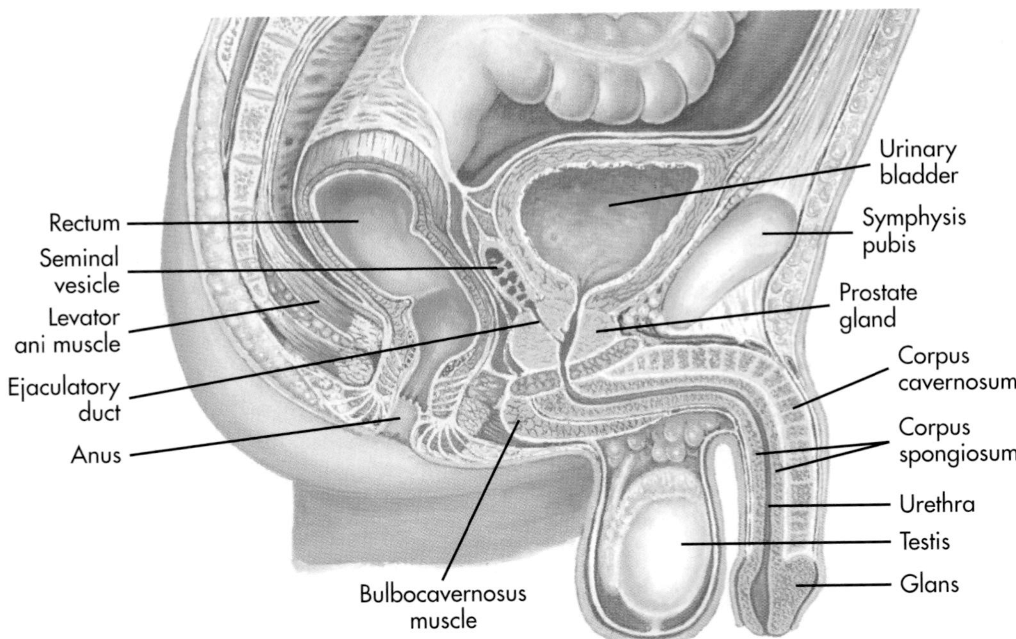

Fig. 22-1 Male pelvic organs. (From Seidel et al, 1999.)

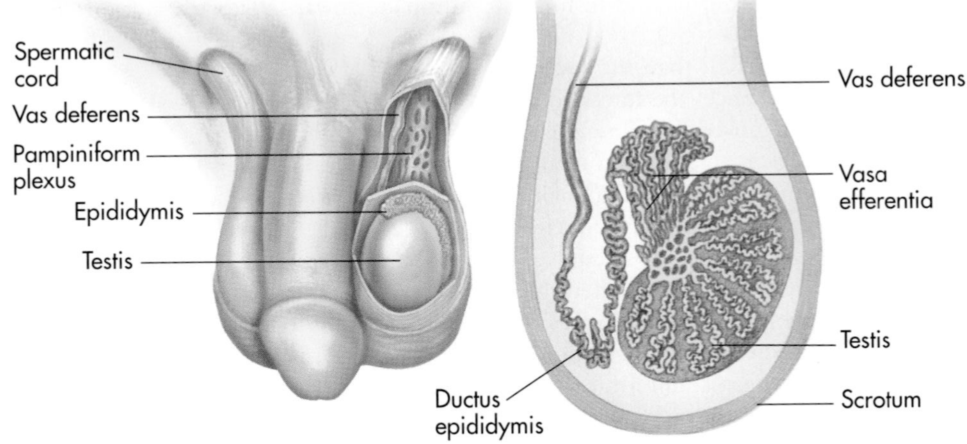

Fig. 22-2 Scrotum and its contents. (From Seidel et al, 1999.)

Prostate Gland

The prostate gland, at the base of the bladder, is approximately the same size as a testis. Its function is not completely understood, but it is assumed to aid sperm motility by producing most of the ejaculatory fluid. The prostate is discussed more thoroughly in Chapter 23.

THE INGUINAL AREA

The vas deferens, along with arteries, veins, and lymph vessels, is encased in the spermatic cord. This cord extends from the scrotum through the abdominal muscles, by way of the inguinal canal (see Fig. 22-2). The cord enters the inguinal canal through the external inguinal ring. The external inguinal ring is vulnerable to hernias, or protrusion of the abdominal contents. See the common problems section later in this chapter for further discussion of hernias.

HEALTH HISTORY

Male Genitalia

QUESTIONS | **RATIONALE**

PRESENT HEALTH STATUS

➤ Do you have any current or chronic illness? If so, describe.

■ Chronic illnesses such as diabetes mellitus, neurologic impairments, vascular insufficiency, and cardiac or respiratory disease can affect sexual function.

➤ Do you take any medications? If so, what do you take?

■ Some medications can cause impotence or decreased libido. Medications that may lead to difficulty with sexual function include diuretics, sedatives, antihypertensives, tranquilizers, and inhibitors of androgen synthesis.

➤ Do you perform testicular self-examinations? If so, how often?

■ Assess self-care behaviors. This provides the opportunity for teaching of self-examination if not performed.

➤ Do you wear a protective device when engaging in contact sports?

■ Failure to protect genitalia while participating in contact sports can lead to injury affecting sexual function, such as scrotal injuries.

PAST MEDICAL HISTORY

➤ Have you ever had infections, injuries, or other condition to your penis, scrotum, or testes? If so, describe.

■ Conditions that could occur include cancer, testicular torsion, hernia, and sexually transmitted infection.

➤ Have you ever had surgery or any procedures done on your penis or scrotum? If so, what was done and for what reason? When did this occur?

■ Surgeries to document include vasectomy, undescended testes, hydrocele, variocele.

SEXUAL ACTIVITY

➤ Are you currently in a relationship that involves sexual intercourse? Do you have one or multiple partners? How frequently do you engage in sexual activities? What type of sex do you engage in (penile-vaginal; penile-rectal, recipient rectal, oral)? Are you and your partner(s) satisfied with the sexual relationship?

■ It is important to determine the type of sexual activity the individual has, as well as the client's satisfaction regarding that activity. The rationale for asking about the type of activity is to determine if the client has one or numerous sexual partners and what type of contraception is used. This may, in turn, lead to more information about the client's risk for sexually transmitted infections. The rationale for asking about client satisfaction is to determine whether the client is satisfied with his sexuality and the sexual practices he is engaging in.

➤ Do you and/or your partner(s) frequently use drugs or alcohol before you engage in sexual activity?

■ Drug and alcohol use leads to high-risk sexual behavior.

➤ Do you and your partner(s) use a protective barrier such as a condom? If so, how often do you use this? When was the last time you used a protective barrier?

■ Determine level of understanding and practice regarding safe sex and sexually transmitted infection. Many times individuals may not have accurate information.

QUESTIONS

RATIONALE

➤ If partner(s) are female: Do you and your partner(s) use a contraceptive? Which one? Is it satisfactory to you? Do you have any questions about the method? Have you ever created or been part of a pregnancy? How does that/did that make you feel? What has been the outcome of that situation?

■ Determine level of understanding and practice regarding pregnancy prevention. Clients may need clarification of information. Determine if pregnancy has occurred and what level of involvement exists.

➤ How many sexual partners have you had in the last 6 months? Do you prefer relationships with men, women, or both? (If the client is gay, inquire if he is in a significant relationship and has a partner.)

■ Gay men need to feel acceptance to discuss their health concerns. If the examiner seems genuinely interested and concerned, the client may appreciate the opportunity to discuss sexuality issues or problems.

➤ Have you ever been physically abused or forced into a sexual act against your will?

■ Men as well as women can be victims of physical and sexual abuse. It is often very difficult for men to admit to such abuse.

PROBLEM-BASED HISTORY

The most commonly reported problems related to the male genitalia are pain or discharge, lesions, problems with urination, and problems with erection or ejaculation. As with symptoms in all areas of health assessment, a symptom analysis is completed, which includes the location, quality, quantity, chronology, setting, associated manifestations, alleviating factors, and aggravating factors. (See Box 4-2 in Chapter 4.)

Pain

➤ Where do you have pain? Lower back? Bladder? Testicle? Groin? When did it begin? On a scale of 1 to 10, how intense is the pain at this time?

■ Identify onset, location, and intensity of the pain. A sudden onset of pain may signal a serious problem. If it occurs in the lower back along the costovertebral angle, it may be related to pyelonephritis. If it is a spasmodic, colicky pain from upper ureteral dilation, it may cause referred pain to the testis on the same side. If it is pain from lower ureteral dilation, the client may feel pain referred to the scrotum. Either of these ureteral pains are very severe, and the client will usually appear very restless and uncomfortable.

➤ Has the pain become worse over the past 24 hours? If so, what seems to make it worse? Is the pain constant or just at certain times? Is it associated with movement or lifting? Is the pain associated with nausea or vomiting? Abdominal distention? Fever or chills?

■ Assess for associated symptoms or problems.

QUESTIONS

➤ Have you noticed any pain, lumps, or swelling in your groin, testicle, or scrotum? Does the scrotum seem to have changed in size? Any bulges? How long has the bulge been there? Have you ever been diagnosed with a hernia? Have you noticed a dragging or heavy feeling in the scrotum?

RATIONALE

■ Pain in the groin may occur from a number of causes, including problems in the spermatic cord; testicles; prostate gland; or lymph nodes; hernia; herpes zoster; or a number of neurologic problems.

Testicular pain can occur secondary to almost any problem of the testis or epididymis. Such problems include epididymitis; orchitis; hydrocele; spermatic cord torsion; and tumor, such as testicular cancer.

Priapism (a persistent erection of the penis that does not occur secondary to sexual excitement) causes pain secondary to a thrombosis of the corpora cavernosa.

Problems With Urination

➤ Do you think you are urinating more frequently than you consider normal? Do you ever feel that you cannot wait to urinate? Do you awaken at night because you have to urinate? How often? For how long has this been occurring?

■ The normal adult male urinates 5 to 6 times each day, with variations depending on fluid intake, activity, and individual habits. When the client has a urinary tract disorder or prostate problem, there is usually an increase in nocturia (awakening at night to urinate), urinary frequency, and urgency. Medications, especially those for cardiovascular problems, diuretics, and antihistamines, may also cause changes in urination.

➤ Have you experienced any pain or burning with urination? Is the urine clear or cloudy? Discolored? Bloody? Foul smelling? Have you had a urinary tract infection before? (A more detailed history of the possibility of urinary tract infection is found in Chapter 20.)

■ These symptoms may accompany problems such as infection, acute cystitis, prostatitis, and urethritis. Urethritis in the young sexually active male may be indicative of sexually transmitted infections such as chlamydia or gonorrhea.

➤ Do you have any trouble initiating a urine stream? Do you strain to get started or to maintain the stream? Is the stream narrower or weaker than usual? Have you noticed that you must stand closer to the toilet because there is dribbling of urine? Do you have to press on your abdomen to start your urine flow? Afterward, do you feel that you still have to urinate? (See Chapter 23 for a complete discussion of prostate problems.)

■ Hesitancy, straining, loss of force or decreased caliber of the stream, terminal dribbling, sensation of residual urine, and recurrent episodes of acute cystitis may be symptoms of a progressive prostatic obstruction.

Penile Lesions or Discharge

➤ Do you notice any discharge from the penis? Do you have any staining in the front of your underwear? If so, how much? Is it increasing or decreasing? What color is it? Does it have a particular odor? Do you notice it when you are urinating? Is there pain?

■ Lesions on the shaft or head of the penis or discharge from the penis may indicate an inflammation or sexually transmitted infection.

QUESTIONS

➤ Have you had any sexual contact with a partner who has a sexually transmitted infection (STI) (for example, gonorrhea, acquired immunodeficiency syndrome [AIDS], syphilis, herpes, chlamydia, or venereal warts) or a partner who has high risk factors for sexually transmitted infections (such as a prostitute, individual who trades sex for drugs, intravenous [IV] drug abuser)? When? Were you infected? How has it been treated? Have there been any complications?

RATIONALE

■ Questions concerning sexual activity should be professional and a routine part of the examination. Help the client to feel comfortable discussing sexual issues by beginning with an open-ended question, showing your acceptance of him. Then ask questions that seem appropriate in light of what he communicates to you. Remember that your comfort with the topics being discussed will prompt the client's comfort in responding.

Difficulty With Erection

➤ Do you ever have difficulty maintaining an erection? Do you have a prolonged erection, is it painful? If so, describe details.

➤ Does your penis ever erect at times when there is no sexual stimulation? Does your penis curve in any direction when you have an erection?

Difficulty With Ejaculation

➤ Do you have painful or premature ejaculation? If so, what have you done about this problem? Has it helped? When you ejaculate, what is the color, consistency, and amount of fluid? (Box 22-1.)

■ Impotence, prolonged erection, and premature ejaculation are all important but delicate topics. Impotence may be a sign of a sexual dissatisfaction or deep-seated emotional problems. If you identify a client who has difficulty with erection or ejaculation, it is generally best to refer the client to a health care professional who specializes in those areas.

Box 22-1 Incidence of Male Sexual Dysfunction

- Sexual dysfunction in the male may be noted anytime after the onset of puberty. The incidence of men who seek treatment for erectile dysfunction increases with age.
  - By age 40, 1.5% of all men have sought treatment for sexual dysfunction.
  - By age 70, 25% of all men have sought treatment for sexual dysfunction.
- The relative incidence of impotence from psychogenic versus organic causes has received great attention. Some investigators have reported that 90% to 95% of the cases of impotence result from psychogenic causes (Smith, 1981; Libertino, 1982).
- More recent data using more sophisticated diagnostic techniques reveal an increased percentage of men whose erectile dysfunction has organic as well as psychogenic components (Libertino, 1991).

EXAMINATION

Equipment

- Examination gloves for palpation
- ❖ Penlight or transilluminator to transilluminate the scrotum

PROCEDURES AND TECHNIQUES WITH NORMAL FINDINGS

ABNORMAL FINDINGS

Start by positioning the client. He may be positioned in one of two ways, either standing or lying down. If the client is lying down, he will need to stand later for adequate evaluation of possible hernia. If the client is standing, the examiner should be seated facing the client wearing gloves (Box 22-2).

Box 22-2 Clinical Note

Men usually feel apprehensive about having their genitalia examined, especially if the examiner is female. This may be seen as an invasion of privacy rather than accepted as a part of the physical examination. The examiner must approach the examination of a male patient in a professional, matter-of-fact way. Always start with the client's history. This should be taken before, not during, the examination.

As the examiner, you must be aware of these concerns and any of your own apprehension in the situation. It is normal for you to feel embarrassment, lack confidence, fear causing pain, or worry about "causing" an erection. Use a firm, deliberate touch. If an erection occurs, reassure the client that this is a normal physiologic response to touch and that he could not have prevented it. Do not stop the evaluation or leave the room; this will focus further on the erection and reinforce the client's embarrassment.

PUBIC HAIR

➤**INSPECT pubic hair for distribution and general characteristics.** Hair distribution varies widely but is normally in a diamond-shaped pattern that may extend to the umbilicus. The hair should appear coarser than scalp hair. The hair should be free of parasites, and the skin should be smooth and clear.

■ Note patchy growth, loss, or absence of hair; distribution of hair in a female pattern (triangular, with the base over the pubis); nits or pubic lice; scars; lower abdominal or inguinal lesions; or a rash.

Tinea cruris ("jock itch") is a common fungal infection found in the groin that appears as large, clearly marginated, reddened patches that are pruritic and often associated with "athlete's foot."

Monilial infections are red, eroded patches with scaling and pustules and are associated with immobility and disability, systemic antibiotics, and immunologic deficits.

PENIS

➤**INSPECT and PALPATE the penis for general characteristics, color, tenderness, and discharge.**

➤The dorsal vein should be apparent on the dorsal surface of the shaft of the penis. The skin is usually dark and hairless, with a wrinkled surface and frequently apparent vascularity. In uncircumcised men, the prepuce is present and folded over the glans (Fig. 22-3); in circumcised men the amount prepuce is often variable (Fig. 22-4). If the client has not been circumcised, ask him to retract the foreskin. The foreskin should retract easily and completely over the glans (Box 22-3).

■ Failure of the ability to retract the foreskin, discomfort on retraction, or difficulty of returning the foreskin to the original position should be considered abnormal.

Phimosis is a very tight foreskin that cannot be retracted over the glans. (See Fig. 22-13 later in this chapter.)

Paraphimosis is the inability to return the foreskin over the glans. (See Fig. 22-14 later in this chapter.)

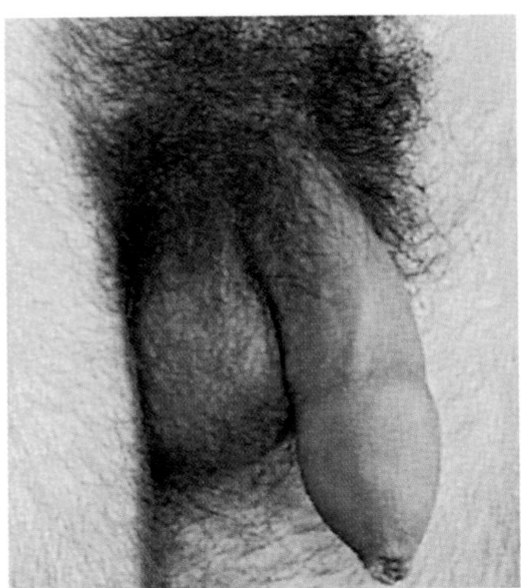

Fig. 22-3 Uncircumcised penis. (From Seidel et al, 1999.)

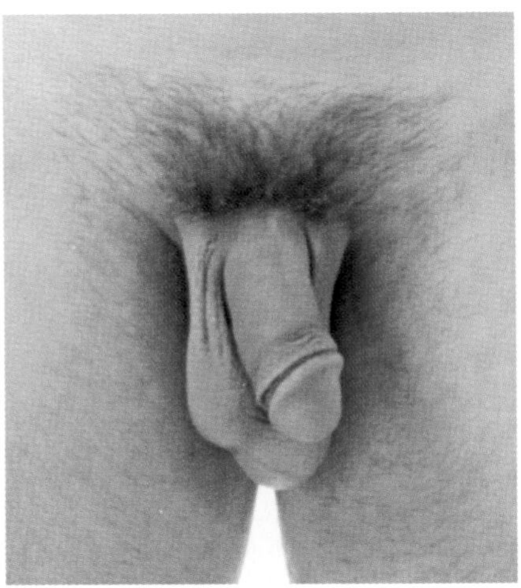

Fig. 22-4 Circumcised penis.

Box 22-3 Clinical Note

Circumcision has been a common practice of the dominant American culture. There have been several identified rationales for circumcision, which include the following:

- Prevention of phimosis
- Decreased incidence of glans penis inflammation
- Decreased incidence of cancer of the penis
- Decreased incidence of urinary tract infections in infants
- Decreased incidence of sexually transmitted infection (particularly syphilis, gonorrhea, and warts)

However, the decision to circumcise a newborn infant is based largely on cultural practice. Judaism and Islam incorporate circumcision as part of their belief systems. Most American Indians, Alaskan natives, and Hispanics, on the other hand, are uncircumcised, as it does not conform to their belief system.

PROCEDURES AND TECHNIQUES WITH NORMAL FINDINGS

ABNORMAL FINDINGS

➤Inspect the glans and under the fold of the prepuce. The glans should be smooth, pink, and bulbous. Note any redness, lesions, swellings, nodules, or presence of discharge. (If discharge or smegma is present, obtain a specimen on a slide for microscopic examination.) The prepuce fold is wrinkled and loosely attached to the underlying glans; it is darker than the glans. Note: Circumcised penises have varying lengths of foreskin remaining; some have multiple folds, and others have none.

■ *Balanitis* is inflammation of the glans that commonly occurs in clients with phimosis. (See Fig. 22-15 later in this chapter.)

➤Inspect the urethral meatus. It should be located centrally at the distal tip of the glans, and no discharge should be present. The meatus should appear as a slit-like opening.

■ Note if the meatus is located either on the upper surface of the penis (epispadias) or on the bottom of the penis (hypospadias) and if there is a discharge present. The discharge may be yellow-green or milky-white or have a foul odor.

➤Palpate the glans anteroposteriorly to open the distal end of the urethra (Fig. 22-5). The surface should be pink and smooth, and no discharge should be present.

■ Report any reddening, swelling, discharge, or crusting.

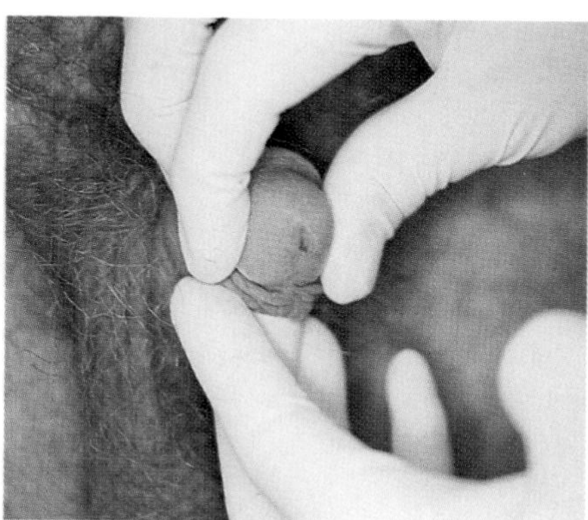

Fig. 22-5 Examination of urethral meatus.

➤Palpate the entire shaft of the penis between the thumb and first two fingers. The penis shaft should be nontender and smooth, with a semifirm consistency.

■ Note tenderness, swelling, nodules, or induration.

SCROTUM AND TESTES

➤**INSPECT the scrotum for texture and general characteristics, color, and asymmetry.** Hold the penis out of the way with the back of your hand (or ask the client to hold the penis out of the way) while you inspect the scrotum (Fig. 22-6). The sac should be divided in half by the septum; the left sac may be larger than the right. Size varies, and the scrotum may appear pendulous. It should appear more deeply pigmented than the body skin. The surface should feel coarse and free of lesions. Small lumps on the scrotal skin known as sebaceous cysts or sebaceous glands are considered a normal finding.

■ Scrotal lesions or either generalized or isolated redness are considered abnormal and may indicate an infection.

PROCEDURES AND TECHNIQUES WITH NORMAL FINDINGS

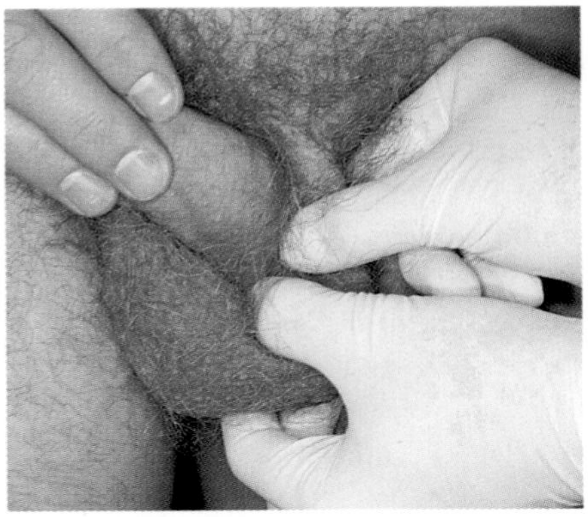

ABNORMAL FINDINGS

Fig. 22-6 Inspection of scrotum and ventral surface of penis.

➤The thickness of the skin of the scrotum changes with temperature and age. In cold or cool temperatures, the scrotal skin feels thickened. As the individual ages, the skin thins.

■ Temperature affects the position of the testes in the scrotum. When the environmental temperature is very cold, the testes slightly retract upward. Likewise, when the temperature is hot or if the client has a fever, the testes will extend more downward.

➤Lift the scrotum to examine its underside (be sure to spread the rugated surface for a better view). This area is deeply pigmented, hairless, and has a rugous surface.

■ Report any redness, edema, absence of rugae, rash, or lesions.

➤**PALPATE the scrotum for presence of testes.** Palpate each half of the scrotum (Fig. 22-7). It should be nontender with thin, loose skin over a muscular layer.

■ Note any marked tenderness or swelling.

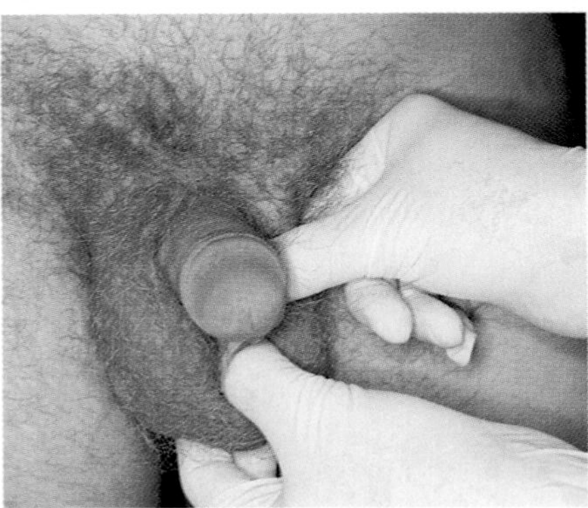

Fig. 22-7 Palpating contents of scrotum and testes.

➤**PALPATE the testes, epididymides, and vas deferens for location, consistency, tenderness, and nodules.**

➤Palpate the testes simultaneously with both hands, using the thumb and the first two fingers. Note that the testes are present in each sac; they should be equal in size, mildly sensitive but nontender to moderate compression, smooth and ovoid, and movable.

■ Note if the testes have not distended into the sac, are enlarged (unilaterally or bilaterally), atrophied, markedly tender, nodular or irregular, or fixed.

PROCEDURES AND TECHNIQUES WITH NORMAL FINDINGS

ABNORMAL FINDINGS

➤Palpate the epididymides. On the posterolateral surface of each testes, palpate the epididymis—it will feel like a tubular, comma-shaped structure, which collapses when gently compressed between your fingers and thumb. This area should be smooth and nontender.

■ If a problem is noted, determine its position in relation to the testes (i.e., proximal or distal); whether it can be moved with your fingers; if it disappears when the client lies down. Report any tenderness, irregular placement, enlargement, induration, or nodules.

➤Palpate the vas deferens. The vas deferens lies within the spermatic cord. To palpate, grasp both spermatic cords between the thumb and forefinger and palpate, starting at the base of the epididymides, moving upward to the inguinal ring. Since the vas deferens lies within the spermatic cord along with arteries and veins, it is difficult to specifically identify with palpation. The vas deferens feels like a smooth cordlike structure. It should be nontender and discretely palpable from the epididymis to the external inguinal ring.

■ Report any tenderness, tortuosity, thickened or beaded area, or induration.

❖ ➤**TRANSILLUMINATE the scrotum for evidence of fluid and masses.** If a mass, fluid, or irregularity is suspected, transilluminate each scrotal sac. There should be no additional contents or fluid. The testes and epididymides do not transilluminate.

■ Note any mass that is distal or proximal to the testis. It may or may not be tender. Hydroceles and spermatoceles are fluid-filled and therefore transilluminate; tumors, hernias, and epididymitis do not.

INGUINAL REGION

Evaluate the inguinal region for hernia. Note: The client should stand and the examiner sit if possible.

➤**INSPECT both inguinal regions and femoral area for bulges.** Ask the client to bear down. While he is straining, inspect the ingunial canal area and femoral area (area just above where the femoral artery is palpated) for presence of a bulge. There should be no bulges.

■ Note any bulges in the area of the external ring, the Hesselbach triangle, or the femoral area. Presence of bulges suggests a hernia. See Common Problems Conditions section later in this chapter.

❖ ➤**PALPATE the inguinal canal for evidence of indirect hernia or direct hernia.** Palpate both the right and left inguinal rings. Use your index finger or middle finger (for adults) of the hand corresponding to the client's side (Fig. 22-8) (e.g., right hand for right side). Insert the your finger into the lower aspect of the scrotum. The finger should follow the spermatic cord upward through the triangular, slit-like opening of the inguinal ring into the inguinal canal. Ask the client to bear down or cough. You should not feel any bulging against your fingertip.

■ Note any palpable mass that touches your fingertip or pushes against the side of your finger (Table 22-1).

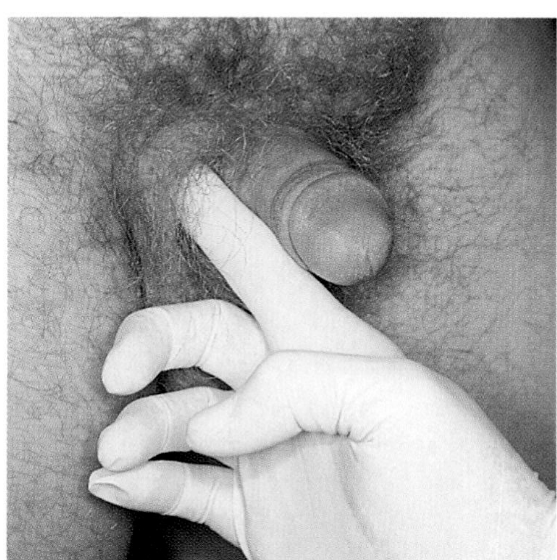

Fig. 22-8 Checking for inguinal hernia; gloved finger inserted through inguinal canal.

Table 22-1 Hernia Evaluation

	INDIRECT HERNIA	DIRECT HERNIA	FEMORAL HERNIA
Description	The sac herniates through the internal inguinal ring. It can remain in the inguinal canal, exit through the external canal, or actually pass into the scrotum.	The sac herniates through the external inguinal ring. Hernia is located in the Hesselbach triangle region. It rarely enters the scrotum.	The sac extends through the femoral ring, canal, and below the inguinal ligament.
Clinical signs	Hernia comes down to meet examiner's fingertip with feeling of soft swelling. Client complains of pain on straining. May decrease when client lies down.	Client has a bulge in the Hesselbach triangle area. Usually feels no pain. Hernia pushes against examiner's fingertip when client bears down. May decrease when client lies down.	Pain in inguinal area. Right side more likely to have hernia than left. Pain may be severe.
Occurrence	The most frequent type of hernia. May occur in both sexes and in children (mostly males).	Less common. Occurs most frequently in males over 40 years of age. Uncommon in women.	The least common type of hernia. Occurs most frequently in women.

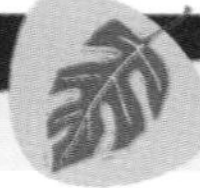

AGE-RELATED VARIATIONS

INFANTS

Anatomy and Physiology

Until the eighth week of gestation, male and female genitalia are indistinguishable; fetal insult during the eighth or ninth gestational week may lead to anomalies of the external genitalia. By 12 weeks' gestation, differentiation is notable. Testes descend from the retroperitoneal space into the scrotum during the third trimester. Separation of the glans and inner preputial epithelium also begins during the third trimester.

At birth, one or both testes may still lie in the inguinal canal; final descent may not occur until the early postnatal period and may be arrested at any point. Complete separation of the glans and inner preputial epithelium will usually not be complete until the age of 3 to 6 years.

Health History

- Has the infant been diagnosed with any problems, such as malpositioning of the opening at the end of the penis (hypospadias or epispadias), swelling of the scrotum, undescended testes, or difficulty telling the child's sex by looking at the genitalia (ambiguous genitalia)?

  Rationale It is important to identify congenital problems that may have been corrected following birth or problems that may still remain.
- Have you noticed the child having any difficulty with urinating? Does the infant cry or hold his genitals? Does the urinary stream seem straight? Has he had any urinary tract infections?

  Rationale It is important to ask screening questions that may provide information about possible infection or urinary tract problems.
- Does the baby's scrotum ever swell when he cries?

  Rationale Scrotal swelling, with or without crying, may indicate the presence of a hydrocele.
- Has the child been circumcised? Were there any problems following the circumcision?

  Rationale Identification of problems that may have occurred either during or following the circumcision may provide information related to current problems or parent concerns.
- If the child has not been circumcised, ask: How do you clean the end of the child's penis? Are you able to retract the foreskin? Does the foreskin ever seem to interfere with the infant's ability to urinate?

  Rationale If the infant is not circumcised, it is important to assess how the parent cleans under the foreskin. If the foreskin is not retracted routinely for cleaning, the skin may retract down around the end of the penis and may make cleaning the penis difficult.

Examination

Procedures and Techniques The examination of the male infant's genitalia is straightforward. The child should be undressed so that the genitalia are completely exposed. When the infant is not actually being examined, he should have his genitalia covered in case of unexpected urination. Inspect the urinary meatus; however, do not attempt to retract the foreskin more than necessary to see the meatus. Force may actually tear the prepuce from the glans, which in turn could cause binding adhesions to form between the prepuce and the glans.

When a mass other than a testicle or spermatic cord is palpated in the scrotum, transillumination is indicated to determine the presence of fluid (hydrocele) or mass (possible hernia) in the testicle. This technique is performed by using a bright penlight or transilluminator and pressing the light source up against the scrotal sac. A hydrocele will transilluminate and will most likely become bigger as the child cries or becomes stressed. A mass (such as a hernia) will not transilluminate.

Normal and Abnormal Findings The penis should measure 1⅛ to 1¾ inches (3 to 4 cm) in length and ⅜ to ½ inch (1 to 1.3 cm) in width. If the infant is uncircumcised, the foreskin (prepuce) should cover the glans. The foreskin will have little mobility. As the infant becomes older, the foreskin will have more mobility. The foreskin should retract enough to permit a good urinary stream and general cleaning. The urinary meatus should be at the tip of the penis. If possible, observe the infant's urine stream. It should be full and strong. A weak stream with dribbling is an abnormal finding and may indicate stenosis of the urethral meatus. The infant should void within 24 hours of birth.

The full-term infant has pendulous scrotum with deep rugae; the scrotum may be edematous, but this is considered normal. The scrotum appears pink in white infants and dark brown in dark-skinned infants. The size of the scrotum in the infant usually appears large when compared to the penis. Palpation of the scrotum should indicate the presence of one or both testes (Fig. 22-9). If either or both testicles are not palpable, gently place a finger over the upper inguinal ring and gently push downward toward the scrotum. If the testicle can be pushed into the scrotum, it is considered descended even though it retracts into the inguinal canal. A hydrocele is a common finding in infants.

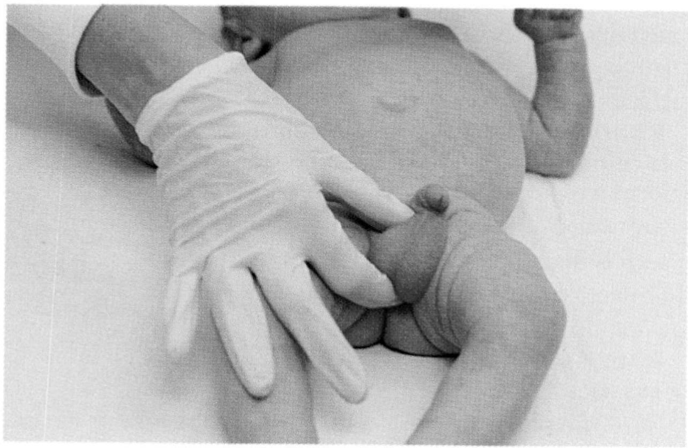

Fig. 22-9 Palpation of the scrotum in an infant.

■ CHILDREN

Anatomy and Physiology

During the prepubertal years of childhood, the only anatomic change is a slight increase in the size of the scrotum and penis.

Health History

- Does the child have any lesions, swelling, or discoloration on the penis or scrotum? Does he ever cry when he urinates?

  Rationale This screens for possible infection, hydrocele, hernia, or injury/abuse.
- Does the child explore his own genitalia? How do you react to this? Does your child know the correct anatomic names for his genitalia?

  Rationale Exploration of the genitalia is a normal behavior. It is important to assess how the parents feel about it and how they interact with the child regarding the self-play.
- For preschool or young school-age children, ask the following: Have you ever been touched on your penis or between your legs by someone when you did not want them to? Has anyone ever asked you to touch them? If so, when did this happen? Who did it? Did you tell anyone? See Box 21-5 on p. 552 for guidelines on talking with children who reveal abuse.

  Rationale These are screening questions for sexual abuse.

Examination

Procedures and Techniques The techniques of examining the male child's genitalia are the same as for the infant. The major difference in the examination is the approach. In many cultures, children are taught at a very early age that the genitalia should not be exposed or touched. In the presence of the child's parent, reassure him that you must examine his genitalia just as you have examined all of his other body areas. Whenever possible, reassure the child that he is growing up normally. Because children are now taught that touching of the genitalia by strangers is not "okay," it is important that the parent reassure the child that you need to examine him to make sure that he is healthy.

The examination is easiest to perform if the child is sitting in either a slightly reclining position with his knees flexed and heels near the buttock (Fig. 22-10) or sitting with his knees spread and ankles crossed.

If the child has not been circumcised, do not force the foreskin to be retracted. Retract the foreskin only to the point of tightness. Then evaluate whether it is retracted far enough to permit adequate urination and cleaning. Determine if the child has any discharge, crusting, or lesions around or under the foreskin. In addition, examine the scrotum for shape, size, and color and to determine the presence of testicles in the scrotum.

Normal and Abnormal Findings The basic findings are the same as for the infant. By age 6, the foreskin

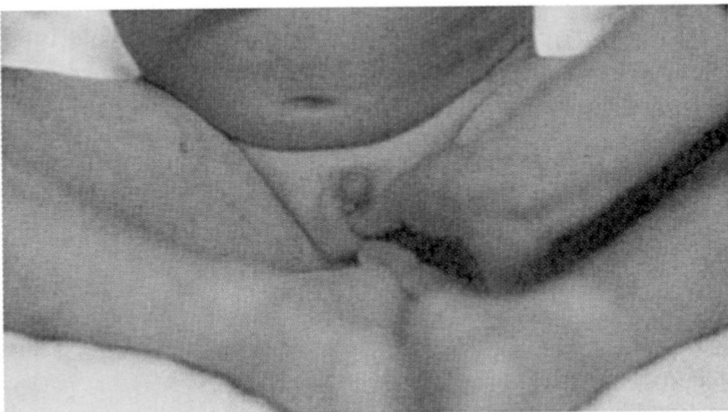

Fig. 22-10 Position of young child for examination of genitalia. (From Wong et al, 1999.)

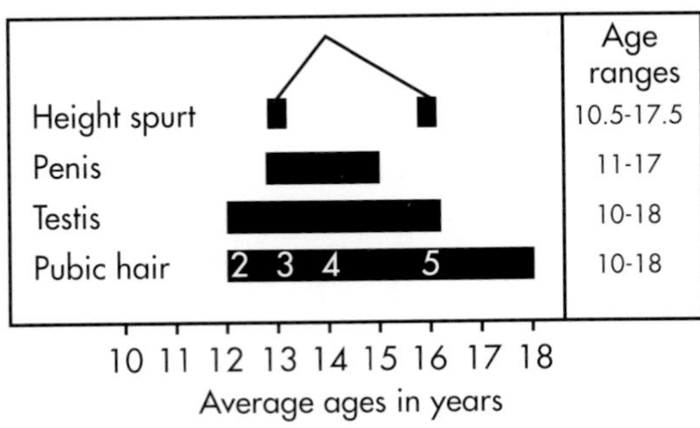

Fig. 22-11 Development of male genitalia and pubic hair. (From Tanner, 1962.)

should be easily retracted. If the scrotum has well-formed rugae, it indicates that the testes have descended into the scrotum, even if the testes are not apparent in the scrotum. When palpated, the testes should be about ⅜ inch (1 cm) in diameter. If the scrotum remains small, flat, and underdeveloped, it is considered an abnormal finding and may indicate cryptorchidism (undescended testes).

■ PREADOLESCENTS AND ADOLESCENTS

Anatomy and Physiology

Puberty begins at some time between age 9 ½ and 13 ½ years. The first sign is an enlargement of the testes, followed by pubic hair development, and finally, an increase in penis size. See Fig. 22-11 and Table 22-2 for Tanner's classic sexual maturity rating chart for males (Tanner, 1962). Sparse, downy hair appears at the base of the penis, and the scrotal skin reddens, thins, and expands at the onset of puberty. At the same time, the testes and penis enlarge. Later, pubic hair darkens and extends until it is dense, coarse, and curly, forming a diamond-shaped pattern from the umbilicus to the anus. The prostate gland also enlarges in later adolescence.

Health History

When taking a health history on an adolescent, it is important to bear in mind the following: (1) Ask questions appropriate for the boy's age, but be aware that "normal" varies widely; it is better to ask too many questions than to omit anything. (2) Ask questions that are direct and professional; avoid judgmental phrases. Consider beginning by establishing that it is normal to feel or think a certain thing, for example, "Young men your age often feel . . . ." (3) Ask questions that assume rather than ask for an admission (this is referred to as ubiquity approach).

- Have you noticed changes in your body over the last 2 years? How do you feel about these changes?

  Rationale Note the adolescent's attitude toward developmental changes taking place.

- Often a young man about your age (usually 12 or 13) will begin to notice that his penis and scrotum have begun to change and grow. What changes have you noticed? Have you ever seen charts of normal growth patterns for boys? Let's look at these now.

  Rationale This assesses the adolescent's level of information about the changes that are taking place and provides an opportunity for education.

- Young men about your age (age 12 or 13) experience fluid coming out of the penis at night, called nocturnal emissions, or "wet dreams." Have you had this?

  Rationale Boys may believe that this indicates a problem or may feel guilty about it. They need to be assured this is normal.

- Other things guys your age often experience are having an erection at embarrassing times, masturbating, or having sexual fantasies. Do you have any questions about these things? Would you like to talk about any of these concerns?

  Rationale Boys may feel guilty about these things and should be reassured that they are normal.

- Who do you usually talk to about body changes and sexual information? Are you comfortable in these talks? Do you think you get enough information? Have you taken sex education classes in school? Is there someone either in or outside of the family, maybe at school or church, with whom you can discuss these issues?

  Rationale Adolescents need accurate information about their changing body and sexuality issues. It is important to identify where the client gets his current information and how complete that information may be.

- Often young men your age have questions about sexual activity. Do you? Do you have questions about birth control or sexually transmitted infections like AIDS or gonorrhea?

  Rationale Assess the adolescent's level of knowledge. It is common for boys not to admit that they need more information.

- Are you dating someone? Do you and your partner have sex? If so, what method of birth control and/or barrier protection did you use the last time you had sex? What questions do you have?

  Rationale: Assess if birth control or protection is being used.

- Have you been taught by a doctor or nurse how to examine your own testicles to make sure they are healthy?

  Rationale Assess the level of knowledge about self-care.

Table 22-2 Tanner's Sex Maturity Development

STAGES	PUBIC HAIR	PENIS	SCROTUM
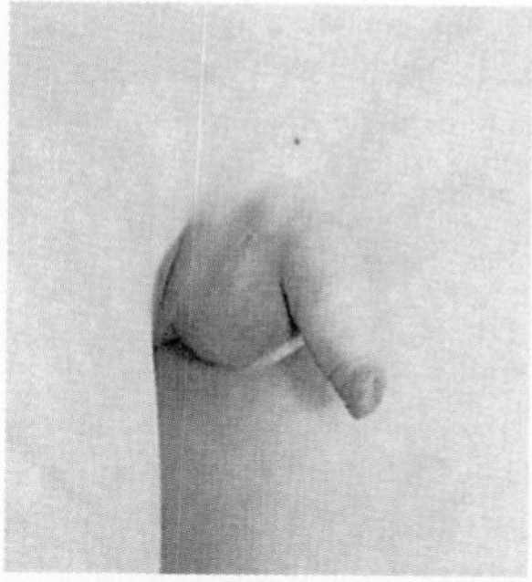	No pubic hair.	Appears like smaller child's penis.	Testes begins to enlarge, but scrotum remains small and undeveloped.
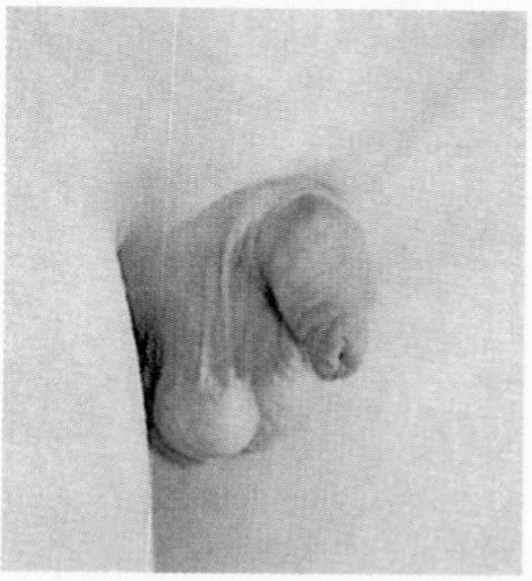	Pubic hair starting to develop. Appears as straight, long, and downy texture.	Little enlargement.	Both testes and scrotum enlarge. The scrotum begins to acquire darker skin tone and change in texture.
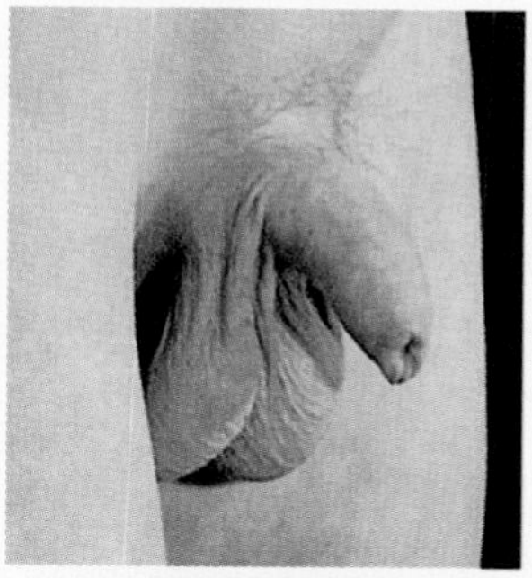	Increasing hair growth over entire pubic region. Hair is darker, curly, and beginning to become coarse.	Penis begins to enlarge. Enlargement is more in length than general size.	Growth and skin texture continue to develop.
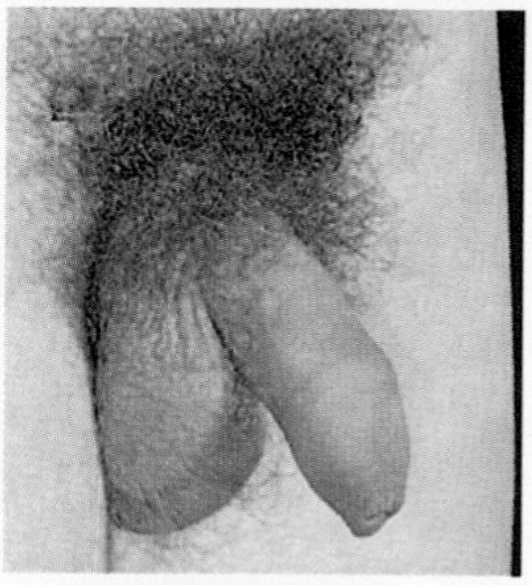	Hair is thick and coarse over entire pubic area.	Penis grows in both length and diameter. The glans also develops.	The scrotum is like the adult, with darker tone, and the testes are almost adult size.
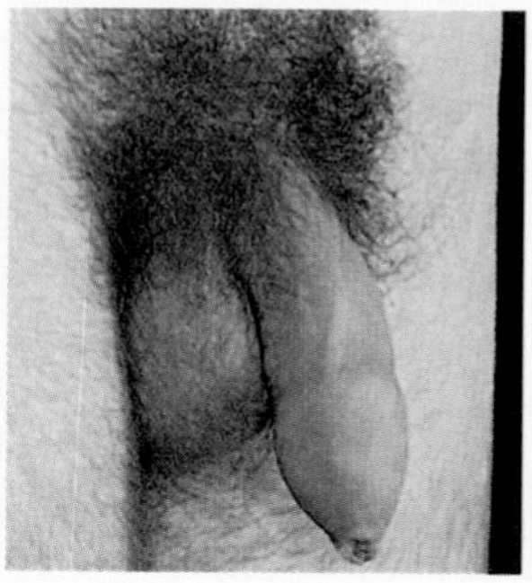	Mature pubic hair distribution, including on upper medial thighs.	Adult appearance of penis.	Full development and adult-appearing testes.

Photographs from Van Wieringen JC: *Growth diagrams 1965 Netherlands, second national survey on 0-24-year-olds*, Groningen, Netherlands, 1971, Wolters-Noordhoff. Reprinted by permission of Kluwer Academic Publishers.

Examination

Procedures and Techniques Genitalia assessment of the adolescent male is very important to ensure that the maturational development is progressing according to schedule. This is also the time when teen modesty is at its peak. The examiner must take time to develop a relationship with the client and reassure him in a matter-of-fact manner that the examination of the genitalia is an essential part of a complete examination. It is also vitally important to ensure privacy and adequate draping when the genitalia are not being examined. It is usually best to defer the examination of the genitalia to the last procedure of the examination.

To actually examine the genitalia and assess the inguinal area for a hernia, the client should be standing as instructed for the adult.

Normal and Abnormal Findings The normal findings are dependent on the maturational stage of the client. Review Table 22-2 for the expected and normal findings of the maturing male.

■ OLDER ADULTS

Anatomy and Physiology

Sexual activity tends to decline in frequency, correlating, as a rule, with the individual's frequency of sexual activity in youth. Erection may develop more slowly, and ejaculation may be less intense. Sperm viability is assumed to decrease, since the rate of conception has been observed to decline with age.

Hypertrophy of the prostate is the major change in the prostate associated with aging. If the prostate enlargement is significant, a decrease or obstruction of urinary flow will occur.

Health History

The older adult should be asked all of the same questions as for adult. In addition, ask the following questions that deal with issues specific to his age.

- As men get older, they may notice a change in sexual relationships or sexual response. It is normal for an erection to develop more slowly. It is not a sign of impotence. Have you noticed any changes you would like to discuss?

Rationale Sexual function continues throughout life, although aging and illness may produce changes. Most men welcome the opportunity to discuss sexual issues; this can be a time of education and encouragement. Some drugs depress sexual function—for example, antihypertensives, sedatives, tranquilizers, and alcohol.

Examination

Procedures and Techniques The approach to examining the male genitalia of the older adult is the same as for the younger adult.

Normal and Abnormal Findings Externally, pubic hair becomes finer and less abundant, sometimes leading to pubic alopecia. In addition, the scrotum becomes more pendulous. The scrotal sac of the client may appear elongated or pendulous. The client may actually have injury or excoriation of the scrotal sac surface secondary to sitting on the scrotum. The testes may feel slightly smaller and softer than in the younger client.

EXAMINATION SUMMARY

Male Genitalia

PROCEDURE

Pubic hair

- Inspect the pubic hair for:
  Distribution
  General characteristics

Penis

- Inspect and palpate the penis for:
  General characteristics
  Color
  Tenderness
  Discharge

Scrotum and Testes

- Inspect the scrotum for:
  Texture and general characteristics
  Color
  Asymmetry
- Palpate the scrotum for:
  Presence of testes
- Palpate the testes, epididymides, and vas deferens for:
  Location
  Consistency
  Tenderness
  Nodules
- ❖ Transilluminate the scrotum for evidence of:
  Fluid
  Masses

Inguinal Region

- Inspect both inguinal regions for:
  Bulges
- ❖ Palpate the inguinal canal for evidence of:
  Direct hernia
  Indirect hernia

SUMMARY OF FINDINGS

Age Group	Normal Findings	Typical Variations	Findings Associated With Disorders
Infants and children	• Transitory penile erections: Common in infants. • *Edema of newborn external genitalia:* Common, especially after breech delivery. • *Testicle of newborn:* Usually 1 cm in diameter. • *Newborn nonerect penis:* 2-3 cm in length. • Newborn scrotum: Without rugae and testes indicates preterm birth. • *Separation of prepuce from glans:* occurs between ages 3 and 6 years. • *Foreskin of noncircumcised males:* fully retractable by 3-4 years of age.	• *Small penis in infants:* May mean organ anomalies.	• *Bulge in inguinal area:* Suggests hernia. Mass may mean hydrocele. • In children, an enlarged penis without testicular enlargement may mean precocious puberty, adrenal hyperplasia, or central nervous system lesions. • *Hypospadias:* Congenital defect on ventral surface of glans, penile shaft, or perineal area. • *Epispadias:* defect on dorsum of penis.
Adolescents	• *Hormonal changes at puberty:* Cause straight hair to appear at base of penis, red scrotal skin color, and increased pendulous movement of scrotum.	• *During puberty:* The scrotum becomes more red and pen-dulous.	• Groin, inguinal, or testicular pain may be associated with masses due to sports injury or testicular cancer.
Adults	• *Pubic hair:* Darkens and curls and covers pubic area. • Prostate gland enlarges. • *Penis:* Enlarges in length and breadth. • *Pubic hair:* Diamond pattern. Dorsal vein apparent. • No masses or abnormalities visible.	• *Scrotum:* Normally more red in red-haired persons. • *Scrotal lumps:* May be caused from sebaceous cysts.	• Uncircumcised males may have balanoposthitis caused by unretractable foreskin. • *Balanitis:* Results from infection. • *Penile discharge:* Suggests inflammation or infection. • Pinpoint opening: suggests meatal stenosis. • Priapism is prolonged penile erection. It is often painful. • Thick scrotum from fluid is associated with disease. • *Irregular testis texture:* Sign of infection, cyst, or tumor. • *Beaded or lumpy vas deferens:* Suggests diabetes, tuberculosis, or inflammatory changes.
Older adults	• *Pubic hair:* With age, becomes finer and less abundant. • *Erection:* May develop more slowly, and ejaculation may be less intense.	• *Scrotum:* Becomes more pendulous.	

HEALTH PROMOTION

GENITAL SELF EXAMINATION (GSE)

There are two main reasons for teaching GSE. The first is that testicular cancer is the most common type of cancer in young men. The second is that it is an excellent way to identify sexually transmitted infection, especially for clients who are frequently sexually active or who have multiple sexual partners. Every man from puberty onward should be asked if he routinely examines his own genitalia and, if so, what he actually does and how he does it. Following are the guidelines:

1. Instruct the client to take his penis in his hand and examine the tip for any evidence of swelling, sores, blisters, or discharge from the tip. If the client is not circumcised, instruct him to retract the foreskin so that the glans may be adequately examined. Uncircumcised males should also be instructed to especially examine the area of the junction between the foreskin and the glans.

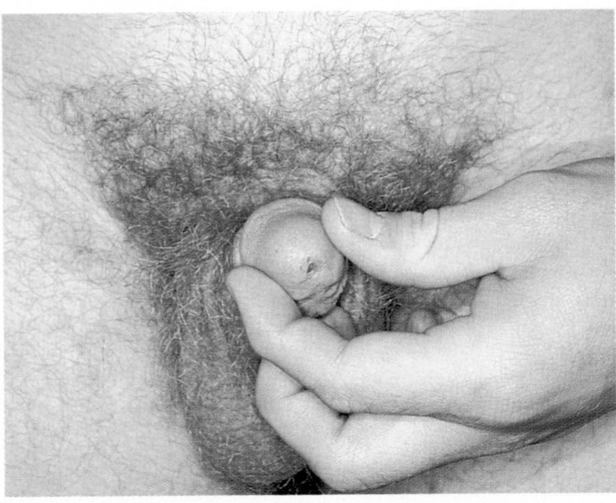

2. Next, instruct the client to palpate the entire shaft of the penis. Instruct him to examine all areas and all surfaces around the entire shaft from the base to the tip. He should feel for lumps, tenderness, and swelling.

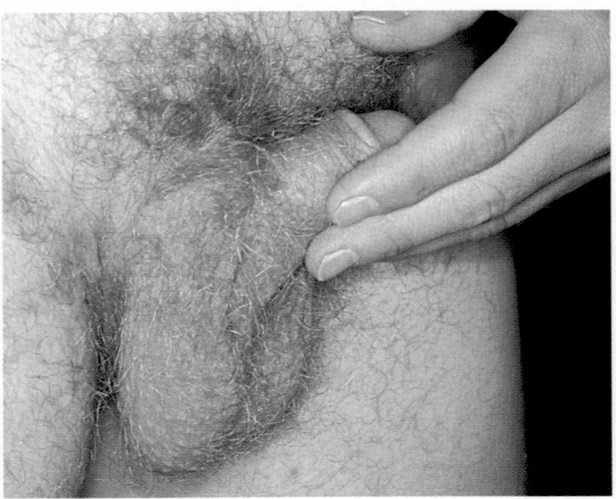

3. Finally, instruct the client to examine his scrotum and testes. To do this, tell him to use the hand on the opposite side from the testicle being examined to lift his penis up and out of the way. First inspect the scrotum for color, texture, and evidence of swelling. Then, with the available hand, gently palpate the scrotum for evidence of lumps, tenderness, or swelling.

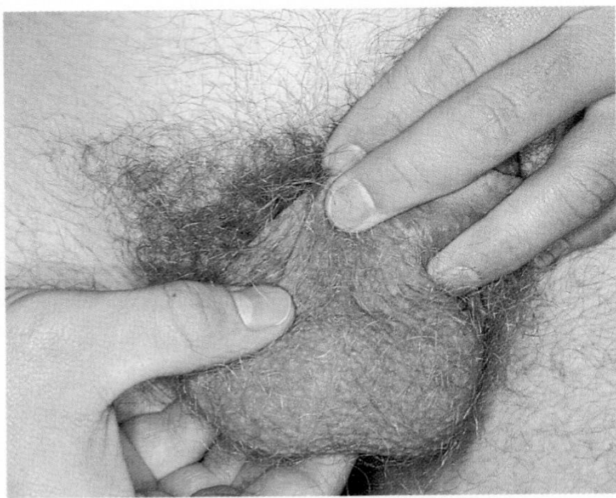

4. Instruct the client to change hands and palpate the other side of the scrotum with the other hand.

Instruct the client to examine himself when he is in the shower or in front of the mirror. The frequency of examination should be at least monthly. If the client is sexually active and is at high risk for infection, he should examine himself more frequently.

PERSONAL PROTECTION FOR SEXUALLY ACTIVE MALES

Personal protection for men is just as important as it is for women. First, a condom will function as a barrier to prevent the transmission of semen and seminal fluid to the client's sexual partner. Second, it will protect the client, as well as the client's partner, from direct tissue-to-tissue contact, thus decreasing the chance of the exposure of sexually transmitted infection, including AIDS.

The client should be educated about the transmission of sexually transmitted infection and the risk of acquiring such an infection if no personal protection is used. All sexually active males, especially young men, should be taught of their equal responsibility during sexual relations to prevent an unwanted pregnancy.

Assess the client's knowledge about how to apply a condom and, if necessary, use a penis model to actually demonstrate the method of putting a condom on the erect penis. In addition, teach the client that the condom is a single-use item that should be discarded after use.

COMMON PROBLEMS AND CONDITIONS

Male Genitalia

INGUINAL AREA

Hernia

A hernia is a protrusion of part of the peritoneal-lined sac through the abdominal wall. Three types of hernias are commonly found when examining the inguinal area of the genitalia. These are the indirect inguinal hernia (Fig. 22-12, *A*), the direct inguinal hernia (Fig. 22-12, *B*), and the femoral hernia (Fig. 22-12, *C*). See Table 22-1 (earlier in this chapter) for comparison of the common types of hernias.

PENIS

Urethritis

Urethritis is a condition characterized by painful burning during urination and purulent urethral discharge. The edges of the urethra are often swollen and reddened; the urine may appear cloudy. Asymptomatic urethritis may occur as well. This condition has significance because many of these cases are caused by STI. Gonorrhea and chlamydia should be ruled out in men with symptoms.

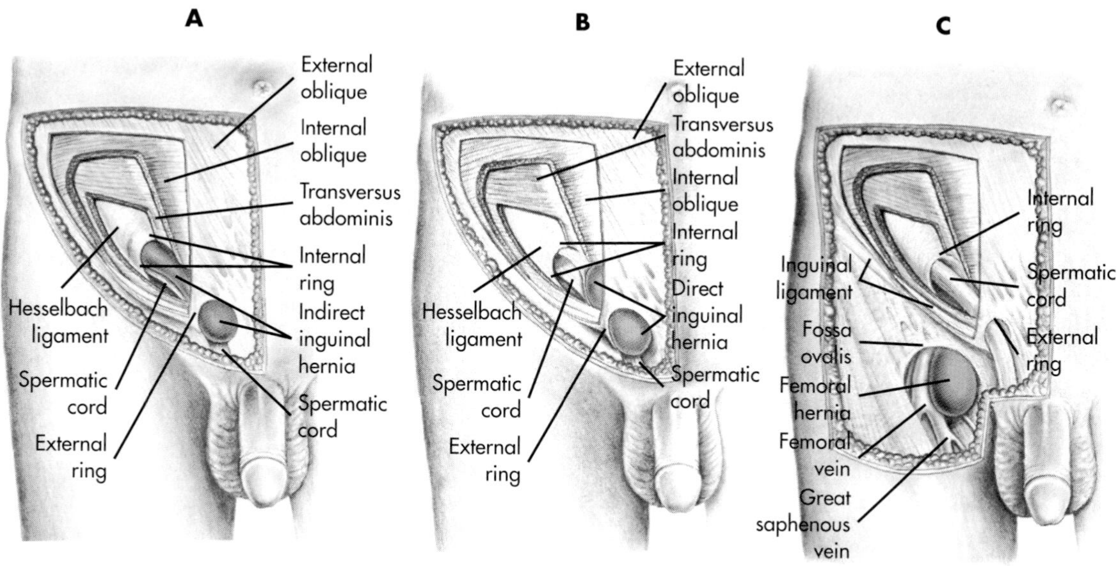

Fig. 22-12 Anatomy of region of common pelvic hernias. **A,** Indirect inguinal hernia. **B,** Direct inguinal hernia. **C,** Femoral hernia. (From Seidel et al, 1999.)

Phimosis

This is a condition in which the foreskin of the penis is constricted at the opening, making retraction difficult or impossible (Fig. 22-13). In an adult, it is frequently associated with adhesions secondary to recurrent inflammation and infection, although in some individuals, this is congenital. Prolonged phimosis caused by chronic inflammation and irritation is associated with penile cancer.

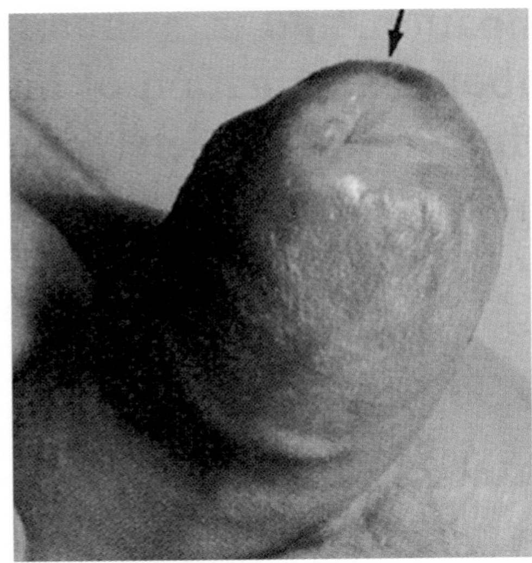

Fig. 22-13 Phimosis. (From *400 Self-assessment picture tests in clinical medicine,* 1984. By permission of Mosby International.)

Paraphimosis

In this painful condition, the foreskin of the penis is retracted at the base of the glans and it cannot be relaxed into its normal position (Fig. 22-14). It may occur after sexual intercourse, masturbation, after rigorous cleaning, or after insertion procedures such as catheter insertion or cystoscopy if the foreskin is not returned to normal position. If the foreskin remains retracted, the glans swells in response to impeded circulation.

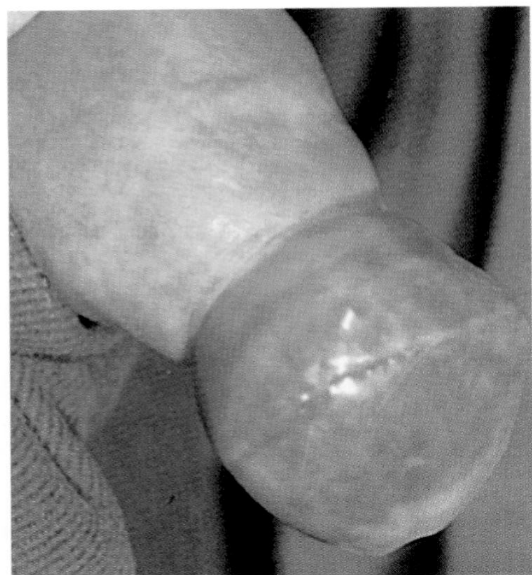

Fig. 22-14 Paraphimosis. (From Lloyd-Davies et al, 1994.)

Balanitis

Balanitis is an inflammation of the glans penis and the mucous membrane beneath it (Fig. 22-15). This condition is commonly associated with phimosis. It is a condition only seen in uncircumcised men. It is caused by bacterial or fungal infections and most commonly affects men with diabetes mellitus.

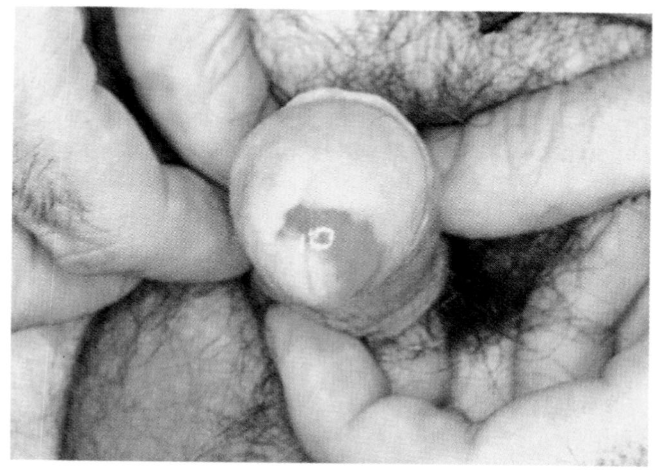

Fig. 22-15 Balanitis. (From Lloyd-Davies et al, 1994.)

Carcinoma

Cancer of the penis is a rare skin cancer occurring most often in older, uncircumcised males who have suffered chronic irritation and who have had poor hygiene habits. Early lesions may appear as dry, wartlike painless lesions on the penis or foreskin; as the lesion progresses it may appear as an ulceration (Fig. 22-16).

RISK FACTORS

COMMON RISK FACTORS ASSOCIATED WITH Cancer of the Penis

- Not circumcised
- Chronic poor hygiene care
- Repeated infections, including condyloma acuminatum (genital warts)

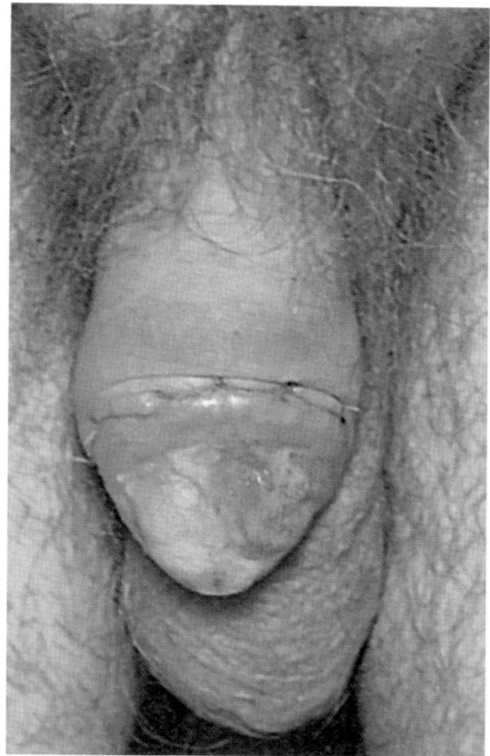

Fig. 22-16 Cancer of the penis. (From Lloyd-Davies et al, 1994.)

SCROTUM/TESTICLES

Testicular torsion

This condition occurs when a testicle and spermatic cord twist, cutting off blood supply. It occurs most frequently in children and adolescents and is considered a surgical emergency. It is not associated with any physical activity or trauma; common history includes a sudden onset of scrotal swelling and severe pain. The testicle becomes very tender, and the scrotum becomes swollen and often slightly discolored.

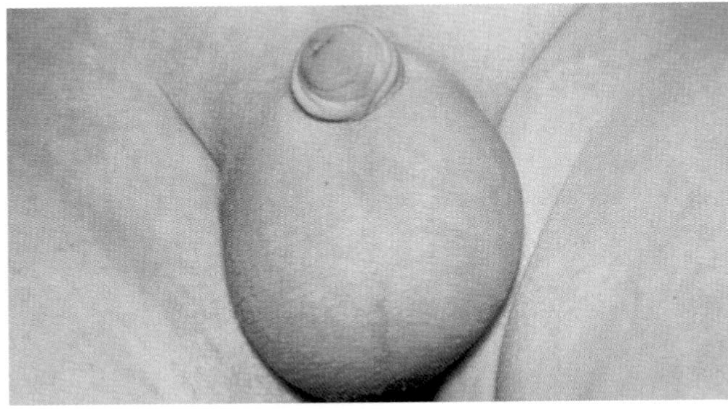

Fig. 22-17 Bilateral congenital hydroceles. Groin swellings are absent, distinguishing them from hernias. (From Zitelli and Davis, 1997.)

Hydrocele

A hydrocele results from fluid accumulation in the tunica vaginalis (Fig. 22-17). The scrotum appears enlarged and, when transilluminated, will have a light red glow that indicates the presence of fluid. The condition is most frequent during early infancy and will usually resolve on its own. If it fails to resolve, surgical correction may be necessary.

Spermatocele

A spermatocele is a sperm-containing cyst that occurs in the epididymis (Fig. 22-18). It will cause significant swelling in the involved testicle. Because the lesion is a cyst, it will transilluminate.

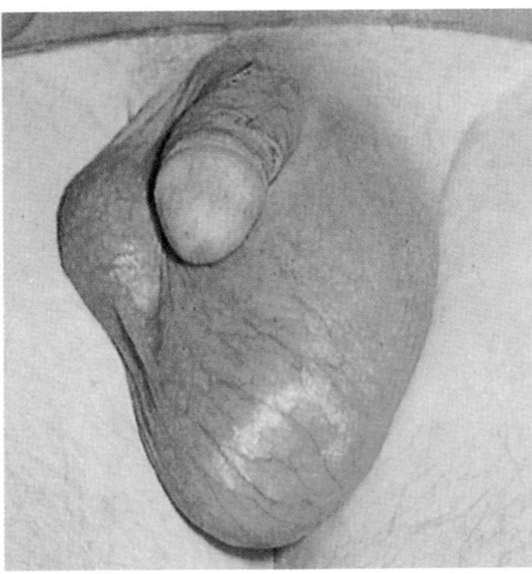

Fig. 22-18 Spermatocele. (From Lloyd-Davies et al, 1994.)

Varicocele

This condition is caused by an abnormal dilation and tortuosity of the veins along the spermatic cord (Fig. 22-19). The client may describe a pulling sensation or a dull ache or have scrotal pain. It occurs in boys and young men and most often affects the left side. If untreated, this condition causes reduced fertility secondary to increased testicular pressure.

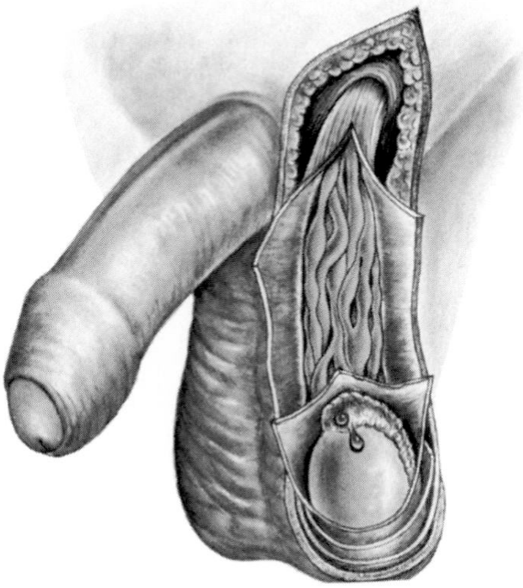

Fig. 22-19 Varicocele. (From Seidel et al, 1999.)

Epididymitis

Epididymitis is a condition, associated with inflammation to the epididymis and vas deferens. It is usually caused by infection, although other causes such as trauma or urinary reflux have been reported. This condition causes the scrotum to become erythematous and the epididymis to become very edematous and tender (Fig. 22-20). Among sexually active men under the age of 35, this condition is most commonly associated with sexually transmitted infections (chlamydia and gonorrhea). Among homosexual men who are insertive partners in anal intercourse, *Escherichia coli* is commonly the identified organism causing infection (CDC, 1998).

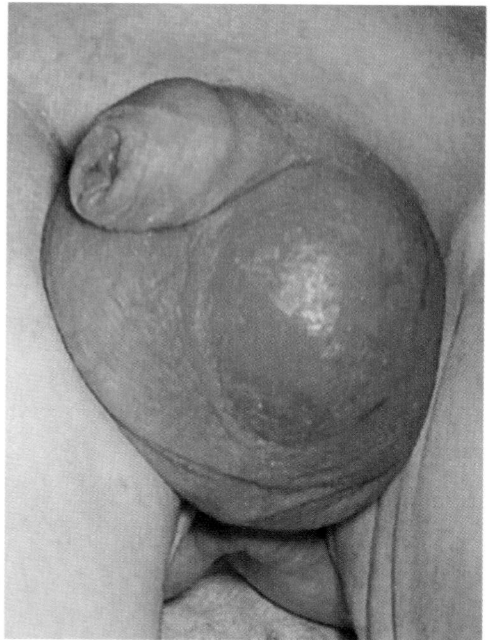

Fig. 22-20 Epididymitis. (From Lloyd-Davies et al, 1994.)

SEXUALLY TRANSMITTED INFECTION

Herpes Genitalis

Herpes is a sexually transmitted viral infection caused by the herpes simplex virus. Herpes simplex virus 1 (HSV1) and herpes simplex virus 2 (HSV2) are two different antigen subtypes of the herpes simplex virus. HSV1 is more commonly associated with gingivostomatitis and oral ulcers whereas HSV2 is usually associated with genital lesions. However, both virus types can be transmitted to both sites through sexual and oral-sexual contact (Box 22-4). This is a chronic, noncurable condition with exacerbation and relapses. The typical clinical manifestations for males include lesions that appear anywhere along the shaft of the penis or near the glans (Fig. 22-21). The lesion is identified because of the red superficial vesicles that are frequently quite painful. It is important to note that many individuals with HSV2 are unaware they have an infection because they have very mild symptoms. Many times transmission of this infection occurs unknowingly by either partner. Use of condoms may significantly reduce transmission of this infection (CDC, 1998).

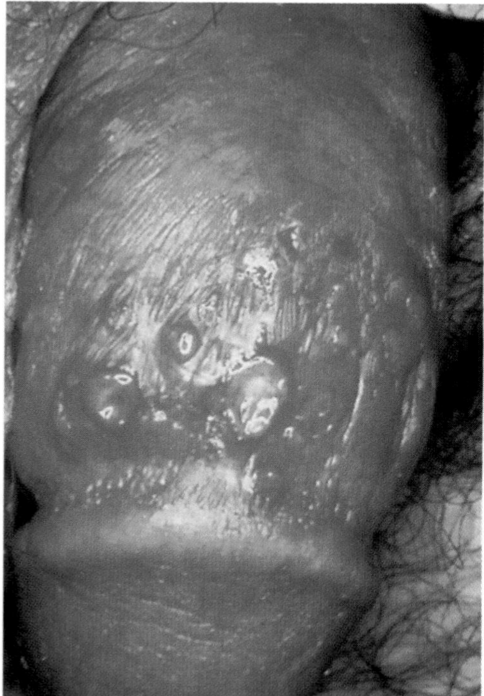

Fig. 22-21 Genital herpes on the penis. (From Grimes, 1991.)

Box 22-4 Clinical Note

Sexually transmitted infection can occur on the genitalia and rectum and in the oral cavity. Furthermore, an STI can concurrently occur in more than one location. Therefore, if an STI is suspected, examination in the other areas is also warranted.

Condyloma Acuminatum (Genital Warts)

This condition is characterized by lesions caused by the human papillomavirus (HPV) commonly found on the glans, the shaft of the penis, within the urethra, or around the anus (Fig. 22-22). As with females, HPV infection in males is associated with early onset of sexual activity, multiple sex partners, and infrequent use of barrier protection. The individual may acquire carcinoma of the penis as a secondary change of these lesions.

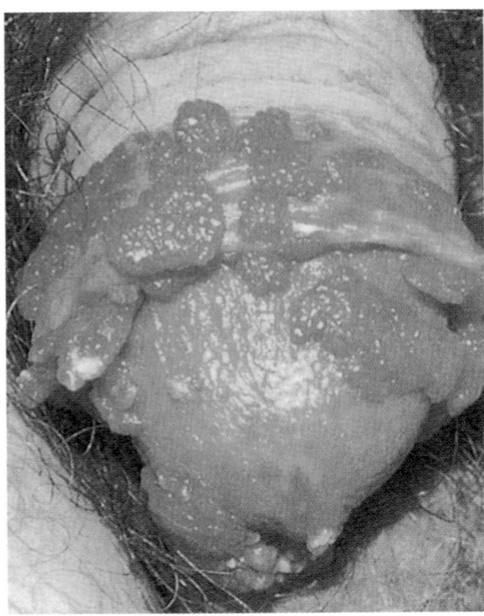

Fig. 22-22 Condyloma acuminatum (genital warts). (From *Diagnostic picture tests in clinical medicine,* 1984. By permission of Mosby International.)

Chlamydia Trachomatis

Chlamydia is the most common sexually transmitted infection in the United States. Men and women under the age of 25 account for the majority of individuals with chlamydia infections. In men, this infection usually occurs in the urethra, but it can also affect the rectum. The most common symptoms with urethral infection include dysuria, discharge, and urethral itch. If untreated, urethral infection can spread to the epididymis and cause epididymitis (Ferreira, 1997). Diagnosis can be made by culture, by Gram's stain of urethral discharge, or from DNA probes used for screening.

Gonorrhea

Gonorrhea is caused by the aerobic, gram-negative diplococcus *Neisseria gonorrhoeae.* It is currently the most frequently reported sexually transmitted disease in the United States. If untreated, gonorrhea can lead to epididymitis. Most infections among men produce symptoms causing them to seek medical attention. The common clinical manifestation of gonorrhea is urethritis. Specific clinical findings include mucopurulent or purulent discharge and dysuria (CDC, 1998). A microscopic examination of Gram's-stained urethral secretions can detect gonorrhea infections with a high degree of accuracy. As an alternative, many clinics are using DNA probes and enzyme immunoassays for diagnostic screening (U.S. Preventive Services Task Force, 1996).

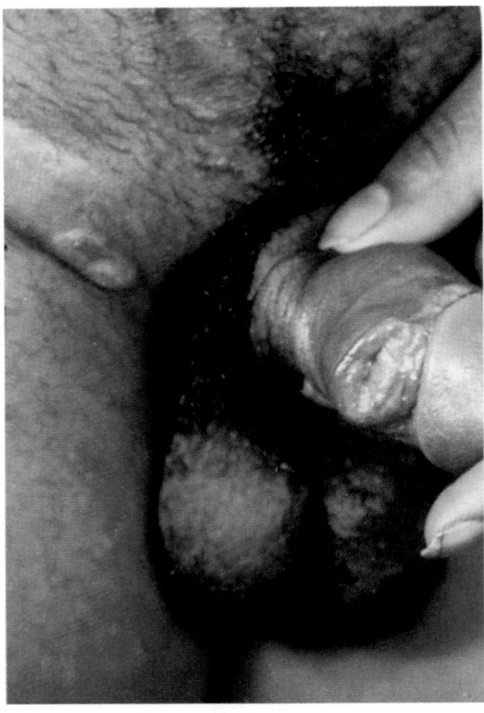

Fig. 22-23 Syphilis chancre on the penis. (From Grimes, 1991.)

Syphilis

This STI is caused by *Treponema pallidum,* which is transmitted congenitally or by sexual contact. Syphilis lesions may occur during the primary or secondary phase. The primary syphilis lesion is called a chancre (Fig. 22-23). It occurs about 2 weeks after exposure and appears as a painless ulcerated lesion with indurated borders. The most frequent location for the lesion is on the glans of the penis, although it can also occur in the mouth or anus. Diagnosis during these stages may be made based on clinical findings and by direct fluorescent antibody test of lesion exudate or by serologic tests for syphilis.

Pediculosis Pubis (Crabs, Pubic Lice)

Pubic lice is a parasitic infection transmitted by close physical contact. Infection is characterized by complaints of severe pruritus in the perineal area. Clients may also notice the lice and/or nits (eggs) in the pubic hair. Examination findings include excoriation and area of erythema; on close inspection the lice and nits can be seen—they will appear as small dark spots.

CLINICAL APPLICATION and CRITICAL THINKING

SAMPLE DOCUMENTATION

CASE 1

A.R. is a 1-month-old male infant with swollen scrotum.

Subjective Data

Mother states infant's scrotum swollen. Swelling first noticed a few days ago. The mother indicates the baby does not seem to be in pain, but is worried that something is seriously wrong. Mother reports no problems with urination; uses 6 to 8 diapers per day. There is no history of injury. Mother verbalizes guilt that this may be a serious problem, and she did not bring baby in for evaluation sooner. States she is feeling overwhelmed with new infant and trying to also care for two other young children.

Objective Data

Weight, 8 ½ lb (birth weight 7 lb, 4 oz); Temperature, 98.4° F (36.9° C). Pulse, 112 beats/min; Respiratory rate, 32.

General appearance: Uncircumcised penis without lesions or discoloration. Urethral opening centered. Foreskin retracts slightly over glans without difficulty. Hygiene—clean. Right scrotum enlarged, firm, and smooth.

Transillumination of scrotum: Scrotal sac has moderate amount of illumination around shadowing of testes; appears to be fluid accumulation in the tunica vaginalis.

Palpation: Penis and scrotum nontender to palpation. Testicles present in scrotal sac bilaterally. No evidence of masses.

Functional Health Patterns Involved

- Role–relationship
- Cognitive–perceptual

Medical Diagnosis

Hydrocele.

Nursing Diagnosis and Collaborative Problems

- *Altered parenting* related to perceived ability to parent as manifested by:
  - Statements by mother regarding inability to take care of baby
  - Newborn baby with two other young children in home
- *Knowledge deficit* related to treatment for hydrocele as manifested by:
  - Mother verbalizes guilt regarding failure to seek medical attention immediately
  - Mother verbalizes fear this is a very serious problem

CASE 2

J.F. is a 24-year-old man with complaint of dysuria and discharge from penis.

Subjective Data

J.F. states yesterday noticed small amount of yellow staining in undershorts, then noted a small amount of discharge from penis just before urination. Urination is described as painful. Had sexual intercourse with prostitute 3 days ago. Does not use personal protection during intercourse; states he finds condoms uncomfortable. Has several female partners sexually involved with; four different partners in last month. No previous infections or problems associated with the genitalia.

Objective Data

General characteristics: Pubic hair distribution is diamond shaped with hair extension to umbilicus. Skin intact and without lesions.

Penis: Circumcised penis with urethral opening centered at distal tip. Penis without lesions. Small amount milky discharge noted when tip of penis was compressed. Specimen taken for Gram's stain and DNA probe screening. No masses or tenderness identified with penis shaft palpation.

Scrotum/Testes: Scrotum well shaped; left side slightly lower than right. Skin is even, dark rose color without lesions. Scrotum and testes are smooth and without tenderness, swelling, or masses.

Inguinal region: No lymph nodes are palpable. Inguinal canals without bulges or tenderness bilaterally.

Functional Health Patterns Involved

- Health perception–health management
- Nutrition–metabolic
- Cognitive–perceptual

Medical Diagnosis

Gonorrhea.

Nursing Diagnosis and Collaborative Problems

- *Pain* related to inflammation of urethra as manifested by:
  - Discomfort with urination.
- *Altered health maintenance* related to lack of barrier protection as manifested by:
  - Statement that he does not use condoms
- *Risk for infection transmission* related to highly contagious pathogens as manifested by:
  - Multiple sex partners
  - High-risk sex partners.
  - Lack of use of barrier protection.
- *PC:* Epididymitis

CRITICAL THINKING QUESTIONS

1. A 30-year-old man requests information regarding self-examination of his genitalia. What information should the examiner share with him?
2. When the examiner attempts to examine the genitalia of a 5-year-old boy, the boy refuses to take off his pants and says, "You can't see my privates." What measures can the examiner take to facilitate this part of the exam?
3. A college student is seen at the student health service for a sexually transmitted infection. What information should be shared with him regarding use of barrier protection?
4. The parents of a newborn infant request information regarding circumcision. What information should be shared with them to help them make a decision regarding their infant?

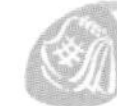

CASE STUDY

Mr. Corazza is a 43-year-old man who presents to the urgent care center. Listed below are data collected by the examiner.

Interview Data

Mr. Corazza tells the nurse, "Yesterday I noticed a painful area in my groin. When I looked, I saw this area of swelling." The examiner asks about recent activity. Mr. Corazza replies, "We have been in the process of moving, and I have been picking up heavy boxes, moving furniture, and have been up and down ladders all weekend."

Examination Data

- **General survey**: Healthy-appearing man.
- **Examination**: Bulge noted in area of Hesselbach triangle that is painless. Inguinal area on right side with palpable mass. Pushes against side of finger on examination.

1. What data deviate from normal findings, suggesting a need for further investigation?
2. What additional information should the nurse ask or assess for?
3. In what functional health patterns does data deviate from normal?
4. What nursing diagnosis and/or collaborative problems should be considered for this situation?

23 Anus, Rectum, and Prostate

REMEMBER to check out your companion CD-ROM

www.mosby.com/MERLIN/wilson/assessment/

ANATOMY AND PHYSIOLOGY

The anus, rectum, and prostate are dealt with as a unit in this chapter because the prostate gland is examined in conjunction with the anus and rectum in the male. In the female, the rectum is usually examined in conjunction with the pelvic examination.

RECTUM, ANAL CANAL, AND ANUS

The rectum and anus are the terminal structures of the gastrointestinal (GI) tract (Fig. 23-1). The rectum lies anterior to the sacrum and coccyx. The proximal end of the rectum lies at the distal end of the sigmoid colon and extends down for approximately 4 ¾ inches (12 cm) to the anorectal junction. The anal canal extends 1 to 1½ inches (2.5 to 4 cm) from the anorectal junction to the exterior opening, the anus.

The rectum is lined with columns of epithelium. Three semilunar folds called rectal valves lie within the rectal wall and extend across half the circumference of the rectal lumen. The function of these valves is not well understood but is thought to support feces while allowing flatus to pass. The lowest of these valves can be palpated with digital examination.

The anal canal is lined with mucous membranes arranged in longitudinal folds called anal columns that contain a network of arteries and veins (frequently referred to as the internal hemorrhoidal plexus). Between each of the columns is a recessed area called the anal crypt into which the perianal glands empty. Surrounding the anal canal are two concentric rings of muscle, the internal and external sphincters. The internal sphincter consists of smooth muscle and is under involuntary control. The external sphincter consists of skeletal muscle and is under voluntary control. The external sphincter allows for control of defecation. The lower portion of the anal canal is sensitive to painful stimuli, whereas the upper half is relatively insensitive.

The anus is hairless, moist mucosal tissue surrounded by hyperpigmented perianal skin. Normally the anus is closed except during defecation.

PROSTATE

The prostate gland of the male contributes to the production of ejaculatory fluid. It lies inferior to (below) the urinary bladder and surrounds the upper portion of the urethra (Fig. 23-2). It is approximately the size of a chestnut ($4 \times 2.5 \times 2$ cm or $1\frac{1}{2} \times 1\frac{1}{4} \times \frac{3}{4}$ inches).

The posterior surface of the prostate lies adjacent to the anterior rectal wall. Two of the three prostate lobes are palpable through the rectum (right and left vertical lobes). These lobes are divided by a slight groove known as the median sulcus.

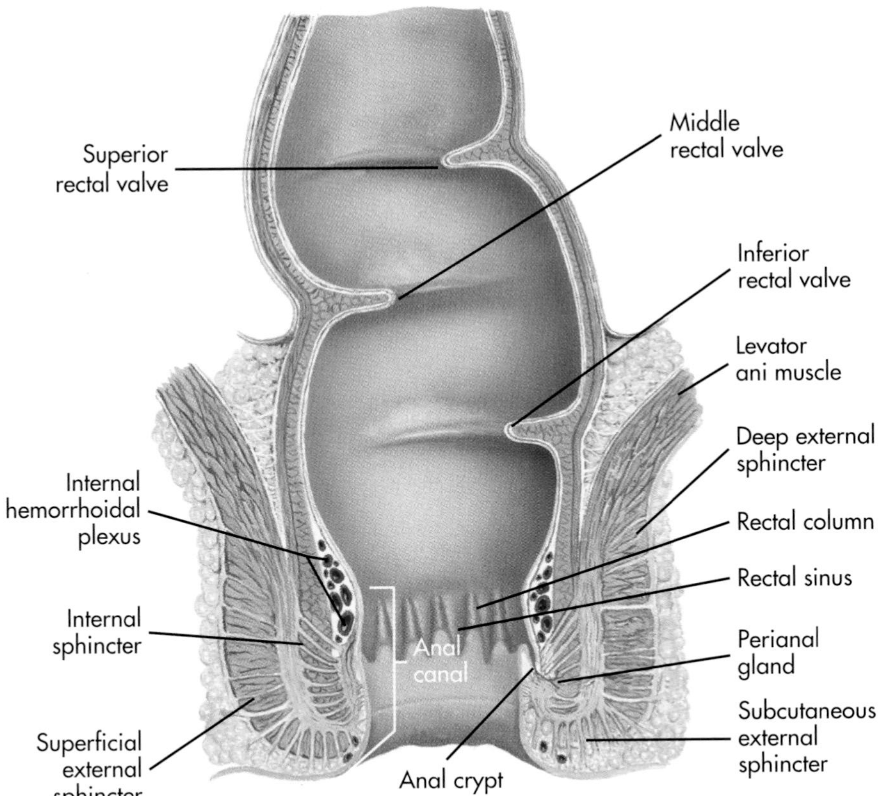

Fig. 23-1 Anatomy of the anus and rectum. (From Seidel et al, 1999.)

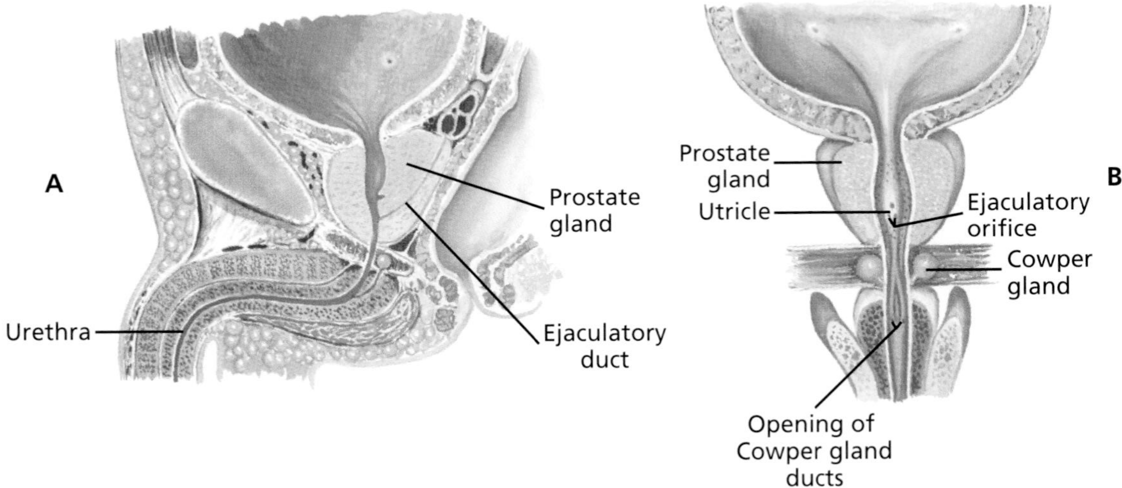

Fig. 23-2 Anatomy of the prostate gland and seminal vesicles. **A,** Lateral view. **B,** Cross section. (From Seidel et al, 1999.)

HEALTH HISTORY

Anus, Rectum, and Prostate

QUESTIONS | RATIONALE

PRESENT HEALTH STATUS

➤ How would you describe your overall health?

■ Determine clients' perception of their overall health. This may provide clues as to diagnosed or undiagnosed chronic conditions.

➤ Do you have any chronic illnesses? If so, describe.

■ Some chronic illness such as ulcerative colitis or Crohn's disease may cause rectal bleeding accompanied by increased mucus production and abdominal cramping.

➤ What medication are you currently taking? Do you use laxatives or stool softeners? How often? Which ones? Do you take iron supplements?

■ Many medications have side effects that can affect bowel elimination patterns and/or the characteristics of the stool. Use of stool softeners or laxatives is common. Assess for chronic use or reliance on laxatives to have a bowel movement.

➤ Briefly describe your diet. Do you routinely eat high-fiber foods such as apples or other fruits, cereals and whole-grain breads, and vegetables? What types of beverages do you drink? Approximately how much fluid do you drink each day?

■ Bowel function is affected by variables, including fluid or bulk in the diet. Note that high-fiber foods should be encouraged to lower cholesterol levels, fight obesity, stabilize blood sugar levels, and relieve certain gastrointestinal disturbances. Insoluble-fiber foods (e.g., cereals and wheat germ) reduce the risk of colon cancer.

Bowel Elimination Pattern

➤ Describe your pattern of bowel movements. How often do you have a bowel movement? Are your bowel movements regular? How would you describe your stool? Hard? Soft? Usual color?

■ Establish what the regular bowel routine is for the client. Remember, frequency and consistency of stool varies among individuals, so it is important to determine what is "normal" for each individual client.

➤ Do you ever use an assistive device such as enema to help you move your bowels? If so, what product do you use? How often?

■ Occasional use of an enema to assist with bowel elimination is common. Assess for chronic use or reliance on enemas to have a bowel movement.

➤ Do you rely on morning coffee, tea, or nicotine to stimulate a bowel movement?

■ Many individuals rely on morning coffee, tea, or nicotine to stimulate a bowel movement.

Anal Sex

➤ Do you ever engage in anal sex? If so, how often? Men: Are you the recipient? Does this include oral-anal or genital-anal sex?

■ Determine pattern of sexual behavior. Cross infections from mouth, anus, and genitalia can occur.

QUESTIONS

RATIONALE

➤ How many partners have you had in the last year? Do you use lubrication? Condoms?

■ Identify clients who are at high risk for STI (see Chapters 21 and 22). Clients should be questioned about safe-sex practices. Those engaging in anal sex should always use lubricant. Condom breakage may occur with anal sex, especially when lubricant is not used.

➤ Does the sex include use of inanimate objects inserted into the anus/rectum? If so, what types of objects are used?

■ Foreign objects can contribute to loss of anal sphincter tone, especially with frequent use of large objects. If foreign objects become stuck, the client may seek medical care with a chief complaint of rectal pain.

PAST MEDICAL HISTORY

➤ Have you ever had a digital rectal examination? Visual examination of the rectum (sigmoidoscopy)? If yes, when? What was the purpose of the examination? What were the results?

■ Establish health care practice by assessing for routine screening and/or examination. Consider cancer risk factors.

➤ Have you ever been diagnosed with a medical condition related to your rectum? (e.g., hemorrhoids, warts, polyp, infection) If so, what was this? When? How was it treated?
➤ Have you ever had cancer? If so, when? Where? How was it treated?
➤ Men: Have you ever had a prostate-specific antigen (PSA) blood test? If so, when was this done last? What were the results?
➤ Men: Have you ever had a problem with your prostate, such as an enlarged prostate, infection of the prostate (prostatitis), or cancer?

■ Identify preexisting or previous problems. Determine what treatment the client received, if any. Assess for risk factors for colorectal cancer and prostate cancer (see Risk Factors box).

RISK FACTORS

COMMON RISK FACTORS ASSOCIATED WITH Colorectal and Prostate Cancer

COLORECTAL CANCER

Age: Risk significantly increases with age after 55
Race: Alaskan native
Diet: High in fat, low in fiber
Personal history: Cancer (metastasis most frequently from ovarian, breast, endometrial cancers), polyps in the rectum or colon, inflammatory bowel disease (ulcerative colitis for longer than 10 years) and Crohn's disease.
Family history: One or more first degree relatives with colorectal cancer. (American Cancer Society, 1998; U.S. Department of Health and Human Services, 1998.)

PROSTATE CANCER

Age: Risk increases with age; highest incidence between 60 and 80 years
Race: African American
Diet: High in fat, low in fiber
Family history: Prostate cancer
(Goolsby, 1998; Parker et al, 1998)

Data from American Cancer Society: *Cancer facts and figures,* Atlanta, 1998, The Society; Goolsby MJ: Screening, diagnosis, and management of prostate cancer: improving primary care outcomes, *Nurse Pract* 23(3):11, 1998; Parker SL et al: Cancer statistics by race and ethnicity, *CA Cancer J Clin* 48(1):31, 1998.

QUESTIONS

RATIONALE

FAMILY HISTORY

➤ Has anyone in your family had colon or rectal cancer? Polyps in the rectum or colon? Inflammatory bowel disease?

■ A family history of colon cancer increases a person's risk of colon cancer.

➤ Men: Has anyone in your family had prostate cancer?

■ A family history of prostate cancer increases a person's risk of prostate cancer.

PROBLEM-BASED HISTORY

The most commonly reported problems related to the rectum, anus, and prostate include constipation/diarrhea, pain, bleeding, and changes in urinary flow. As with symptoms in all areas of assessment, a symptom analysis is completed, which includes the location, quality, quantity, chronology, setting, associated manifestation, alleviating factors, and aggravating factors (see Box 4-2 in Chapter 4).

Change in Bowel Function

➤ Have you noticed a change in your bowel movements? If so, when did it start? Did it start suddenly or gradually? Have you had a dietary change? Activity change? Stressful life change? Recently stopped smoking?

■ Changes in bowel function can be related to a large number of factors, including changes in diet, activity, stress, and medications the client may be taking. In all cases, it is important to sort out the variables involved in the bowel habit changes.

➤ Describe the change in your bowel function. Has it been a change in number of stools per day? Consistency? Presence of mucus or blood? Odor? Color? Frothy-appearing stool? Pain associated with your bowel movements?

■ Complete a symptom analysis to best understand the problem. Stools that are clay colored indicate a lack of bile pigment, suggesting obstruction of bile flow from the gallbladder or liver disease. Frothy-appearing stool is referred to as steatorrhea and is caused by malabsorption of fat.

➤ Have you had other symptoms such as increased gas (flatus), pain, fever, nausea, vomiting, abdominal pain or cramping, diarrhea, or discomfort after eating? Have you noted any connection with specific foods? Does anyone else in your family have the same symptoms?

■ Change in bowel elimination is often related to foods eaten. Some foods are commonly associated with increased flatus. Some foods can cause GI symptoms in individuals because of food intolerance. If nausea, vomiting, fever, and/or diarrhea occur, particularly if concurrent with other family members, this may suggest a virus or food poisoning.

Rectal Bleeding

➤ Do you have, or have you ever had, bloody or black stools? If so, when did you first become aware of this?

■ Determine onset and duration of the problem.

QUESTIONS | **RATIONALE**

➤ Describe the color of the blood. Bright red? Dark red? Black and tarry? How much blood have you noticed? Just a spot? A great deal? Did it fill the toilet bowl with red? Have you noticed an odd odor accompanying the bloody stool?

■ Determine characteristics of the bleeding. Bleeding from high in the intestinal tract will produce black, tarry stools, whereas bleeding near the rectum will produce bright red bleeding. Black stools may result from occult blood or melena caused by gastrointestinal bleeding; these stools are generally tarry. Black, nontarry stools may occur with certain medications such as iron supplementation. Red blood in stools usually occurs with gastrointestinal bleeding or bleeding in the area around the rectum and anus.

➤ Have you noticed the presence of mucus in the stools in addition to the blood? Have you had accompanying abdominal cramping or pain?

■ Identify associated symptoms. Some conditions such as ulcerative colitis can cause rectal bleeding accompanied by increased mucus production and abdominal cramping.

➤ Have you experienced any other symptoms such as fatigue?

■ Fatigue is a significant finding in clients complaining of rectal bleeding as this may indicate an anemic condition secondary to the rectal bleeding.

Rectal Pain

➤ Do you ever experience rectal pain? If so, when did you first notice this? Is the pain constant, or does it come and go? Is the pain localized in the rectal area, or does it occur elsewhere?

■ Complete a symptom analysis. Determine onset, location, and duration of the pain.

➤ How severe is the pain? On a scale of 1 to 10, how would you rate the pain? Does the rectal pain interfere with your routine daily activities?

■ Determine the client's perception of the severity of the pain.

➤ Does anything seem to make the pain worse? Activity or having a bowel movement? What seems to reduce the pain—if anything?

■ Rectal pain associated with bowel movements suggests hemorrhoids, fissures, or constipation. Also consider the possibility of a foreign object causing pain. Determine if certain positions or self-treatment have been effective in pain relief.

➤ Do you think you have hemorrhoids? If so, do they bleed? What have you done, if anything, to treat them?

■ Hemorrhoids are a very common cause of rectal pain. Clients who have had them before may recognize the symptoms. It is important to determine what the client has done for self-treatment.

➤ Do you have or have you had sores on your anus or on the skin around your anus? If so, what does it (did it) look like?

■ Some sexually transmitted infections may produce sores or lesions causing rectal pain. Many clients will inspect their own perineal area and notice sores or lesions.

Rectal Itching, Burning, Stinging

➤ Do you currently have any rectal burning, itching, or stinging? If so, what is it associated with? Bowel movements? Hemorrhoids? Bathing? Use of medications such as hemorrhoid preparations? Do you ever notice that there is bleeding associated with the problem?

■ Rectal burning, itching, or stinging may also be associated with a number of factors, including poor hygiene, hemorrhoids, and parasites such as pinworms.

➤ What have you done to decrease the problem? Has it helped?

■ Most clients will attempt self-treatment before seeking professional care.

QUESTIONS | RATIONALE

Fecal Incontinence

➤ Do you ever soil your underwear? If so, how often does this occur? When did it begin?

■ Determine onset of the problem.

➤ Why do you think that it is happening? Is it that you cannot make it to the restroom in time, or is it that you are unaware that you are becoming incontinent of stool? Does it interfere with routine activities?

■ Client may have understanding of the problem. Incontinence of stool may be associated with neurologic dysfunction, or it may be due to poor sphincter control or a gastrointestinal bowel problem. Prolapsed hemorrhoids may cause the client to have mucoid discharge and soiled underwear.

➤ What have you done about it?

■ Assess self-treatment measures. This may impact future treatment strategies.

Prostate-Related Discomfort (Male Clients)

➤ Have you noticed a change in your urinary function? If so, describe. When did this begin?

■ Prostate problems are common in men, especially as they become older. An enlarged prostate obstructs the urethra and thus urinary flow Determine onset of the problem.

➤ Is it difficult for you to begin to urinate? Is your urine stream weak? Do you dribble urine? Does this come and go, or is it constant problem?

➤ Do you feel as though you have to urinate but can't? Do you have to get up in the middle of the night to urinate?

■ If benign prostatic hyperplasia is suspected, use the symptom index tool (see Table 23-1, later in the chapter).

EXAMINATION

Equipment

- Examination gloves to palpate rectum and prostate
- Water-soluble lubricant to aid in palpation of rectum and prostate
- Guaiac test reagents to test stool for occult blood
- Light source (penlight or examination lamp) for inspection of the anus

PROCEDURES AND TECHNIQUES WITH NORMAL FINDINGS | ABNORMAL FINDINGS

The examination of the rectum and anus is done on all adults. The techniques of the examination include inspection and palpation. Examination gloves are worn throughout the entire examination procedure. Essentially, anal and rectal examination is the same for males and females. In the male client, the prostate should also be examined in conjunction with the rectal examination.

Positioning the client for the rectal examination usually depends on the client's gender and age. The male client should assume either the left lateral position with the hips and knees flexed, a knee-chest position, or the standing position with the hips flexed, and the client bending over the examination table with feet pointed together. The female client should assume a lithotomy position, if the examination is being done in conjunction with the genitalia examination, or the left lateral position just described if only a rectal examination is done (Fig. 23-3).

PROCEDURES AND TECHNIQUES WITH NORMAL FINDINGS

ABNORMAL FINDINGS

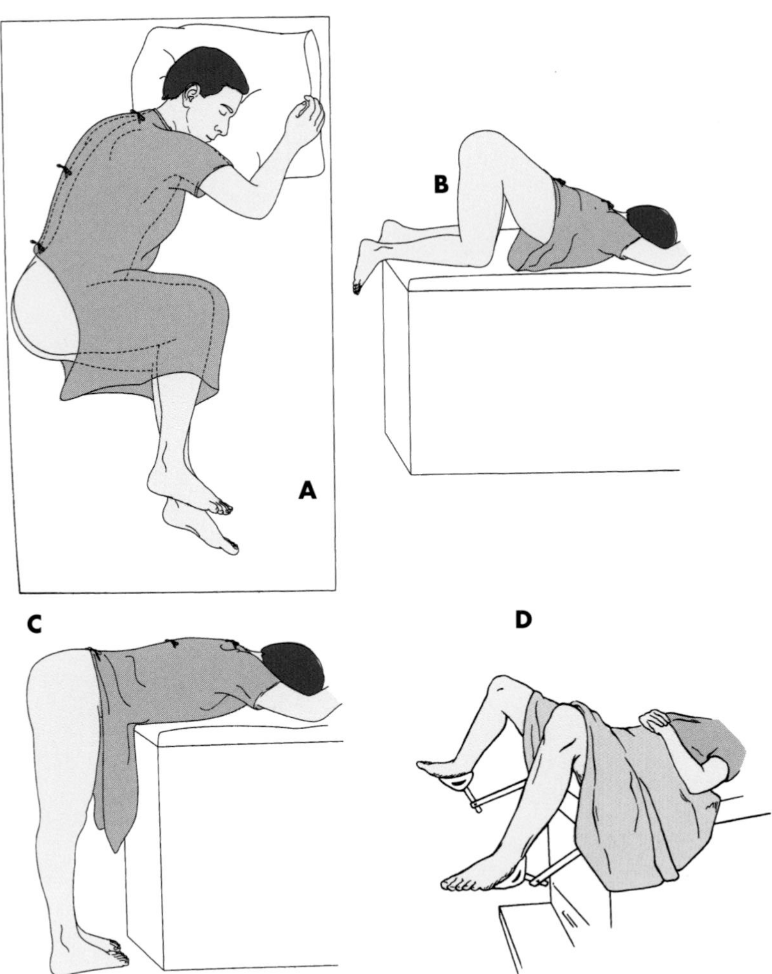

Fig. 23-3 Positions for rectal examination. **A,** Left lateral or Sims' position. **B,** Knee-chest position. **C,** Standing position. **D,** Lithotomy position. (From Barkauskus et al, 1998.)

ANUS AND RECTUM

➤INSPECT and PALPATE the sacrococcygeal areas for surface characteristics and tenderness. The skin surface should be smooth and clear, and there should be no tenderness to palpation.

■ A dimple with a tuft of hair with inflammation and/or a tender palpable cyst in the sacrococcygeal area suggests a pilonidal cyst or sinus (see the Common Problems and Conditions section at the end of the chapter).

PROCEDURES AND TECHNIQUES WITH NORMAL FINDINGS

➤INSPECT the perianal area and anus for pigmentation and surface characteristics. Spread the buttocks with both hands to inspect this area. (Tell the client what is going to happen *before* the buttocks are spread.) The perianal skin is darker than general skin tone. The anus is coarse, moist, hairless, and more deeply pigmented than the perianal skin. The anus should be tightly closed. No lesions or inflammation should be present. Ask the client to bear down and repeat the inspection of the anal area. Again, no lesions should be observed.

➤PALPATE the anus for sphincter tone. To perform an adequate internal rectal examination, the client's hips should be in a flexed position.

Ask the client to bear down again. Place the finger pad surface of a gloved and lubricated index finger at the anal opening; as the sphincter relaxes, slowly insert the finger, pointing toward the client's umbilicus (Fig. 23-4). (Tell the client what is going to happen *before* the finger is inserted.) Ask the client to tighten the anus around your examining finger. The sphincter should tighten evenly around your finger with minimum discomfort to the client.

ABNORMAL FINDINGS

■ Note the presence and location of inflammation and/or lesions. Identify the location of the abnormality in terms of the position of a clock, with the 12 o'clock position being toward the symphysis pubis and the 6 o'clock position toward the sacrococcygeal area. Lesions that may be seen include external hemorrhoids, ulcerations, warty growths (condylomata acuminta), skin tags, inflammation, fissures, and fistulas. While the client is straining, note for the presence of internal hemorrhoids, polyps, tumors, and rectal prolapse (see the Common Problems and Conditions section at the end of the chapter).

■ Report if the client is unable to tighten the sphincter around your finger, has excessive sphincter tightening, or experiences discomfort. A hypotonic sphincter can occur with neurologic deficits, following rectal surgery, or with anal/rectal trauma—especially associated with frequent anal sex. Hypertonic sphincter may be associated with lesions, inflammation, scarring, or anxiety related to the examination. Extreme pain with anal palpation almost always indicates a local inflammation such as a fissure, fistula, or cyst.

PROCEDURES AND TECHNIQUES WITH NORMAL FINDINGS

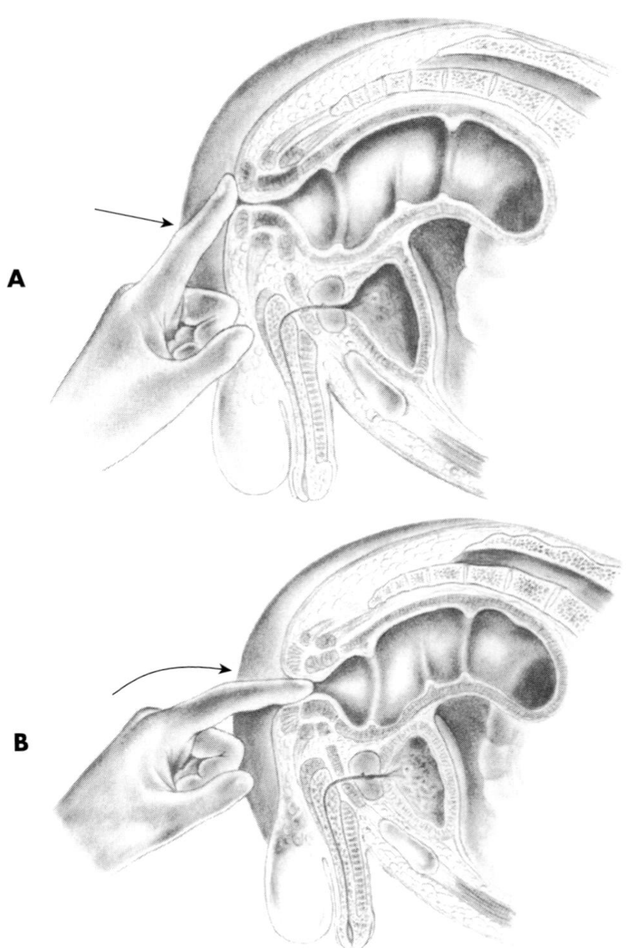

Fig. 23-4 Correct procedure for introducing finger into rectum. **A,** Press pad of finger against the anal opening. **B,** As external sphincter relaxes, slip the fingertip into the anal canal. Note that client is in the hips-flexed position. (From Seidel et al, 1999.)

➤**PALPATE the anal canal and rectum for surface characteristics.** Rotate the finger around the musculature of the anal ring to palpate the surface characteristics. The area should be smooth, with even pressure on your finger. Insert the finger as far as possible into the rectum (2⅜ to 4 inches, or 6 to 10 cm) to palpate all four rectal walls. There should be a continuous smooth surface, and the client should experience only minimal discomfort.

ABNORMAL FINDINGS

■ Note any nodules, irregularities, masses, presence of hard stool, or tenderness. (Note: In females, occasionally the cervix may be palpable on the anterior wall; this could be mistaken for a mass.) Always report an anal or rectal mass.

PROCEDURES AND TECHNIQUES WITH NORMAL FINDINGS

❖ PROSTATE GLAND (FOR MALE CLIENTS)

➤**PALPATE the anterior rectal surface to evaluate the prostate for size, contour, consistency, mobility, and tenderness.** Palpate the posterior surface of the prostate gland by palpating the anterior surface of the rectum (Fig. 23-5). (Note: The client may state that he has the urge to urinate during the prostate examination. Reassure him that this is only a sensation and that he will not urinate.) Note the size, contour, consistency, and mobility of the gland. It should be about 1½ inches (3.8 cm) in diameter and project less than ½ inch (1 cm) into the rectum. The contour is symmetric and bilobed, with a palpable groove in the center (referred to as the sulcus). The prostate should feel firm, smooth, and slightly mobile. Palpation should not produce tenderness.

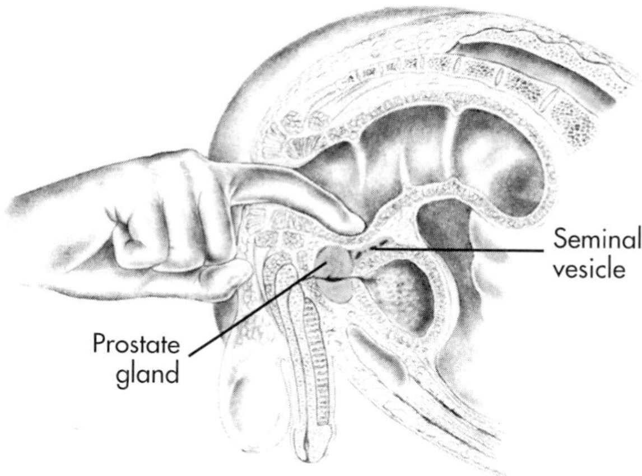

Fig. 23-5 Palpation of the anterior surface of the prostate gland. Feel for the lateral lobes and median sulcus. (From Seidel et al, 1999.)

STOOL EXAMINATION

➤**INSPECT and EXAMINE fecal material for characteristics and presence of occult blood.** Slowly remove the gloved finger from the client's rectum. Inspect the gloved finger for color and consistency of stool. It should be brown and soft. Use a guaiac test to evaluate for occult blood on all stool specimens (Box 23-3). A negative response is normal.

ABNORMAL FINDINGS

■ Note if the prostate projects more than ½ inch (1 cm) into the rectum. Estimate classification of prostate enlargement (Box 23-1).

Box 23-1 Classifications of Prostate Enlargement

GRADE	PROTRUSION INTO RECTUM
Grade I	⅜ to ¾ inch (1 to 2 cm)
Grade II	¾ to 1⅛ inches (2 to 3 cm)
Grade III	1⅛ to 1¾ inches (3 to 4 cm)
Grade IV	greater than 1¾ inches (4 cm)

■ Note if there is asymmetry or if the median sulcus is obliterated; also note any tenderness, a boggy feeling, irregularity, or nodules. A rubbery or boggy consistency may be indicative of benign hyperplasia. A stony-hard or nodular prostate may indicate carcinoma, prostate calculi, or fibrosis.

■ Note the presence of blood, pus, mucus, or abnormal color of stool (Box 23-2). Report any positive guaiac test, which indicates the presence of occult blood.

Box 23-2 Stool Colors and Significance

COLOR	SIGNIFICANCE
Bright red	Hemorrhoidal or lower rectal bleeding
Tarry black	Upper intestinal tract bleeding or excessive iron or bismuth ingestion
Light tan or gray	Obstruction of the biliary tract (obstructive jaundice)
Pale yellow	Malabsorption syndrome

Box 23-3 Guaiac Testing

If stool is present on your gloved finger, check the stool for occult blood.

1. Obtain a guaiac slide and developer (Fig. 23-6, *A*).
2. Open the flap of the cardboard guaiac slide.
3. Dab the gloved finger containing stool on the paper in the boxes of the slide (Fig. 23-6, *B*).
4. Close the flap and remove soiled gloves. Don clean examination gloves.
5. Turn the slide to the reverse side and open the cardboard flap.
6. Apply 2 drops of developing solution on each box of guaiac paper (Fig. 23-6, *C*).
7. Wait 30 to 60 seconds and note the color of the paper. A bluish discoloration of the paper indicates presence of occult blood and is documented as guaiac positive.

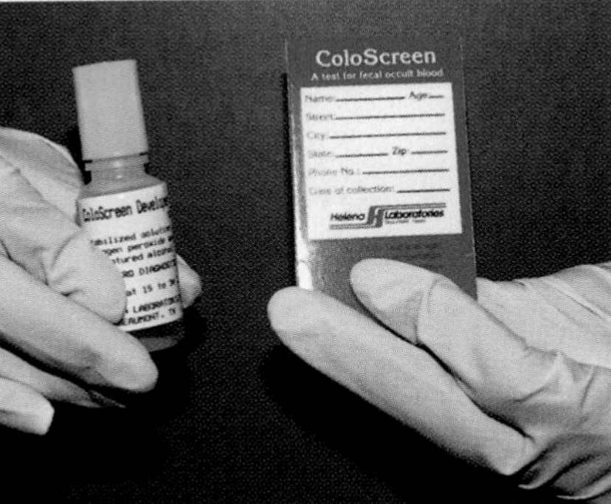

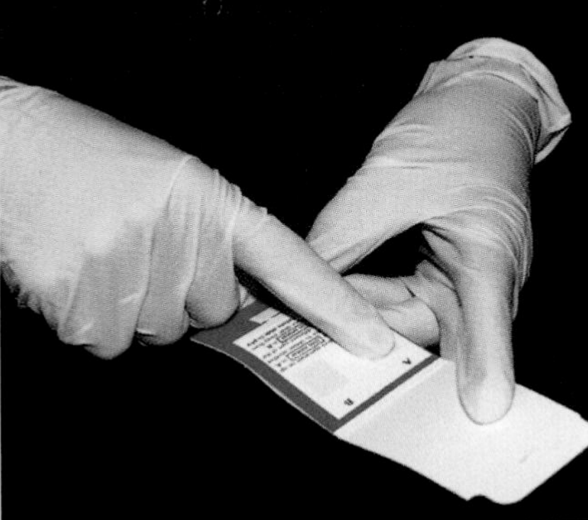

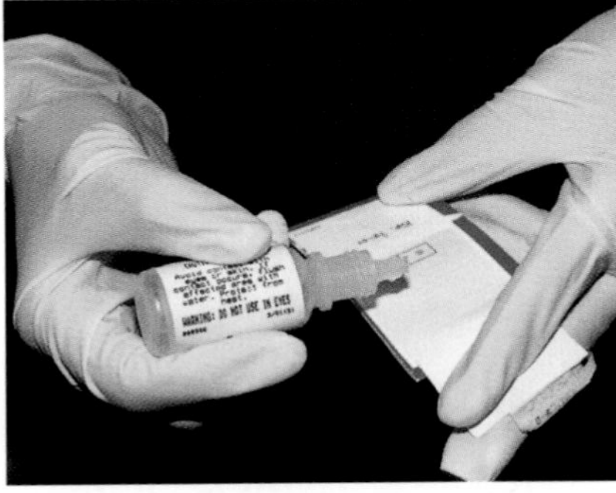

Fig. 23-6 **A,** Guaiac slide and developer. **B,** Apply stool onto slide as indicated. **C,** Add developer to other side of slide.

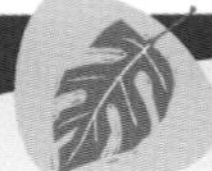

AGE-RELATED VARIATIONS

■ INFANTS

Anatomy and Physiology

At birth, meconium stool is passed within 24 to 48 hours; this indicates anal patency. After this first stool, newborns commonly experience gastrocolic reflex, which causes a stool production after each feeding. At this age, because myelination of the spinal cord is incomplete, both the internal and external sphincters are under involuntary reflexive control; control of the external anal sphincter will not be achieved until sometime between the ages of 18 and 24 months. By the end of the first year, bowel movements will occur once or twice per day.

In males, the prostate will be undeveloped, unpalpable, and inactive until the androgenic influences of puberty initiate its functions.

Health History

- Describe the infant's diet. Breast-feeding? Bottle? If bottle-feeding, what type of formula? Iron supplementation? Is the infant offered other fluids, such as juices or water? If so, how much?

  Rationale Diet will affect the stool composition and color.
- After the infant was born, did he or she have any problem having a bowel movement? Did anyone at the hospital tell you that they were concerned about the infant's rectum or ability to defecate?

  Rationale This is baseline information regarding the infant.
- Describe the infant's stool characteristics. Color? General texture: diarrhea; formed and soft; formed and hard? Does the baby cry or strain during a bowel movement? How frequently does the infant have a stool?

  Rationale It is important to correlate the infant's stool characteristics with the type of diet and fluid intake. Often, crying or straining with a bowel movement may be indicative of hard stools or constipation.

Examination

Procedures and Techniques The external perianal examination is routinely performed with comprehensive assessment. An internal anal examination is not routinely performed. The infant is generally placed on his or her back with the feet held in the examiner's hand and the infant's knees flexed upward toward the abdomen (Fig. 23-7). In the newborn, inspect the perineum and anal region for presence of anus, lesions, and inflammation. Confirm a patent rectum and anus by noting passing of meconium stool. Confirm anal contraction by lightly stroking the anal opening with a cotton-tipped applicator. Observe the lower back and buttocks for appearance and surface characteristics. If stool is present when the diaper is removed, note the characteristics, color, odor, and consistency (Box 23-4).

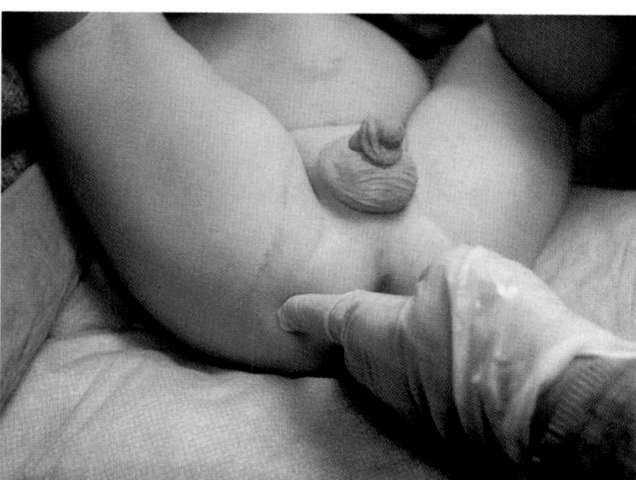

Fig. 23-7 Position for rectal examination of the infant. (From Seidel et al, 1999.)

Normal and Abnormal Findings The perineal and perianal skin should be free of lesions or inflammation, although diaper rash is a common finding with infants. A patent anus is the expected finding; imperforate anus is an abnormal finding (Fig. 23-8). Stroking the anus with the cotton-tipped applicator should produce an "anal wink" or contraction (Wong and Perry, 1998). Lack of anal contraction may indicate a lower spinal cord deformity. The lower back and buttocks should be free of lesions. Normal variations include mongolian spots and birthmarks. Tufts of hair or dimpling in the pilonidal area may indicate a lower spinal deformity or sinus tract. Buttocks should be firm and rounded. Asymmetry of the buttocks may indicate hip dislocation.

■ CHILDREN

Anatomy and Physiology

There are no anatomic differences between the child and the adult.

Box 23-4 Infant Stool Characteristics

BREAST-FED

Stool will be mushy, loose, golden color; frequency varies from after each feeding to daily. The stool is generally not irritating to the skin.

FORMULA-FED

Stool is light colored, with a foul odor; frequency varies from several times a day to daily. The stool is frequently irritating to the skin.

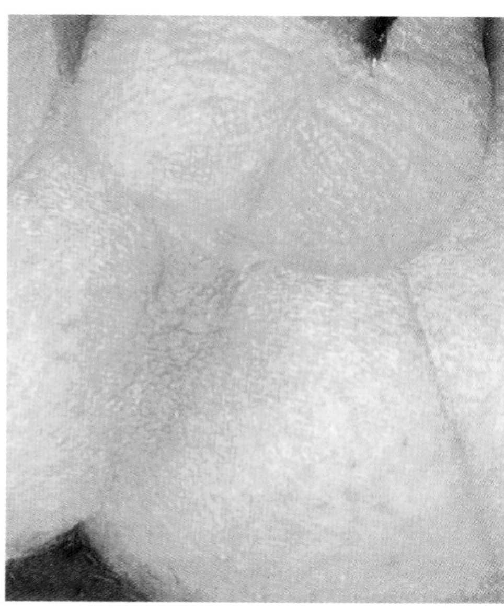

Fig. 23-8 Imperforate anus. (From *Diagnostic picture tests in clinical medicine,* 1984. By permission of Mosby International.)

Health History

In addition to the questions asked for the infant, inquire about self-toileting, anal or rectal itching, and general bowel functioning.

- What are the child's normal bowel habits? Describe the child's stool characteristics. Frequency? Color? General texture?

Rationale Establish what the normal routine is for the child as baseline information.

- Have you noticed that the child has had any problems with his or her bowels? Does the child experience discomfort or strain during a bowel movement? Constipation? Diarrhea? Cramping? If any of these are present, how long has the problem existed? When did it start?
- Are there any current stresses in the family? Please describe them.
- Describe the child's diet for a day. How much food, juice, and water is consumed in a 24-hour period?

Rationale Symptoms of constipation or diarrhea may be indications of problems from inadequate diet to parental punishment if the child has an "accident" to a more serious problem such as megacolon. If any are present, it is important to try to identify the causative factors.

- Have you observed redness or irritation to your child's anal area? Have you observed your child frequently scratching his or her anal area?

Rationale Intense anal itching indicates an irritation. The most common cause of anal itching and irritation in children is pinworms.

- Is the child independent with toileting? If so, when did the child successfully complete toilet training? If not, have you started to toilet train the child? How old was the child when you started?

Rationale There is a wide range of professional opinions about when toilet training should begin and how it should be done. It is most important to learn how the parent is doing the training and how successful it has been. This will provide baseline information should additional education or assistance become necessary.

Examination

Procedures and Techniques External perianal examination is routinely performed during a comprehensive assessment. For the external examination, be sure to respect the child's modesty and apprehension; take the time to explain what is going to happen and what the child can expect. Children should be positioned so that the perianal area is adequately exposed and so that the child is comfortable. The child should be positioned either in a knee-chest position or on the left side with the hips and knees flexed toward the abdomen (the same positioning as for the adult).

Internal rectal examination is not performed in children unless there are specific symptoms such as severe abdominal pain, constipation, or injury. If an internal rectal examination is warranted, the examiner should use the little finger to perform the examination. Even when this is done, there may occasionally be slight rectal bleeding. The parent should be told about this possibility before the examination. The procedure for the internal examination is the same as for the adult.

Normal and Abnormal Findings The findings for external examination are the same for the child as for the adult. Variations are based on developmental maturity. Redness or irritation may be an indication of a bacterial or fungal infection or pinworms. If any pustules or signs of physical or sexual abuse are noted during the examination, such as bruising, anal tearing, rapid anal wink, anal dilation, or extreme or inappropriate apprehension from the child, assess the finding further with the family. If there is suspicion of child abuse or assault, report the findings to the appropriate local health authorities. The findings for the internal examination are the same as for the adult with the exception that the prostate in the small child is not palpable.

■ ADOLESCENTS

Anatomy and Physiology

There are no anatomic differences between the adolescent and the adult. The prostate enlarges and develops with puberty.

Health History

Questions are the same for an adolescent as an adult.

Examination

Procedures and Techniques The rectal and prostate examination should be part of a comprehensive assessment for the older adolescent. It is recommended that males have a baseline rectal and prostate examination by age 18. It will provide baseline information and, for males, will provide an opportunity to discuss the importance of a periodic prostate examination. Because many adolescents may never have had a rectal examination before, it is important to take the time to explain what will be done and reasons for the examination. The procedure is the same as reasons for the examination.

Normal and Abnormal Findings The findings for the adolescent are the same as for the adult.

■ OLDER ADULTS

Anatomy and Physiology

With increasing age, the rectal wall's afferent neurons degenerate, interfering with pressure sensitivity and internal sphincter relaxation in response to rectal distention. Because of this, the older adult may experience stool retention. At the same time, as the internal sphincter loses tone, the external sphincter is not able to control the bowels on its own, so the older adult may experience fecal incontinence instead of retention.

In men, with loss of gland function, the prostate atrophies. A benign enlargement of the prostate frequently occurs associated with aging. Usually this enlargement produces no symptoms. However, the hyperplasia can obstruct the bladder outlet, leading to a number of urinary problems (Matteson et al, 1997) (see the Common Problems and Conditions section at the end of the chapter).

Health History

Older adult clients frequently express numerous problems associated with elimination, and individuals may be preoccupied with bowel movement regularity to the extent that it can alter daily living functions. Clarification of symptoms is needed. If the symptoms are long-standing, ask carefully about the client's method of self-treatment. The questions to be asked are the same as for adults, but care should be taken to pay attention to the client's responses concerning constipation, gas in the stomach, diarrhea, or abdominal cramping. Medications are often more likely to produce changes in bowel motility in older clients and should be carefully evaluated. Additional specific questions to ask include the following:

- Describe your diet. Do any specific foods bother you? If so, which ones and how?

  Rationale Changes in bowel function may be associated with diet changes such as lack of bulk or roughage in the diet, decreased fluid intake, decreased exercise, or more serious problems such as a bowel obstruction secondary to cancer.

The older male may have urinary symptoms caused by an enlarged prostate. It is important to ask all of the questions related to the prostate in the adult question section. Consider using the American Urological Association (AUA) index (Table 23-1).

Examination

Procedures and Techniques The client may need assistance getting into an adequate position for the examination. If the client is lying on his or her back on the ex-

Table 23-1 The American Urological Association Symptom Index for Benign Prostatic Hyperplasia

QUESTIONS	NOT AT ALL	LESS THAN 1 TIME IN 5	LESS THAN HALF THE TIME	ABOUT HALF THE TIME	MORE THAN HALF THE TIME	ALMOST ALWAYS
1. During the last month or so, how often have you had a sensation of not emptying your bladder completely after you finished urinating?	0	1	2	3	4	5
2. During the last month or so, how often have you had to urinate again less than 2 hours after you finished urinating?	0	1	2	3	4	5
3. During the last month or so, how often have you found you stopped and started again several times when you urinated?	0	1	2	3	4	5
4. During the last month or so, how often have you found it difficult to postpone urination?	0	1	2	3	4	5
5. During the last month or so, how often have you had a weak urinary stream?	0	1	2	3	4	5
6. During the last month or so, how often have you had to push or strain to begin urination?	0	1	2	3	4	5
	NONE	1 TIME	2 TIMES	3 TIMES	4 TIMES	5 OR MORE TIMES
7. During the last month, how many times did you most typically get up to urinate from the time you went to bed at night until the time you got up in the morning?	0	1	2	3	4	5

Score:
7 or below indicates mild symptoms
8-19 = moderate symptoms
Above 20 = severe symptoms
From Barry MJ et al: The American Urologic Association symptom index for benign prostatic hyperplasia, *J Urol* 148(11):1549-1557, 1992.

amination table, care should be taken to assist the client into a left lateral lying position. The examination procedure for the older adult is the same as previously discussed.

Normal and Abnormal Findings The examination findings for the older adult are the same as for the adult. Because older male clients are at highest risk for developing prostatic hypertrophy, the prostate gland should be carefully examined. The older adult's prostate is more likely to feel smooth and rubbery. The median sulcus may or may not be palpable. The examiner may also note a relaxation of the client's perianal muscles and decreased sphincter control when the older adult bears down.

EXAMINATION SUMMARY

Anus, Rectum, and Prostate

PROCEDURE

- Inspect and palpate the sacrococcygeal area for:
  Surface characteristics
  Tenderness
- Inspect the perianal area and anus for:
  Pigmentation
  Surface characteristics
- Palpate the anus and rectum for:
  Sphincter tone
  Surface characteristics

❖ Prostate Gland

- In males: Palpate the anterior rectal surface to evaluate the prostate for:
  Size
  Contour
  Consistency
  Mobility

Stool Evaluation

- Inspect and examine the fecal material for:
  Characteristics
  Presence of occult blood

SUMMARY OF FINDINGS

Age Group	Normal Findings	Typical Variations	Findings Associated With Disorders
Infants and children	• Newborns: determine anal patency by noting meconium stool within 24-48 hours of birth. Symmetric rounded buttocks. External findings same as adult; internal examination not routinely done unless specific problem exists.	• Typically, sphincter control is achieved between 18 and 24 months, although in some children this may occur later.	• Lack of stool passage in 24-48 hours may suggest imperforate anus. • Sinuses, tufts of hair, dimpling in pilonidal area suggest pilonidal tract. • Perirectal redness or inflammation may suggest diaper rash, or pin worms.
Adolescents	• Prostate develops with puberty.		Same as for adult.

Age Group	Normal Findings	Typical Variations	Findings Associated With Disorders
Adults	• Perianal skin smooth and intact, without lesions. Anus is coarse, darker pigmentation. Anal sphincter tight around examining finger; rectal walls smooth. • Prostate gland palpable; feels firm, smooth, slightly mobile and is nontender.	• External hemorrhoids common. Internal hemorrhoids are not typically palpable.	• Inflammation and pain of perianal area suggest abscess, anorectal fistula, fissure, or pilonidal cyst. Lesions on or around anus abnormal. • Hypotonic rectal sphincter tone may be associated with rectal trauma or frequent recipient of anal sex. • Mass in rectum may indicate tumor. • Stony hard nodular prostate suggests carcinoma.
Older adults	• Sphincter tone may be decreased. • Median sulcus of the prostate may or may not be obliterated.	• Prostate may be enlarged. • Higher incidence of colorectal polyps.	• Same as for adult; higher incidence of colorectal cancer and prostate cancer with age.

HEALTH PROMOTION

COLORECTAL CANCER

Much can be done to reduce the risk of colon and rectal cancer or to improve its identification.

Dietary Guidelines

- Reduce the amount of fat in your diet to 30% of your total calorie intake.
- Limit the amount of charbroiled, smoked, and salted foods you eat.
- Eat foods high in vitamins and fiber.

Screening Guidelines

The American Cancer Society (Von Eschenbach et al, 1997) and the Agency for Health Care Policy and Research (1998) offer the following baseline recommendations:

- Fecal occult blood testing (FOBT) for all individuals over the age of 50. If client has a positive FOBT, a colonoscopy is recommended.
- Flexible sigmoidoscopy is suggested every 5 years for clients over the age of 50.

Research has shown that early detection by FOBT and other examination reduces mortality from colorectal cancer (Spencer-Cisek, 1998). Unfortunately, one study showed that colorectal screening was performed less often in older clients and less often in females, despite the known risk factors associated with increasing age and despite national screening guidelines (Borum, 1998).

PROSTATE CANCER

There are no prevention guidelines for prostate cancer; however, screening guidelines are recommended.

Screening Guidelines

Both the AUA and the American Cancer Society make the following recommendations:

- Digital rectal examination (DRE) annually starting at age 50, or at age 40 if the client has strong risk factors. The AUA further recommends discontinuing screening at age 70.
- Prostate-specific antigen blood test annually starting at age 50, or at age 40 if the client has strong risk factors.

Early diagnosis with PSA or DRE have yet to show an improvement in outcomes with clients who have prostate cancer.

COMMON PROBLEMS AND CONDITIONS

Anus, Rectum, and Prostate

ANUS AND RECTUM

Pilonidal Cyst or Sinus

Located in the sacrococcygeal area, a pilonidal cyst or sinus is usually seen as a dimpled area with a small sinus opening that may contain a tuft of hair. This is a congenital anomaly that is usually diagnosed in young adulthood, although occasionally it is recognized at birth by a depression in the sacral area. If the cyst develops a sinus that communicates with the skin, an infection results. The area becomes red and tender, and the cyst may become palpable. The client may complain of pain and swelling at the base of the spine (Fig. 23-9). Unless the sinus or cyst becomes infected or abscessed, the client is asymptomatic.

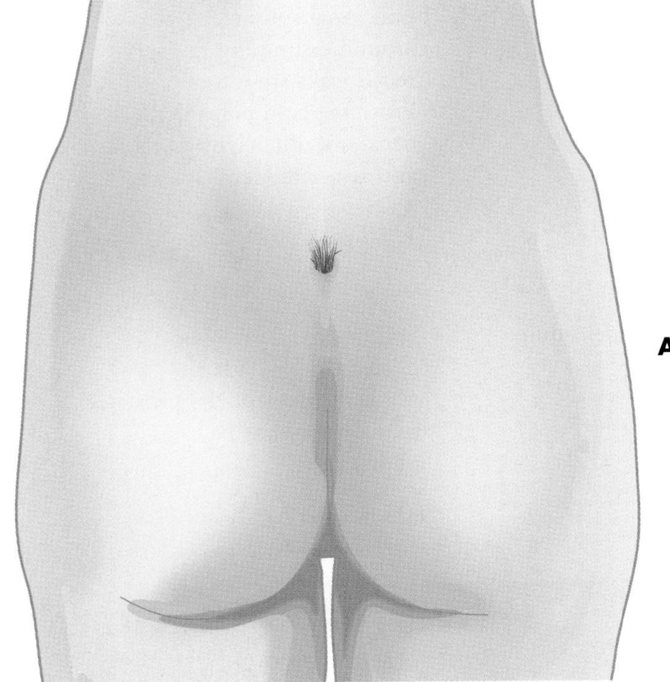

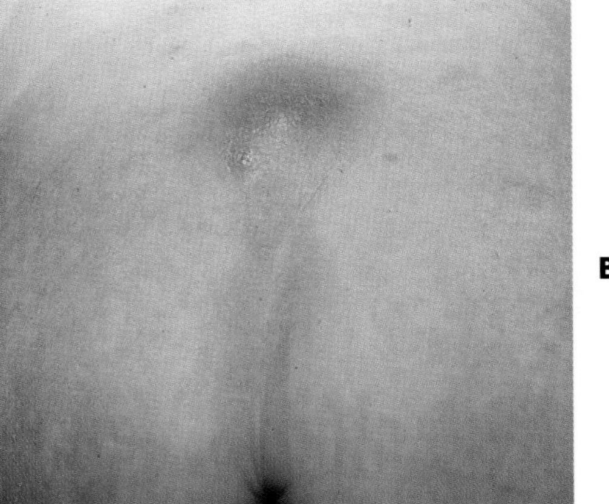

Fig. 23-9 **A,** Pilonidal sinus. **B,** Inflamed pilonidal cyst. (From Zitelli and Davis, 1997.)

Hemorrhoids

Hemorrhoids are varicose veins of the hemorrhoidal plexus resulting from increased portal venous pressure. Pregnancy, constipation, chronic liver disease, and obesity are conditions that frequently are associated with hemorrhoids.

External hemorrhoids originate below the anorectal line and appear as flaps of tissue or skin. If they become irritated or thrombosed, symptoms include localized itching and perhaps bleeding and they may appear as blue shiny masses at the anus.

Internal hemorrhoids originate above the anorectal junction. Although they may be present in the rectum, they may not be identified clinically unless they become thrombosed, prolapsed, or infected (Fig. 23-10).

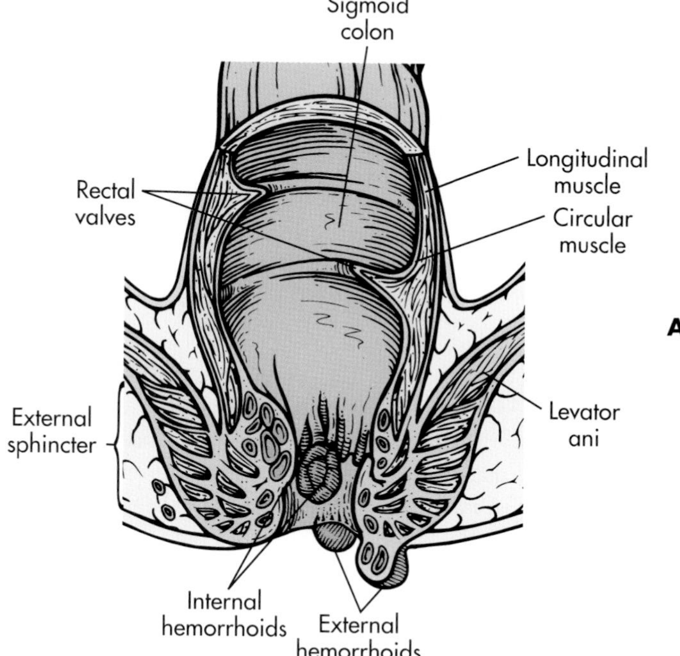

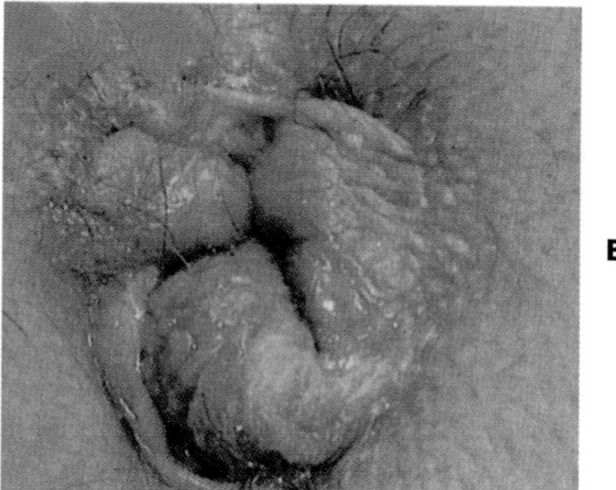

Fig. 23-10 **A,** Internal and external hemorrhoids. **B,** External hemorrhoid. (Courtesy Gershon Efron, MD, Sinai Hospital of Baltimore. **A** From Lewis, Heitkemper, and Dirksen, 2000; **B** from Seidel et al, 1999.)

Box 23-5 Focus on Pain: Anus, Rectum, and Prostate

Rectal fistula, fissure, and perianal abscess are among the most painful problems associated with the anus and rectum. When these problems are acute, walking is very painful, and the client has trouble finding a position of comfort. Oftentimes the client will be observed sitting to the side or frequently shift uncomfortably. The client may prefer to lie prone, avoiding any pressure to the area.

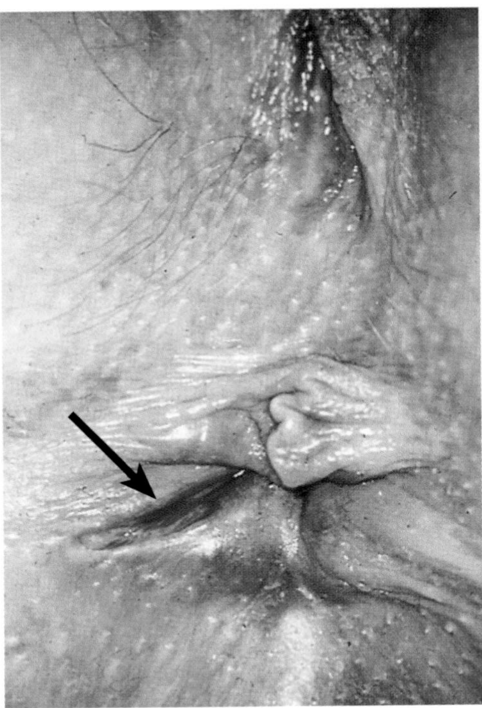

Fig. 23-11 Lateral anal fissure. (Courtesy Gershon Efron, MD, Sinai Hospital of Baltimore. From Seidel et al, 1999.)

Anorectal Fissure

This is a tear of the anal mucosa causing intense pain (Box 23-5). This usually occurs secondary to trauma, such as passing a hard large stool or irritating diarrhea stools (Fig. 23-11). Usually the fissure is located midline in the posterior wall of the rectum. Common symptoms include severe rectal pain, itching, and rectal bleeding.

Anorectal Fistula

An anorectal fistula is an inflamed tract that forms an abnormal passage that runs from within the anus or the rectum and opens to the outside skin surface—usually in the perianal area. The fistula is frequently caused by the drainage of a local abscess, thus the drainage seen is serosanguinous or purulent (Fig. 23-12). The opening on the skin usually appears as red, raised granulation tissue.

Anorectal Abscess

A pus-filled cavity from an infection in the anorectal area is referred to as an anorectal abscess (see Fig. 23-12). The client typically complains of moderate to severe throbbing rectal pain and frequently has a fever. The abscess clinically appears as an area of swelling and erythema and induration in the perianal area.

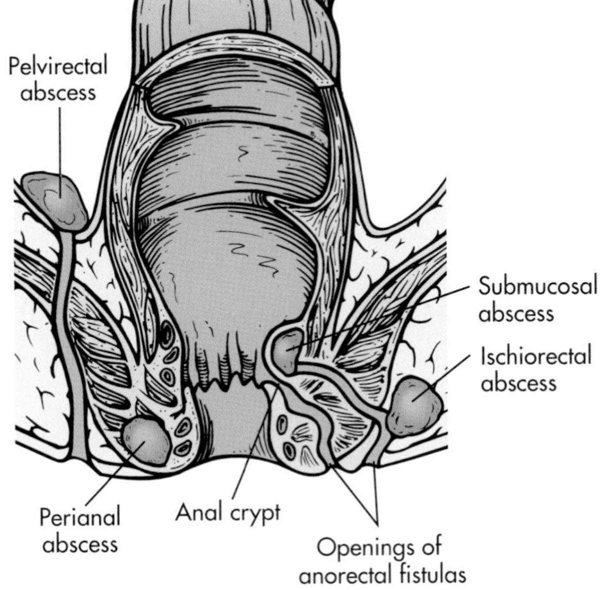

Fig. 23-12 Common sites of anorectal fistula and abscess formation. (From Lewis, Heitkemper, and Dirksen, 2000.)

Rectal Polyp

A rectal polyp is a protruding growth from the rectal mucosa anywhere in the intestinal tract. These growths may grow outward, as on a stalk (pedunculated) or may grow adhering to the mucosa (sessile) (Fig. 23-13). A common symptom is rectal bleeding. Occasionally, they may protrude from the anus and are presenting as small, soft nodules. Polyps may be difficult to palpate. Biopsy is necessary to distinguish the polyp from carcinoma.

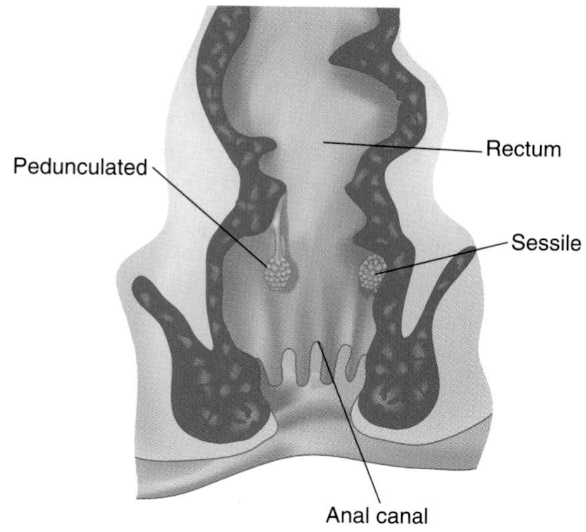

Fig. 23-13 Rectal polyp.

Rectal Carcinoma

A malignant tumor growing on the rectal mucosa is referred to as rectal cancer. It is estimated that nearly 35,000 new cases of rectal cancer will be diagnosed in 1999 (Landis et al, 1999). Of clients diagnosed with colorectal cancer, 10% to 15% have a first-degree relative who also has had this (Hardcastle, 1997).

Clients may or may not present with symptoms. The most important symptom is rectal bleeding because those presenting with rectal bleeding have better long-term outcomes. Rectal bleeding is consistent with a tumor at an early stage because it is more vascularized than an advanced lesion (Jessup et al, 1997). Many clients are asymptomatic; thus a rectal lesion may go undetected until palpated. A malignant rectal tumor presents on palpation as an irregular mass on the rectal wall with nodular, raised edges. The center of the mass often has an area of depression as well (Fig. 23-14).

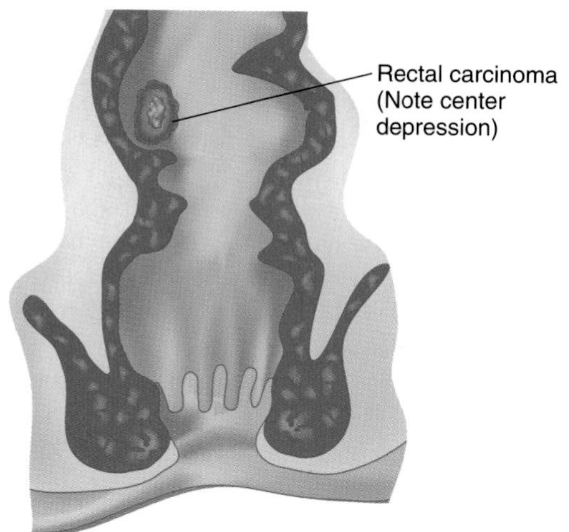

Fig. 23-14 Rectal carcinoma.

CULTURAL NOTE

Ethnicity plays a role in the outcome of colorectal cancers. As a group, African Americans have a higher incidence and mortality rate than other racial groups, (Landis, 1999) and are diagnosed with colorectal cancer at an earlier age compared with whites. This trend is especially notable in males (Thomas et al, 1990). This is concerning because a diagnosis of colorectal cancer at an early age is associated with a worse outcome. In addition, one study found that African-American clients tended to present with more advanced disease than other ethnic groups (Weaver, 1991). This may, in part, reflect a real or perceived limited access to health care.

Rectal Prolapse

Rectal prolapse is an intussusception (turning inside out) of the rectum, so that the rectum protrudes from the anus (Fig. 23-15). Rectal prolapse most commonly occurs either before age 3 or in the older adult. In children, boys and girls are affected equally; however, 80% of adult cases occur in women. The cause of rectal prolapse is not completely understood, although it frequently manifests itself after straining. The client presenting with rectal prolapse frequently reports that an intestine or hemorrhoid is hanging out of the rectum and may also report fecal incontinence or soiling with mucous discharge. Blood staining may also occur, although hemorrhage is uncommon (Jacobs, 1997). The prolapsed rectum appears as a pink mucosal bulge that is described as a "doughnut" or "rosette."

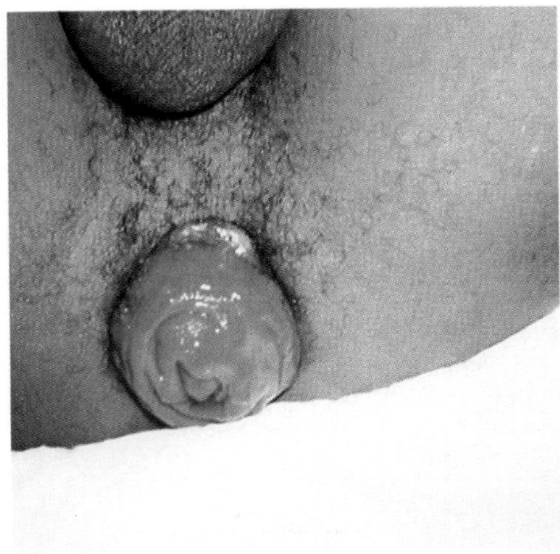

Fig. 23-15 Prolapse of the rectum. (Courtesy Gershon Efron, MD, Sinai Hospital of Baltimore. From Seidel et al, 1999.)

PROSTATE

Benign Prostatic Hyperplasia (BPH)

Benign prostatic hyperplasia is an asymptomatic enlargement of the prostate gland that usually affects older men (Fig. 23-16). At least some degree of BPH will eventually develop in all men with advanced age, although this causes only minor to moderate symptoms in most men (Albertson, 1997). The American Urology Association symptom index is a tool used to assess voiding symptoms associated with obstruction. The higher the score, the more likely BPH is present. In addition to symptoms, prostate examination may reveal hyperplasia. When palpated, the prostate feels smooth, firm, and rubbery, and the prostate will project more than 1 cm into the rectum. There is no association between BPH and cancer of the prostate, although some factors such as age are common to both (Mebust et al, 1992).

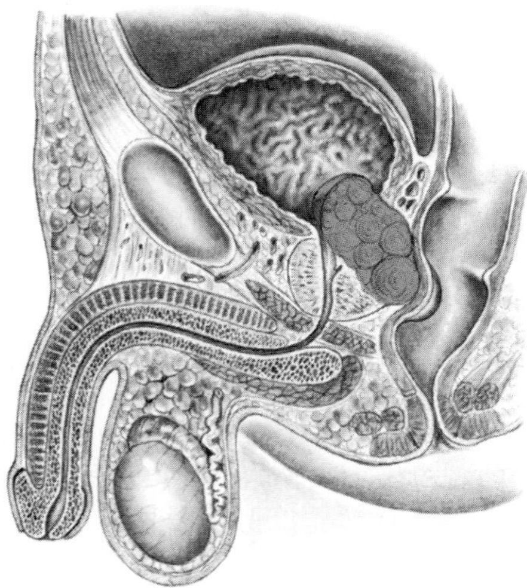

Fig. 23-16 Benign prostatic hyperplasia. (From Seidel et al, 1999.)

Prostatitis

An inflammation of the prostate gland is referred to as prostatitis (Fig. 23-17). Prostatitis can present as acute bacterial prostatitis, chronic prostatitis, and nonbacterial prostatitis—which is has an unknown cause. The client with acute prostatitis classically presents with fever, chills, pain in the back and rectal or perineal area, and obstructive symptoms; examination reveals an enlarged prostate that is usually tender with induration. Chronic prostatitis commonly causes recurrent urinary tract infection, pain, dysuria, and scrotal or penile pain; examination findings may be nonspecific or may reveal an enlarged, tender, and boggy prostate. Nonbacterial prostatitis presents with urinary urgency, frequency, nocturia, dysuria, and pain or discomfort; examination findings may be normal or may include a soft and boggy prostate (Donovan and Nicholas, 1997).

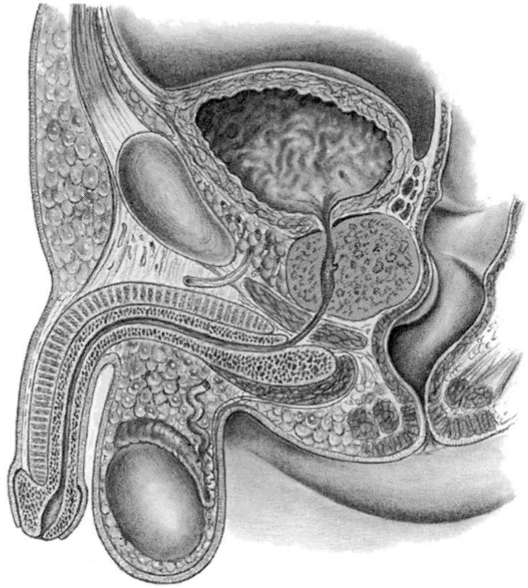

Fig. 23-17 Prostatitis. (From Seidel et al, 1999.)

Prostate Cancer

The leading site of cancer in men (accounting for 29% of new cancer cases in men) is the prostate. It is expected that 179,000 new cases of prostate cancer will be diagnosed in 1999 (Landis et al, 1999). This occurs mostly in men over the age of 50, and the incidence increases significantly with age. It is estimated that 80% of men who reach the age of 90 have in situ carcinoma of the prostate (Gambert, 1997). Urinary obstruction with difficulty urinating may be the first sign of a problem. On palpation, the prostate feels hard and irregular. The median sulcus is obliterated as the prostate tumor grows (Fig. 23-18). Surgery with biopsy is the only method to confirm a diagnosis.

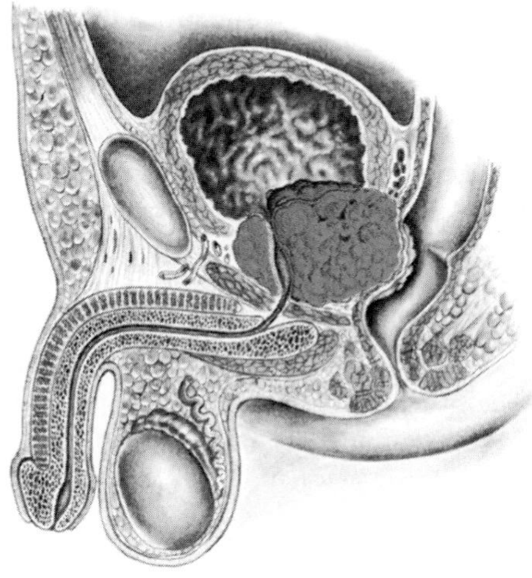

Fig. 23-18 Carcinoma of the prostate. (From Seidel et al, 1999.)

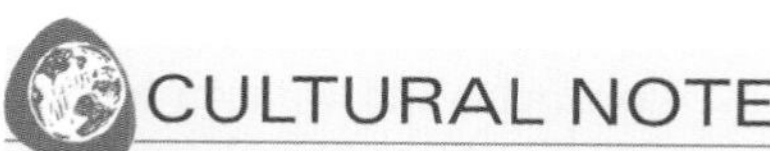

CULTURAL NOTE

Prostate cancer is the most common site for new cancer cases in men, and the second leading cause of cancer-related deaths in men. The incidence varies significantly by racial groups. African-American men are at highest risk for prostate cancer, followed by whites and Hispanics. The risk is much lower for Koreans, Chinese, Alaskan natives, Hawaiians, and American Indians.

Data from National Cancer Institute: *Racial/ethnic patterns of cancer in the United States* 1988-1992, NIH Publication No. 96-4104, 1996.

CLINICAL APPLICATION and CRITICAL THINKING

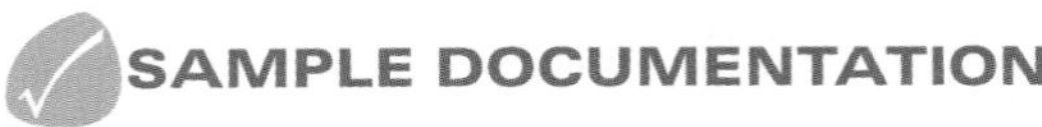

SAMPLE DOCUMENTATION

CASE 1

M.W. is an 81-year-old widow with a presenting complaint of rectal bleeding.

Subjective Data

Mrs. W. reports bright red blood on toilet tissue and underwear for 2 weeks. No previous episodes of rectal bleeding or bowel problems. Frequent constipation; worse than usual last couple weeks. Reports stools are hard, dark brown; experiences pain with defecation. Has bowel movement once per day. Diet limited to soft cooked vegetables, fruits, and bread due to poor dentition. Activity limited; spends most time sitting because of pain in knees from osteoarthritis and is fearful of falling. Denies any other health care problems.

Objective Data

Height, 5′1″ (155 cm); weight, 172 lb (78 kg).

Well-nourished, healthy, obese white woman.

Perianal area: Appears intact, with no evidence of active bleeding, lesions, or excoriation. Multiple external, pale hemorrhoids noted around anus. One hemorrhoid at 9 o'clock position from symphysis pubis is thrombosed and appears dark purple in color. Upon palpation, the hemorrhoid is painful and feels full. Anal sphincter tone is strong around examiner's finger. No evidence of internal rectal wall lesions, masses, nodules, or discomfort to digital palpation; guaiac negative.

Functional Health Patterns Involved

- Elimination
- Cognitive–perceptual
- Activity–exercise

Medical Diagnosis

Hemorrhoids, osteoarthritis

Nursing Diagnosis and Collaborative Problems

- *Pain* related to hemorrhoids as manifested by:
  - Reports pain with bowel movements
  - Hemorrhoids observed, one thrombosed, dark and purple.
  - Pain on palpation on hemorrhoids.
- *Constipation* related to inadequate dietary bulk and exercise as manifested by:
  - History of constipation.
  - Report of hard stools.
  - Eating soft vegetables and fruits.
  - Activity limitation due to arthritis in knee.
- *Impaired walking* related to inflammation and pain within knee joints as manifested by:
  - Reports arthritis prevents her from walking very much.
  - Spends most of her time in chair.
  - Expresses fear of falling.
- *PC*: Anal fissure

CASE 2

C.H. is a 62-year-old man with a history of difficulty urinating.

Subjective Data

Client reports difficulty with urination, especially when starting to urinate. Symptoms have increased over the past 6 months. Reports urine stream is not as strong as it used to be; dribbling occurs following urination. Frequency of urination has increased; gets up at least one or two times during the night to urinate. No pain or discomfort reported with urination; frequently experiences bladder fullness. No difficulty with bowel movements nor any change in bowel movement pattern. No pain or discomfort, no weight change, no dietary changes. Client has not had a physical examination or prostate examination for 4 years.

Objective Data

Height, 5′6″ (168 cm); weight, 142 lb (64.5 kg).

Well-nourished, healthy-appearing man. Slight distention noted with bladder palpation.

Sacrococcygeal and perianal areas: Without lesions, dimpling, or skin discoloration.

Anus: Intact, with dark even pigment, and without lesions, hemorrhoids, polyps, or fissures. Strong anal sphincter tone around examiner's finger.

Rectal walls: Smooth and without evidence of masses, swelling, or tenderness.

Prostate: Palpated on the posterior wall of the rectum, extends into the rectum approximately 1⅛ inches (3 cm). Prostate is symmetric and feels smooth, rubbery, and enlarged. The median sulcus is not evident.

Guaiac testing of fecal material: Negative.

Functional Health Patterns Involved

- Elimination
- Health promotion–health perception

Medical Diagnosis

Benign prostatic hyperplasia

Nursing Diagnosis and Collaborative Problems

- *Altered patterns of elimination* related to bladder outlet obstruction as manifested by:
  - Difficulty initiating urine stream.
  - Decreased urinary stream.
  - Frequency of urination, nocturia.
  - Enlarged prostate palpated.
- *Urinary retention* related to bladder outlet obstruction as manifested by:
  - Postvoiding dribbling.
  - Frequency of urination, nocturia.
  - Enlarged prostate palpated.
  - Bladder fullness.
- *PC*: Urinary tract infection
- *PC*: Prostatitis

CRITICAL THINKING QUESTIONS

1. A 68-year-old man comes to the emergency department with a history of urinary retention. He states, "I know my bladder is full, but I can't seem to pee." This symptom could be caused by prostatitis, benign prostatic hyperplasia, or prostate cancer. How does the examiner differentiate the cause of his symptom?
2. A 70-year-old woman comes to a clinic with a complaint of rectal bleeding. There are multiple causes of rectal bleeding. What kind of interview questions should be asked to help the examiner narrow down the cause of the problem?
3. A 24-year-old man has a chief complaint of rectal soreness. During the course of the interview, you learn he is homosexual, has multiple partners, and is the receptive partner in anal sex. He estimates he has anal sex approximately 1 to 2 times a week. He indicates he uses condoms on occasion. This client is at risk for several problems. List some health problems he is at risk for.
4. You have been asked to speak at a Rotary Club function about dietary measures to reduce the risk of colorectal cancer. Describe what areas you might want to cover.

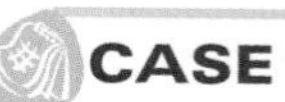

CASE STUDY

Mr. Murphy is a 66-year-old man who presents to his primary care provider complaining of a 3-month history of rectal fullness. Listed below is data collected by the examiner during an interview and examination.

Interview Data

Mr. Murphy tells the examiner he has had rectal discomfort off and on for last several months, but became concerned when he started seeing blood in his stool. The blood is described as "red." Mr. Murphy states he first started to see blood spots on his underwear about 8 weeks ago but ignored it, thinking he had hemorrhoids. Since that time the bleeding has increased and occurs not only when he has a bowel movement, but also throughout the day. Now he states is afraid he might be "more than a little sick." When asked about changes in his diet, Mr. Murphy indicates that he really hasn't been very hungry lately and has lost 10 lb (4.5 kg) over the last several months. He states he has become increasingly tired over this time and feels he has no energy.

Examination Data

- **General survey:** Thin-appearing man who moves slowly into room, appears fatigued.
- **Vital signs:** Respiratory rate, 20; Pulse, 110 beats/min; Blood pressure, 114/78 mm Hg; Temperature, 98.2° F (36.8° C).
- **Rectal examination:** Perineal and anal inspection is unremarkable with no lesions, dimpling, or changes in skin characteristics. Sphincter tone findings unremarkable. A large mass is felt with rectal palpation extending from the posterior to the left lateral rectal wall. The prostate is smooth, firm, and nontender to palpation with a 1-cm protrusion.

1. What data deviate from normal findings, suggesting a need for further investigation?
2. What additional information should the nurse ask or assess for?
3. In what functional health patterns does data deviate from normal?
4. What nursing diagnosis and/or collaborative problems should be considered for this situation?

REMEMBER to check out your companion CD-ROM

24 Musculoskeletal System

www.mosby.com/MERLIN/wilson/assessment/

ANATOMY AND PHYSIOLOGY

The musculoskeletal system provides both support and mobility for the body and protection for internal organs. This system also produces red blood cells and stores minerals such as calcium and phosphorous.

SKELETON

The human skeleton can be divided into two structures. The axial skeleton comprises the skull facial bones, auditory ossicles, vertebrae, ribs, sternum, and hyoid bone; the appendicular skeleton comprises bones of the upper and lower extremities. Each of the skeleton's 206 bones is shaped to facilitate its function. Major bones of the body are shown in Figs. 24-1, 24-2, 24-3, and 24-4.

SKELETAL MUSCLES

Skeletal muscles are composed of muscle fibers that attach to bones to facilitate movement. Although some skeletal muscles move by reflex, all are under voluntary control. Skeletal muscle fibers are arranged parallel to the long axis of bones to which they attach, or they are obliquely attached. Muscles attach at each end to a bone, ligament, tendon, or fascia. Muscles of the arms, legs, trunk, and pelvis are shown in Figs. 24-5, 24-6, and 24-7.

JOINTS

Joints are articulations where two or more bones are joined together or where two bone surfaces come together. They help hold the bones firmly while allowing movement between them.

Joints are classified in two ways. First, they are classified by the type of material between the bones: fibrous, cartilaginous, or synovial. Joints also are classified by their degree of movement: immovable joints are synarthrodial, slightly movable joints are amphiarthrodial, and freely movable joints are diarthrodial.

Diarthrodial joints are further classified by their type of movement. Hinge joints permit extension and flexion; examples are the knee, elbow, and fingers. Some hinge joints allow hyperextension; however, there is variability among clients; not all hinge joints are able to hyperextend. Pivot joints permit movement of one bone articulating with a ring or notch of another bone, such as the head of the radius, which articulates with the radial notch of the ulna. The ends of saddle-shaped bones articulate with each other; the base of the thumb is the only example. Condyloid or ellipsoidal joints consist of the condyle of one bone that fits into the elliptically shaped portion of its articulating bone; for instance, the distal end of the radius articulates with three wrist bones. Ball-and-socket joints are made of a ball-shaped bone that fits into a concave area of its articulating bone, such as the hip and shoulder joints. Gliding joints permit movement along various axes through relatively flat articulating surfaces, such as joints between two vertebrae.

JOINT MOVEMENT AND RANGE OF MOTION

Only the diarthrodial joints have one or more ranges of motion. Table 24-1 shows the type of movement of each joint.

Diarthrodial joints are called synovial joints because they are lined with synovial fluid (Fig. 24-8). Some synovial joints such as the knee also have a disk called the meniscus, which is a pad of cartilage that cushions the joint (Fig. 24-9). These joints have a covering surrounding them, called the joint capsule, which is an extension of the periosteum of the articulating bone. Ligaments also encase the capsule to add strength.

LIGAMENTS AND TENDONS

The difference between ligaments and tendons is more functional than structural. Ligaments are strong, dense, flexible bands of connective tissue that hold bones to bones. They can provide support in several ways: by encircling the joint, by gripping it obliquely, or by lying parallel to the bone ends, across the joint. They can simultaneously allow some movements while restricting others.

Conversely, tendons are strong, nonelastic cords of collagen located at the ends of muscles to attach them to bones. Tendons support bone movement in response to skeletal muscle contractions, transmitting remarkable force at times from the contracting muscles to the bone without sustaining injury themselves. Tendons and ligaments of the knee joint are shown in Fig. 24-9.

CARTILAGE AND BURSAE

Cartilage is a semismooth, gel-like supporting tissue that forms a cap over the ends of bones, providing a smooth surface for articulation (see Fig. 24-8). Cartilage absorbs weight and stress. Because it contains no blood vessels, cartilage re-

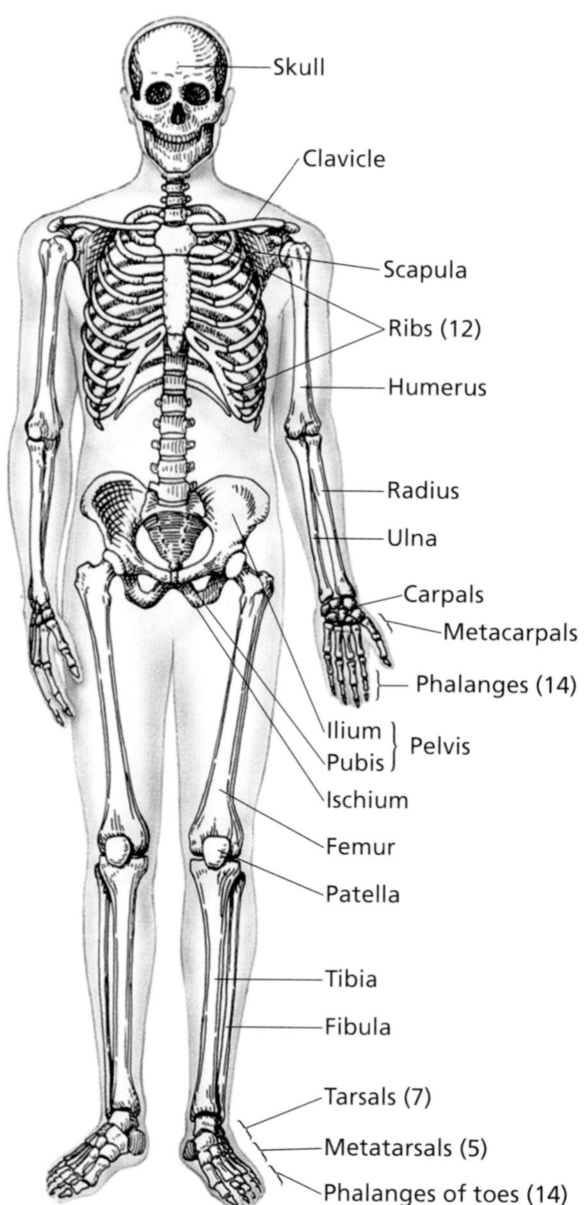

Fig. 24-1 Major bones of the body. (From Mourad, 1991.)

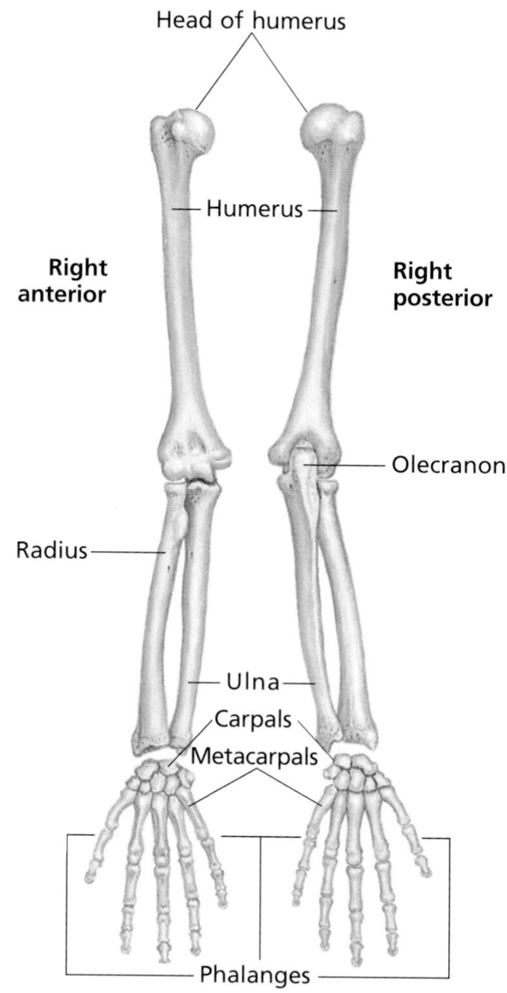

Fig. 24-2 Bones of the arm. (From Mourad, 1991.)

ceives nutrition from the synovial fluid forced into it during movement and weight-bearing activities. For this reason, weight-bearing activity and joint movement are essential to maintaining cartilage health.

Bursae are small sacs or cavities in the connective tissues surrounding or near a joint. Each bursa is lined with synovial membrane containing synovial fluid that acts as a lubricant for the joint. Bursae can form spontaneously as a result of pressure or friction (see Fig. 24-8).

AXIAL SKELETON AND SUPPORTING STRUCTURES

Skull and Neck

The six bones of the cranium—one frontal, two parietal, two temporal, and one occipital—are fused together. The face consists of 14 bones—two nasal, a frontal, two lacrimal, a sphenoid, two zygomatic, two maxillary bones and a mandible, which is movable (Fig. 24-10) (not shown are two nasal conchal and an ethmoid bone, see Fig. 13-2). The neck is supported by the cervical vertebrae, ligaments, and the sternocleidomastoid and trapezius muscles, with its greatest mobility at the level of C4-5 or C5-6. The type of movement permitted includes flexion, extension, and hyperflexion as well as lateral, flexion, and rotation. The sternocleidomastoid muscle stretches from the upper sternum and anterior clavicle to the mastoid process; the trapezius links the scapula, the lateral third of the clavicle, and the vertebrae, extending to the occipital prominence (Fig. 24-11).

Spine

The spine is composed of 7 cervical, 12 thoracic, 5 lumbar, and 5 sacral vertebrae. The cervical, thoracic, and lumbar vertebrae are separated from each other by fibrocartilaginous disks, whereas the sacral vertebrae are fused. The vertebral joints, separated by disks, glide slightly over one another's surfaces, permitting flexion, hyperextension, lateral bending, and rotation. The cervical joints are most active.

Text continued on p. 635

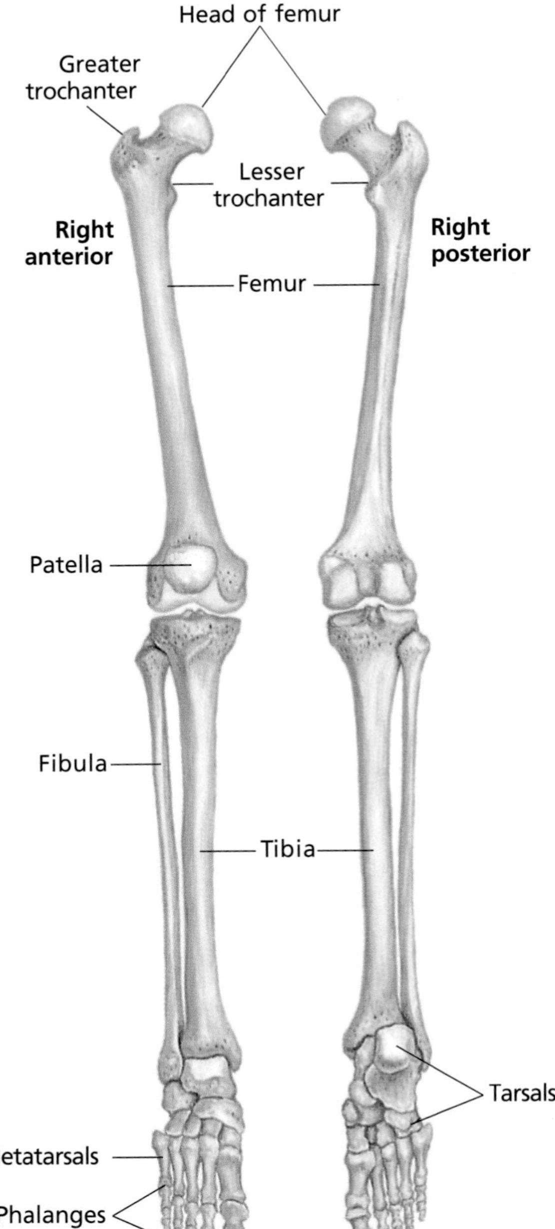

Fig. 24-3 Bones of the leg. (From Mourad, 1991.)

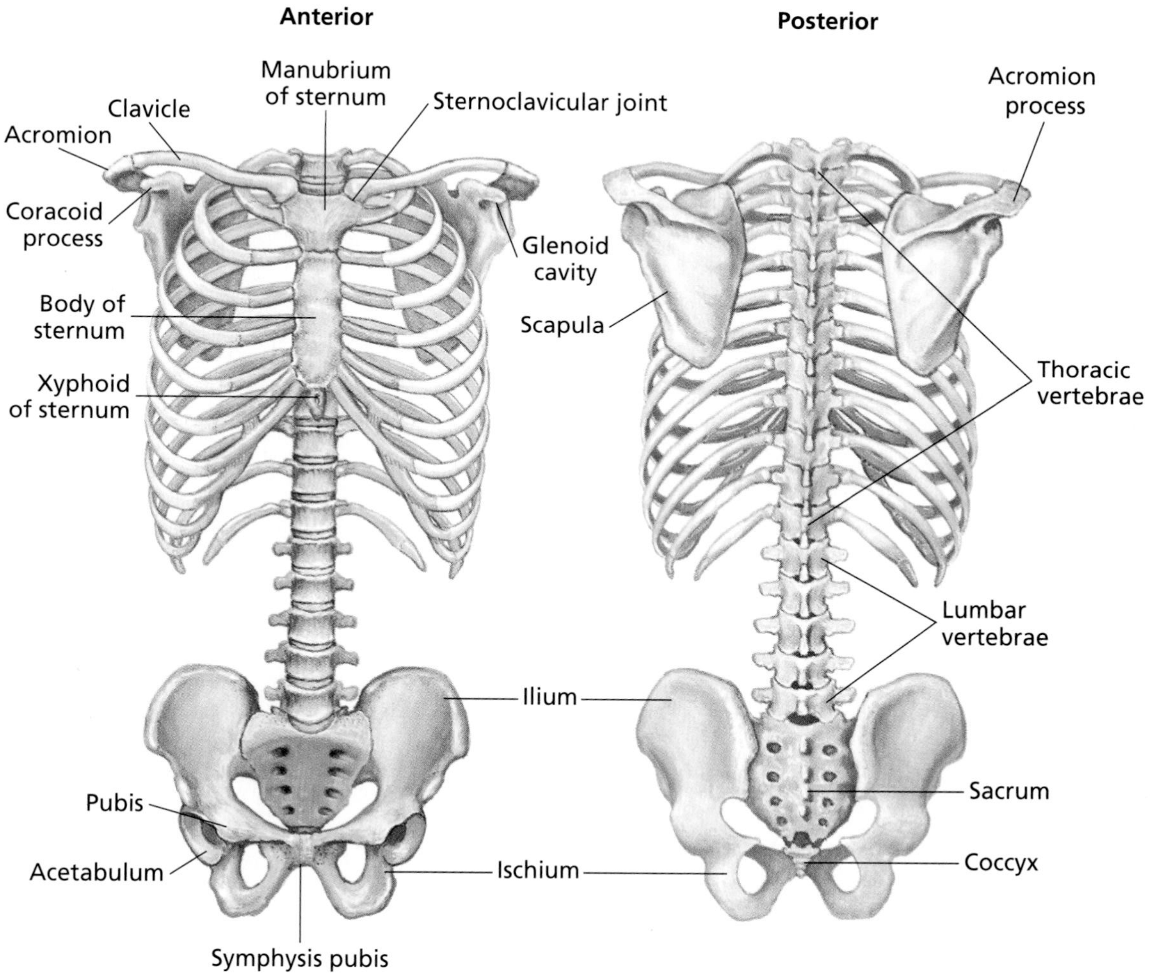

Fig. 24-4 Bones of the trunk and pelvis. (From Mourad, 1991.)

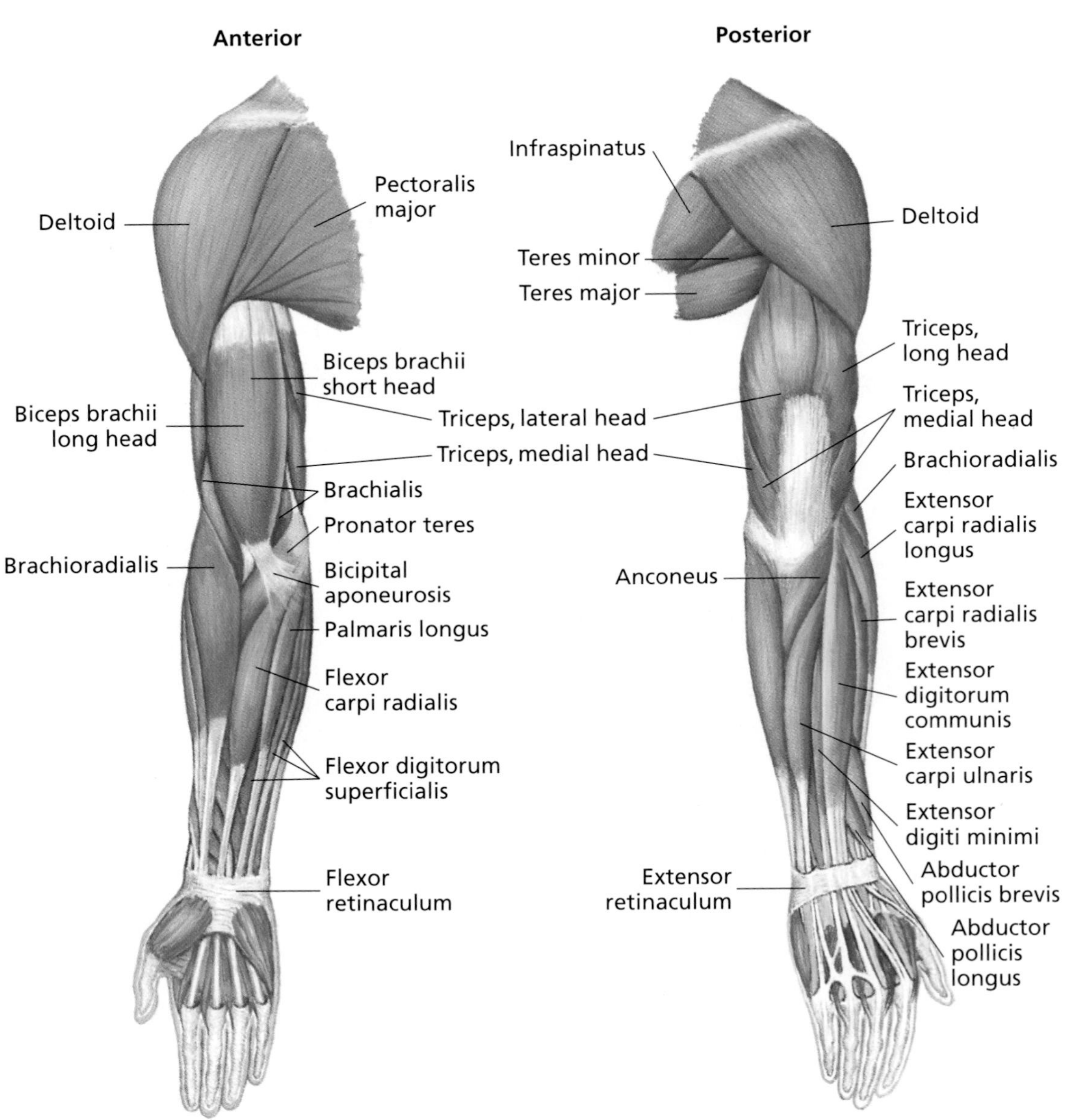

Fig. 24-5 Muscles of the arm. (From Mourad, 1991.)

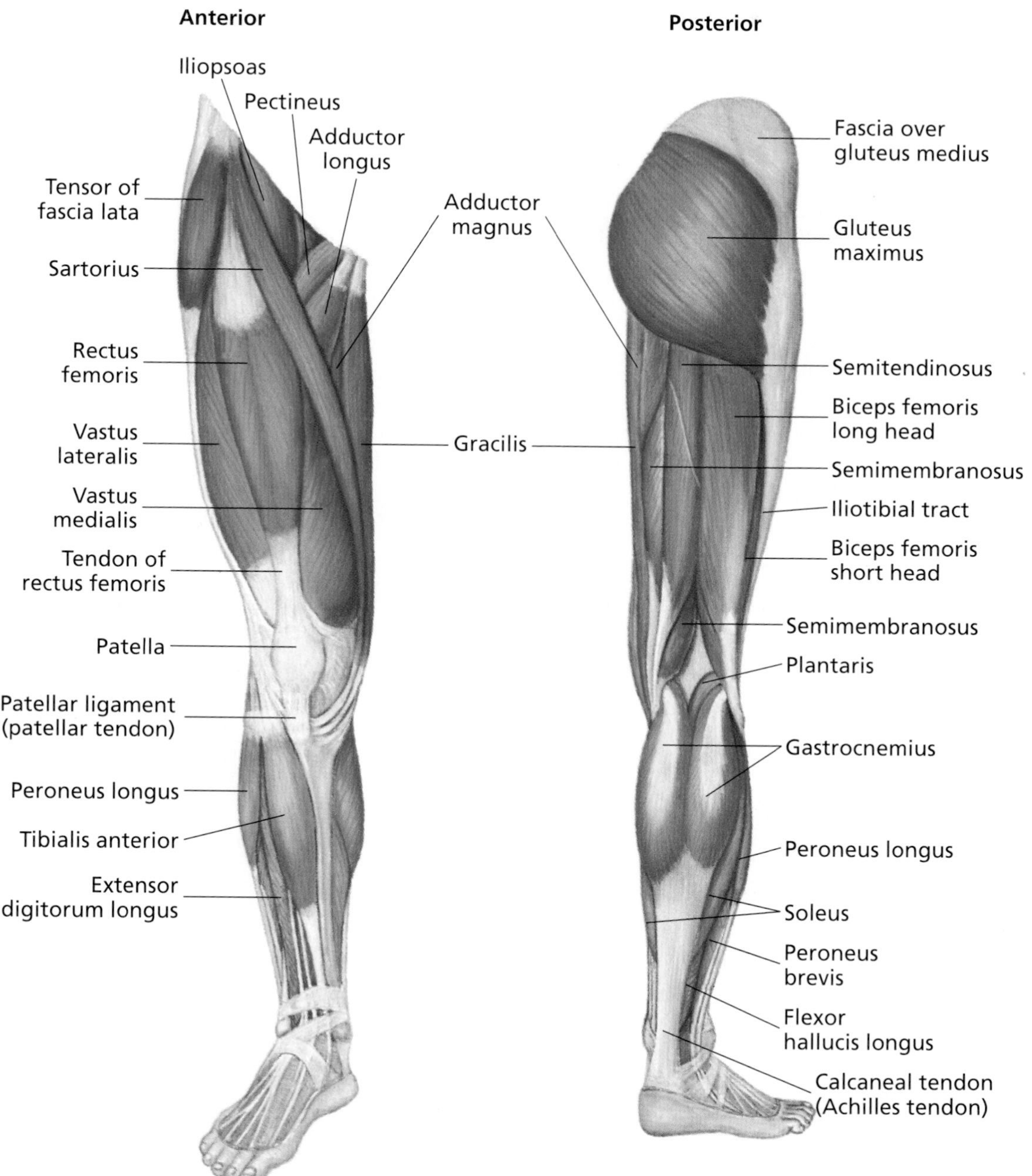

Fig. 24-6 Muscles of the leg. (From Mourad, 1991.)

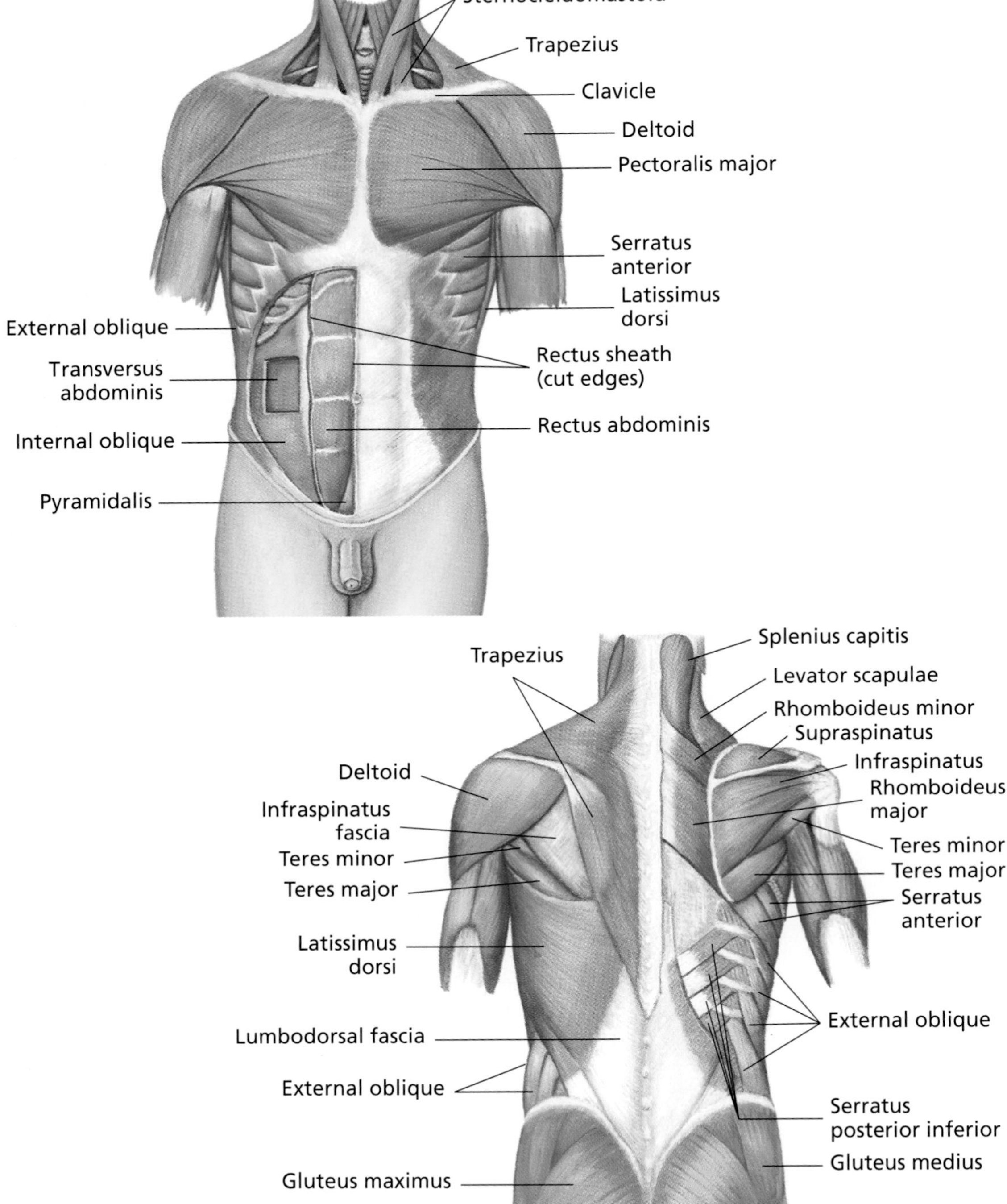

Fig. 24-7 Muscles of the trunk and pelvis. (From Mourad, 1991.)

Table 24-1 Range of Motion for Joints

BODY PART	TYPE OF JOINT	TYPE OF MOVEMENT
Neck and cervical spine	Pivotal 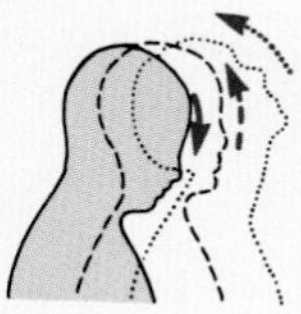	Flexion: bring chin to rest on chest Extension: return head to erect position Hyperextension: bend head back as far as possible
	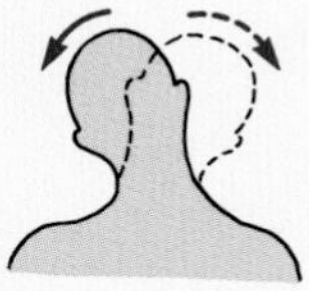	Lateral flexion: tilt head as far as possible toward each shoulder
	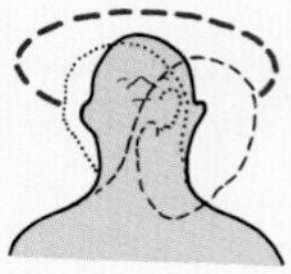	Rotation: turn head as far as possible to right and left
Shoulder	Ball and socket 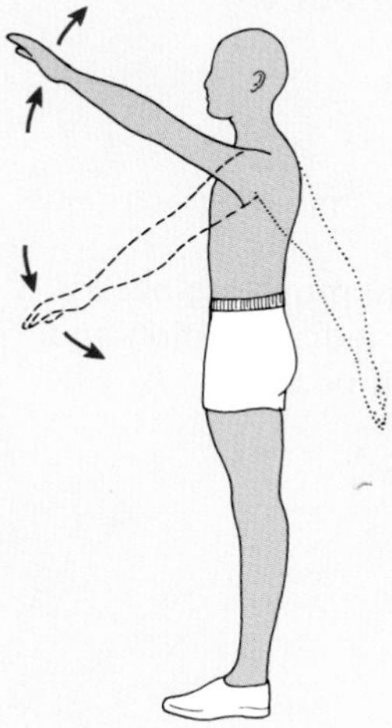	Flexion: raise arm from side position forward to position above head
		Extension: return arm to position at side of the body Hyperextension: move arm behind body, keeping elbow straight
	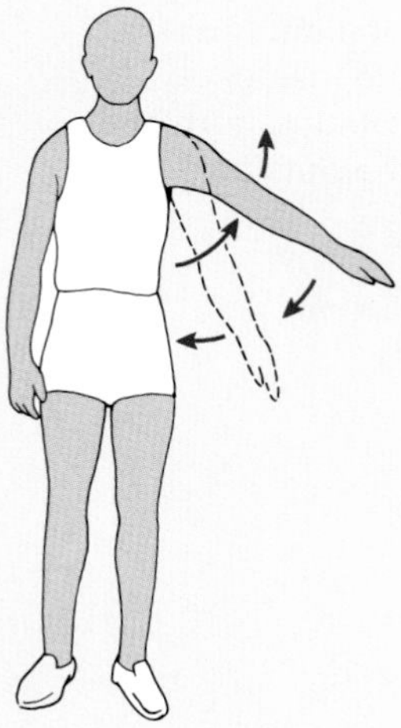	Abduction: raise arm to side to position above head with palm away from head Adduction: lower arm sideways and across body as far as possible
	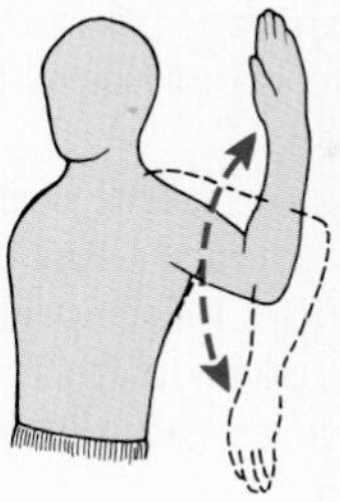	Internal rotation: with elbow flexed, rotate shoulder by moving arm until thumb is turned inward and toward back External rotation: with elbow flexed, move arm until thumb is upward and lateral to head
	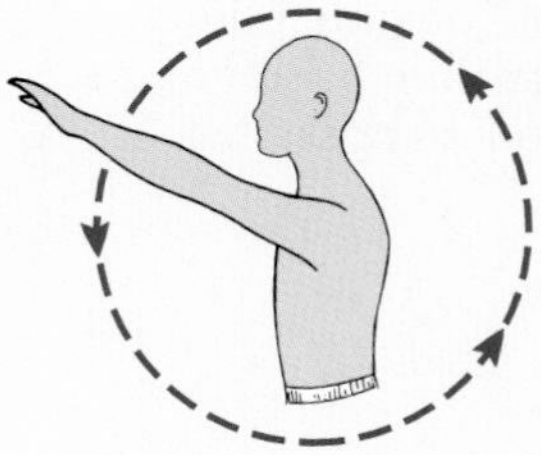	Circumduction: move arm in full circle. Circumduction is combination of all movements of ball-and-socket joint
Elbow	Hinge 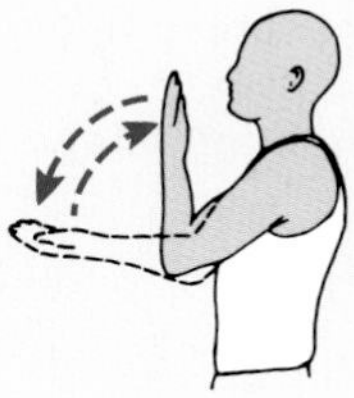	Flexion: bend elbow so that lower arm moves toward its shoulder joint and hand is level with shoulder Extension: straighten elbow by lowering hand Hyperextension: bend lower arm back as far as possible. Not all elbows hyperextend
Forearm	Pivotal 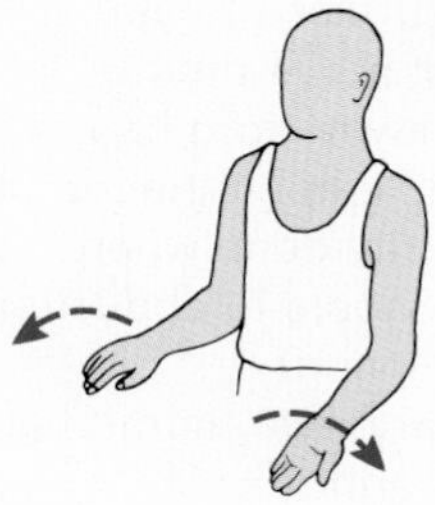	Supination: turn lower arm and hand so that palm is up Pronation: turn lower arm so that palm is down
Wrist	Condyloid 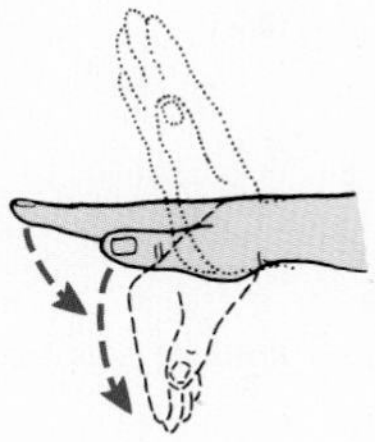	Flexion: move palm toward inner aspect of the forearm Extension: move fingers so that fingers, hands, and forearm are in same plane Hyperextension: bring dorsal surface to hand back as far as possible

From Potter PA, Perry AG: *Basic nursing: A critical thinking approach,* ed 4, St. Louis, 1999, Mosby.

Continued

Table 24-1 Range of Motion for Joints—cont'd

BODY PART	TYPE OF JOINT	TYPE OF MOVEMENT	BODY PART	TYPE OF JOINT	TYPE OF MOVEMENT
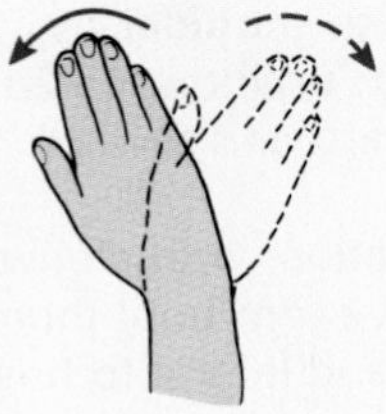		Hyperextension: bring dorsal surface to hand back as far as possible Radial flexion: bend wrist medially toward thumb Ulnar flexion: bend wrist laterally toward fifth finger Referred to as radial/ulnar deviation	Hip 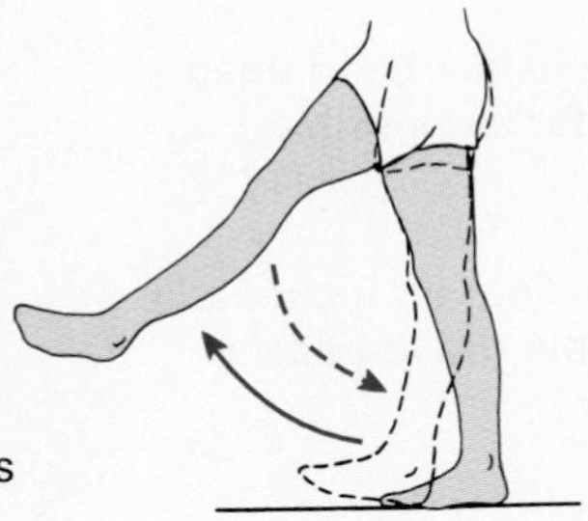	Ball and socket	Flexion: move leg forward and up Extension: move leg back beside other leg
Fingers 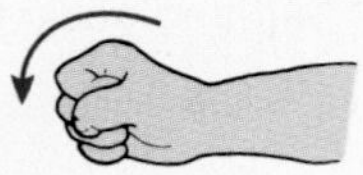 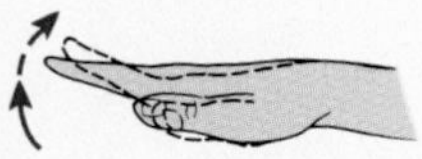	Condyloid hinge	Flexion: make fist Extension: straighten fingers Hyperextension: bend fingers back as far as possible	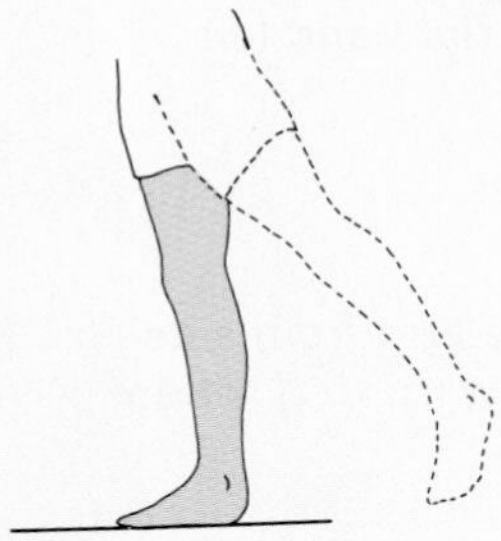		Hyperextension: move leg behind body
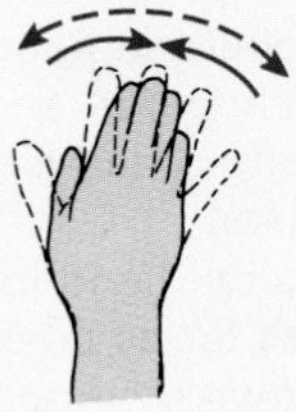		Abduction: spread fingers apart Adduction: bring fingers together	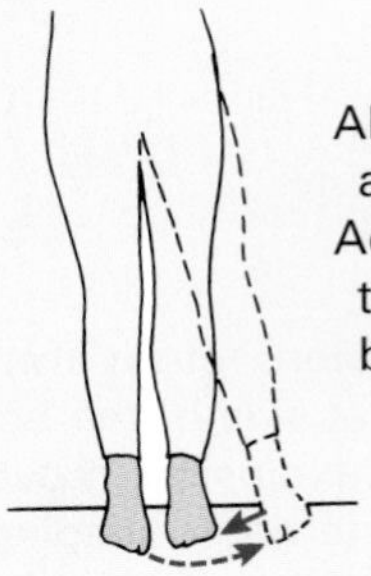		Abduction: move leg laterally away from body Adduction: move leg back toward medial position and beyond if possible
Thumb 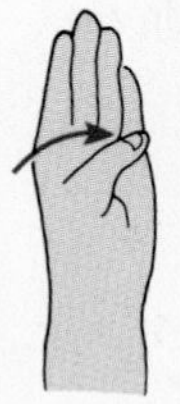 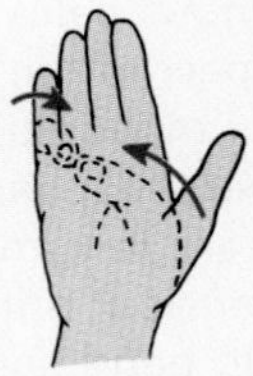	Saddle	Flexion: move thumb across palmar surface of hand Extension: move thumb straight away from hand Abduction: extend thumb laterally (usually done when placing fingers in abduction and adduction) Adduction: move thumb back toward hand Opposition: touch thumb to each finger of same hand	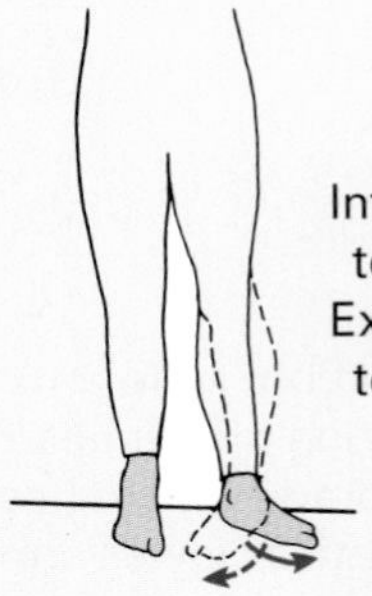		Internal rotation: turn knee toward the inside External rotation: turn knee toward the outside

From Potter PA, Perry AG: *Basic nursing: A critical thinking approach,* ed 4, St. Louis, 1999, Mosby.

Table 24-1 Range of Motion for Joints—cont'd

BODY PART	TYPE OF JOINT	TYPE OF MOVEMENT
		Circumducti move leg in circle
Knee	Hinge	lexion: bring heel back toward back of thigh Extension: return heel to floor
	Hinge	Dorsiflexion: move foot so that toes are pointed upward Plantar flexion: move foot so that toes are pointed downward
Foot	Gliding	Inversion: turn sole of foot medially Eversion: turn sole of foot laterally
Toes	Condyloid	Flexion: curl toes downward Extension: straighten toes Abduction: spread toes apart Adduction: bring toes together

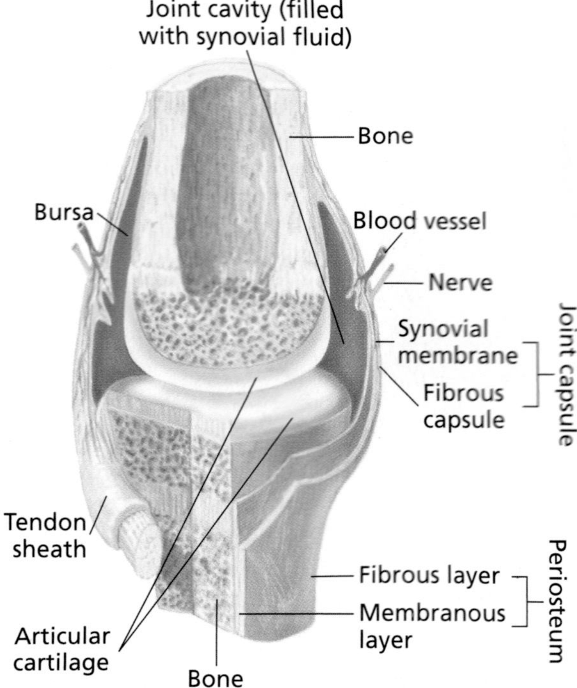

Fig. 24-8 Structures of a synovial joint (the knee). (From Mourad, 1991.)

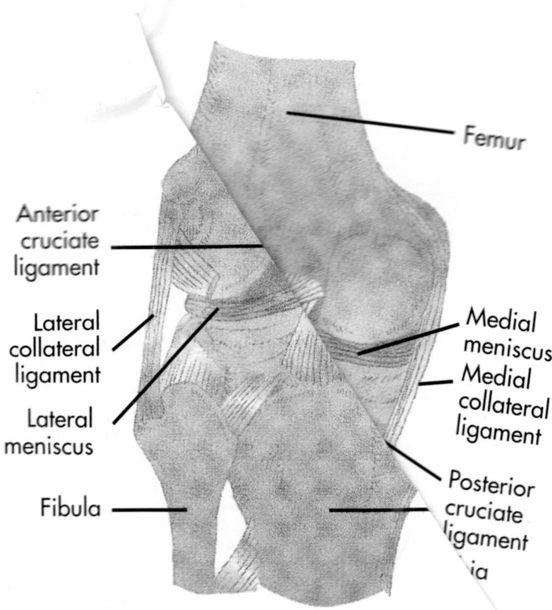

Fig. 24-9 A posterior view of the left knee. The n collateral ligament prevents the knee from going i much valgus during stress (inward). The lateral coll ligament prevents the knee from going into too much varus during stress (outward). (From Black and Matassairin-Jacobs, 1997.)

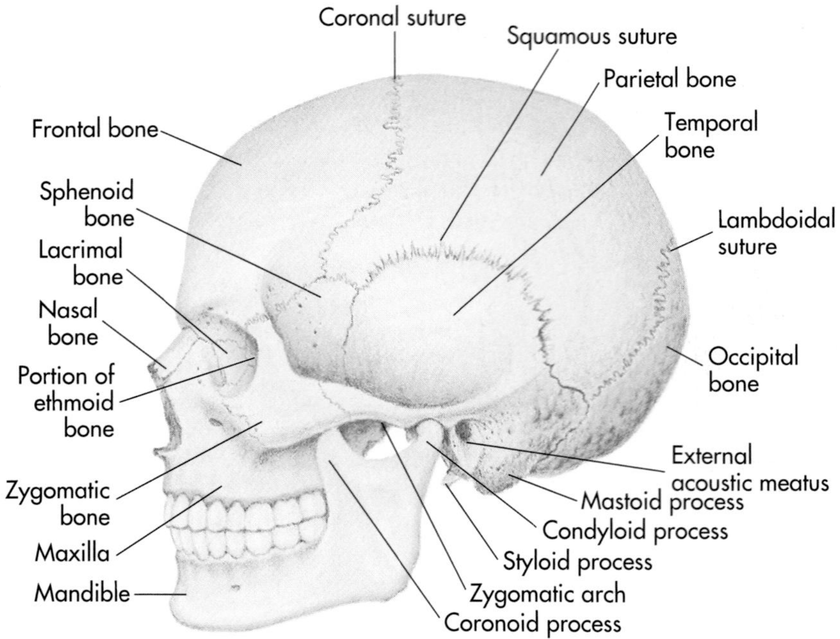

Fig. 24-10 Bones of the skull. (From Seidel et al, 1999.)

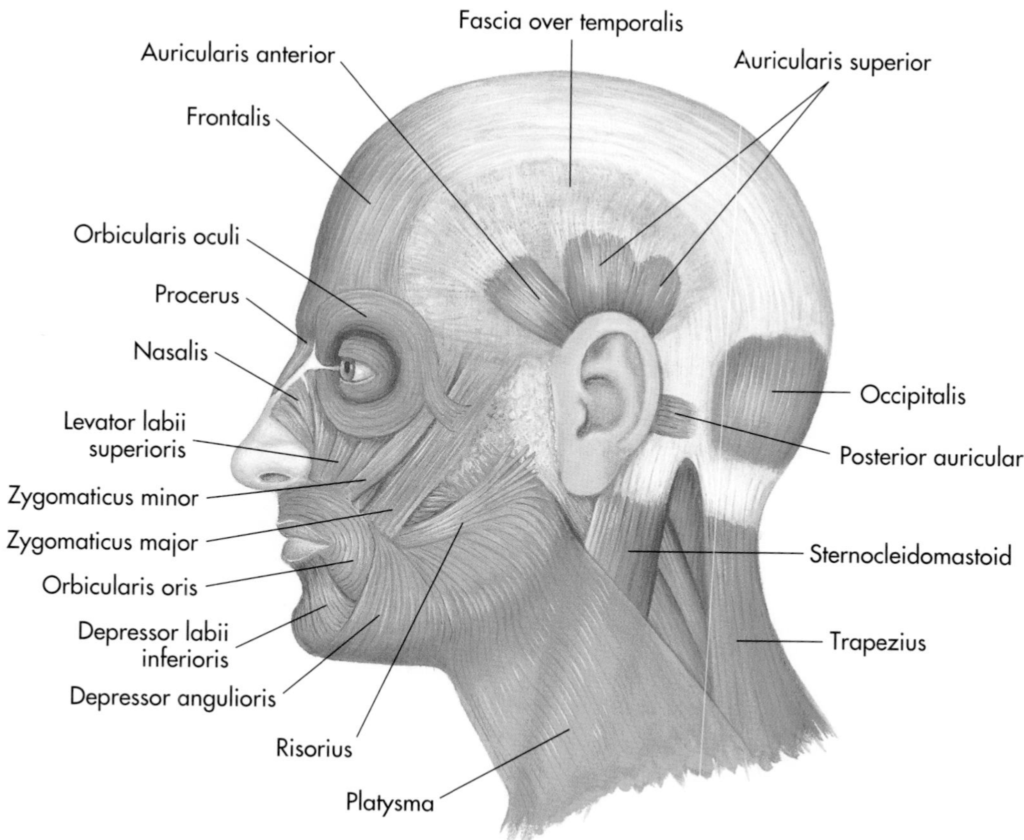

Fig. 24-11 Muscles of the head, face, and neck, left lateral view. (From Seidel et al, 1999.)

APPENDICULAR SKELETON AND SUPPORTING STRUCTURES

Upper Extremities

Shoulder and Arm The shoulder joint, also called the glenohumeral joint, consists of the point where the humerus and the glenoid fossa of the scapula articulate. The acromial and coracoid processes (see Fig. 24-4) and surrounding ligaments protect this ball-and-socket joint and permit flexion, extension and hyperextension, abduction and adduction, and internal and external rotation. Besides the glenohumeral joint, two other joints contribute to shoulder movement: the acromioclavicular joint (between the acromial process and the clavicle) (Fig. 24-12) and the sternoclavicular joint (between the sternal manubrium and the clavicle) (see Fig. 24-4).

Elbow and Wrist The elbow joint consists of the humerus, radius, and ulna enclosed in a single synovial cavity protected by ligaments and a bursa between the olecranon and the skin. The elbow is a hinge joint, permitting extension, flexion, and sometimes hyperextension (see Fig. 24-2). Pronation and supination of the forearm are provided also. The wrist joins the radius and the carpal bones with articular disks of the wrist, ligaments, and a fibrous capsule to form a condyloid joint, permitting flexion, extension, and hyperextension as well as radial and ulnar flexion, also called radial and ulnar deviation.

Hand There are small, subtle movements or articulations within the hand between the carpals and metacarpals, the metacarpals and proximal phalanges, and between the middle and distal phalanges. Ligaments protect the diarthrotic joints, which allow flexion, extension, and hyperextension. The fingers are able to flex and extend as well as abduct and adduct.

Lower Extremities

Hip and Thigh The acetabulum and femur form the hip joint, protected by a fibrous capsule and three bursae. Three ligaments help stabilize the head of the femur in the joint capsule (Fig. 24-13). Like the shoulder, this is a ball-and-socket joint that provides flexion, extension and hyperextension, abduction and adduction, internal and external rotation and circumduction.

Knee and Lower Leg The knee, a hinge joint, is a more complex joint than some joints. It serves as the point of articulation between the femur, the tibia, and the patella, making use of medial and lateral menisci (disk-shaped fibrous cartilage), that cushion the tibia and the femur and connect to the articulated capsule. Ligaments provide stability, whereas the bursae reduce friction on movement between the femur and the tibia (see Fig. 24-8). Movements of this joint include flexion, extension, and sometimes hyperextension.

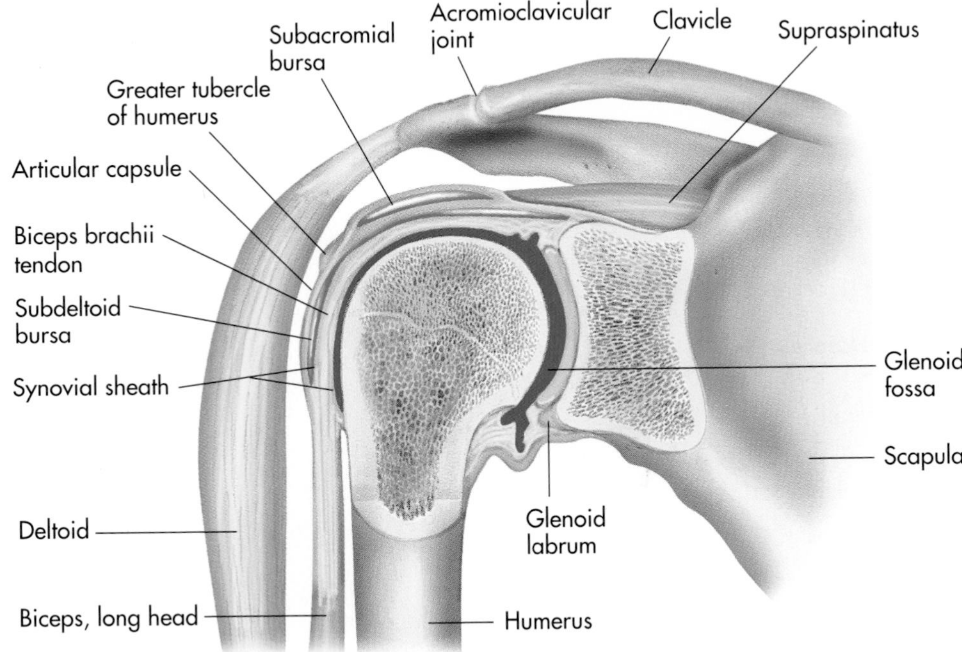

Fig. 24-12 Structures of glenohumeral and acromioclavicular joint of the shoulder. (From Seidel et al, 1999.)

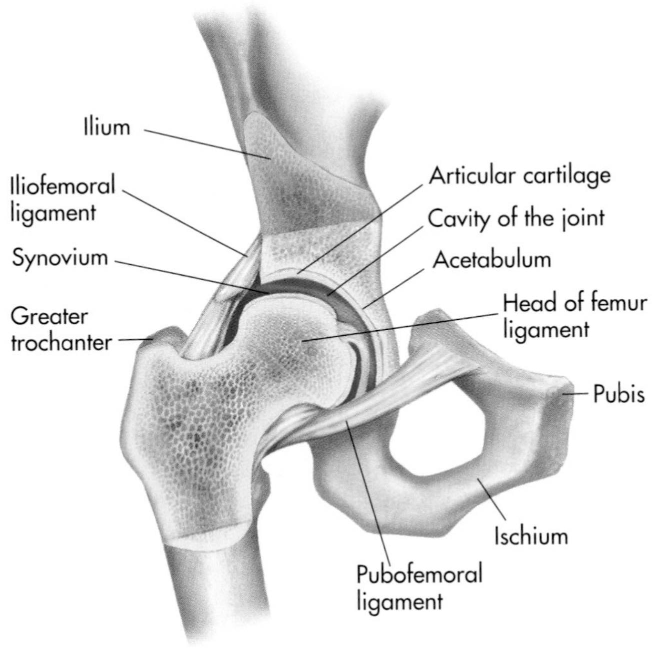

Fig. 24-13 Structures of the hip. (From Thompson et al, 1997.)

Ankle and Foot The ankle joint, or tibiotalar joint, forms a hinge joint, permitting flexion, called dorsiflexion, and extension in one plane, which is called plantar flexion. This joint joins the tibia, the fibula, and the talus with protective medial and lateral ligaments. Smaller joints within the ankle permit a pivot or rotation movement, producing inversion and eversion, as well as adduction and abduction. These are the subtalar (talocalcaneal) joint and the talonavicular joint (transverse tarsal) (Fig. 24-14).

Like the hand, the foot has several smaller articulations occurring between the tarsals and metatarsals, the metatarsal and proximal phalanges, and the middle and distal phalanges. The foot has a gliding joint that allows inversion and eversion of the foot. The toes are condyloid joints that allow flexion and extension, as well as abduction and adduction.

A number of racial variations of the musculoskeletal system have been noted.

ETHNIC & CULTURAL VARIATIONS

A number of racial variations have been noted in the anatomy of the skeleton and of the skeletal muscles. Long bones are generally longer, narrower, and denser in African Americans, particularly African-American males. They are thus less subject to osteoporosis and other diseases involving the loss of bone density. Curvature of the femur tends to be straight in African Americans, convex anterior in Native Americans and Alaskan natives, and intermediate in whites.

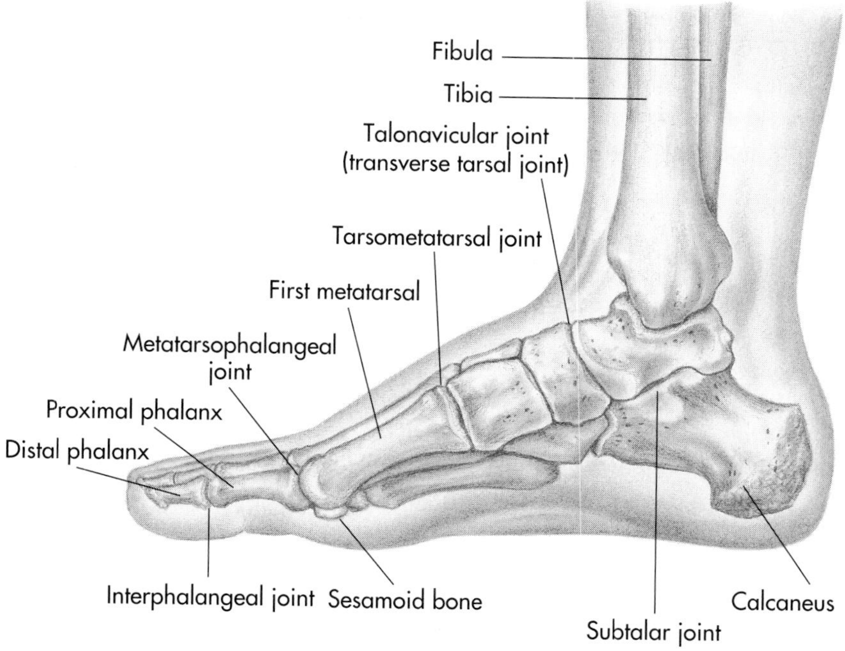

Fig. 24-14 Bones and joints of the ankle and foot. (From Seidel et al, 1999.)

HEALTH HISTORY

Musculoskeletal System

QUESTIONS	RATIONALE
PRESENT HEALTH STATUS	
➤ How would you describe the health of your bones, muscles, and joints?	■ It is important to obtain the client's perception of the health of his or her musculoskeletal system.
➤ Do you have any chronic diseases? Cancer? Arthritis? Loss of bone density or osteoporosis?	■ Chronic diseases may affect the mobility and activities of daily living.
➤ Do you take any medications? If yes, what do you take and how often? Are you taking medications as they were prescribed? Are you taking any medications to prevent loss of bone density?	■ Both prescription and over-the-counter medications should be documented. Clients may not report musculoskeletal problems if they are being successfully treated with medications. Many medications for musculoskeletal problems (aspirin; nonsteroidal antiinflammatory drugs, e.g., ibuprofen; narcotics; tranquilizers, or sleep aids) can cause adverse side effects and may increase risk of injury.

QUESTIONS

RATIONALE

➤ Have you noticed any changes in your ability to move around or participate in your usual activities? Have you noticed any change in your muscle strength? What do you do to deal with these changes in muscle strength?

■ This question focuses the client's attention on any changes that he or she might have noticed that interfere with performance of daily activities. If there are changes, they can be diagnosed and treated at an early stage, or they can generate a discussion of how to prevent further changes. Need to determine how client is adapting to these changes.

➤ What do you do for exercise? How often do you exercise and for what period of time? Do you play sports? If yes, which ones and how often? How do you protect yourself from injury while exercising or playing sports? Do you smoke cigarettes? If yes, how many and how often? Do you drink alcohol? If yes, how much and how often?

■ These questions assess for risk for injury and osteoporosis and identify client's learning needs for health promotion. Adults should protect themselves from injury (e.g., stretching before running, wearing a bike helmet, and wearing elbow pads and wrist guards for roller blading).

➤ Do you lift, push, or pull items or bend or stoop frequently as a part of your daily routine either at home or at work? How do you protect yourself from muscle strain or injury?

■ Musculoskeletal injuries during work are a common cause of on-the-job injuries. Many of these can be prevented with proper body mechanics, appropriate help when lifting, and use of protective equipment. Similar injuries may occur in the home. These activities may cause weakness or pain from repeated stress and strain on bones, muscles, ligaments, and tendons. These questions also provide an opportunity to teach about preventing such injuries.

PAST MEDICAL HISTORY

➤ Have you ever had any accidents or trauma that affected the bones or joints, including fractures, strains of the joints, sprains, and dislocations? When? What was done for the problem? Have you noticed any continuing problems or difficulties that seem related to this previous incident?

■ History of musculoskeletal disorders tells you what type of disorders the client has experienced and may provide insight into findings to anticipate during the assessment. Previous injury can leave residual problems such as stiff joints or decreased range of motion.

➤ Do you have congenital bone or joint problems? If yes, describe. Have these problems altered your activities? If yes, explain how. How have you adapted to these problems?

■ Information about congenital deformities may give you data about what to anticipate during the assessment and about how well the client is adapting (has adapted), if necessary, to the deformity.

➤ Have you ever had surgery on any bones or joints or muscles? If yes, describe the procedure(s), when it (they) occurred and what the outcome was.

■ The incidence of surgery may provide additional information about possible musculoskeletal problems and the findings to anticipate during assessment.

FAMILY HISTORY

➤ In your family is there is history of curvature of the spine or back problems? If yes, describe.

■ Family history may be used to determine client's risk for spinal disorders.

➤ In your family is there a history of arthritis: rheumatoid, osteoarthritis, or gout?

■ Family history may be used to determine client's risk for forms of arthritis.

QUESTIONS

RATIONALE

PROBLEM-BASED HISTORY

The problem-based history gathered when interacting with clients who have musculoskeletal problems should focus on the following: pain, limitation of motion, and self-care behaviors. As with symptoms in all areas of health assessment, a symptom analysis is completed, which includes the location, quality, quantity, chronology, setting, associated manifestations, alleviating and aggravating factors (see Box 4-2 in Chapter 4).

Pain

➤ Where do you feel the pain? When did you first notice the pain? Describe how the pain feels. How severe is the pain on a scale of 1 to 10, with 10 being the worst pain possible?

■ Joint pain is the most common musculoskeletal symptom for which clients seek help. Pain is felt in and around the joint and may be accompanied by edema and erythema, indicating inflammation. Bone pain typically is described as "deep," "dull," "boring," or "intense." Bone pain frequently is not related to movement unless the bone is fractured, in which case the pain is described as sharp. Muscle pain is described as "crampy." Muscle pain in legs that occurs while walking but is relieved by rest is associated with peripheral vascular ischemia. Muscle pain associated with weakness suggests a primary muscular disorder.

➤ Did the pain occur suddenly? When during the day do you feel the pain?

■ Sudden onset of pain and erythema in the great toe, ankle, and lower leg suggests gout (also called gouty arthritis). Pain from rheumatoid arthritis and tendinitis may awaken the client, especially when the client is lying on the affected limb. Clients with rheumatoid arthritis often have morning stiffness lasting 1 to 2 hours. By contrast, clients with osteoarthritis experience pain when weight bearing that is relieved by rest.

➤ Does the pain move from one joint to another? Has there been any injury, overuse, or strain? Were you ill before the onset of pain?

■ Some disorders cause migratory arthritis, in which pain moves among joints (e.g., acute rheumatic fever, leukemia, or juvenile arthritis). Viral illnesses can cause muscle aches and pain (myalgia).

QUESTIONS | **RATIONALE**

➤ What makes the pain worse? Does the pain change according to the weather? Does the pain shoot to another part of your body?

■ Learning what makes the pain worse may help in diagnosing the disorder. Arthritis pain may become worse with changes in the barometric pressure. Movement usually makes joint pain worse except in rheumatoid arthritis, in which movement often reduces pain. Pain caused by compression of nerves may cause a radiating pain (e.g., spinal nerve roots compressed by a herniated disk may cause radiating pain along the sciatic nerve in the leg).

➤ What do you do to relieve the pain? How effective has it been?

■ Knowing what relieves pain may help selection of pain-relief strategies.

Limitation of Motion

➤ Have you had a recent sore throat?

■ Joint pain that occurs 10 to 14 days after a sore throat may be associated rheumatic fever.

➤ Are your joints swollen, red, or hot to the touch? Is the movement in your joints limited?

■ Acute inflammation such as arthritis or gout produces erythema, warmth, and edema. Decreased range of motion occurs in injury to the cartilage or capsule or with muscle contracture or edema.

➤ Do you feel any weakness in your muscles? Where? How long have you had this? Do you have trouble standing up after sitting in a chair? Does the weakness make you limp? Does the weakness become worse as the day progresses?

■ Muscle weakness may be due to altered nerve innervation or muscle contraction disorder. Atrophied muscles may be due to prolonged lack of use (e.g., unilateral atrophy occurs from disuse when an extremity is casted). This is referred to as disuse atrophy. Proximal muscle weakness is usually a myopathy, whereas distal weakness is usually a neuropathy.

➤ Have you noticed your knees or ankles giving way when you put pressure on them? If yes, when does this occur? How long does it last? How often does it occur? What do you think makes this happen?

■ This may indicate joint instability that may occur from chronic inflammation or joint trauma. Safety must be a concern of the client when a joint gives way.

➤ Have your joints felt as if they are locked and will not move? If yes, when does this occur? How long does it last? How often does it occur? What makes the locking better? What makes it worse?

■ This may indicate joint instability that may occur from chronic inflammation or joint trauma. Safety must be a concern of the client when a joint gives way.

QUESTIONS

RATIONALE

RISK FACTORS

COMMON RISK FACTORS ASSOCIATED WITH Osteoarthritis and Osteoporosis

OSTEOARTHRITIS

Over 50 years of age
Family history of osteoarthritis
History of joint trauma
History of rheumatoid arthritis
Obesity

OSTEOPOROSIS

Nonmodifiable risk factors
- Age: Over 35 years
- Gender: Female
- Race: White, Asian
- Body size: Small stature
- Family history of osteoporosis

Modifiable risk factors
- Estrogen deficiency from menopause, surgical removal of ovaries (oophorectomy), or amenorrhea from underweight.
- Heavy cigarette smoking
- Heavy alcohol consumption
- Low-calcium diet
- Lack of weight bearing (e.g., immobility or sedentary lifestyle)
- Prolonged use of corticosteroids

Limitations of Self-Care Behaviors

➤ What activities are limited by your musculoskeletal disorders? To what extent are they limited? How do you compensate for this limitation?
- -Bathing (getting in and out of the tub, turning faucets on or off)?
- -Toileting (urinating, defecating, ability to raise or lower yourself onto or off of the toilet)?
- -Dressing (buttoning, zipping, fastening openings behind your neck, hooking your brassiere, pulling a dress or shirt over your head, pulling up your pants, tying shoes, having shoes fit your feet)?
- -Grooming (shaving, brushing teeth, brushing or combing hair, washing and drying hair, applying makeup)?
- -Eating (preparing meals, pouring, holding utensils, cutting up food, bringing food to your mouth, drinking)?
- -Moving around (walking, going up or down stairs, getting in or out of bed, getting out of the house)?
- -Sleeping?
- -Communicating (writing, talking, using the telephone)?

■ Any impaired mobility or function may cause a self-care deficit. It is important to identify which activities are impaired, to what extent, and how the client compensates. The client may need further treatment or assistance with his or her compensation.

➤ For clients who have chronic disability or a crippling disease: How has your illness affected your interactions with your family? How has it affected your relationships with friends?

■ Assess for disturbance of self-esteem, body image, or role performance; loss of independence; or social isolation. Maintaining social relationships is an important aspect of therapy.

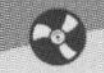

EXAMINATION

Equipment

- Tape measure to record length or circumference of extremities
- Goniometer to measure joint range of motion

PROCEDURES AND TECHNIQUES WITH NORMAL FINDINGS	ABNORMAL FINDINGS
➤Use a cephalocaudal organization with side-to-side comparisons for examining bones, muscles, and joints.	■ Since there are often no "normals" for the musculoskeletal system, the comparison with the other side is the preferred way to establish normality.
➤**OBSERVE gait for conformity, symmetry, and rhythm.** Ask the client to walk across the room and back. Expected findings are conformity (ability to follow gait sequencing of both stance and swing), regular smooth rhythm, symmetry in length of leg swing, smooth swaying, and smooth, symmetric arm swing.	■ An unstable or exaggerated gait, limp, irregular stride length, arm swing that is unrelated to gait, or any other inability to maintain straight posture or asymmetry of body parts will require further assessment when specific musculoskeletal regions are examined. When unequal leg length is suspected, measure the leg from the anterior superior iliac spine to the medial malleolus (see Fig. 24-16, *A*).
➤**INSPECT axial skeleton and extremities for alignment, contour, symmetry, size, and gross deformities.** Observe the client standing upright and straight from the front, back, and sides (Fig. 24-15, *A-C*). He or she should stand erect, with body parts symmetric. The spine should be straight with normal curvatures (cervical concave, thoracic convex, lumbar concave) (see Fig. 24-15, *C*). The knees should be in a straight line between the hips and ankles, and the feet should be flat on the floor and pointing directly forward. No gross deformities should be noted.	■ Irregular posture or any asymmetry or misalignment observed will warrant further assessment when specific musculoskeletal regions are assessed.

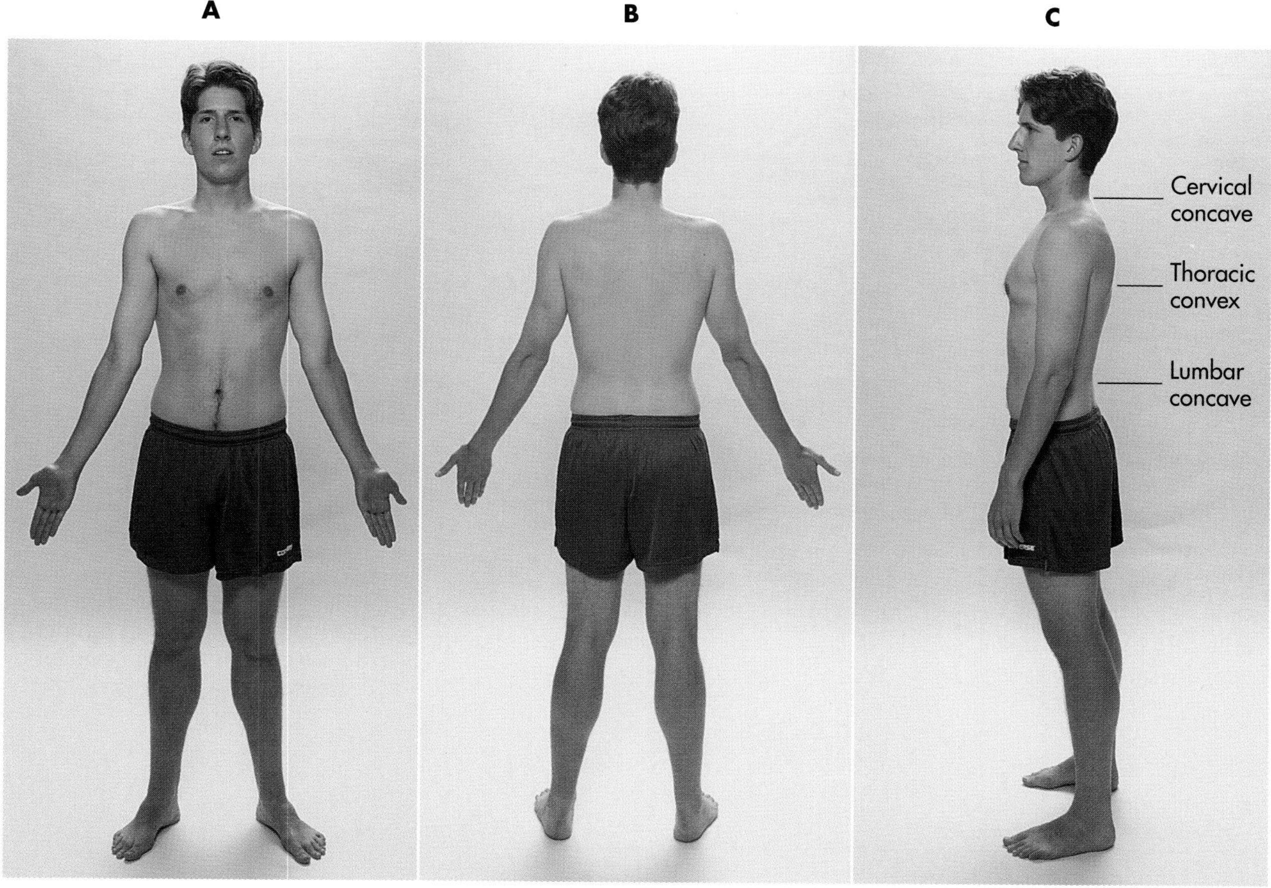

Fig. 24-15 Inspection of overall body posture. Note the even contour of the shoulders, level scapulae and iliac crests, alignment of the head over the gluteal folds, and symmetry and alignment of extremities. **A,** Anterior view. **B,** Posterior view. **C,** Lateral view showing normal cervical concave, thoracic convex, and lumbar concave curves of the spine.

PROCEDURES AND TECHNIQUES WITH NORMAL FINDINGS

OVERVIEW OF THE EXAMINATION OF SPECIFIC MUSCULOSKELETAL REGIONS

For each specific region, you will inspect muscles for symmetry; palpate bones and muscles for tone, tenderness, heat, and edema; observe range of joint motion; and test muscles for strength.

➤**INSPECT muscles for size and symmetry.** Muscle size should appear relatively symmetric bilaterally. (No person has exact symmetry side-to-side.) Muscle circumference can be measured with a cloth or paper tape measure to provide a baseline for future comparisons and to make side-to-side comparisons. Remember that the dominant side usually is slightly larger than the nondominant side. To ensure consistency of measurement, record the number of centimeters or inches above or below the joint where the muscle was measured or include a diagram like the one shown in Fig. 24-16, *B*. Measurement differences less than 1 cm (3/8 inch) usually are not significant.

ABNORMAL FINDINGS

■ Atrophy of muscle mass bilaterally may indicate lack of nerve stimulation, such as a spinal cord injury or malnutrition. Unilateral muscle atrophy may be from disuse, from pain on movement, or after removal of a cast. Fasciculations (muscle twitching of a single muscle group) may be caused by side effects of drugs or sodium deficiency. Fasciculations are localized, whereas spasms (involuntary muscle contractions) tend to be more generalized.

PROCEDURES AND TECHNIQUES WITH NORMAL FINDINGS

ABNORMAL FINDINGS

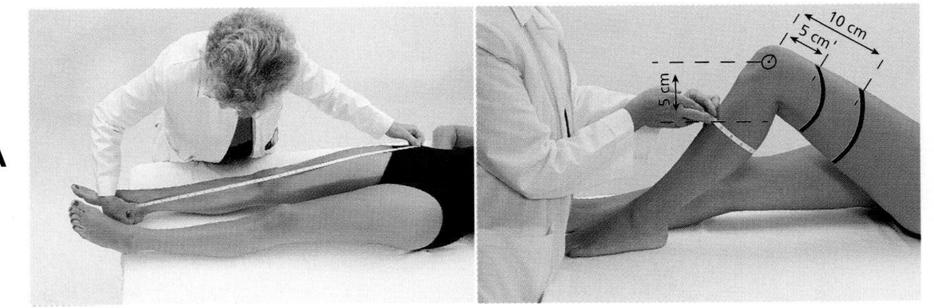

Fig. 24-16 Sites at which a limb is measured. **A,** Measure limb length from the anterior superior iliac spine to the medial malleolus. **B,** Measurement of midgastrocnemius at 5 cm below patella and 5 and 10 cm above the patella. Exact location of measurement should be noted for future comparison.

➤**PALPATE bones for tenderness and muscles for tenderness, heat, edema, and tone.** Muscles should feel firm, not hard or soft. No tenderness, heat, or edema should be detected. Table 24-2 contains a subjective scale for defining the degree of tenderness.

■ Tenderness, heat, or edema over bones or muscles may indicate tumor, inflammation, or trauma. Muscle atrophy may be evident by a decrease in muscle tone.

Table 24-2 Grading Scale to Quantify Tenderness

GRADE	DEFINITION
No tenderness	
1+	Client says it is tender.
2+	Client complains of pain and winces.
3+	Client complains of pain, winces, and pulls back.
4+	Client will not allow palpation.

From Greenberger NJ, Hinthorn DR: *History taking and physical examination,* St. Louis, 1993, Mosby.

PROCEDURES AND TECHNIQUES WITH NORMAL FINDINGS

➤OBSERVE and PALPATE each major joint and adjacent muscles for range of motion, tenderness on movement, joint stability, and deformity. Ask the client to perform range of motion actively. You may need to demonstrate active range of motion for the client. When you move the client's joints passively through the full range of motion, do not force movement of a joint when it is painful or spastic. There should be full range of motion actively and passively with joint stability but without tenderness, heat, edema, crepitus, deformity, or contracture.

When a joint seems to have increased or decreased range of motion, use a goniometer to measure the angle (Fig. 24-17, Box 24-1). With the joint in neutral position or fully extended, flex the joint as far as possible and measure the angles of greatest flexion and extension.

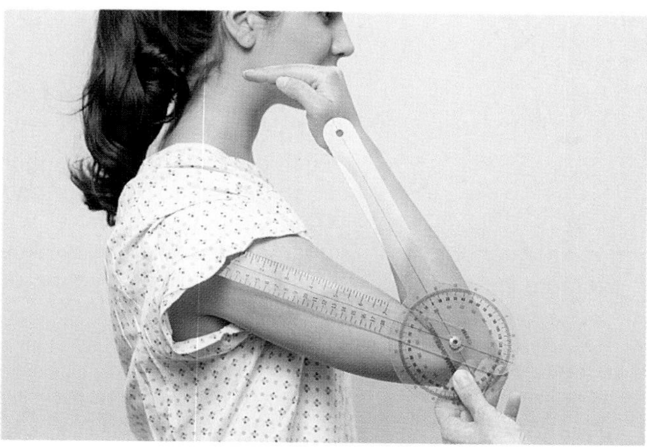

Fig. 24-17 Use of goniometer to measure joint range of motion.

Box 24-1 How to Use a Goniometer

A goniometer looks like a protractor with two long arms (see Fig. 24-17). Place the 0 setting of the goniometer over the middle of a joint that is in neutral position. The middle of one arm of the goniometer is aligned with the extremity proximal to that joint and the other arm is aligned with the middle of the distal joint. Keeping the 0 at the middle of the joint, move the distal joint through its range of motion and notice the degrees of flexion, extension, or hyperextension on the goniometer.

➤TEST muscle strength and compare contralateral sides. Testing muscle strength may be performed as part of the musculoskeletal or neurologic system examinations. Ask the client to flex the muscle being evaluated and then to resist when you apply opposing force against the muscles. Screening tests for strength are listed in Table 24-3. There are three scales used to determine the functional level (or "measure") of muscles, and each requires a subjective assessment of muscle strength. These scales are the Lovett scale, grading, and percent of normal. Grading is commonly used. Criteria for grading and recording muscle strength using these scales are described in Table 24-4. Expect muscle strength to be 5/5, bilaterally symmetric, with full resistance to opposition. The numerator reflects the client's muscle strength, while the denominator reflects the highest possible score, 5.

ABNORMAL FINDINGS

- Differences between active and passive range of motion may indicate an actual muscle weakness or a joint disorder (e.g., arthritis or joint effusion). Tenderness, heat, or edema over joints may indicate inflammation. Limited range of motion may indicate inflammation such as arthritis; fluid in the joint; or contracture of muscle, ligament, or capsule. By contrast, increased mobility of a joint may indicate connective tissue disruption, tear of a ligament, or a fracture.
- *Crepitus* is a crackling sound produced by bone fragments or articular surfaces rubbing together (e.g., osteoarthritis). Crepitus is also heard in chondromalacia patellae that occurs after knee injury.
- Joint instability or deformity may indicate a number of disorders, including muscle weakness, fracture, inflammation, strained ligaments, or meniscus tear.
- Muscle weakness may indicate a muscular or joint disease or atrophy from disuse.

Table 24-3 Screening Tests for Muscle Strength

MUSCLES TESTED	CLIENT ACTIVITY	EXAMINER ACTIVITY
Ocular musculature		
Lids	Close eyes tightly	Attempt to resist closure
Eye muscles	Track object in six cardinal positions	
Facial musculature	Blow out cheeks	Assess pressure in cheeks with fingertips
	Place tongue in cheek	Assess pressure in cheek with fingertips
	Stick out tongue, move it to right and left	Observe strength and coordination of thrust and extension
Neck muscles	Extend head backward	Push head forward
	Flex head forward	Push head backward
	Rotate head in full circle	Observe mobility, coordination
	Touch shoulders with head	Observe range of motion
Deltoid	Hold arms upward	Push down on arms
Biceps	Flex arm	Pull to extend arm
Triceps	Extend arm	Push to flex arm
Wrist musculature	Extend elbow	Push to flex
	Flex elbow	Push to extend
Finger muscles	Extend fingers	Push dorsal surface of fingers
	Flex fingers	Push ventral surface of fingers
	Spread fingers	Hold fingers together
Hip musculature	In supine position raise extended leg	Push down on leg above knee
Hamstring, gluteal, abductor, and adductor muscles of leg	Sit and perform alternate leg crossing	Push in opposite direction of crossing limb
Quadriceps	Extend leg	Push to flex leg
Hamstring	Bend knees to flex leg	Push to extend leg
Ankle and foot muscles	Bend foot up (dorsiflexion)	Push to plantar flexion
	Bend foot down (plantar flexion)	Push to dorsiflexion
Antigravity muscles	Walk on toes	
	Walk on heels	

From Barkauskas VH et al: *Health and physical assessment,* ed 2, St. Louis, 1998, Mosby.

Table 24-4 Criteria for Grading and Recording Muscle Strength

FUNCTIONAL LEVEL	LOVETT SCALE	GRADE	PERCENT OF NORMAL
No evidence of contractility	Zero (0)	0	0
Evidence of slight contractility	Trace (T)	1	10
Complete range of motion with gravity eliminated	Poor (P)	2	25
Complete range of motion with gravity	Fair (F)	3	50
Complete range of motion against gravity with some resistance	Good (G)	4	75
Complete range of motion against gravity with full resistance	Normal (N)	5	100

From Barkauskas VH et al: *Health and physical assessment,* ed 2, St. Louis, 1998, Mosby.

PROCEDURES AND TECHNIQUES WITH NORMAL FINDINGS

ABNORMAL FINDINGS

EXAMINATION OF SPECIFIC MUSCULOSKELETAL REGIONS

➤**INSPECT musculature of the face and neck for symmetry.** Client is in a sitting position. Ask client to open and close his or her mouth.

■ Asymmetric facial or neck musculature may indicate musculoskeletal disorders. For example, previous or current facial fractures or previous facial surgery may make the face asymmetric.

➤**PALPATE each temporomandibular joint in front of the tragus of each ear for movement, sounds, and tenderness.** The mandible should move smoothly and painlessly. An audible or palpable snapping or clicking in the absence of other symptoms is not unusual (see Fig. 24-18, *A*).

■ Pain, limited range of motion, or crepitus of the temporomandibular joint (TMJ) with locking or popping may indicate a temporomandibular joint disorder.

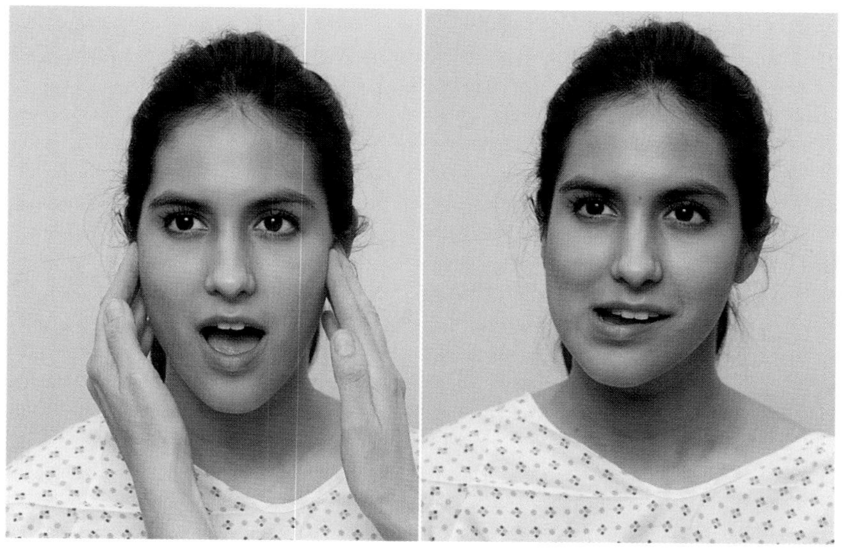

Fig. 24-18 **A,** Palpation of temporomandibular joint. **B,** Lateral range of motion in the temporomandibular joint.

➤**OBSERVE jaw for range of motion.** Ask the client to open and close the mouth. It should open between 1 ¼ and 2 ½ inches (3 to 6 cm) between upper and lower teeth. Ask the client to move the jaw side to side; the mandible should move ⅜ to ¾ inch (1 to 2 cm) in each direction (Fig. 24-18, *B*). Motion should be smooth without pain. Finally, the client should be able to protrude and retract the chin without difficulty or pain.

■ Difficulty opening the mouth may result from injury or arthritic changes. Pain in the TMJ may indicate malocclusion of teeth or arthritic changes.

➤**PALPATE neck for pain.** The neck is soft and firm without masses, pain, or spasms.

■ Pain on palpation may indicate inflammation of the muscle (myositis). Masses may be enlarged lymph nodes, indicating inflammation or neoplasm. Neck spasm may indicate nerve compression or psychologic stress.

PROCEDURES AND TECHNIQUES WITH NORMAL FINDINGS

➤OBSERVE neck for range of motion. Ask the client to flex chin to the chest. It should move to a point 45° from midline.

Ask the client to hyperextend the head, if possible; it should reach 55° from midline (Fig. 24-19, *A*).

Have the client laterally bend his or her head to the right and the left. Range should be 40° from midline in each direction (Fig. 24-19, *B*).

Have the client rotate the chin to the shoulders, first to the right and then to the left. It should reach 70° from midline (Fig. 24-19, *C*).

ABNORMAL FINDINGS

■ Range of motion may be impaired by pain or muscle spasms. Hyperextension and flexion may be limited because of cervical vertebral disk herniation or osteoarthritic changes. Changes in sensation may indicate compression of cervical spinal root nerves.

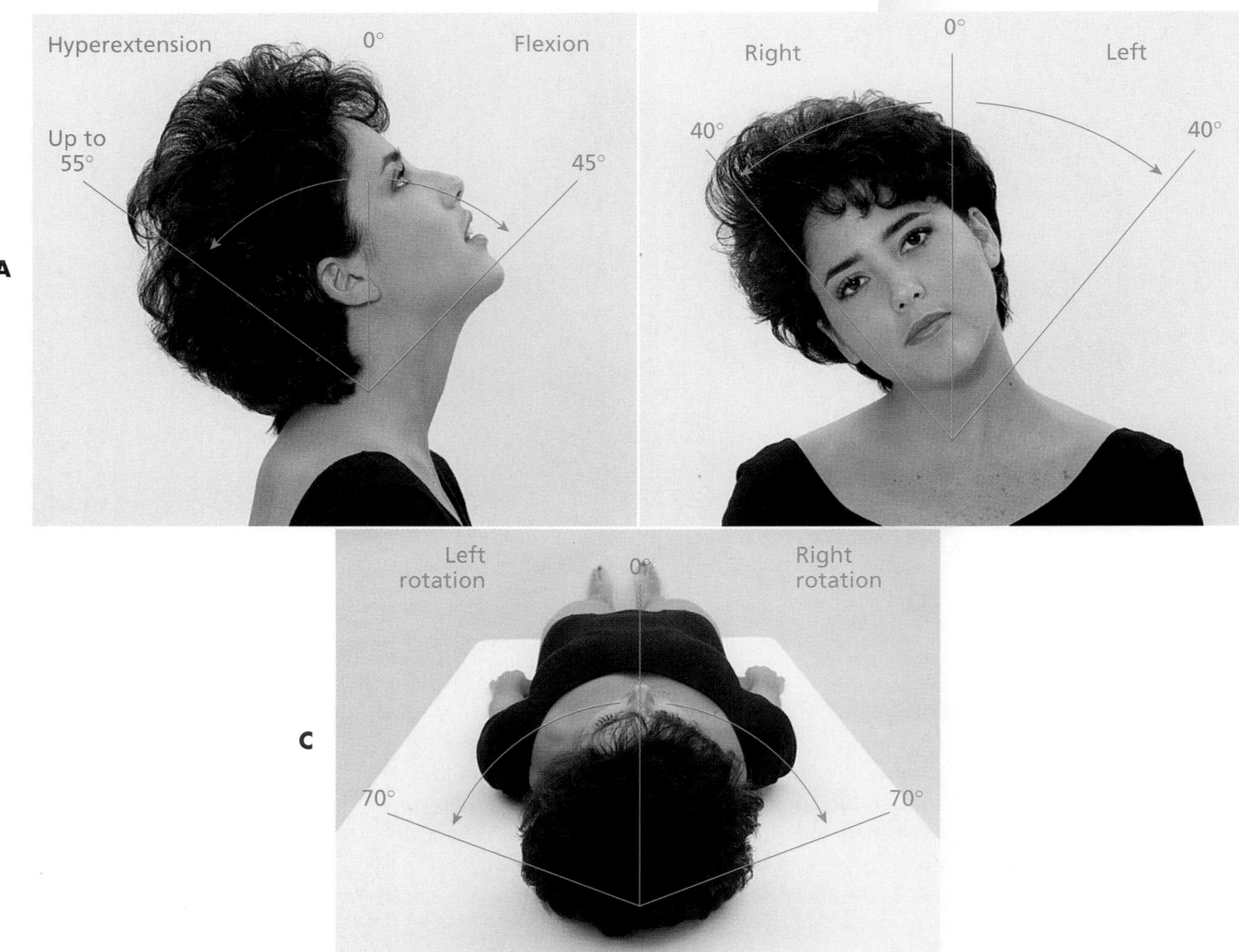

Fig. 24-19 Range of motion of the cervical spine. **A,** Flexion and hyperextension. **B,** Lateral bending. **C,** Rotation.

PROCEDURES AND TECHNIQUES WITH NORMAL FINDINGS

ABNORMAL FINDINGS

➤TEST neck muscles for strength. To assess muscle strength of the neck, ask client to repeat the rotation of the head against resistance of your hand to test strength of the sternocleidomastoid muscle (Fig. 24-20, *A*). Ask client to flex chin to the chest and maintain the position while you palpate the sternocleidomastoid muscle and try to manually force the head upright. If muscle strength is present, you should be unable to force the head upright (Fig. 24-20, *B*).

Have the client extend the head and maintain position while you try to manually force the head upright to assess the trapezius muscle strength (Fig. 24-20, *C*). If muscle strength is 5/5, you should be unable to force the head upright.

■ If you can break the muscular flexion before the anticipated point, then client has muscle weakness.

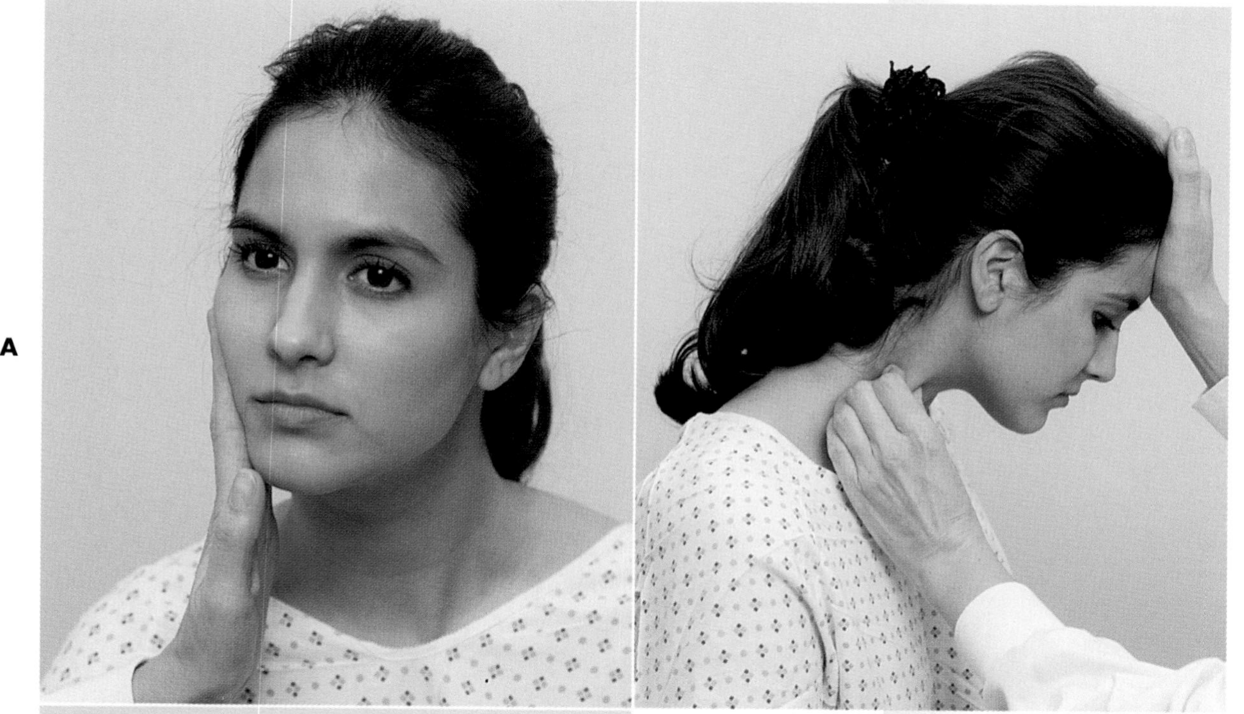

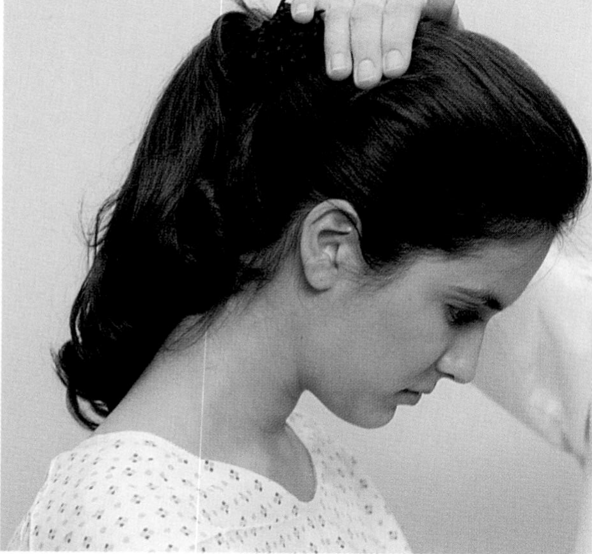

Fig. 24-20 Examining the strength of the sternocleidomastoid and trapezius muscles. **A,** Rotation against resistance. **B,** Flexion with palpation of the sternocleidomastoid muscle. **C,** Extension against resistance.

PROCEDURES AND TECHNIQUES WITH NORMAL FINDINGS

➤INSPECT the shoulders and cervical, thoracic, and lumbar spine for alignment and symmetry. Ask the client to stand and you stand to the side of the client, observe the cervical concave, the thoracic convex, and the lumbar concave (see Fig. 24-15). Ask the client to touch the toes. Move behind the client to inspect spine. Vertebrae should be aligned, indicating a straight spine. Shoulders should be level or at equal heights (Fig. 24-21). (While the client is bending forward, you will perform the next assessment.)

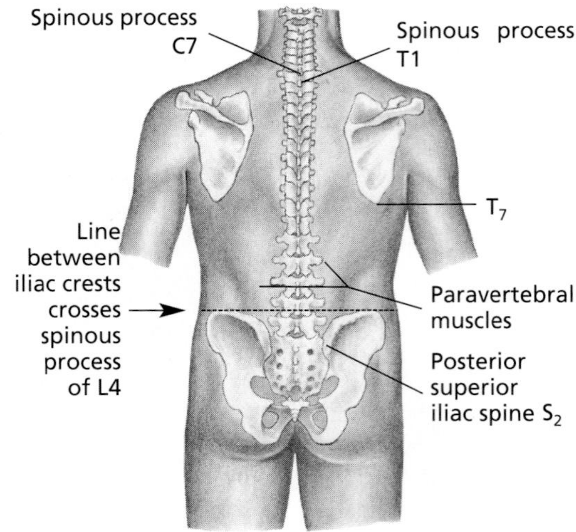

Fig. 24-21 Landmarks of the back. (From Seidel et al, 1999.)

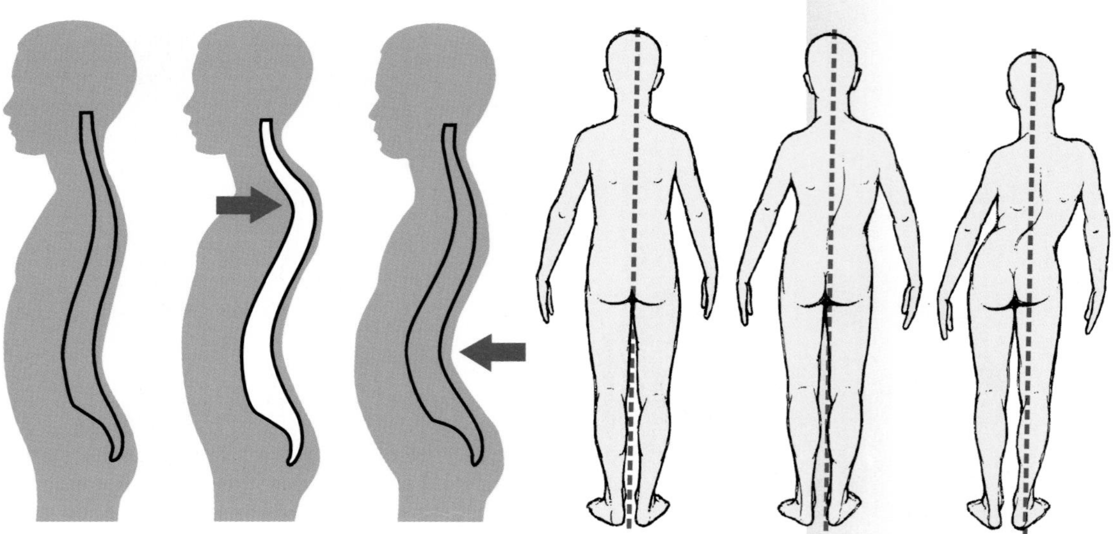

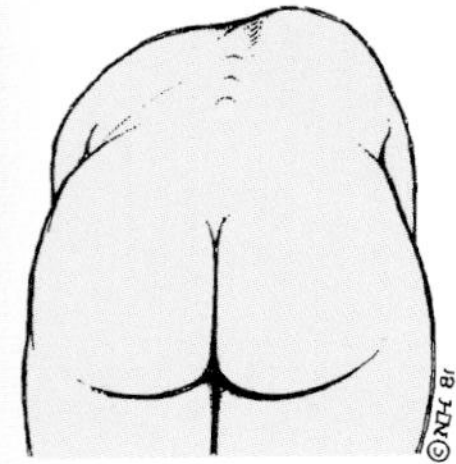

Fig. 24-22 Defects of the spinal column. **A,** Normal spine. **B,** Kyphosis. **C,** Lordosis. **D,** Normal spine in balance. **E,** Mild scoliosis. **F,** Severe scoliosis, not in balance. **G,** Rib hump and flank asymmetry seen in flexion. (Modified from Hilt and Schmitt, 1975. In Wong et al, 1999.)

ABNORMAL FINDINGS

■ Deviation of the spine or asymmetry of shoulder or iliac height is an abnormal finding. *Kyphosis* is a posterior curvature (convexity) of the thoracic spine, *lordosis* is an anterior curvature (concavity) of the spine, and *scoliosis* is a lateral curvature of the spine (Fig. 24-22). Curvature of the spine may create asymmetry of the shoulders.

PROCEDURES AND TECHNIQUES WITH NORMAL FINDINGS

➤**OBSERVE range of motion of thoracic and lumbar spine.** While the client is touching toes; he or she should be able to reach 75° of flexion (Fig. 24-23, *A*). Document how close the client gets to the floor by measuring from fingertips to the floor (e.g., 6 inches from the floor). Some clients will be unable to touch the floor due to tight hamstrings and leg muscles or due to obesity. These are considered normal variations.

➤Observe for range of motion as client hyperextends the spine; it should reach 30° back from the neutral position (extension) (Fig. 24-23, *B*).

➤Ask the client to bend laterally right and left. (Note: It may be necessary to stabilize the client's hips.) He or she should be able to reach 35° of flexion both ways from midline (Fig. 24-23, *C*).

➤Have the client rotate the upper trunk (you may need to stabilize pelvis) to the right and left; he or she should achieve 30° of rotation in both directions from a directly forward position (Fig. 24-23, *D*).

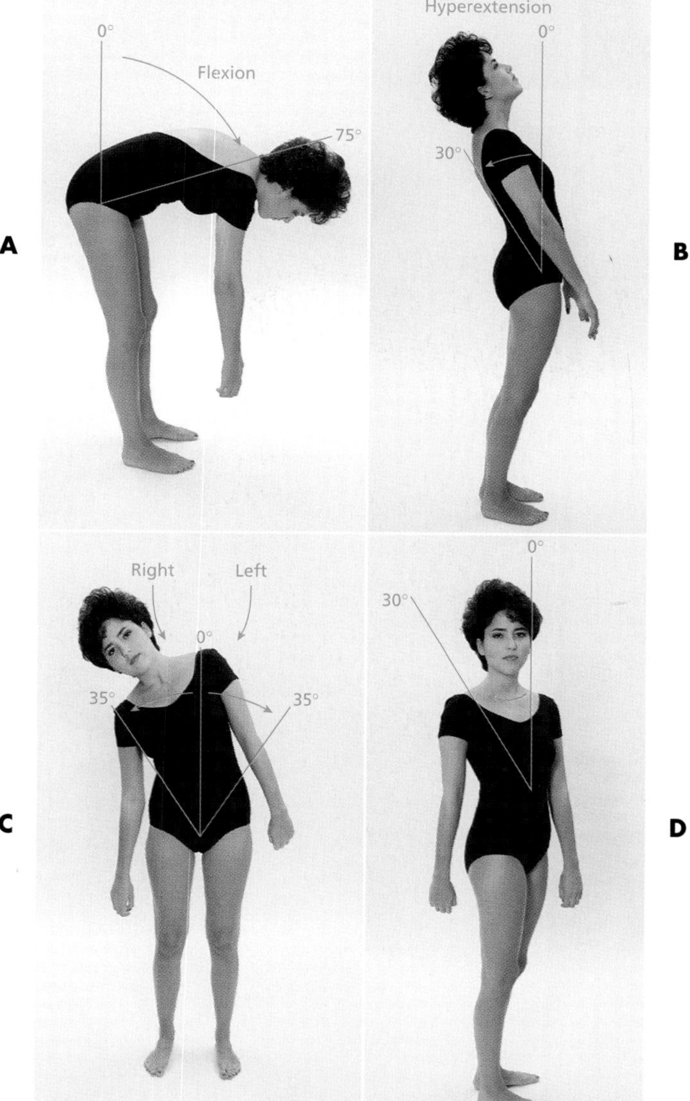

Fig. 24-23 Range of motion of the thoracic and lumbar spine. **A,** Flexion. **B,** Hyperextension. **C,** Lateral bending. **D,** Rotation of the upper trunk.

ABNORMAL FINDINGS

- Flexion less than 75° with pain or muscle spasm is abnormal.
- Impaired range of motion during hyperextension may be due to pain from muscle strain or spasms or herniated vertebral disk.
- Impaired range of motion during lateral flexion may be due to pain from muscle strain or spasms or herniated vertebral disk.
- Impaired range of motion during rotation may be due to pain from muscle strain or spasms.

PROCEDURES AND TECHNIQUES WITH NORMAL FINDINGS

➤PALPATE posterior neck, spinal processes, and paravertebral muscles for alignment and tenderness. Stand behind the client. The spine should be straight and nontender. (Note: It may be helpful to have the client hunch his or her shoulders forward and slightly flex the neck [Fig. 24-24]).

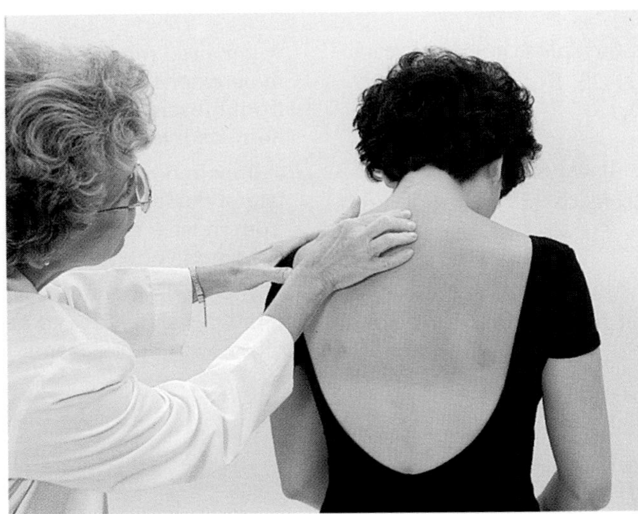

Fig. 24-24 Palpation of the spinal processes of the vertebrae.

ABNORMAL FINDINGS

- Misalignment may be due to muscle weakness. Tenderness may be due to inflammation such as myositis or herniated vertebral disk.

PROCEDURES AND TECHNIQUES WITH NORMAL FINDINGS

➤**PERCUSS spinal processes for tenderness.** First tap each process with one finger, and then lightly tap each side of the spine with the ulnar surface of your fist. No muscle spasm or tenderness should be noted to palpation or percussion.

➤**INSPECT the shoulders and shoulder girdle for equality of height and contour.** Facing the client who is in a seat position, inspect scapulae and clavicles, as well as the acromioclavicular junction, for equality of height and symmetry.

Observe the trapezius muscle for shape and size. All structures should be smooth, regular, and bilaterally symmetric. Right and left shoulders should be level, rounded, and firm, with smooth contour and no bony prominences. Each shoulder should be equidistant from the vertebral column and located over thoracic ribs two through seven. Note any erythema, edema, or nodules.

➤**PALPATE the shoulders for firmness, fullness, tenderness, and masses.** This includes the acromioclavicular joint and humerus as well as the trapezius, biceps, triceps, and deltoid muscles. Compare one side to the other side. These areas should be nontender, smooth, firm and full without masses, and bilaterally symmetric. The muscles of the dominant arm may be slightly larger.

ABNORMAL FINDINGS

- Tenderness may be due to inflammation such as myositis or herniated vertebral disk. Muscle spasm may be due to muscle strain.
- Shoulder joints may have some deformity from trauma, arthritic changes, or scoliosis.
- Tenderness may be due to inflammation of the muscles, overwork of unconditioned muscles, or sports injuries.

PROCEDURES AND TECHNIQUES WITH NORMAL FINDINGS

➤TEST trapezius muscles for strength. Ask the client to shrug shoulders while you attempt to push them down (Fig. 24-25). This also tests function of cranial nerve XI (spinal accessory).

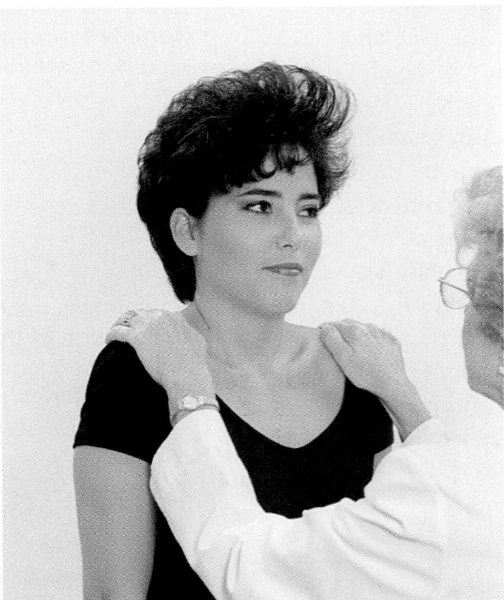

Fig. 24-25 Test strength of the trapezius muscle with the shrugged shoulder movement.

➤OBSERVE the shoulders for range of motion. Ask the client to extend arms straight up beside the ears. Arms should reach 180° from resting neutral position, be bilaterally equal, and show no discomfort (Fig. 24-26, *A*).

Ask the client to hyperextend the arms backward. They should reach 50°, be bilaterally equal, and cause no discomfort.

Ask the client to lift both arms laterally over head. Expected shoulder abduction is 180°. Then ask the client to swing each arm across the front of the body. Expected adduction is 50° (Fig. 24-26, *B*).

To test external rotation, have the client place the hands behind the head with elbows out. A range of 90° is normal; movement should be bilaterally equal and without discomfort (Fig. 24-26, *C*).

To test internal rotation, ask the client to place the hands at the small of the back. Range should be 90°, with movements bilaterally equal and without discomfort (Fig. 24-26, *D*).

ABNORMAL FINDINGS

- Weakness of the trapezius muscles may indicate compressed spinal nerve root or compression of spinal accessory cranial nerve (CN XI).

- Limited range of motion, pain with movement, crepitations, and asymmetry are abnormal findings. Degenerative joint changes or sports injuries may impair range of motion.

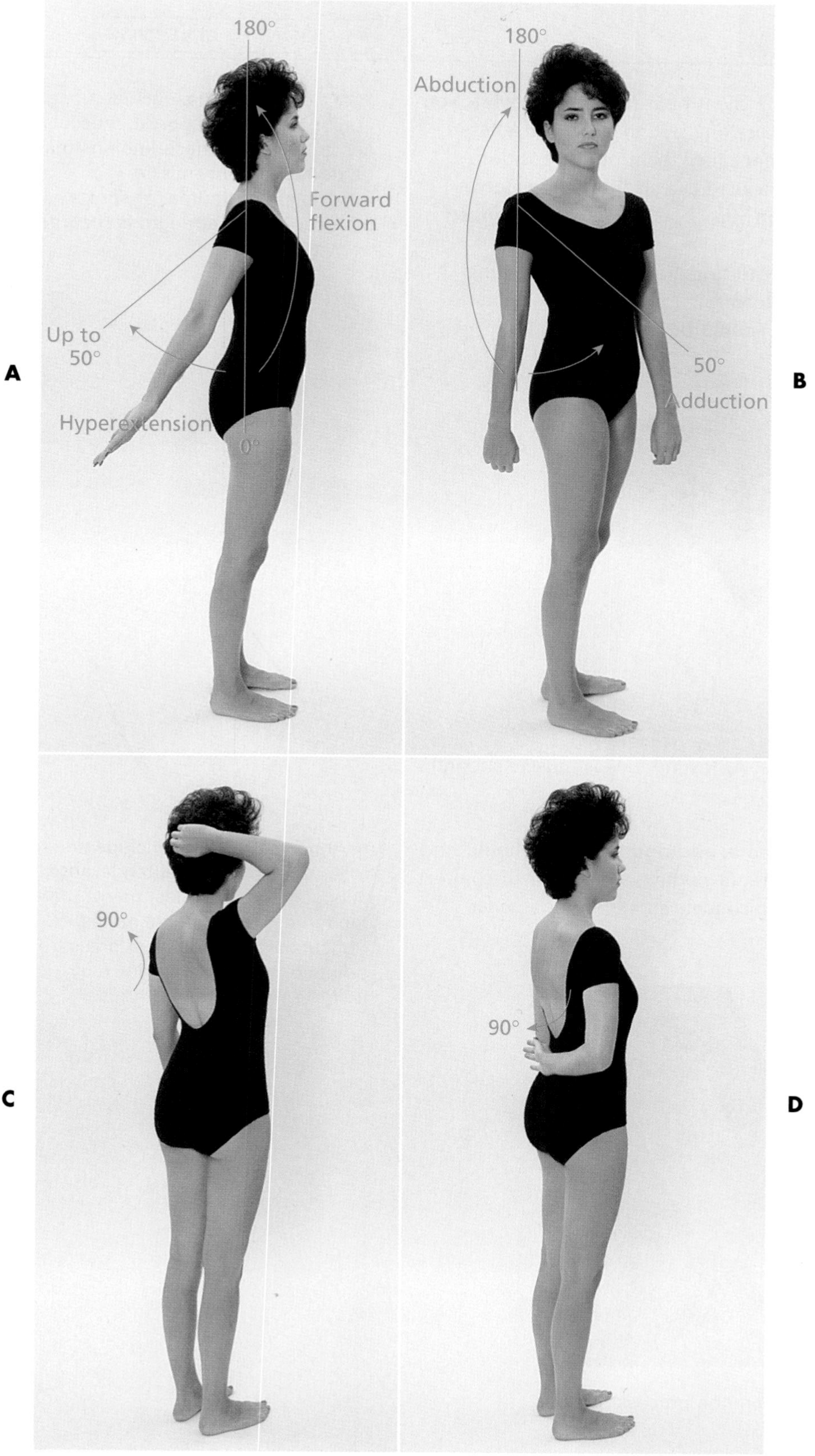

Fig. 24-26 Range of motion of the shoulders. **A,** Forward flexion and hyperextension. **B,** Abduction and adduction. **C,** External rotation and abduction. **D,** Internal rotation and adduction.

PROCEDURES AND TECHNIQUES WITH NORMAL FINDINGS

➤TEST arms for muscle strength. Have the client hold the arms up while you try to push them down. Remember to compare one side to the other. They should be strong bilaterally so that you cannot move them out of position.

To test triceps muscle strength, ask the client to extend the arm while you resist by pushing the arm to a flexed position (Fig. 24-27, *A*). Expected muscle strength is recorded as 5/5 (see Table 24-4).

To test biceps strength, have the client try to flex the arm into a fighting position while you try to extend his or her forearm. You should be unable to move the arm out of position, and strength should be equal bilaterally (Fig. 24-27, *B*).

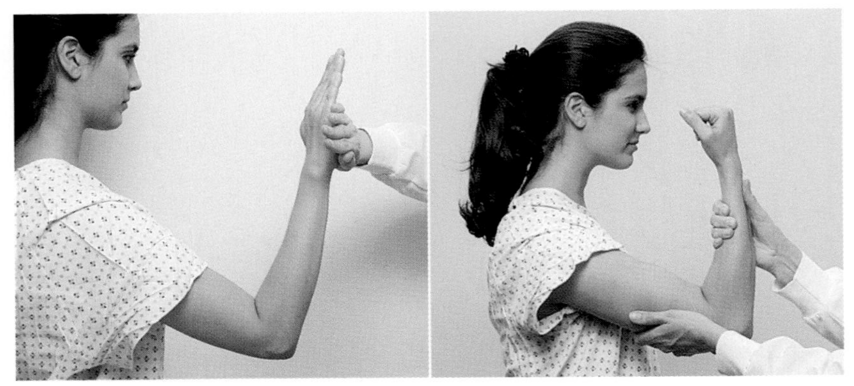

Fig. 24-27 Testing muscle strength of arms. **A,** Testing triceps muscle strength. **B,** Testing biceps muscle strength.

➤PALPATE the elbows for tenderness, edema, and nodules. You should find smooth olecranon processes (Fig. 24-28) without nodules, edema, or discomfort over the groove on either side. The lateral epicondyle should be nontender without edema.

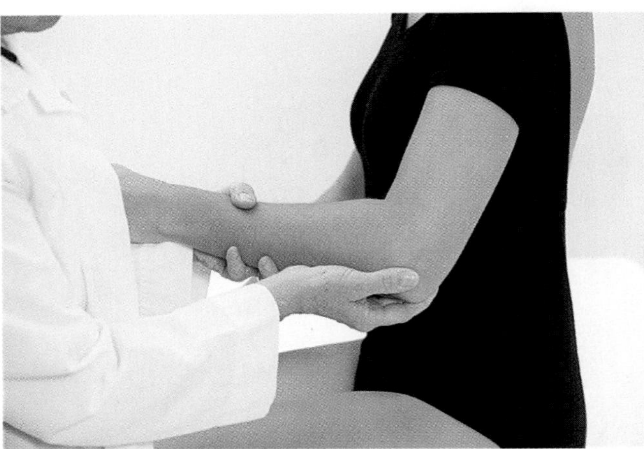

Fig. 24-28 Palpation of the olecranon process grooves.

ABNORMAL FINDINGS

■ Abnormal findings include unequal response, weak response, muscular spasm, or pain. These findings may be due to joint or muscle inflammation, trauma, or sports injuries. Muscle strength is recorded as 4/5 to 5/5.

■ Abnormal findings include edema, inflammation, general tenderness, subcutaneous nodules, point tenderness, or palpable nodes. Subcutaneous nodules at pressure points of the ulnar surface may indicate rheumatoid arthritis.

PROCEDURES AND TECHNIQUES WITH NORMAL FINDINGS

➤**OBSERVE the elbows for range of motion.** Ask the client to flex and extend the elbow; 160° of full movement should be present bilaterally without discomfort (Fig. 24-29, *A*).

Assess pronation and supination of the elbow by having the client rotate the hands palms up and palms down (pronate and supinate); 90° should be achieved in each direction, and the movements should be bilaterally equal and without discomfort (Fig. 24-29, *B*).

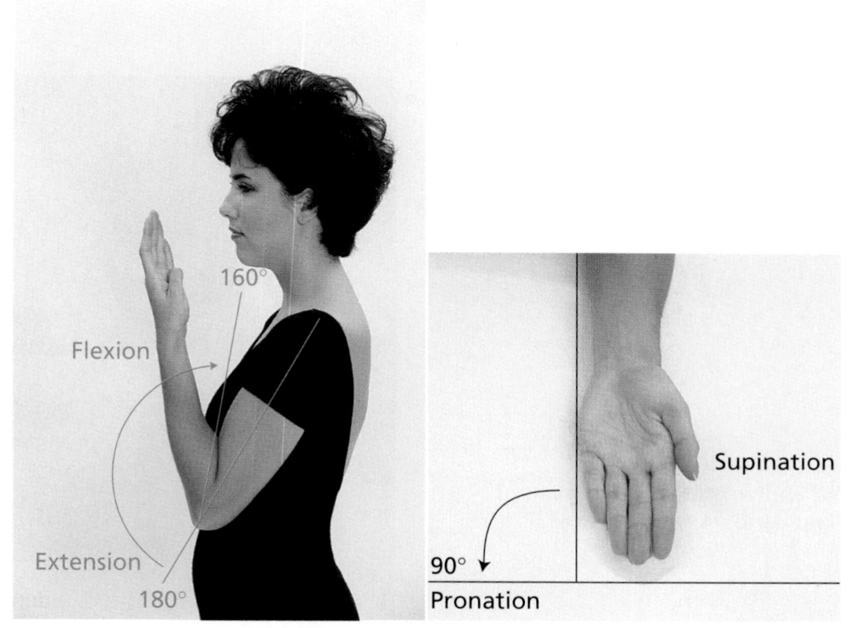

Fig. 24-29 Range of motion of the elbow. **A,** Flexion and extension. **B,** Palm up, supination; palm down, pronation.

ABNORMAL FINDINGS

■ Note any limitation of motion, asymmetry of movement, or pain at the elbow. Subcutaneous nodules just inferior to olecranon process (elbow joint) may indicate rheumatoid arthritis. Tenderness or pain with pronation and supination of the elbow and point tenderness on the lateral epicondyle may indicate lateral tendonitis or epicondylitis (tennis elbow), whereas point tenderness on the medial epicondyle may indicate medial tendonitis (golfer's elbow).

PROCEDURES AND TECHNIQUES WITH NORMAL FINDINGS

➤**INSPECT the joints of both wrists and hands for position, contour, and number of digits.** Compare the right wrist and hand with the left. They should be smooth, firm, and symmetric, with no edema or deformities. The hand with five digits is aligned with the wrist, and fingers are aligned with wrist and forearm (Fig. 24-30, *A, B*).

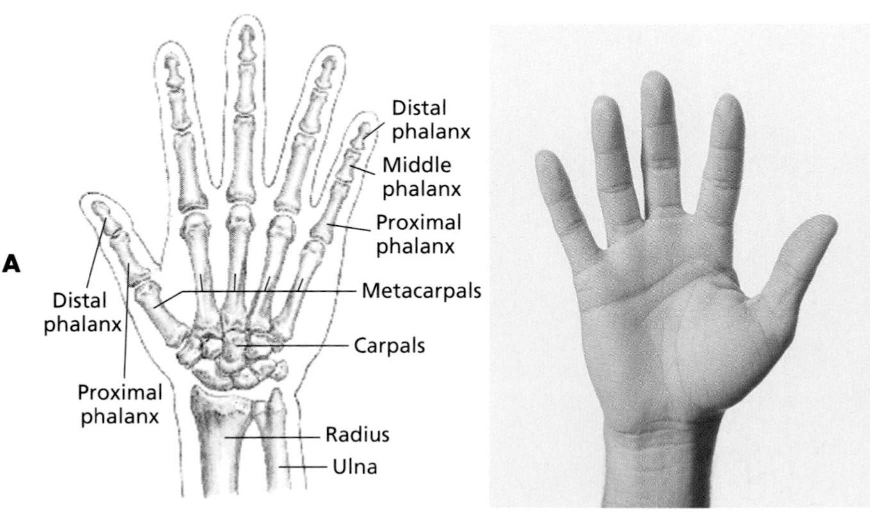

Fig. 24-30 **A,** Bony structures of the right hand and wrist. Note alignment of fingers with the radius. **B,** Palmar aspect of right hand. (**A** From Seidel et al, 1999.)

ABNORMAL FINDINGS

■ Missing fingers are recorded. Swan-neck and boutonnière deformities of interphalangeal joints may be related to rheumatoid arthritis (Fig. 24-31). Osteoarthritis may cause Bouchard's nodes in proximal interphalangeal (PIP) joints, whereas Heberden's nodes form in the distal interphalangeal (DIP) joints (Fig. 24-32).

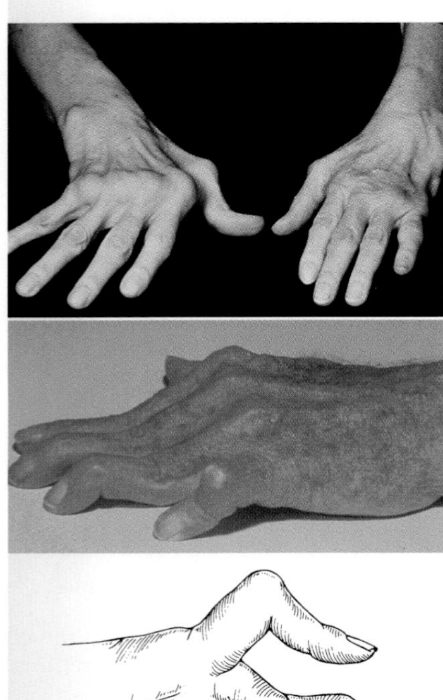

Fig. 24-31 **A,** Ulnar deviation and subluxation of metacarpophalangeal joints. **B,** Swan-neck deformities. **C,** Boutonnière deformity. (**A** and **B** Reprinted from the Clinical Slide Collection of the Rheumatic Diseases, copyright 1991, 1995, 1997. Used with permission of the American College of Rheumatology. **C** From Seidel et al, 1999.)

PROCEDURES AND TECHNIQUES WITH NORMAL FINDINGS

ABNORMAL FINDINGS

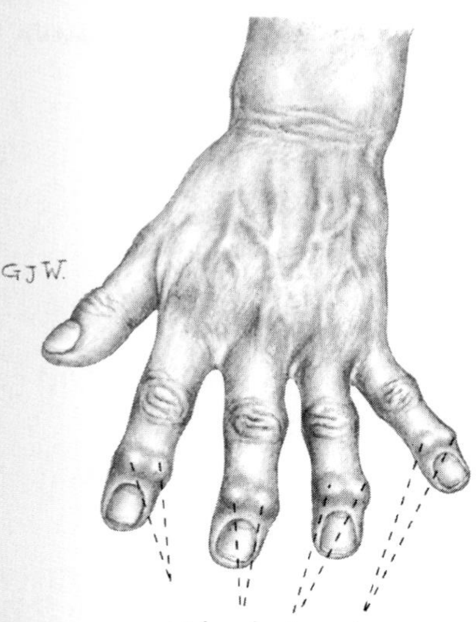

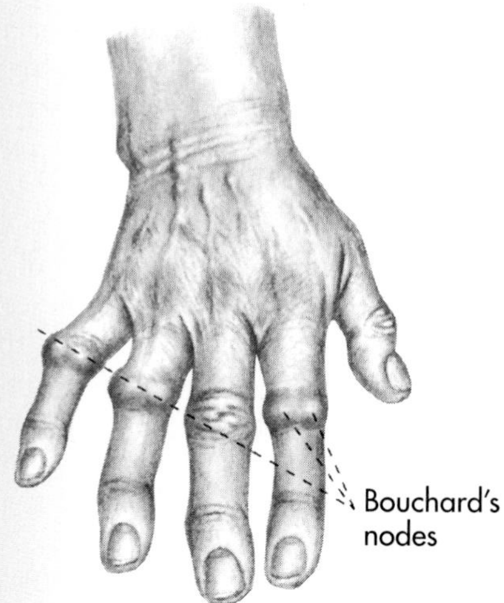

Fig. 24-32 Osteoarthritis. Heberden's nodes and Bouchard's nodes. (From Mourad, 1991.)

➤**PALPATE each joint of the hand and wrist for surface characteristics and tenderness.** Palpate interphalangeal joints with your thumb and index finger. Palpate metacarpophalangeal joints with both thumbs. Palpate the wrist and radiocarpal groove with your thumbs on the dorsal surface and your fingers on the palmar surface. Joint surfaces should be smooth without nodules, edema, or tenderness (Fig. 24-33, *A, B, C*).

■ Painful, edematous joints are found in osteoarthritis. A firm mass over the dorsum of the wrist may be a ganglion. Rheumatoid arthritis may cause wrists and interphalangeal joints to appear hot, tender, painful, deformed, and edematous.

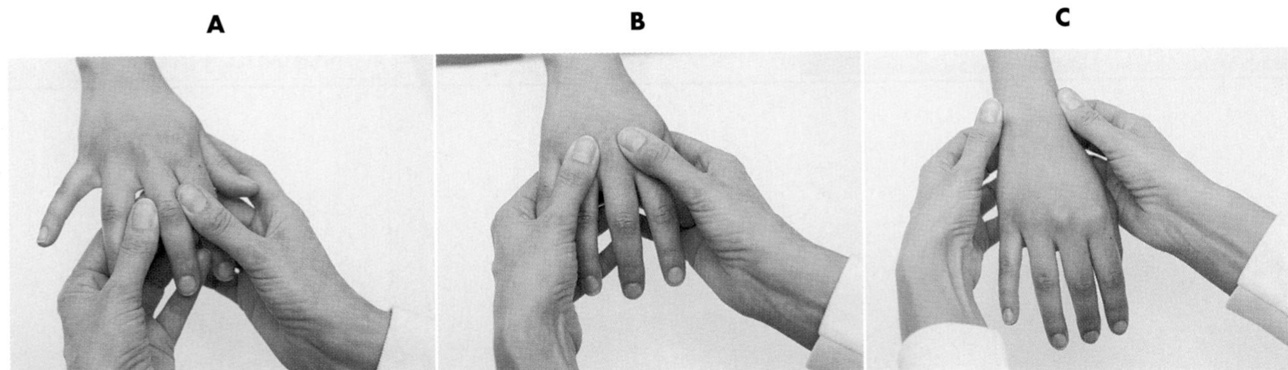

Fig. 24-33 Palpation of joints of the hand and wrist. **A,** Interphalangeal joints. **B,** Metacarpophalangeal joints. **C,** Radiocarpal groove.

PROCEDURES AND TECHNIQUES WITH NORMAL FINDINGS

➤TEST for muscle strength and OBSERVE for range of motion of wrists and fingers. First, ask the client to extend and spread the fingers (both hands) while you attempt to push the fingers together (Fig. 24-34, *A*). The response should be symmetric, to full flexion and extension, without discomfort, and with sufficient muscle strength to overcome the resistance you apply.

Next, have the client grip your first two fingers on each hand. The response should be bilaterally equal and the grip tight and full flexion (Fig. 24-34, *B*).

Observe the range of motion of wrists as the client bends the hand up at the wrist (hyperextension to 70°), flexes the hand down at the wrist (palmar flexion of 90°) (Fig. 24-35, *A*), and flexes the fingers up and down at the metacarpophalangeal joints (flexion of 90°, hyperextension of 30°) (Fig. 24-35, *B*). Then, with the client's palms flat on the table, ask the client to turn them outward and inward (ulnar deviation of 50° to 60°, radial deviation of 20°) (Fig. 24-35, *C*), spread the fingers apart (Fig. 24-35, *D*), and then make a fist (abduction of 20°, fist tight) (Fig. 24-35, *E*), and touch the thumb to each finger (opposition) and to the base of the fifth finger (able to perform all motions) (Fig. 24-35, *F*). These findings should be bilaterally equal.

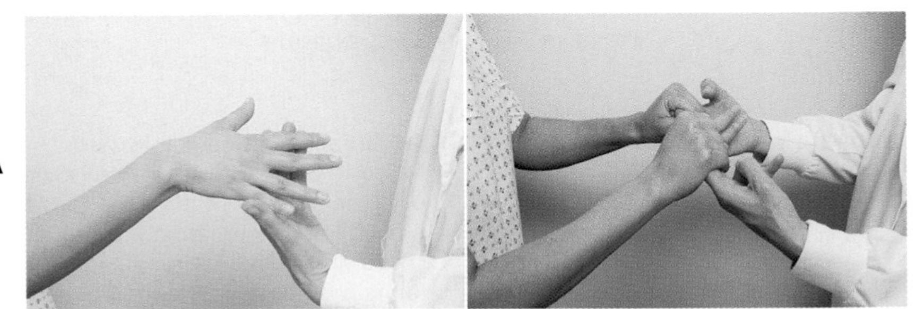

Fig. 24-34 **A,** Assessment of finger strength. **B,** Assessment of grip strength.

ABNORMAL FINDINGS

- Weak muscle strength and impaired range of motion may accompany rheumatoid arthritis and osteoarthritis. Fractures of metatarsals or phalanges may weaken the muscle strength.

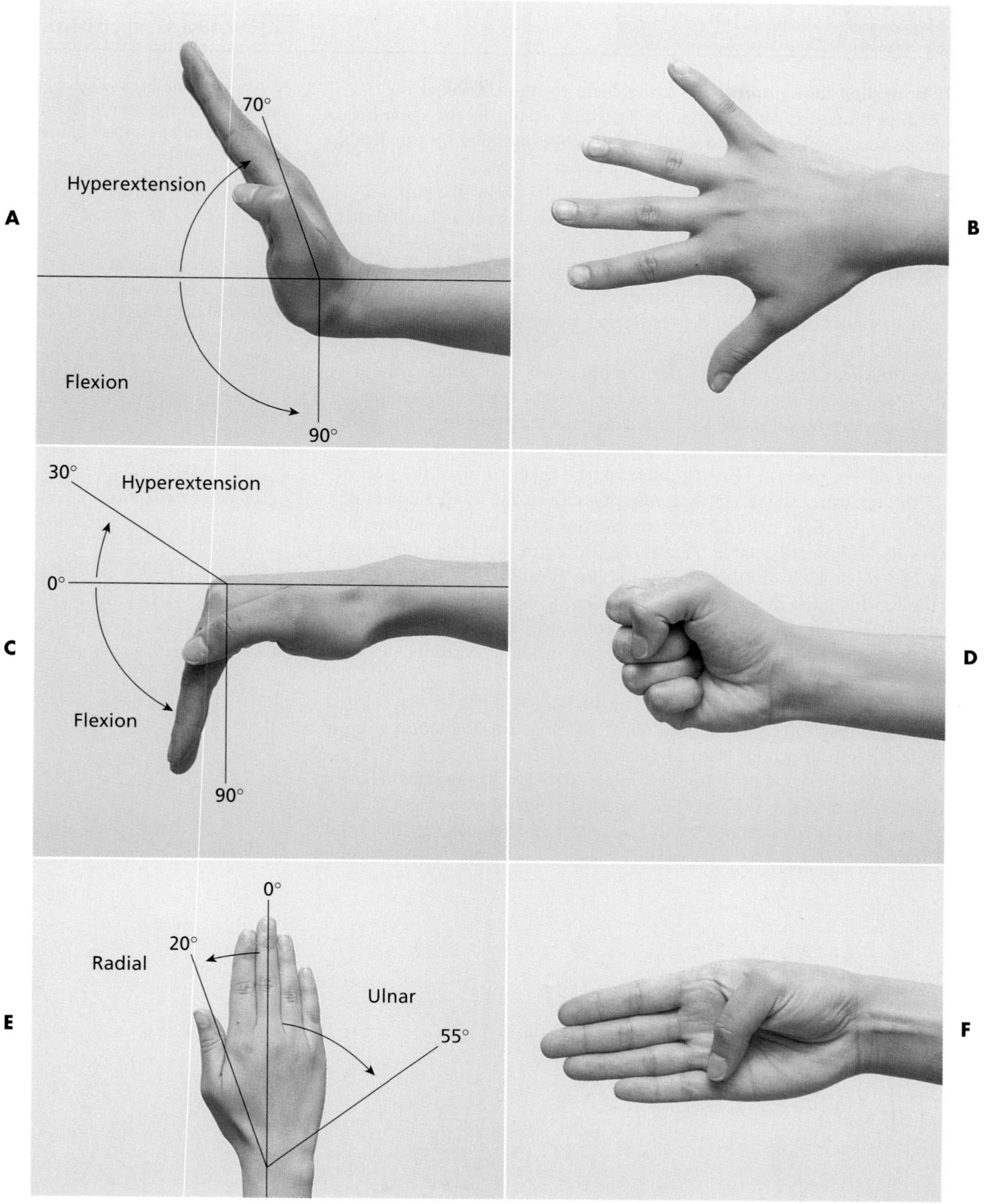

Fig. 24-35 Range of motion of hand and wrist. **A,** Wrist flexion and hyperextension. **B,** Metacarpophalangeal flexion and hyperextension. **C,** Wrist radial and ulnar deviation. **D,** Finger abduction. **E,** Finger flexion: fist formation. **F,** Finger extension: thumb to each fingertip and to base of little finger.

PROCEDURES AND TECHNIQUES WITH NORMAL FINDINGS

➤INSPECT both hips for symmetry. Ask the client to stand. Look at the symmetry of hips anteriorly and posteriorly. The hips should be the same height and symmetric. You may need to move the client's clothing aside to visualize the hips.

➤PALPATE hips for stability and tenderness. Assist the client to a supine position. Use the iliac crests and greater trochanter of the femur as landmarks. Findings should be bilaterally symmetric hips that are stable and painless.

➤OBSERVE hips for range of motion. Assist the client to a supine position. To evaluate hip range of motion, ask the client to alternately pull each knee up to the chest. Client should achieve 120-degree flexion from the straight, extended position (Fig. 24-36, *A*).

Next, have the client raise the leg to flex the hip as far as possible without bending the knee. Results should be 90° from the straight extended position (Fig. 24-36, *B*). An extension of 60° to 70° is a normal variation in adults with tight hamstrings, especially in men.

To test external hip rotation (Patrick test), ask the client to place the heel of one foot on the opposite patella. Apply gentle pressure to the medial aspect of the flexed knee as the client externally rotates the hip until the knee or lateral thigh touches the examination table. Repeat the procedure with the other hip. Rotation should reach 45° from the straight midline position (Fig. 24-36, *C*).

To test the hip for internal rotation, ask the client to flex the knee and turn medially (inward) as you pull the heel laterally (outward) to test internal hip rotation. Rotation should reach 40° from the straight midline position (Fig. 24-36, *D*).

Ask the client to move one leg laterally with the knee straight to test abduction and medially to test adduction. Expected range for abduction is up to 45°, and for adduction up to 30° (Fig. 24-36, *E*).

Assist the client to a prone position. Test hyperextension of the hip by raising the leg upward with the knee straight. The expected range of movement is up to 30° (Fig. 24-36, *F*). This assessment can also be performed with the client in the standing position.

ABNORMAL FINDINGS

■ Asymmetric hips may occur from curvature of the spine. Osteoarthritis or hip dislocation may cause pain and hip instability.

■ Osteoarthritis and hip dislocation also impair hip range of motion. Vertebral compression of spinal nerves may cause back or leg pain during hip flexion with leg extension.

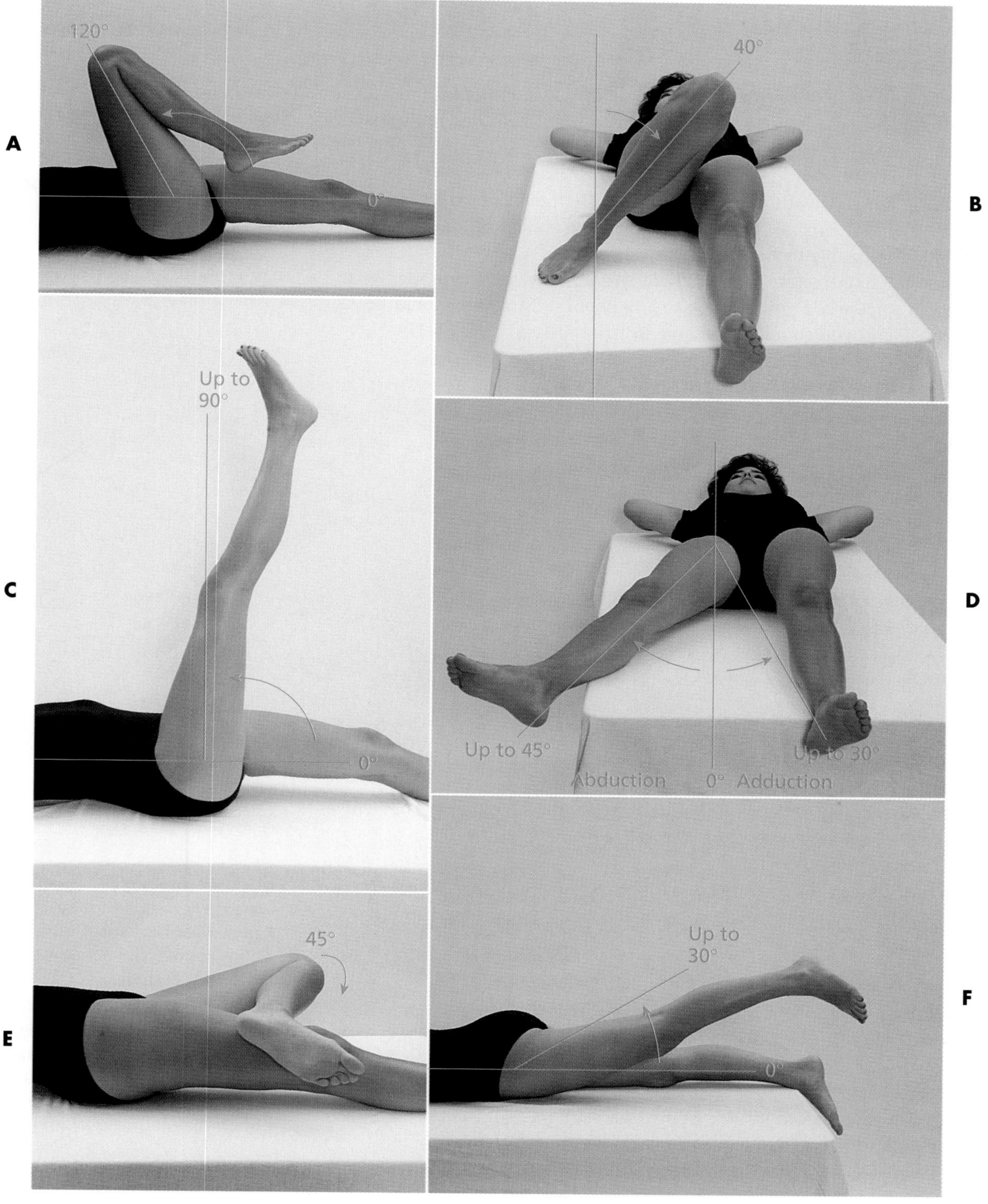

Fig. 24-36 Range of motion of hips. **A,** Hip flexion, knee flexed. **B,** Hip flexion, leg extended. **C,** External rotation of hip. **D,** Internal rotation of hip. **E,** Abduction and adduction of hip. **F,** Hyperextension of hip, leg extended.

PROCEDURES AND TECHNIQUES WITH NORMAL FINDINGS

➤TEST hips for muscle strength. Assist the client to a supine position. Ask him or her to attempt to raise the legs while you try to hold them down. Evaluate one leg at a time, noting if the response is bilaterally strong and if you are unable to interfere with the movement.

To test the quadriceps with the client sitting, have the client extend the legs at the knee while you attempt to flex the knee. Strength should be bilaterally equal, and you should be unable to flex the knee.

To evaluate the hamstrings with the client sitting, have the client attempt to bend his or her knee while you attempt to straighten it. Strength should be bilaterally equal, and you should be unable to flex the knee (Fig. 24-37).

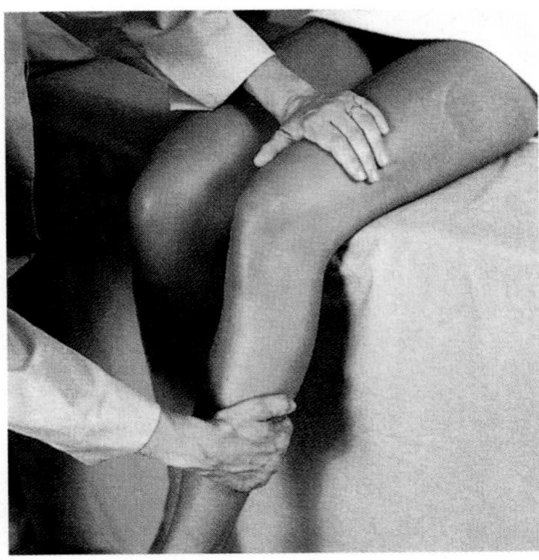

Fig. 24-37 Assessment of hamstring muscle strength. Client flexes knee while examiner tries to straighten it. (From Barkauskas et al, 1998.)

➤INSPECT both knees for symmetry, alignment, or erythema. Knees should be lined up with the tibia and ankle without medial or lateral deviation.

➤PALPATE knees for contour and tenderness. First, palpate the suprapatellar pouch on each side of the quadriceps with the thumb and fingers of one or both hands. Compare one side to the other. Knees should feel smooth, nonedematous, and nontender.

Next, with the knee flexed to 90°, palpate over the medial and lateral aspects of the tibiofemoral joint space. These areas should be nonedematous and nontender. Palpate the popliteal space for contour, tenderness, and edema. It should be smooth and nontender.

ABNORMAL FINDINGS

- Abnormal findings include unequal response, weak response, muscular spasm, or pain. These findings may be due to joint or muscle inflammation, trauma, or sports injuries.
- Knees that appear edematous and warm, bowlegged (genu varum), knock-kneed (genu valgum), thick, boggy (spongy), or inflamed are abnormal findings.
- Abnormal findings include bogginess, thickening, tenderness, or pain that may occur from rheumatoid arthritis, osteoarthritis, or joint effusion. Edema of the suprapatellar pouch may indicate synovitis.

PROCEDURES AND TECHNIQUES WITH NORMAL FINDINGS

➤OBSERVE knees for range of motion. Evaluate the range of motion by having the client flex the knees (Fig. 24-38). Flexion should reach 130° from the straight extended position without discomfort or difficulty. If the knee is able to hyperextend, it should reach 15° from the extended position (midline).

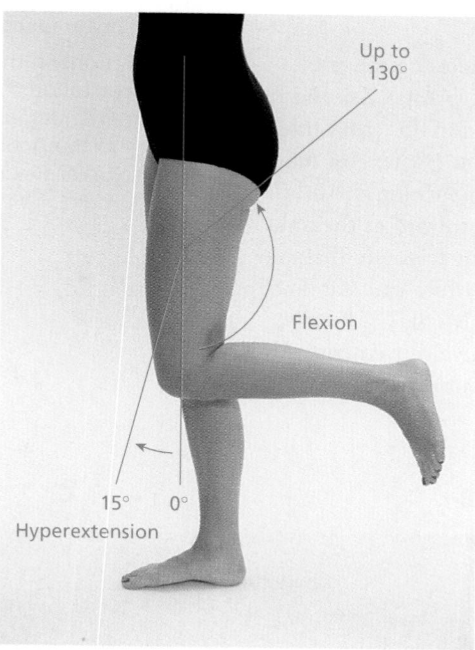

Fig. 24-38 Flexion and hyperextension of knee.

➤TEST leg muscles for strength. Apply opposing force while client tries to maintain flexion and extension. Compare one side to the other.

➤INSPECT feet and ankles for contour, alignment, and number of toes. They should be smooth, with no deformity; five toes maintain extended and straight position on each foot, and feet maintain straight position aligned with long axis of lower leg.

ABNORMAL FINDINGS

■ A decrease in the range of motion may occur as a result of a form of arthritis, trauma, or ligament, tendon, or meniscus injury.

■ Abnormal findings include unequal response, weak response, muscular spasm, or pain. These findings may be due to joint or muscle inflammation, trauma, or sports injuries.

■ Abnormal findings include misalignment of the feet with the ankle or leg or amputation or deformity of toes. Medial deviation of the toes, hallux valgus (Fig. 24-39), claw toes, hammer toes, or calluses are abnormal findings as well.

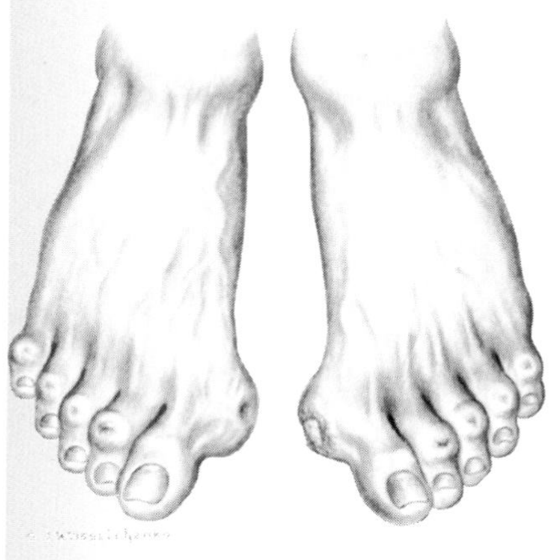

Fig. 24-39 Hallux valgus with bunions and hammer toes. (From Mourad, 1991.)

PROCEDURES AND TECHNIQUES WITH NORMAL FINDINGS

ABNORMAL FINDINGS

➤**PALPATE feet and ankles for contour and tenderness.** These structures should be smooth, nonedematous, and nontender.

■ Abnormal findings include tenderness (diffuse versus pinpoint), inflammation, ulcerations, or nodules. Localized pain in one heel may indicate a bone spur. Pain in both feet that is worse on arising may indicate plantar fasciitis.

➤**OBSERVE feet and ankles for range of motion.** To evaluate the range of motion of both feet and ankles, have the client dorsiflex and plantar flex the foot. Dorsiflexion should reach 20° from midline, and plantar flexion 45° from midline (Fig. 24-40, *A*). Then have the client invert and evert the foot. (Note: You may need to stabilize the heel during these maneuvers.) Eversion (turning the foot outward at the ankle) is 20° and inversion (turning the foot inward at the ankle) 30° from midline position (Fig. 24-40, *B*). Next, ask the client to rotate the ankle, turning the foot away from and then toward the other foot while you stabilize the leg. Expect abduction of 10° and adduction of 20° (Fig. 24-40, *C*). Finally, have the client flex and extend the toes. These should be active movements. All movements should be bilaterally equal and performed without discomfort.

■ Limitations in the range of motion, pain, crepitations, and asymmetry are abnormal findings. Tightening or trauma to the Achilles tendon may cause plantar flexion.

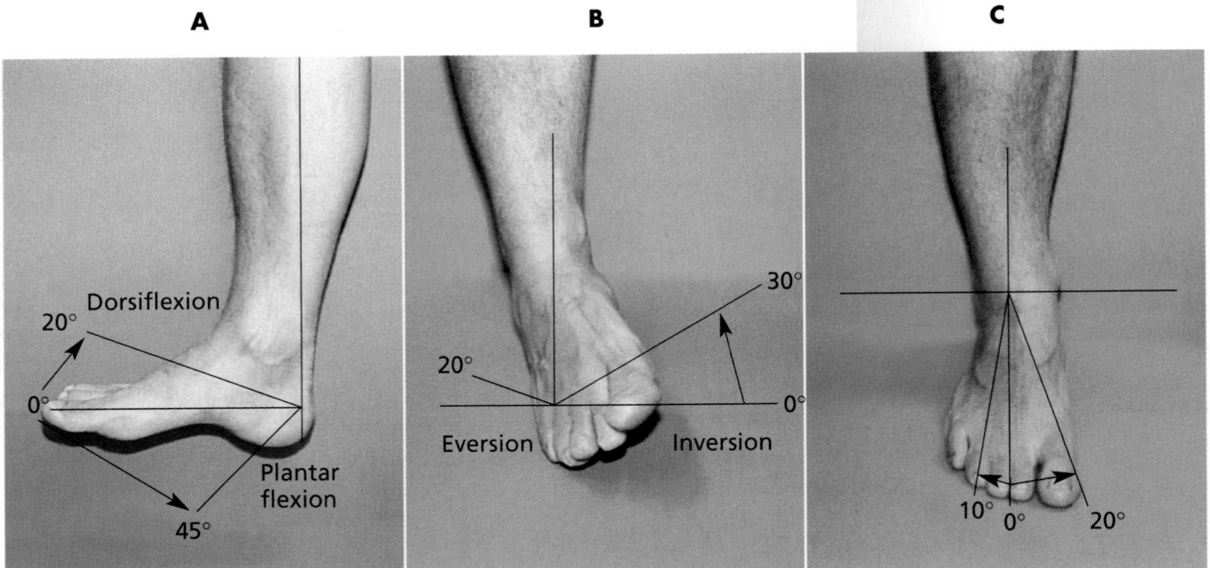

Fig. 24-40 Range of motion of the ankle. **A,** Dorsiflexion and plantar flexion. **B,** Inversion and eversion. **C,** Abduction and adduction. (From Seidel et al, 1999.)

PROCEDURES AND TECHNIQUES WITH NORMAL FINDINGS

ABNORMAL FINDINGS

➤**TEST feet and ankle muscles for strength.** Ask the client to walk on his or her toes, then heel followed by walking on the inside of the feet (eversion) and finally walking on the outside of the feet (inversion).

■ Abnormal findings include unequal response, weak response, muscular spasm, or pain. These findings may be due to joint or muscle inflammation, trauma, or sports injuries.

ADDITIONAL ASSESSMENT TECHNIQUES FOR SPECIAL CASES

Assessing for Carpal Tunnel Syndrome

❖ ➤The test for Phalen's sign is performed by asking the client to flex both wrists and press the dorsum of the hands against each other for 1 minute (Fig. 24-41). No report of numbness, tingling, or pain is a negative test.

■ A positive Phalen's sign occurs if the client complains of numbness, pain, or paresthesia over the palmar surface of the hand and the first three fingers and part of the fourth. This positive finding may indicate carpal tunnel syndrome.

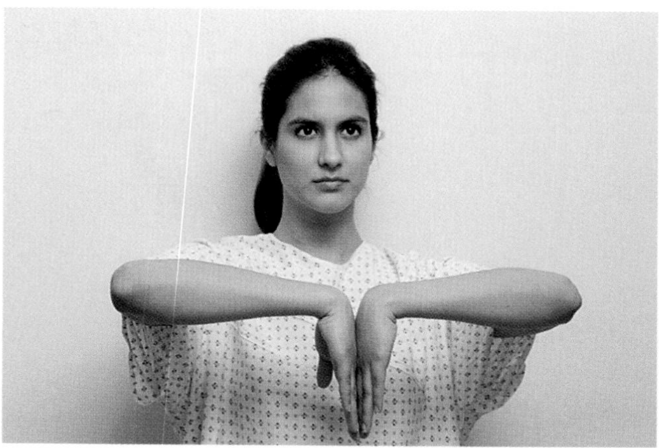

Fig. 24-41 Phalen's test for carpal tunnel syndrome.

❖ ➤The test for Tinel's sign is performed by tapping on the median nerve where it passes through the carpal tunnel under the flexor retinaculum (carpal ligament) and volar carpal ligament. No report of tingling sensation is a negative Tinel's sign (Fig. 24-42).

■ A positive Tinel's sign occurs when the client reports a tingling sensation or pain radiating from the wrist to the hand along the median nerve. This positive finding may indicate carpal tunnel syndrome.

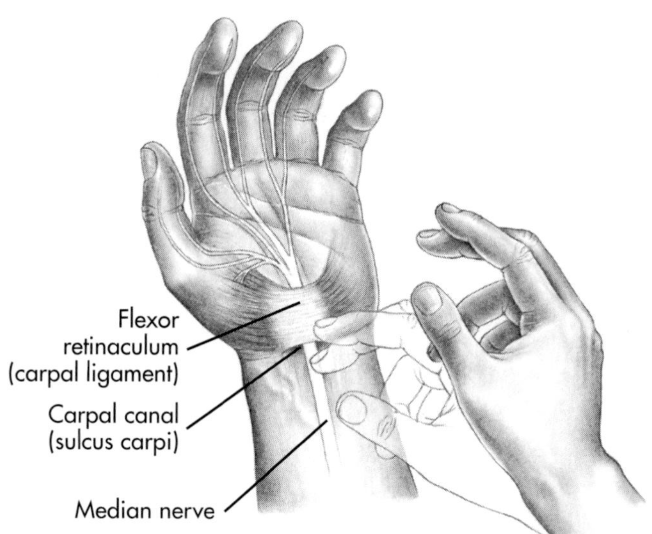

Fig. 24-42 Tinel's sign for carpal tunnel syndrome. (From Seidel et al, 1999.)

PROCEDURES AND TECHNIQUES WITH NORMAL FINDINGS

ABNORMAL FINDINGS

Assessing for Rotator Cuff Damage

❖ ➤Rotator cuff damage can be determined with the drop arm test. Abduct the client's affected arm and ask client to lower arm slowly. The expected response is a slow, controlled adduction of the arm.

■ Inability to lower the arm slowly and smoothly or severe shoulder pain while adducting the arm may indicate rotator cuff damage.

Assessing for Knee Effusion

❖ ➤Two tests evaluate the presence of fluid in the knee joint. The bulge sign tests for small effusions of the knee. Assist the client to a supine position. Elicit the bulge sign by extending the knee and milking the medial aspect upward two or three times. Then tap on the lateral side of the patella. No fluid waves or bulging should be seen on the opposite side of the joint (Fig. 24-43, *A, B*).

■ If fluid is present, fluid waves are palpable on the opposite side of the joint. Fluid in a joint (effusion) is an accumulation of serous exudate as part of an inflammatory process.

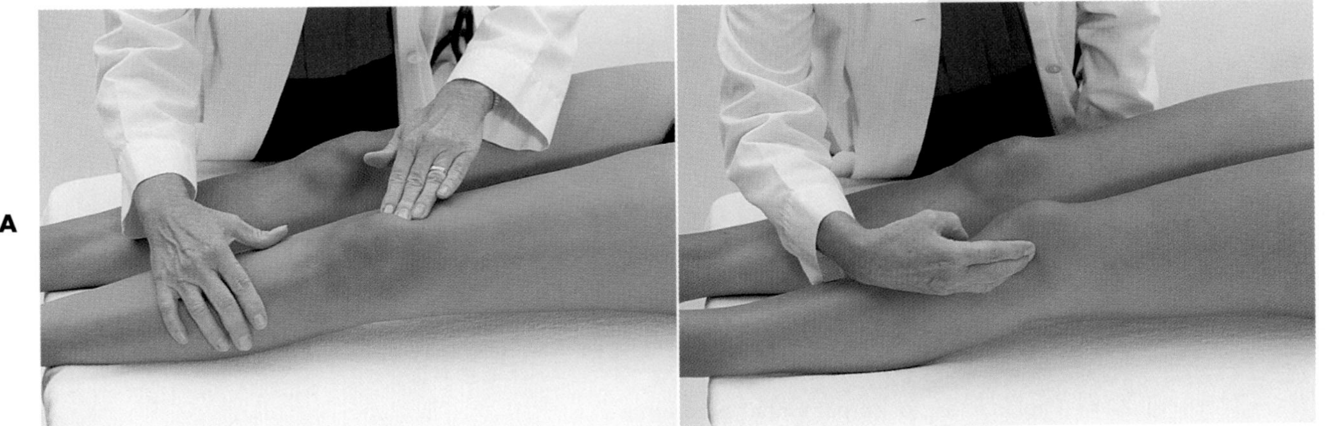

Fig. 24-43 Bulge sign to detect small effusion in knee joint. **A,** Milk the medial aspect of the knee two or three times. **B,** Then tap the lateral side of the patella.

PROCEDURES AND TECHNIQUES WITH NORMAL FINDINGS

❖ ➤The second test, ballottement, is used for larger effusions. With the knee extended, apply downward pressure on the suprapatellar pouch with the thumb and fingers of one hand, and with the other hand push the patella firmly against the femur. Release the pressure from the patella, but leave fingers in contact with the knee to detect any fluid wave (Fig. 24-44).

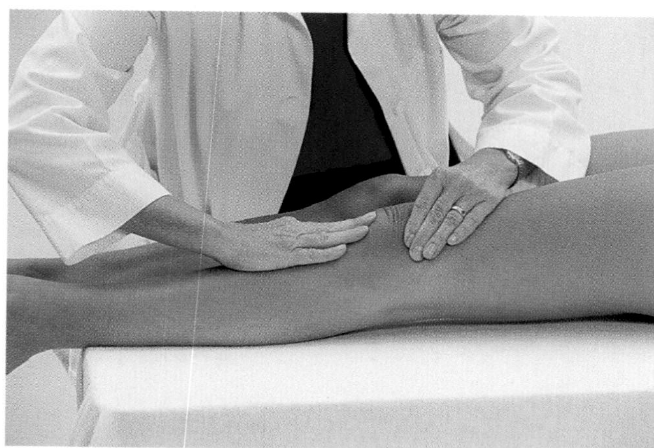

Fig. 24-44 Ballottement procedure to detect large effusion in knee joint.

Assessing for Knee Stability

❖ ➤With the client in supine position, assess knee stability provided by collateral and cruciate ligaments (see Fig. 24-9). Assess the lateral collateral ligament by placing one hand against medial aspect knee joint to keep it from moving and using your other hand to grasp the ankle. Adduct the lower leg (Fig. 24-45, *A*). Normally there is little lateral motion at the knee. To test the medial collateral ligament, place your hand on the lateral aspect of the knee, grasp the ankle, and abduct the lower leg. Repeat the procedure on the other knee if indicated.

❖ ➤Assess the anterior and posterior cruciate ligaments using the drawer test. The client remains in supine position with the hip flexed 45° and the knee flexed with the foot flat on the examination table. Sit on the client's foot to stabilize it. Instruct the client to relax muscles in the flexed leg. It is important to be sure that the hamstrings are relaxed by palpating them at the back of the knee. Using both hands, pull the head of the tibia forward (open drawer) to assess the posterior cruciate ligament and push backward (closed drawer) to assess the anterior cruciate ligament (Fig. 24-45, *B*). Repeat the procedure on the other knee if indicated. You should not be able to displace the knee from its position.

ABNORMAL FINDINGS

■ Palpation of a fluid wave after release of pressure against the patella is ballottement, indicating excess fluid in the knee joint.

■ Movement of the knee medially or laterally suggests collateral ligament damage, which often results from trauma to the knee.

■ When the tibia can be pulled anteriorly more than 6 mm from the femur, injury to the anterior cruciate ligament may be indicated. When the tibia can be pushed posteriorly from the femur, an injury to the posterior cruciate ligament may be indicated.

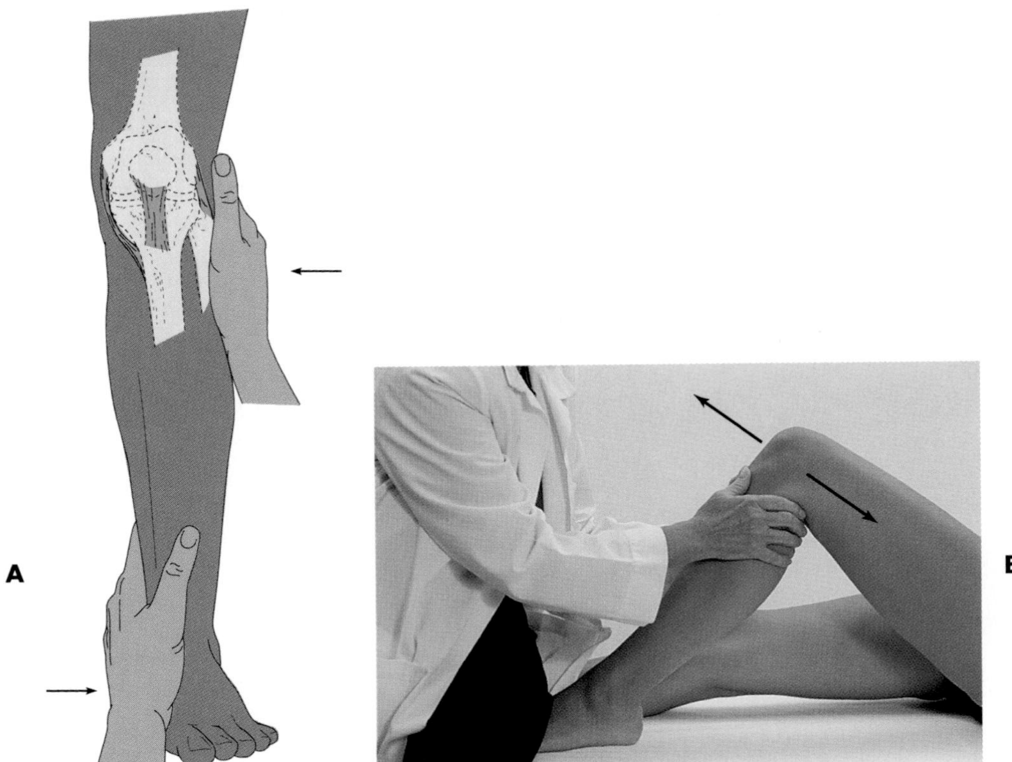

Fig. 24-45 Assessing knee stability. **A,** Assessing collateral ligaments. **B,** Drawer test for assessing anterior and posterior cruciate ligaments. (**A** From Greenberger and Hinthorn, 1993.)

PROCEDURES AND TECHNIQUES WITH NORMAL FINDINGS

❖ ➤Perform McMurray's test to evaluate the presence of a damaged medial or lateral meniscus. Ask the client to lie supine with one foot flat on the table near the buttocks. This flexes the knee. Place the thumb and index finger of one hand on either side of the joint space to maintain flexion and stabilize the knee. With the other hand, grasp the client's heel, raise the lower leg parallel with the table (knee will be flexed 90°), and rotate the knee. External rotation tests the lateral meniscus, and internal rotation tests the medial meniscus (Fig. 24-46).

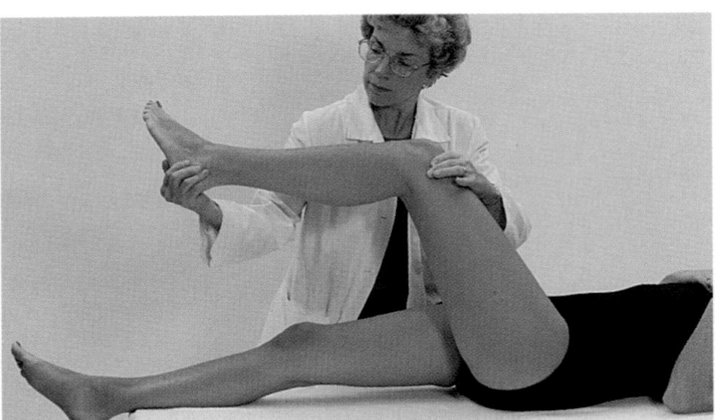

Fig. 24-46 Examination of the knee with McMurray's test. Knee is flexed, stabilized with thumb and index finger; with the other hand rotate and extend the lower leg.

ABNORMAL FINDINGS

■ A positive McMurray's test in the presence of meniscal damage are pain on the medial or lateral surfaces of the knee, audible click or locking of the knee on movement, or pain reproduced along the joint lines. If meniscal tear is present, the client will be unable to bear weight or flex the knee. Medial meniscus tear is more common than lateral meniscus tear. A meniscal tear frequently occurs with twisting of the knee playing sports.

PROCEDURES AND TECHNIQUES WITH NORMAL FINDINGS

❖ ➤When the client complains of knee locking, perform the Apley test to detect meniscal tear. With the client in prone position, flex the knee 90°. Press down on the client's foot so that the tibia is firmly against the femur; then rotate the knee externally. No pain or locking is a negative test (Fig. 24-47).

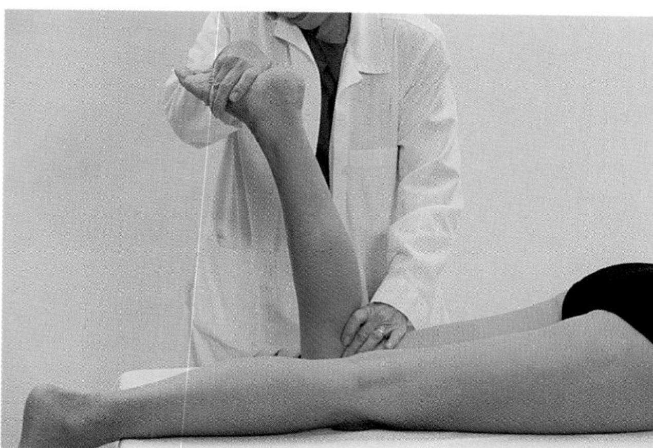

Fig. 24-47 Examination of the knee with the Apley test.

Assessing for Hip Flexion Contractures

❖ ➤Perform the Thomas test to evaluate flexion contractures of the hip. Have the client lie supine and ask him or her to fully extend one leg on the table and flex the other knee up to the chest as far as possible. Observe if the extended leg remains flat on the table when the other leg is flexed. The extended leg should remain flat on the table, a negative Thomas test (Fig. 24-48).

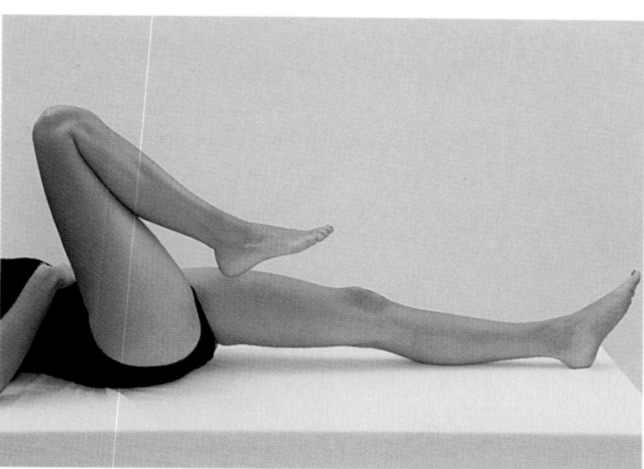

Fig. 24-48 Examination of the hip with the Thomas test. Response is negative in this client since the extended leg remains flat on the table.

ABNORMAL FINDINGS

■ Pain, locking of the knee, or clicking during rotation of the knee is a positive Apley test, indicating meniscal tear.

■ Lifting of extended leg off the table in response to the other leg being flexed indicates a hip flexion contracture. Record the degree of flexion.

PROCEDURES AND TECHNIQUES WITH NORMAL FINDINGS

ABNORMAL FINDINGS

Assessing for Nerve Root Compression

❖ ➤To evaluate for nerve root irritation or lumbar disk herniation, perform straight leg raises. With the client supine, raise one leg, keeping the knee straight. Tightness of the hamstring may be reported, but there should be no pain felt (Fig. 24-49).

■ Pain in back of the leg with 30° to 60° of elevation indicates pressure on a peripheral nerve by a intervertebral disk.

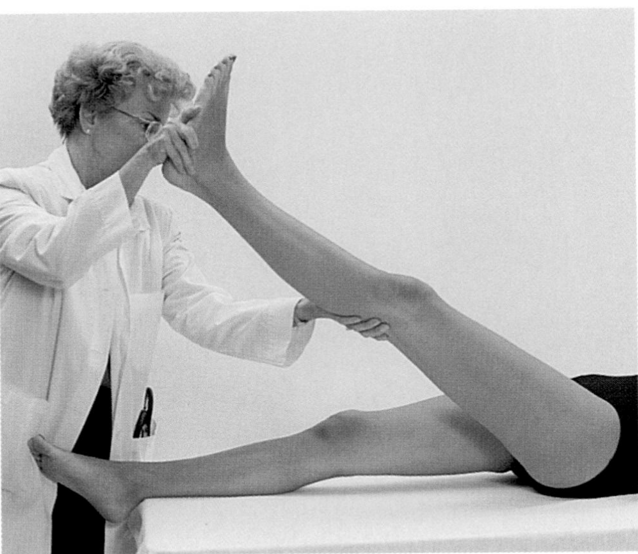

Fig. 24-49 Straight leg raising test.

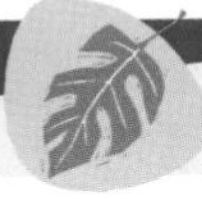

AGE-RELATED VARIATIONS

■ INFANTS

Anatomy and Physiology

At birth the cranial bones are soft; they are separated by the frontal, sagittal, coronal, and lambdoid sutures. During vaginal births, the skull may be molded when the skull is elongated with the cranial bones to overlap at the suture lines. The skull resumes its appropriate size and shape within several days. At about 6 years of age, when brain growth declines, these sutures will begin to ossify, a process completed by adulthood.

Health History

- Was the delivery difficult? Were forceps used? Did the infant cry soon after birth?

  Rationale Injury during delivery increases the risk for fractures and other injuries to the musculoskeletal system. A period of anoxia can cause hypotonia of the muscles (floppy infant syndrome).

- Did the infant develop movement and skills as expected for his or her age?

  Rationale Developmental delays may indicate musculoskeletal disorders.

Examination

Procedures and Techniques Examine the infant undressed and lying on his or her back. Palpate clavicles for stability. Extend both arms to compare muscle tone and length. Extend both legs to compare muscle tone and length. Inspect the back and spine for alignment, tufts of hair, or bulges.

Assess hip location by performing the Barlow-Ortolani maneuver for infants age birth to 2 months (Fig. 24-50, *A*, *B*). With the infant supine, flex the knees, holding your thumbs on the inner midthighs and your fingers outside on the hips touching the greater trochanters. Adduct the legs until your thumbs touch. Then abduct, moving the knees apart and down to touch the table with their lateral aspects. Allis' sign is another assessment of hip location. With the infant supine, flex the knees with the feet flat on the table, and align the femurs. Observe the height of the knees (Fig. 24-51).

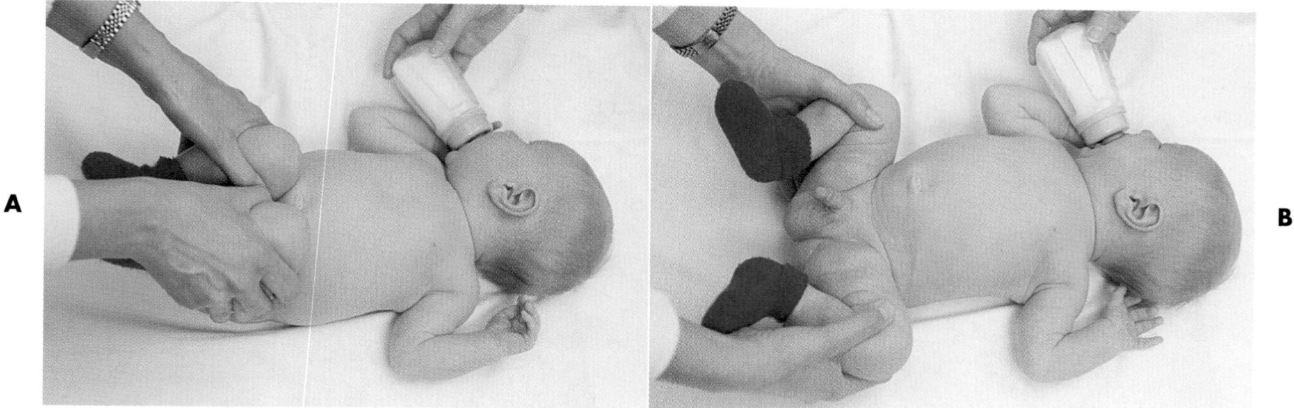

Fig. 24-50 Barlow-Ortolani maneuver to detect hip dislocation. **A,** Phase I, adduction. **B,** Phase II, abduction. This is a negative findings since no dislocation is found.

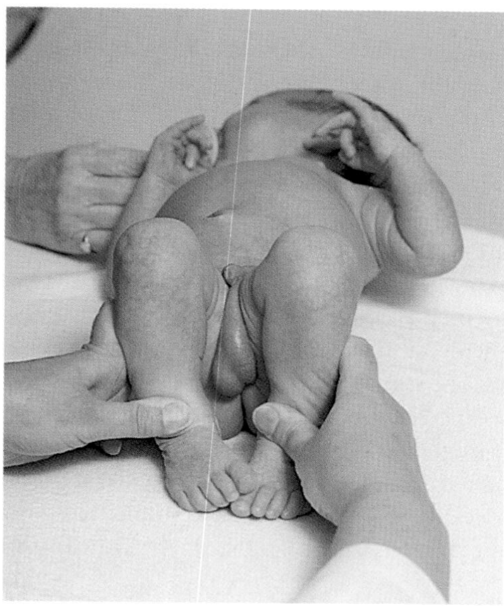

Fig. 24-51 Positive Allis' sign shows the left leg is shorter than the right leg, indicating left hip dysplasia. (From Seidel et al, 1999.)

Assess the feet for position. Scratch the outside and inside borders of the foot or immobilize the heel with one hand and gently push the forefoot to neutral position with the other hand.

Normal and Abnormal Findings Normal findings include stable and smooth clavicles, without crepitus. Arms and legs should have strong muscle tone and have equal length bilaterally. The Barlow-Ortolani maneuver should feel smooth and produce no clicking. When both knees are the same height, Allis' test is negative. The spine should be flexible with convex dorsal and sacral curves, no masses, and easy movement in and out of fetal position. A newborn's feet are often held in varus or valgus position. They should be flexible and not fixed. If the deformity is self-correctable, the foot assumes a normal right angle to the lower leg (moves into neutral position). Note the relationship of the forefoot to the hindfoot. The hindfoot aligns with the lower leg and the forefoot turns inward slightly.

Abnormal findings include limited shoulder range of motion and deformity that can be palpated if clavicle is fractured. Erb's palsy (paralysis of shoulder and upper arm muscles) may be noted. Asymmetry of extremities, limited movement, syndactyly (fused digits), and polydactyly (extra digits) are abnormal findings. Proliferation of cartilage at the growth plates increases the length of long bones, whereas in smaller bones ossification forms calcified cartilage. Note asymmetric back curve, masses (hair tufts, dimples), and abnormal posturing perhaps indicating malformation of vertebrae and/or spinal column.

Note any click that occurs when you perform external hip rotation. This is a positive Barlow-Ortolani's sign. Uneven gluteal folds is another sign of hip dislocation (Fig. 24-52). When one knee is lower than the other, Allis' sign is positive (see Fig. 24-51). Stages of developmental dysplasia of the hip (DDH) vary by severity. Dysplasia occurs when there is a shallow acetabulum; subluxation, when there is an incomplete dislocation; and dislocation, when the head of the femur is completely out of the acetabulum. About 20% of the cases involve both hips. When only one hip is involved, the left hip is involved 3 times more often than the right (Wong et al, 1999). Metatarsus varus (toeing in or pigeon-toed) or talipes equinovarus (clubfoot) may be noted.

CHILDREN

Anatomy and Physiology

Throughout childhood long bones increase in diameter and length. Ligaments are stronger than bones until adolescence, increasing the risk of fracture. Muscle fibers lengthen during childhood as the skeletal system grows.

Health History

- Have your ever noticed any bone deformity such as curved back or abnormally shaped knees, feet, or toes? How old was the child when these deformities were noted? What treatment was received?

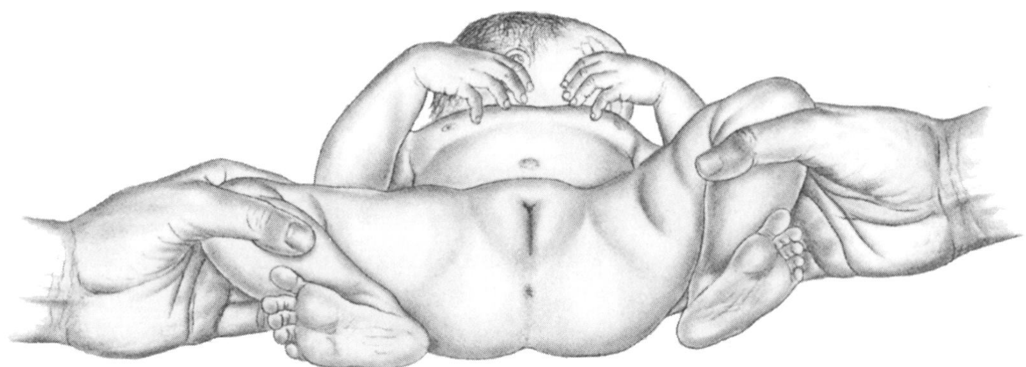

Fig. 24-52 Sign of hip dislocation: the three skin folds on the left upper leg and limited abduction indicate left hip dysplasia. (Seidel et al, 1999.)

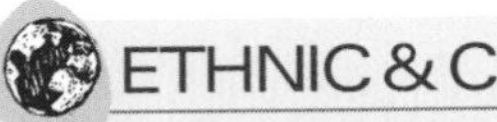

ETHNIC & CULTURAL VARIATIONS

Navajo Indians and Canadian Eskimos are among the cultures with the highest incidence of hip dislocation. In these cultures newborns are tightly wrapped in blankets or strapped to cradle boards. Hip dislocation is virtually unknown in cultures where infants are carried on their mother's backs or hips in the widely adducted straddle position such as in the Far East and Africa (Wong et al, 1999).

Rationale Growth may be affected by bone injury or deformity. Walking may be affected by knee or foot deformities. A curved spine, if severe, displaces ribs so that they may impair respiratory expansion.

Examination

Equipment Scale for measuring height and weight.

Procedures and Techniques When evaluating children, compare data obtained with tables of normal age and sequence of motor development. (Chapter 2 discusses expected motor development for children.) Weigh and measure the child and compare values to tables of percentiles for growth and weight. (See Appendix F for height and weight tables.) Observe the gait for steadiness. Inspect the spine for alignment. Inspect the knees for symmetric alignment.

❖ Trendelenburg's sign (or gait) tests for hip dysplasia and the function of the gluteus medius muscle (see Fig. 24-7), which normally acts to abduct and rotate the thigh. Assist the client to stand. You stand behind the client to observe the tilt of the pelvis as the client stands on one foot and then the other.

Normal and Abnormal Findings Toddlers have a wide stance and a wide-waddle gait pattern, which tends to disappear by age 2 to 2½ years. The gait should become progressively stronger, steadier, and smoother as the child matures. The spine should be straight. By 12 to 18 months the lumbar curve develops as the child learns to walk; lumbar lordosis is common in toddlers; after 18 months, the cervical spine is concave, the thoracic spine convex (although less than that of adults), and the lumbar spine is concave like an adult's. There should be no bulges or dimpling along the spine. Lordosis is seen more frequently in African-American children but should not be seen in children over the age of 6 years. Knees should be in a direct straight line between the hip, the ankle, and the great toe. Valgus rotation (medial malleolus greater than 1 inch [2.5 cm] apart with knees touching) is normal in children 2 to 3½ years of age and may be present up to age 12 years. Varus rotation (medial malleolus touching, with knees greater than 1 inch [2.5 cm] apart) requires further evaluation for tibial torsion; it may be normal until 18 to 24 months of age. The expected finding of Trendelenburg's sign is that the opposite thigh and hip elevate because the pelvic muscles to the greater trochanter are sufficient to elevate the hip not bearing weight (Fig. 24-53). For example, when the client stands on the left leg, the right thigh and hip should tilt upward.

Any deviation from the pattern or a history of increasing falls or balance problems should be considered abnormal. A positive Trendelburg's sign indicates hip dysplasia. When standing on the affected leg, no pelvic tilt is noted in the opposite thigh and hip. The client with a Trendelenburg sign shortens the step on the unaffected leg and has a lateral deviation of the entire trunk and affected side. This is one of the more common gait deviations.

■ ADOLESCENTS

Anatomy and physiology, health history, and examination of the adolescent are the same as for the adult. Emphasis is needed in assessing for scoliosis and risk factors for injury from sports and other extracurricular activities.

■ OLDER ADULTS

Anatomy and Physiology

The aging process may be accompanied by a number of musculoskeletal changes such as a decrease in bone mass, making the client increasingly vulnerable to stress in weight-bearing areas and resultant fractures. Intervertebral

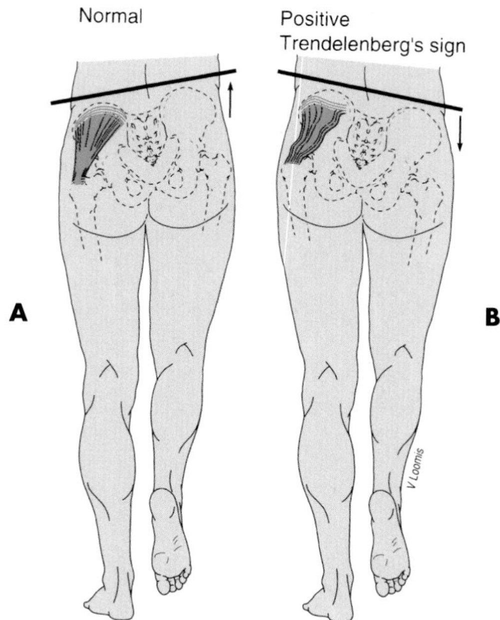

Fig. 24-53 Trendelenburg's test or sign. **A,** Normally when standing on the left foot, right pelvis rises. **B,** Lack of pelvic tilt when standing on affected leg indicates hip dysplasia, a positive Trendelenburg's test.
(From Greenberger and Hinthorn, 1993.)

disks become thin and sometimes collapse, whereas cartilage and ligaments are prone to calcification. Tendons and muscles decrease in elasticity and tone, with the muscles losing both mass and strength, although this decrease usually does not exceed a 10% to 20% loss at 60 years of age. This alteration in muscle tone and strength means the person may be less able to perform sudden, intense exercise or to endure exercise for extended periods of time; there may be loss of agility.

Health History

- What activities do you do each day to take care of yourself, such as bathing, dressing, eating, and exercising? Do you need assistance in taking care of yourself? If so, who provides that care?

  Rationale This assesses the degree of independence in activities of daily living (ADL) that may be interrupted by muscle weakness or joint pain.
- Do you use any gadgets to help you throughout the day (e.g., mobility aids, elevated commode seat)? Describe which gadgets you use.

  Rationale This provides information about how clients maintain independence or suggests ways that these devices could be used. Mobility aids can prevent falls and improve independence.
- What have you done to prevent falls in your residence (Box 24-2)?

  Rationale It is important to discuss fall prevention with older adults. Falls injure the musculoskeletal system by straining ligaments and tendons and bruising tissues, and they also may cause fractures.

Examination

Procedures and Techniques Examination of the older adult is the same as the adult. They may be slower at performing range-of-motion and muscle-strength assessments.

Normal and Abnormal Findings Normal findings are the same as for the younger adult. Abnormal findings include osteoarthritic changes in joints and muscle atrophy from disuse. Many joints may not have the expected degree of movement or range of motion. When asking the client to hyperextend the neck to assess the cervical spine, he or she may experience dizziness or visual changes from altered carotid circulation. Provide safety to prevent injury to the client.

Box 24-2 Risk of Falls Assessment Tool

FALL ASSESSMENT SCORING SYSTEM — **POINTS**

I. AGE

65-79 Years	1	
80 & Above	2	I. ☐

II. MENTAL STATUS

A. Oriented at all times or comatose	0	
Confusion at all times	2	II.A ☐
Intermittent confusion	4	
B. Agitated/uncooperative/anxious-moderate	2	
Agitated/uncooperative/anxious-severe	4	II.B ☐

III. ELIMINATION

Independent and continent	0	
Catheter and/or ostomy	1	
Elimination with assistance	3	
Ambulatory with urge incontinence or episodes of incontinence	5	III. ☐

IV. HISTORY OF FALLING WITHIN SIX MONTHS

No history	0	
Has fallen one or two times	2	
Multiple history of falling	5	IV. ☐

V. SENSORY IMPAIRMENT

Sensory impairment (Blind, deaf, cataracts, not using corrective device)	1	V. ☐

VI. ACTIVITY

Ambulation/transfer without assistance	0	
Ambulation/transfer with assist of one or assistive device	2	VI. ☐
Ambulation/transfer with assist of two	1	

VII. MEDICATIONS

❑ Narcotics ❑ Tranquilizers ❑ Sleeping aids
❑ Diuretics ❑ Chemotherapy ❑ Antiseizure/antiepileptic

For the above medications, check how many the patient is taking currently at home or that the patient will be taking in the hospital.

No medications	0	
1 medication	1	
2 or more medications	2	VII. ☐

Add one more point if there has been a change in these medications or dosages in the past 5 days.

A score of 10 or more indicates a high risk for falling. TOTAL ☐

Indicate high risk and care plan. SCORE ☐

If the patient does not meet a score of 10, but in the nurse's judgement is at risk to fall, initiate the high-risk fall protocol.

From MacAvoy S, Skinner T, Hines M: Clinical methods: fall risk assessment tool, *Appl Nurs Res* 9(4):213, 218, 1996. In Phipps WJ, Sands JK, Marek JF: *Medical-surgical nursing: concepts and clinical practice,* ed 6, St. Louis, 1999, Mosby.

EXAMINATION SUMMARY

Musculoskeletal System

PROCEDURE

Routine Examination (p. 642)

- Observe gait for:
  Conformity
  Symmetry
  Rhythm
- Inspect skeleton and extremities for:
  Alignment
  Contour
  Size
  Symmetry
  Gross deformities
- Inspect muscles for:
  Size
  Symmetry
  Fasciculations
  Spasms
- Palpate bones for:
  Tenderness
- Palpate muscles for:
  Tenderness
  Heat
  Edema
  Tone
- Observe and palpate joints and adjacent muscles for:
  Active and passive range of motion
  Tenderness on motion
  Joint stability
  Deformity
  Contracture
- Test muscles for strength and compare contralateral sides

Specific Musculoskeletal Regions (pp. 643-647)

- Inspect musculature of face and neck for symmetry

Temporomandibular Joint (p. 647)

- Palpate for:
  Movement
  Sounds (clicking or popping)
  Tenderness
- Observe range of motion
- Test muscle strength

Cervical Spine (pp. 647-649)

- Palpate for:
  Pain
- Observe range of motion of neck:
  Forward flexion
  Hyperextension
  Lateral bending
  Rotation
- Test strength of sternocleidomastoid and trapezius muscles

Thoracic and Lumbar Spine (pp. 650-651)

- Inspect spine, iliac crest, and shoulders for:
  Alignment
  Symmetry
- Observe range of motion:
  Forward flexion and hyperextension
  Lateral bending
  Rotation
- Palpate spinal processes and paravertebral muscles for:
  Alignment
  Tenderness
- Percuss spinal processes for:
  Tenderness

Shoulders (pp. 652-655)

- Inspect shoulders and shoulder girdle for:
  Equality of height
  Contour
- Palpate shoulders for:
  Firmness and fullness
  Tenderness
  Masses
- Test muscle strength of trapezius muscles
- Observe range of motion:
  Forward flexion and hyperextension
  Abduction and adduction
  External and internal rotation

Arms (p. 656)

- Test muscle strength and compare contralateral side of triceps and biceps muscles

Elbows (pp. 656-657)

- Palpate elbows for:
  Tenderness
  Edema
  Nodules
- Observe range of motion:
  Flexion and extension
  Pronation and supination

Hands and Wrists (pp. 658-661)

- Inspect joints for:
  Position

Contour
Number of digits
- Palpate each joint for:
  Surface characteristics
  Tenderness
- Test muscles for strength
- Observe range of motion:
  Wrist hyperextension and flexion
  Metacarpophalangeal flexion and hyperextension
  Ulnar and radial deviation
  Abduction and adduction of fingers
  Finger flexion (forming fist)
  Thumb opposition

Hips (pp. 662-664)

- Inspect for symmetry
- Palpate for stability and tenderness
- Observe range of motion:
  Flexion and hyperextension
  Internal and external rotation
  Abduction and adduction
- Test muscle strength

Knees (pp. 664-665)

- Inspect knees for:
  Symmetric alignment
  Erythema
- Palpate knees for:
  Contour
  Tenderness
- Observe range of motion for:
  Flexion
  Hyperextension
- Test muscle strength around the knee

Feet and Ankles (pp. 665-667)

- Inspect feet and ankles for:
  Contour
  Alignment
  Number of toes
- Palpate feet and ankles for:
  Contour
  Tenderness
- Observe range of motion:
  Dorsiflexion and plantar flexion
  Inversion and eversion
  Abduction and adduction
  Flexion and extension of toes
- Test muscles for strength

Additional Assessment Techniques for Special Cases (pp. 667-672)

❖ *Assess for Carpal Tunnel Syndrome*

Phalen's sign
Tinel's sign

❖ *Assess for Rotator Cuff Damage*

Drop arm test

❖ *Assess for Knee Effusion*

Bulge sign
Ballottement

❖ *Assess for Knee Stability*

Collateral ligament test
Drawer test
McMurray's test
Apley test
Thomas test

❖ *Assess for nerve root compression*

Straight leg raises

SUMMARY OF FINDINGS

Age Group	Normal Findings	Typical Variations	Findings Associated With Disorder
Infants and children	• Head circumference is within expected limits for age. Fontanels, if present, are soft. Posterior fontanel closes by 2 months, anterior fontanel closes by 24 months. Clavicles of newborn are stable, smooth without crepitus. The spine is flexible and straight. Hips are firmly in the acetabulum. Extremities are bilaterally symmetric. Joints have full range of motion. Five digits appear on each hand and foot. • Gait of toddlers is a wide-waddle gait, but gait should be stronger and steadier by age 2 ½ years. Feet are at right angles with leg.	• Lumbar lordosis is common in toddlers.	• Shoulder range of motion is limited and deformity can be palpated if clavicle is fractured. Erb's palsy (paralysis of shoulder and upper arm muscles) may be noted. Asymmetry of extremities, limited movement, syndactyly (fused digits), polydactyly (extra digits) are abnormal findings. Proliferation of cartilage at the growth plates increases the length of long bones, whereas in smaller bones ossification forms calcified cartilage. Note asymmetric back curve, masses (hair tufts, dimples), and abnormal posturing perhaps indicating malformation of vertebrae and/or spinal column. • A positive Barlow-Ortolani's sign, uneven gluteal folds, and hip clicks with abduction should be reported. When one knee is lower than the other, Allis' sign is positive. Dysplasia occurs when there is a shallow acetabulum; subluxation, when there is an incomplete dislocation; and dislocation, when the head of the femur is completely out of the acetabulum. Metatarsus varus (toeing in or pigeon-toed) or talipes equinovarus (clubfoot) may be noted. • Positive Trendelburg's sign indicates hip dysplasia.
Adolescents	Same as for adult.		• Chronic poor posture can cause kyphosis or scoliosis. Pain, edema, and erythema of extremities may occur as a result of sports injuries.

Age Group	Normal Findings	Typical Variations	Findings Associated With Disorder
Adults	• Gait rhythmic, symmetric; stands erect, spine straight, knees in straight line between hips and ankles. Extremities are symmetric bilaterally. • Muscles are toned, strength with opposition. Full range of motion in all joints. No joint, muscle or bone tenderness to palpation.	• Arm muscles of dominant arm may be larger than the non-dominant arm. • Not all people are able to hyperextend their joints. • Some are unable to touch their toes because of tight hamstrings and leg muscles or obesity. An extension from 60° to 70° is a normal variation for adults with tight hamstrings, especially men.	• Unsteady gait or limb may indicate muscle weakness, uneven leg length, or pain in lower extremities. Curvature of the spine may be scoliosis, lordosis, or kyphosis depending on the angle of the curve. Muscle atrophy and weakness unilaterally may be due to disuse from casted extremity or hemiparesis from head injury or stroke; bilaterally it may be due to malnutrition or spinal cord disorder. Hot, erythematous, edematous, and painful joints indicates inflammation, e.g., arthritis, gout, or trauma. • Inpaired range of motion may be due to contracture, joint pain, muscle spasticity, or weakness. • Tenderness or pain with pronation or supination of the elbow and point tenderness on the lateral epicondyle may be lateral tendonitis (tennis elbow); but on the medial epicondyle it may be medial tendonitis (golfer's elbow). • Positive Phalen's or Tinel's sign with numbness, tingling, and pain of palmar surface of hand may indicate carpel tunnel syndrome. • Fluid on the knee, impaired range of motion or pain may indicate an effusion from inflammation. • Positive drawer test may indicate injury to the anterior or posterior cruciate ligament. • Positive McMurray's or Apley test may indicate damaged medial or lateral meniscus. • Positive Thomas test may indicate a hip flexion contracture. • Pain on straight leg raise may indicate a herniated disk.
Older adults	Same as for younger adult. • These clients may perform range of motion slower and have less muscle strength.		• Osteoarthritic changes in joints and muscle atrophy from disuse. Osteoporosis increases risk for fractures.

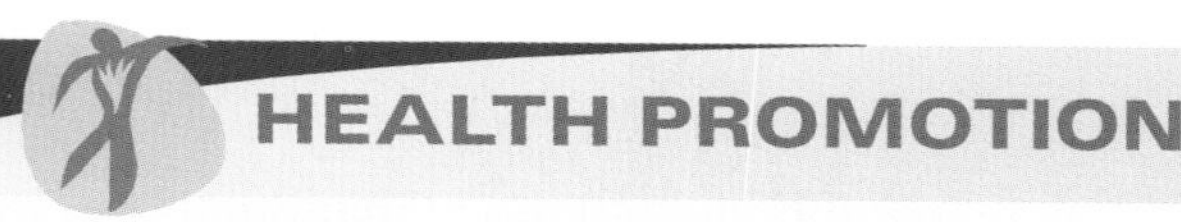

HEALTH PROMOTION

PREVENTING OSTEOPOROSIS

Osteoporosis can be prevented by regular exercise to stress bones, which maintains deposition of calcium in the bones, and adequate intake of calcium. The daily amount of calcium recommended is 1 g for premenopausal woman and 1.2 to 1.5 g for postmenopausal women. Also, based on the risk factors for osteoporosis, limiting alcohol consumption, stopping smoking, and using estrogen replacement therapy are other preventive strategies for osteoporosis.

MAINTAINING HEALTHY BODY WEIGHT AND EXERCISING REGULARLY

Obesity strains bones, muscles, and joints. While weight-bearing on bones is needed to maintain calcium deposition, excessive weight can exert too much stress on bones, as well as on ligaments, tendons, and muscles. Regular exercise (at least walking) for 30 minutes 3 times a week is recommended to provide sufficient stress on bones and to help maintain weight. The other side of the equation to maintaining body weight is a sensible diet following recommendations from the food pyramid (see Chapter 10).

PREVENTING INJURIES

Injuries related to exercise can be prevented by stretching muscle, tendons, and ligaments before exercising. Starting an exercise program gradually is also recommended; for example, begin with 5 minutes of walking and increase the exercise time by 5 minutes each week. Using proper body mechanics when pushing, pulling, or lifting prevents strain of back muscles. By using the longest and strongest muscles, those in the legs, rather than those in the back, individuals can prevent back injuries. Falls can be prevented by maintaining a safe environment, for example, using handrails and night-lights, removing throw rugs, and applying non-slip mats in the bathtub.

COMMON PROBLEMS AND CONDITIONS

Musculoskeletal System

CARPAL TUNNEL SYNDROME

Compression of the medial nerve causes a common painful disorder called carpal tunnel syndrome. The medial nerve is compressed between the inelastic flexor retinaculum (also called transverse ligament) and other structures within the carpal tunnel. It may be caused by repetitive movements of hands and arms, microtrauma, or vibration as well as rheumatoid arthritis, gout, hypothyroidism, and with fluid retention that occurs with pregnancy and menopause. Symptoms include burning, numbness, and tingling in the hands, often at night. It occurs more frequently in women. Use Phalen's sign or Tinel's sign to assess for this disorder (see Figs. 24-41 and 24-42).

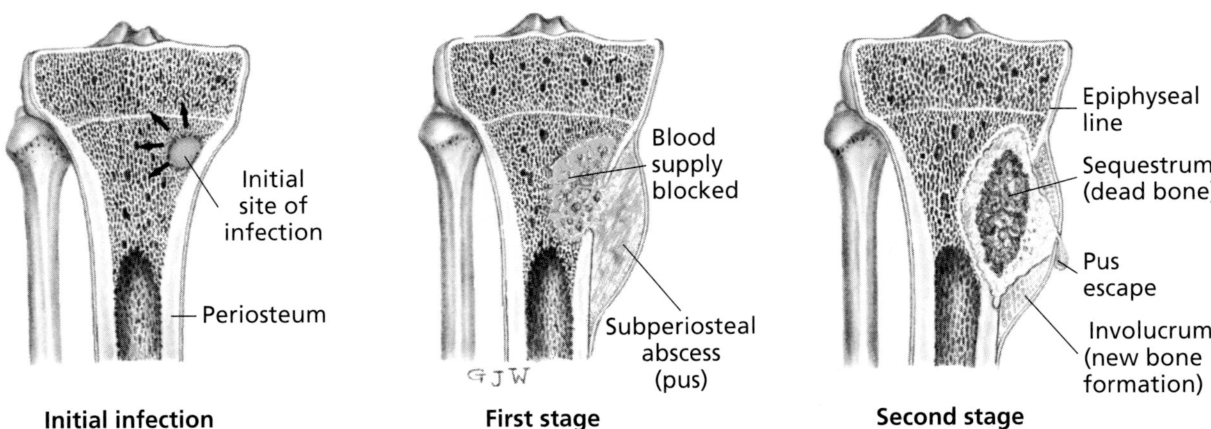

Fig. 24-54 Osteomyelitis. (From Mourad, 1991.)

OSTEOMYELITIS

An infection of the bone and its marrow is called osteomyelitis. It is often due to systemic infection or an open wound contaminated by bacteria introduced by trauma or surgery, by direct extension from a nearby infection, or via the bloodstream (Fig. 24-54). Purulent exudate spreads through the cortex of the bone and into the soft tissues. Assessment findings include signs of localized inflammation (edema, erythema, warmth at the site of infection, pain on movement) and signs of systemic inflammation (fever).

TEMPOROMANDIBULAR JOINT SYNDROME

This joint syndrome results in painful jaw movement due to congenital anomalies, malocclusion, trauma, arthritis, and other joint diseases. Unilateral jaw pain is worse with jaw movement. Pain may be referred to the face or neck. Clients complain of muscle spasm and clicking; popping or crepitus can be palpated.

GOUT

An increase in serum uric acid may result in gout. It is a hereditary disease in which there is either an overproduction or decreased excretion of uric acid and urate salts. The disease is thought to be caused by lack of an enzyme needed to completely metabolize purines for renal excretion. Uric acids accumulate commonly in the great toe but also in other joints such as wrists, hands, ankles, and knees. The symptoms include erythema and edema of joints that are very painful to move and thus limited in the range of motion. Tophi are a sign of gout; these are round, pealike deposits of uric acid in ear cartilage or large, irregularly shaped deposits in other joints (Fig. 24-55). This disorder primarily affects men over 40 years of age.

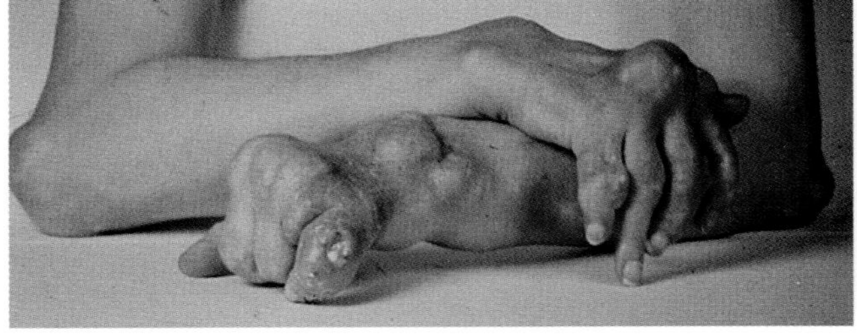

Fig. 24-55 Gout with many tophi present on the hands, wrists, and in both olecranon bursae. (Reprinted from the Clinical Slide Collection of the Rheumatic Diseases, copyright 1991, 1995, 1997. Used by permission of the American College of Rheumatology.)

BURSITIS

An inflammation of a bursa is called bursitis. The bursa is the connective tissue structure surrounding a joint; it becomes inflamed by constant friction around joints (Fig. 24-56). It may be precipitated by arthritis, infection, injury, or excessive exercise. Common sites of bursitis are the shoulder, elbow, hip, and knee. Assessment findings include limited and painful range of motion, edema, point tenderness, and erythema.

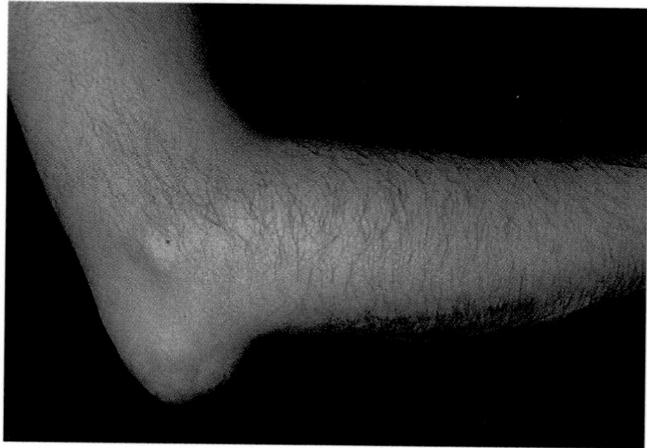

Fig. 24-56 Olecranon bursitis. (Reprinted from the Clinical Slide Collection of the Rheumatic Diseases, copyright 1991, 1995, 1997. Used by permission of the American College of Rheumatology.)

RHEUMATOID ARTHRITIS

A chronic, systemic autoimmune inflammatory disease of the connective tissue of the body is a description of rheumatoid arthritis. Even though this is a systemic disease, the synovial lining of joints is one of the major tissues initially inflamed. Joint pain, edema, and stiffness of the fingers, wrists, ankles, feet, and knees are common symptoms. Joints are symmetrically and bilaterally inflamed. Inflammation leads to deterioration of cartilage and erosion of surfaces, causing bone fissures, cysts, and bone spurs. Ligaments and tendons around inflamed joints become fibrotic and shortened, causing contractures and subluxation (partial dislocation) of joints (Fig. 24-57). Women have rheumatoid arthritis 3 times more often than men. The incidence is lower in Asians and Hispanics than in whites and African Americans.

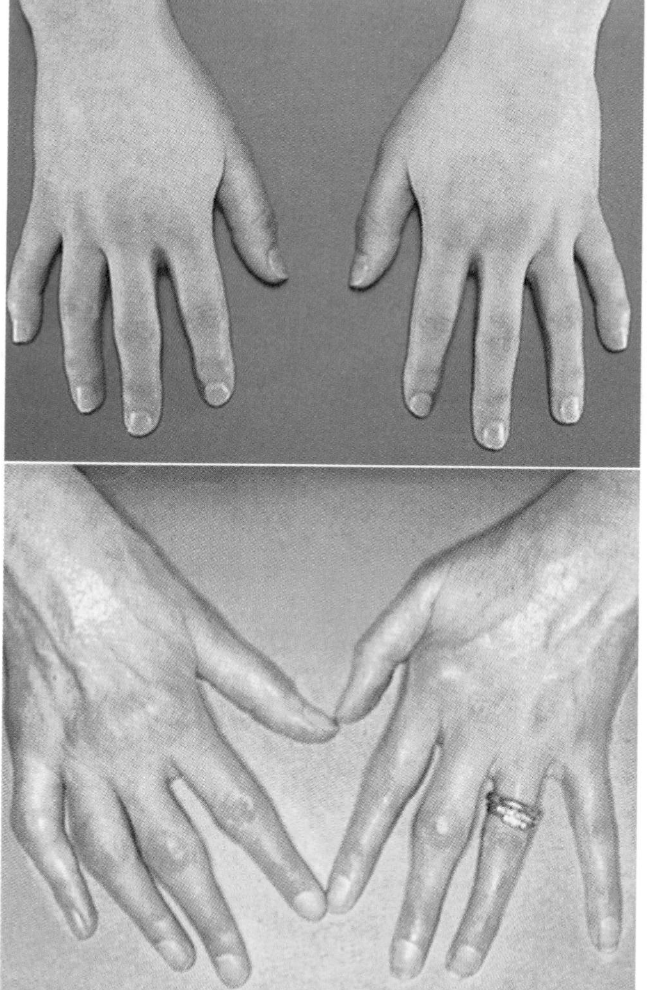

Fig. 24-57 Rheumatoid arthritis of hands. **A,** Early stage. **B,** Moderate involvement. (From Shipley, 1993.)

HERNIATED NUCLEUS PULPOSUS (HERNIATED DISK)

The intervertebral disk provides a cushion between two vertebrae and contains a nucleus pulposus encased in fibrocartilage. When the fibrocartilage surrounding an intervertebral disk ruptures, the nucleus pulposus is displaced from lying between two vertebrae to the pressing on the adjacent spinal nerve (Fig. 24-58). This rupture frequently occurs in lumbar vertebrae when there is increased strain on the vertebrae such as lifting a heavy object improperly. Pressure on the spinal nerve may cause pain that radiates down the leg on the involved side. Straight leg raises cause pain in the involved leg.

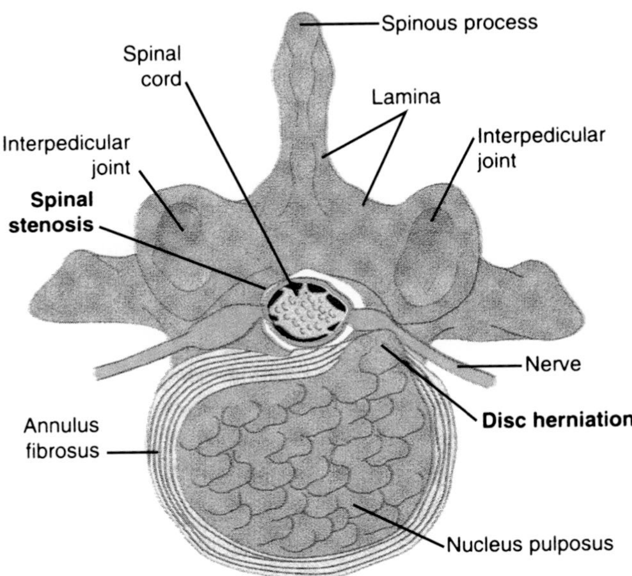

Fig. 24-58 Herniated intervertebral disk. (From Black and Matassarin-Jacobs, 1997.)

INJURIES

Overuse of the musculoskeletal system resulting from sports, exercise, or repetitive trauma can result in the following disorders; muscle strain, sprain, dislocation, and fracture.

Muscle strain develops from stretching, tearing, or forceful contraction of a muscle beyond its functional capacity. Severity ranges from a mild intrafibrinous tear to a total rupture of a single muscle. Signs include temporary weakness, edema, and echymosis.

Sprain is a stretching or tearing of a ligament by forced movement beyond its normal range, characterized by pain, edema, discoloration of the skin over the joint, and loss of function. The duration and severity of symptoms vary with the extent of damage to supporting tissue. Severe sprains may rupture ligaments, causing joint instability if not treated.

Dislocation is a displacement of a bone from its normal articulation, often caused by pressure or force pushing the bone out of the joint. Signs and symptoms include deformity, edema, pain, and loss of function.

Fracture is a traumatic injury in which there is a partial or complete break in the continuity of a bone. This injury results in muscle spasm and shortening of tissue around the bone, causing deformity. Additional signs and symptoms are edema, pain, loss of function, and changes in skin color. A pathologic fracture is a break in the continuity of the bone due to weakness in the bone such as osteoporosis or a neoplasm.

AGE-RELATED VARIATIONS
Infants and Children
Skeletal Disorders

Myelomeningocele/spina bifida. This developmental defect of the central nervous system results from a hernial sac protruding through a congenital cleft in the vertebral column (Fig. 24-59). This hernial sac contains a portion of the spinal cord, its meninges, and cerebrospinal fluid. The defect of the vertebra (spina bifida) may range from displacement of a lamina to complete absence of lamina. The condition is primarily caused by failure of the neural tube to close during embryonic development. Signs vary, depending on the damage to the spinal cord, and may include paralysis, anesthesia, and loss of bowel and bladder function.

Spina bifida occulta is a defective closure of the laminae of the vertebrae in the lumbosacral area. There is no herniation of the spinal cord or meninges. This defect is recognized by a tuft of hair or dimple over the site.

Meningocele is a defective closure of the skull or vertebrae with a saclike protrusion of meninges through the defect that creates a cyst filled with cerebrospinal fluid. The cyst does not contain neural tissue. This defect is recognized by observation of the sac at the cervical or lumbar site.

Myelomeningocele is a defective closure of the skull or vertebrae with a saclike protrusion of meninges, cerebrospinal fluid, and neural tissue (spinal cord) through the defect. Functions below the level of the spinal cord are impaired, which may include paralysis of legs and loss of bowel and bladder control, depending on where along the vertebral column the defect occurs. This defect is caused by failure of the neural tube to close during embryonic development. It is recognized by observation of the sac and by abnormal to no movement of lower extremities.

Congenital dislocation of the hip. This congenital defect, also called developmental dysplasia, occurs when the head of the femur does not articulate with the acetabulum because of an abnormal shallowness of the acetabulum. This dislocation is assessed using the Barlow-Ortolani maneuver and/or Allis' sign (see Figs. 24-50, 24-51, and 24-52).

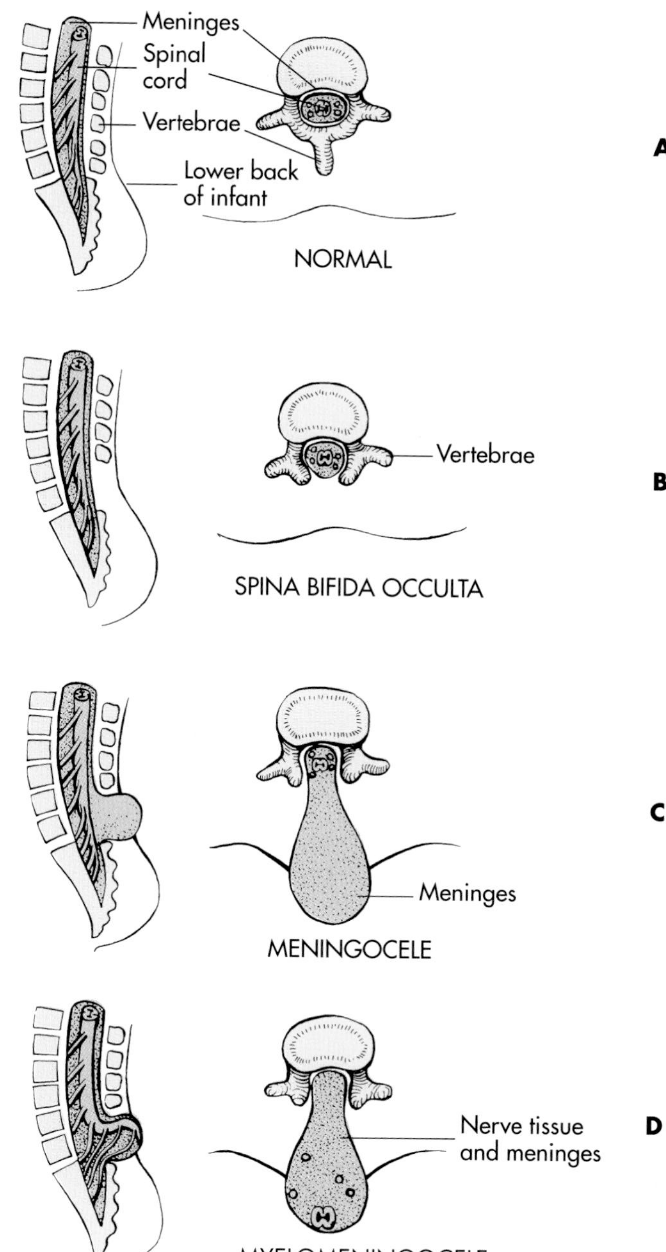

Fig. 24-59 Midline defects of osseous spine with varying degrees of neural herniations. **A,** Normal. **B,** Spina bifida occulta. **C,** Meningocele. **D,** Myelomeningocele. (From Wong et al, 1999.)

Talipes equinovarus (clubfoot). This congenital deformity of the ankle and foot is caused by intrauterine constriction. It is characterized by unilateral or bilateral deviation of the metatarsal bones of the forefoot. Most deformities are equinovarus, in which there is a medial deviation and plantar flexion of the forefoot, but a few cases may be calcaneovarus, in which there is lateral deviation and dorsiflexion of the forefoot (Fig. 24-60).

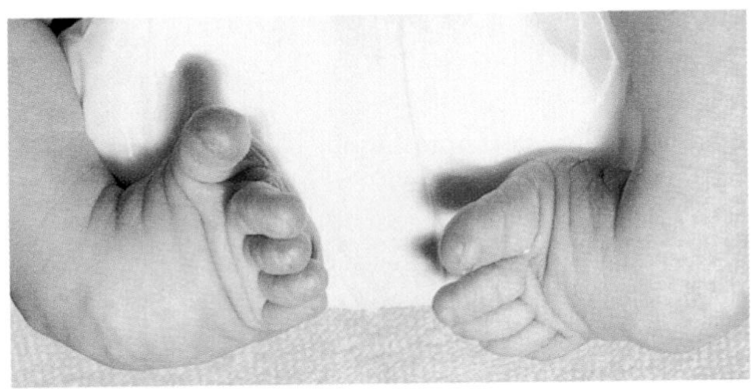

Fig. 24-60 Bilateral deviation. (From Zitelli and Davis, 1992.)

Metatarsus adductus (metatarsus varus). This common foot deformity is also called pigeon-toed or toeing in. It involves medial adduction of the toes and forefoot from angulation at the tarsometatarsal joint (Fig. 24-61, *A*, *B*).

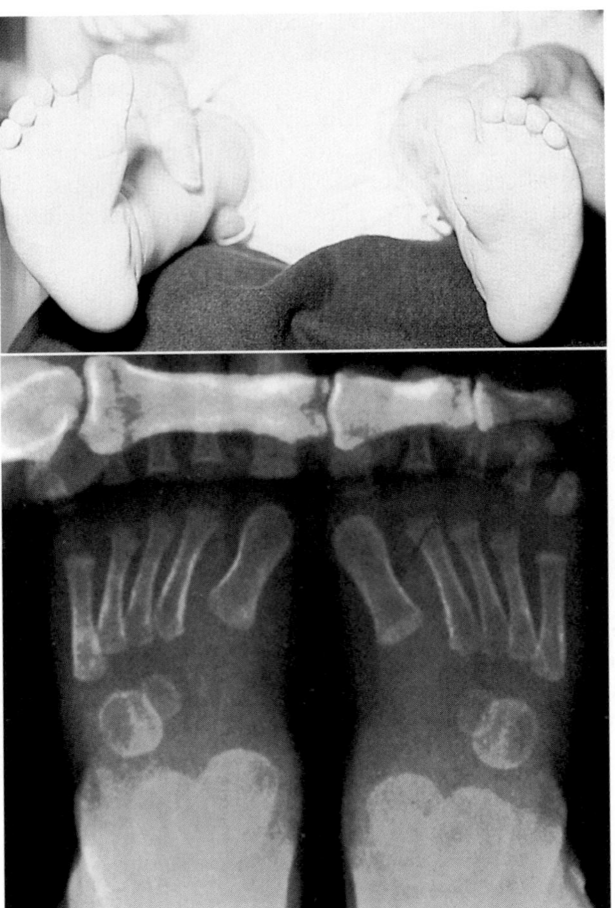

Fig. 24-61 Bilateral metatarsus adductus. **A,** When viewed from the planar aspect, rounding of the lateral border of the feet can be appreciated. **B,** The metatarsals are deviated medially with respect to the remainder of the foot; otherwise, the bony structures are normal. (From Zitelli and Davis, 1997.)

Scoliosis. An S-shaped deformity of the vertebrae is called scoliosis. It is a skeletal deformity with a concave curvature of the anterior vertebral bodies, convex curvature of posterior vertebral bodies, and lateral rotation of the thoracic spine (Fig. 24-62). Causes include congenital malformations of the spine, poliomyelitis, skeletal dysplasia, spastic paralysis, and unequal leg length. Scoliosis produces uneven shoulders and hip levels. Rotation deformity also may cause a rib hump and flank asymmetry on forward flexion. Depending on the severity of the curve, physiologic function of lungs, spine, and pelvis may be compromised. Structural scoliosis affects girls more often than boys and progresses during early adolescence.

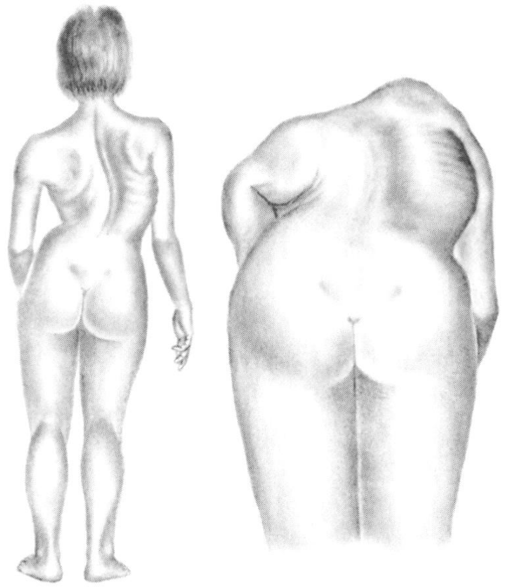

Fig. 24-62 Scoliosis. (From Mourad, 1991.)

Muscular Disorders

Muscular dystrophy (MD). A group of genetically transmitted diseases characterized by atrophy of muscles is a description of muscular dystrophy. It is characterized by progressive atrophy of symmetric groups of skeletal muscle fibers without evidence of degeneration of neural tissue. In all forms of muscular dystrophy there is a progressive muscle atrophy or pseudohypertrophy from fatty infiltration. Each type differs in the group of muscles affected, age of onset, rate of progression, and mode of genetic inheritance. Duchenne type, limb-girdle, and facioscapulohumeral are commonly seen in children, and these children rarely live past 25 years of age (Marek, 1999).

Older Adults

Osteoporosis Loss of bone density is a way to describe osteoporosis. It is a systemic condition of overall reduction in bone mass or density in which bone reabsorption is greater than bone deposition (Fig. 24-63). Lack of bone density increases risk of fractures. An increase in the thoracic kyphotic curve and lumbar lordotic curve develops, which decreases height. Scoliosis occurs in about 30% of all women over the age of 45.

Osteoarthritis (Degenerative Joint Disease [DJD]) This form of arthritis is caused by degenerative changes in articular cartilage. It affects weight-bearing joints such as vertebrae, hips, knees, and ankles but also is noted in hands and fingers. As the cartilage wears away, the bones move against each other, causing joint inflammation. Joint involvement may be unilateral or bilateral. Symptoms include joint edema and aching joint pain. Joint deformities of fingers develop (Heberden's nodes in distal interphalangeal joints and Bouchard's nodes in proximal interphalangeal joints) (see Fig. 24-32). The incidence increases with age, affecting about 90% of people over 60 years of age.

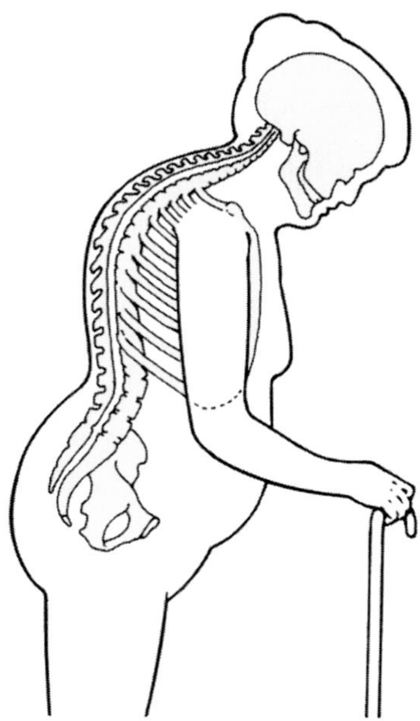

Fig. 24-63 Hallmark of osteoporosis: dowager's hump. (From Seidel et al, 1999.)

CLINICAL APPLICATION and CRITICAL THINKING

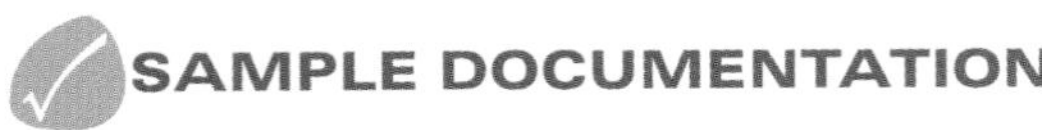

SAMPLE DOCUMENTATION

CASE 1

S.C. is a 33-year-old man complaining of right wrist pain.

Subjective Data

Pain in right wrist noticed 1 week ago; slowly getting worse; hand swollen; painful on movement, 6 on a scale of 10. Some pain relief after taking ibuprofen. No history of trauma to wrist. Does not participate in sports. Unable to perform job as computer programmer; painful to tie necktie, shave face, and button shirt.

Objective Data

Alert, cooperative client in no apparent distress.

Right wrist: Edema over right distal radius and medial carpals; no redness or heat noted. Pain on flexion and hyperextension of radiocarpal joint; grip strength 3/5 with pain on contraction; able to perform thumb opposition, but slowly and with pain; negative Tinel's sign; sensation present in all fingers.

Left wrist: No pain on range of motion, grip strength 5/5, thumb opposition brisk without pain; negative Tinel's sign; sensation present in all fingers.

Functional Health Patterns Involved

- Cognitive–perceptual
- Activity–exercise

Medical Diagnosis

Tendonitis

Nursing Diagnosis and Collaborative Problems

- *Pain* related to inflammation of tendons as manifested by:
  - Report of 6/10 pain.
  - Right wrist edema.
  - Pain on range of motion of right wrist.
- *Impaired physical mobility* related to limitation of joint function and pain as manifested by:
  - Unable to perform job as computer programmer due to pain and edema.
  - Report of pain with activities (tie necktie, shave face, and button shirt).

CASE 2

A 76-year-old woman complains of "arthritis pain."

Subjective Data

Stiffness of left hip and knee getting worse, gradual change over the past several months; stiff when arising in morning, lasts 15 to 20 minutes; joints painful when walking, cleaning, or ironing, but relieved by rest; pain is an ache, cannot localize pain precisely. No fatigue reported. Unable to walk in evening with husband because of pain.

Objective Data

Temperature, 98.2° F (36.8° C); Pulse, 88 beats/min; Respiratory rate, 16. Blood pressure, 148/88 mm Hg.

Height, 5′5″ (165 cm); weight, 175 lb (79 kg).

Ambulates independently, slowing, symmetrically.

Left hip and knee: Pain on palpation, no heat or edema; crepitus on movement, positive ballottement and bulge signs. Peripheral pulses 2+; sensation to sharp, dull, and vibratory sense present.

Range of motion: Hip flexion, knee extended 75°; hip flexion, knee flexed 90°, internal rotation 30°, abduction 35°.

Right hip and knee: No pain on palpation, no heat, edema, or crepitus. Peripheral pulses 2+; sensation to sharp, dull, and vibratory sense present.

Range of motion: Hip flexion, knee extended 85°; hip flexion, knee flexed 100°, internal rotation 35°, abduction 45°.

Functional Health Patterns Involved

- Activity–exercise
- Cognitve–perceptual
- Nutrition–metabolic

Medical Diagnosis

Osteoarthritis

Nursing Diagnosis and Collaborative Problems

- *Impaired physical mobility* related to joint degeneration as manifested by:
  - Left knee and hip joints painful when walking, cleaning, or ironing.
  - Pain relieved by rest; reduced range of motion of affected joints.
- *Pain* related to joint degeneration as manifested by:
  - Client complains of pain relieved by rest.
  - Painful left hip and knee joint on palpation.
  - Unable to walk because of pain.
- *Altered nutrition: more than body requirements* related to lack of exercise as manifested by:
  - Height is 5′5″ (165 cm); weight 175 lb (79 kg)
  - Unable to walk due to joint pain and stiffness.

CRITICAL THINKING QUESTIONS

1. Mark is a 17-year-old who presents with pain to the ankle. He states he twisted it during his soccer game earlier in the afternoon, and now the pain seems to be getting worse. The ankle is very swollen with a bluish discoloration. How does the examiner differentiate muscle strain, sprain, or a fracture?
2. You are observing the range of motion of a 58-year-old client who is obese. When assessing his knees, you notice that the right knee flexion is 125° and the left knee is 90°. What additional data are needed to determine the reasons for the discrepancy in the flexion between the right and left knees?
3. A 16-year-old client comes to the clinic for cast removal after a fracture of the right arm. The cast is successfully removed. What differences would you anticipate comparing the right and left arm?

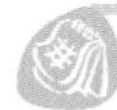

CASE STUDY

Mrs. Simmons is a 46-year-old woman with rheumatoid arthritis (RA). Listed below are data collected by the examiner during an interview and examination.

Interview Data

According to the medical record, Mrs. Simmons was diagnosed with RA at age 30. She complains of a great deal of pain in her joints, particularly in her hands, and says she has just learned to live with the pain because it will always be there. She states that the stiffness and pain in her joints is always worse in the morning or if she sits around too much. She denies muscle weakness other than the fact that her stiffness and soreness prevent her from doing much. Mrs. Simmons reports that the RA is progressing to the point where she is having difficulty doing things requiring fine motor dexterity such as changing clothes, holding utensils to eat, and cutting up her food. She had different faucet handles placed in her home so she could turn the water on and off. Mrs. Simmons says she rarely goes out because she feels ugly.

Examination Data

- Client is able to stand, but standing up erect is not possible. Gait is slow and purposeful.
- Significant inflammation, swelling, and tenderness noted with inspection and palpation at wrists, hands, knees, and ankles bilaterally. Hand grips are weak bilaterally. Subcutaneous nodules noted at ulnar surface of elbows bilaterally.

1. What data deviate from normal findings, suggesting a need for further investigation?
2. What additional information should the nurse ask or assess for?
3. In what functional health patterns does data deviate from normal?
4. What nursing diagnosis and/or collaborative problems should be considered for this situation?

REMEMBER to check out your **companion CD-ROM**

25 Neurologic System

www.mosby.com/MERLIN/wilson/assessment/

ANATOMY AND PHYSIOLOGY

The nervous system controls all body functions through voluntary and autonomic responses to external and internal stimuli. Structural divisions of the nervous system are the central nervous system, which consists of the brain and spinal cord; the peripheral nervous system; and the autonomic nervous system.

CENTRAL NERVOUS SYSTEM

Protective Structures

The brain is protected by the skull. At the base of the skull in the occipital bone is a large oval opening called the foramen magnum, through which the spinal cord extends off the medulla oblongata in the brainstem. Also at the base of the skull are a series of openings (foramina) for the entrance and exit of paired cranial nerves and cerebral blood vessels.

Between the skull and the brain lie three layers called meninges. The outer layer is a fibrous, double layer called the dura mater. The middle meningeal layer is called the arachnoid. It is a two-layer, fibrous, elastic membrane that covers the folds and fissures of the brain. The inner meningeal layer is called the pia mater. It contains small vessels to supply blood to the brain (Fig. 25-1). Between the arachnoid and the pia mater is the subarachnoid space, where the cerebrospinal fluid (CSF) circulates.

The falx cerebri is a vertical fold of dura mater that separates the two cerebral hemispheres. The tentorium cerebelli is a horizontal double fold of dura that supports the temporal and occipital lobes and separates the cerebral hemispheres from the cerebellum. Structures above the tentorium are referred to as supratentorial and those below as infratentorial (see Fig. 25-1).

Cerebral Ventricular System and Cerebrospinal Fluid

The cerebral ventricular system consists of four interconnecting chambers or ventricles that produce and circulate CSF (see Fig. 25-1). There is one lateral ventricle in each hemisphere, with a third ventricle adjacent to the thalamus and a fourth adjacent to the brainstem.

Cerebrospinal fluid is a colorless, odorless fluid containing glucose, electrolytes, oxygen, water, and carbon dioxide, a small amount of protein, and a few leukocytes. It is produced in the choroid plexus of the ventricles. It circulates around the brain and spinal cord to provide a cushion, maintain normal intracranial pressure, provide nutrition, and remove metabolic wastes.

Brain

The brain, consisting of the cerebrum, diencephalon, cerebellum, and brainstem, is made up of gray matter (cell bodies) and white matter (myelinated nerve fibers). Blood flows to the brain from two internal carotid arteries, two vertebral arteries, and the basilar artery (Fig. 25-2) and drains away from the brain through venous sinuses that empty into the jugular veins (see Fig. 25-1 for superior sagittal sinus).

Cerebrum The cerebrum is the largest part of the brain and is composed of two hemispheres. Each hemisphere is divided into four lobes: frontal lobe, parietal lobe, temporal lobe, and occipital lobe (Fig. 25-3).

The frontal lobe contains the primary motor cortex and is responsible for functions related to motor activity. The location in the frontal lobe motor cortex that provides motor nerves to specific parts of the body is shown in Fig. 25-4, *B*. The left frontal lobe contains Broca's area (see Fig. 25-3), which is involved in formulation of words. The frontal lobe also controls higher intellectual function, awareness of self, and autonomic responses related to emotion.

The parietal lobe contains the primary sensory cortex. One of its major functions is to process sensory input such as position sense, touch, shape, and consistency of objects. The location in the parietal lobe sensory strip that receives sensory nerves from specific parts of the body is adjacent to the motor strip and shown in Fig. 25-4, *A*.

The temporal lobe contains the primary auditory cortex. Wernicke's area (see Fig. 25-3), located in the left temporal lobe, is responsible for comprehension of spoken and written language. The temporal lobe also contains the interpretative area where auditory, visual, and somatic input are integrated into thought and memory.

The occipital lobe contains the primary visual cortex and is responsible for receiving and interpreting visual information.

Diencephalon The thalamus, hypothalamus, epithalamus, and subthalamus make up the diencephalon (Fig. 25-5). The thalamus is a relay and integration station from the spinal cord to the cerebral cortex and other parts of the brain. The hypothalamus has an important function in maintaining homeostasis. Some of these functions include

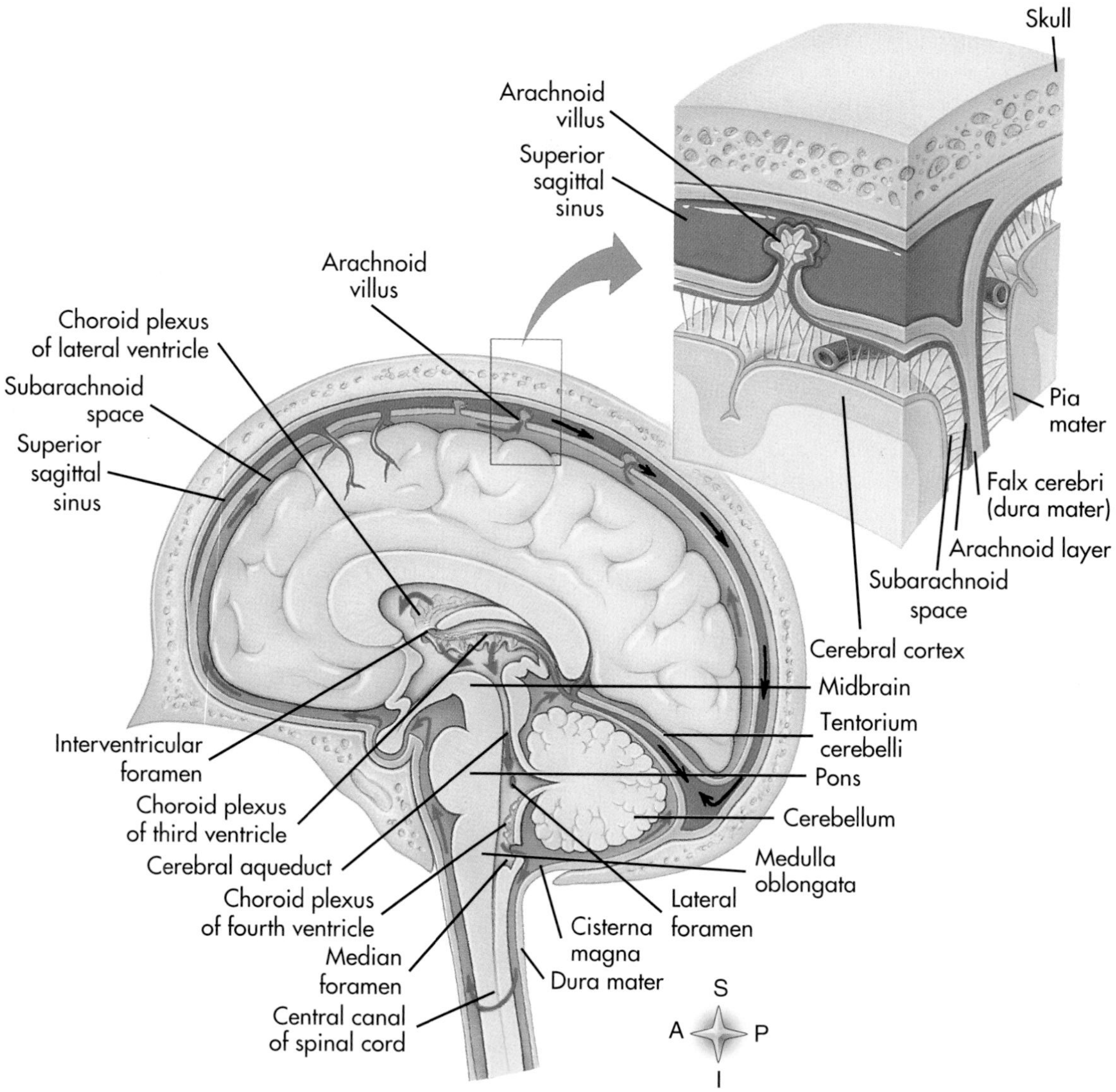

Fig. 25-1 Structures of the brainstem and cerebrospinal fluid (CSF) circulation. *White arrows* represent the route of the CSF. *Black arrows* represent the route of blood flow. Cerebrospinal fluid is produced in the ventricles, exits the fourth ventricle, and returns to the venous circulation in the superior sagittal sinus. The *inset* depicts the arachnoid granulations in the superior sagittal sinus, where the CSF enters the circulation. (Modified from Thibodeau and Patton, 1999.)

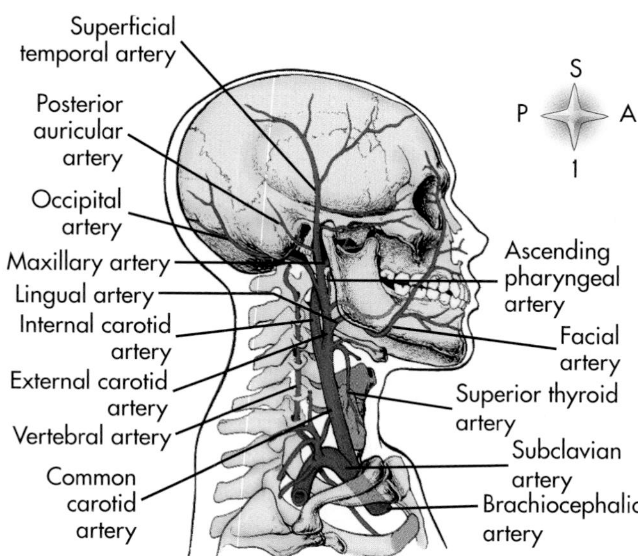

Fig. 25-2 Arteries of the head and neck, including the brachiocephalic artery, the right common carotid artery, the right subclavian artery, and their branches. The major arteries to the head are the common carotid and vertebral arteries. (From Thibodeau and Patton, 1999.)

regulation of body temperature, hunger, and thirst; formation of autonomic nervous system responses; and storage and secretion of hormones from the pituitary gland. The epithalamus contains the pineal gland, which is believed to have a role in physical growth and sexual development. The subthalamus is part of the extrapyramidal system of the autonomic nervous system and the basal ganglia.

Basal Ganglia Between the cerebral cortex and midbrain and adjacent to the diencephalon lie the structures that form the basal ganglia (Fig. 25-6). The basal ganglia's function is the refinement of voluntary motor activity via a balanced production of the neurotransmitters acetylcholine and dopamine.

Brainstem The midbrain, pons, and medulla oblongata make up the brainstem. Ten of the twelve cranial nerves (CN) originate from the brainstem (Fig. 25-7). The major function of the midbrain is to relay stimuli concerning muscle movement to other brain structures. It contains part of the motor tract pathways that control reflex motor movements in response to visual and auditory stimuli. The oculomotor nerve (CN III) and trochlear nerve (CN IV) originate in the midbrain.

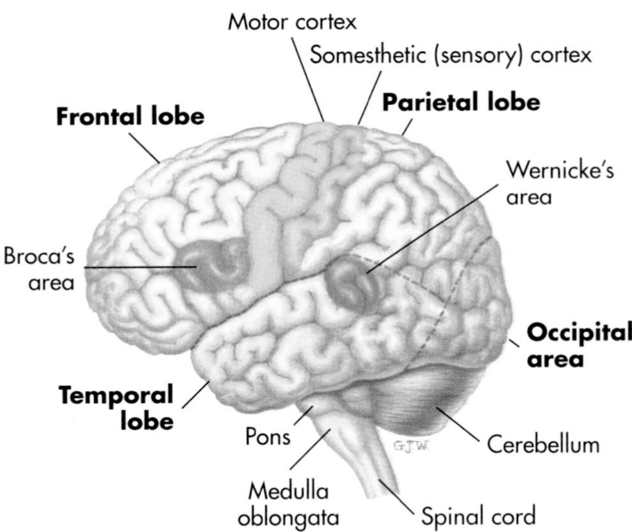

Fig. 25-3 Cerebral hemispheres. Lateral view of the brain. The motor cortex in the frontal lobe is depicted in pink, and the somesthetic cortex in the parietal lobe is depicted in blue. (Modified from Chipps, Clanin, and Campbell, 1992.)

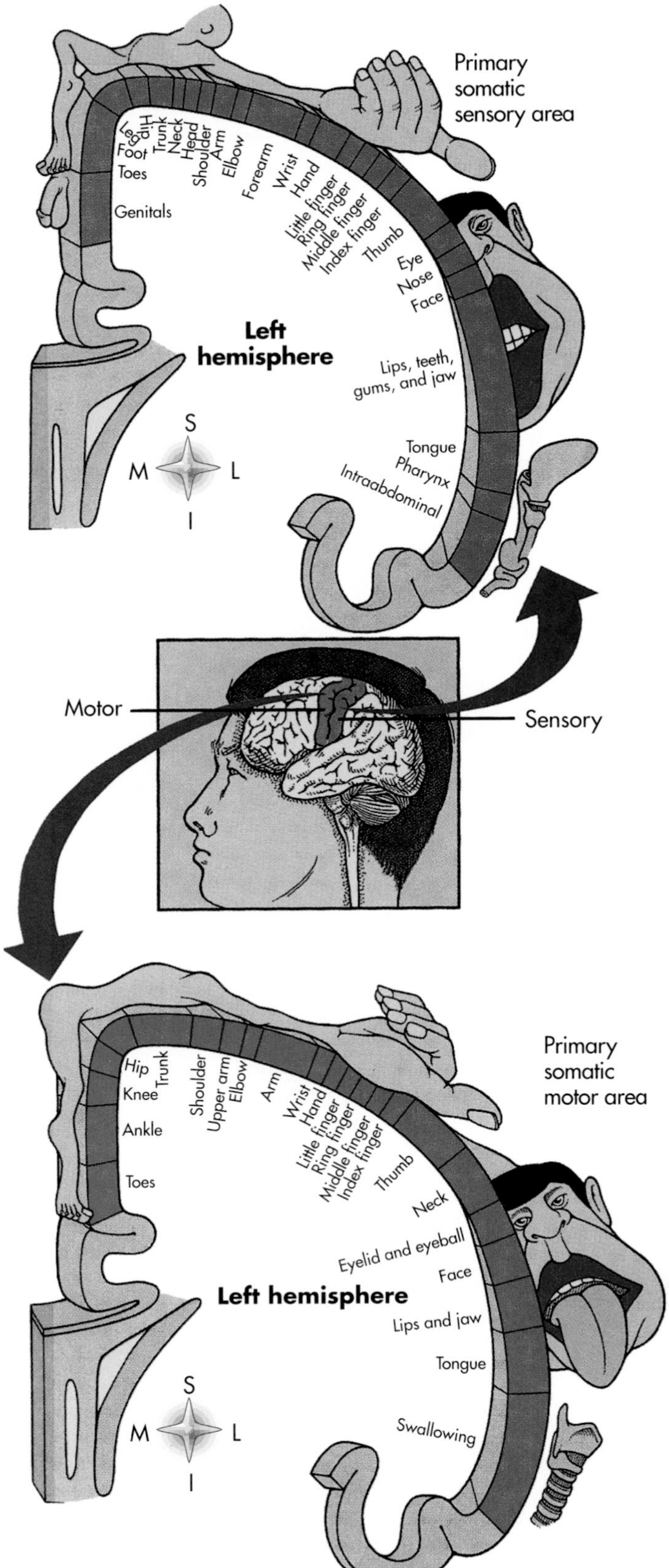

Fig. 25-4 Topography of the somesthetic and motor cortex. Cerebral cortex seen in coronal section on the left side of the brain. The figure of the body (homunculus) depicts the relative nerve distributions; the size indicates relative innervation. Each cortex occurs on both sides of the brain but appears on only one side in this illustration. The inset shows the motor and somesthetic regions of the left hemisphere. **A,** Somesthetic cortex. **B,** Motor cortex. (From Thibodeau and Patton, 1999.)

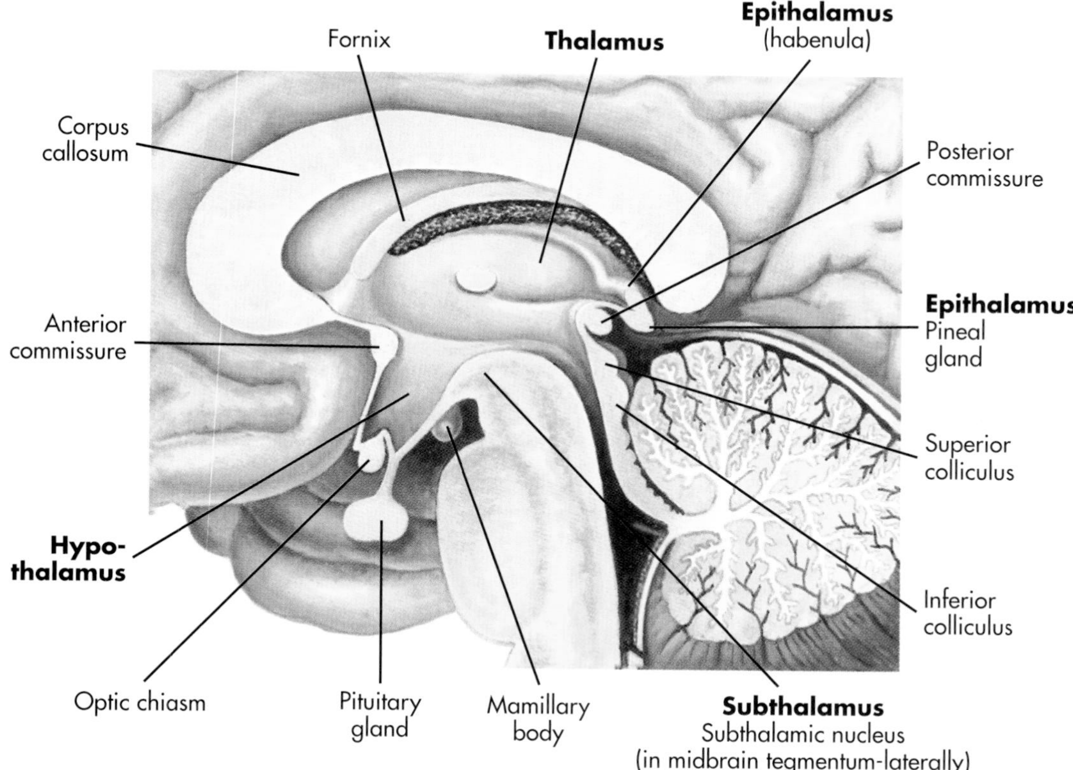

Fig. 25-5 Diencephalon. Lateral view of the brain. (From Chipps, Clanin, and Campbell, 1992.)

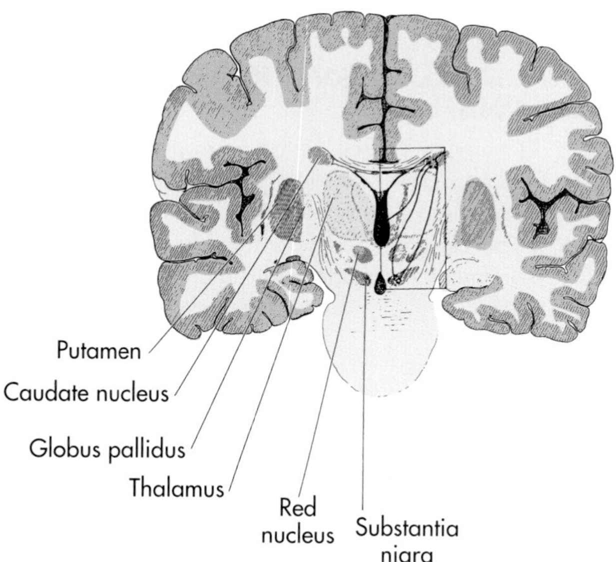

Fig. 25-6 Coronal section of the brain shows six ganglia that make up the basal ganglia. (From Cutler WP: *Degenerative and hereditary diseases.* Scientific American Medicine, Rubenstein E, Federman D, Eds. Scientific American, Inc., New York, 1998. All rights reserved.)

The pons relays impulses to the brain centers and lower spinal nerves. The CNs that originate in the pons are trigeminal (CN V), abducens (CN VI), facial (CN VII), and acoustic (CN VIII).

The medulla oblongata contains reflex centers for controlling involuntary functions such as breathing, sneezing, swallowing, coughing, vomiting, and vasoconstriction. The cranial nerves that originate in the medulla are glossopharyngeal (CN IX), vagus (CN X), spinal accessory (CN XI), and hypoglossal (CN XII).

Cerebellum The cerebellum is separated from the cerebral cortex by the tentorium cerebelli (see Fig. 25-1). Functions of the cerebellum include coordinating movement, equilibrium, muscle tone, and proprioception. Each of the cerebellar hemispheres controls movement for the same (ipsilateral) side of the body.

Spinal Cord The spinal cord is a continuation of the medulla oblongata that begins at the foramen magnum and ends at the first and second lumbar (L1 and L2) vertebrae. At L1 and L2 the spinal cord branches into lumbar and sacral nerve roots called the cauda equina. The spinal cord consists of 31 segments, each giving rise to a pair of spinal nerves (Fig. 25-8). Nerve fibers, grouped into tracts, run through the spinal cord transmitting sensory, motor, and autonomic impulses between the higher centers in the brain and the body (Fig. 25-9, *A*). The myelinated nerves making up white matter of the spinal cord contain ascending and descending tracts of nerve fibers. The descending or motor tracts (e.g., anterior and lateral corticospinal or pyramidal tracts) carry impulses from the frontal lobe to muscles for voluntary movement (Fig. 24-9, *A, B*). They also play a role in muscle tone and posture.

The ascending or sensory tracts carry sensory information from the body to the parietal lobe. The fasciculus grac-

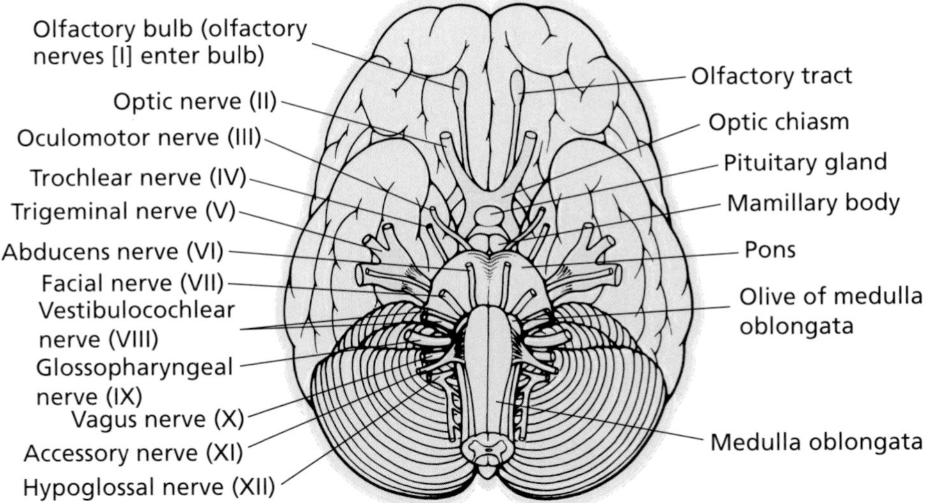

Fig. 25-7 Inferior surface of the brain showing the origin of the cranial nerves. (From Seeley, Stephens, and Tate, 1995.)

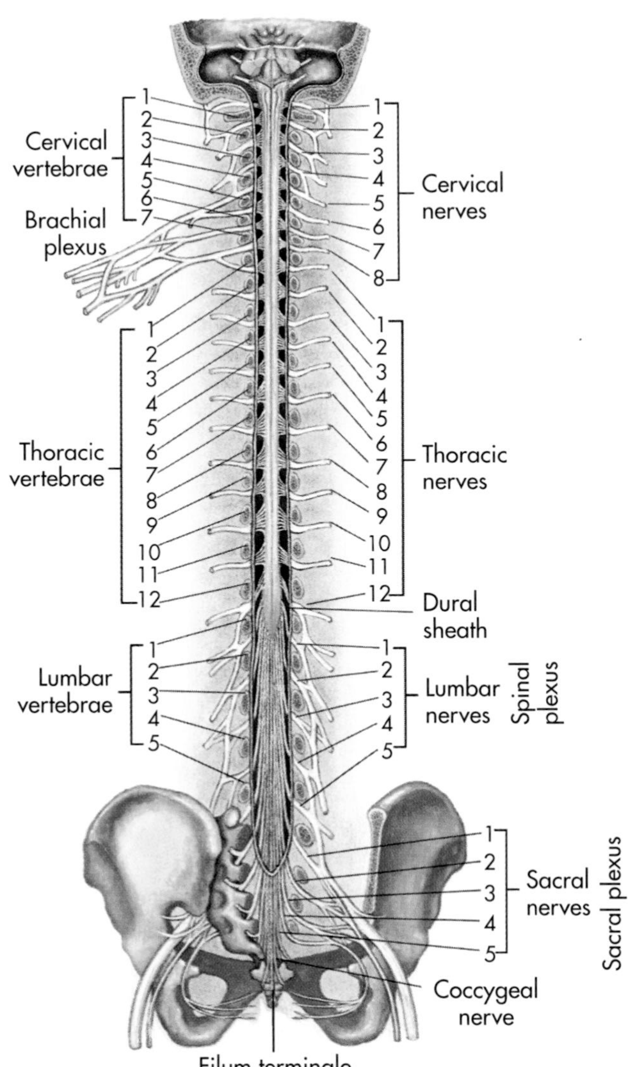

Fig. 25-8 View of the spinal column showing vertebrae, spinal cord, and spinal nerves exiting. (From Chipps, Clanin, and Campbell, 1992.)

ilis and fasciculus cuneatus in the posterior (dorsal) column spinal tract carry fibers for the sensations of touch, deep pressure, vibration, position of joints, stereognosis, and two-point discrimination (Fig. 25-9, *B*). The lateral spinothalamic tract carries fibers for sensations of light touch, pressure, temperature, and pain. The gray matter, which contains the nerve cell bodies, is arranged in a butterfly shape with anterior and posterior horns.

PERIPHERAL NERVOUS SYSTEM

Cranial Nerves

Of the 12 pairs of cranial nerves some nerves have only motor fibers (5 pairs) or only sensory fibers (3 pairs), whereas others have both (4 pairs). Table 25-1 lists the 12 cranial nerves and their functions. Box 25-1 describes ways to remember the names and functions of the cranial nerves.

Spinal Nerves

The 31 pairs of spinal nerves emerge from different segments of the spinal cord. There are 8 pairs of cervical nerves, 12 pairs of thoracic nerves, 5 pairs of lumbar nerves, 5 pairs of sacral nerves, and 1 pair of coccygeal nerves. The first 7 cervical nerves exit above their corresponding vertebrae. The remaining spinal nerves exit below the corresponding vertebrae (see Fig. 25-8).

Each pair of spinal nerves is formed by the union of an efferent or motor (ventral) root and an afferent or sensory (dorsal) root. The motor fibers carry impulses from the brain through the spinal cord to muscles and glands, whereas sensory fibers carry impulses from the sensory receptors of the body through the spinal cord to the brain. Each pair of spinal nerves and its corresponding part of the spinal cord make up a spinal segment and innervates specific body segments. The dorsal root of each spinal nerve supplies the sensory innervation to a segment of the skin known as a dermatome. Refer to the dermatome map to de-

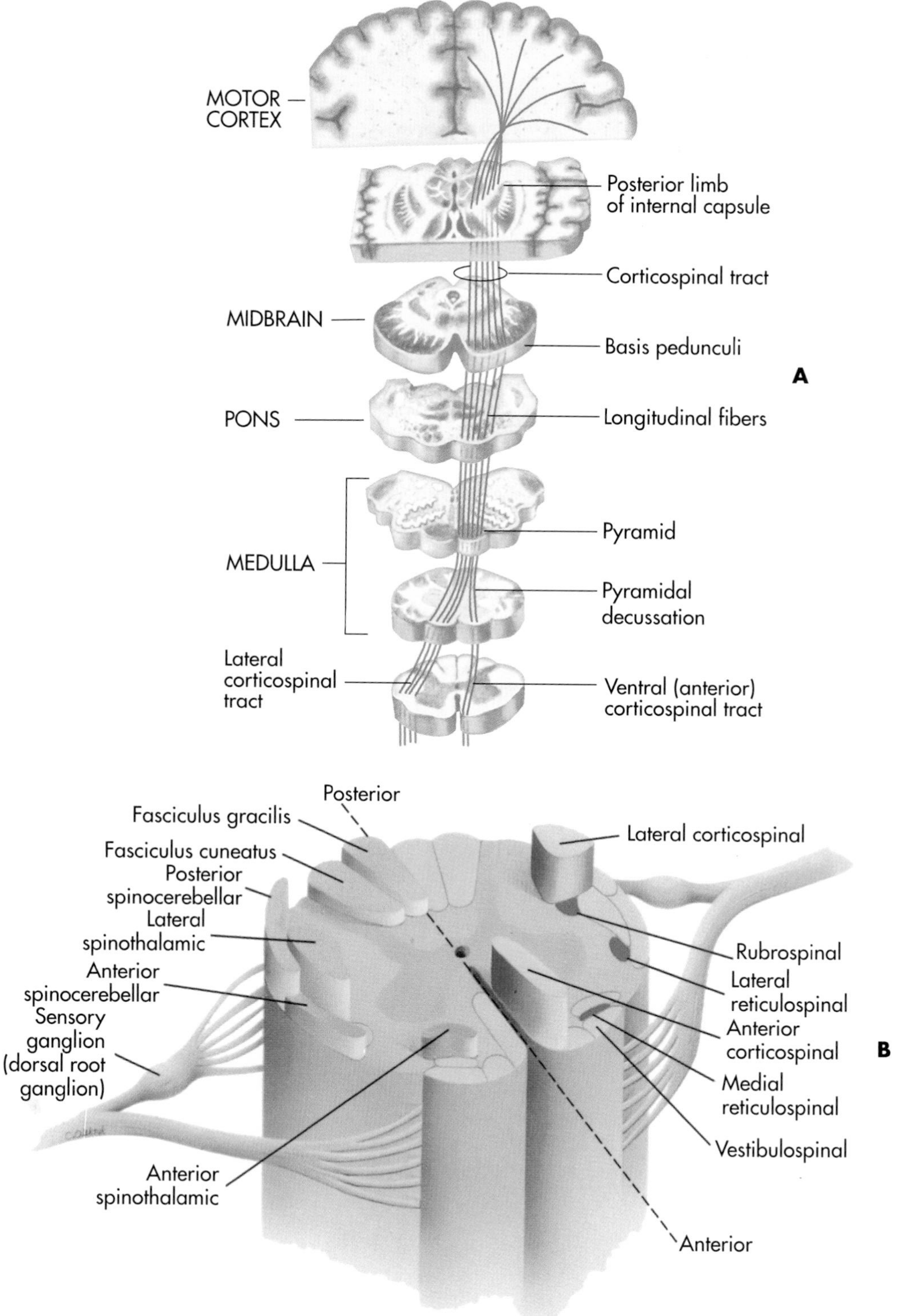

Fig. 25-9 Tracts of the spinal cord. **A,** Pathway of spinal tracts from the spinal cord to motor cortex. **B,** Major ascending (sensory) tracts of the white matter, shown here only on the left, are highlighted in blue. Major descending (motor) tracts, shown here only on the right, are highlighted in red. (**A** Modified from Rudy, 1984; **B** from Thibodeau and Patton, 1999.) the spinal nerves innervating a given region of skin. (From Rudy, 1984.)

Table 25-1 The Cranial Nerves and Their Functions

CRANIAL NERVE	FUNCTION
Olfactory (I)	Sensory: smell reception and interpretation
Optic (II)	Sensory: visual acuity and visual fields
Oculomotor (III)	Motor: raise eyelids, most extraocular movements
	Parasympathetic: pupillary constriction, change lens shape
Trochlear (IV)	Motor: downward, inward eye movement
Trigeminal (V)	Motor: jaw opening and clenching, chewing and mastication
	Sensory: sensation to cornea, iris, lacrimal glands, conjunctiva, eyelids, forehead, nose, nasal and mouth mucosa, teeth, tongue, ear, facial skin
Abducens (VI)	Motor: lateral eye movement
Facial (VII)	Motor: movement of facial expression muscles except jaw, close eyes, labial speech sounds (b, m, w, and rounded vowels)
	Sensory: taste—anterior two thirds of tongue, sensation to pharynx
	Parasympathetic: secretion of saliva and tears
Acoustic (VIII)	Sensory: hearing and equilibrium
Glossopharyngeal (IX)	Motor: voluntary muscles for swallowing and phonation
	Sensory: sensation of nasopharynx, gag reflex, taste—posterior one third of tongue
	Parasympathetic: secretion of salivary glands, carotid reflex
Vagus (X)	Motor: voluntary muscles of phonation (guttural speech sounds) and swallowing
	Sensory: sensation behind ear and part of external ear canal
	Parasympathetic: secretion of digestive enzymes; peristalsis; carotid reflex; involuntary action of heart, lungs, and digestive tract
Spinal accessory (XI)	Motor: turn head, shrug shoulders, some actions for phonation
Hypoglossal (XII)	Motor: tongue movement for speech sound articulation (l, t, n) and swallowing

From Seidel HM et al: *Mosby's guide to physical examination*, ed 3, St Louis, 1995, Mosby.

Box 25-1 How to Remember Names and Nerve Type of Cranial Nerves

Read the words in the column on the left from top to bottom. The first letter of each word is the same as the first letter in the name of the cranial nerve. The fourth column gives the type of impulses carried by the nerve—sensory, motor, or both sensory and motor. The last column is a phrase to remember the type of nerve for each cranial nerve.

MEMORY WORD	CN NUMBER	CN NAME	TYPE	MEMORY WORD
On	CN I	Olfactory	Sensory	Some
Old	CN II	Optic	Sensory	Say
Olympic's	CN III	Oculomotor	Motor	Marry
Towering	CN IV	Trochlear	Motor	Money
Top	CN V	Trigeminal	Both	But
A	CN VI	Abducens	Motor	My
Fin	CN VII	Facial	Both	Brother
And	CN VIII	Acoustic	Sensory	Says
German	CN IX	Glossopharyngeal	Both	Bad
Viewed	CN X	Vagus	Both	Business to
Some	CN XI	Spinal accessory	Motor	Marry
Hops	CN XII	Hypoglossal	Motor	Money

termine the spinal nerve that corresponds to the area where the client reports sensory alteration (Fig. 25-10).

Reflex Arc

Some sensory stimuli may initiate a reflex response that involves a sensory nerve synapsing immediately with a motor nerve, such as a tap on a stretched tendon. Structures needed for a reflex arc include a receptor, an afferent (sensory) nerve, an efferent (motor) nerve, and an effector muscle or gland (Fig. 25-11). Deep tendon reflexes are segmental responses to stimulation of a tendon, stretching the neuromuscular spindles of a muscle group. Table 25-2 shows the deep tendon reflexes and superficial reflexes and the segments of the spinal cord that innervate each reflex.

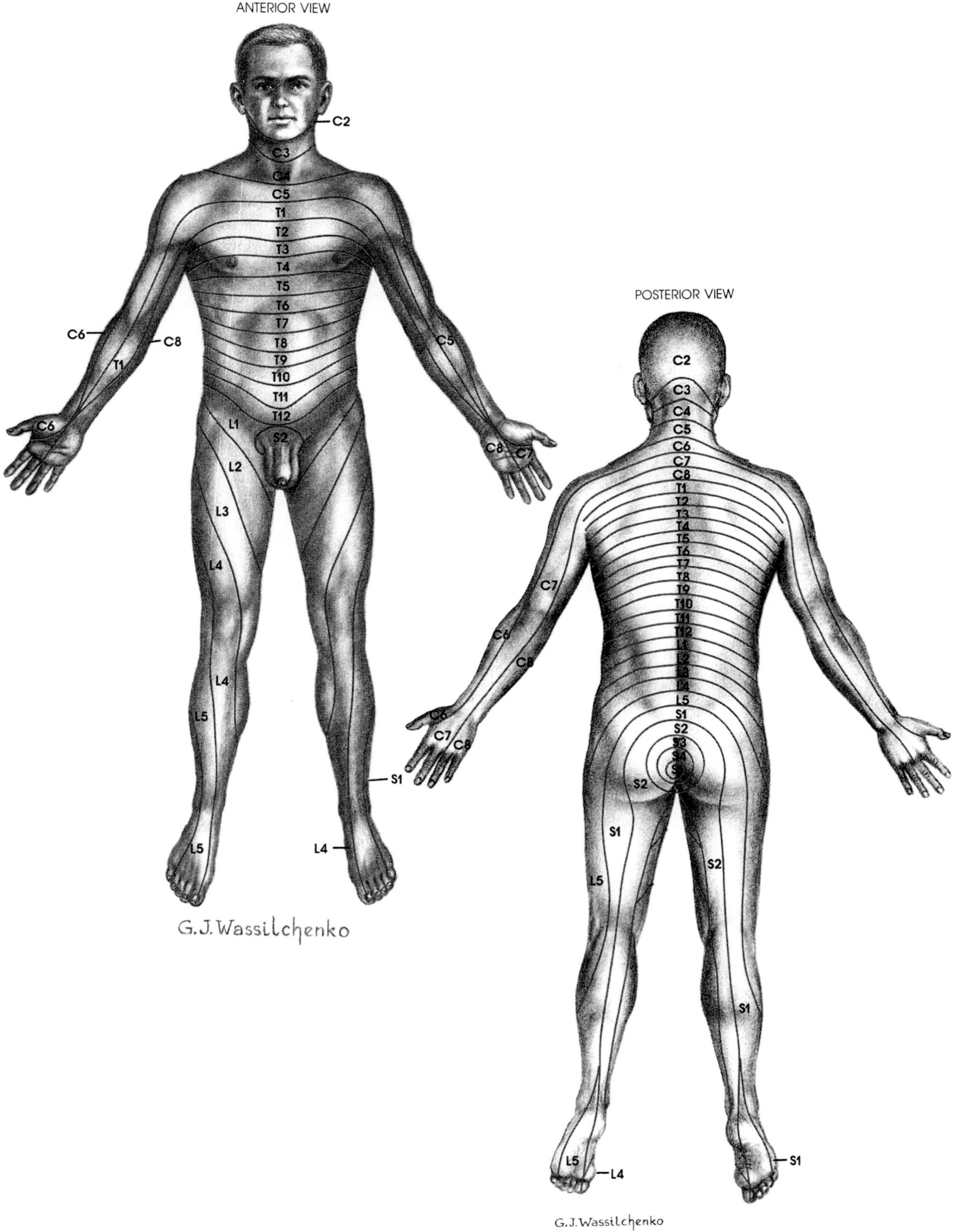

Fig. 25-10 Dermatomal map. Letters and numbers indicate the spinal nerves innervating a given region of skin. (From Rudy, 1984.)

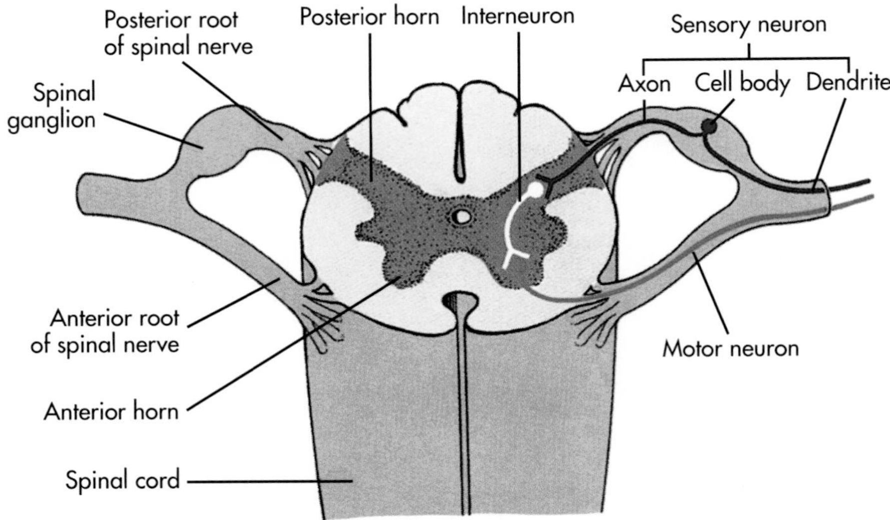

Fig. 25-11 Cross section of the spinal cord showing three-neuron reflex arc. (From Chipps, Clanin, and Campbell, 1992.)

Table 25-2 Superficial and Deep Tendon Reflexes

REFLEX	SPINAL LEVEL
SUPERFICIAL	
Upper abdominal	T7, T8, and T9
Lower abdominal	T10 and T11
Cremasteric	T12, L1, and L2
Plantar	L4, L5, S1, and S2
DEEP	
Biceps	C5 and C6
Brachioradial	C5 and C6
Triceps	C6, C7, and C8
Patellar	L2, L3, and L4
Achilles	S1

Modified from Seidel HM et al: *Mosby's guide to physical examination,* ed 4, St. Louis, 1999, Mosby; and Rudy EB: *Advanced neurological and neurosurgical nursing,* St. Louis, 1984, Mosby.

AUTONOMIC NERVOUS SYSTEM

The autonomic nervous system (ANS) regulates the body's internal environment in conjunction with the endocrine system. The ANS has two components: the sympathetic nervous system and the parasympathetic nervous system (Fig. 25-12). The sympathetic nervous system (SNS) arises from the thoracolumbar segments of the spinal cord and is activated during stress (the fight-or-flight response). The SNS actions include increasing blood pressure and heart rate, vasoconstricting peripheral blood vessels, inhibiting gastrointestinal peristalsis, and dilating bronchi. By contrast, the parasympathetic nervous system (PNS) arises from craniosacral segments of the spinal cord and controls vegetative functions (breed and feed). The PNS actions are involved in functions associated with conserving energy such as decreasing heart rate and force of myocardial contraction, decreasing blood pressure and respiration, and stimulating gastrointestinal peristalsis.

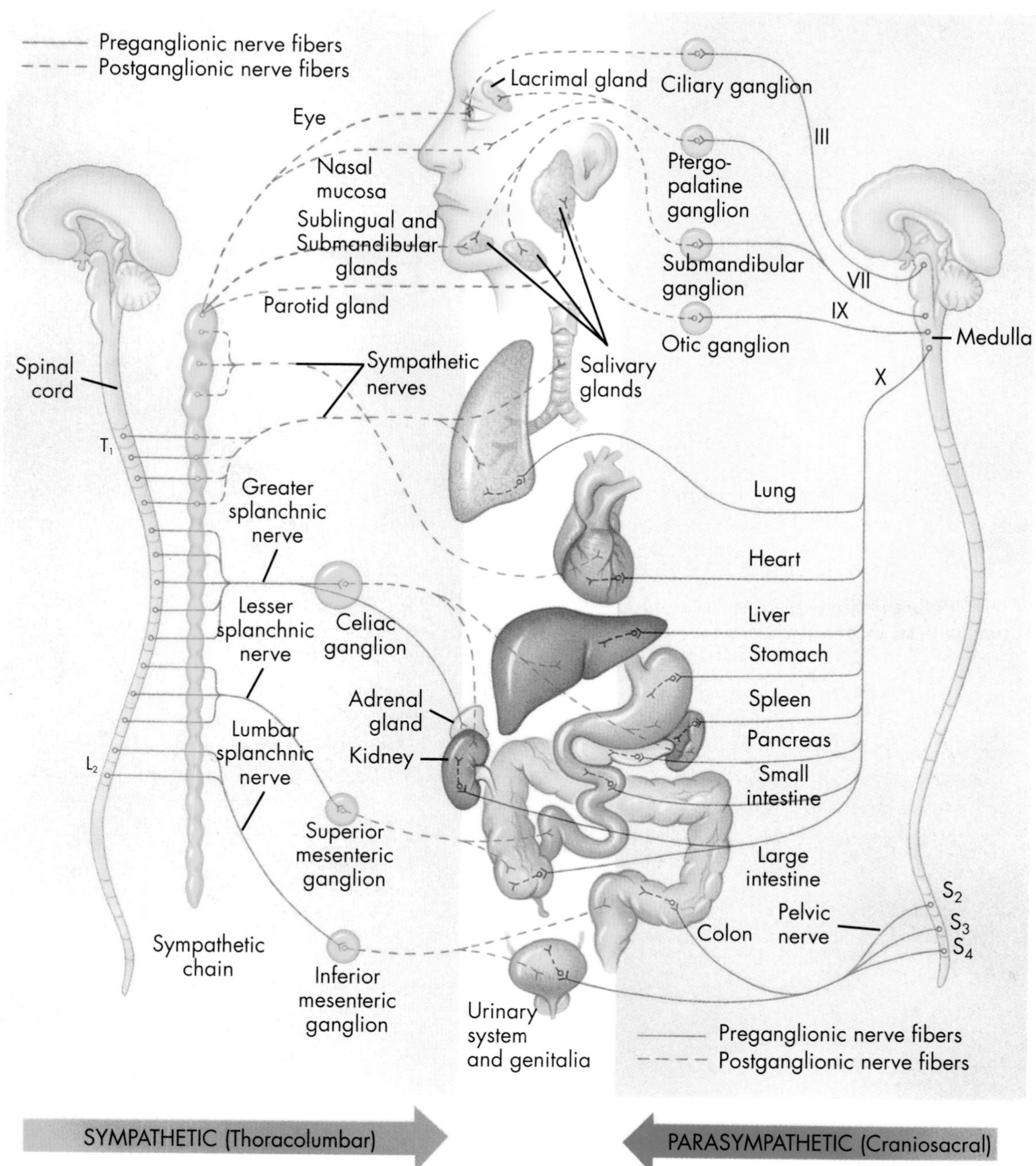

Fig. 25-12 Innervation of organs by the autonomic nervous system. Preganglionic fibers are indicated by solid lines, and postganglionic fibers are indicated by broken lines. (From Thibodeau and Patton, 1999.)

HEALTH HISTORY

Neurologic System

QUESTIONS | RATIONALE

PRESENT HEALTH STATUS

➤ Have you noticed any changes in your ability to move around or participate in your usual activities?

■ It is important to obtain the client's perception of the functioning of his or her nervous system. Difficulty moving due to weakness or spasticity may indicate a neuromuscular problem. Often clients can identify they are have difficulty in performing usual activities, but may not associate it with a neurologic disorder.

➤ Do you have any chronic diseases? High blood pressure? Myasthenia gravis? Multiple sclerosis? If yes, describe it (them). In what ways does this chronic disease keep you from maintaining a healthy lifestyle?

■ Chronic diseases may affect mobility and daily living. These questions may help identify risks for injury and opportunities for teaching.

➤ Do you take any medications? If yes, what do you take and how often? Are you taking medications as prescribed?

■ Both prescription and over-the-counter medications should be documented. Side effects of medications may influence the nervous system. Drugs (prescription or street drugs) or alcohol may interfere with the functioning of the nervous system. Note especially any anticonvulsant medications, antitremor drugs, antivertigo agents, or pain medications that could alter a client's neurologic examination.

➤ How much alcohol do you drink per week? Do you use or have you ever used substances such as marijuana, cocaine, barbiturates, tranquilizers, or any other mood-altering drugs?

■ Documentation of these substances is necessary since they may alter the cognitive or neuromuscular function. Also the actions of these substances may interfere with medications that may be prescribed.

PAST MEDICAL HISTORY

➤ Have you ever had injury or trauma to your head or spinal cord? If yes, describe when this happened. What residual changes have you experienced since the injury or trauma?

■ Previous trauma or injury to the central nervous system may leave residual deficits such as weakness or spasticity that you can anticipate during the examination.

➤ Have you ever had a stroke? If yes, describe when and what residual changes you have as a result of the stroke (see risk factors box).

■ Previous stroke (cerebrovascular accident [CVA] or brain attack) may leave residual deficits such as aphasia that affect your subjective data collection or hemiparesis that you will examine further during the health assessment.

➤ Have you ever had surgery on your brain, spinal cord, or any of your nerves? If yes, when was the surgery? What was the outcome of the surgery?

■ A history of surgery may provide additional information about possible neurologic problems and the findings to anticipate during the examination.

➤ Have you ever had a seizure? If yes, describe the kind of seizure, how often you had them, and what you do to prevent the seizures.

■ Although seizure will probably not be evident during the examination, you need to determine if the client is caring for this disorder to maintain his or her safety and prevent recurrence of seizures.

QUESTIONS

RATIONALE

FAMILY HISTORY

➤ In your family has anyone ever had a stroke, seizures, or tumor of the brain or spinal cord? If yes, what was the outcome?

■ Family history may be used to determine the client's risk for these conditions.

RISK FACTORS

COMMON RISK FACTORS ASSOCIATED WITH Cerebrovascular Accident (Stroke) or Brain Attack

PRIMARY RISK FACTORS

- Increasing age: Chance of brain attack doubles for each decade of life after age 55.
- Gender: Men have a 19% greater chance of stroke than women.
- Heredity (family history) and race: The chance of stroke is greater in people who have a family history of brain attack. African Americans have a high risk of death and disability from strokes due in part to the high incidence of hypertension.
- Hypertension: High blood pressure is the most important risk factor for stroke. Brain attack risk varies directly with blood pressure.
- Cigarette smoking: The nicotine in cigarette smoke constrict arteries, increasing blood pressure. The use of oral contraceptive increases risk of thrombus formation and, combined with cigarette smoking, greatly increases risk for brain attack.
- Diabetes mellitus: This is an independent risk factor for brain attack and is strongly correlated with hypertension. Chronic elevated blood glucose levels tend to thicken the capillary membrane of arteries, making them more narrow.
- Carotid artery disease: Carotid arteries that supply blood to the brain can become blocked by a thrombus from accumulation of plaque. The sound detected by auscultation of a narrowed carotid artery is called a bruit.
- Heart disease: People with heart disease have more than twice the risk of brain attack than those without heart disease. Atrial fibrillation is one heart disease that increases risk for brain attack because small emboli form in the atria and can be released into the cerebral circulation, occluding a cerebral vessel and causing a brain attack.
- Polycythemia: A high erythrocyte count makes the blood thicker than usual so that blood clots form more readily. Polycythemia can occur as a result of chronic hypoxia because the bone marrow provides more red blood cells to carry needed oxygen, even though the oxygen needed is not available.

OTHER FACTORS THAT AFFECT THE RISK OF BRAIN ATTACK

- Geographic location: Brain attacks are more common in the southeastern United States than in other areas. This area of the country is referred to as the "stroke belt."
- Season and climate: More brain attack deaths occur during periods of extremely hot or cold temperatures.
- Socioeconomic factors: There is some evidence that people in lower income and educational levels have a higher risk of brain attacks.
- Excessive alcohol intake: Excessive drinking or binge drinking can raise the blood pressure, contribute to obesity, increase triglycerides, cause heart failure, and lead to brain attack. Excessive drinking is defined as more than one drink daily for women and two drinks daily for men.
- Certain kinds of drug abuse: Intravenous drug abuse carries a high risk of brain attack from cerebral emboli. Cocaine use has been closely related to brain attacks, heart attacks, and other cardiovascular complications such as endocarditis.

Data from *http://www.amhrt.org/* Select heart and stroke A-Z guide, 1999.

QUESTIONS | RATIONALE

PROBLEM-BASED HISTORY

The disorders involving neurologic system impairment are headache, dizziness or vertigo, seizures, changes in consciousness, altered mobility (tremors, weakness, or incoordination), altered sensation (numbness or tingling), dysphagia, and aphasia. As with symptoms in all areas of health assessment, a symptom analysis is completed, which includes the location, quality, quantity, chronology, setting, associated manifestations, and alleviating and aggravating factors (see Box 4-2 in Chapter 4).

Headache

➤ Have you had any unusually frequent or severe headaches? For a more complete headache history outline, see Chapter 13.

■ Headaches may be an indication of impaired circulation to the brain or a mass in the brain (Smith and Schumann, 1998).

➤ Have you had any recent surgeries or medical procedures such as spinal anesthesia or lumbar puncture?

■ Transient headache can occur after some diagnostics tests for neurologic disorders, such as a lumbar puncture to diagnosis meningitis. When the client is in an upright position, the loss of cerebrospinal fluid causes tension on the meninges, causing a headache.

Dizziness or Vertigo

➤ Do you feel dizzy or light-headed, as if you cannot keep your balance and may fall? Do you feel as if you may faint? When do you feel this way? How often? Is it associated with a change in position or with activity? What makes the dizziness worse? What relieves the dizziness?

■ Distinguish between dizziness and vertigo by questioning the client about these symptoms. Fainting (syncope) is a loss of consciousness caused by decreased cerebral blood flow.

➤ Have you ever experienced vertigo when the room seemed to spin (objective vertigo), or do you feel that you are spinning (subjective vertigo)? Does this happen suddenly or gradually? What makes the vertigo worse? What relieves the vertigo?

■ Vertigo (when the room seems to be spinning) may be caused by a neurologic dysfunction (usually with a gradual onset) or a problem with the vestibule apparatus such as an inner ear infection (labyrinthitis) or Ménière's disease (usually with a sudden onset).

Seizures

➤ Are you having seizures or convulsions? When? What were they like? How often did they occur?

■ Seizure may be caused by idiopathic epilepsy or result from a pathologic process, endogenous or exogenous poison, metabolic disturbances, or fever (see the Common Problems and Conditions section at the end of the chapter).

➤ Do you have any warning signs before the seizure starts? Describe what happens.

■ An aura can precede a seizure; it can involve auditory, gustatory, olfactory, visual, or motor sensations. The area in the brain that corresponds to the aura provides information about seizure origin.

QUESTIONS

RATIONALE

➤ (Refer these questions to the person who observed client's seizure.) Describe how the seizure proceeds through the body. Where does it begin? Does it travel? If yes, to where? Have you observed the client performing repeated, automatic movements (e.g., lip smacking or eyelid fluttering)? Have you noted any other signs, such as a change in color of the face or lips; loss of consciousness (note how long)? Does the client urinate or have a bowel movement during the seizure? How long after the seizure until the client is back to normal self?

■ Responses to these questions help identify the areas of the brain involved in the seizure activity. Figure 25-4, *B* is helpful in understanding the path a seizure may move. For example, if the seizure begins in the wrist and travels to the head, neck, and trunk, you can follow the path of the excessive nervous discharge of the seizure along the motor cortex. This is an example of a simple seizure in which the client maintains consciousness.

➤ After the seizure, are you confused? Have a headache or aching muscles? Feel weak? Do you spend time sleeping?

■ Affirmative answers to these questions may indicate the expected recovery phase of a generalized seizure.

➤ Are there any factors that seem to start these seizures, such as stress, fatigue, activity, or discontinuing medication? Do you take any actions to prevent hurting yourself during seizures?

■ Answers to these questions help plan prevention strategies for seizures or any injury experienced during the seizure.

➤ How have the seizures affected your life? Your occupation? Do you wear any identification that indicates you have seizures?

■ Since seizures may be a chronic disease that affects driving, personal relationships, and employment, it is important to learn how seizures have affected the client's life and if the client has adapted to the seizure condition. Carrying identification about seizures helps those who may help the client during a seizure.

Changes in Consciousness

➤ Have you recently lost consciousness? Had a blackout? Fainted? Felt you were not aware of your surroundings? Did the change occur suddenly? Can you describe what happened to you just before you lost consciousness? Were there other symptoms associated with the change of consciousness? Do you have diabetes mellitus, liver failure, or kidney failure?

■ Loss of consciousness may be due to cardiovascular disorders, which tend to cause symptoms more rapidly, or neurologic disorders. Changes in consciousness are also associated with drugs, psychiatric illness, or metabolic diseases such as liver or kidney failure or diabetes mellitus.

Altered Mobility

➤ Have you noticed any tremors or shaking of the hands or face? When did they start? Do they seem worse when you are anxious or at rest? When you focus on doing something (intention)? What relieves the tremors—rest, activity, or alcohol? Do they affect your performance of daily activities? Do you have thyroid disease?

■ Answers to these questions may help identify the cause of the altered mobility. Parkinson's disease causes tremor at rest, and cerebellar disorders cause tremor with intentional movement. Hyperthyroidism can also cause tremors.

➤ Have you noted any twitches or sudden jerks? Where? When did these begin? Does anything seem to make the twitches worse? What relieves twitching?

■ Answers to these questions may help identify the cause of the altered mobility. These symptoms are related to a variety of neurologic disorders that may impair innervation to selected muscles.

QUESTIONS

RATIONALE

➤ Have you felt any sense of weakness in or difficulty moving parts of your body? Is this confined to one area or generalized? Is it associated with anything in particular (e.g., activity)? Do you do anything to prevent the weakness? To relieve the weakness?

■ Decreased circulation to the brain can cause these symptoms. Some types of transient ischemic attack (TIA) or CVA may have occurred. Other conditions to be ruled out include multiple sclerosis.

➤ Do you have problems with coordination? Do you have difficulty keeping your balance when you walk? Do you lean to one side or fall? Which direction? Do you feel clumsy? Do your legs suddenly give way?

■ A CVA may be the cause, but dysfunction of the cerebellum or inner ear should also be considered when balance is impaired. Multiple sclerosis, Parkinson's disease, or brain tumor may also be causes. If a client reports falls in one direction, such as to the right, that may indicate that muscle weakness is due to impaired nerve function on the left side of the brain.

Altered Sensation

➤ Are you experiencing any numbness or tingling? Where? How does it feel? Like pins and needles? Is it associated with any activity in particular?

■ These questions relate to some types of central nervous system disorder (e.g., multiple sclerosis or CVA) or peripheral nerve disorder (e.g., diabetics may develop peripheral neuropathy). Paresthesias often fluctuate with posture, activity, rest, edema, congestion, or underlying disease. Hypoesthesia is decreased sensation that may indicate a sensory problem from impaired circulation or nerve compression. Identifying the location of the abnormal sensation may help identify the cause of altered sensation.

Dysphagia

➤ Have you noted any problems swallowing? Do these problems involve liquids or solids? Both? Do you have excessive saliva or drooling? Do you cough or choke when trying to swallow?

■ These may be due to dysfunction of cranial nerves IX, X, and/or XI or muscle weakness, (e.g., from a stroke). Parkinsonism and myasthenia gravis may cause excessive salivation that may increase the need to swallow.

Aphasia

➤ Have you had any problems speaking? With forming words or finding the right words? Have you had difficulty understanding things that are said to you? Has your handwriting changed? When did this begin? How long did it last? Note: these questions may need to asked of the person accompanying the client when the client is unable to respond.

■ Aphasia is the term for defective or absent language function, whereas dysphasia is an impairment of speech not as severe as aphasia. Aphasia may be associated with dysfunction in the temporal lobe by tumor, head injury, or stroke. Parkinson's disease may create difficulty forming words because of bradykinesia of facial muscles.

EXAMINATION

Equipment

- Aromatic materials to test sense of smell (CN I)
- Penlight to test pupillary reaction (CN III)
- Tuning fork (200 to 400 Hz) to test vibratory sensation
- Cotton-tipped applicator to test corneal reflex (CN V) and apply condiments to tongue to test taste (CNs VII and IX)
- Tongue blade to test uvula (CNs IX and X)
- ❖ Examination gloves to test strength of tongue
- ❖ Reshaped paper clip or broken tongue blade to test sharp and dull sensation
- ❖ Cotton ball to test sensation of light touch
- ❖ Cotton-tipped applicator or reshaped paper clip to test two-point discrimination
- Percussion hammer to test deep tendon reflexes

PROCEDURES AND TECHNIQUES WITH NORMAL FINDINGS

ABNORMAL FINDINGS

As with the musculoskeletal system, use a cephalocaudal organization with side-to-side comparison to assess the neurologic system. A complete neurologic system assessment is performed when problems are found during the history, otherwise a neurologic screening examination is performed as described in Box 25-2.

Box 25-2 Procedures of the Neurologic Screening Examination

The shorter screening examination is commonly used for health visits when no known neurologic problem is apparent.

CRANIAL NERVES

Cranial nerves II through XII are routinely tested; however, taste and smell are not tested unless some aberration is found (pp. 706-710).

PROPRIOCEPTION AND CEREBELLAR FUNCTION

One test is administered for each of the following: rapid rhythmic alternating movements, accuracy of movements, balance (Romberg test is given), and gait and heel-toe walking (pp. 711-712).

SENSORY FUNCTION

Superficial pain and touch at a distal point in each extremity are tested; vibration and position senses are assessed by testing the great toe (pp. 714-717).

DEEP TENDON REFLEXES

All deep tendon reflexes are tested, excluding the plantar reflex and the test for clonus (pp. 714-719).

From Seidel HM et al: *Mosby's guide to physical examination,* ed 4, St. Louis, 1999, Mosby.

PROCEDURES AND TECHNIQUES WITH NORMAL FINDINGS

ABNORMAL FINDINGS

➤EVALUATE speech for articulation and voice quality and conversation for comprehension of verbal communication. Voice should have inflections and sufficient volume with clear speech. The client's responses should indicate an understanding of what is said.

■ Errors in choice of words or syllables; difficulty in articulation, which could involve impaired thought processes or dysfunction of the tongue or lips; slurred speech (tone sounds slurred); poorly coordinated or irregular speech; monotone or weak voice; nasal tone, rasping, or hoarseness; whispering voice; and stuttering are abnormal responses.

➤TEST nose for smell. Evaluate olfactory cranial nerve (CN I). Have client close eyes and properly identify common aromatic substance held under the nose; test one nostril at a time. Examples include coffee, toothpaste, orange, or oil of cloves (Fig. 25-13).

■ Inability to smell anything or incorrect identification of odors is abnormal. Allergic rhinitis, sinusitis, excessive smoking, cocaine use may interfere with ability to distinguish odors (O'Hanlon-Nichols, 1999). Loss of smell may be caused by an olfactory tract lesion. *Anosmia* is the term used for loss or impaired sense of smell.

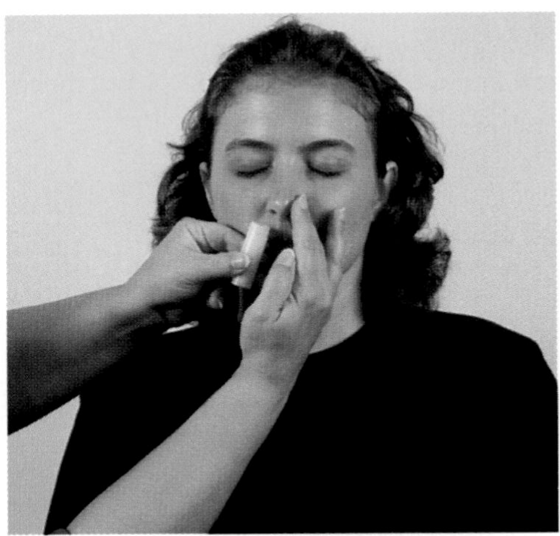

Fig. 25-13 Examination of the olfactory cranial nerve (CN I). (From Chipps, Clanin, and Campbell, 1992.)

➤TEST eyes for visual acuity. Test the optic nerve (CN II) for visual acuity using Snellen's chart (see Chapter 16).

■ Refer client to an optometrist or ophthalmologist for further evaluation if vision is worse than 20/20. Chapter 16 provides more detail.

➤TEST eyes for peripheral vision. (See Chapter 16 for the confrontation test for peripheral vision.)

■ If the client cannot see the pencil or finger at the same time you see it, peripheral field loss is suggested. Refer the client for more precise testing. Lesions in the central nervous system (e.g., tumors) may cause peripheral visual defects such as loss of vision in one half or one quarter of the visual field, either medially or laterally.

➤OBSERVE eyes for extraocular muscle movement. The oculomotor (CN III), trochlear (CN IV), and abducens (CN VI) nerves are tested together since they control muscles that provide eye movement (see Chapter 16).

■ Eye movements that are not parallel indicate extraocular muscle weakness or dysfunction of cranial nerve III, IV, or VI. Report nystagmus other than that noted as normal. Report ptosis (eyelid droop) that may occur with ocular myasthenia gravis.

PROCEDURES AND TECHNIQUES WITH NORMAL FINDINGS

ABNORMAL FINDINGS

➤**OBSERVE eyes for pupillary size, shape, equality, constriction, and accommodation.** *P*upils should appear *e*qual, *r*ound and *r*eactive to *l*ight and *a*ccommodation (documented as PERRLA [see Chapter 16]).

■ Increased intracranial pressure on or trauma to the midbrain may exert pressure on CN III, resulting in diminished to absent pupillary constriction, ptosis of the eye, and altered superior and inferior movement of the eyeball. Pupil size can be changed by drug effects, constricted by heroin or morphine and dilated by cocaine.

■ Clients with diabetes or syphilis may lose pupillary constriction to light, but retain accommodation.

➤**EVALUATE face for movement and sensation.** Evaluate the trigeminal nerve (CN V) for facial movement and sensation.

➤Test motor function by having the client clench his or her teeth, then palpate the temporal and masseter muscles for muscle mass and strength. There should be bilaterally strong muscle contractions (Fig. 25-14, *A*).

■ Inequality in muscle contractions, pain, twitching, or asymmetry is abnormal. Disorders of the pons, (e.g., a tumor) may cause altered function of CN V, VI, VII, or VIII.

A

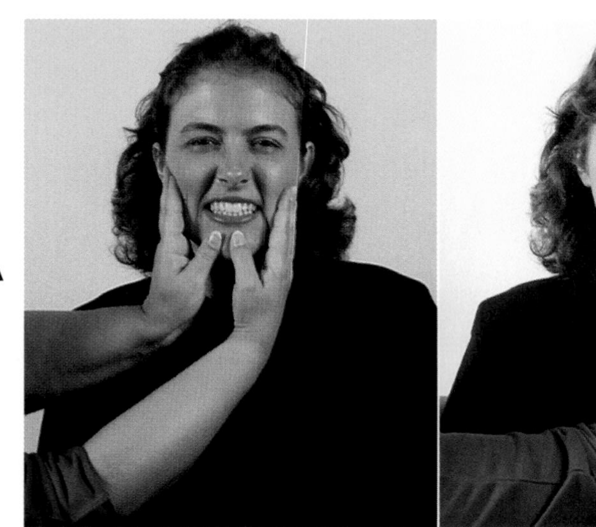

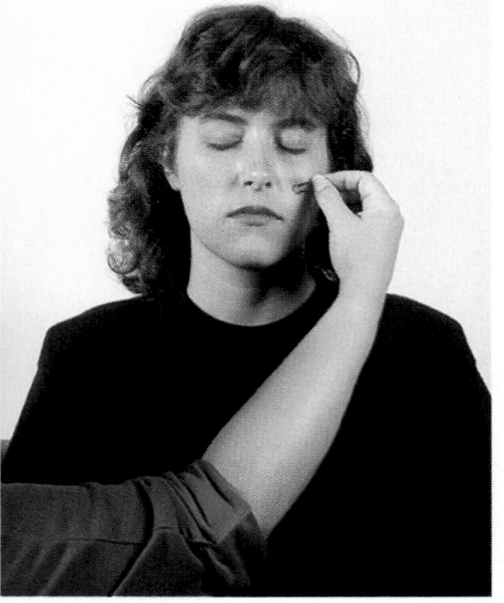

B

Fig. 25-14 Examination of the trigeminal nerve (CN V) for motor function, **A,** and sensory function, **B,** (From Chipps, Clanin, and Campbell, 1992.)

❖ ➤To test sensation of light touch supplied by the three branches of CN V, have the client close his or her eyes, then wipe cotton lightly over the anterior scalp (ophthalmic branch), paranasal sinuses (maxillary branch), and jaw (mandibular branch). A tickle sensation should be present equally over the three areas touched. Repeat the procedure on the other side of the face.

■ Decreased or unequal sensation is abnormal. Record the extent of the involved areas of the face.

❖ ➤To test deep sensation, use alternating blunt and sharp ends of a paper clip over the client's forehead, paranasal sinuses, and jaw. He or she should be able to feel pressure and pain equally throughout these areas and should be able to differentiate between sharp and dull (Fig. 25-14, *B*). Repeat the procedure on the other side of the face.

■ Decreased or unequal sensation is abnormal. Trigeminal neuralgia is characterized by stab-like pain radiating along the trigeminal nerve, caused by degeneration of or pressure on the nerve.

PROCEDURES AND TECHNIQUES WITH NORMAL FINDINGS

ABNORMAL FINDINGS

❖ ➤Test the ophthalmic branch (sensory) of CN V and motor function of CN VII by testing for the corneal reflex. Ask client to remove contact lenses if applicable and to look up and away from you. Approach the client from the side and lightly touch the cornea with a wisp of cotton. There should be a bilateral blink to corneal touch. Clients who wear contact lenses regularly may have diminished or absent reflex. *This test may be omitted when client is alert and blinking naturally.*

■ Absence of a blink is abnormal. Be sure to check that this abnormal response is not caused by the presence of contact lenses.

➤Evaluate the facial nerve (CN VII) for facial movement. Inspect the face both at rest and during conversation. Have the client raise the eyebrows, purse lips, close the eyes tightly, show the teeth, smile, and puff out the cheeks. He or she should be able to correctly follow each command, and the results should be symmetric (Fig. 25-15, *A-F*).

■ Asymmetry, unequal movements, facial weakness, drooping of one side of the face or mouth, or inability to maintain position until instructed to relax is abnormal.

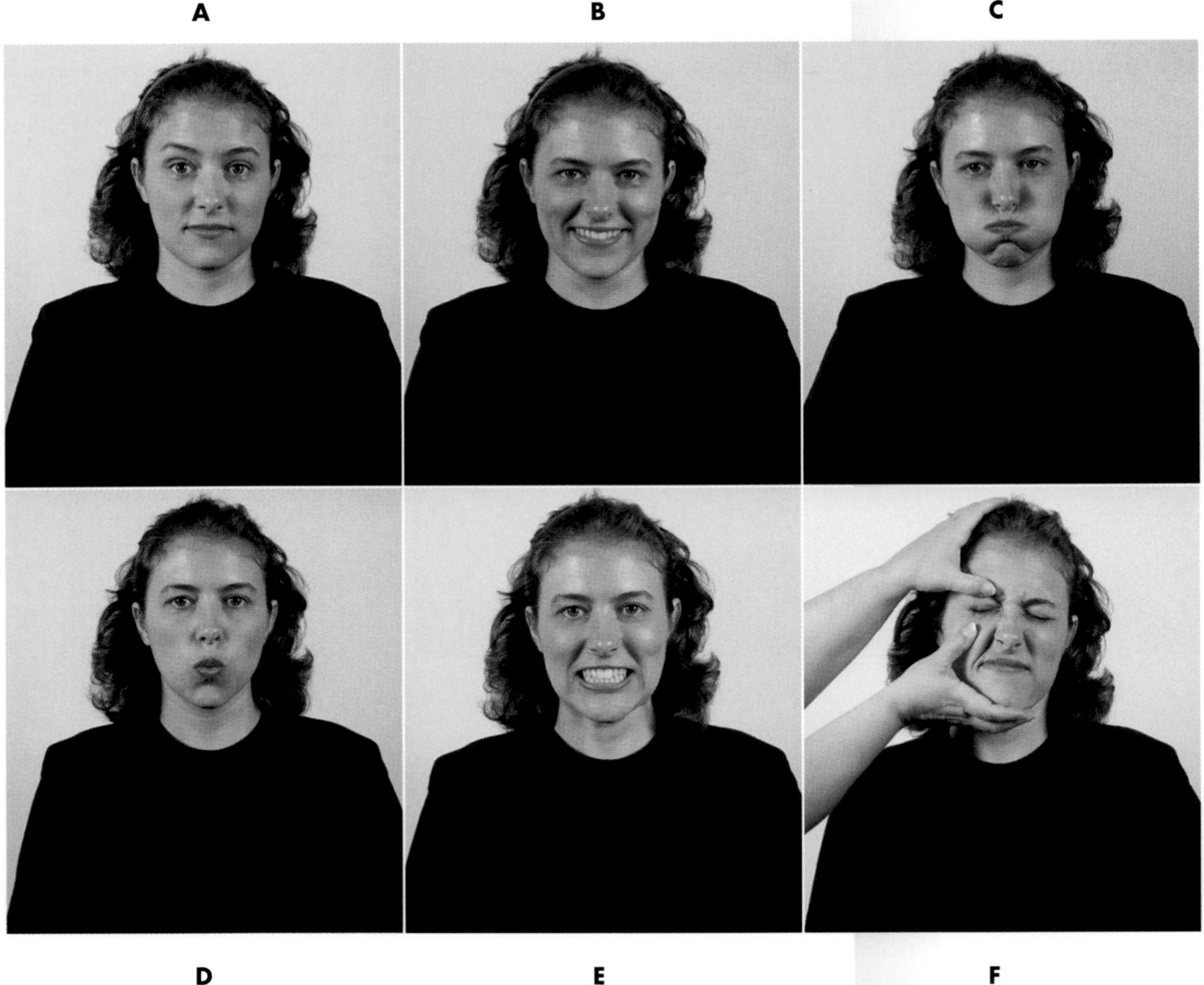

Fig. 25-15 Examination of the facial nerve (CN VII). Ask the client to make the following movements: **A,** Raise eyebrows and wrinkle forehead. **B,** Smile. **C,** Puff out cheeks. **D,** Purse lips and blow out. **E,** Show teeth. **F,** Squeeze eyes shut while you try to open them. (From Chipps, Clanin, and Campbell, 1992.)

PROCEDURES AND TECHNIQUES WITH NORMAL FINDINGS

➤TEST ears for hearing. Evaluate acoustic nerve (CN VIII) for hearing and balance. Hearing initially can be screened while taking the history. Assessment of hearing using the whispered voice, finger-rubbing, Rinne, and Weber's tests are described in Chapter 15.

➤TEST tongue for taste. Evaluate taste over the anterior two thirds of the tongue (CN VII, facial). Instruct the client to stick out the tongue and leave it out during the testing process. Use a cotton applicator to place on the client's anterior tongue small quantities of salt, sugar, and lemon one at a time. The client should be able to correctly identify salty and sweet tastes (Fig. 25-16). Taste, the sensory component of CN VII, usually is not tested unless the client reports a problem (O'Hanlon-Nichols, 1999).

Test glossopharyngeal nerve for taste of the posterior one third of the tongue or pharynx (CN IX). The client should be able to taste bitter and sour tastes. Taste, the sensory component of CN IX), is rarely tested (O'Hanlon-Nichols, 1999).

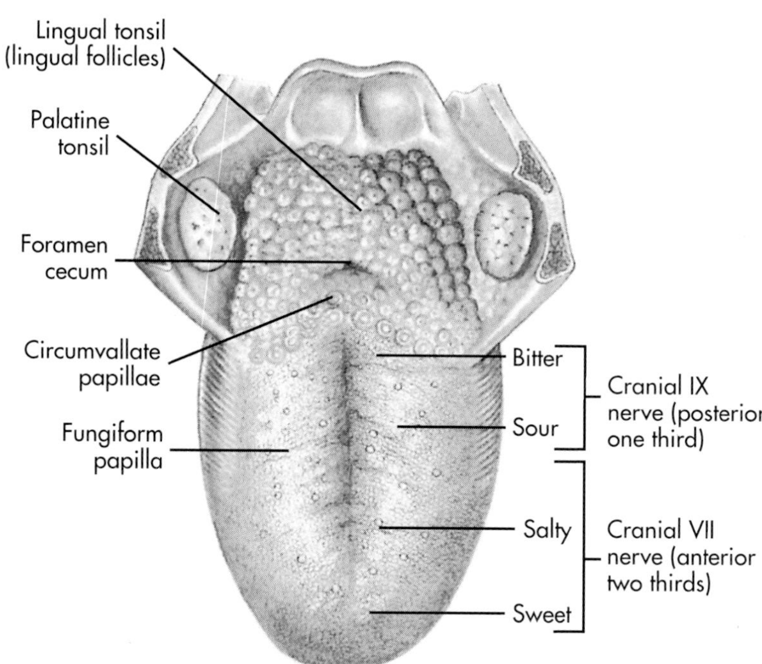

Fig. 25-16 Location of the taste bud regions tested for the sensory function of the facial and glossopharyngeal cranial nerves. (From Seidel et al, 1999.)

➤INSPECT oropharynx for gag reflex and movement of soft palate. Evaluate glossopharyngeal nerve (CN IX) and vagus nerve (CN X) together for movement and gag reflex. Instruct the client to say "Ah" to test CN X. There should be bilaterally equal upward movement of the soft palate and uvula; touch the posterior pharynx with the end of a tongue blade, client should gag momentarily. Movement of the posterior pharynx and gag reflex test CN IX.

ABNORMAL FINDINGS

■ For hearing, refer to Chapter 15.

■ Inability to identify tastes or consistently identifying a substance incorrectly is abnormal. Loss of smell and taste may occur together. Clients who are chronic smokers may have decreased taste.

■ Asymmetry of the soft palate or tonsillar pillar movement, any lateral deviation of the uvula, or absence of the gag reflex may indicate disorders of the medulla oblongata. For example, tumors may cause pressure on glossopharyngeal cranial nerve (CN IX) and vagus cranial nerve (X).

PROCEDURES AND TECHNIQUES WITH NORMAL FINDINGS

ABNORMAL FINDINGS

❖ ➤**INSPECT tongue for movement, symmetry, strength, and absence of tumors; test for muscle strength.** Evaluate hypoglossal nerve (CN XII) for symmetry and movement. Client protrudes tongue. Note symmetry, atrophy, and absence of tumors. Then ask client to move tongue toward nose, chin, and side to side. Don examination gloves to test strength of tongue by pressing it against your gloved index finger (Fig. 25-17).

■ Asymmetric movement or weakness of the tongue may indicate impairment of the hypoglossal cranial nerve (XII). The tongue deviates toward the impaired side. Tumors of the tongue may develop from alcohol, tobacco, or chronic irritation.

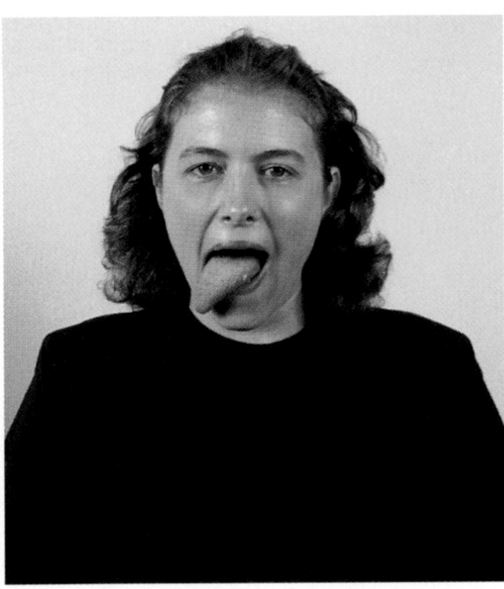

Fig. 25-17 Examination of the hypoglossal nerve (CN XII). (From Chipps, Clanin, and Campbell, 1992.)

➤**TEST shoulders and neck muscles for strength and movement.** Evaluate spinal accessory nerve (CN XI) for movement. Ask client to shrug his or her shoulders upward against your hands. Contraction of the trapezius muscles should be strong and symmetric.

■ Unilateral or bilateral muscle weakness on any pain or discomfort is abnormal.

➤Have the client turn his or her head to the side against your hand; repeat with the other side. Observe the contraction of the opposite sternocleidomastoid muscle, and note the force of movement against your hand. Movement should be smooth, and muscle strength should be strong and symmetric.

■ Weakness or pain when pushing against your hand or asymmetry is abnormal.

➤**TEST cerebellar function for balance and coordination.** To test proprioception (awareness of position and movement) and cerebellar function, use at least two techniques for each area assessed (e.g., balance and coordination of upper and lower extremities). Choose these techniques based on the client's age and overall physical ability. For example, not every client should have to perform deep knee bends.

■ Abnormal findings may be due to a variety of causes, such as cerebellar tumors, stroke, Parkinson's disease, or inner ear problems.

General Observe gait by having the client walk across the room, turn, and walk back. He or she should be able to maintain upright posture, walk unaided, maintain balance, and use opposing arm swing.

■ Poor posturing, ataxia, unsteady gait, rigid or absent arm movements, wide-based gait, trunk and head held tight, legs bent from hips only, lurching or reeling, scissors gait, or parkinsonian gait (stooped posture, flexion at hips, elbows, and knees) is abnormal.

PROCEDURES AND TECHNIQUES WITH NORMAL FINDINGS

ABNORMAL FINDINGS

Balance Perform the Romberg test. Have the client stand with feet together, arms resting at sides, eyes open, then eyes closed. Stand close to the client with arms ready to "catch" client if he or she begins to fall off balance. There will be slight swaying, but the upright posture and foot position should be maintained.

- If client sways with eyes closed but not open, the problem is probably proprioceptive. If client sways with eyes open and closed, the problem is probably cerebellar.

❖ ➤Have the client close his or her eyes and stand on one foot, then the other. He or she should be able to maintain position for at least 5 seconds.

- Inability to maintain single-foot balance for 5 seconds is abnormal.

➤Have the client walk in tandem, placing the heel of one foot directly against the toes of the other foot. The client should be able to maintain this heel-toe walking pattern along a straight line (Fig. 25-18).

- Inability to walk heel-to-toe or using a wide-based gait to maintain the upright posture is abnormal.

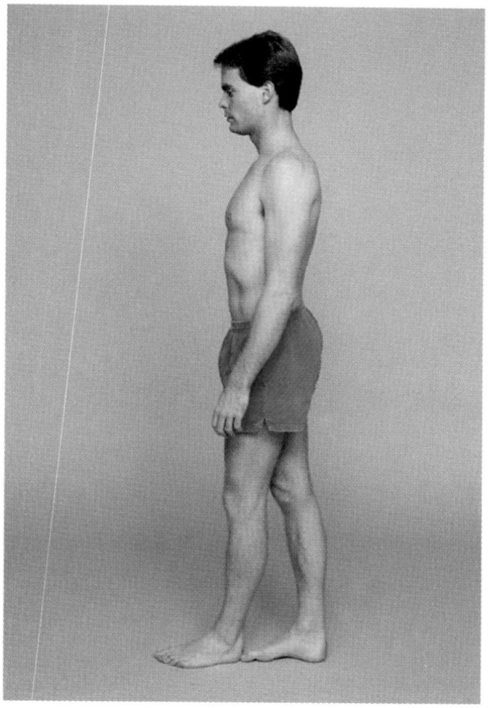

Fig. 25-18 Evaluation of balance with heel-toe walking on a straight line. (From Seidel et al, 1999.)

❖ ➤Have the client hop first on one foot and then on the other. The client should be able to follow directions successfully and have enough muscle strength to accomplish the task (Fig. 25-19).

- Inability to hop or maintain single-leg balance is abnormal.

PROCEDURES AND TECHNIQUES WITH NORMAL FINDINGS

ABNORMAL FINDINGS

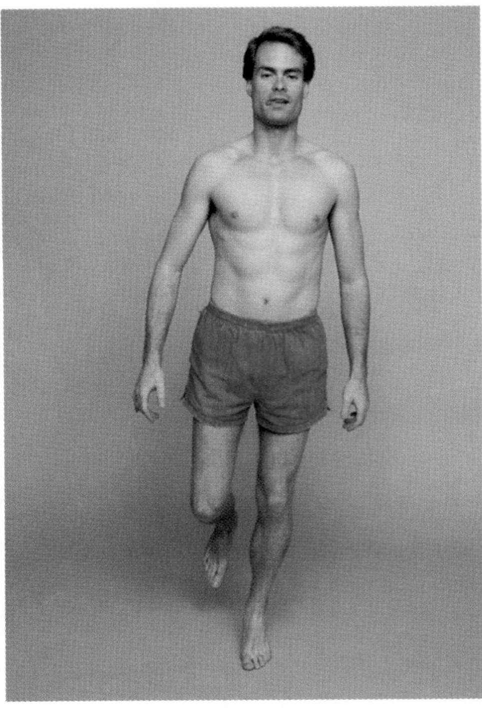

Fig. 25-19 Evaluation of balance with the client hopping in place on one foot. (From Seidel et al, 1999.)

❖ ➤Have the client hold a hand outward and perform several shallow or deep knee bends. He or she should be able to follow directions successfully, with muscle strength adequate to accomplish the task.

■ Inability to perform activity because of difficulty with balance or lack of muscle strength is abnormal.

❖ ➤Have the client walk on toes, then heels. The client should be able to follow directions, walking several steps on the toes and then on the heels. He or she may need to use the hands to maintain balance.

■ Inability to retain balance, poor muscle strength, or inability to complete the activity is abnormal.

Upper Extremity Have the client alternately tap thighs with hands using rapid pronation and supination movements. Timing should be equal bilaterally and movement purposeful; the client should have no problem maintaining a rapid pace (Fig. 25-20, *A, B*).

■ Inability to maintain rapid pace is abnormal and may indicate cerebellar dysfunction.

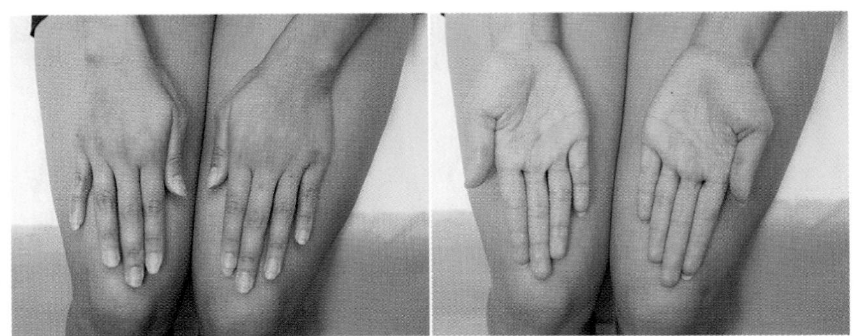

Fig. 25-20 Examination of coordination with rapid alternating movements. Ask client to tap top of thighs with both hands, alternately with **A,** palms down, and **B,** palms up.

PROCEDURES AND TECHNIQUES WITH NORMAL FINDINGS

❖ ➤Have the client close eyes and stretch arms outward. Use index fingers to alternately touch the nose rapidly. The client should be able to repeatedly touch the nose in a rhythmic pattern.

❖ ➤Evaluate the client's ability to perform rapid, rhythmic, alternating movement of fingers by having the client touch each finger to the thumb in rapid sequence. Test each hand separately. The client should have no problem rapidly and purposefully touching each finger to thumb (Fig. 25-21).

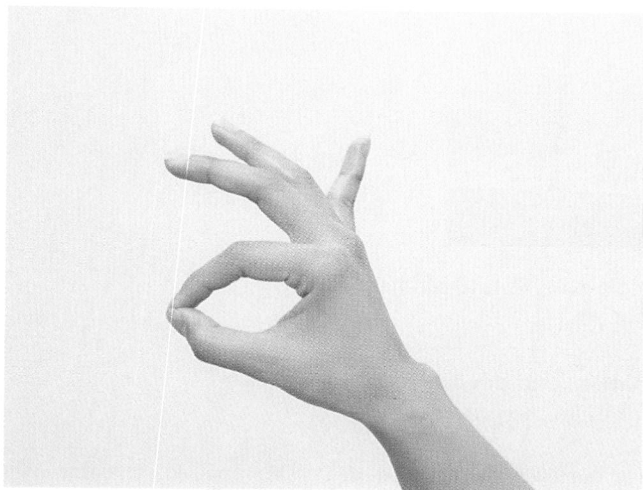

Fig. 25-21 Examination of finger coordination. Ask client to touch each finger to thumb in rapid sequence.

❖ ➤Have the client rapidly move his or her index finger back and forth between his or her nose and your finger 18 inches (46 cm) apart. Test one hand at a time. The client should be able to maintain the activity with a conscious coordinated effort (Fig. 25-22).

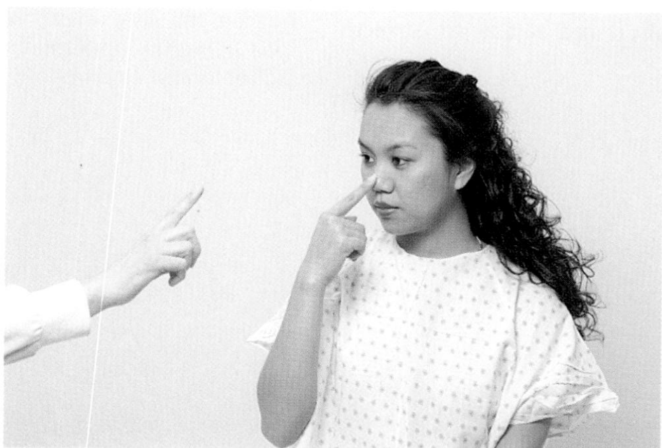

Fig. 25-22 Examination of fine motor function. Ask client to alternately touch own nose and the examiner's index finger with the index finger of one hand.

ABNORMAL FINDINGS

■ Cerebellar dysfunction may cause the client to miss touching his or her nose several times or cause the arms to drift downward.

■ Inability to coordinate fine, discrete, rapid movement is abnormal.

■ Inability to maintain continuous touch with both his or her own nose and your finger, inability to maintain the rapid movement, or obvious difficulty coordinating these is abnormal.

PROCEDURES AND TECHNIQUES WITH NORMAL FINDINGS

❖ ***Lower Extremity*** With the client lying supine, ask him or her to place the heel of one foot to the knee of the other leg, sliding it all the way down the shin (Fig. 25-23). Repeat on the other leg. The client should be able to run the heel down the opposite shin purposefully, with equal coordination.

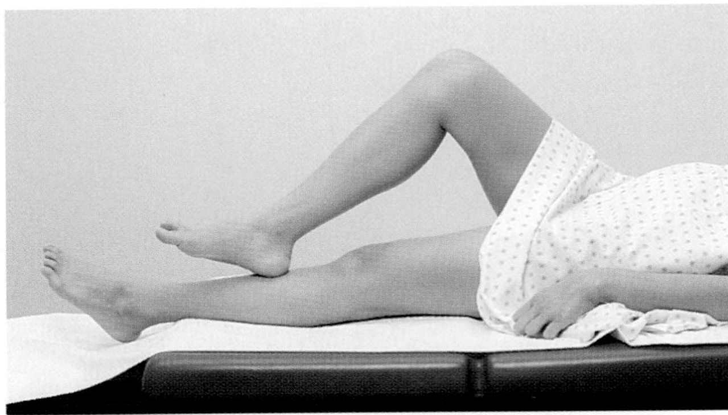

Fig. 25-23 Examination of lower extremity coordination. Ask client to run heel of one foot down shin of other leg. Repeat with opposite leg.

➤**EVALUATE extremities for muscle strength, sensation, and deep tendon reflexes.** Muscle strength: Test muscle strength according to the procedures outlined in Chapter 24.

Sensory Function Ask the client to close his or her eyes during the tests of sensory function. Areas routinely assessed are the hands, lower arms, abdomen, lower legs, and feet. If sensation is intact, then no further evaluation is needed; if impaired, move up extremities, testing periodically until a level or area of sensation is identified. If a deviation is identified, try to map out the area involved. Compare bilateral responses in each sensory testing area. Refer to dermatome map (see Fig. 25-10) to identify the spinal nerve providing sensation to that area of the body.

➤To test sensation to light touch (superficial touch), use a cotton wisp and the lightest touch possible to test each designated area (client's eyes are closed) (Fig. 25-24, *A*). The client should perceive light sensation and be able to correctly point to or name the spot touched.

ABNORMAL FINDINGS

■ Clients with cerebellar disease may overshoot the knee and oscillate back and forth. With loss of position sense, the client may lift the heel too high and have to look to ensure the heel is moving down the shin.

■ Impaired sensation or absence of sensation is abnormal. Absence of sensation may be due to compression of the nerve, whereas inflammation of the nerve may cause abnormal sensation.

■ Abnormal findings include the client reporting that he or she does not feel the light touch, incorrectly identifying the area touched, or exhibiting an asymmetric response.

PROCEDURES AND TECHNIQUES WITH NORMAL FINDINGS

ABNORMAL FINDINGS

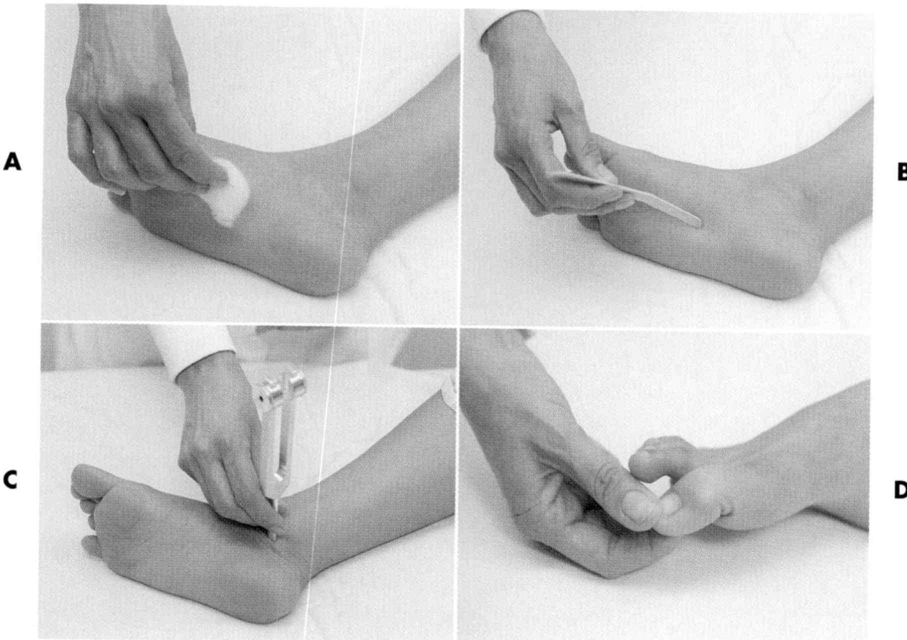

Fig. 25-24 Evaluation of peripheral nerve sensory function. **A,** Superficial tactile sensation. **B,** Superficial pain sensation. **C,** Vibratory sensation. **D,** Position sense of joints.

❖ ➤Test sharp and dull sensation by using the pointed tip of a paper clip (or broken tongue blade) to lightly prick each designated area (client's eyes are closed) (Fig. 25-24, *B*). Alternate sharp and dull sensations to more accurately evaluate the client's response. The client should perceive sensation and be able to identify the area touched.

■ Abnormal findings include client reporting that he or she does not feel the sharp or dull touch, cannot distinguish between sharp and dull, or exhibiting an asymmetric response.

➤Ask the client to close his or her eyes for the test of vibratory sense. Place a vibrating tuning fork on a bony area of the styloid process of the radius (wrist), medial or lateral malleolus (ankle), and sternum (chest) and ask the client to describe the sensation (Fig. 25-24, *C*). He or she should feel a sense of vibration. Repeat the procedure in the same location. Ask client when he or she no longer feels vibration, then stop vibration with tuning fork by touching it with your fingers but without moving it from its location on the bony prominence.

■ Unequal or decreased vibratory sensation is abnormal. Client may not be able to distinguish the change in sensation from vibration to nonvibration or may not feel the vibration in one or more locations. Referring to the dermatome drawing (see Fig. 25-10) will help identify the spinal nerve supplying this area. This may be found in clients with diabetes and those who have had a stroke or spinal cord injury.

➤Test kinesthetic sensation by grasping the client's finger or toe and moving its position ⅜ inch (1 cm) up or down (client's eyes are closed) (Fig. 25-24, *D*). The client should be able to describe how the position has changed.

■ If client cannot distinguish the change in position, it may indicate impairment of sensory (afferent nerves) or parietal lobe.

❖ ➤Test stereognosis by asking client to close eyes. You place a small familiar object in client's hand and ask him or her to identify it (Fig. 25-25, *A*). The object should be properly identified.

■ Altered stereognosis may indicate a parietal lobe dysfunction or sensory nerve tract.

PROCEDURES AND TECHNIQUES WITH NORMAL FINDINGS

ABNORMAL FINDINGS

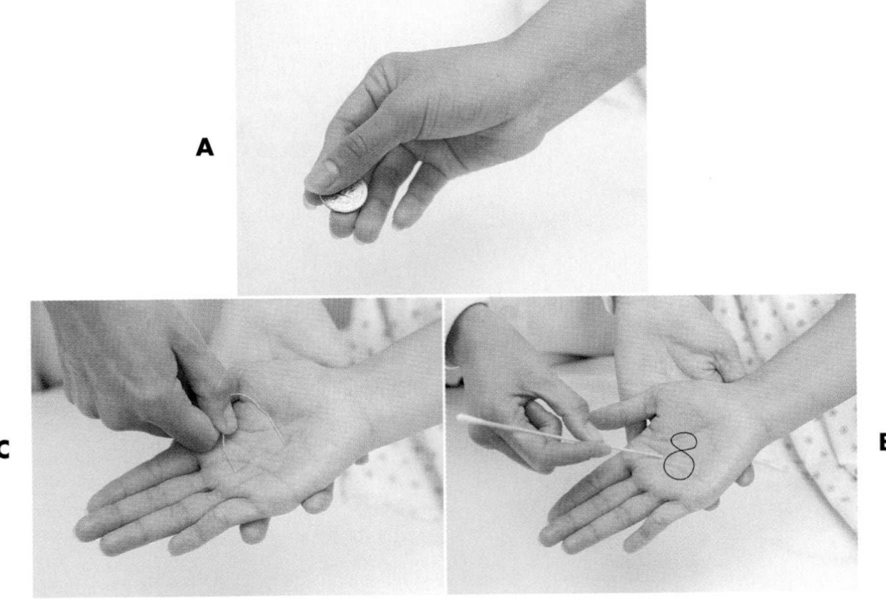

Fig. 25-25 Evaluation of cortical sensory function. **A,** Stereognosis: identification of a familiar object by touch. **B,** Two-point discrimination. **C,** Graphesthesia: draw letter or number on palm and ask client to identify by touch.

❖ ➤Test two-point discrimination by touching selected parts of the body simultaneously while the client's eyes are closed (Fig. 25-25, *B*). Use the points of two cotton-tipped applicators or reshape a paper clip so that two prongs can be lightly pressed against client's skin simultaneously. Ask the client how many points he or she detects. The expected values for two-point discrimination are listed in Box 25-3.

■ Inability to distinguish two-point discrimination is abnormal. Report the anatomic location of the sensory alteration.

Box 25-3 Minimal Distances for Distinguishing Two Points

LOCATION	MINIMAL DISTANCE
Tongue	1 mm or 1/32 inch*
Fingertips	2-8 mm or 2/32* to 5/16 inch
Toes	3-8 mm or 3/32* to 5/16 inch
Palm of hand	8 to 12 mm or 5/16 to ½ inch
Chest and forearms	40 mm or 1 ½ inches
Back	40-70 mm or 1 ½ to 2 ¾ inches
Upper arms and thighs	75 mm or 3 inches

*Too small to measure with conventional inch ruler.

❖ ➤Evaluate graphesthesia using a blunt instrument to draw a number or letter on the client's hand, back, or other area (client has eyes closed) (Fig. 25-25, *C*). The end of a reflex hammer can be used. He or she should be able to recognize the number or letter drawn.

■ If client cannot distinguish the number or letter, it may indicate a parietal lobe lesion.

PROCEDURES AND TECHNIQUES WITH NORMAL FINDINGS

ABNORMAL FINDINGS

➤Reflexes: Test deep tendon reflexes for muscle contraction in response to direct or indirect percussion of a tendon. See Box 25-4 for the scoring system. Hold reflex hammer between your thumb and index finger, and briskly tap the tendon with a flick of the wrist.

■ Abnormal response may range from a hyperactive to a diminished response. Observe whether the abnormal reflex response is unilateral or bilateral. See Table 25-2 for the spinal level of each reflex.

Box 25-4 Scoring Deep Tendon Reflexes

Test the five deep tendon reflexes (triceps, biceps, brachioradial, patellar, and Achilles) using a reflex hammer. Compare the reflexes bilaterally. Reflexes are graded on a scale of 0 to 4+, with 2+ being the expected findings. Findings are recorded as follows:

0 = no response
1+ = sluggish or diminished
2+ = active or expected response
3+ = slightly hyperactive, more brisk than normal; not necessarily pathologic
4+ = brisk, hyperactive with intermittent clonus associated with disease

The client must be relaxed and sitting or lying down. To elicit the triceps reflex, ask the client to let a relaxed arm fall onto your arm. Hold his or her arm, with elbow flexed at a 90° angle, in one hand. Palpate and strike the triceps tendon just above the elbow with either end of the reflex hammer (Fig. 25-26, *A*). (Some examiners prefer the flat end because of the wider striking surface.) The expected response is the contraction of the triceps muscle that causes visible or palpable extension of the elbow. An alternate arm position is to grasp the upper arm and allow the lower arm to bend at the elbow and hang freely, and then to strike the triceps tendon.

The biceps reflex is elicited by asking the client to let his or her relaxed arm fall onto your arm. Hold the arm with elbow flexed at a 90° angle, and place your thumb over the biceps tendon in the antecubital fossa and your fingers over the biceps muscle. Using the pointed end of the reflex hammer, strike your thumb instead of striking the tendon directly (Fig. 25-26, *B*). The expected response is the contraction of the biceps muscle that causes visible or palpable flexion of the elbow.

The brachioradial reflex is elicited by asking the client to let his or her relaxed arm fall into your hand. Hold the arm with the hand slightly pronated. Using either end of the reflex hammer, strike the brachioradialis tendon directly about 1 to 2 inches (2.5 to 5 cm) above the wrist (Fig. 25-26, *C*). The expected response is pronation of the forearm and flexion of the elbow.

The patellar reflex is tested with the client sitting with legs hanging free. Flex the client's knee at a 90° angle and strike the patellar tendon just below the patella (Fig. 25-26, *D*). The expected response is the contraction of the quadriceps muscle, causing extension of the lower leg. When no response is found, divert the client's attention to another muscular activity by asking him or her to pull the fingers of each hand against the other. While the client is pulling, strike the patellar tendon.

The Achilles tendon is tested by flexing the client's knee and dorsiflexing the ankle 90°. Hold the bottom of the client's foot in one hand while you use the flat end of the reflex hammer to strike the Achilles tendon at the level of the ankle malleolus (Fig. 25-26, *E*). The expected response is the contraction of the gastrocnemius muscle, causing plantar flexion of the foot.

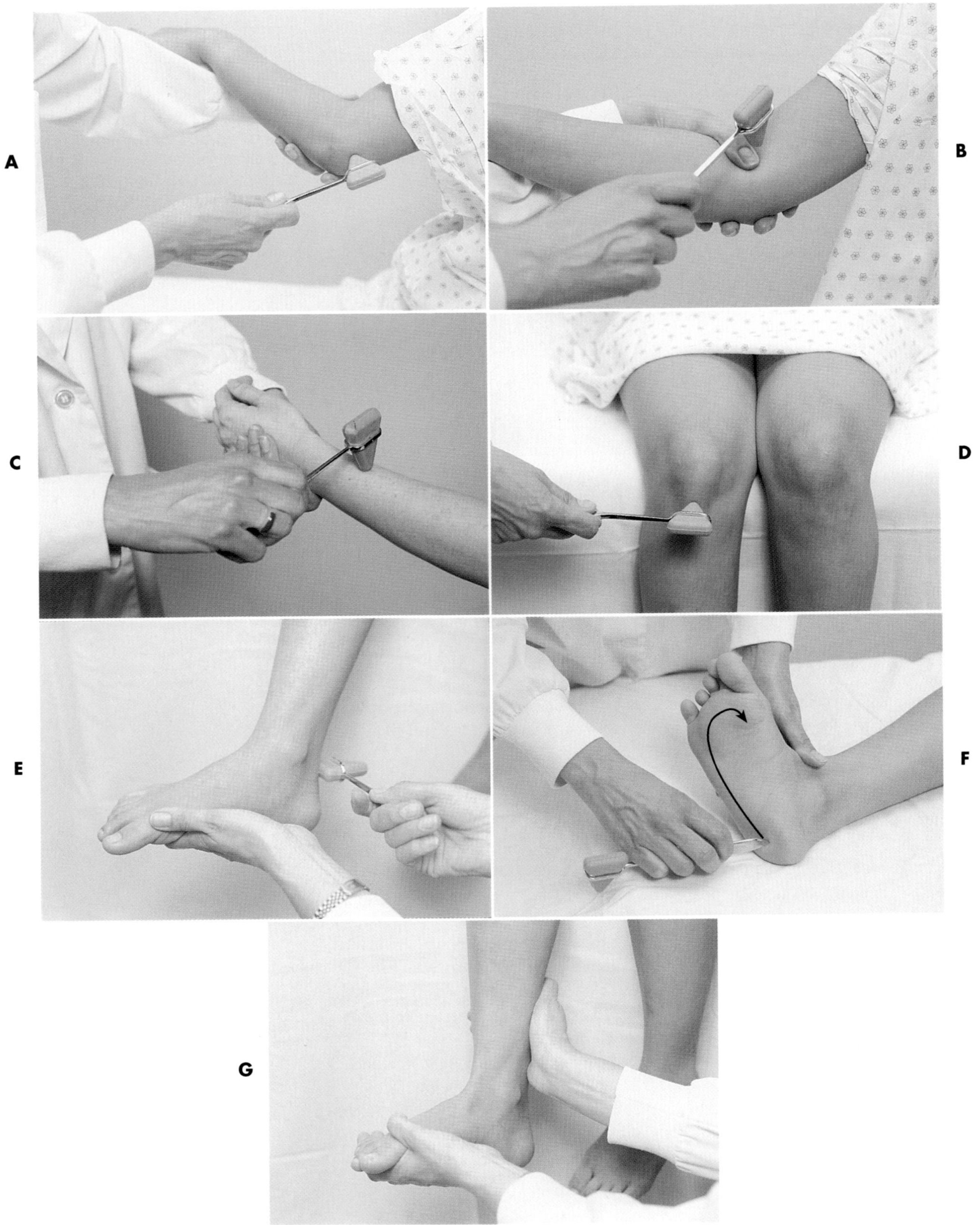

Fig. 25-26 Location of tendons for evaluation of deep tendon reflexes. **A,** Triceps reflex. **B,** Biceps reflex. **C,** Brachioradialis reflex. **D,** Patellar reflex. **E,** Achilles reflex. **F,** Babinski's reflex. **G,** Ankle tonus.

PROCEDURES AND TECHNIQUES WITH NORMAL FINDINGS

❖ ➤Check for the plantar (Babinski's) reflex. Using the end of the handle on the reflex hammer, stroke the lateral aspect of the sole of the foot from heel to ball, curving medially across the ball of the foot (Fig. 25-26, *F*). The expected findings should be plantar flexion of all toes; this is a negative Babinski's sign.

❖ ➤Test for ankle clonus if reflexes are hyperactive. Support the client's knee in partly flexed position. With the other hand, sharply dorsiflex the foot and maintain it in flexion (Fig. 25-26, *G*). There should be no movement of the foot.

❖ ➤**INSPECT abdomen for superficial reflexes.** Testing this reflex is described in Chapter 20 (see Fig. 20-21). The expected response is twitching of the umbilicus toward the quadrant stimulated. The response should be equal bilaterally. In assessing the neurologic system, you correlate the expected response with the spinal level involved. See Table 25-2 for the spinal level of these reflexes.

➤For male clients: Check the cremasteric reflex. Lightly stroke the upper, inner aspect of the thigh with the reflex hammer or tongue blade. The ipsilateral testicle should rise slightly.

ADDITIONAL ASSESSMENT TECHNIQUES FOR SPECIAL CASES

❖ ➤Meningeal signs are assessed when meningitis is suspected. These include tests for Kernig's sign and Brudzinski's sign. Kernig's sign is tested by flexing one of the client's legs at the hip and knee, then extending the knee (Fig. 25-27, *A*). No pain reported is a negative Kernig's sign. Brudzinski's test is performed with the client supine. The examiner flexes the client's neck (Fig. 25-27, *B*). The client should report no pain or resistance to neck flexion.

ABNORMAL FINDINGS

■ Extension of the great toe, with fanning of the other toes is an abnormal response and may indicate pyramidal (motor) tract disease.

■ Rhythmic oscillations between dorsiflexion and plantar flexion are abnormal responses.

■ Hyperactive or diminished response or responses that are unequal bilaterally are abnormal responses.

■ Absence of the cremasteric reflex is seen in disorders of the pyramidal (motor) tract above the level of the first lumbar vertebrae.

■ If a client has inflammation of the meninges, he or she will report pain along the vertebral column when the leg is extended, a positive Kernig's sign indicating irritation of the meninges.

■ A positive Brudzinski's sign occurs when the client passively flexes the hip and knee in response to head flexion and reports pain along vertebral column.

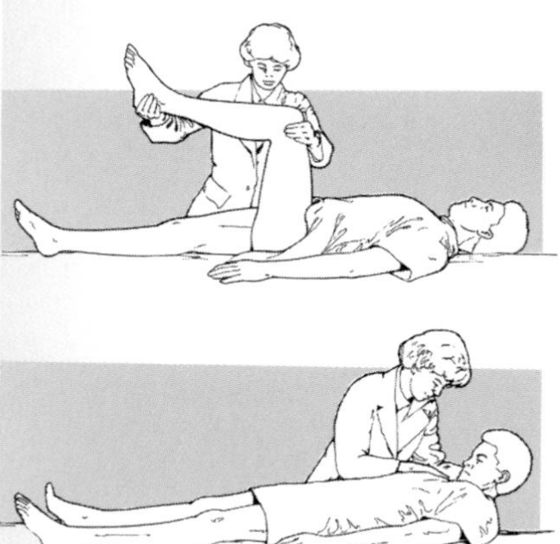

Fig. 25-27 Kernig's sign and Brudzinski's sign are tests of meningeal irritation. **A,** *Kernig's sign.* Flex one of the client's legs at the hip and knee. Note resistance or pain. **B,** *Brudzinski's sign.* With the client recumbent, place your hands behind the client's head and flex the neck forward. Note resistance or pain. Watch also for flexion of the client's hips and knees in reaction to your maneuver. (From Chipps, Clanin, and Campbell, 1992.)

PROCEDURES AND TECHNIQUES WITH NORMAL FINDINGS	ABNORMAL FINDINGS

➤The Glasgow Coma Scale assesses level of consciousness using a 15-point scale (Fig. 25-28). Client is assessed for the best response to eye opening, motor response, and verbal response. For example, when a client who is paralyzed on one side due to a stroke is assessed, the best motor response is assessed on the client's unaffected side.

■ A score from 14 to 3 is considered abnormal. The lower the score, the deeper the coma.

Pain is one descriptor used in the assessment of best eye opening and best motor response. You want to determine how much stimulation or pain is required to elicit a response from the client. This is the only situation when it is acceptable for the nurse to inflict pain on a client. The first stimulation you begin with is touch and a normal tone of voice. If this does not create a response, then you shake the client such as on the shoulder or leg and shout at him or her. If this does not produce a response, then you resort to painful stimuli beginning peripherally and moving centrally. You may begin with depressing the nail bed at the cuticle with your fingernail or with an object such as the length of a pen or pencil. If this does not elicit a response, then squeeze the trapezius muscle very hard and observe for any movement. If this does not yield a response, then push upward on the supraorbital notch above the eye. Do not push inward on the eyeball, but on the bony orbit above the eyeball.

The best motor response describes and assigns an arbitrary number to the levels of movement. The response observed from the client may be a localization of pain (score of 5) when he or she moves as if trying to remove the stimulus, an attempt to withdraw from the stimulus (score of 4), abnormal flexion (formerly called decorticate posturing) (score of 3), abnormal extension (formerly called decerebrate posturing) (score of 2), or no response at all to any painful stimuli (score of 1).

When the client is unable to speak because of an endotracheal or tracheostomy tube placement, then the best verbal response of the Glasgow Coma Scale cannot be assessed. Each institution has its specific way of documenting this. For example, if the client is comatose, the score may be recorded as 2T, meaning 1 for best eye response, 1 for best motor response, and the T meaning "tube," indicating that verbal response cannot be assessed.

Glasgow Coma Scale

Best eye-opening response	Spontaneously	4
	To verbal command	3
	To pain	2
	No response	1
Best verbal response	Oriented, converses	5
	Disoriented, converses	4
	Inappropriate words	3
	Incomprehensible sounds	2
	No response	1
Best motor response		
To verbal command	Obeys	6
To painful stimulus	Localizes pain	5
	Flexion-withdrawal	4
	Flexion-decorticate	3
	Extension-decerebrate	2
	No response	1
	TOTAL	(3-15)

Abnormal flexion (Decorticate) Rigid flexion; upper arms held tightly to the sides of body; elbows, wrists, and fingers flexed; feet are plantar flexed, legs extended and internally rotated; may have fine tremors or intense stiffness

Abnormal extension (Decerebrate) Rigid extension; arms fully extended; forearms pronated; wrists and fingers flexed; jaws clenched, neck extended, back may be arched; feet plantar flexed; may occur spontaneously, intermittently, or in response to a stimulus

Fig. 25-28 Glasgow Coma Scale. (Modified from Chipps, Clanin, and Campbell, 1992.)

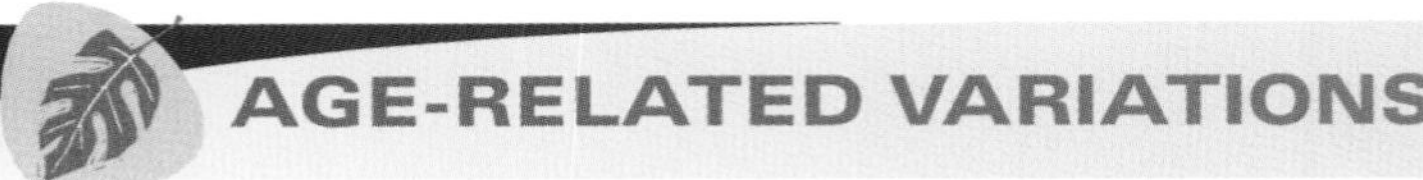

AGE-RELATED VARIATIONS

INFANTS

Anatomy and Physiology

Major growth of the nervous system occurs during the first year of life. Initial reflexes that should be evident in the newborn are shown in Table 25-3. Motor control develops in a cephalocaudal direction, from head and neck to trunk and extremities. Functions generally develop in an orderly sequence but may vary considerably in timing from one child to the next. The posterior fontanel closes by age 2 months, and the anterior closes between 18 and 24 months.

Health History

- Did you (or the mother) have any health difficulties while you were pregnant? Any infections or illnesses? Toxemia? Hypertension (high blood pressure)? Did you take any medications? Use alcohol or drugs? Do you have diabetes?

  Rationale Any of the above factors can impair fetal development of the neurologic system.
- Was the infant born at term or prematurely? What was the infant's birth weight? Were there any problems with the birth? Trauma? Did the infant breathe right away? Do you remember the newborn's Apgar scores? Were any congenital defects found?

  Rationale Problems during delivery such as birth trauma or delayed crying at birth can cause cerebral anoxia that can result in neurologic deficits.
- Does the infant seem to have coordinated sucking and swallowing reflexes? When you touch his or her cheek, does the infant turn toward the touch? Does the infant startle when there is a loud noise or when the crib is shaken? Does the infant hold onto your finger when you place it in his or her palm? Has the infant sneezed, hiccupped, and yawned?

  Rationale Absence of any of these expected behaviors can indicate absence of one or more reflexes.
- Has the infant had any seizures? Was this associated with a high fever? Describe the seizure. How long did it last? Did the infant lose consciousness? How many seizures did the infant have with this illness (if the seizures were associated with a high fever)?

  Rationale Seizures can occur in infants and children with high fevers or may be evidence of a neurologic disorder.

Examination

Equipment Tape measure for measuring head circumference.

Procedures and Techniques Palpate the infant's fontanels for presence and contour. Measure the infant's head circumference and compare it with previous measurements if available. Observe the infant's response to touch and pressure. Determine the presence of the Moro's, tonic neck, rooting, sucking, palmar grasp, Babinski's, clonus, and plantar reflexes as applicable (see Table 25-3). Cra-

Table 25-3 Infantile Reflexes

REFLEX	TECHNIQUE FOR EVALUATION	APPEARANCE AGE	DISAPPEARANCE AGE	NORMAL RESPONSE
REFLEXES TO EVALUATE POSITION AND MOVEMENT				
Moro's	Startle infant by making loud noise, jarring examination surface, or slightly raising infant off examination surface and letting him fall quickly back onto examining table	Birth	1 to 4 months	Infant abducts and extends arms and legs; index finger and thumb assume C position; then infant pulls both arms and legs up against trunk as if trying to protect self
Tonic neck	Infant supine; rotate head to side so that chin is over shoulder	Birth to 6 weeks	4 to 6 months	Arm and leg on side to which head turns extend; opposite arm and leg flex; infant assumes fencing position (some normal infants may never show this reflex)
Plantar grasp	Touch object to sole of infant's foot	Birth	8 to 10 months	Toes will flex tightly downward in attempt to grasp
Palmar grasp	Touch object against ulnar side of infant's hand; then place finger in palm of hand	Birth	3 to 4 months	Infant will grasp finger; grasp should be tight, and examiner may be able to pull infant into sitting position by infant's grasp

nial nerves are assessed by observing eye movements, wrinkling of the forehead, turning the head toward a sound, swallowing, and sucking. Flex the infant's head forward. With the infant supine, pull to a sitting position holding the wrists; observe head control. Observe spontaneous motor activity. Evaluate resting posture for muscle tone. Flex the infant's knees onto the abdomen and quickly release them.

Normal and Abnormal Findings Normal findings begin with fontanels that are soft and flat, if they are present. Between 5 months and 2 years the head circumference should closely approximate the chest circumference. The infantile reflexes are present but disappear during the first year as the infant's nervous system matures. Babinski's reflex is an exception; it disappears by 18 months. Infant's neck should flex without difficulty or apparent pain. Some head flexion (head lag) is normally present. Three-month-old infants raise the head and arch the back; this reflex persists until 18 months of age. Spontaneous movement should be smooth and symmetric. Infant's knees should unfold gradually after being flexed to chest.

Abnormal findings may include fontanels that feel full and distended. This finding together with head circumference greater than expected with lethargy, irritability, weakness, and "sunset eyes" may indicate hydrocephalus. Sunken fontanels may be a sign of dehydration. Motor activity delays may indicate brain damage, mental retardation, peripheral neuromuscular damage, illness, or neglect. The infant will resist head movement and push back against the exam-

Table 25-3 Infantile Reflexes

REFLEX	TECHNIQUE FOR EVALUATION	APPEARANCE AGE	DISAPPEARANCE AGE	NORMAL RESPONSE
Babinski's	Stroke lateral surface of infant's sole, using inverted J-curve from sole to great toe	Birth	18 months	Infant response: positive response showing fanning of toes
		Starting 18 months		Adult response: occurs after child has been walking for some time; flexion of great toe with slight fanning of other toes
Step in place	Infant in upright position, feet flat on surface	Birth	3 months	Will pace forward using alternating steps
Clonus	Dorsiflex foot; pinch sole of foot just under toes	Birth	4 months	May get clonus movement of foot (not always present)
FEEDING REFLEXES				
Rooting response (awake)	Brush infant's cheek near corner of mouth	Birth	3 to 4 months	Infant will turn head in direction of stimulus and will open mouth slightly
Sucking	Touch infant's lips	Birth	10 to 12 months	Sucking motion follows with lips and tongue

iner's hand. Note any head lag, which could indicate brain damage. Any continued asymmetry of posture is also abnormal. Note any spasticity, which may be an early sign of cerebral palsy. If present, the legs quickly extend and adduct, possibly even in a scissoring pattern.

CHILDREN

Anatomy and Physiology

This is the same as in the adult.

Health History

In addition to the questions asked concerning infants, ask the parent or guardian the following:

- Does the child participate in activities you would expect for a child this age? Does he or she seem to be growing and maturing like other children the same age?

  Rationale If the child did not achieve motor and developmental milestones, he or she could have neurologic deficits.

- Have you been notified of any problems the child has in school, such as short attention span, lack of concentration, or hyperactivity?

  Rationale Parental report of hyperactivity is usually the first sign of an attention deficit hyperactivity disorder (ADHD).

- Does the child appear to have problems with balance? Does he or she seem to fall unexpectedly, be clumsy or unsteady in gait, have progressive muscular weakness, have problems going up and down stairs, or getting up from a lying position?

Rationale These symptoms may indicate impairment with innervation of muscles or cerebral or cerebellar anomaly.

Examination

Procedures and Techniques Follow the same sequence of evaluation as for adults when dealing with children. Observe the child carefully during spontaneous activity, since the child may not be able to cooperate with requests as an adult would. Making the examination a game helps in data collection.

Observe the child for achievement of expected developmental milestones for fine- and gross-motor, social/adaptive, and language skills described in Chapter 2. Evaluate the child's general behavior while he or she is at play, interacting with parents, and cooperating with parents and with the examiner.

In testing cranial nerves, sense of smell usually is not tested; if it is, use a scent familiar to the child, such as orange or peanut butter. In testing visual fields and gaze (CN II, III, IV, and VI), gently immobilize the head so that the child cannot follow objects with the whole head but only with the eyes. When testing CN VII, approach it like a game, asking the child to make "funny faces" as the examiner models them.

Use the Denver II to assess fine-motor coordination in children under 6 years of age. For children older than 6 years, use the finger-to-nose test, with the examiner's finger held 1 to 2 inches (2.5 to 5 cm) away from the child's nose.

Sensory function is not normally tested before age 5. Carefully explain what is being done when children are tested, and use descriptions that the child can understand, such as "this will feel like a tickle or a mosquito bite." Use simple numbers for graphesthesia testing (such as 0, 7, 5, 3, or 1) and X and O for younger children.

The screening for neurologic "soft" signs in school-age children is used to describe vague and minimal dysfunction signs, such as clumsiness, language disturbances, motor overload, mirroring movement of extremities, or perceptual development difficulties (Table 25-4).

Normal and Abnormal Findings Normal findings should be the same as those for adults with the following exceptions. It is not necessary to test reflexes if the child shows all other expected neurologic signs. Soft neurologic signs may be considered normal in the young child, but as the child matures, the signs should disappear.

Abnormal findings are the same as for the adult. Spasticity, paralysis, seizures with mental retardation, or impaired vision, speech, or hearing may indicate cerebral palsy. The identification of soft signs indicates failure of the child to perform age-specific activities (see Table 25-4), and the child should be referred to a health care professional for further evaluation. Inattention, motor restlessness, and easily distractibility may indicate attention deficit hyperactivity disorder.

■ ADOLESCENTS

Anatomy and Physiology

Anatomy and physiology for adolescents is the same as for the adult.

Health History

Health history for adolescents is the same as for the adult.

Examination

Examination procedures and techniques as well as normal and abnormal findings are the same as for the adult.

■ OLDER ADULTS

Anatomy and Physiology

The effects of normal aging of the nervous system are gradual. "An abrupt decline is always due to disease" (Crigger and Forbes, 1997, p. 37). Starting as early as age 30, the velocity of the conduction of nerve impulses—and thus responses—diminishes by about 10%.

The sense of smell declines. Expected changes in vision include presbyopia, reduced ability to distinguish blues and greens, miosis, reduced upward gaze, and slower adjustment to lighting changes. The corneal reflex and the sense of taste may be diminished. Presbycusis alters hearing of middle- to high-frequency sounds. Finally, the gag reflex is reduced (Crigger and Forbes, 1997).

The Achilles tendon and abdominal reflexes may be decreased without any pathologic condition. Speed and agility are reduced as is range of motion of joints and neck. Proprioception declines with normal aging. Balance may be altered with the degeneration of the cochlea (Crigger and Forbes, 1997).

Health History

Health history is the same as for the younger adult.

Examination

Procedures and Techniques The neurologic examination for older adults is the same as for younger adults. Older adults may have difficulty relaxing their limbs and may require reinforcement when you are eliciting deep tendon reflexes.

Normal and Abnormal Findings For indications of the client's ability to perform activities of daily living (ADL), note his or her personal hygiene, appearance, and dress. Be aware that some older adults have slowed responses, move more slowly, or show a decline in function (for example, the sense of taste). Other expected changes with aging may include senile tremors or dyskinesias (defects in voluntary movements); deviation of gait from midline; difficulty with rapidly alternating movements; and some loss of reflexes and sensations (for example, the knee jerk or ankle jerk reflexes and light touch and pain sensations). Often a normal flexor response is indistinct, and the plantar reflex may be missing or hard to interpret. Superficial abdominal reflexes may be missing (Lueckenotte, 1996). Abnormal findings are the same as for younger adults.

Table 25-4 Screening Assessment of Neurologic "Soft" Signs

INSTRUCTIONAL TECHNIQUE	IMPORTANT OBSERVATIONS	VARIABLES AND CONSIDERATIONS
1. Evaluation of fine motor coordination: observe child during:		
a. Undressing, unbuttoning	Note child's general coordination	
b. Tying shoe		
c. Rapidly touching alternate fingers with thumb	Note if similar movement on opposite side	For items *c* to *e* and *h* and *i*, movement of other side noted as associated motor movements, adventitious overflow movements, or synkinesis
d. Rattling imaginary doorknob	Note if similar movement on other side	
e. Unscrewing imaginary light bulb	Note if similar movement on other side	
f. Grasping pencil and writing	Note excessive pressure on pen point; fingers placed directly over point, or placed greater than 1 inch (2.5 cm) up shaft	May indicate difficulty with fine-motor coordination
g. Moving tongue rapidly		
h. Demonstrating hand grip	Note if similar movement on opposite side	
i. Inverting feet	Note if similar movement on opposite side	
j. Repeating several times "pa, ta, ka" or "kitty, kitty, kitty"	Accurate reproduction of these sounds indicates auditory coordination	
2. Evaluation of special sensory skills		
a. Dual simultaneous sensory tests (face-hand testing): first demonstrate technique, then instruct child to close eyes; examiner performs simultaneously:		
(1) Touch both cheeks (2) Touch both hands (3) Touch right cheek and right hand (4) Touch left cheek and right hand (5) Touch left cheek and left hand (6) Touch right cheek and left hand	Failure to perceive hand stimulus when face simultaneously touched referred to as *rostral dominance*	About 80% of normal children able to perform this test by age 8 years without rostral dominance
b. Finger localization test (finger agnosia test): touch two spots on one finger or two fingers simultaneously; child has eyes closed; ask, "How many fingers am I touching, one or two?"	Evaluate number of correct responses with four trials for each hand Six out of eight possible correct responses passes	About 50% of all children pass test by age 6 years About 90% of all children pass by age 9 years This test reflects child's orientation in space, concept of body image, sensation of touch, and position sense

Data from McMillan J, Nieburg P, Oski F: *The whole pediatrician catalog,* Philadelphia, 1977, WB Saunders.

Continued

Table 25-4 Screening Assessment of Neurologic "Soft" Signs—cont'd

INSTRUCTIONAL TECHNIQUE	IMPORTANT OBSERVATIONS	VARIABLES AND CONSIDERATIONS
3. Evaluation of child's laterality and orientation in space		
a. Imitation of gestures: instruct child to use same hand as examiner and to imitate the following movements ("Do as I do"): (1) Extend little finger (2) Extend little and index fingers (3) Extend index and middle fingers (4) Touch two thumbs and two index fingers together simultaneously (5) Form two interlocking rings—thumb and index finger of one hand, with thumb and index finger of other hand (6) Point index finger of one hand down toward cupped finger of opposite hand held below	Note difficulty with fine finger movements, manipulation, or reproduction of correct gesture Note any marked right-left confusion regarding examiner's right and left hands	This test helps to evaluate child's finger discrimination and awareness of body image, right, left, front, back, and up and down orientation Especially important after age 8 years if there continues to be marked right-left confusion
b. Following directions: ask child to: (1) Show me your left hand (2) Show me your right eye (3) Show me your left elbow (4) Touch your left knee with your left hand (5) Touch your right ear with your left hand (6) Touch your left elbow with your right hand (7) Touch your right cheek with your right hand	Note any incorrect response Note any difficulty with following sequence of directions	Items *1* through *7* mastered by approximately age 6 years
(8) Point to my left ear (9) Point to my right eye (10) Point to my right hand (11) Point to my left knee		Items *8* through *11* mastered by age 8 years

CLIENTS WITH SITUATIONAL VARIATIONS

CLIENTS WITH APHASIA

Clients with aphasia have difficulty receiving or sending communication. Those with expressive aphasia are able to receive information but may have difficulty answering questions about their history. When answering questions, these clients may require more time to respond. Patience is needed on the part of the examiner to determine how this person communicates best.

Clients with receptive aphasia appear alert but are unable to process the information. Thus, they can neither understand what is said to them nor verbally communicate. Subjective data about these clients may be obtained from caregivers and/or family members. (See section on Common Problems and Conditions for more information about aphasia.)

CLIENTS TAKING ANTICONVULSANTS

Clients taking medications, for example, anticonvulsants, may be slow to answer questions due to the medications they take to reduce seizures. These clients may include those diagnosed with epilepsy and those who have had craniotomy or head injury. One of the side effects of slowing neuronal responses to reduce seizures may be a slowed thought process, requiring additional time and patience from the examiner.

CLIENTS IN A WHEELCHAIR

Clients who use a wheelchair full time will require some modification in the examination procedure. If their wheelchair cannot be moved close to the assessment equipment mounted on the wall such as an otoscope or sphygmomanometer, then handheld equipment will be needed. If the chief complaint involves moving him or her out of the wheelchair, then assistance will be needed for transferring from chair to examination table.

CLIENTS WHO ARE UNCONSCIOUS

Modified neurologic assessment is needed for the unconscious client since he or she cannot actively participate. When interacting with an unconscious client ALWAYS assume that he or she can hear *everything* you say; thus, you tell the client what action you are going to do before you do it. For example, "I am going to lift your right leg to make sure your joints bend." You must assess the pupillary reaction by holding the eyelid open while shining the light in the eye.

Tests of sensation are changed for the unconscious client since they cannot voluntarily respond. The sensation that is assessed is tactile stimulation or pain. The Glasgow Coma Scale is used for this assessment (see Fig. 25-28).

EXAMINATION SUMMARY

Neurologic System

PROCEDURE

- Evaluate speech (p. 706) for:
  Articulation
  Voice quality
  Comprehension
- Test nose (p. 706) for:
  Smell (olfactory nerve, CN I)
- Test eyes (p. 706) for:
  Visual acuity and peripheral vision (optic nerve, CN II)
- Observe eyes (pp. 706-707) for:
  Extraocular movement (oculomotor nerve, CN III; trochlear nerve, CN IV; and abducens nerve, CN VI)
  Pupillary size, shape, equality, constriction and accommodation (oculomotor nerve, CN III)
- Evaluate face (pp. 707-708) for:
  Movement (trigeminal nerve, CN V, and facial nerve, CN VII)
  ❖ Sensation (trigeminal nerve, CN V)
- Test ears (p. 709) for:
  Hearing (acoustic nerve, CN VIII)
- Test tongue (p. 709) for:
  Taste (anterior tongue: facial nerve, CN VII; posterior tongue: glossopharyngeal nerve, CN IX)
- Inspect oropharynx (p. 709) for:
  Movement of soft palate (glossopharyngeal nerve, CN IX) and gag reflex
- ❖ Inspect tongue (p. 710) for:
  Movement, symmetry, strength, and absence of tumors (hypoglossal nerve, CN XII)
- Test shoulders and neck muscles (p. 710) for:
  Strength (spinal accessory nerve, CN XI)
  Movement
- Test cerebellar function (p. 710) for:
  ❖ Balance and coordination (also tests CN VIII)
- Evaluate extremities (pp. 714-719) for:
  Muscle strength

- ❖ Sensation
  Deep tendon reflexes
- Inspect abdomen (p. 719) for:
- ❖ Superficial reflexes

Additional Assessment Techniques for Special Cases (pp. 719-721)

- ❖ • Meningeal signs: Kernig's and Brudzinski's signs
- Glasgow Coma Scale

SUMMARY OF FINDINGS

Age Group	Normal Findings	Typical Variations	Findings Associated With Disorders
Infants and children	• Fontanels, if present, are soft and flat. Head circumference closely equal to chest circumference by age 2. Infantile reflexes (Moro's, tonic neck, rooting, sucking, palmar grasp, Babinski's, clonus, and plantar) are present and brisk but disappear as nervous system matures. Neck flexion is present with some head lag in infants. Fine and gross motor, social/adaptive, and language skills are age appropriate. • Movement is smooth and symmetric. Soft neurologic signs may be considered normal in the young child, but as the child matures, the signs should disappear.		• Widening fontanel and increased head circumference with lethargy, irritability, weakness, and sunset eyes may indicate hydrocephalus. Sunken fontanels may indicate dehydration. Spasticity, paralysis, seizures with mental retardation, impaired vision, speech, or hearing may indicate cerebral palsy. Developmental delay or lag in the sensory or motor system may indicate cerebral impairment The identification of soft signs indicates failure of the child to perform age-specific activities (see Table 25-4). Inattention, motor restlessness, and easy distractibility may indicate attention deficit hyperactivity disorder.
Adolescents older adults	Same as for adult. • Some older adults have slowed responses, move more slowly, or show a decline in function (for example, the sense of taste). Occasionally senile tremors or dyskinesias, deviation of gait from midline, difficulty with rapidly alternating movements, and some loss of reflexes and sensations (for example, the patellar or plantar reflexes and light touch and pain sensations). Normal flexor response may be indistinct, and the plantar reflex may be missing or hard to interpret.	Same as for adult. • Superficial abdominal reflexes may be missing.	Same as for adult. • Abnormal findings are the same as younger adult.

Age Group	Normal Findings	Typical Variations	Findings Associated With Disorders
Adults	• Speech is clear and comprehensible. CN I-XII intact. Cerebellar function intact bilaterally, muscles 5/5 bilaterally with light and deep sensation and vibration intact. • Kinesthetic sensation, stereognosis, two-point discrimination and graphesthesia intact. Reflexes 2+ bilaterally. Superficial reflexes of abdomen present. (For males cremasteric reflex intact.)	• Mild nystagmus at extreme gaze during extraocular muscle assessment is a normal variation. • Clients who wear contact lenses may have diminished or absent corneal reflex.	• Errors in choice of words, difficulty in articulation may indicate aphasia. Dysfunction of the tongue or lips; slurred speech (tone sounds slurred); poorly coordinated or irregular speech; monotone or weak voice; nasal tone, rasping, or hoarseness; whispering voice; and stuttering may indicate compression of cranial nerves or brainstem lesion. • Allergic rhinitis, sinusitis, excessive smoking, cocaine use, or olfactory tract lesion may interfere with ability to smell. • Vision > 20/20, decreased peripheral visual fields, asymmetric eye movements, nystagmus other than that expected at extreme gaze, or unequal pupils may indicate dysfunction of cranial nerve III, IV, or VI. • Asymmetric muscle contractions, twitching, or loss of movement may indicate disorders of motor nerves, whereas pain or decreased or abnormal sensation or vibration may indicate disorders of sensory nerves. Loss of equilibrium may indicate inner ear or cerebellar disorder. Positive Kernig's or Brudzinski's sign with headache, fever, and stiff neck may indicate meningitis. A Glasgow Coma Scale 3-14 indicates a decrease in consciousness.

Below is sample documentation of expected findings for CN I to CN XII: Sense of smell intact, vision 20/20, peripheral vision and extraocular muscles (EOM) intact, PERRLA. Face is symmetric with strong muscles bilaterally, sensation and movement present and symmetric. Hears 50% of words whispered, air conduction (AC) greater than bone conduction (BC), lateralization of sound is equal. Able to taste; gag reflex present; tongue movement symmetric; and shoulder muscles strong and symmetric bilaterally.

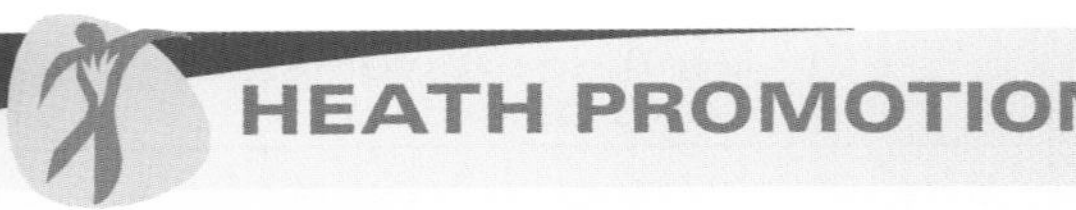

HEATH PROMOTION

SAFE TRAVEL

The number of central nervous system injuries from motor vehicle accidents (MVA) can be reduced by wearing seat belts and helmets in addition to using a designated driver program to prevent those under the influence of alcohol or drugs from driving. Approximately 15,000 to 20,000 people sustain spinal cord injuries each year in the United States. Vehicular accidents account for 48% of these injuries.

According to the Centers for Disease Control and Prevention, an estimated 2 million traumatic brain injuries (TBI) occurred in 1990. Of these, 51,600 deaths occurred, and 20% to 30% of the survivors sustained severe enough injury to result in lifelong disability. Young males are the highest risk group and are usually injured in motor vehicle accidents. Infants and older adults are the second highest group and usually are injured in falls (Waxweiler et al, 1995).

SAFE RECREATION

The number of nervous system injuries from recreational activities can be reduced in a variety of ways. Helmets are recommended for skateboarding and riding bicycles, motorbikes, and motorcycles. Sports injuries also account for 14% of the spinal cord injuries, with diving injuries accounting for 66% of those injuries. The highest incidence occurs in men between the ages of 16 and 32. Diving accidents can be reduced by using the strategy of "Feet first, first time" to encourage divers to get into water feet first to determine the water depth before diving in. Near-drowning accidents can be reduced when all occupants of a boat wear life jackets, swimmers swim with a buddy, and young children are closely supervised around swimming pools.

Many unintentional injuries from firearms in the home and while hunting involve children, adolescents, and young adult men. Strategies to prevent firearm injuries include keeping guns stored unloaded and in a locked compartment. When hunting, preventive strategies are supervising children and adolescents and wearing fluorescent orange clothing to increase visibility (Report of the U.S. Preventive Services Task Force, 1996).

COMMON PROBLEMS AND CONDITIONS

Neurologic System

DISORDERS OF THE CENTRAL NERVOUS SYSTEM

Multiple Sclerosis

Progressive demyelination of nerve fibers of the brain and spinal cord may result in multiple sclerosis. It is thought to be an autoimmune disorder initiated by a virus that attacks the myelin at various sites of the central nervous system. Since the sites of demyelination are varied, the signs and symptoms of the disease are varied. It is the most common neurologic disorder in young adults, striking between ages 15 and 60, with the highest incidence between 20 and 40 years of age. Common symptoms are fatigue, depression, and paresthesias; common signs are focal muscle weakness; ocular changes (diplopia, nystagmus); bowel, bladder, and sexual dysfunction; gait instability and spasticity.

Seizure Disorder

A hyperexcitation of neurons in the brain leading to a sudden involuntary series of muscle contractions describes seizures. A seizure involving the entire brain (generalized seizure) may render the client unconscious for several minutes with tonic and clonic movements and incontinence. Conversely, a seizure in a small part of the brain (local or focal) may produce slow repetitive movement without loss of consciousness.

Meningitis

Inflammation of the meninges that surround the brain and spinal cord is called meningitis. It may result from invasion of bacteria, viruses, fungi, parasites, or other toxins. Bacterial meningitis is most common and can result in death if not treated promptly. By contrast, viral meningitis is a self-limiting infection with full recovery. Symptoms of meningitis include severe headache, fever, and generalized malaise. Signs of meningeal irritation are common; these include stiff neck and positive Brudzinski's and Kernig's signs. Level of consciousness may decrease with drowsiness and reduced attention span, which may progress to stupor and coma. Confusion, agitation, and irritability may occur.

Encephalitis

Inflammation of the brain tissue and meninges is called encephalitis. It is caused by bacteria, viruses, fungi, and parasites; with viral encephalitis being most common. Symptoms of encephalitis are variable, depending on the invading organism and the part of the brain involved. The onset may be gradual or sudden with symptoms of headache, lethargy, irritability, and nausea and signs of fever, nuchal rigidity, and vomiting. Over several days the client may develop reduced consciousness, motor weakness, tremors, seizures, aphasia, and positive Babinski's sign.

Spinal Cord Injury

A spinal cord injury may be any traumatic disruption of the spinal cord. Common spinal cord injuries are vertebral fractures and dislocations, such as those suffered by individuals involved in car accidents, sports injuries, and other violent impacts. Injury to the cervical spinal cord may result in quadriplegia, whereas injury to the thoracic and lumbar spinal cord may result in paraplegia. Symptoms include paresthesia or anesthesia, and signs are paralysis below the level of injury with loss of bowel and bladder control. When the injury to the spinal cord is incomplete, the signs and symptoms are variable with perhaps some sensation and movement that correlates to the location and extent of injury.

Head Injury

Craniocerebral injury, or head injury, can result from primary or secondary injury to the head. Primary injury occurs when the head is subjected to traumatic forces. Head injuries may be open or closed. Open head injuries result from fractures or penetrating wounds; closed head injuries result from blunt head injury producing cerebral concussion, contusion, or laceration. Manifestations of head injury are variable depending on the severity of the trauma and the areas of the brain involved.

Parkinson's Disease

Degeneration of the brain's dopamine-producing neurons in the substantia nigra of the basal ganglia may lead to Parkinson's disease. It is a chronic, slowly progressive disease characterized by resting tremor, bradykinesia, and rigidity. Other manifestations include masklike facies, trunk-forward flexion, muscle weakness, shuffling gait, and finger pill-rolling tremor (Fig. 25-29; see Fig. 25-6 earlier in this chapter).

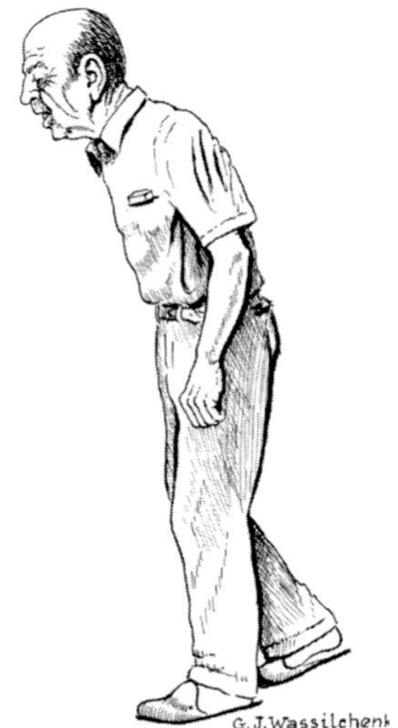

Fig. 25-29 Posture and shuffling gait associated with Parkinson's disease. (From Rudy, 1984.)

Cerebrovascular Accident

Stroke or brain attack are other names for CVA. It occurs when a cerebral blood vessel is occluded by a thrombus or embolus or when cerebrovascular hemorrhage occurs. These mechanisms result in ischemia of the brain tissue. Manifestations depend on which areas of the brain are involved and the extent of ischemic area. For example, ischemia to the frontal lobe on the left side of the brain may result in paralysis of the right arm or leg.

Aphasia

Injury to the speech areas of the left hemisphere of the brain may result in absent or impaired language. Damage often occurs as a consequence of a CVA but may also occur following head injury or intracranial surgery, depending on the area of the procedure. When Broca's area in the frontal lobe (see Fig. 25-3) is affected, the client may develop a type of aphasia called expressive or motor, in which the client can understand what is said but cannot express or formulate a response. When Wernicke's area in the temporal lobe (see Fig. 25-3) is affected, the client may develop a type of aphasia called receptive or sensory, in which the client cannot understand spoken or written words. Most aphasias are mixed with some impairment of both understanding and speaking. Global aphasia may occur when a large area of the brain is involved and the client is unable to understand or speak. The term dysphasia is used to describe impaired communication that is not as severe as aphasia.

DISORDERS OF THE PERIPHERAL NERVOUS SYSTEM

Myasthenia Gravis

This neuromuscular disease is characterized by abnormal weakness of voluntary muscles that improves with rest and administration of anticholinesterase drugs. The receptor sites for acetylcholine at the myoneuronal junctions are destroyed by autoantibodies against them, resulting in the muscle weakness. Signs and symptoms vary with the type of myasthenia. Ocular myasthenia produces muscle weakness confined to the muscles of the eye. Ptosis and diplopia are common clinical manifestations. Generalized myasthenia produces weakness of face, limbs, and trunk, including the muscles of breathing. Bulbar myasthenia involves cranial nerves IX, X, XI, and XII, which involves muscles needed for swallowing. Clients often aspirate saliva and other fluids due to impaired swallowing.

Guillain-Barré Syndrome

This acute syndrome is characterized by widespread demyelination of nerves of the peripheral nervous system due to a cell-mediated autoimmune response. Clients usually have a viral infection weeks before onset. Symptoms often begin with weakness and paresthesia in the lower extremities and ascend the body to the upper extremities and face. When paralysis reaches the thorax, respiratory depression may result.

DISORDERS OF CHILDREN

Hydrocephalus

When flow of cerebrospinal fluid is obstructed (usually between the third and fourth ventricles) the build-up of fluid increases intracranial pressure, resulting in hydrocephalus. Since the cranial bones are malleable during infancy, the head circumference increases. The infant is irritable, lethargic, and has a shrill cry. *Sunset eyes* is a term used to describe the paresis of upward gaze (Fig. 25-30). With surgical intervention, deficits may be reversed.

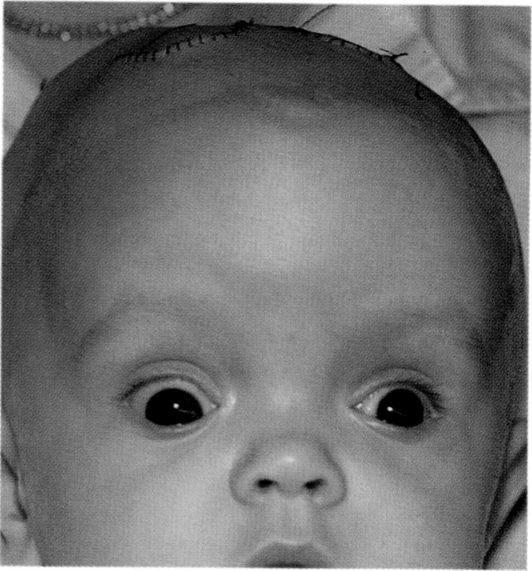

Fig 25-30 Infantile hydrocephalus. Paresis of upward gaze is seen in the infant with hydrocephalus due to stenosis of the aqueduct between the third and fourth ventricles. This finding is often called sunset eyes. (From Zitelli and Davis, 1997. Courtesy Dr. Albert Biglan, Children's Hospital, Pittsburgh.)

Cerebral Palsy

This is a motor function disorder caused by a permanent, nonprogressive brain defect or lesion present at birth or shortly thereafter. It is usually associated with premature or abnormal birth and intrapartum asphyxia, causing damage to the central nervous system. The neurologic deficits vary widely from involvement of one extremity to all extremities and mental deficit. Deficits may include spasticity, paralysis, seizures, varying degrees of mental retardation, and impaired vision, speech, and hearing.

Attention Deficit Hyperactivity Disorder

This disorder is a combination of behavior problems that interfere with a child's ability to learn. It is characterized by impulsivity, inattention, and motor restlessness. Because these signs are typically seen in preschoolers, a diagnosis usually cannot be made until at least 5 years of age. Indications of inattention include frequent forgetfulness, distractibility, poor attention to detail, and difficulty in maintaining attention. Indications of hyperactivity include excessive talking, motor restlessness, difficulty remaining seated, interrupting others, and impatience. These manifestations may continue into adulthood.

CLINICAL APPLICATION and CRITICAL THINKING

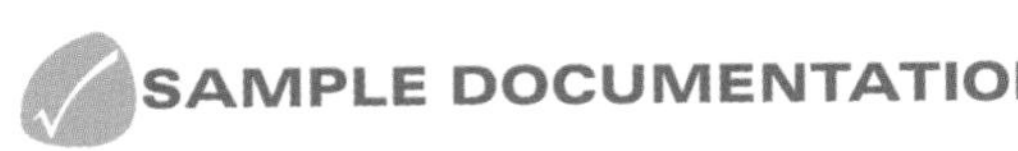

SAMPLE DOCUMENTATION

CASE 1

H.S. is a 60-year-old woman presenting with foot injury.

Subjective Data

H.S. dropped hammer on left foot yesterday helping her husband with repairs to their one-story home. Applied ice and elevated foot. Had cerebrovascular accident 18 months ago with left-sided paralysis. History of multiple accidents since then; H.S. states she will not give up her independence. History of hypertension; family history of CVA.

Objective Data

Blood pressure, 138/88 mm Hg; Pulse, 88 beats/min; Respiratory rate, 14; Temperature, 98.8° F (37.1° C).

Cooperative, alert woman in wheelchair accompanied by husband. Communicates and dresses appropriately. CN I-XII intact.

Upper extremity (UE): Voluntary, symmetric, coordinated movement with full range of motion, sensation to vibration, cotton, sharp object bilaterally.

Lower extremity (LE): Right, voluntary, symmetric, coordinated movement with full range of motion, sensation to vibration, cotton, sharp object. Left, paralysis and anesthesia; dorsum of foot edematous, erythematous, no sensation.

Cerebellum: Alternating movement both arms; right heel down left leg. Deep tendon reflexes 2+ bilaterally.

Functional Health Patterns Involved

- Health perception–health management
- Activity–exercise

Medical Diagnosis

Hematoma dorsum left foot; previous right CVA

Nursing Diagnosis and Collaborative Problems

- *Impaired physical mobility* related to altered sensory and neuromuscular status as manifested by:
  - Paralysis and loss of sensation of left leg from stroke.
  - Uses wheelchair.
- *Risk for injury, trauma* related to desire to be as independent as possible.

CASE 2

M.G. is an 8-year-old girl presenting with seizures.

Subjective Data

Mother states M.G. was at home watching television when she started "shaking and jerking all over." Mother estimates this lasted several minutes. M.G. slept an hour after the seizure. This incident occurred several hours ago. Mother states that M.G. has had a seizure before but not in 4 years. M.G. states she feels "fine." Expresses fear about M.G.'s safety at school. Denies history of recent headaches or problems with balance.

Objective Data

Blood pressure, 110/68 mm Hg; Pulse, 84 beats/min; Respiratory rate, 18; Temperature, 98.6° F (37° C).

Cooperative, alert child with flat affect. Communicates slowly but appropriately. PERRLA; CN I-XII intact.

Extremities (upper and lower): Voluntary, symmetric, coordinated movement with full range of motion, sensation to vibration, cotton, pinprick bilaterally. Deep tendon reflexes 2+ bilaterally.

Functional Health Patterns Involved

- Health perception–health management

Medical Diagnosis

Seizure disorder

Nursing Diagnosis and Collaborative Problems

- *Risk for injury* related to tonic-clonic movements secondary to seizures.
- *Fear* related to child's safety when at school as manifested by:
  - Fear verbalized.
  - Child had seizure today.

CRITICAL THINKING QUESTIONS

1. Kevin uses an unfolded paper clip to test peripheral two-point discrimination. He adjusts the paper clip so that the points are 1 inch apart. With this instrument, he tests the client's fingertips, palm, toe, and abdomen. He reports that the client fails to discriminate between one and two points in each of these areas. Kevin concludes that the client has some sort of peripheral sensory deficit. What is incorrect in Kevin's methods and/or conclusion?
2. You are performing a neurologic assessment on a client who has a brain tumor in the central nervous system. Your findings reveal that this client has the following deficits: inability to taste in posterior tongue; when the client says "ah," the uvula does not rise; when he protrudes his tongue, it does not move; and when he shrugs his shoulders, they feel weak. Which part of the nervous system do these abnormal findings represent? What is your rationale for this conclusion?
3. The following objective data were documented on a client. Sense of smell intact, vision 20/20, peripheral vision and EOM intact, PERRLA. Face is symmetric with strong muscles bilaterally; sensation and movement present and symmetric. Hears 25% of words whispered, BC > AC, lateralization of sound is to the left. Able to taste; gag reflex present; tongue movement symmetric; and shoulder muscles strong and symmetric bilaterally.
   a. What are the abnormal findings?
   b. Which cranial nerve is impaired?
4. You are performing an assessment of an adolescent who has an incomplete spinal cord injury (the spinal cord is not totally severed). In assessing sensation, you discover that this client has sensation to deep stimuli on the right upper outer thigh but not on the medial aspect of the lower thigh. On the left leg the client has sensation on the upper outer thigh and medial aspect of the lower thigh but not on the medial aspect of the left lower leg. Use the dermatome map (see Fig. 25-10) to determine the location of the spinal cord lesion.

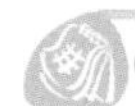

CASE STUDY

Leroy Thomas is a 64-year-old man admitted to the hospital with a diagnosis of acute CVA. Listed below are data collected by the examiner during an interview and examination.

Interview Data

Mr. Thomas's wife tells the examiner that he was fine until this morning when he suddenly had a headache, fell to the floor, and could not get up. Mrs. Thomas adds that her husband only made mumbling noises, and she could not understand him.

Examination Data

Neurologic examination: Awake, alert man. Unable to talk, but able to follow commands. Client cries and avoids eye contact with his wife and the examiner.

Cranial nerves I, II, III, IV, V, VI, VII, VIII intact. Client has asymmetry and unequal movements of face, with a drooping of the left side of face. Has asymmetry of shoulder shrug, with weakness noted on left side. Supination and pronation of right hand, unable to perform with left hand. Light touch with sharp and dull sensation present on right arm and leg, no sensation of left arm or leg. Right arm and leg muscle strength $\frac{5}{5}$, left arm muscle tone $\frac{0}{5}$, left leg $\frac{1}{5}$. Unable to move around in bed unassisted at this time. Assessment of balance deferred.

1. What data deviate from normal findings, suggesting a need for further investigation?
2. What additional information should the nurse ask or assess for?
3. In what functional health patterns does data deviate from normal?
4. What nursing diagnoses and/or collaborative problems should be considered for this situation?

REMEMBER to check out your companion CD-ROM

26 Assessment of the Pregnant Client

www.mosby.com/MERLIN/wilson/assessment/

The health assessment of the pregnant client warrants special attention because of the multiple hormonal, structural, and physiologic changes associated with pregnancy. Physical changes that occur during pregnancy are noted with both a history and an examination. This chapter builds on previous chapters regarding taking a health history and the sequence of examination.

ANATOMY AND PHYSIOLOGY

The maternal physiologic adaptations occurring during pregnancy are a result of hormones of pregnancy and mechanical pressures caused by the enlarging uterus and other tissues. These changes affect most body systems. They protect the woman's physiologic functioning with the increased metabolic demands associated with pregnancy and also provide a protective environment for the growing fetus.

ENDOCRINE SYSTEM

Elevated levels of estrogen and progesterone occur throughout pregnancy. These hormones have pronounced effects throughout the body. Early in pregnancy, the corpus luteum is the primary producer of hormones; after 10 to 12 weeks, the placenta takes over this role. Progesterone is essential to maintaining the endometrium for implantation and in preventing shedding of the endometrium (with the loss of the embryo) after implantation. Progesterone also relaxes smooth muscles in the uterus to prevent uterine contractility. Estrogen stimulates growth of the uterus and breasts, increases vascularity to these tissues, and promotes relaxation of the pelvic ligaments and joints later in pregnancy.

In addition to estrogen and progesterone, a number of other hormones are involved during pregnancy. Prolactin, a hormone from the anterior pituitary, is responsible for lactation. Oxytocin, a hormone from the posterior pituitary, stimulates uterine contractions as the fetus matures and stimulates the milk ejection reflex after delivery. Human placental lactogen (hPL) acts as a growth hormone, contributes to changes within the breast, and increases maternal metabolism of glucose and fatty acids to ensure adequate glucose supply to the mother and fetus. The parathyroid gland increases parathormone production slightly, increasing calcium and vitamin D absorption to meet the fetal requirements during skeletal development. Glandular tissue hyperplasia and increased vascularity cause a slight enlargement of the thyroid gland (Cunningham et al, 1997). Although thyroid function tests are slightly altered, thyroid function remains unchanged.

REPRODUCTIVE SYSTEM

Uterus

The most noticeable change during pregnancy is uterine growth. This growth is demonstrated by an increase in size, weight, and capacity. During the first trimester of pregnancy uterine enlargement is due to the increased levels of estrogen and progesterone. After the third month, uterine growth is largely due to the growth of the fetus.

As the uterus becomes larger and more ovoid, the muscular walls become thicker and more elastic, and the uterus rises out of the pelvic area. The fundus (top of the uterus) is usually palpated above the symphysis pubis around the twelfth week of gestation (Lowdermilk et al, 1999). By 22 to 24 weeks the fundus is at the umbilicus, and by 36 to 38 weeks, the fundus is at the level of the xiphoid process. Fundal height generally decreases slightly during the last 2 weeks of gestation as the fetus begins to descend or engage into the pelvis. This fetal descent is also referred to as lightening (Fig. 26-1).

An increase in the blood flow to the uterus causes other significant changes. Within the first few weeks of pregnancy, the cervix turns a bluish color (known as Chadwick's sign). At approximately the sixth week of gestation, the cervix undergoes slight hypertrophy and softening (known as Goodell's sign). By 7 to 8 weeks of gestation, increased blood flow causes the lower segment of the uterus (known as the isthmus) to become soft and easily compressed with bimanual examination (known as Hegar's sign).

After delivery, the uterus returns to a nonpregnant state—a process known as involution. This process begins with expulsion of the placenta and occurs rapidly over several days after delivery. By the ninth postpartum day, the uterus should not be palpable abdominally and should lie within the true pelvis once again (Wong and Perry, 1998).

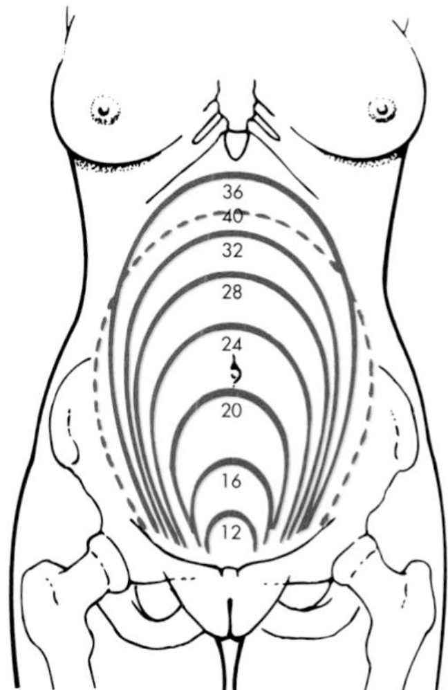

Fig. 26-1 Changes in fundal height with pregnancy. Weeks 10-12, uterus within pelvis; Week 12, uterus palpable just above symphysis pubis; Week 16, uterus palpable halfway between symphysis and umbilicus; Week 20, uterine fundus at lower border of umbilicus; Weeks 24-26, palpable just above the umbilicus, fetus palpable; Week 28, uterus approximately halfway between umbilicus and xiphoid; fetus easily palpable; Week 34, uterine fundus just below xiphoid; Week 36, fundus reaches maximum height; Weeks 36-40, fundal height drops as fetus begins to engage in pelvis (lightening). (From Seidel et al, 1999.)

Female Genitalia

An increase in blood flow causes a bluish violet color change to the vagina and vulva, similar to the color changes of the cervix. Hormone production stimulates the vaginal walls to thicken and vaginal secretions to increase. Leukorrhea, a grayish white mucoid vaginal discharge, is produced. The pH of vaginal secretions increases from 4 to 6.5 (Lowdermilk et al, 1999).

After delivery, vaginal discharge (lochia) is dark red for 1 to 3 days (lochia rubra), then pink-brown with no clots for 5 to 7 days (lochia serosa), then yellow-brown or yellow-white and odorless for 1 to 3 weeks (lochia alba). Breast-feeding may accelerate the progress through these stages.

BREASTS

The breasts undergo significant changes during the course of pregnancy in response to hormonal stimulation. During the early weeks of pregnancy, the woman notices fullness or heaviness of the breasts with increased sensitivity. As the pregnancy continues, the lactiferous ducts multiply rapidly, and the alveoli increase greatly in size and number; as a result, the breasts enlarge. As the size of the breast increases, striae (also known as stretch marks) may appear. During this time, the nipples and areolae become more prominent and deeply pigmented. Montgomery's glands or tubercles often become more apparent as sebaceous glands hypertrophy. Increased mammary vascularization causes veins to become engorged and visible as a blue network beneath the skin's surface. Colostrum, a creamy yellow-white fluid is formed by the breasts during pregnancy. It may be expressed from the nipples as early as 16 weeks; however, most of it is produced near the end of pregnancy.

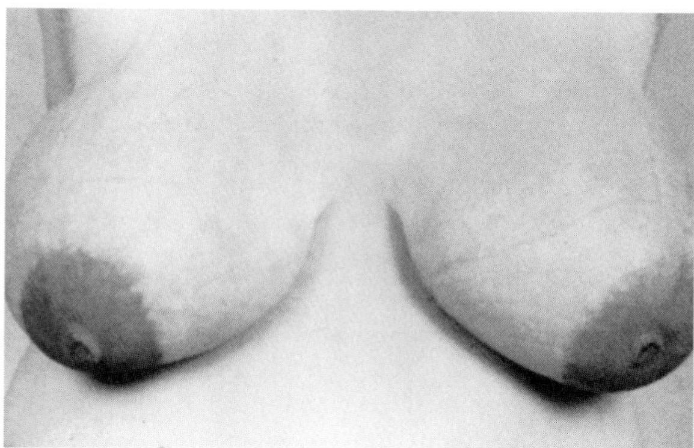

Fig. 26-2 Breast engorgement. (From Isaacs, 1992.)

Small amounts of colostrum are secreted from the breasts during the first few days after delivery. Colostrum contains more minerals and proteins than mature milk, as well as antibodies and other host resistance factors. Between 2 and 4 days after delivery, mature milk production begins to replace colostrum. The breasts may become full, tense, and edematous, resulting in breast engorgement (Fig. 26-2).

Breasts undergo involution—a process in which the breast returns to a nonpregnant or nonlactating state. Involution occurs over a period of about 3 months after the termination of lactation, or after delivery in women who do not breast-feed their infants.

INTEGUMENT SYSTEM

An increase in blood flow to the skin increases vasodilation and the number of capillaries. The hands and feet may take on a reddened appearance, and vascularities may be noted on the skin. Sweat and sebaceous gland activities also increase to help relieve the extra heat caused by increased metabolic activity. The skin thickens, and there is an increase in subcutaneous fat. As the skin stretches, connective tissues may separate, causing characteristic stretch marks (striae).

Hormonal changes, stimulated by the anterior pituitary hormone melanotropin, is responsible for increased pigmentation of the skin, particularly to the nipples, areolae, axillae, and vulva. This change is referred to as chloasma, or the "mask of pregnancy." Another common pigmentation change is linea nigra, a dark pigmented line on the abdomen extending from the top of the fundus to the symphysis pubis (Lowdermilk et al, 1999) (Fig. 26-3).

A change in hair and nail growth may occur during pregnancy. Some women experience faster hair growth or excessive growth of fine hair in unusual places such as on the face

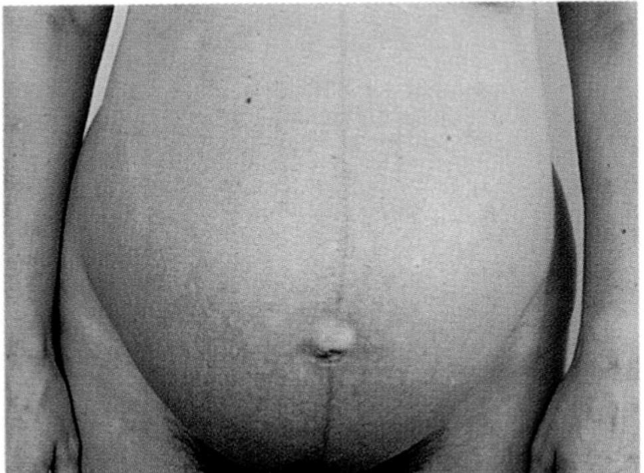

Fig. 26-3 Linea nigra on abdomen. (From Seidel et al, 1999.)

or chest, but this usually disappears after pregnancy. Other women may notice a decrease in hair growth or may notice an increase in hair loss. Changes in rates of hair growth or hair loss are not universal as many women do not notice any such changes.

LUNGS AND RESPIRATORY SYSTEM

Changes in the pregnant woman's respiratory function are due to both mechanical and hormonal alterations. Most of these changes are not evident in the early months of pregnancy. However, as the uterus enlarges, it pushes the diaphragm upward, putting pressure on the lungs and causing, in some cases, shortness of breath and an increased respiratory rate. Breathing becomes more thoracic than abdominal, and the thoracic cage widens. The effects of estrogen allow the ligaments of the ribs to relax, allowing an increase in chest size. The transverse diameter of the thoracic cage increases by 2 cm (¾ inch), causing the costal angle to increase (Cunningham, 1997). An increase in the level of progesterone may stimulate an increased tidal volume (deeper inspiration). After delivery, the chest wall may remain wider, not returning to its prepregnancy state, although all respiratory characteristics should return to their prepregnancy states.

Elevated levels of estrogen may cause increased vascularity of the upper respiratory tract, engorging the capillaries of the nose, pharynx, and eustachian tubes.

HEART AND PERIPHERAL VASCULAR SYSTEM

During pregnancy, the volume of blood increases to meet the blood needs of the enlarged uterus, as well as the fetal tissues. The degree of blood-volume expansion is variable, but typically the volume will increase by 1500 ml, or 40% to 50% above nonpregnancy levels (Cunningham et al, 1997). The increase in blood volume peaks between weeks 32 and 34.

The workload of the heart increases because of the increased blood volume and increased tissue demands of the maternal and fetal tissues. Heart rate and cardiac output increase, but these compensatory changes do not occur until sometime during the second trimester.

Another notable change to the heart during pregnancy is its position. As the uterus increases in size, it pushes up

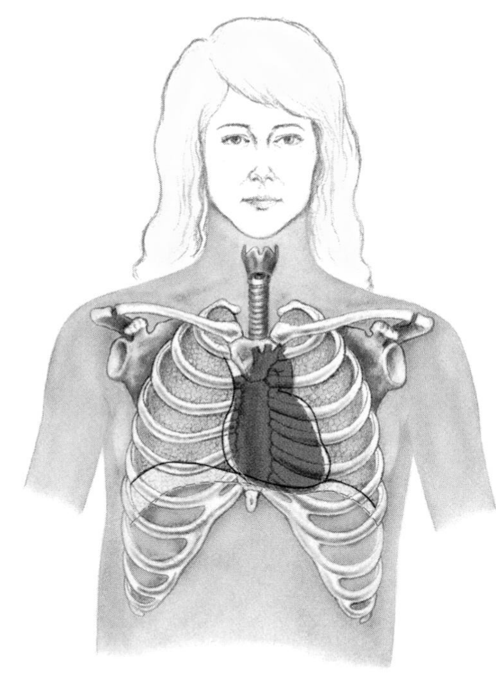

Fig. 26-4 Changes in position of heart, lungs, and thoracic cage during pregnancy. *Broken line,* nonpregnant; *solid line,* changes during pregnancy. (From Lowdermilk, Perry, and Bobak, 1999.)

on the diaphragm, shifting the heart upward and forward and rotating the heart so the apex moves slightly laterally (Fig. 26-4).

Maternal blood pressure remains constant throughout most of the pregnancy. During the second trimester, blood pressure may drop slightly, due to peripheral vasodilation, but it should return to normal ranges by the third trimester. Maternal anxiety and position can affect the blood pressure. Blood pressure is highest when the woman is sitting and lowest when lying in a lateral recumbent position (Reeder et al, 1997).

Edema of the lower extremities and varicosities in the legs frequently occur during pregnancy. These are caused by blood pooling in the lower extremities because of occlusion of pelvic veins and inferior vena cava from pressure created by the enlarged uterus.

GASTROINTESTINAL SYSTEM

Changes in hormone levels contribute to a number of gastrointestinal symptoms. Early in pregnancy, a rise in human chorionic gonadotropin (HCG) causes nausea and vomiting, often referred to as morning sickness. Heartburn, constipation, and increased flatus are common symptoms later in the pregnancy, all caused by a combination of progesterone and displacement of abdominal contents by the growing uterus. Progesterone causes decreased tone and motility of smooth muscles. The colon and appendix are pushed toward the back of the abdomen, and the stomach is displaced

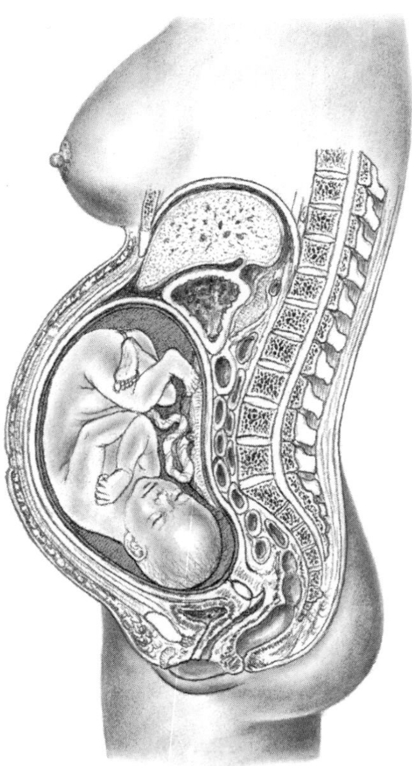

Fig. 26-5 Displacement of abdominal organs in last month of pregnancy. (From Lowdermilk, Perry, and Bobak, 1999.)

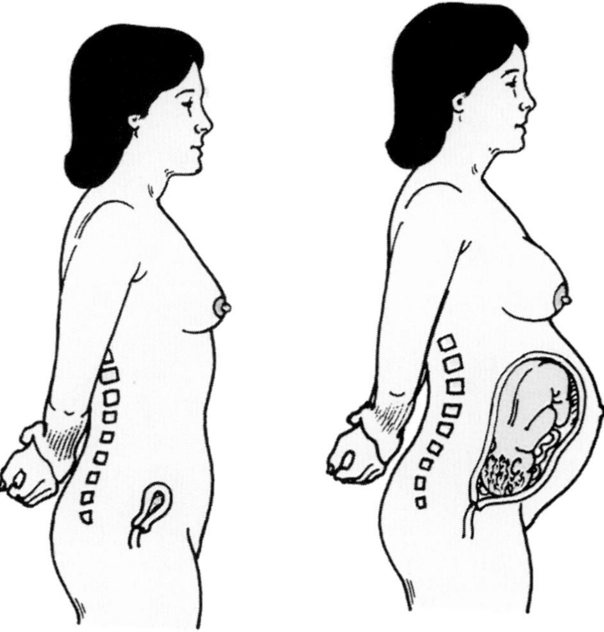

Fig. 26-6 Lordosis during pregnancy. (From Lowdermilk, Perry, and Bobak, 1999.)

upward. These factors cause a decrease in peristalsis and esophageal regurgitation (Fig. 26-5).

In the mouth, connective gum tissue increases in vascularity and proliferation, causing many women to experience bleeding gums.

Hemorrhoids are another common problem reported by pregnant women, caused by increased pelvis vascularity and pressure as well as constipation. Increased incidence of gallstones during pregnancy may be due to a combination of gallbladder distention, decreased emptying time, bile thickening, and hypercholesterolemia.

RENAL SYSTEM

The kidney, ureters, and bladder undergo changes during pregnancy caused by estrogen, progesterone, and pressure from the growing uterus and changes in blood volume.

The size of the kidney increases slightly, and the increase in blood volume and hormonal influences result in an increase in renal blood flow and glomerular filtration rate (Cunningham et al, 1997). Nocturia and urinary frequency are commonly reported symptoms caused by pressure of the uterus on the urinary bladder. The renal pelvis and ureters dilate, resulting in a larger volume of accumulated urine within the pelvis and ureters and slowing urine flow. This urinary stasis increases the woman's risk of urinary tract infection. For reasons not well understood, tubular reabsorption of glucose is impaired, causing a mild glycosuria (glucose in the urine).

MUSCULOSKELETAL SYSTEM

Like other body systems, the musculoskeletal system undergoes changes during pregnancy because of hormonal influences and changes caused by a growing fetus. Changes in spinal curvature occur with a tipping of the pelvis forward and a shift of the center of gravity forward. The increased spinal curvature is known as lordosis (Fig. 26-6).

Hormonal activity also contributes to a softening and strengthening of the pelvic ligaments, allowing the pelvic joints to separate slightly for increased mobility. In addition, ligaments and joints of the spine soften under hormonal influence, causing more strain and pelvic instability. Many women experience back discomfort and gait and balance problems, especially with advanced pregnancy. Young well-muscled women may adapt to these changes without any discomfort, whereas older women, those with a previous back disorder, or women who are obese prior to pregnancy may have a considerable amount of back pain during pregnancy (Lowdermilk et al, 1999).

As the uterus enlarges, the abdominal muscles stretch and lose some of their tone. During the third trimester, the recti abdominis muscles may separate, allowing the abdominal contents to protrude at the midline, creating a condition known as diastasis recti abdominis (Fig. 26-7). Although the muscles gradually regain their tone after pregnancy, diastasis recti abdominis may persist.

In the second half of pregnancy, temporary blood shunting and hypocalcemia may cause muscle cramps, usually in the calf, thigh, or gluteal muscles, especially at night or after awakening and initiating movement. After delivery, posture and comfort should soon return to the prepregnancy state.

CHANGES IN NUTRITIONAL NEEDS

Weight gain during pregnancy is a marker of adequate calorie intake. A weight gain of 25 to 35 lb can be expected as the fetus grows, with 3 lb expected in the first trimester, 12 lb in the second, and 12 lb in the third. The weight gain is attributed to the fetus 7.5 lb (3.4 kg), placenta and membranes 1.5 lb (.7 kg), amniotic fluid 2 lb (.9 kg), uterus 2.5 lb (1.1 kg), breast enlargement 3 lb (1.4 kg), increased blood volume 2 to 4 lb (.9 to 1.8 kg), and extravascular fluid volume and fat reserves (4 to 9 lb). Using prenatal weight and height values, a body mass index can be calculated (see Fig. 10-4 in Chapter 10). Based on the client's body mass index, an appropriate weight gain goal for the pregnancy can be determined.

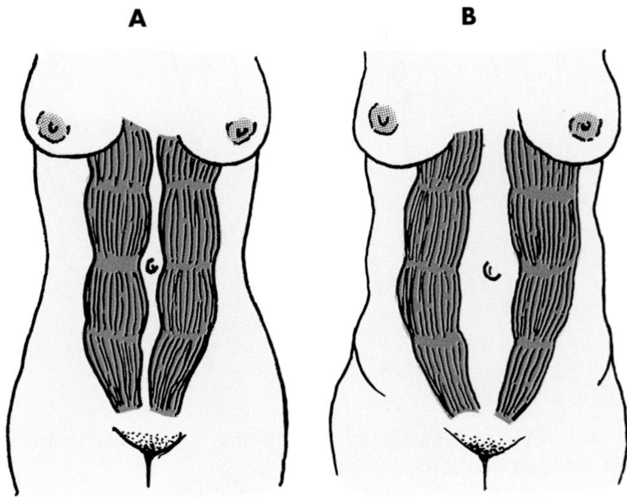

Fig. 26-7 Possible changes in rectus abdominis muscles during pregnancy. **A,** Normal position in nonpregnant woman. **B,** Diastasis recti abdominis in pregnant woman. (From Lowdermilk, Perry, and Bobak, 1999.)

To achieve ideal weight gain goals, an extra 300 calories per day is recommended for the second and third trimesters of pregnancy. Additional protein, calcium, phosphorus, folate, and iron intake is essential for a healthy pregnancy. Nutrient needs are actually greater with lactation than with pregnancy. The lactating woman must consume an additional 500 calories per day over nonpregnant requirements. Significant increases in protein, vitamins A and C, niacin, folate, calcium, phosphorus, and iodine are necessary. Specific nutritional recommendations during pregnancy and lactation are presented in Table 10-2 in Chapter 10.

Biochemical tests are frequently used to assess the nutritional status of pregnant women. Hematocrit and hemoglobin level should be assessed to screen for iron deficiency anemia. A pregnant woman is considered anemic if the hemoglobin level is less than 11.0 g/dl and hematocrit is less than 33 g/dl in the first and third trimesters. A normal value for serum albumin is greater than or equal to 3.0 g/dl in pregnancy. Laboratory values below normal may reflect protein-calorie malnutrition. There are multiple causes of decreased albumin levels. Low albumin should be interpreted cautiously as a reflection of malnutrition.

Fluid status may affect the accuracy of the laboratory value because excess fluid causes hemodilution, which lowers the hemoglobin, hematocrit, and albumin levels. Alter-

Table 26-1 Signs of Pregnancy

CATEGORY	SIGN	TIME OF OCCURRENCE (GESTATION)
Presumptive signs	Breast fullness/tenderness	3-4 weeks
	Amenorrhea	4 weeks
	Nausea, vomiting	4-12 weeks
	Urinary frequency	6-12 weeks
	Quickening	16-20 weeks
Probable signs	Goodell's sign	5 weeks
	Chadwick's sign	6-8 weeks
	Hegar's sign	6-12 weeks
	Positive pregnancy test	
	Serum	4-12 weeks
	Urine	6-12 weeks
	Ballottement	16-28 weeks
Positive signs	Visualization of fetus by ultrasound	5-6 weeks
	Auscultation of fetal heart tones	
	Doppler	8-17 weeks
	Fetoscope	17-19 weeks
	Palpation of fetal movements	19-22 weeks
	Observable fetal movements	Late pregnancy

ations in lipoprotein metabolism occur normally with pregnancy. Elevated cholesterol and triglyceride values do not require dietary intervention during pregnancy.

SIGNS OF PREGNANCY

Many of the physiologic changes discussed in the previous section are recognized as signs and symptoms of pregnancy. Traditionally, signs and symptoms of pregnancy have been placed in three categories: (1) presumptive symptoms—symptoms experienced by the woman, (2) probable signs—changes observed by an examiner, and (3) positive signs—findings that prove the presence of a fetus. Table 26-1 lists the signs of pregnancy by category and when they may become evident.

A combination of laboratory tests and the signs of pregnancy usually make the clinical diagnosis. The laboratory tests most commonly used detect an antigen-antibody reaction between HCG hormone and an antiserum. These tests are very sensitive and are available for use by both health professionals and laypersons.

HEALTH HISTORY

Pregnant Client

The history of the pregnant client is similar to that of the adult (see Chapter 4). The general physical and psychologic health of the mother and the presence of chronic diseases could affect her health and that of the fetus. The health history should also assess for prenatal risk factors. A health history should be conducted on the client at the first prenatal visit to establish a baseline; it can then be updated as needed with subsequent visits. Prenatal visits are recommended every 4 weeks up to 28 weeks' gestation, every 2 weeks from 28 to 36 weeks' gestation, and weekly after 36 weeks' gestation.

BIOGRAPHIC DATA

- *Age:* Note if woman is under 18 or over 40 years of age.
- *Culture:* Include beliefs, customs, and expectations regarding pregnancy and the birthing process.
- Occupation and socioeconomic factors, including health insurance information.
- Persons living in home: number of other children in the home, presence of partner, name of support persons for labor, delivery, and child rearing.

RISK FACTORS

COMMON RISK FACTORS ASSOCIATED WITH High-Risk Pregnancy

MATERNAL CHARACTERISTICS

Age: Under 18 or over 40
Marital status: Single (or lack of supporting relationship)
Height: Short stature (less than 5 feet tall or 150 cm)
Weight: Weigh less than 100 lb (4.5 kg), or over 200 lb (91 kg)
Socioeconomic: Poverty, low education level

MATERNAL HABITS

Alcohol consumption
Drug use
Failure to obtain prenatal care
Smoking
High-risk sexual behaviors

OBSTETRIC HISTORY

Previous birth to infant weighing less than 2500 g
Previous birth to infant weighing more than 4000 g
Previous pregnancy ending in perinatal death
More than two previous abortions
Birth to infant with congenital or perinatal disease
Birth to infant with isoimmunization or ABO incompatibility

CURRENT MEDICAL PROBLEMS

Chronic illnesses, including diabetes mellitus, endocrine disorder, heart disease, hypertension, pulmonary disease, renal failure, sickle cell disease
Sexually transmitted infection
Infectious disease (such as rubella or cytomegalovirus)

SYMPTOMS WITH CURRENT PREGNANCY

Anemia
Bleeding
Pregnancy-induced hypertension (PIH)
Eclampsia or preeclampsia
Fetal position breech or transverse at term
Polyhydramnios
Multiple pregnancy
Postmaturity
Premature rupture of membranes
Weight gain that is inadequate or excessive

Table 26-2 Determining Gravidity and Parity Using a Five-Digit (GTPAL) System

CONDITION	G GRAVIDA	T TERM BIRTH	P PRETERM BIRTH	A ABORTIONS	L LIVING CHILDREN
Woman pregnant for the first time.	1	0	0	0	0
Woman who has carried her first pregnancy to term, and the infant survives.	1	1	0	0	1
Woman who is currently pregnant for the second time; has one child from the first pregnancy born full term.	2	1	0	0	1
Woman who has been pregnant twice; has one child who was born preterm and had one miscarriage.	2	0	1	1	1
Woman who has been pregnant once and delivered full-term twins.	1	1	0	0	2

Modified from Lowdermilk DL, Perry SE, Bobak IM: *Maternity and women's health care,* ed 7, St. Louis, 2000, Mosby.

REASON FOR SEEKING CARE

The pregnant woman may be seeking prenatal care or may have a specific problem. Prenatal visits are needed to monitor the health of the mother and the growth of the fetus, as well as to educate the mother and family about the care of mother and neonate during the delivery process and neonatal period.

PRESENT HEALTH STATUS

Data collected are the same as was discussed in Chapter 4. Data specific to the pregnant woman include her present general physical and psychologic well-being and motherhood coping abilities. Also, it is essential to determine what medications (both prescriptive and over-the-counter) the client uses.

PAST HEALTH HISTORY

Data collected in this section are the same as was discussed in Chapter 4. It is especially important to note any chronic illness such as diabetes, thyroid or cardiovascular conditions, renal disease, and depression, in addition to other current risks the pregnant client may have.

FAMILY HISTORY

In addition to the family history described in Chapter 4, a pregnant woman's family history should specifically address the childbearing history of her mother and sister(s), including multiple births; chromosome abnormalities such as Down syndrome; genetic disorders; congenital disorders; and chronic illness such as diabetes mellitus or renal disease and cancer.

Gynecologic and Obstetric History

General information regarding the reproductive system, such as problems with menstruation, infections, painful intercourse, and sexual patterns, should be included. See Chapter 21 for specific information.

Information regarding the current pregnancy and past pregnancies is included in the history. Determine the exact date of the last menstrual period (LMP). This date is used to estimate expected delivery date.

Two systems are used to document an obstetric history, one using two digits and another using five digits. The two-digit system documents a woman's obstetric history by gravidity (G) (number of pregnancies, including current pregnancy) and parity (P) (number of pregnancies in which the fetus has reached viability or after 20 weeks). If a woman has one child and is now pregnant for the second time, one would document G 2, P1 (Wong and Perry, 1998). The five-digit system is more much more detailed. The first digit is for gravidity (as discussed above); the second is for full-term births (T); the third indicates the number of preterm births (P); the fourth is for abortions (A) (both spontaneous "miscarriages" and "therapeutic" pregnancy interruptions); and finally, the fifth digit indicates the number of living children (L) (Wong and Perry, 1998; Lowdermilk et al, 1999). The acronym GTPAL may be of help in remembering this system of documentation (Table 26-2).

The obstetric history also includes specific data regarding each pregnancy. Document the following information for each pregnancy:

- The course of the pregnancy (including the duration of gestation, date of delivery, significant problems or complications)
- The process of labor (including manner in which labor was started [i.e., spontaneous or induced], length of labor, complications associated with labor)
- The delivery (presentation of the infant, the method of delivery [i.e., vaginal or cesarean section], and pain management strategies used for delivery, if any)
- Condition of the infant at birth (including weight)
- Postpartum course (including any maternal or infant problems)

CULTURAL NOTE

Cultural diversity should be taken into account with dietary assessment. An understanding of how different foods are viewed is important. Specific foods may be considered healthful or harmful during pregnancy and lactation by some cultures. For instance, in some cultures, eating hot foods is believed to provide warmth for the fetus and enable the baby to be born into a warm, loving environment. Additionally, many cultural groups believe certain cravings for foods should be met while pregnant to avoid harm to the baby (Purnell and Paulanka, 1998).

Box 26-1 Focus on Pain: Childbirth

Most women have some concerns about pain during the childbirth process. Green (1993) reported that 67% of women were a "bit worried" about such pain, 12% were "very worried," and 23% were "not at all worried." The discomfort and pain associated with childbirth are unique not only to each woman, but also as a pain experience in itself. Compared with other known painful events or experiences, the potential for achieving satisfactory pain relief is high because of the uniqueness of this pain experience (Reeder et al, 1997). Unique points include:

- The woman knows the pain will happen.
- The woman knows approximately when (within a week or so) the pain will happen.
- The woman knows there will be a predictable pattern to the pain.
- The woman knows there is a time limit to the pain experience (hours as opposed to days or weeks) and that it will end.
- The woman knows there is a tangible end product associated with the birth (i.e., the birth of her child).

Nutritional History

A woman's nutritional status during pregnancy affects maternal and fetal health. An understanding of the women's normal dietary practices is essential for nutritional assessment. Cultural diversity should be taken into account when evaluating dietary practices. The use of a nutrition questionnaire as a screening tool for dietary assessment is helpful. A 24-hour recall, food frequency, food checklists, and diet records are all useful tools for obtaining nutrient intake information.

Clients should be interviewed regarding food allergies or intolerance. Development of an individualized meal pattern may be necessary to ensure nutrient needs are met if the client must avoid particular foods or food groups. Lactose intolerance is a commonly reported problem.

Dietary assessment should also include questions regarding ingestion of nonnutritive substances known as pica. Clay, starch, baking soda, and dirt are some of the reported cravings during pregnancy. It is important to determine what is being ingested, the quantity, and the frequency in order to assess potentially harmful effects.

Psychosocial History

The nurse should collect psychologic and sociologic data as described in Chapter 4.

Attitude Toward This Pregnancy Inquire how the woman and her partner feel about the pregnancy. Was it planned? What kind of expectations does she have regarding being pregnant, the process of labor, childbirth, and parenthood? Explore if the client has any fear regarding the process. Adjustments to parenthood should be assessed. Emotional stability data should be collected, which would include the incidence of excessive crying, social withdrawal, or decisions related to infant care.

Maternal Habits Habits of the mother help identify risk factors for pregnancy and guide the nurse in areas of needed teaching. Some of the specific habits to discuss are tobacco use, alcohol use, and drug use.

Tobacco use should be assessed. Smoking during pregnancy is associated with premature and underweight infants. Furthermore, smoking increases the need for vitamin C, a nutrient that has increased intake requirements during pregnancy.

All pregnant women should be questioned about alcohol intake. No safe level of alcohol ingestion has been identified for the pregnant woman (Cerrato, 1992). Advise the woman to avoid drinking alcoholic beverages entirely while pregnant. Fetal alcohol syndrome (FAS) is a major public health problem.

The use of street drugs should also be explored with pregnant women. Many drugs are known teratogens, others have significant long-term effects on the infant after birth. Stimulants may affect the client's appetite and therefore lead to decreased nutrient intake. Barbiturates and opiates may impair the client's desire and ability to obtain food; in fact, in some cases the client's resources for food may be used to obtain drugs. Clients who admit to drug use should be counseled and referred to a drug treatment program.

Safety Pregnant women should also be questioned about safety issues, including activities at work and in the home, routine safety practices such as use of seat belts while in a car, and the presence of physical abuse and violence in the home.

Environmental Health

Environmental factors are particularly important to evaluate during childbearing because of the risks of teratogens. Exposure to toxins should be assessed, and preventive steps taken if warranted.

Review of Systems

The health history should also include questions related to body systems. Below is an outline, organized by body systems, of common symptoms you would ask a pregnant client about. If a client reports a symptom of concern, you should conduct a symptom analysis, which includes the location, quality, quantity, chronology, setting, associated manifestations, alleviating factors, and aggravating factors (see Box 4-2 in Chapter 4).

Fetal assessments
- Report of fetal movements; frequency, time of day

Integumentary system
- Skin marks, lines, varicosities
- Pruritis

Nose and mouth
- Nose bleeding
- Nasal stuffiness
- Gum bleeding or swelling

Ears
- Changes in hearing
- Sense of fullness in ears

Eyes
- Excessive dryness
- Visual changes

Respiratory system
- Shortness of breath

Cardiovascular system
- Palpitations
- Edema of extremities
- Orthostatic hypotension

Breasts
- Enlargement, engorgement, tenderness
- Nipple discharge

Gastrointestinal system
- Nausea, vomiting (morning sickness)
- Food aversions
- Heartburn (gastric reflex), epigastric pain (second and third trimesters)
- Constipation (second and third trimesters)
- Hemorrhoids (second and third trimesters)

Genitourinary system
- Urinary pain, frequency, and urgency
- Vaginal discharge or bleeding

Musculoskeletal system
- Backache
- Leg cramps
- Ankle edema

Neurologic system
- Headaches

EXAMINATION

Equipment

Utilize equipment discussed in previous chapters for general examination including pelvic examination. Equipment needed for specific pregnancy examination techniques include the following:

- Fetoscope to auscultate fetal heart tones
- Measuring tape (calibrated in centimeters) to measure fundal height

PROCEDURES AND TECHNIQUES WITH NORMAL FINDINGS	ABNORMAL FINDINGS
Positioning of the pregnant client for examination purposes is the same as discussed in previous chapters with one exception: be sure not to position the pregnant woman flat on her back for an extended length of time.	

PROCEDURES AND TECHNIQUES WITH NORMAL FINDINGS

VITAL SIGNS AND BASELINE MEASUREMENTS

➤MEASURE temperature, blood pressure, pulse, and respiration. The vital signs and weight should be measured with every visit. Height should be measured on the first visit.

Pulse The heart rate increases as much as 10 to 15 beats per minute.

Respiration Respiratory rate increases, especially during the third trimester; the client may also experience shortness of breath.

Blood Pressure Document blood pressure trends throughout pregnancy. Blood pressure should remain fairly consistent during pregnancy. It may decrease slightly in the second trimester and then return to the usual level during the third trimester. Since position affects blood pressure readings, it is essential to use a consistent method and position of blood pressure measurement throughout pregnancy (O'Day, 1997).

➤MEASURE height and weight. Prepregnancy weight may give the clinician insight into the woman's nutritional status. On an initial visit, complete a weight-for-height assessment to determine if the weight is within or outside ideal weight range. Calculate a body mass index to determine an appropriate weight gain goal for pregnancy.

The examiner should evaluate the rate of weight change at each prenatal visit in addition to assessment of overall weight change. Generally, a total weight gain of between 25 and 35 lb (11.4 to 16 kg) is associated with positive pregnancy outcome for women with normal prepregnancy weight. Underweight women should gain more weight, whereas overweight women should gain somewhat less weight (Institute of Medicine, 1991).

EXAMINATION OF THE EXTREMITIES

➤INSPECT the hands and nails for color and surface characteristics, movement, and sensation. Pinkish red blotches or diffuse mottling of the hands is known as palmar erythema and is considered a normal finding. The client's nails may become thin and brittle. Women who take prenatal vitamins may report fast-growing, strong nails. Movement and sensation of fingers and hands should remain the same.

ABNORMAL FINDINGS

■ Excessive shortness of breath and dyspnea is of concern and may indicate pulmonary complications such as embolus. Hypertension in pregnancy contributes significantly to preterm delivery and infant mortality. Pregnancy-induced hypertension is a serious disorder that requires prompt and close medical management. It is characterized by systolic blood pressure of at least 140 mm Hg or a rise of 30 mm Hg or more above the usual level in two readings 6 hours apart or diastolic blood pressure of 90 mm Hg or more or a rise of 15 mm Hg above baseline in two readings done 6 hours apart.

■ A rapid weight increase or significant weight decrease indicates the need for additional evaluation by the examiner. A rapid weight increase could indicate multiple gestation, preeclampsia, or diabetes associated with pregnancy (gestational diabetes). If a woman gains more than 2 lb (.9 kg) in any one week or more than 6 lb (2.7 kg) in a month, preeclampsia should be suspected (Cunningham et al, 1997). Poor weight gain or weight loss may indicate a small for gestational age (SGA) infant, maternal smoking, or more serious complications such as placental dysfunction or fetal death in utero. A weight loss of up to 5 lb (2.3 kg) during the first trimester may be caused by nausea and vomiting.

■ Some pregnant clients may periodically report numbness of the fingers, caused by a brachial plexus traction syndrome (caused by drooping shoulders associated with increased breast size and weight). A carpal tunnel syndrome caused by compression of the median nerve in the arm and the hand may lead to symptoms of numbness, tingling, burning, and impaired finger movement. This most typically affects the thumb and the second and third fingers.

PROCEDURES AND TECHNIQUES WITH NORMAL FINDINGS

➤**INSPECT and PALPATE the lower extremities for edema, surface characteristics, redness, and tenderness.** Edema in the lower extremities occurs in over half of women during late pregnancy. Most typically, women notice the swelling late in the day or after long periods of standing. Palpation of the legs will help to determine the extent and severity of the edema. Vascular spiders or varicosities may appear on the lower legs and thighs and are considered normal findings. The legs should be free from redness and tenderness.

EXAMINATION OF THE HEAD AND NECK

➤**INSPECT the head and face for skin characteristics, pigmentation, and edema.** Blotchy, brownish pigmentation of the face—chloasma, or the mask of pregnancy—is a normal finding. There should be no facial edema. Fine lanugo type of hair may be observed on the face and is a normal finding.

➤**TEST vision for acuity.** Visual acuity should be tested with the first visit to establish a baseline. Visual checks should be repeated if the client verbalizes a change in vision during the pregnancy. Contact lenses may be uncomfortable to wear due to increased dryness. Both eyesight and the corrective prescription may change.

➤**EXAMINE the eyes.** The eye examination should proceed as discussed in Chapter 16. Findings generally remain the same; however, the eyelids of some women may darken from melanin pigment.

➤**EXAMINE the ears, nose, and mouth.** The examination of the ears, nose, and mouth should proceed as discussed in Chapters 14 and 15. Findings generally are the same as previously discussed for the adult. However, the examiner may note an increase in vascularization of the external ear, the auditory canal, and the tympanic membrane while examining the ear. The nose and mouth of the pregnant woman also are associated with an increase in vascularization, causing redness in the nose, pharynx, and gums; the gums become swollen, spongy, and may bleed easily. A hypertrophied gum lesion, known as an epulis, is a raised nodule that may be seen toward the end of the third trimester.

➤**INSPECT and PALPATE the neck.** The examination of the neck and thyroid should proceed as discussed in Chapters 13. Findings generally are the same as previously discussed. There may be transient thyroid enlargement that makes the thyroid more easily palpable, but this will disappear following delivery.

ABNORMAL FINDINGS

■ Although some edema is considered normal, excessive edema (particularly if noted in the hands and face in addition to the lower extremities) is considered pathologic and may be an indication of PIH (Branch and Porter, 1999). Edema not associated with preeclampsia or normal lower-extremity swelling should be evaluated for adequate protein intake. Redness in the legs, particularly if accompanied by tenderness, may be an indication of thrombophlebitis.

■ Facial edema is considered an abnormal finding and should be reported.

■ Pregnancy-induced hypertension may cause blurred vision. Chromatopsia may be noted, characterized by unusual color perception, seeing spots, or blindness in the lateral visual field. This requires immediate follow-up.

■ Retinal arteriole constriction, disc edema, or retinal detachment (which is an emergency) are a concern; these may be caused by pregnancy-induced hypertension. Pale conjunctivae may indicate anemia.

■ Some women develop a pregnancy-induced tumor in the mouth. Any growth in the mouth is an abnormal finding.

■ Excessive or asymmetric enlargement of the thyroid gland or nodules on the thyroid gland are abnormal findings.

PROCEDURES AND TECHNIQUES WITH NORMAL FINDINGS

EXAMINATION OF THE ANTERIOR AND POSTERIOR CHEST

➤**INSPECT, AUSCULTATE, PERCUSS, and PALPATE the anterior and posterior chest.** The examination of the anterior and posterior chest proceeds as discussed in Chapters 17 and 18. If the client is near term or has difficulty breathing when lying down, be sure to perform chest examination when the client is in a sitting position.

The breathing pattern changes from abdominal to costal or lateral; likewise, the breathing pattern may be shallow with an increased respiratory rate. A wide thoracic cage and increased costal angle may be noted. Diaphragmatic excursion may decrease secondary to the growing fetus.

The heart shifts laterally in response to the positions of the uterus and diaphragm. The point of maximum impulse also shifts up and laterally 1 to 1.5 cm. Murmurs, splitting of S_1, S_2, and the presence of S_3 may be heard after the twentieth week of gestation.

ABNORMAL FINDINGS

■ Abnormal findings as discussed in Chapters 17 and 18 also apply to the pregnant client. Dyspnea, orthopnea, fatigue, and palpitations may be attributed to the pregnancy but should be evaluated for other causes. Preexisting cardiac conditions may have pronounced symptoms due to the increased blood volume. Note any signs of heart failure. Note low blood pressure or tachycardia occurring during this period.

EXAMINATION OF THE BREAST

➤**INSPECT and PALPATE the breast for surface and tissue characteristics.** Examine the breasts as described in Chapter 19. The woman should perform breast self-examination at regular times during pregnancy, just as when she is not pregnant.

During the first trimester the breasts will become fuller and tender, increase in size, and may have a tingling sensation. A subcutaneous venous pattern may be seen as a network of blue tracings across the breasts.

As pregnancy advances, striae may be present. Palpation of the breasts reveal fullness and coarse nodularity (Fig. 26-8). Following delivery, breast engorgement will be at its peak about the third to fifth day. Engorged breasts may be very uncomfortable and actually painful. This is most pronounced in women who are not breast-feeding.

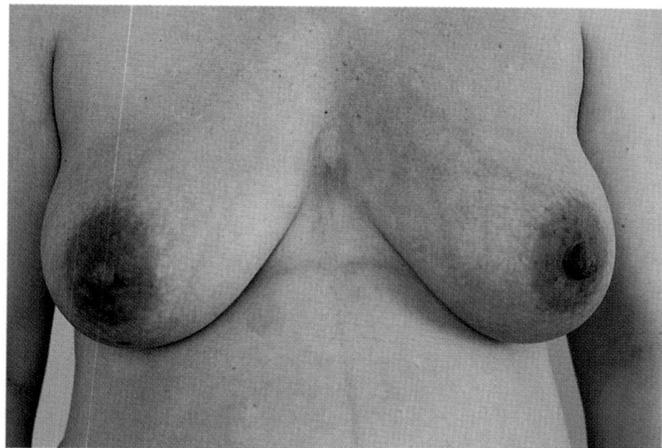

Fig. 26-8 Enlarged breasts in pregnancy with venous network and darkened areolae and nipples. (From Seidel et al, 1999.)

■ Engorgement or breast pain that lasts beyond 4 days, or breasts that become engorged or painful after that time, must be assessed for possible infection or mastitis. Other clinical signs of mastitis include fever, headache, malaise, chills, and other flulike symptoms. An isolated tender spot or lump on the breast may be a clogged milk duct. If this is the case, frequent nursing or expression of milk, along with the application of moist heat and massage, may help to unclog the duct. A clogged duct may occur secondary to inadequate emptying of the breast or a bra that is too tight. If the clogged duct is left unattended, it may result in mastitis.

PROCEDURES AND TECHNIQUES WITH NORMAL FINDINGS

ABNORMAL FINDINGS

➤INSPECT and PALPATE the nipples for surface characteristics and nipple shape. During the first trimester the nipples may become somewhat flattened or inverted. The areolae become darker and Montgomery's tubercles may appear. The nipples should be assessed in preparation for breast-feeding. Press on the nipple just behind the areola to express any discharge and note whether the nipple protracts or inverts. Following the first trimester, colostrum may be expressed from the breast (a yellowish discharge).

The nipples of lactating women require careful assessment, especially during the early period following delivery of the infant and the beginning of breast-feeding. Nipples should be smooth and without lesions or cracks.

■ Breast-feeding may cause the client's nipples to become irritated, red, and tender. If left unattended, they may become blistered and actually crack. If this is evident, it must be attended to and healed so that successful breast-feeding may continue.

EXAMINATION OF THE ABDOMEN

➤INSPECT the abdomen for surface characteristics and fetal movement. Common changes to the skin on the abdomen are linea nigra, striae gravidarum, and venous patterns. After the twenty-eighth week, fetal movements may be observed with inspection.

■ Absence of fetal movement is of concern and could indicate fetal demise.

■ Note scars from previous abdominal surgeries.

➤PALPATE the abdomen for fetal movement and uterine contraction. The mother should report fetal movements (also known as quickening) by approximately 20 weeks' gestation. Fetal movement and uterine contraction can be evaluated by placing the hands directly on the abdomen.

❖ **➤MEASURE the fundus for height.** Measure fundal height from the top of the symphysis pubis to the top of the fundus (Fig. 26-9). From the twentieth to thirty-sixth week of gestation, the expected pattern of uterine growth is an increase in fundal height of about 1 cm (3/8 inch) per week. Uterine size should roughly correlate with gestational age. Any discrepancy greater than 2 cm between fundal height and the estimate of gestational age (based on last menstrual period) should be evaluated further. It is important to note that measurement of fundal height is an estimate and may vary among examiners by 1 to 2 cm.

■ A uterus that is larger than expected may be due to inaccurate dating of the pregnancy, more than one fetus, gestational diabetes, or polyhydramnios. A uterus that is smaller than expected for gestational age may be due to inaccurate dating of the pregnancy or growth retardation of the fetus.

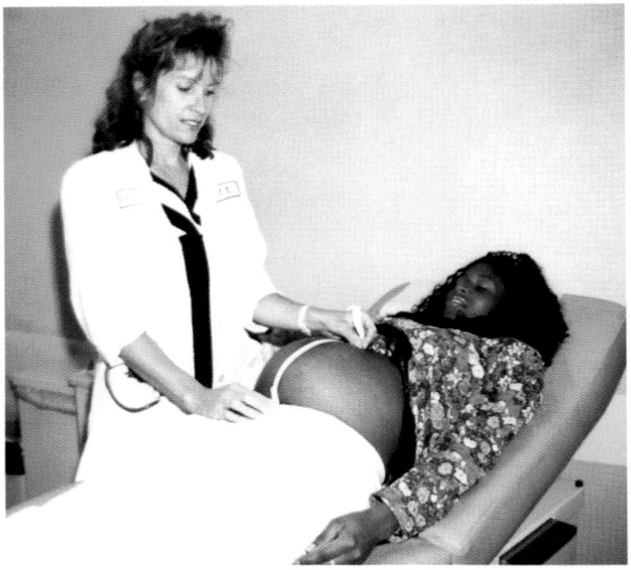

Fig. 26-9 Measuring fundal height. (Courtesy Marjorie Pyle, RNC, Lifecircle.)

PROCEDURES AND TECHNIQUES WITH NORMAL FINDINGS	ABNORMAL FINDINGS
❖ ➤**AUSCULTATE the abdomen for fetal heart sounds.** Auscultation of fetal heart tones is performed by use of a Doppler ultrasonic stethoscope after 10 to 12 weeks' gestation or with a fetoscope after 17 to 19 weeks. (The Doppler and fetoscope are discussed in Chapter 5.) The fetal heart rate is expected to be heard over the lower abdomen for fetuses that are in a head-down position. The expected fetal heart rate ranges between 120 and 160 beats/min.	■ Increases and decreases in fetal heart rate can be caused by multiple factors. A fetal heart rate over 160 beats/min or below 120 beats/min requires further investigation. Absence of fetal heart tones is always abnormal and usually indicates fetal demise.
❖ ➤**PALPATE fetal position for fetal lie and presentation, position, and attitude.** The outline of the fetus can be determined after 26 to 28 weeks. Palpate the fundus using Leopold's maneuvers. The client should be lying supine, with head slightly elevated and knees flexed slightly. Leopold's maneuvers help to determine the fetus's presentation (the part presenting in the mother's pelvis) and the lie (longitudinal, transverse, or oblique within the uterus), the position of the presenting fetal part, and the attitude (or the relationship of the fetal head to the limbs and body) (Table 26-3).	■ Inability to palpate the fetal position could be associated with polyhydramnios. A fetus with breech presentation or a transverse lie prior to delivery is of concern due to higher risks during the labor and delivery process. Breech presentation occurs in 3% to 4% of cases at term (Reeder et al, 1997).

Table 26-3 Fetal Assessment Terms

TERM	PICTURE
FETAL LIE The lie is the relationship of the long axis of the fetus to the long axis of the uterus. **PRESENTATION** The presentation is determined by the fetal lie and by the body part of the fetus that enters the pelvic passage first. The presentation may be vertex, brow, face, shoulder, or breech.	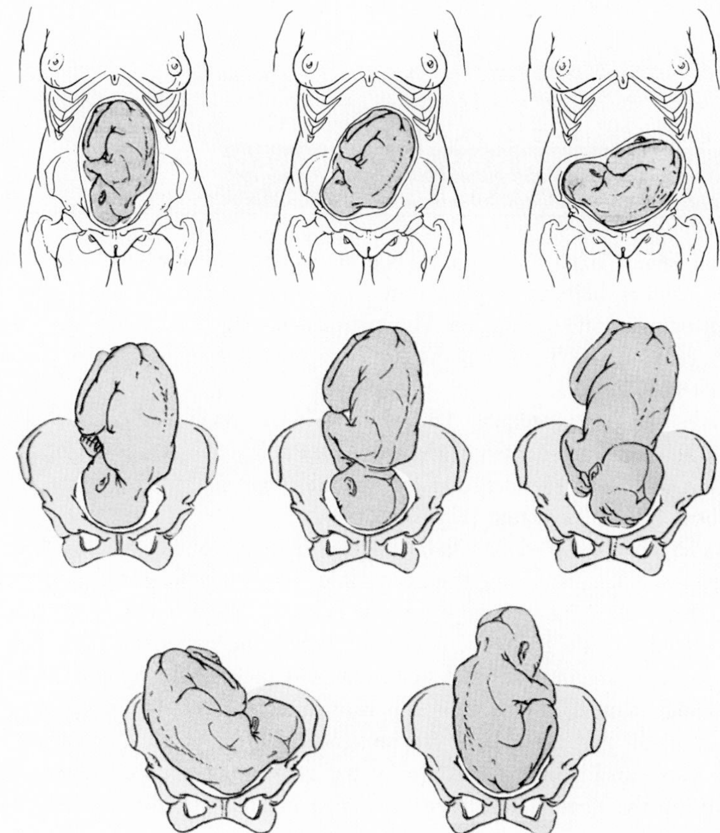

Continued

Table 26-3 Fetal Assessment Terms—cont'd

TERM	PICTURE
POSITION Position refers to the relationship of the landmark on the presenting fetal part to the front, sides, or back of the maternal pelvis. The landmark on the fetal presenting part is related to four imaginary quadrants of the pelvis: left anterior, right anterior, left posterior, and right posterior. These quadrants indicate whether the presenting part is directed toward the front, back, left, or right of the pelvic passage.	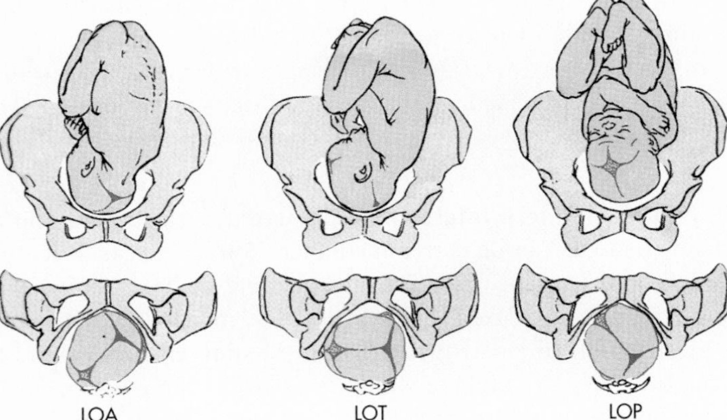
ATTITUDE The attitude is the relationship of the fetal head and limbs to the body. The expected attitude is moderate flexion of the head, flexion of the arms onto the chest, and flexion of the legs.	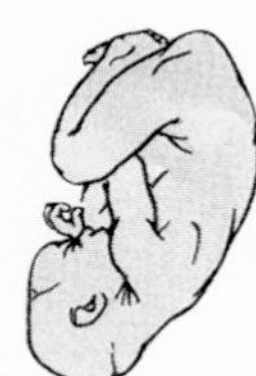 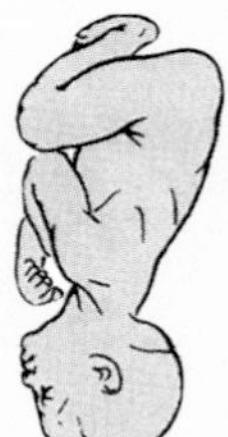 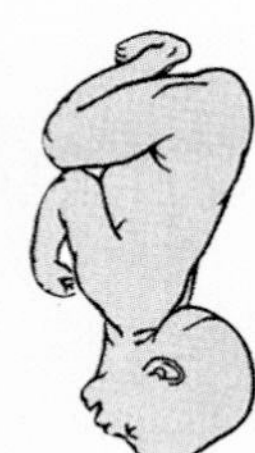

PROCEDURES AND TECHNIQUES WITH NORMAL FINDINGS

ABNORMAL FINDINGS

Fundal Palpation This is done to determine what part of the fetus is at the fundus, helping to determine fetal presentation. Most typically, the feet or buttocks are at the fundus. The buttocks feel firm, but not hard, and slightly irregular. If the head is at the fundus, you will palpate a firm, movable part (Fig. 26-10, *A*).

Lateral Palpation This is done to determine the *fetal lie.* Palpate the sides of the uterus to identify the spine of the fetus. It is smooth and convex, compared with the irregular feel on the other side of the fetus—the hands, elbows, knees, and feet (Fig. 26-10, *B*).

Symphysis Pubis Palpation This is done to assess which part of the fetus is in or just above the pelvic inlet. This (along with fundal palpation) confirms the fetal presentation and helps to assess if the presenting part is engaged. Gently grasp the presenting anatomic part over the symphysis pubis using your dominant hand. If the head is the presenting part, it will feel very smooth, round, and firm. If it is movable from side to side and you are able to palpate all the way around it, the head is not engaged. If engaged, the head is not movable and is below the level of the symphysis, preventing palpation all the way around the head. The presenting part could also be the buttocks. The buttocks feel softer and irregular (Fig. 26-10, *C*).

Deep Pelvic Palpation If the head is the presenting part, palpation allows you to determine the position and attitude (Fig. 26-10, *D*). Use both hands to identify the outline of the fetal head. Depending on the fetal position, the cephalic prominence can be either the forehead or the occipit.

PROCEDURES AND TECHNIQUES WITH NORMAL FINDINGS

ABNORMAL FINDINGS

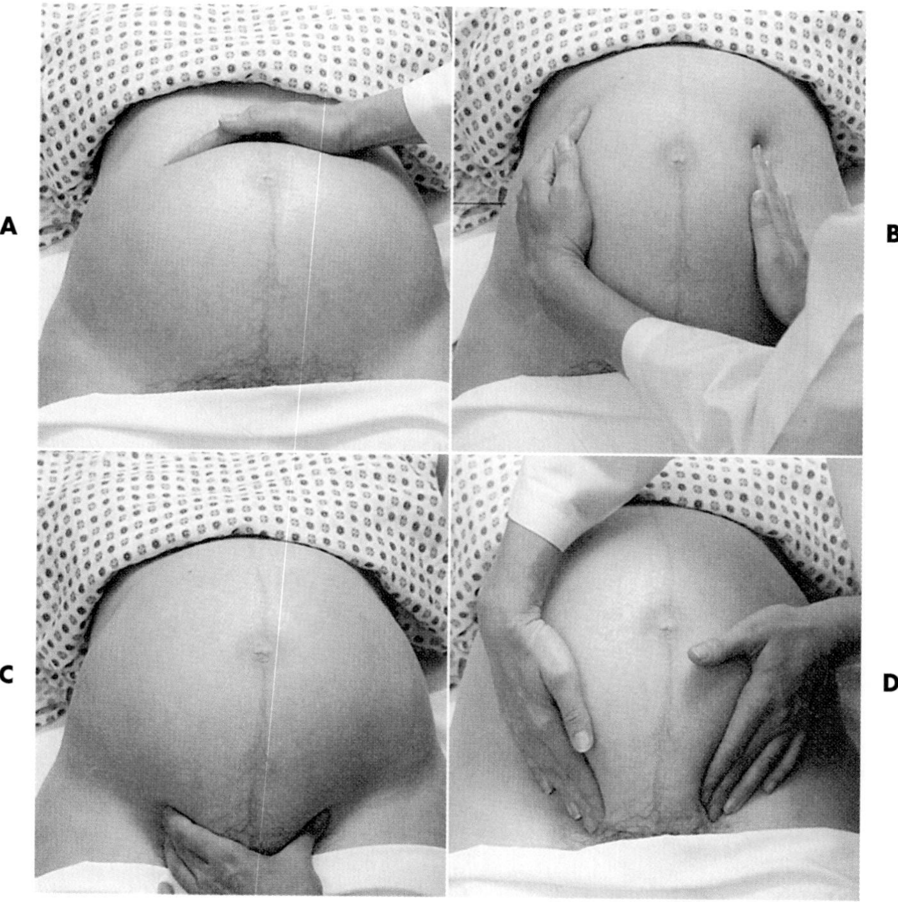

Fig. 26-10 Leopold maneuvers. **A,** First maneuver. Place hand(s) over fundus and identify the fetal part. **B,** Second maneuver. Use the palmar surface of one hand to locate the back of the fetus. Use the other hand to feel the irregularities such as hands and feet. **C,** Third maneuver. Use thumb and third finger to grasp presenting part over the symphysis pubis. **D,** Fourth maneuver. Use both hands to outline the fetal head. With a head presenting deep in the pelvis, only a small portion may be felt. (From Seidel et al, 1999.)

EXAMINATION OF THE GENITALIA

❖ ➤**INSPECT the external and internal genitalia.** Follow the guidelines described in Chapter 21. By the second month of pregnancy, the cervix, vagina, and vulva take on a bluish color, and there will be increased vaginal secretions.

■ Note presence of infection of genitalia, including vaginal discharge with a foul odor and/or lesions. Vaginal bleeding or leakage of watery fluid associated with preterm labor are abnormal findings.

PROCEDURES AND TECHNIQUES WITH NORMAL FINDINGS

❖ **➤PALPATE the cervix to determine length (effacement) and dilation.** This procedure is done near the expected date of delivery and once labor begins. The cervix typically maintains its usual length of 1.5 cm to 2 cm until the last month of pregnancy. During these last 4 weeks the cervix shortens (known as effacement) as the fetal head descends. The cervical os softens and is pulled upward, becoming incorporated into the isthmus of the uterus. As the cervix shortens, it also begins to dilate. Cervical dilation is measured in centimeters from 0 cm, when completely closed, to 10 cm, when it is completely open. The effacement and dilation of the cervix is estimated by palpation of the cervix (Fig. 26-11).

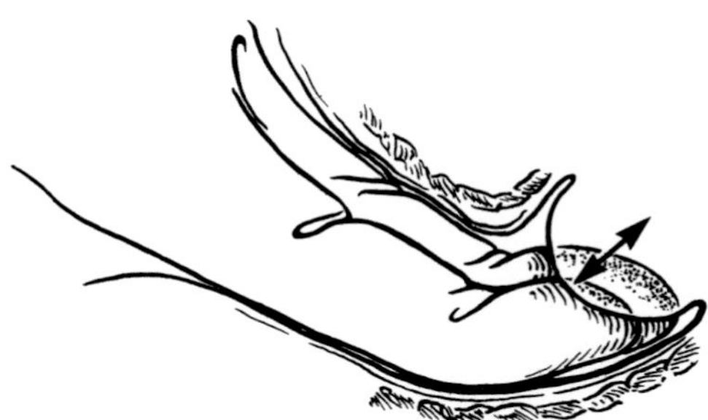

Fig. 26-11 Measurement of cervical length (effacement) and dilation. (From Barkauskus et al, 1998.)

EXAMINATION OF THE RECTUM AND ANUS

❖ **➤INSPECT and PALPATE the anus and rectum.** The perianal and rectal examination should be carried out in the pregnant woman as described in Chapter 23. The rectum and anus are most commonly examined while the client is in the lithotomy position with her legs up in stirrups. Early during pregnancy, the client should have minimal difficulty attaining and maintaining the position for the examination. Later in pregnancy, however, positioning for the rectal examination could be uncomfortable.

The presence of hemorrhoids is the most common variation usually considered normal with pregnancy. The client may not have hemorrhoids during the early phase of pregnancy, but toward the last trimester the hemorrhoids may appear secondary to pressure on the pelvic floor or possible constipation with straining when having a bowel movement. The hemorrhoids may be either internal in the lower segment of the rectum or prolapsed as external hemorrhoids.

EXAMINATION OF THE MUSCULOSKELETAL SYSTEM

➤INSPECT and PALPATE the spine, extremities, and joints. Examination of the musculoskeletal system proceeds as described in Chapter 24. Changes that are expected during pregnancy include progressive lordosis, anterior cervical flexion, kyphosis, and slumped shoulders. A characteristic "waddling" gait develops at the end of pregnancy. Backache is a symptom that is reported in 50% of pregnant women (Cunningham et al, 1997).

ABNORMAL FINDINGS

■ The cervix should not efface until about the thirty-sixth week. The cervical os should remain closed until near delivery. Effacement and dilation of the cervix prior to the thirty-sixth week may result in premature delivery. Failure of the cervical os to efface and dilate impedes the progression of labor. If the cervix has inadequate effacement and dilation at the onset of delivery, trauma to the cervix often results.

■ Presence of lesions or rectal bleeding are considered abnormal findings.

■ Exaggerated posture or excessive activity can cause muscle strains. Preexisting conditions may become worse both during the pregnancy and after delivery. Muscle cramps, numbness, or weakness of the extremities are considered abnormal findings.

PROCEDURES AND TECHNIQUES WITH NORMAL FINDINGS

ABNORMAL FINDINGS

EXAMINATION OF THE NEUROLOGIC SYSTEM

➤**EXAMINE the client for neurologic changes.** Examine the client as described in Chapter 25. Although the examination proceeds as for other adults, pregnancy alters balance. Reflexes may also provide valuable information if the examiner suspects pregnancy-induced hypertension (PIH).

■ Seizures or increased frequency of seizures associated with pregnancy is abnormal. Other abnormal findings are signs of multiple dystrophy or myasthenia gravis, carpal tunnel syndrome (burning, pain, tingling in hand, wrist, or elbow), or hand numbness as a result of brachial plexus traction. These conditions return to prepregnant state after delivery. Hyperreflexia is an abnormal finding that may indicate PIH.

EXAMINATION SUMMARY

Pregnancy

PROCEDURE

Vital Signs and Baseline Measurements

- Measure temperature, blood pressure, pulse, and respiration.
- Measure height and weight.

Examination of the Extremities

- Inspect the hands and nails for color and surface characteristics movement and sensation.
- Inspect and palpate the lower extremities for edema, surface characteristics, redness, and tenderness.

Examination of the Head and Neck

- Inspect the head and face for skin characteristics, pigmentation, and edema.
- Test vision for acuity.
- Examine the eyes.
- Examine the ears, nose, and mouth.
- Inspect and palpate the neck.

Examination of the Anterior and Posterior Chest

- Inspect, auscultate, percuss, and palpate the anterior and posterior chest.

Examination of the Breast

- Inspect and palpate the breast for surface and tissue characteristics.
- Inspect and palpate the nipples for surface characteristics and nipple shape.

Examination of the Abdomen

- Inspect the abdomen for surface characteristics and fetal movement.
- Palpate the abdomen for fetal movement and uterine contraction.
- ❖ Measure the fundus for height.
- ❖ Auscultate the abdomen for fetal heart sounds.
- ❖ Palpate fetal position for fetal, lie, presentation position, and attitude.

Examination of the Genitalia

- ❖ Inspect the external and internal genitalia.
- ❖ Palpate the cervix to determine length (effacement) and dilation.

Examination of the Rectum and Anus

- ❖ Inspect and palpate the anus and rectum.

Examination of the Musculoskeletal System

- Inspect and palpate the spine, extremities, and joints.

Examination of the Neurologic System

- Examine the client for neurologic changes.

SUMMARY OF FINDINGS

Body System	Normal Findings	Typical Variations	Findings Associated With Disorders
Reproductive system	• Uterus increases in size, most notably during second and third trimester. • Cervix turn bluish color within first few weeks; cervix softens by sixth week. • Increase in vaginal secretions—mucus with a high pH. • Fetal heart tones (FHTs) auscultated. • Fetal movements reported by mother.	• More than one fetus will cause increase in uterine size more than expected.	• Excessive uterine growth may be due to polyhydramnios or gestational diabetes. Inadequate uterine growth may be indicate a poorly growing fetus or fetal demise. • Purulent or malodorous discharge may indicate infection. • FHT over 160 or below 120 beats/min indicates fetal distress. Lack of FHT indicates fetal demise.
Breasts	• Breast fullness and tenderness early during pregnancy. • Nipples and areolae become more darkly pigmented. • Colostrum production. • Breast engorgement occurs 2-3 days after delivery.	• Dried colostrum or slight colostrum drainage may be noted on nipples during pregnancy. • Nodularity to breasts.	• Red, inflamed, painful breasts could indicate mastitis or clogged milk duct.
Integument	• Increased pigmentation to the skin, especially on tissue that is more darkly pigmented. • Increased vascularization to hands and feet. • Accelerated hair and nail growth.	• Chloasma and linea nigra. • Striae to abdomen and breasts. • Palmar erythema and spider telangiectases. • Hair falling out and increased oiliness to hair—excessive fine hair growth to face/chest.	• Any abnormal skin lesion for nonpregnant adult is also abnormal for pregnant woman.
Respiratory system	• Shortness of breath with activity in late pregnancy. • Thoracic breathing more common than abdominal.	• Wide chest. • Increased costal angle. • Nasal stuffiness.	• Severe dyspnea could indicate cardiovascular compromise.
Cardiovascular system	• Heart shifts upward and laterally. • Increased cardiac output with increased pulse rate in last trimester.	• Edema and varicosities in lower extremities. • Splitting of S_1, S_2; presence of S_3; murmurs.	• Increases in blood pressure. • Excessive edema in lower extremities, as well as face and trunk.
Gastrointestinal system	• Hormones of pregnancy cause nausea—usually resolves after twelfth week.	• Gastric reflux. • Constipation. • Increased proliferation of gum tissue.	• Excessive nausea could interfere with proper nutrition. • Mouth tumors.
Renal system	• Increased pressure on bladder.	• Nocturia. • Slight glycosuria. • Slight proteinuria.	• Excessively high glucose levels could indicate gestational diabetes.
Musculoskeletal system	• Hormones of pregnancy causes a loosening of ligaments throughout the body. • Center of gravity changes.	• Lordosis. • Waddling gait. • Recti abdominis. • Muscle cramps.	• Excessive protruding of abdominal contents through recti abdominis. • Hypocalcemia (cramps).
Neurologic system	• No specific changes noted.	• Headaches.	• Seizures.

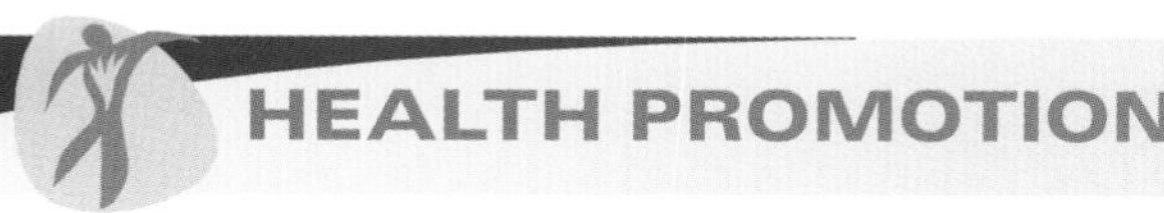

HEALTH PROMOTION

PREGNANCY AND NUTRITION

All women should be screened for nutritional risks and counseled on the nutritional needs of pregnancy.

Protein

The pregnant woman should increase the total grams of protein by 10 g/day while pregnant. Adequate protein is essential to facilitate fetal tissue development.

Calcium and Phosphorus

The developing fetus places an additional need for calcium and phosphorus on the mother. Requirements for both minerals increase from 800 to 1200 mg/day. These minerals are crucial for appropriate skeletal development of the fetus.

Iron

The recommended dietary allowance (RDI) for iron during pregnancy is 30 mg/day, twice the RDA for nonpregnant women. Adequate iron intake is difficult to achieve by diet alone. To prevent iron deficiency anemia, the National Academy of Sciences (NAS) recommends a 30-mg ferrous iron supplement daily for all pregnant women in the second and third trimesters in addition to a well-balanced diet (IOM, 1990).

Folate

The Centers for Disease Control and Prevention recommends that all women of childbearing age consume 400 mcg of folic acid per day to decrease the chance of neural tube defects. (Centers for Disease Control and Prevention, 1992). However, women should keep their total daily folic acid consumption under 1 mg to avoid potential risks associated with oversupplementation. Increased folate intake in pregnant women may cause problems ranging from nausea to serious neurologic damage secondary to the masking of B_{12} deficiency (Giotta, 1993).

Caffeinated Beverages

Advise the pregnant woman to limit caffeine intake to no more than 2 to 3 servings per day. Excessive caffeine may cause increased maternal and fetal heart rates and has been possibly linked to low-birth-weight infants.

LACTATION

The Healthy People 2010 campaign has established as a national goal that 75% of postpartum women will be breast-feeding at the time of hospital discharge, and 50% of these mothers will still be breast-feeding when their babies are 6 months old (HPWebsite@osophs.dhhs.gov). To accomplish this goal health care providers of women and babies will be responsible for educating parents and their families about the advantages of breast-feeding versus formula-feeding to make an informed choice for their baby's nutrition.

Endorsements for breast-feeding have been formally made by the American Dietetic Association (ADA, June 1997), the American Academy of Pediatrics, the American College of Obstetricians and Gynecologists (ACOG), the Association of Women's Health Organization (WHO), the American Public Health Association, and UNICEF (Bell and Rawlings, 1998).

REDUCING RISK FACTORS DURING PREGNANCY

Smoking Cessation

Cigarette smoking during pregnancy poses problems resulting in placental abnormalities and fetal complications, including prematurity and low birth weight (Williams, 1999). Pregnant women should be strongly advised to stop smoking during pregnancy.

Abstinence from Alcohol

Alcohol use or abuse during pregnancy damages the fetus. Advise pregnant women about the harmful effects of drug and alcohol use during pregnancy. Because of the damaging effects of alcohol on the fetus, and the wide variability in alcohol tolerance and effect, no alcohol should be used during pregnancy; abstinence is the only safe policy.

Drug Use

During pregnancy, drug use (whether it be prescriptive, over-the-counter, or illicit drug abuse) poses numerous problems. Women should be advised to take medications only under the supervision of their physician or nurse practitioner. Abstinence from illicit street drugs is imperative.

COMMON PROBLEMS AND CONDITIONS

Pregnancy

BLEEDING

Bleeding from the vagina during pregnancy is a significant finding. During early pregnancy, slight bleeding may occur for unknown reasons and be of no consequence, or it could indicate an impending abortion. During late pregnancy, bleeding could be caused by abruptio placentae or placenta previa. Bleeding should never be considered a normal finding in pregnancy and should always be investigated thoroughly.

Abruptio placentae is the premature separation of the implanted placenta before the birth of the fetus—usually during the third trimester, but it could occur as early as 20 weeks. It is the most common cause of intrapartum fetal death. Symptoms in addition to bleeding include abdominal pain and uterine contractions. This is considered an obstetric emergency (Scott, 1999).

Placenta previa occurs when the placenta overlies the cervix or lies near the cervix as opposed to a more typical attachment higher within the uterus. The symptom is painless vaginal bleeding in the third trimester (Scott, 1999).

HYDRAMNIOS (POLYHYDRAMNIOS)

Hydramnios is an excessive quantity of amniotic fluid, which can range from 2 to 15 L. Hydramnios is common in pregnancies with more than one fetus. In single-fetus pregnancies, it is associated with fetal malformation of the central nervous system and gastrointestinal tract. Clinical findings suggesting hydramnios include excessive uterine size, tense uterine wall, and difficulty palpating fetal parts, and hearing fetal heart tones. Maternal symptoms include dyspnea, edema, and discomfort and are attributed to pressure on the surrounding organs. Hydramnios may result in perinatal mortality from premature labor and fetal abnormalities.

PREGNANCY-INDUCED HYPERTENSION

Preeclampsia

Eclampsia

These are a group of hypertensive conditions that develop as a direct result of pregnancy. Hypertension that precedes pregnancy or occurs prior to 20 weeks' gestation is considered chronic hypertension (Chari et al, 1995).

- PIH is a condition of hypertension caused by the pregnancy.
- Preeclampsia refers to a condition of PIH with proteinuria and pathologic edema.
- Eclampsia is the occurrence of seizures precipitated by PIH.
- Hypertension in pregnancy is defined as follows:
  Systolic blood pressure is 140 mm Hg or higher
  or
  There is an increase of more than 30 mm Hg of systolic blood pressure from baseline in the first half of pregnancy
  or
  Diastolic blood pressure is more than 90 mm Hg
  or
  There is an increase of more than 15 mm Hg of diastolic blood pressure from baseline.

PREMATURE RUPTURE OF MEMBRANES

Premature rupture of membranes (PROM) is the spontaneous rupture of uterine membranes prior to the onset of labor. It can occur at any time during the pregnancy, but this is mostly seen with term pregnancy. This situation is associated with a high risk of perinatal and maternal morbidity and mortality. The symptom of PROM is passage of amniotic fluid from the vagina prior to labor. The cause of PROM is not known, although infection and hydramnios are thought to be associated factors (Parsons and Spellacy, 1999).

PROLAPSED CORD

Prolapsed cord is an emergency situation in which the umbilical cord precedes the fetus's presenting part, causing compression of the cord and an interruption of blood flow to the fetus. The incidence of prolapsed cord is low – occurring in only 0.2% to 0.6% of births (Cruikshank, 1999). Predisposing factors include excessive cord length, premature labor, breech presentation at birth, hydramnios, and multiple pregnancy. Prolapsed cord can present either visually, with a loop of cord protruding from the vagina, or by palpation of the pulsating cord on vaginal examination. Another clue to prolapsed cord is variable deceleration of the fetal heart rate. This situation results in fetal death if measures to relieve cord compression are not taken.

CLINICAL APPLICATION and CRITICAL THINKING

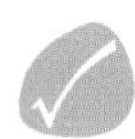

SAMPLE DOCUMENTATION

CASE 1

J.G. is a 23-year-old woman at her first prenatal visit.

Subjective Data

J.G. is a 23-year-old woman who reports that she is pregnant. Her LMP was 10 weeks ago; she performed a home pregnancy test 2 weeks ago, and this was positive. J.G. is married and has a healthy 3-year-old son at home. She indicates this is a planned pregnancy. G2, T1, P0, A0, L1. She reports having a great deal of nausea and loss of appetite since becoming pregnant and has had 2-lb weight loss in last 2 weeks. J.G. smokes one-half pack of cigarettes a day and indicates a desire to quit smoking to improve the health of her baby. She admits to occasional alcohol intake but reports that during pregnancy she avoids alcohol completely; denies drug use.

Objective Data

Temperature, 98.3° F (36.8° C); Pulse, 82 beats/min; Respiration rate, 18; Blood pressure, 114/76 mm Hg.
Height, 5′5″ (165 cm); Weight, 132 lb (60 kg); LMP March 4.
Skin: Warm, dry, no lesions; hair clean, full head of hair, good turgor.
Mouth: No lesions, mucous membranes dry.
Abdomen: Positive bowel sounds, soft, nontender, unable to palpate uterus.
Vaginal examination: Within normal limits; positive Chadwick's; positive Goodell's.

Functional Health Patterns Involved

- Health perception–health management
- Sexuality–reproductive
- Nutrition–metabolic

Medical Diagnosis

Pregnancy

Nursing Diagnosis and Collaborative Problems

- *Health-seeking behaviors:* desire for smoking cessation.
- *Altered comfort* related to nausea and vomiting associated with pregnancy as manifested by:
  - Reports of nausea.
- *Risk for fluid volume deficit* related to nausea.
- *Risk for altered nutrition: less than body requirements* related to nausea, loss of appetite, and increased metabolic demands.

CASE 2

A 31-year-old woman comes in for routine prenatal visit; 36 weeks' gestation.

Subjective Data

Client reports that since last visit 2 weeks ago, has had problems catching her breath and getting tired easily. She has had problems sleeping due to discomfort and having to urinate during the night—reports that she feels tired in the morning when she wakes up. Reports problems having regular bowel movements (BMs)—last bowel movement 2 days ago, hard, dark brown. Other than that, has been feeling good.

Objective Data

Vital signs: Temperature, 98.8° F (37.1° C); Pulse, 104 beats/min; Respiration rate, 22; Blood pressure, 118/72 mm Hg.
Height, 5′ 6″ (167 cm); Weight, 160 lb (72.6 kg); (Prepregnant weight, 138 lb [62.6 kg]); Weight at last visit, 158 lb (71.6 kg).
Urine: +1 glucose, negative for albumin and ketones.
Abdomen: Fundal height, 38 cm; Fundal height at last visit, 37 cm; FHT = 134; fetal movement palpable; fetus palpated in longitudinal lie, vertex presentation.
Breasts: Enlarged with palpable glandular nodularities; small amount of fluid expressed from nipples bilaterally.
Extremities: 1+ edema to ankles and feet.

Functional Health Patterns Involved

- Elimination
- Activity-exercise
- Sleep-rest

Medical Diagnosis

Pregnancy—36 weeks

Nursing Diagnosis and Collaborative Problems

- *Constipation* related to decreased peristalsis secondary to pregnancy as manifested by:
  - Client reports having difficulty having bowel movement.
  - Last BM 2 days ago.
  - 36 weeks pregnant.
- *Sleep pattern disturbance* related urinary frequency and discomfort as manifested by:
  - Client reports difficulty sleeping.
  - Client reports does not feel rested after sleeping.
- *Activity intolerance* related to compromised lung expansion secondary to pregnancy as manifested by:
  - Client reports having trouble "catching breath."
  - Client reports getting tired easily.
  - Shortness of breath occurs with activity.

CRITICAL THINKING QUESTIONS

1. A 35-week pregnant woman comes to the clinic for prenatal care. Her vital signs are as follows: temperature, 98.1° F (36.7° C); pulse, 110 beats/min; blood pressure, 152/94 mm Hg; respiratory rate, 20. What are expected changes in vital signs during pregnancy? Are these findings within typical parameters?
2. A 43-year-old woman comes to the clinic and announces she is pregnant, which places her in a "high-risk" pregnancy category. Consider the physiologic changes that occur with pregnancy, and rationalize why women over age 40 are considered high risk.
3. Consider all of the signs of pregnancy. Which are clinically useful? Which are most accurate?

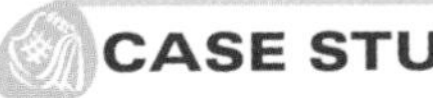

CASE STUDY

Kristin is a 17-year-old pregnant client (P1, G0) who is in her thirtieth week of pregnancy. She comes to the clinic for a routine prenatal visit. Listed below are data collected by the nurse.

Interview Data

Kristin tells the nurse, "I have been feeling pretty good the last few weeks, but I have noticed I'm getting so puffy in my feet, hands, and face. I feel like I'm full of water." When asked about other symptoms or problems, Kristin responds, "I have a backache sometimes." Kristin indicates she feels the baby move "all the time now." She conveys to the nurse that she is excited about the baby but is very worried about how bad the labor pain will be. "My friend Shawna told me that the pain was so bad that I will want to be knocked out when it is time to have the baby."

Examination Data

- **Vital signs:** Blood pressure, 154/96 mm Hg; Pulse, 92 beats/min; Respiration rate, 18; Temperature, 98.3° F (36.8° C); (prepregnancy blood pressure reading, 114/70 mm Hg—within normal limits up until this visit).
- **Weight:** 152 lb (prepregnancy weight, 116 lb). She has had an increase of 10 lb in last month.
- **Fundal height:** 31 cm.
- **Urine dipstick:** 3+ protein.

1. What data deviate from normal findings, suggesting a need for further investigation?
2. What additional information should the nurse ask or assess for?
3. In what functional health patterns does data deviate from normal?
4. What nursing diagnosis and/or collaborative problems should be considered for this situation?

REMEMBER to check out your companion CD-ROM

27 Head-to-Toe Examination and Documentation

www.mosby.com/MERLIN/wilson/assessment/

Now that you have studied and practiced assessing all of the body systems separately, it is time to put everything together. This is tricky, because you start with your knowledge and techniques for each single system, but the client presents to you as a whole person. You must then organize your approach and techniques to examine the person, literally from "head to toe." This means that when you start at the top with the head, you should examine the facial characteristics, skin, hair, eyes, ears, mouth, throat, and range of motion of the neck in a systematic manner. When you have done this, you have assessed the neurologic, integumentary, musculoskeletal, visual, and auditory systems, and the head, neck, nose, and mouth regions. Then you must move on to the next area of the body and do the same. After all body regions are examined, you must then take the information apart again so that it may be systematically analyzed and accurately documented on the client's record.

How each nurse approaches a head-to-toe assessment is usually unique. No two nurses do things in exactly the same way, nor are any two clients exactly the same. Therefore it is important that, as a student, you take time to determine what total examination method works best for you. It is of utmost importance to try to learn a systematic method so that you do not leave things out. When performing a focused assessment, you refer only to those regions needed.

SPECIAL CONSIDERATIONS

Even after you spend hours, days, weeks, and months learning how to do a complete health assessment in a systematic and thorough manner, the unexpected always occurs:

- The baby is crying so hard that there is no way you can listen to the infant's heart or lungs during the examination of the chest. Also, when a baby is crying hard, the tympanic membranes may appear red in the absence of a pathologic condition.
- Every time the client tries to lie down for the abdominal examination, he becomes short of breath.
- The client is paralyzed and confined to a wheelchair, but she needs her annual examination and Papanicolaou (Pap) smear.
- The client arrived in the United States 2 weeks ago from Puerto Rico and does not speak a word of English.

In each of these cases, an examination must be performed. In each case you must individualize your approach and perhaps the order of the actual assessment procedures. Think about each situation just described and plan your approach.

For the baby you can try to quiet the baby by making sure he or she is warm enough and does not have a wet diaper. Have the mother hold and comfort him or her, and try a pacifier or a bottle to provide sucking for comfort or food if hunger is causing the crying.

When a client becomes short of breath when lying supine, raise the head of the examination table to a 45° angle or higher or add pillows behind the client's head and back for elevation. Note the degree of elevation or number of pillows needed to relieve the shortness of breath.

For the client who needs a Pap smear and is confined to a wheelchair, use two or three people to lift the client onto the examination table and assist her to the lithotomy position. Using a mechanical lift device may be another option. If the client has spasms of the lower extremities, one person may need to ensure the client's feet stay in the stirrups during the examination.

For the client who speaks a language you do not know, use an interpreter or family member. This is essential for obtaining a history. If this is not possible, then there are no subjective data for the client. When an interpreter is not available, use gestures to show the client what you are going to do. For example, before auscultating the chest, place the stethoscope on your own chest and take a deep breath, showing the client what you are going to do him or her and what he or she needs to do to assist you.

THE MODEL INTEGRATED HEALTH ASSESSMENT

In the model situation, the assessment should begin as you first meet the client. During this introductory period, watch the client enter the room, noting gait, posture, and ease of movement. Shake hands with the client, and note eye contact and firmness of the hand grip. Introduce yourself to the client, and conduct introductory conversation. Note the language spoken, as well as initial hearing and speech capability. In addition, observe such characteristics as obvious vision difficulties or blindness; difficulty standing, sitting, or rising; obvious musculoskeletal difficulties; general affect; appearance of interest and involvement; dress and posture; general mental alertness, orientation, and integration of thought processes; obvious shortness of breath or posture that would facilitate breathing; and obesity, emaciation, or malnourishment.

After the initial observations, obtain the history, assess vital signs, assess vision, and prepare the client for the examination. Instruct the client to first empty the bladder

Box 27-1 Equipment for Health Examination in a Suggested Order of Use

Writing surface for examiner
Scale with height measurement
Thermometer
Watch with second hand
Vision charts—Snellen's or Jaeger card
Sphygmomanometer
Stethoscope with bell and diaphragm
Client gown
Drape sheet
Examination table (with stirrups for female clients)
Otoscope with pneumatic bulb
Tuning fork
Ophthalmoscope
Nasal speculum
Tongue blade
Penlight
Gauze pads
Nonsterile examination gloves
Cup of water
Ruler and tape measure
Marking pen
Goniometer
Aromatic items
Cotton balls
Sharp and dull testing items
Objects for stereognosis such as a key or comb
Percussion hammer
Lubricant
❖Vagina speculum (for female clients)
❖Pap smear materials (for female clients)
Gooseneck light

(collect specimen if necessary based on client history) and then remove all clothing (including shoes, socks, and underwear), put on a gown, and sit on the table in the examination room. You are now ready to conduct the model assessment as follows, or use the components of the model assessment to conduct an individualized assessment that accommodates the client's special circumstances.

Use the following information only as a guide. It was developed to show how each body system must now be taken apart and integrated with other body systems to permit comprehensive regional assessment. Note in the following example that all relevant body systems in one region are assessed. For example, when the nurse is examining the client's anterior chest, he or she must think about the other body systems in that region that must be assessed at that time and incorporate them into an individual but integrated assessment. Body systems that should be assessed during the anterior chest examination include skin, thorax and lungs, lymphatic, cardiovascular, musculoskeletal, and breast.

Exactly how the assessment and documentation will be formatted depends on the purpose of the assessment, the needs of the client, and the nurse's ability. It is anticipated that, as you actually assess the client, the sample format described below will need to be modified, expanded, or simplified to meet the client's situational needs. Equipment for a health assessment is listed in Box 27-1.

The purpose of providing this guide is to make the point that every time you assess a client, you should regiment your mind and your methods so that you think about each individual and all of what needs to be assessed in a single, systematic, head-to-toe evaluation (Box 27-2). Nothing is worse for a client than having a disorganized nurse who jumps around the client's body assessing areas that were previously forgotten.

Most important are the following points:

- Be organized.
- Develop a routine. This will help with consistency.
- Before you ever begin the actual assessment, have a clear picture in your mind of what you plan to do in what order.
- Practice, practice, practice so that you will learn to become systematic and inclusive.
- Imagine yourself as the client, and prepare as you would want a nurse prepared if he or she were to assess you.

INTEGRATION OF THE INFANT AND PEDIATRIC EXAMINATION

The procedure for integrating the pediatric examination depends entirely on the age and cooperation of the child. By the time the child reaches school age, he or she should be able to participate fully in a cooperative manner. It is the younger child who will present the challenge. The sample format changes in Box 27-3 should facilitate a thorough assessment.

HEALTH ASSESSMENT DOCUMENTATION

Information collected during the health assessment must be organized and documented. The components of the documentation are (1) subjective data (history), (2) objective data (health assessment), (3) risk profile, and (4) problem list/nursing diagnoses. Before the actual documentation, the nurse must decide whether to record the data on plain paper or on a predesigned form. Each has advantages and disadvantages, which are listed in Box 27-4.

Once the style of documentation is determined, the nurse must decide how to synthesize the client's history and health data and then document the information. **The nurse is urged to document what is observed, heard, percussed, or palpated and to avoid using vague and nondescriptive terms such as *normal, negative, good,* or *poor.* Always be specific and descriptive.**

The following documentation model should be viewed as a guide to the comprehensiveness of the types of information that are recorded. The information presented here is not intended to be an exhaustive list of all content areas in-

Text continued on p. 772

Box 27-2 Clinical Guidelines for Adult Head-to-Toe Examination

PROCEDURE	BODY PART OR SYSTEMS INVOLVED	CLINICAL STRATEGIES (ADULT AND OLDER ADULT)
Begin examination with client fully dressed (client may remove shoes for height measurement).		
1. Assess vital signs and other baseline measurements before asking client to get undressed		
Temperature Blood pressure (both arms) Radial pulse Respirations Height Weight Vision testing Snellen's chart or Jaeger card		If deviation from normal discovered, reevaluate when associated system assessed
Instruct client to undress, put on a gown, and sit on the examination table.		
2. Examine client's hands		
Inspect and palpate skin surface characteristics, temperature and moisture of hands	Skin, hair, and nails Heart and peripheral vascular	Both examiner and client will be at ease if examiner starts with client's hands
Inspect and palpate characteristics of nails		
Observe clubbing	Lungs and respiratory	
Inspect and palpate skeletal characteristics and/or deformities of fingers and hands Test range of motion and motor strength of fingers and hands Test muscle strength Inspect symmetry	Musculoskeletal	Fine motor neurologic assessment may be included at this point; others find it more convenient to perform neurologic assessment as a clustered procedure toward end of evaluation period
3. Examine client's arms from wrists to shoulders		
Inspect and palpate skin surface characteristics	Skin, hair, and nails	Examine each arm separately
Test muscle strength Inspect symmetry	Musculoskeletal	
Palpate radial pulses: compare one arm to another	Heart and peripheral vascular	May have already been done during vital signs evaluation
Test range of motion of wrists, elbows, arms, shoulders	Musculoskeletal	
Palpate epitrochlear lymph nodes	Lymphatic	
4. Examine client's head and neck		
Inspect facial characteristics and symmetry Inspect and palpate skin surface characteristics Inspect symmetry and external characteristics of eyes and ears Palpate hair: texture, distribution, quantity	Head and neck Neurologic Skin and hair	Observe head and neck, gathering as much information as possible Do not touch skin until after thorough observation
Palpate scalp		Palpate thoroughly; do not be intimidated by hair spray or dirty hair (may need to wash hands before progressing)

Continued

Box 27-2 Clinical Guidelines for Adult Head-to-Toe Examination—cont'd

PROCEDURE	BODY PART OR SYSTEMS INVOLVED	CLINICAL STRATEGIES (ADULT AND OLDER ADULT)
4. Examine client's head and neck—cont'd		
Palpate facial bones	Musculoskeletal	
Test temporomandibular joint		
Clench teeth	Neurologic—CN V (trigeminal nerve)	
Palpate sinus regions	Paranasal sinuses	
Clench eyes tight, wrinkle forehead, smile, stick out tongue, and puff out cheeks	Neurologic—CN VII, XII (facial, hypoglossal nerves)	Be straightforward; provide client with step-by-step instructions
Assess near vision	Eyes and visual	
Inspect external eye: eyebrows, eyelids, eyelashes, surface characteristics, lacrimal apparatus, corneal surface, anterior chamber, iris		
Assess near vision and eye function: pupillary response, accommodation, cover-uncover test	Neurologic—CN II, III (optic, oculomotor nerves)	
Test extraocular eye movements; vision field testing	Neurologic—CN III, IV, VI, (oculomotor, trochlear, abducens nerves)	Hold chin if head movement occurs
❖Internal eye examination: inspect red reflex, disc, cup margins, vessels, retinal surface, vitreous	Eye and visual	Room must be darkened; should have small amount of secondary light Instruct client to focus on single object at distance
Inspect external ear: alignment, surface characteristics, external canal	Ears and auditory	
Use whisper test to evaluate hearing	Neurologic—CN VIII (acoustic nerve)	Room must be quiet
❖Otoscopic examination: inspect characteristics of external canal, cerumen, eardrum (landmarks)		Use largest speculum that will fit into canal; if necessary, review technique guidelines for using otoscope
Perform Rinne and Weber's tests	Ears and auditory; neurologic—CN VIII (acoustic nerve)	
Inspect nasal structure, septum position; use nasal speculum or otoscope to evaluate patency, turbinates, meatuses	Nose, paranasal sinuses, mouth, and oropharynx	Even though uncomfortable, should be part of every thorough assessment
Evaluate sense of smell	Neurologic—CN I (olfactory nerve)	
Inspect gingivobuccal fornices, buccal mucosa, and gums	Nose, paranasal sinuses, mouth, and oropharynx	
Inspect teeth: number, color, surface characteristics		If client has dentures, they should be removed
Inspect and palpate tongue: symmetry, movement, color, surface characteristics		
Inspect floor of mouth: color, surface characteristics		
Inspect hard and soft palates: color, surface characteristics		

Box 27-2 Clinical Guidelines for Adult Head-to-Toe Examination—cont'd

PROCEDURE	BODY PART OR SYSTEMS INVOLVED	CLINICAL STRATEGIES (ADULT AND OLDER ADULT)
4. Examine client's head and neck—cont'd		
Inspect oropharynx: note mouth odor, anterior and posterior pillars, uvula, tonsils, posterior pharynx		
Palpate tongue and gums		
Evaluate gag reflex	Neurologic—CN IX, X (glossopharyngeal, vagus nerves)	
Test range of motion of head and neck: instruct client to shrug shoulders against resistance; head movement positions, neck flexion and hyperextension, ear-to-shoulder flexion, chin-to-shoulder rotation	Musculoskeletal Neurologic—CN XI (accessory nerve)	
Observe symmetry and smoothness of neck and thyroid region	Head and neck	Client's gown should be lowered slightly so that examiner may fully inspect neck
Palpate carotid pulses	Heart and peripheral vascular	
Observe for jugular venous distention		
❖Palpate trachea, thyroid (isthmus and lobes), lymph nodes (preauricular, postauricular, occipital, parotid, retropharyngeal, submandibular, submental, sublingual, suprahyoid, and thyrolinguofacial as well as the deep and superficial cervical, posterior cervical spinal nerve chain, posterior superficial cervical chain, anterior jugular, and supraclavicular nodes	Head and neck; lymphatic	Client may need drink of water to facilitate swallowing during thyroid evaluation
Auscultate carotid for bruits	Heart and peripheral vascular	
❖Complete assessment of cranial nerves: use cotton swab to evaluate sensitivity of forehead to light touch, cheeks, chin	Neurologic—CN V (trigeminal nerve)	Client should be instructed to close eyes and identify where and when light touch felt
5. Assess posterior chest: examiner moves behind client; client seated; gown to waist for men; gown removed but pulled up to cover breasts for women		
Observe posterior chest: symmetry of shoulders, muscular development, scapular placement, spine straightness, posture	Musculoskeletal	
Observe skin: intactness, color, lesions	Skin	

Continued

Box 27-2 Clinical Guidelines for Adult Head-to-Toe Examination—cont'd

PROCEDURE	BODY PART OR SYSTEMS INVOLVED	CLINICAL STRATEGIES (ADULT AND OLDER ADULT)
5. Assess posterior chest—cont'd		
Observe respiratory movement: excursion, quality, depth, and rhythm of respirations	Lungs and respiratory	
Palpate posterior chest: evaluate muscles and bone structure, palpate excursion of chest expansion; palpate down vertebral column; note straightness	Musculoskeletal Lungs and respiratory	
Palpate posterior chest for fremitus ❖Percuss posterior chest for resonance, respiratory excursion		Palpate with pads of fingers while client says "one-two-three" During excursion evaluation, demonstrate to client how to take deep breath and hold it Measure amount of excursion with ruler
Percuss with fist along costovertebral angle for kidney tenderness	Kidney	
Inspect, bilaterally palpate, and percuss along lateral axillary chest walls	Lungs and respiratory	
Auscultate posterior and lateral chest walls for breath sounds; note quality of sounds heard and presence of adventitious sounds ❖Assess for bronchophony, egophony, and whispered pectoriloquy if adventitious sounds are present	Lungs and respiratory	Instruct client to breathe deeply by mouth
6. Assess anterior chest: move to front of client; client should lower gown to waist		
Inspect skin color, intactness, presence of lesions, muscular symmetry, bilaterally similar bone structure	Skin Musculoskeletal	
Observe chest wall for pulsations or heaving	Heart and peripheral vascular	
Observe movement during respirations Observe client's ease with respirations, posture, pursing lips	Lungs and respiratory	
Female breasts: Inspect size, symmetry, contour, moles or nevi, breast or nipple deviation, dimpling, or lesions; test range of motion of shoulders and regularity of breast tissue during various movements: a. Client's arms extended over head; inspect axillae for rashes, lesions	Musculoskeletal Breasts and axillae	It is helpful to explain to client basically what she will be expected to do and why before actual examination; may help to alleviate client's anxiety as well facilitate active participation

Box 27-2 Clinical Guidelines for Adult Head-to-Toe Examination—cont'd

PROCEDURE	BODY PART OR SYSTEMS INVOLVED	CLINICAL STRATEGIES (ADULT AND OLDER ADULT)
6. Assess anterior chest—cont'd **Female breasts—cont'd** b. Client's arms behind head c. Client's hands behind small of back d. Client's hands pushed tightly against each other at shoulder level e. Client leaning forward slightly so that breasts hang away from chest wall; note symmetry and pull on suspensory ligaments		During examination, it may be helpful to discuss what is being observed; breast self-examination instruction should follow at some point to reiterate these and other aspects of breast examination
Male breasts: Inspect size, symmetry, breast enlargement, nipple discharge, or lesions		
All clients: Palpate anterior chest wall for stability, crepitations, muscular or skeletal tenderness	Musculoskeletal	
Palpate precordium for thrills, heaves, pulsations	Heart and peripheral vascular	Evaluate chest while client is sitting upright and then leaning forward
Palpate left chest wall to locate point of maximum impulse (PMI)	Heart	
Palpate chest wall for fremitus, as with posterior chest Percuss anterior chest for resonance	Lungs and respiratory	If examiner has difficulty percussing woman's anterior chest because of large breasts, percuss downward until breast tissue reached; then postpone further percussion until client lies down
All clients: Palpate lymph nodes associated with lymphatic drainage of breasts and axillae, including lateral axillary, posterior axillary, central axillary, anterior and apical axillary nodes, as well as the mammary, internal mammary, and external mammary nodes of the breast; palpate the epitrochlear node of both arms		
For male clients: Palpate breasts, note swelling or presence of excessive tissue or lumps, nipple discharge, or lesions		
All clients: Auscultate breath sounds of anterior chest from apex to base; note quality, rate, type, presence of adventitious sounds	Lungs and respiratory	Instruct client to breathe deeply through mouth

Continued

Box 27-2 Clinical Guidelines for Adult Head-to-Toe Examination—cont'd

PROCEDURE	BODY PART OR SYSTEMS INVOLVED	CLINICAL STRATEGIES (ADULT AND OLDER ADULT)
6. Assess anterior chest—cont'd		
Auscultate heart: aortic area, pulmonic area, Erb's point, tricuspid area, apical area; note rate, rhythm, location, intensity, frequency, timing, and splitting of S_1, S_2, S_3, S_4 murmurs	Heart and peripheral vascular	Examiner must decide whether to start at apical area and work upward or start at aortic area and work downward; examiner should develop routine method of procedure If examining large-breasted woman, part of auscultatory evaluation may be deferred until client lying down
Assist client to lying or low Fowler position		
7. Assess anterior chest in recumbent position		
Inspect and measure jugular venous pressure for height seen above sternal angle	Heart and peripheral vascular	Extend footrest for client's legs
Female breast inspection: Note symmetry, contour, venous pattern, skin color, areolar area (note size, shape, surface characteristics), nipples (note direction, size, shape, color, surface characteristics, possible crusting)	Breasts and axillae	Provide drape for legs and abdomen Place towel under shoulder of the breast to be evaluated Instruct client to abduct arm overhead Explain procedures to client as performed After breast palpation, may teach client to palpate own breasts
Female breast palpation: Note firmness, tissue qualities, lumps, areas of thickness, or tenderness; areolar and nipple area (note elasticity, tissue characteristics, discharge)		
All clients: Palpate anterior chest wall for cardiac movements or thrills, heaves, pulsations	Heart and peripheral vascular	
Provide chest drape for females; expose abdomen from pubis to epigastric region		
8. Assess abdomen		
Observe skin characteristics from pubis to midchest region; note scars, lesions, vascularity, bulges, navel	Skin and hair	Client should be comfortably positioned with pillow under head and knees slightly flexed to relax abdominal muscles
Observe abdominal contour	Abdomen and gastrointestinal	
Observe movement of abdomen, peristalsis, pulsations	Heart and peripheral vascular	
Auscultate abdomen (all quadrants); note bowel sounds, bruits, venous hums	Abdomen and gastrointestinal Heart and peripheral vascular	
❖Percuss abdomen (all quadrants) and epigastric region for tone	Abdomen and gastrointestinal	
❖Percuss upper and lower liver borders and estimation of liver span		
❖Percuss left midaxillary line for splenic dullness		
Lightly palpate all quadrants; note tenderness, guarding, masses		Allow client to become accustomed to examiner's hands

Box 27-2 Clinical Guidelines for Adult Head-to-Toe Examination—cont'd

PROCEDURE	BODY PART OR SYSTEMS INVOLVED	CLINICAL STRATEGIES (ADULT AND OLDER ADULT)
8. Assess abdomen—cont'd		
Deeply palpate all quadrants; note tenderness, guarding, masses		Gently but firmly move palpation deeper and deeper until examiner convinced that abdomen sufficiently assessed
❖Deeply palpate right costal margin for liver border		Decide whether to use one-hand or two-hand approach
❖Deeply palpate left costal margin for splenic border		
❖Deeply palpate abdomen for right and left kidneys		
Deeply palpate midline epigastric area for aortic pulsation	Heart and peripheral vascular	Tenderness in epigastric area normal
❖Test abdominal reflexes with pointed instrument	Neurologic	
Client raises head to evaluate flexion and strength of abdominal muscles	Musculoskeletal	Note use of arms or hand to assist; older client may have difficulty with this technique
Lightly palpate inguinal region for lymph nodes, femoral pulses, and bulges that may be associated with hernia	Lymphatic Heart and peripheral vascular Abdomen and gastrointestinal	
Client remains lying; abdomen and chest should be draped		
9. Assess lower limbs and hips		
Inspect client's feet and legs for skin characteristics, vascular sufficiency, pulses; note deformities of toes, feet, nails, ankles, legs	Skin, hair, and nails Heart and peripheral vascular Musculoskeletal	
Palpate feet and lower legs; note temperature, pulses, tenderness, deformities	Heart and peripheral vascular Musculoskeletal	
Test range of motion and motor strength of toes, feet, ankles, and knees	Musculoskeletal Neurologic	Motor strength testing may be postponed until patient seated
Test range of motion and motor strength of hips		
Palpate hips for stability	Musculoskeletal	
Client is lying and adequately draped		
10. Assess genitalia, pelvic region, and rectum		
For males: Inspect and palpate external genitalia, including pubic hair, penis and scrotum, testes, epididymides, and vas deferens	Genitalia and reproductive	If mass in scrotal sac suspected, transilluminate
Inspect sacrococcygeal and perianal areas and anus for surface characteristics	Anus, rectum, and prostate	Position client lying on left side with right hip and knee flexed
❖Palpation of anus, rectum, and prostate gland with lubricated gloved finger		Lubricate gloved finger and slowly insert; wait for sphincter to relax before advancing finger
Note characteristics of stool when gloved finger removed	Anus, rectum, and prostate	

Continued

Box 27-2 Clinical Guidelines for Adult Head-to-Toe Examination—cont'd

PROCEDURE	BODY PART OR SYSTEMS INVOLVED	CLINICAL STRATEGIES (ADULT AND OLDER ADULT)
10. Assess genitalia—cont'd		
For females (client should be lying in lithotomy position): With gloved hands inspect and palpate external genitalia, including pubic hair, labia, clitoris, urethral and vaginal orifices, perineal and perianal area and anus for surface characteristics	Genitalia and reproductive Urinary	Wear nonsterile gloves to assess female genitalia
❖Insert vaginal speculum and inspect surface characteristics of vagina and cervix		
❖Collect Pap smear and culture specimen		
❖Perform bimanual palpation to assess form, size, and characteristics of vagina, cervix, uterus, adnexa		Lubricate first two fingers of gloved hand to be inserted internally; other hand should be positioned on abdomen directly above internal hand
❖Perform vaginal-rectal examination to assess rectovaginal septum and pouch, surface characteristics, broad ligament tenderness		When examination completed, client should be offered tissue for drying of genital area
❖Perform rectal examination to assess anal sphincter tone, surface characteristics (anal culture may be obtained)	Anus and rectum	
Note characteristics of stool when lubricated gloved finger removed		
Client resumes seated position; client should have gown on and be draped across lap		
11. Assess neurologic system		
Observe client moving from lying to sitting position; note use of muscles, ease of movement, and coordination	Neurologic Musculoskeletal	
❖Test sensory function by using light and deep (dull and sharp) sensation on forehead, paranasal sinus area, hands, lower arms, feet, lower legs	Neurologic	Client's eyes should be closed; instruct client to either point to or verbally report area that has been touched Alternate light, dull, and pinprick sensations
Bilaterally test and compare vibratory sensations of ankle, wrist, sternum		
❖Test two-point discrimination of palms, thighs, back	Neurologic	
❖Test stereognosis or graphesthesia		
❖Test fine-motor functioning and coordination of upper extremities by instructing client to perform at least two of following: a. Alternating pronation and supination of forearm	Neurologic	Perform technique bilaterally and compare responses

Box 27-2 Clinical Guidelines for Adult Head-to-Toe Examination—cont'd

PROCEDURE	BODY PART OR SYSTEMS INVOLVED	CLINICAL STRATEGIES (ADULT AND OLDER ADULT)
11. Assess neurologic system—cont'd		
b. Touching nose with alternating index fingers		
c. Rapidly alternating finger movements to thumb		
d. Rapidly moving index finger between nose and examiner's finger		
Test and bilaterally compare fine-motor functioning and coordination of lower extremities by instructing client to run heel down tibia of opposite leg		
Alternately cross legs over knee	Musculoskeletal	
Test proprioception by moving the toe up and down	Neurologic	If client shows any neurologic problems, evaluate by Babinski's and ankle clonus tests.
Test and bilaterally compare deep tendon reflexes, including: a. Biceps tendon b. Triceps tendon c. Brachioradialis tendon d. Patellar tendon e. Achilles tendon		
Instruct client to stand		
12. Palpate scrotum and inguinal region (male)	Genitalia	
Palpate scrotum and inguinal region for characteristics and hernias	Genitalia	Instruct client to bear down or cough during hernia evaluation
13. Assess neurologic and musculoskeletal system		
Assessment of client's gait: observe and palpate straightness of client's spine as client stands and bends forward to touch toes	Musculoskeletal Neurologic	Older adult clients may not be able to do this Client's age and general ability may help define which technique to use
With client's waist stabilized, evaluate hyperextension, lateral bending, rotation of upper trunk	Musculoskeletal	
❖Assess proprioception and cerebellar and motor functions by using at least two of the following: a. Romberg's test (eyes closed) b. Walking straight heel-to-toe formation c. Standing on one foot and then other (eyes closed) d. Hopping in place on one foot and then other e. Knee bends	Neurologic	Protect client from falling by remaining close and ready to catch him or her if necessary Older adult clients may not be able to do this

Box 27-3 Clinical Guidelines for Neonatal and Pediatric Examination

AGE AND PREPARATION	ASSESSMENT PROCEDURES	BODY PART OR SYSTEM INVOLVED
Newborn to 6 months: infant undressed, lying on examination table	Check vital signs: temperature, pulse, respiration	
	Record weight, length, chest and head circumference	
	Observe child lying on examination table; note color, general health, body symmetry, gross motor movement, alertness, gross and fine motor development, language development, social adaptive development, skin characteristics, and response to sound and vision stimulation	Heart and peripheral vascular, neurologic, musculoskeletal, skin, eyes and visual, ears and auditory
	Palpate and inspect external characteristics of head, neck, face, axillary region	Lymphatic, head and neck, eyes and visual, ears and auditory, nose, mouth, and oropharynx
	Examine eyes with ophthalmoscope	Eyes and visual
	Examine mouth, teeth (development), tongue, posterior pharynx, nose	Nose, mouth, and oropharynx
	Examine ears with otoscope; test hearing	Ears and auditory
	Palpate thorax, abdomen, and umbilical area	Lungs and respiratory, abdomen and gastrointestinal
	Auscultate thorax, lungs, heart, abdomen	Lungs and respiratory, heart and peripheral vascular, abdomen and gastrointestinal
	Inspect and manipulate hands, arms, shoulders, hips, feet, legs; note range of motion and tone	Musculoskeletal, neurologic
	Inspect skin over extremities, chest, abdomen, and back	Skin, hair, nails
	Observe and palpate external genitalia, inguinal area, and hip stability	Genitalia, musculoskeletal
Six months to 2 years: child in diaper, sitting on parent's lap; examiner's chair should be in front of parent's chair, and during supine examination, child may lie on parent's and examiner's laps	Perform developmental, social, vision, speech, hearing, and fine and gross motor assessment during play and initial "get acquainted" period	Neurologic, eyes and visual, ears and auditory, musculoskeletal
	Record weight, length, and chest and head circumferences	

Box 27-3 Clinical Guidelines for Neonatal and Pediatric Examination—cont'd

AGE AND PREPARATION	ASSESSMENT PROCEDURES	BODY PART OR SYSTEM INVOLVED
Six months to 2 years—cont'd	Check vital signs, including blood pressure in children over 18 months of age (may be postponed until later if child becomes agitated)	
	Inspect and palpate external characteristics of head, neck, and face	Skin, hair, head, neck
	Examine ears with otoscope; test hearing	Ears, auditory
	Examine eyes with ophthalmoscope	Eyes, visual
	Examine nose, mouth, teeth (development), tongue, and posterior pharynx	Nose, mouth, oropharynx
	Inspect skin over chest, abdomen, and back	Skin
	Palpate chest and axillae	Lungs, respiratory, lymphatic, axillae
	Auscultate heart and lungs	Lungs, respiratory
	Auscultate abdomen with child in supine position	Heart
	Palpate abdomen	Abdomen, gastrointestinal
	Inspect and manipulate hands, arms, shoulders, hips, legs, and feet	Skin, nails, musculoskeletal, neurologic, peripheral vascular
	Inspect and palpate external genitalia, inguinal area, and hip stability	Genitalia, musculoskeletal
Two to 4 years: Child undressed to underpants; may be examined either on parent's lap or examination table; much of assessment may be informal as examiner observes and plays with child	Same assessment procedures as for child age 6 months to 2 years	
Four to 6 years: child undressed to underpants, sitting on examination table; assessment should move toward adult format; child's developmental immaturity may necessitate that examiner alter various examination techniques to facilitate child's participation and correct response	Same assessment procedures as for child age 6 months to 2 years	
Over 6 years old: child in gown on examination table	Same assessment procedures and approach as for adult client	

Box 27-4 Comparison of Documentation Forms

PLAIN PAPER	PREDEVELOPED FORM
Advantages	**Advantages**
Documentation space is not a problem. Specific data for individual client may be emphasized as necessary.	Departmental continuity is maintained. Data will be easy to locate by other examiners. Preprinted forms serve as reminder for completeness.
Disadvantages	**Disadvantages**
The examiner must be organized; if not, rambling and insignificant data may be a problem. All examiners in the agency may not use the same format.	Individual situations may be difficult to emphasize. Examiner may not have adequate space for documentation. If form was developed without examiner's input, it may not include all data the examiner wants to collect. Separate forms necessary for different types of clients (e.g., children, older adults).

cluded in the text. For complete and detailed descriptions of the information that may be recorded, refer to the individual body system chapters.

DOCUMENTATION FORMAT

Subjective Database (History)

- Biographic data
- Reason for seeking care
- Present health status
  - Current health promotion activities
  - Client's perceived level of health
  - Current medications
- Past health history
  - Allergies
  - Childhood illnesses
  - Surgeries
  - Hospitalizations
  - Accidents or injuries
  - Chronic diseases
  - Immunizations
  - Last examinations
  - Obstetric history
- Family history with genogram
- Review of physiologic systems
  - Sleep and rest
  - Nutritional status
  - Skin, hair, nails
  - Head
  - Eyes
  - Ears, nose, mouth, and oropharynx
  - Neck
  - Breasts
  - Cardiovascular
  - Respiratory
  - Gastrointestinal
  - Urinary
  - Genitalia
  - Musculoskeletal
  - Neurologic
  - Endocrine
- Psychosocial status
  - General statement about feelings about self
  - Activities
  - Cultural/religious practices
  - Occupational history
  - Recent changes or stresses
  - Changes in personality, behavior, mood
  - Habits
  - Financial status
- Environmental health
  - General assessment
  - Employment
  - Home
  - Neighborhood
  - Community

Objective Database (Health Examination)

- Baseline measurements
  - Height
  - Weight
  - Body mass index (BMI)
- Vital signs
  - Temperature
  - Pulse
  - Blood pressure (both arms, lying and sitting)
  - Respiration
- Communication skills
- General appearance
- Integumentary system (skin, hair, and nails)
  - Color
  - Integrity, moisture, temperature, and texture of skin
  - Distribution, surface characteristics, and texture of hair
  - Shape, contour, thickness, and cleanliness of nails
- Head and neck
  - Contour and intactness of skull
  - Size and symmetry of head and face
  - Description of lymph nodes
  - ❖Size and consistency of thyroid gland
  - ❖Position of trachea
  - Range of motion of neck

- Nose
  Position, including septum
  Nasal patency
  Appearance of turbinates
- Mouth and pharynx
  Condition and alignment of teeth
  Color and characteristics of tongue, mucosa, pharynx, gums
  Position and appearance of tonsils and palate
  Symmetry and movement of tongue and uvula
  Presence of taste and gag reflex
- Ears and auditory system
  Position and alignment of auricles
  Surface characteristics of external ear and canal
  ❖ Characteristics of auditory canal and tympanic membrane
  Tests of hearing
  Rinne and Weber's tests
- Eyes and visual system
  Visual acuity and visual fields
  Symmetry of extraocular movements
  Distribution and symmetry of eyebrows
  Position and symmetry of eyelids and eyelashes
  Color and patency of lacrimal puncta
  Clarity and color of conjunctiva and sclera
  Transparency of cornea and anterior chamber
  Color and shape of iris
  Reaction of pupils to light
  Presence of consensual response to light
  ❖ Findings from ophthalmoscopic examination
- Lungs and respiratory system
  Chest wall configuration and anteroposterior diameter
  Respiratory depth and rhythm
  Symmetry and tactile fremitus of chest wall
  ❖ Sound tones on percussion and diaphragm excursion
  Description of breath sounds
- Heart and peripheral vascular system
  Location and characteristics of the apical impulse
  Description of S_1 and S_2 to note location, pitch, intensity, timing, splitting, systole, and diastole
  Description of jugular veins
  Description of peripheral pulses: quality of pulses, bilaterally equal
- Breasts and axillae
  Size, shape, symmetry, and color of breasts
  Surface characteristics of breasts and axillae
  Description of tissue consistency
  Description of lymph nodes of breast and axillae
- Abdomen and gastrointestinal system
  Color, surface characteristics, and contour
  Presence of visible aortic pulsations
  Description of bowel sounds in all quadrants
  Response to light and deep palpation of all quadrants
  ❖ Palpation of liver and spleen
  ❖ Palpation of kidneys
  ❖ Percussion of liver borders and spleen
  Description of inguinal lymph nodes
- Female genitalia and reproductive system
  Characteristics of external genitalia
  ❖ Speculum examination: surface characteristics of vagina and cervix
  ❖ Bimanual examination: size and position of uterus and ovaries
- Male genitalia
  Characteristics of external genitalia
  Location and consistency of testes, epididymides, and vas deferens
  ❖ Patency of inguinal canal
- Anus, rectum, and prostate
  Color and surface characteristics of perianal area and anus
  Description of anal sphincter tone
  ❖ Characteristics of rectal wall, contents of rectum
  ❖ Size and surface characteristics of prostate
- Musculoskeletal system
  Steadiness of gait
  Alignment and symmetry of extremities and spine
  Range of motion of joints
  Muscle development, symmetry, and strength
- Neurologic system
  Cranial nerve assessment
  Presence of fine and gross motor function
  Balance and coordination
  Sensory evaluation
  Presence of deep tendon reflexes

Risk Profile The risk profile should include those items from the client's history and health assessment that might indicate risk to the overall health status. They are potential problems. After you have determined any risk factors that the client may have, you should discuss with the client how some or all of these may be modified. (Remember that not all risk factors are modifiable.) The history and health assessment provides an excellent opportunity to discuss health promotion with the client (see Health Promotion boxes in Chapters 11-26).

Problem List or Nursing Diagnoses The problem list or nursing diagnoses should be selected based on your synthesis of data that are identified as stressors for the client. The stressors may be physiologic, sociologic, psychologic, or a combination. The problems are those items that reduce the client's overall level of health. Cluster subjective and objective data to identify problems or nursing diagnoses. Current nursing diagnoses are listed in Appendix B. Once the problems or nursing diagnoses are listed and assigned a priority, then you decide which are within your scope of practice to complete and which must be referred to other health care providers.

Always remember to document accurately and completely subjective and objective findings. Your record will be the basis for subsequent care and health promotion delivered to the client.

Two examples of health assessment documentation, one for an adult and one for a neonate, follow in Appendix A.

APPENDIX

REMEMBER to check out your companion CD-ROM

A Sample Documentation

www.mosby.com/MERLIN/wilson/assessment/

ADULT CLIENT

Note: This health assessment documentation is for the client whose history appears in Chapter 4, "Interviewing to Obtain a Health History"; thus the documentation begins with the examination.

Physical Examination

General: Cooperative, oriented, alert woman; maintains eye contact; appropriately groomed.

Vital signs: BP 110/78; P 78; R 14; T 98° F (36.7° C); Wt 137 lb (62 kg); Ht 5′7″ (170 cm).

Skin, hair, nails: Smooth, soft, moist, tanned, warm, intact skin with elastic turgor. Hair brown with female distribution, soft texture; nails smooth, rounded, manicured.

Head and neck: Skull symmetric; scalp intact; face and jaw symmetric; trachea midline; thyroid smooth, soft, size of thumb pad; full ROM of neck.

Eyes: Vision 20/20 each eye with contact lenses; near vision, able to read magazine at 13″ with contacts. Peripheral vision present; EOM intact; brows, lids, and lashes symmetric; eyeball indents with slight pressure; lacrimal ducts pink and open without discharge. Conjunctiva clear, sclera white, moist and clear; cornea smooth and transparent, iris transparent and flat, PERRLA.

Ophthalmic exam: red reflex present, disc margins distinct, round, yellow; artery to vein 2:3, retina red uniformly; macula and fovea slightly darker.

Ears: Auricles aligned with eyes, ears symmetric, ear lobes pierced once. Moderate creamy cerumen in auditory canal, TM pearly gray, cone of light reflex present. Able to hear whispered voice 2 ft to side.

Nose and sinuses: Septum midline, nasal cavity patent, able to identify lemon scent. Turbinates pink with moderate serous exudate, no pain on sinus palpation.

Mouth and throat: TMJ moves without difficulty, no halitosis. Lips symmetric moist, smooth; 32 white, smooth, and aligned teeth. Mucous membranes pink and moist, symmetric pillars, clear saliva. Tongue symmetric, pink, moist, and movable. Hard palate smooth, pale; soft palate smooth, pink and rises, uvula midline; posterior pharynx pink, smooth, tonsils pink with irregular texture.

Chest and lungs: AP diameter ½ lateral, muscle and respiratory effort symmetric, equal excursion, tactile fremitus equal, resonant percussion tones throughout, diaphragm excursion 3 cm bilaterally, vesicular breath sounds throughout with no adventitious sounds; even, quiet breathing.

Breasts: Moderate size R slightly > L; granular consistency bilaterally, fibrocystic changes in both breasts, more pronounced in outer quadrants; nipples erect without discharge, areolas symmetric with Montgomery's tubercles; symmetric venous pattern; no palpable axillary lymph nodes, no dimpling.

Heart: Apical pulse palpated at fifth LICS, MCL; no lifts, heaves, or thrills or abnormal pulsations, S_1 and S_2 heard without splitting, no murmurs; S_1 heard best at apex, S_2 at base.

Peripheral vascular: Pulse rate and rhythm regular; smooth contour, jugular venous pulsation visible at 30° elevation, no carotid, renal, or abdominal bruits; no edema or tenderness; lower extremities warm and pink with symmetric hair distribution, pulse amplitude 2+ in all pulses, except dorsalis pedis 1+.

Abdomen: Rounded, striae noted; skin smooth with no lesions; bowel sounds in all quadrants; tympanic percussion tones, liver span 6 cm at RMCL; abdomen soft, nontender; liver, spleen, and kidney not palpable; no CVA tenderness, no inguinal lymphadenopathy; superficial abdominal reflexes intact.

Musculoskeletal: Full ROM in all joints without tenderness; muscle strength 5/5 bilaterally, extremities aligned and symmetric, vertebral column straight.

Neurologic: Oriented to time, place, person; coordinated, smooth gait; cranial nerves I to XII grossly intact; negative Romberg's sign; alternating rapid movement and sensory function intact.

Gynecologic: Pubic hair in female distribution; labia smooth and soft; urethral meatus midline; perineum smooth without lesions; Skene's and Bartholin's glands nontender; vaginal tone firm; cervix pink, midline, posterior pointed; parous os with regular shape, pliable, smooth; no discharge noted in vagina or cervical os; vaginal wall smooth, homogenous, moist, and nontender; anteverted uterus, pear-shaped, firm, smooth, movable, nontender; ovaries smooth, firm, movable. Rectal wall smooth, nontender, sphincter tone tight, 2 small hemorrhoids. Specimen for Pap smear collected.

Problem List

- Seasonal allergies.
- Needs tetanus immunization.
- Concerned about fibrocystic disease.
- Conflict with mother over discipline of children.
- Concerned about relationship with new principal.

Functional Health Patterns

- Health perception–health management: Pap smear, tetanus immunization, prevention of fibrocystic disease.
- Activity–exercise: seasonal allergic response.
- Role-relationship: conflict with mother, concern about principal.

Nursing Diagnosis

- *Risk for altered health maintenance* related to preventive health services (tetanus immunization and preventive behavior for fibrocystic disease).
- *Ineffective airway clearance* related to allergic reaction.
- *Decisional conflict* related to mother's interaction with children.
- *Anxiety related to changes* associated with new principal.

Outcomes

- Client will consent to tetanus immunization.
- Client will continue vitamin E and reduction in caffeine for fibrocystic disease.
- Client will be relieved of seasonal nasal allergy reaction.
- Client will discuss feelings about conflict with mother and decide a plan of action.
- Client will discuss feelings about new principal and options available.

Nursing Interventions

- Assist with Pap smear.
- Administer tetanus toxoid 0.5 ml SQ right deltoid.
- Encourage client to continue vitamin E and caffeine reduction, discuss fibrocystic disease, provide pamphlet. Client voiced understanding of the condition and prevention.
- Teach client action and side effects of medication for rhinorrhea, expressed understanding.
- Discuss feelings about mother and children. Identify social support resources available to assist with a plan for action.
- Discuss feelings about new principal and options available if relationship becomes positive or negative.

OLDER ADULT CLIENT

Date: 1-8-00

Biographic Data

Name: Sara Jane Borden
Address: 1001 S. Gloucester St.
Richland, TX 76092-2415
Telephone: (214) 650-7650.
Date of birth: 7-5-21.
Birthplace: Topeka, Kansas.
Gender: Female.
Race: Black.
Religion: Protestant.
Marital status: Widow.
Soc. security no.: 459-67-9980.
Occupation: Retired.
Source of referral: Daughter: Karen Marsh.
Usual source of health care: Dr. Murphy, who retired.
Source and reliability of information: Self; reliable.
Advance directive: Yes, copy in file.
Health Insurance: Medicare and private insurance.

Reason for Seeking Health Care

Pain in right leg and knee when walking for last 2 months.

Present Illness

Pain is burning and radiates from right hip to knee, worse when getting up in the morning; has to hobble to bathroom; after up for a few hours, pain is better, but never completely relieved; tried water exercise and ibuprofen to relieve pain; pain sometimes prevents grocery shopping, because pain is worse the longer she stands; pain relieved somewhat by sitting; unable to take daily walks since pain occurred.

Present Health Status

Current health promotion activities: Walks with a friend 1½ miles around track at local high school 4 to 5 times each week. Eats diet consistent with food pyramid. Stopped drinking coffee and eating chocolate because of fibrocystic breast disease.

Client's perceived level of health: "I feel pretty healthy for someone my age. I take care of myself and can still live alone and play bridge."

Current medications: Dyazide 1 tab daily
Lanoxin 0.25 mg daily
Captopril 50 mg bid
Premarin 0.625 mg daily
Vitamin E 400 units daily
Calcium supplement daily

Past Health History

Allergies: Morphine and codeine "make me deathly ill."
Sulfa drugs "break me out in a rash."

Childhood illness: Chicken pox, measles, mumps.

Surgeries: Tonsillectomy as a child
Cholecystectomy 1993
Carpal tunnel 1991
C-section 1945, 1949
Appendectomy 1940
Total hysterectomy with anterior/posterior repair 1954

Hospitalizations: Chest pain 1993.

Accidents or injuries: None.

Chronic diseases: Hypertension for 30 years
Type 2 diabetes controlled with diet for 25 years
Fibrocystic breast disease for 7 years

Immunizations: Tetanus—doesn't remember date
Annual flu shot
Pneumonia immunization 1999

Last exams: Eyes—3 months ago
Ears—wears hearing aid R ear since 1970, nerve deafness
Dental—8 months ago
Physician—for annual physical
ECG—today
Mammogram—10 years ago

Review of Systems

In good health until 2 months ago.

Mental health status: Appropriate responses to all questions, short- and long-term memory intact, positive outlook, able to cope with stress.

Sleep and rest: Daily nap—2 hr. Sleeps 9:30 PM to 6:00 AM. Gets up once in night for bathroom. Pain in R leg sometimes keeps her awake.

Nutritional status: Eats according to food pyramid. Daughter sometimes shops for groceries when client's leg and knee hurt.

Skin, hair, nails: Skin itches on feet because of diabetic neuropathy; skin thin, bleeds easily when she bumps her arm or her cat scratches her while playing; bathes daily; applies body lotions; has hair fixed weekly; keeps nails manicured and polished.

Head: Reports no headaches unless her blood pressure is elevated.

Eyes: Wears bifocals, has black floaters, photophobia; able to see to read, watches television, drives; reports no blurred vision, itching, drainage.

Ears: Wears hearing aide R ear because of nerve deafness; reports no tinnitus, pain, drainage.

Nose and sinuses: Reports no congestion, drainage, sinus pain.

Throat and mouth: Reports no sore throat, hoarseness, dysphagia, bleeding gums, or difficulty in chewing; no dental appliances, brushes and flosses teeth twice daily, no slipping or crepitation of temporomandibular joint.

Genogram

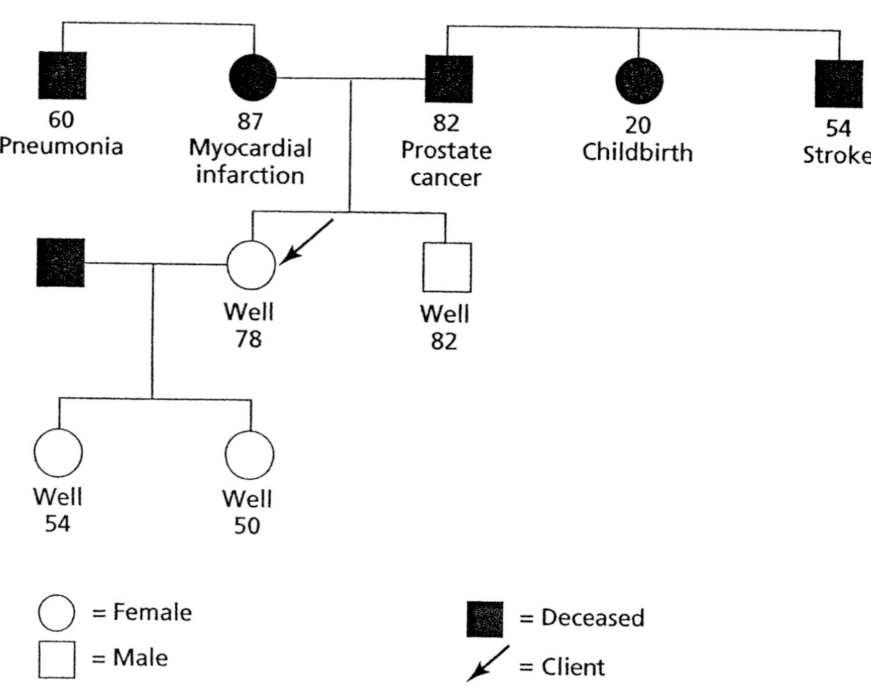

Neck: Reports no stiffness or tenderness.

Breasts: Reports no tenderness or nipple drainage; performs breast self-exam when she remembers, about every 6 months; has fibrocystic disease that has improved since she started taking vitamin E and decreased coffee and chocolate.

Cardiovascular: Last blood pressure was normal, chest pain 1993, hospitalized, palpitation 2 years ago, feet swell; no report of shortness of breath, dyspnea, or chest pain; extremities warm and with no discoloration.

Respiratory: Had pneumonia last year, treated at home with antibiotics; no reports of wheeze, cough, dyspnea, SOB, or hemoptysis.

Hematolymphatic: No report of excess bruising; bleeds easily when bumps arm or cat scratches her "due to thinner skin since I'm getting old." No swollen lymph nodes reported.

Gastrointestinal: No report of diarrhea, constipation, rectal bleeding, nausea, or emesis; has bowel movement each morning after breakfast, formed brown stool; no report of laxative use, eats fresh vegetables instead.

Genitourinary: Voids about 5 times each day, clear light yellow; reports no nocturia, dysuria, itching, or discharge.

Musculoskeletal: No report of weakness, spasms, or pain until 2 months ago when hip and leg pain began.

Neurologic: No report of difficulty performing activities of daily living until pain in hip and leg began; has tingling in her feet periodically from diabetic neuropathy, rubbing her feet helps.

Endocrine: No report of changes in thyroid function, skin, or hair. Has polyuria when she goes off her diet; occurs several times per year, usually during holidays.

Psychosocial Status

Feelings about self: Feels she helps with grandchildren and contributes to family. Has a positive outlook. Enjoys playing bridge.

Significant others: Brother, daughters, and grandchildren.

Cultural/religious practices: Born in U.S., black, belongs to Methodist church, not active.

Occupational history: High school teacher until retirement.

Educational level: Master's degree.

Activities of daily living: All self-care, prepares meals, shops for groceries, plays bridge twice a week at churches.

Habits: Smokes ½ pack of cigarettes/day, drinks one bourbon with water nightly while fixing dinner.

Financial: Lives on social security, teacher retirement, and investments.

Environmental Health

Home: Lives alone in a two-story, three-bedroom, two-bath apartment with a cat.

Neighborhood: Lives in a suburban neighborhood with stores and service station nearby. She drives wherever she needs to go.

Commu
service
declini

Physical

General: C
contact, a
Vital signs:
130 lb (59
Skin, hair, na
ecchymosis
trauma, no
hair, gray wi
Head: Scalp int
Neck: Trachea m ... ble or
tender, no lyr ... full range of motion
with strong m ... ment, no tenderness or masses; carotid arteries full, round, rate = 88, jugular veins flat at 45°.

Nose and sinuses: Septum midline, patent bilaterally, mucous membranes moist and pink without exudate, no pain on palpation of sinuses; correctly identified coffee and orange odors bilaterally.

Mouth and throat: Mucosa and gingiva pink and moist without lesions, 28 teeth in good repair, tongue midline without lesions or tremor, uvula midline with elevation of soft palate, gag reflex intact, pharynx pink, moist without exudate, no hoarseness.

Ears: Auricles aligned with eyes without lesions, masses, or tenderness; tympanic membranes gray, translucent with light reflex and bony landmarks present; no perforations. Weber's lateralizes to right ear, negative Rinne (BC>AC) right ear; repeats whispered words at ½ foot bilaterally (with hearing aid).

Eyes: Snellen 20/20 each eye with glasses, near vision, able to read newspaper at 14 inches with glasses; brows, lids, and lashes intact with no crusting; no tearing; conjunctiva pink without discharge, sclera white; corneal light reflex symmetric; pupils equal, round, and react to light and accommodation; extraocular movement intact, peripheral vision bilaterally, discs with well-defined borders bilaterally, vessels present in all quadrants without crossing defects, no hemorrhages or exudates; retina pink, macula present; cornea, lens, and vitreous clear.

Chest and lungs: AP diameter < lateral, muscle and respiratory effort symmetric, equal excursion, tactile fremitus equal, resonant percussion throughout, diaphragmatic excursion 4 cm bilaterally, vesicular breath sounds throughout with no adventitious sounds; even, quiet breathing.

Heart: Apical pulse full and round fifth L, ICS MCL; no L, lifts, heaves, thrills, or abnormal pulsations; S_1 and S_2 present with regular rate and rhythm without murmurs.

Breasts: Symmetric, moderate size, nodular, granular consistency bilaterally; nipples soft without discharge, areolas equal in size, no dimpling, masses, tenderness, or lesions; no lymphadenopathy.

, skin smooth with no le- , bowel sounds in all quad- ic percussion tones over most of 6 cm at right MCL; abdomen soft, kidney not palpable, no abdominal ten- VA tenderness, no inguinal lymphadenop- rficial abdominal reflexes intact.

: Female hair distribution, sparse amount of r; external genitalia dark pink, dry, no lesions or discharge; vaginal walls nontender; anus, no hemorrhoids, fissures, or lesions; rectal wall no tenderness, no masses, strong sphincter tone, stool soft brown, guaiac negative.

Peripheral vascular: Extremities black, no edema, clubbing; pulses strong, round, warm, no tenderness.

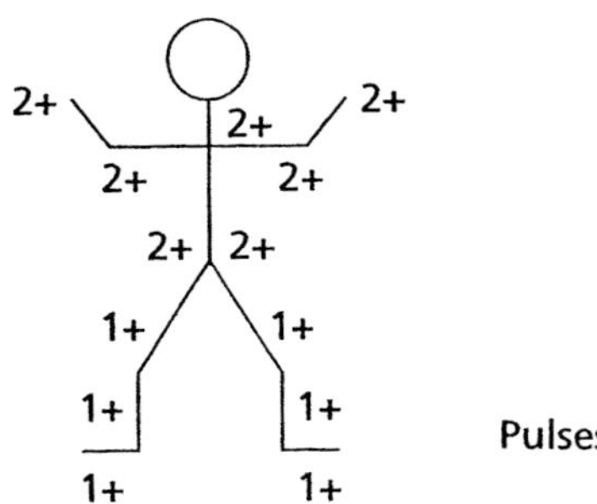

Musculoskeletal: Vertebral column symmetric, no tenderness or curvature; full extension, lateral bending and rotation; arms and left leg symmetric, range of motion without pain or crepitation; right leg pain with hip and knee flexion and straight leg raises; muscle strength 4/5.

Neurologic: Cranial nerves I-XII intact; upper extremity (UE) sensation intact to pinprick, vibration, and light touch bilaterally; lower extremity (LE) sensation decreased to pinprick and vibration and absent to light touch; deep tendon reflexes 2+ UE and 1+ LE; Babinski's negative bilaterally, no clonus; negative Romberg's, cerebellum finger to nose intact, unable to walk on toes of right foot.

Problem List

- Pain in right leg.
- Type 2 diabetes mellitus controlled with diet.
- Health promotion behaviors: BSE q 6 months; smoking.
- Anticipatory guidance: plans for transportation when no longer able to drive due to visual impairment.

Functional Health Patterns

- Activity–exercise
- Nutrition–metabolic
- Health perception–health management
- Coping–stress tolerance

Nursing Diagnosis

- *Pain* related to ineffective comfort measures.
- *Risk for ineffective management of therapeutic regimen: individual* related to dietary control of type 2 diabetes mellitus.
- *Altered health maintenance* related to smoking behavior and frequency of BSE.
- *Anticipatory grieving for loss of independence* when no longer able to drive due to visual impairment.

CHILD CLIENT

Date: 1-5-00

Biographic Data

Name: Roberto Aquera
Address: 912 West Rochelle, Apt. 101
Fort Worth, TX 76129
Telephone: (817) 921-7659
Date of birth: 12-1-99.
Birthplace: Medical Center Hospital
Fort Worth, Texas
Race: Hispanic.
Culture: Mexican-American.
Religion: Catholic.
Marital status: Single.
Family in home: Lives with parents and older brother.
Soc. security no.: 693-42-8309.
Occupation: Not applicable.
Parents employed full time: mother as teacher aide, father as plumber.
Contact person: Arturo and Esther Aquero.
Advance directive: Not applicable.
Dual power of attorney: Not applicable.
Usual source of health care: Private.
Health insurance: Yes—health maintenance organization.
Description of home: Two-bedroom apartment, ground floor.
Source of data: Parents, reliable sources.

Reason for Seeking Health Care

"Cough and runny nose for 3 days."

Present Health Status

He was well until 3 days ago. Nasal drainage is slightly thick and yellow, cough is productive. No fever, sneezing, or rash reported. He coughs more when lying down, nose runs more when he is sitting up. No medications have been given due to his age.

Past Health History

Health of mother:

Prenatal care: In second and third trimesters.

Complications during pregnancy: None.

Planned pregnancy: Yes.

Mother's attitude: Pleased with healthy baby, wanted a girl.

Father's attitude: Pleased with healthy baby.

Hospitalizations: Vaginal delivery with epidural anesthesia 4 weeks ago, breech presentation, 38 weeks' gestation, no complications during labor or delivery.

Health of neonate:

Birth weight: 7 lb 13 oz; length: 22½ inches.

Allergies: None.

Immunizations: First hepatitis B at birth.

Family history: Father, alive and well, age 26
Mother, alive and well, age 23
Brother, alive and well, age 5

Genogram

Review of Systems

Sleep: 6 to 7 hours at night, several naps during the day; sleeps on side or back.

Nutrition: Bottle feeding, Similac formula 4 to 5 oz per feeding, 7 to 8 feedings per day.

Skin, hair, nails: Reports no changes in skin, hair, or nails; has darker area over buttocks.

Eyes: Opens eyes to sounds, follows movement.

Ears: Turns head to noises, no discharges reported.

Nose: Has had moderately thick yellow discharge, previously able to breath without difficulty.

Throat: No difficulty reported, swallows formula without difficulty, strong suck.

Neck: No swollen areas reported, turns head to noises.

Cardiovascular: No difficulty reported.

Genogram

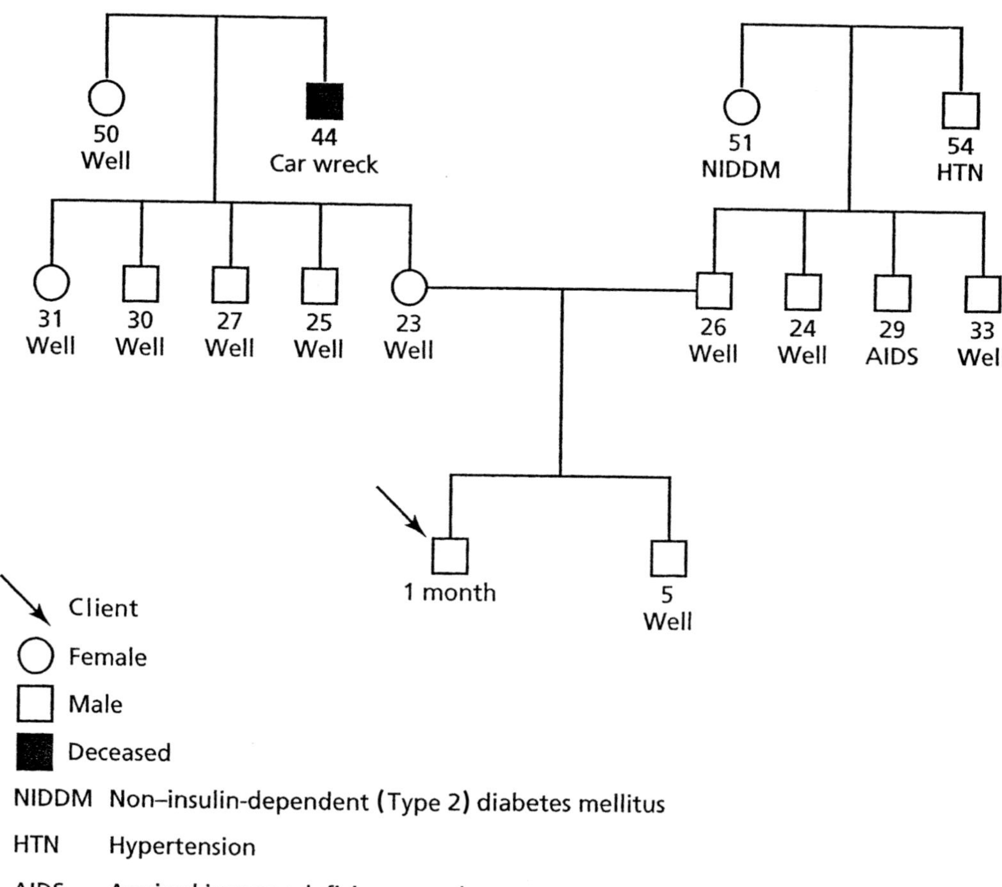

Respiratory: Cough for 3 days, no sneezing, wheezing. Stops frequently to take breaths during feeding.
Gastrointestinal: See nutrition above; has 1 to 2 soft stools each day, no abdominal distention reported.
Genitourinary: Urinates 7 to 8 times a day.
Musculoskeletal: Moves all extremities symmetrically.
Neurologic: Cry is normal, parents able to console him; likes to be held.

Psychosocial Status

Sibling rivalry: Older child is adjusting to new brother; was jealous at first, now helps with care of younger brother.
Return to work: Mother returns to work in 2 weeks; baby's aunt will keep him while parents work.

Environmental Health

Safety: Using infant car seat and seat belts, parents supported baby's head appropriately, neither parent smokes.
Home: Lives in two-bedroom, centrally heated and air-conditioned home with parents and 5-year-old brother. House on 3 acres. Use septic tank and well water.
Neighborhood: Lives in small town (5,000 people) outside major metropolitan area. Know many people in the town, parents grew up there.
Community: School and parks available, major hospital 30 miles in next town. Community clinic for periodic check-ups.

Physical Examination

General: Alert, active infant—age 1 month, 4 days.
Vital signs: T 98.2° F (36.8° C); P 130 bpm; R 40 rpm; Ht (length): 22½″ (57 cm) (90th percentile); Wt: 11 lb 12 oz (5.3 kg) (90th percentile); Head circumference: 14¾″ (37 cm) (90th percentile); Chest circumference: 13½″ (34 cm).
Skin: Light brown, smooth, soft; turgor elastic; mongolian spot over buttocks.
Head: Anterior fontanel soft, diamond-shaped 1¼″ (3.2 cm); posterior fontanel soft, triangular-shaped ½″ (1.25 cm); skull symmetric, hair evenly distributed.
Eyes: Symmetric, sclera white, conjunctiva moist, pink, no tears; red reflex bilaterally; pupils equal, round, and react to light, symmetric corneal light reflex, able to follow to midline.
Ears: Lateral edge of eye aligned with top of pinna, pinna flexible, cartilage present; startle reflex elicited by loud noise; tympanic membrane pearly gray bilaterally.
Nose: Symmetric, patent, small amount yellow exudate.
Mouth and throat: Mucous membranes moist, uvula midline, sucking, rooting, and gag reflexes present.
Neck: Short, thick neck.
Chest and lungs: Anteroposterior and lateral diameters equal, no retraction noted; abdominal respirations, bilateral bronchial breath sounds.
Heart: Apex fourth ICS, MCL, S_2 slightly sharper and higher in pitch than S_1.
Abdomen: Round; bowel sounds in all quadrants; liver, spleen, kidneys not palpable; equal bilateral femoral pulses.
Genitalia: Urethral opening at tip of glans penis, circumcised; testes palpable in scrotum.
Musculoskeletal: Hands closed, full range of motion, nail beds pink; spine intact, vertebral column straight, patent; hips stable.
Neurologic: Extension of extremity followed by some degree of flexion, head lag while sitting, able to turn head side to side when prone, grasp reflex strong, tonic neck reflex present.

Problem List

- Nasal congestion, purulent rhinorrhea.
- Remind parents of immunizations due at 2 months: Hep B, IPV, Hib, DPT.

Nursing Diagnosis

- *Ineffective airway clearance* related to nasal congestion.
- *Health-seeking behaviors of parents* related to immunization schedule.

Functional Health Patterns

- Activity–exercise
- Health perception–health management

APPENDIX B

NANDA Nursing Diagnoses

www.mosby.com/MERLIN/wilson/assessment/

Activity intolerance
Activity intolerance, risk for
Adaptive capacity, decreased: intracranial
Adjustment, impaired
Airway clearance, ineffective
Anxiety
Anxiety, death
Aspiration, risk for
Body image disturbance
Body temperature, altered, risk for
Bowel incontinence
Breastfeeding, effective
Breastfeeding, ineffective
Breastfeeding, interrupted
Breathing pattern, ineffective
Cardiac output, decreased
Caregiver role strain
Caregiver role strain, risk for
Communication, impaired verbal
Community coping, ineffective
Community coping, potential for enhanced
Confusion, acute
Confusion, chronic
Constipation
Constipation, perceived
Constipation, risk for
Coping, defensive
Coping, family: potential for growth
Coping, ineffective family: compromised
Coping, ineffective family: disabling
Coping, ineffective individual
Decisional conflict (specify)
Denial, ineffective
Dentition, altered
Development, altered, risk for
Diarrhea
Disuse syndrome, risk for
Diversional activity deficit
Dysreflexia
Dysreflexia, autonomic, risk for
Energy field disturbance

From *NANDA nursing diagnoses: definitions and classification 1999-2000*, Philadelphia, 1999, North American Nursing Diagnosis Association.

Environmental interpretation syndrome, impaired
Failure to thrive, adult
Family processes, altered
Family processes, altered: alcoholism
Fatigue
Fear
Fluid volume deficit
Fluid volume deficit, risk for
Fluid volume excess
Fluid volume imbalance, risk for
Gas exchange, impaired
Grieving, anticipatory
Grieving, dysfunctional
Growth, altered, risk for
Growth and development, altered
Health maintenance, altered
Health-seeking behaviors (specify)
Home maintenance management, impaired
Hopelessness
Hyperthermia
Hypothermia
Incontinence, stress
Incontinence, total
Incontinence, urge
Incontinence, urinary, functional
Incontinence, urinary, reflex
Incontinence, urinary urge, risk for
Infant behavior, disorganized
Infant behavior, disorganized, risk for
Infant behavior, organized, potential for enhanced
Infant feeding pattern, ineffective
Infection, risk for
Injury, perioperative positioning, risk for
Injury, risk for
Knowledge deficit (specify)
Latex allergy
Latex allergy, risk for
Loneliness, risk for
Management of therapeutic regimen, community: ineffective
Management of therapeutic regimen, families: ineffective
Management of therapeutic regimen, individual: effective
Management of therapeutic regimen, individuals: ineffective
Memory, impaired
Mobility, impaired bed
Mobility, impaired physical
Mobility, impaired wheelchair
Nausea
Noncompliance (specify)
Nutrition, altered: less than body requirements
Nutrition, altered: more than body requirements
Nutrition, altered: risk for more than body requirements
Oral mucous membrane, altered
Pain
Pain, chronic
Parent/infant/child attachment, altered: risk for
Parental role conflict
Parenting, altered
Parenting, altered, risk for
Peripheral neurovascular dysfunction, risk for
Personal identity disturbance
Poisoning, risk for
Posttrauma syndrome
Posttrauma syndrome, risk for
Powerlessness
Protection, altered
Rape-trauma syndrome
Rape-trauma syndrome: compound reaction
Rape-trauma syndrome: silent reaction
Relocation stress syndrome
Role performance, altered
Self-care deficit, bathing/hygiene
Self-care deficit, dressing/grooming
Self-care deficit, feeding
Self-care deficit, toileting
Self-esteem disturbance
Self-esteem, chronic low
Self-esteem, situational low
Self-mutilation, risk for
Sensory/perceptual alterations (specify: visual, auditory, kinesthetic, gustatory, tactile, olfactory)
Sexual dysfunction

Sexuality patterns, altered
Skin integrity, impaired
Skin integrity, impaired, risk for
Sleep deprivation
Sleep pattern disturbance
Social interaction, impaired
Social isolation
Sorrow, chronic
Spiritual distress (distress of the human spirit)
Spiritual distress, risk for
Spiritual well-being, potential for enhanced
Suffocation, risk for
Surgical recovery, delayed
Swallowing, impaired
Thermoregulation, ineffective
Thought processes, altered
Tissue integrity, impaired
Tissue perfusion, altered (specify type: renal, cerebral, cardiopulmonary, gastrointestinal, peripheral)
Trauma, risk for
Unilateral neglect
Urinary elimination, altered
Urinary retention
Ventilation, inability to sustain spontaneous
Ventilatory weaning response, dysfunction (DVWR)
Violence, risk for: directed at others
Violence, risk for: self-directed
Walking, impaired
Wheelchair transfer ability, impaired

APPENDIX C

Health History Using Functional Health Patterns

www.mosby.com/MERLIN/wilson/assessment/

1. HEALTH PERCEPTION–HEALTH MANAGEMENT

- How would you describe your health overall?
- How would you describe your health at this time?
- What is the reason for this health care visit? What are your expectations?
- If ill, describe your illness. What do you think caused this illness?
- What treatments, health care practices, folk remedies have you used to treat your illness?
- Are you usually able to follow prescribed instructions given by a health care professional?
- Do you anticipate problems caring for yourself or others? If so, describe.
- Describe what you do to keep healthy and prevent disease in yourself and/or family, including exercise, leisure activities, regular dental care; routine professional examinations, self-examinations, nutrition, weight control, immunizations.
- What medications (prescribed and over-the counter) do you take?
- Do you use tobacco products? Alcohol? If so, how much and how frequently?
- What safety measures do you take? (Smoke alarms in home? Use of helmets when cycling, skiing, or roller blading? Weapons in home? Use of seat belt in automobile? Storage of poison in home?)
- Describe the health of your family (maternal grandparents, mother, paternal grandparents, father, siblings, spouse, children).
- Are you aware of any risk factors you have for disease?

2. NUTRITION–METABOLIC

- Describe what you usually eat. Breakfast? Lunch? Dinner? Snacks?
- What is your typical fluid intake? (Name the type of fluids and amounts.)
- Describe your appetite. Do you have any problems that affect your appetite? (such as nausea, fullness, indigestion)
- Are you on, or have you been on any special prescribed diet?
- Describe your food preferences.
- Do you take any nutritional supplements? (such as vitamin or protein)
- Do you have any food restrictions? Any food allergies?
- Have you experienced any difficulties with eating such as chewing or swallowing?
- How much do you think you weigh?
- Have you experienced weight changes (loss or gains) in the last 6 to 9 months?
- Have you noticed problems with your skin? (such as dryness, swelling, lesions, itching)
- When you have a wound, do you heal quickly?
- Do you have any risk factors making you susceptible to skin ulcers? (decreased circulation, sensory deficits, decreased mobility)

3. ELIMINATION

- How many times a day do you urinate?
- What color is your urine?
- Do you experience any problems with urination? (pain or burning, dribbling, incontinence, retention, frequency)
- Are any assistive devices used for urinating? (incontinence pads, intermittent or indwelling catheter, cystostomy)
- Describe your normal bowel elimination pattern, including time and frequency.
- What does your stool look like? (color, consistency)
- Are any assistive devices used for bowel elimination? (laxative, suppositories, enemas, colostomy/ileostomy)

4. ACTIVITY–EXERCISE

- Describe your activity level.
- Do you exercise? If so, describe the type, frequency, intensity, and duration of exercise.
- What do you do for leisure activities?
- Do you experience any of the following: shortness of breath, fatigue or weakness, cough, chest pain, palpitations, leg pain, pain in muscles or joints? If so, describe.
- To what extent to you require assistance for the following daily activities:

Feeding ___	Grooming ___
Bathing ___	General mobility ___
Toileting ___	Cooking ___
Bed mobility ___	Home maintenance ___
Dressing ___	Shopping ___

Level 0: Full self-care
Level I: Requires use of equipment or device
Level II: Requires assistance or supervision from another person
Level III: Requires assistance from another person (and equipment or device)
Level IV: Is dependent and does not participate

Modified from Gordon M: *Nursing diagnosis: process and application,* ed 3, St Louis, 1994, Mosby.

5. SLEEP–REST

- How many hours of night do you generally sleep?
- What time do you usually go to bed? Wake up?
- Do you generally feel rested after sleep?
- Do you have any sleep rituals? If so, describe.
- Do you experience any problems associated with sleeping? (difficulty falling asleep, difficulty remaining asleep, early awakening) If so, describe.

6. COGNITIVE–PERCEPTUAL

- Are you able to read and write?
- What languages do you speak?
- How do you learn best?
- Do you experience any problems with hearing? Do you use a hearing aid?
- Do you wear glasses or contact lenses? Do you experience any problems with vision?
- When was your last visual examination?
- Do you experience problems with dizziness? If so, describe.
- Have you noticed any insensitivity to cold, heat, or pain? If so, describe.
- Do you experience pain? If so, describe.

7. SELF-PERCEPTION–SELF-CONCEPT

- How would you describe yourself?
- Has anything occurred recently that has made you feel differently about yourself? If so, describe.
- What are you most concerned about?
- Do you frequently have feelings of anger? Anxiety? Depression? Fearfulness? If so, describe.

8. ROLE–RELATIONSHIP

- Describe your living arrangements. Do you live alone? If not, with whom?
- Do you have a significant other? If yes, is this relationship satisfying?
- What are the different roles within your family? Do others depend on you? If so, explain.
- Describe how relationships are among your family members. (close, marital difficulties, estrangement)
- How are family decisions made in your family?
- When there is a conflict in your family, how is this resolved?
- Are finances adequate to meet family needs?
- Outside the family, do you have close friends, or do you belong to any social groups? If so, describe.

9. SEXUALITY–REPRODUCTIVE

- Are you sexually active? If yes, how many partners do you have?
- Do you routinely use protection against sexually transmitted infections and/or pregnancy? If yes, describe.
- Are you comfortable with your sexual functioning?
- Are you experiencing any difficulties with sexual activity? If yes, describe.
- Do you anticipate a change in your sexual activity or relations with illness?
- Women: date of last menstruation, description of menstrual flow, age of menarche, age of menopause (if applicable), pregnancy history, problems associated with menstruation.

10. COPING–STRESS TOLERANCE

- Have there been any major changes in your life within the last couple of years? If so, describe.
- When a big problem arises in your life, how do you handle it? Is this effective most of the time?
- Is there an individual who is helpful to talk problems over with? Is this person available to you now?
- Would you describe yourself as tense or relaxed most of the time? If tense, how do you relieve the tension?
- Do you use medications, drugs, or alcohol to help you relax? If yes, describe.

11. VALUE–BELIEF

- Do you generally get what you want out of life?
- Do you have any plans or goals for the future?
- Are there any personal beliefs or values you feel may be compromised?
- Is religion an important part of your life? If so, describe.

APPENDIX D

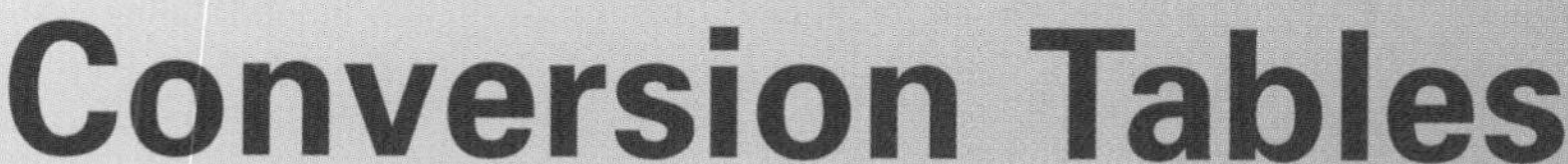

Conversion Tables

www.mosby.com/MERLIN/wilson/assessment/

Table D-1 Length

IN	CM	CM	IN
1	2.54	1	0.4
2	5.08	2	0.8
4	10.16	3	1.2
6	15.24	4	1.6
8	20.32	5	2.0
10	25.40	6	2.4
20	50.80	8	3.1
30	76.20	10	3.9
40	101.60	20	7.9
50	127.00	30	11.8
60	152.40	40	15.7
70	177.80	50	19.7
80	203.20	60	23.6
90	228.60	70	27.6
100	254.00	80	31.5
150	381.00	90	35.4
200	508.00	100	39.4

1 in = 2.54 cm
1 cm = 0.3937 inch

Table D-2 Weight

LB	KG	KG	LB
1	0.5	1	2.2
2	0.9	2	4.4
4	1.8	3	6.6
6	2.7	4	8.8
8	3.6	5	11.0
10	4.5	6	13.2
20	9.1	8	17.6
30	13.6	10	22
40	18.2	20	44
50	22.7	30	66
60	27.3	40	88
70	31.8	50	110
80	36.4	60	132
90	40.9	70	154
100	45.4	80	176
150	66.2	90	198
200	90.8	100	220

1 lb = 0.454 kg
1 kg = 2.204 lb

Table D-3 Temperature

To *convert Centigrade or Celsius degrees to Fahrenheit degrees:* multiply the number of Centigrade degrees by 9/5 and add 32 to the result. To *convert Fahrenheit degrees to Centigrade degrees:* Subtract 32 from the number of Fahrenheit degrees and multiply the difference by 5/9

Fahrenheit and Celsius equivalents: body temperature range

F°	C°	F°	C°	F°	C°	F°	C°	F°	C°
94.0	34.44	97.0	36.11	100.0	37.78	103.0	39.44	106.0	41.11
94.2	34.56	97.2	36.22	100.2	37.89	103.2	39.56	106.2	41.22
94.4	34.67	97.4	36.33	100.4	38.00	103.4	39.67	106.4	41.33
94.6	34.78	97.6	36.44	100.6	38.11	103.6	39.78	106.6	41.44
94.8	34.89	97.8	36.56	100.8	38.22	103.8	39.89	106.8	41.56
95.0	35.00	98.0	36.67	101.0	38.33	104.0	40.00	107.0	41.67
95.2	35.11	98.2	36.78	101.2	38.44	104.2	40.11	107.2	41.78
95.4	35.22	98.4	36.89	101.4	38.56	104.4	40.22	107.4	41.89
95.6	35.33	98.6	37.00	101.6	38.67	104.6	40.33	107.6	42.00
95.8	35.44	98.8	37.11	101.8	38.78	104.8	40.44	107.8	42.11
96.0	35.56	99.0	37.22	102.0	38.89	105.0	40.56	108.0	42.22
96.2	35.67	99.2	37.33	102.2	39.00	105.2	40.67		
96.4	35.78	99.4	37.44	102.4	39.11	105.4	40.78		
96.6	35.89	99.6	37.56	102.6	39.22	105.6	40.89		
96.8	36.00	99.8	37.67	102.8	39.33	105.8	41.00		

APPENDIX E

Abbreviations

www.mosby.com/MERLIN/wilson/assessment/

A & W Alive and well
abd Abdomen; abdominal
$\overline{ac}$ Before meals
ADL Activities of daily living
AJ Ankle jerk
AK Above knee
ANS Autonomic nervous system
AP Anteroposterior
bid Twice a day
BK Below knee
BP Blood pressure
BPH Benign prostatic hyperplasia
BS Bowel sounds; breath sounds
$\bar{c}$ With
CC Chief complaint
CHD Childhood disease; congenital heart disease; coronary heart disease
CHF Congestive heart failure
CNS Central nervous system
c/o Complains of
COPD Chronic obstructive pulmonary disease
CV Cardiovascular
CVA Costovertebral angle; cerebrovascular accident
CVP Central venous pressure
Cx Cervix
D & C Dilation and curettage
D/C Discontinued
DM Diabetes mellitus
DOB Date of birth
DOE Dyspnea on exertion
DTRs Deep tendon reflexes
DUB Dysfunctional uterine bleeding
Dx Diagnosis
ECG, EKG Electrocardiogram; electrocardiograph
EENT Eye, ear, nose, and throat
ENT Ear, nose, and throat
EOM Extraocular movement
FB Foreign body
FH Family history
FROM Full range of motion
FTT Failure to thrive
Fx Fracture
GB Gallbladder
GE Gastroesophageal
GI Gastrointestinal
GU Genitourinary
GYN Gynecologic
HA Headache
HCG Human chorionic gonadotropin
HEENT Head, eyes, ears, nose, and throat
HOPI History of present illness
HPI History of present illness
Hx History
ICS Intercostal space
IOP Intraocular pressure
IUD Intrauterine device
IV Intravenous
JVP Jugular venous pressure
KJ Knee jerk
KUB Kidneys, ureters, and bladder
lat Lateral
LCM Left costal margin
LE Lower extremities
LLL Left lower lobe (lung)
LLQ Left lower quadrant (abdomen)
LMD Local medical doctor
LMP Last menstrual period
LOC Loss of consciousness; level of consciousness
LS Lumbosacral; lumbar spine
LSB Left sternal border
LUL Left upper lobe (lung)
LUQ Left upper quadrant (abdomen)
M Murmur
MAL Midaxillary line
MCL Midclavicular line
MGF Maternal grandfather
MGM Maternal grandmother
MSL Midsternal line
MVA Motor vehicle accident
N & T Nose and throat
N & V Nausea and vomiting
NA No answer; not applicable
NKA No known allergies
NKDA No known drug allergies
NPO Nothing by mouth
NSR Normal sinus rhythm
OD Oculus dexter; right eye
OM Otitis media
OS Oculus sinister; left eye
OTC Over the counter
OU Oculus uterque; each eye
$\bar{p}$ After
$\overline{pc}$ After meals
PE Physical examination
PERRLA Pupils equal, round, react to light and accommodation
PGF Paternal grandfather
PGM Paternal grandmother
PI Present illness
PID Pelvic inflammatory disease
PMH Past medical history
PMI Point of maximum impulse; point of maximum intensity
PMS Premenstrual syndrome

prn As necessary
Pt Patient
PVC Premature ventricular contraction
q Every
qd Every day
qh Every hour
qid Four times a day
qod Every other day
RCM Right costal margin
REM Rapid eye movement
RLL Right lower lobe (lung)
RLQ Right lower quadrant (abdomen)
RML Right middle lobe (lung)
ROM Range of motion
ROS Review of systems
RSB Right sternal border
RUL Right upper lobe (lung)
RUQ Right upper quadrant (abdomen)
s̄ Without
SCM Sternocleidomastoid
SQ Subcutaneous
Sx Symptoms
T & A Tonsillectomy and adenoidectomy
tid Three times a day
TM Tympanic membrane
TPR Temperature, pulse, and respiration
UE Upper extremities
URI Upper respiratory infection
UTI Urinary tract infection
WD Well developed
WN Well nourished
x Times; by (size)

APPENDIX

F Growth Charts

www.mosby.com/MERLIN/wilson/assessment/

BOYS: BIRTH TO 36 MONTHS
PHYSICAL GROWTH
NCHS PERCENTILES*

NAME ______________________ RECORD # __________

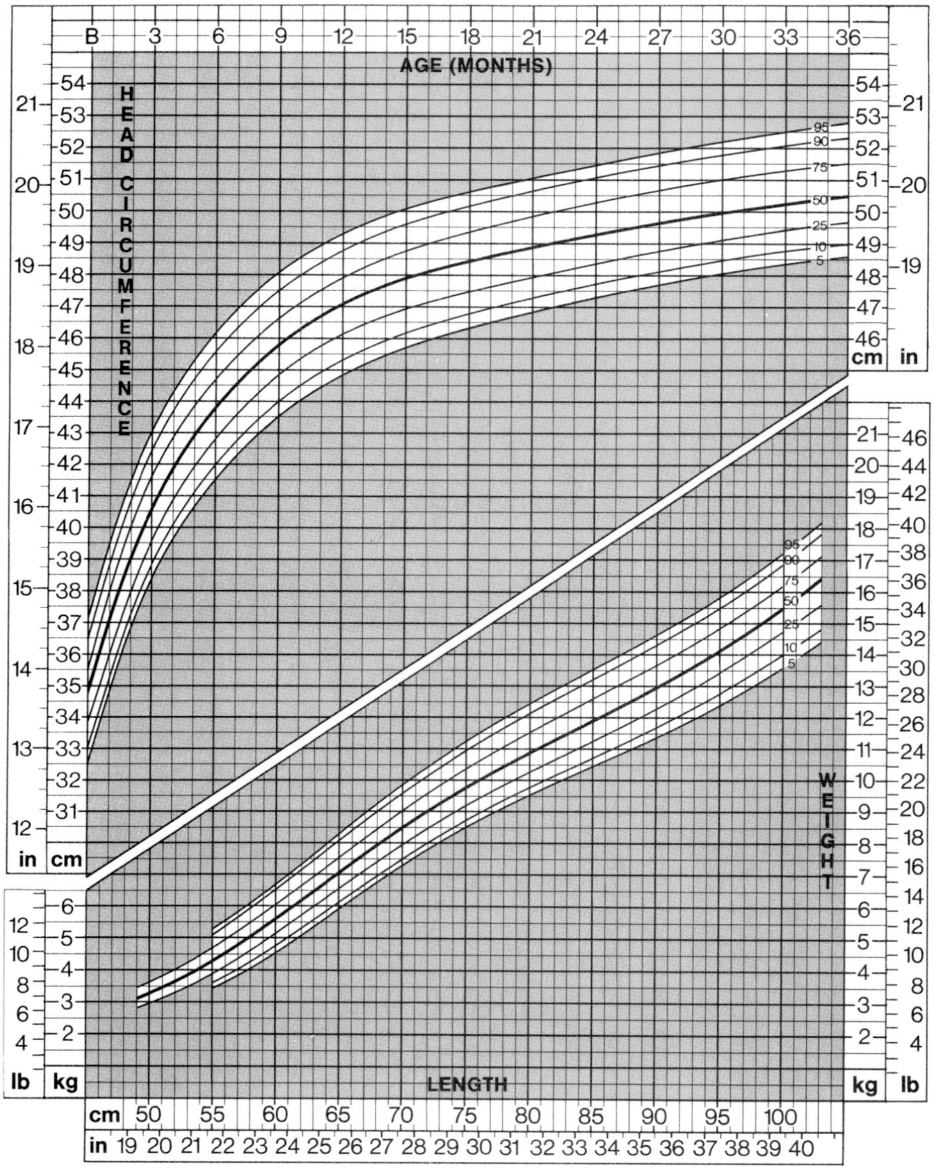

*Adapted from: Hamill PVV, Drizd TA, Johnson CL, Reed RB, Roche AF, Moore WM: Physical growth: National Center for Health Statistics percentiles. AM J CLIN NUTR 32:607-629, 1979. Data from the Fels Longitudinal Study, Wright State University School of Medicine, Yellow Springs, Ohio.

DATE	AGE	LENGTH	WEIGHT	HEAD CIRC.	COMMENT

SIMILAC® WITH IRON
Infant Formula

ISOMIL®
Soy Protein Formula with Iron

Reprinted with permission of Ross Laboratories

Fig. F-1 Growth curves for boys: birth to 36 months. (Courtesy Ross Laboratories, Columbus, Ohio.)

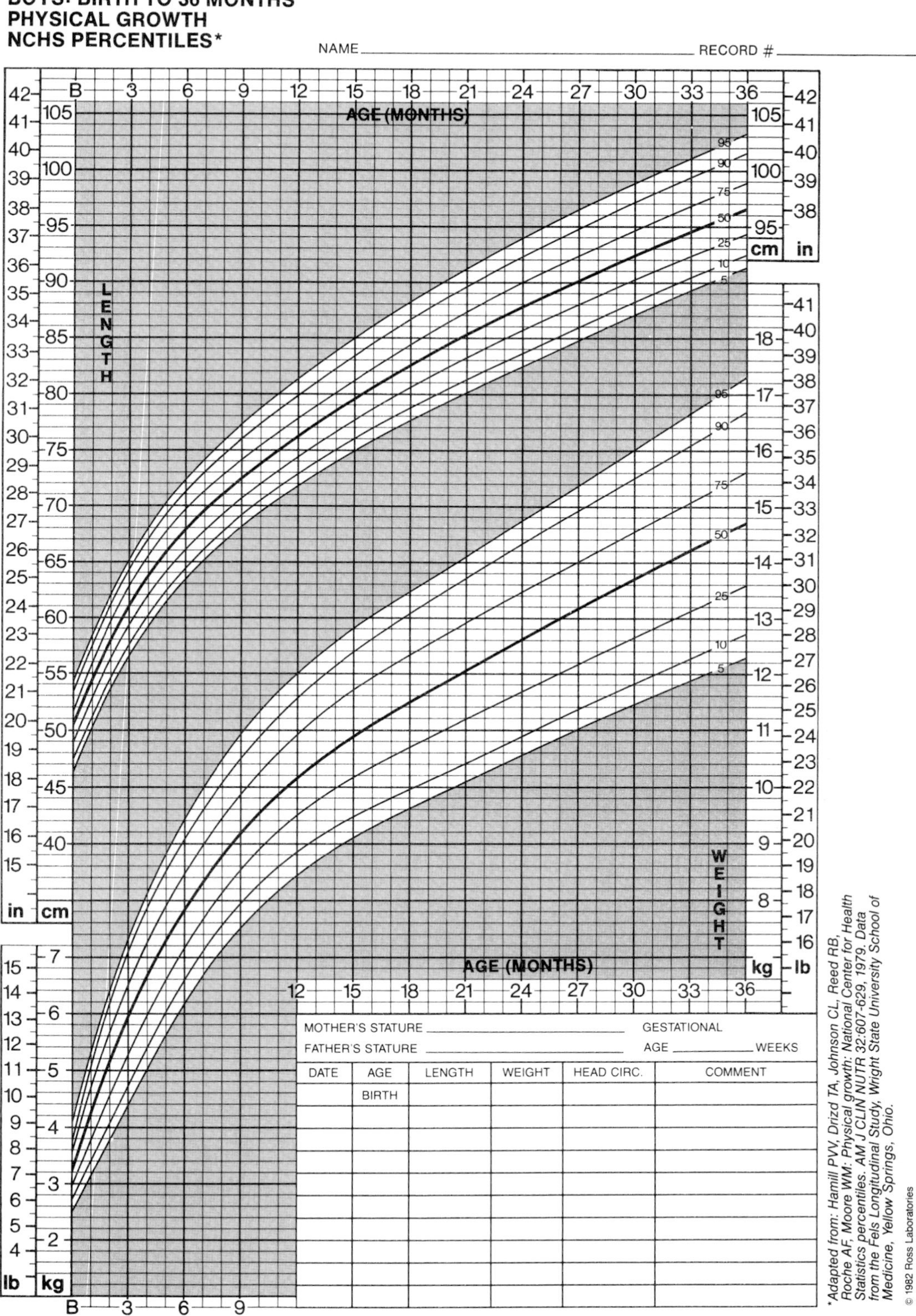

Fig. F-1, cont'd Growth curves for boys: birth to 36 months. (Courtesy Ross Laboratories, Columbus, Ohio.)

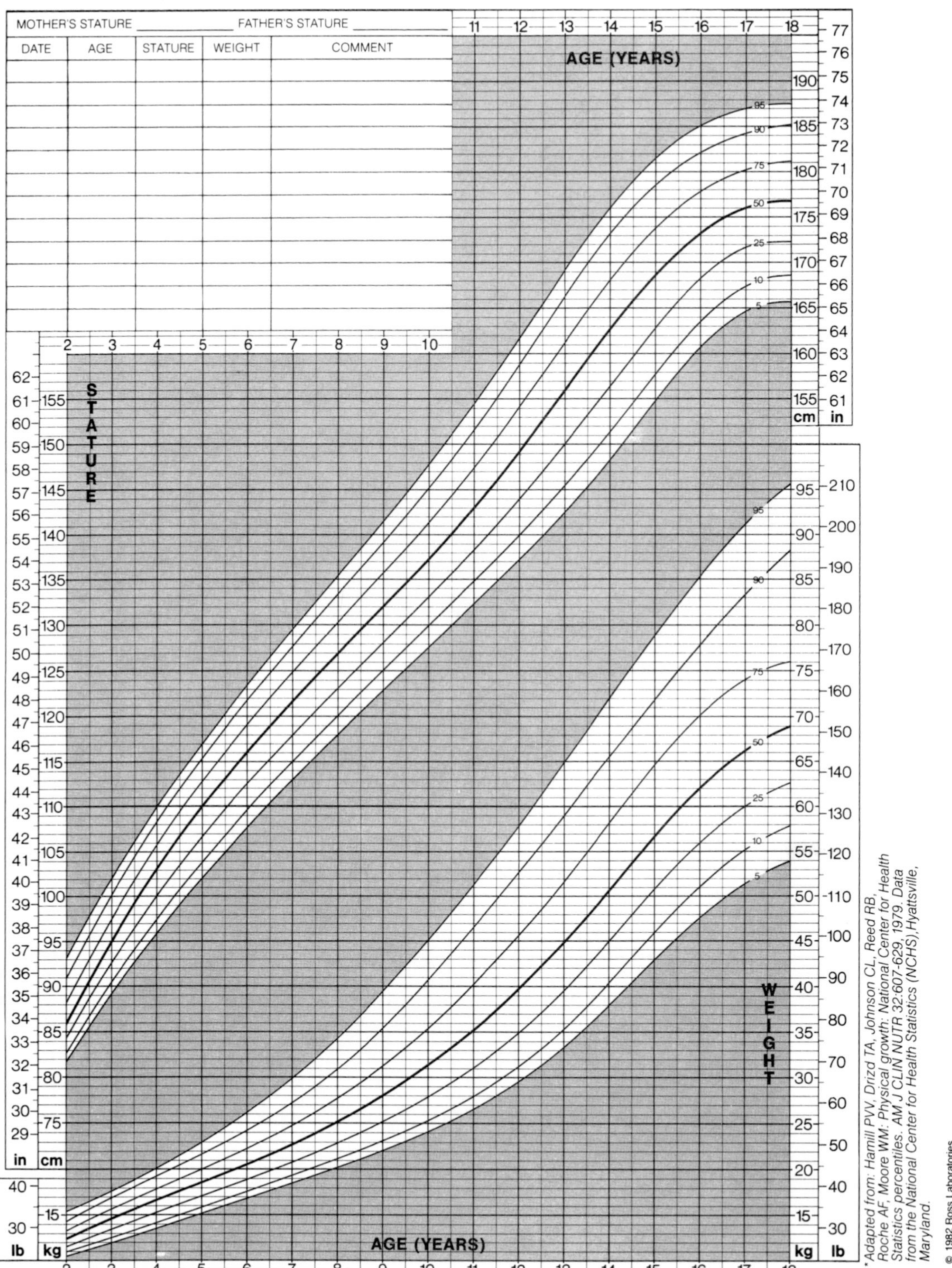

Fig. F-2 Growth curve for boys: ages 2 through 18 years. (Courtesy Ross Laboratories, Columbus, Ohio.)

GIRLS: BIRTH TO 36 MONTHS PHYSICAL GROWTH NCHS PERCENTILES*

NAME ______________________ RECORD # ______________

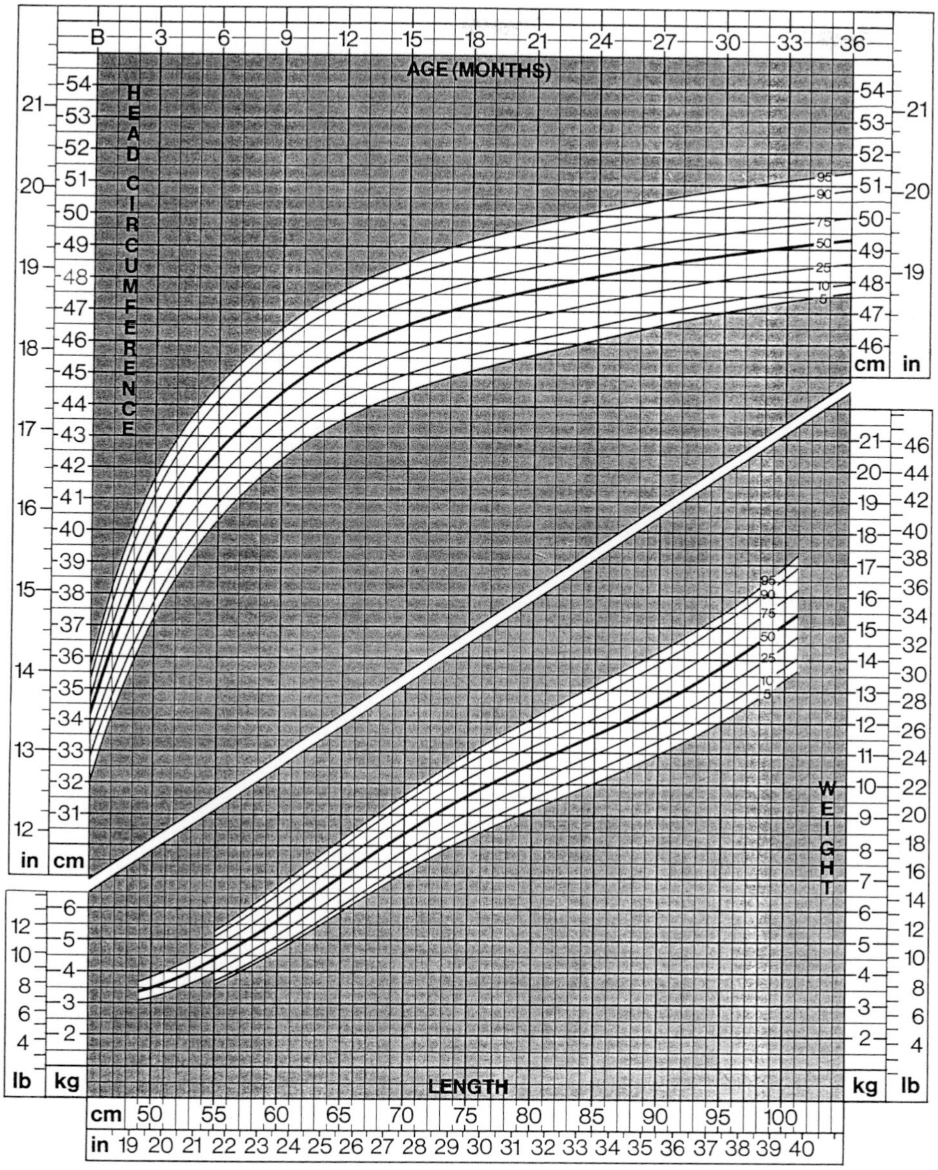

AGE (MONTHS)

HEAD CIRCUMFERENCE

WEIGHT

LENGTH

DATE	AGE	LENGTH	WEIGHT	HEAD CIRC.	COMMENT

*Adapted from: Hamill PVV, Drizd TA, Johnson CL, Reed RB, Roche AF, Moore WM: Physical growth: National Center for Health Statistics percentiles. AM J CLIN NUTR 32:607-629, 1979. Data from the Fels Longitudinal Study, Wright State University School of Medicine, Yellow Springs, Ohio.

Fig. F-3 Growth curve for girls: birth to 36 months. (Courtesy Ross Laboratories, Columbus, Ohio.)

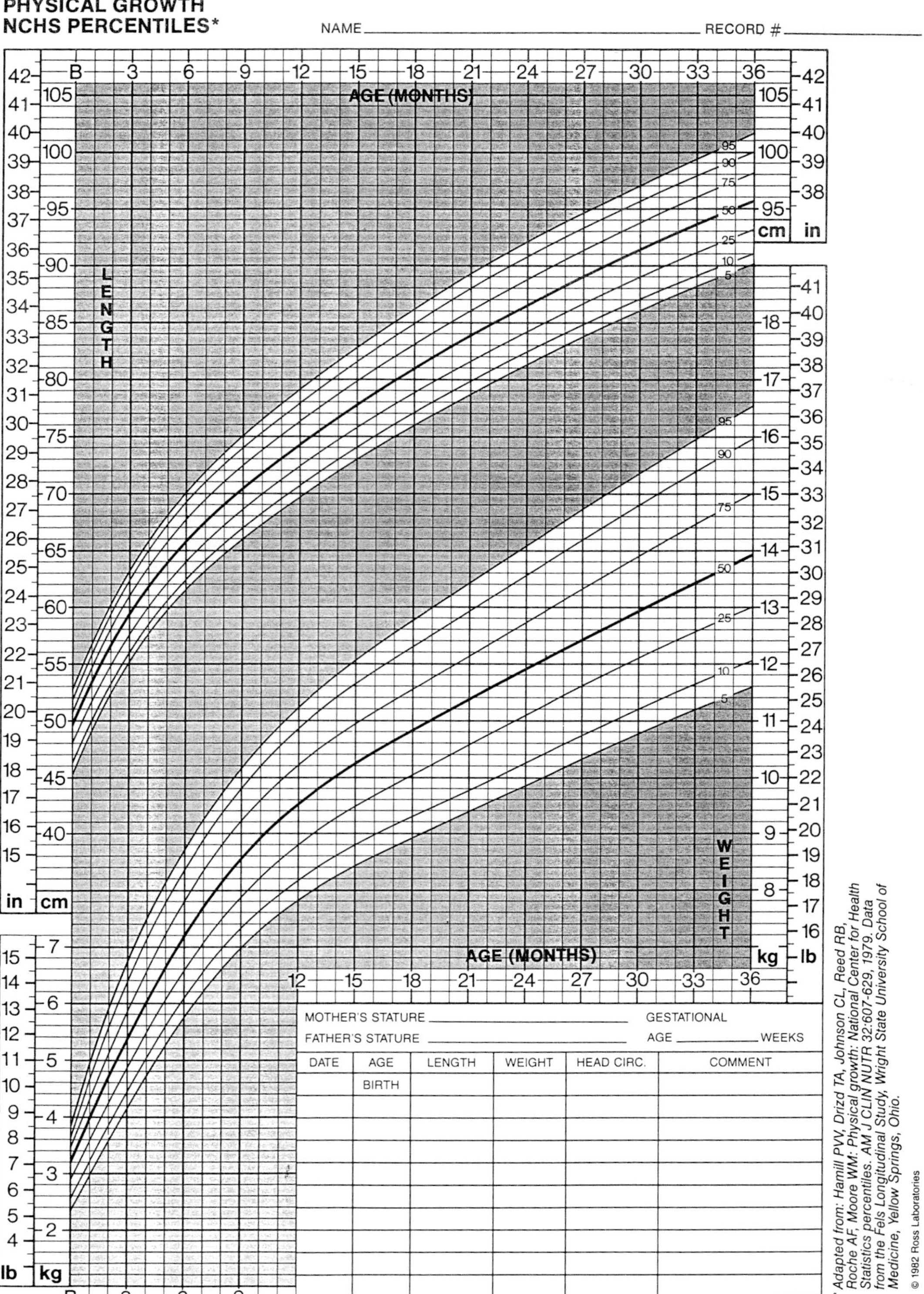

Fig. F-3, cont'd Growth curve for girls: birth to 36 months. (Courtesy Ross Laboratories, Columbus, Ohio.)

GIRLS: 2 TO 18 YEARS
PHYSICAL GROWTH
NCHS PERCENTILES*

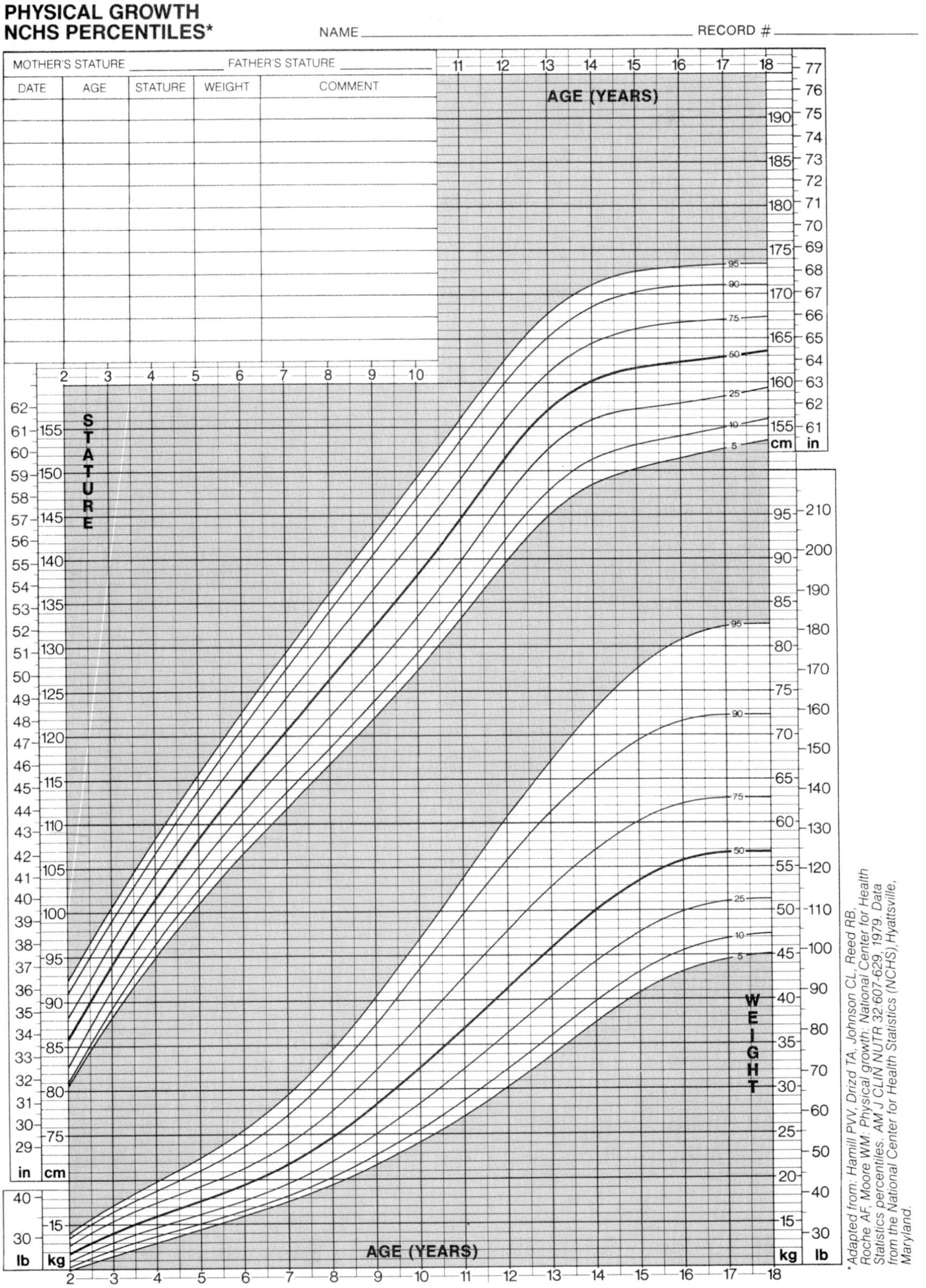
NAME
RECORD #
MOTHER'S STATURE
FATHER'S STATURE
DATE
AGE
STATURE
WEIGHT
COMMENT
AGE (YEARS)
STATURE
WEIGHT
95
90
75
50
25
10
5
cm
in
kg
lb
*Adapted from: Hamill PVV, Drizd TA, Johnson CL, Reed RB, Roche AF, Moore WM: Physical growth: National Center for Health Statistics percentiles. AM J CLIN NUTR 32:607-629, 1979. Data from the National Center for Health Statistics (NCHS), Hyattsville, Maryland.
© 1982 Ross Laboratories

Fig. F-4 Growth curve for girls: ages 2 through 18 years. (Courtesy Ross Laboratories, Columbus, Ohio.)

APPENDIX

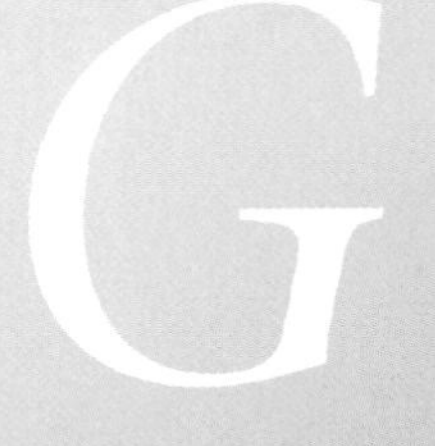

G Nutrition Screening Forms

www.mosby.com/MERLIN/wilson/assessment/

Level I Screen

Body Weight

Measure height to the nearest inch and weight to the nearest pound. Record the values below and mark them on the Body Mass Index (BMI) scale to the right. Then use a straight edge (ruler) to connect the two points and circle the spot where this straight line crosses the center line (body mass index). Record the number below.

Healthy adults should have a BMI between 22 and 27.

Height (in):________________
Weight (lbs):________________
Body Mass Index:________________
(number from center column)

Check any boxes that are true for the individual:

- ❑ Has lost or gained 10 pounds (or more) in the past 6 months.
- ❑ Body mass index <22
- ❑ Body mass index >27

For the remaining sections, please ask the individual which of the statements (if any) is true for him or her and place a check by each that applies.

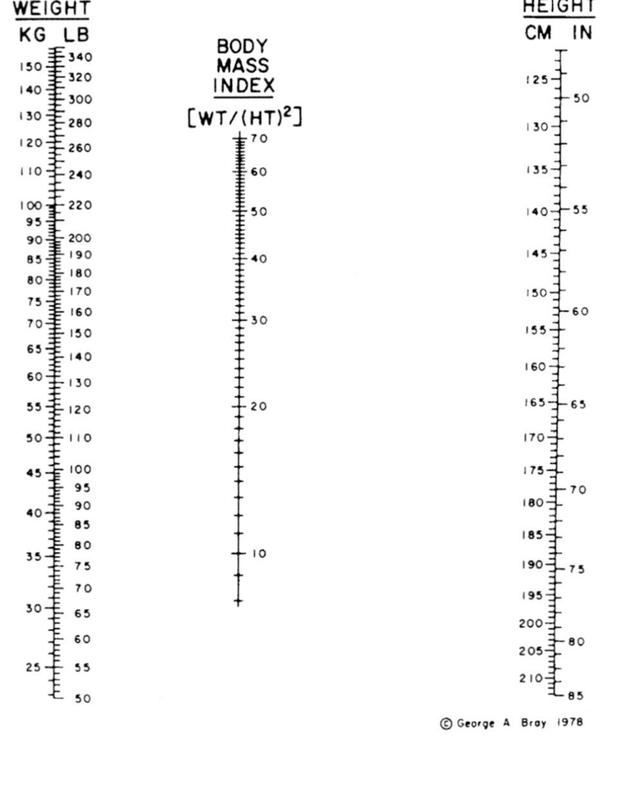

Eating Habits

- ❑ Does not have enough food to eat each day
- ❑ Usually eats alone
- ❑ Does not eat anything on one or more days each month
- ❑ Has poor appetite
- ❑ Is on a special diet
- ❑ Eats vegetables two or fewer times daily
- ❑ Eats milk or milk products once or not at all daily
- ❑ Eats fruit or drinks fruit juice once or not at all daily
- ❑ Eats breads, cereals, pasta, rice, or other grains five or fewer times daily
- ❑ Has difficulty chewing or swallowing
- ❑ Has more than one alcoholic drink per day (if woman); more than two drinks per day (if man)
- ❑ Has pain in mouth, teeth, or gums

LEVEL I SCREEN

Name:

Date:

A health care provider should be contacted if the individual has gained or lost 10 pounds unexpectedly or without intending to during the past 6 months. A health care provider should also be notified if the individual's body mass index is above 27 or below 22.

Living Environment

- ☐ Lives on an income of less than $6000 per year (per individual in the household)
- ☐ Lives alone
- ☐ Is housebound
- ☐ Is concerned about home security
- ☐ Lives in a home with inadequate heating or cooling
- ☐ Does not have a stove and/or refrigerator
- ☐ Is unable or prefers not to spend money on food (<$25-30 per person spent on food each week)

Functional Status

Usually or always needs assistance with (check each that apply):

- ☐ Bathing
- ☐ Dressing
- ☐ Grooming
- ☐ Toileting
- ☐ Eating
- ☐ Walking or moving about
- ☐ Traveling (outside the home)
- ☐ Preparing food
- ☐ Shopping for food or other necessities

If you have checked one or more statements on this screen, the individual you have interviewed may be at risk for poor nutritional status. Please refer this individual to the appropriate health care or social service professional in your area. For example, a dietitian should be contacted for problems with selecting, preparing, or eating a healthy diet, or a dentist if the individual experiences pain or difficulty when chewing or swallowing. Those individuals whose income, lifestyle, or functional status may endanger their nutritional and overall health should be referred to available community services: home-delivered meals, congregate meal programs, transportation services, counseling services (alcohol abuse, depression, bereavement, etc.), home health care agencies, day care programs, etc.

Please repeat this screen at least once each year--sooner if the individual has a major change in his or her health, income, immediate family (e.g., spouse dies), or functional status.

LEVEL II SCREEN Name: Date:

Level II Screen

Complete the following screen by interviewing the patient directly and/or by referring to the patient chart. If you do not routinely perform all of the described tests or ask all of the listed questions, please consider including them but do not be concerned if the entire screen is not completed. Please try to conduct a minimal screen on as many older patients as possible, and please try to collect serial measurements, which are extremely valuable in monitoring nutritional status. Please refer to the manual for additional information.

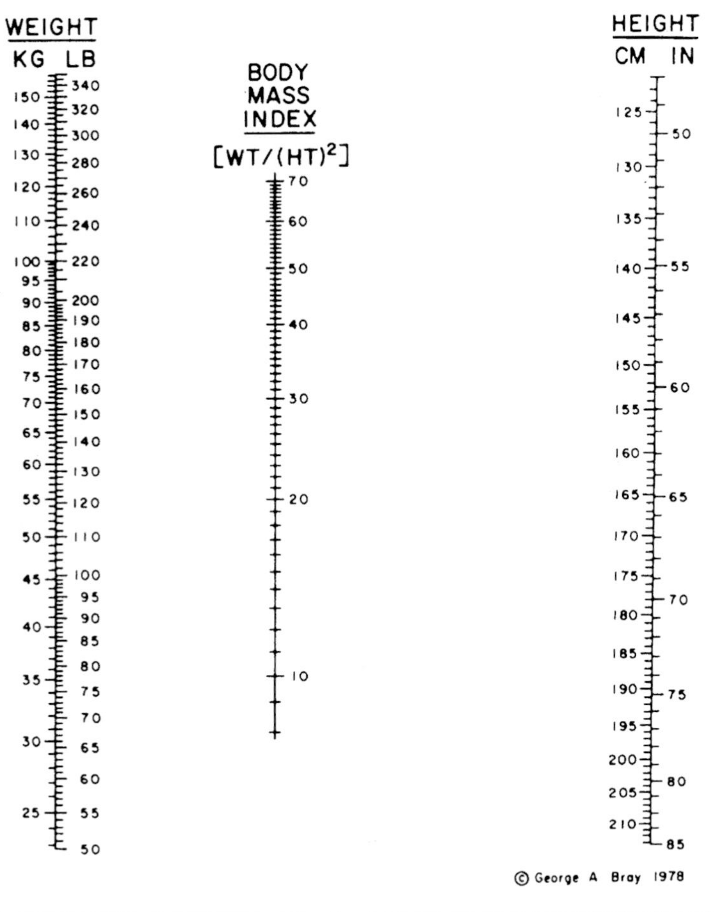

Anthropometrics

Measure height to the nearest inch and weight to the nearest pound. Record the values below and mark them on the Body Mass Index (BMI) scale to the right. Then use a straight edge (paper, ruler) to connect the two points and circle the spot where this straight line crosses the center line (body mass index). Record the number below; healthy older adults should have a BMI between 22 and 27; check the appropriate box to flag an abnormally high or low value.

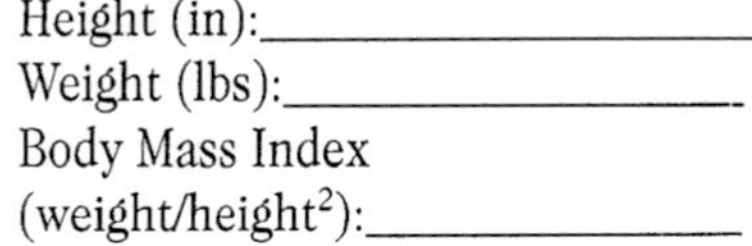

Height (in):________________
Weight (lbs):________________
Body Mass Index (weight/height^2):________________

Please place a check by any statement regarding BMI and recent weight loss that is true for the patient.

- ❑ Body mass index <22
- ❑ Body mass index >27
- ❑ Has lost or gained 10 pounds (or more) of body weight in the past 6 months

Record the measurement of mid-arm circumference to the nearest 0.1 centimeter and of triceps skinfold to the nearest 2 millimeters.

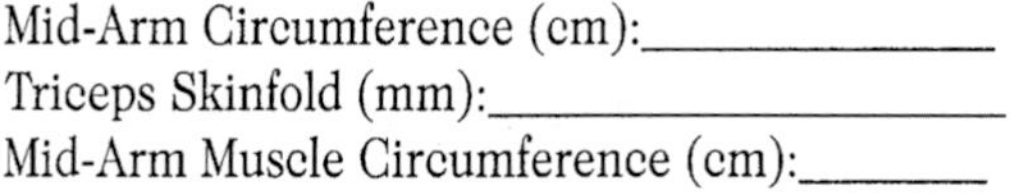

Mid-Arm Circumference (cm):________________
Triceps Skinfold (mm):________________
Mid-Arm Muscle Circumference (cm):________

Refer to the table and check any abnormal values:

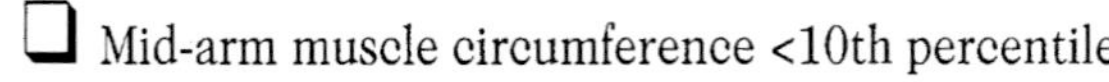

- ❑ Mid-arm muscle circumference <10th percentile
- ❑ Triceps skinfold <10th percentile
- ❑ Triceps skinfold >95th percentile

Note: mid-arm circumference (cm) - {0.314 x triceps skinfold (mm)}= mid-arm *muscle* circumference (cm)

For the remaining sections, please place a check by any statements that are true for the patient.

Laboratory Data

- ❑ Serum albumin below 3.5 g/dl
- ❑ Serum cholesterol below 160 mg/dl
- ❑ Serum cholesterol above 240 mg/dl

Drug Use

- ❑ Three or more prescription drugs, OTC medications, and/or vitamin/mineral supplements daily

Clinical Features

Presence of (check each that apply):

- ❑ Problems with mouth, teeth, or gums
- ❑ Difficulty chewing
- ❑ Difficulty swallowing
- ❑ Angular stomatitis
- ❑ Glossitis
- ❑ History of bone pain
- ❑ History of bone fractures
- ❑ Skin changes (dry, loose, nonspecific lesions, edema)

Percentile	Men 55-65 y	Men 65-75 y	Women 55-65 y	Women 65-75 y
Arm circumference (cm)				
10th	27.3	26.3	25.7	25.2
50th	31.7	30.7	30.3	29.9
95th	36.9	35.5	38.5	37.3
Arm muscle circumference (cm)				
10th	24.5	23.5	19.6	19.5
50th	27.8	26.8	22.5	22.5
95th	32.0	30.6	28.0	27.9
Triceps skinfold (mm)				
10th	6	6	16	14
50th	11	11	25	24
95th	22	22	38	36

From: Frisancho AR. New norms of upper limb fat and muscle areas for assessment of nutritional status. Am J Clin Nutr 1981; 34:2540-2545. © 1981 American Society for Clinical Nutrition.

Eating Habits

- ❑ Does not have enough food to eat each day
- ❑ Usually eats alone
- ❑ Does not eat anything on one or more days each month
- ❑ Has poor appetite
- ❑ Is on a special diet
- ❑ Eats vegetables two or fewer times daily
- ❑ Eats milk or milk products once or not at all daily
- ❑ Eats fruit or drinks fruit juice once or not at all daily
- ❑ Eats breads, cereals, pasta, rice, or other grains five or fewer times daily
- ❑ Has more than one alcoholic drink per day (if woman); more than two drinks per day (if man)

Living Environment

- ❑ Lives on an income of less than $6000 per year (per individual in the household)
- ❑ Lives alone
- ❑ Is housebound
- ❑ Is concerned about home security
- ❑ Lives in a home with inadequate heating or cooling
- ❑ Does not have a stove and/or refrigerator
- ❑ Is unable or prefers not to spend money on food (<$25-30 per person spent on food each week)

Functional Status

Usually or always needs assistance with (check each that apply):

- ❑ Bathing
- ❑ Dressing
- ❑ Grooming
- ❑ Toileting
- ❑ Eating
- ❑ Walking or moving about
- ❑ Traveling (outside the home)
- ❑ Preparing food
- ❑ Shopping for food or other necessities

Mental/Cognitive Status

- ❑ Clinical evidence of impairment, e.g. Folstein<26
- ❑ Clinical evidence of depressive illness, e.g. Beck Depression Inventory>15, Geriatric Depression Scale>5

Patients in whom you have identified one or more major indicator (see pg 944) of poor nutritional status require immediate medical attention; if minor indicators are found, ensure that they are known to a health professional or to the patient's own physician. Patients who display risk factors of poor nutritional status should be referred to the appropriate health care or social service professional (dietitian, nurse, dentist, case manager, etc.).

GLOSSARY

A

abduction Movement of the limbs or the trunk and head away from the median plane of the body.

accommodation Process of visual focusing from far to near; accomplished by contraction of the ciliary muscle, which thickens and increases the convexity of the crystalline lens.

active listening State of selective attention and awareness that encompasses the skill of observation so that verbal and nonverbal cues are registered and clarified in an interaction; involves data absorption, retention, and exchange for clarification.

adduction Movement of the limbs or the trunk and head toward the median plane of the body.

adnexa General term meaning adjacent or related structures. *Example:* The ovaries and fallopian tubes are adnexa of the uterus.

adolescent Refers to a person between the ages of 12 and 20 years.

adventious sounds Sounds within the lungs that are not normal.

adulthood Stage of life that can be divided into several recognized categories:

Young adult	ages 20 to 35 years
Middle adult	ages 35 to 65 years
Young-old adult	ages 65 to 74 years
Middle-old adult	ages 75 to 84 years
Old-old adult	ages 85 and up

affect Observable behaviors indicating an individual's feelings or emotions.

ageusia Absence or impairment of the sense of taste.

alopecia Absence or loss of hair.

alveolar ridge Bony prominences of the maxilla and mandible that support the teeth; in edentulous clients these structures support dentures.

amblyopia Reduced vision that occurs after deprivation of visual stimulation during visual maturation (birth to 2 years); the eye appears normal during examination. Also called *suppression amblyopia.*

amenorrhea Absence of menstruation.

ametropia General term denoting a condition involving a refractive error. *Example:* Myopia, hyperopia.

anesthesia Partial or complete loss of sensation.

angina pectoris Paroxysmal chest pain, often associated with myocardial ischemia; pain patterns and severity vary among individuals; pain sometimes radiates to the neck, jaw, or left arm; may be accompanied by choking or smothering sensations.

angle of Louis Visible and palpable angulation between the sternum and manubrium; also referred to as the *manubriosternal junction.*

ankylosis Fixation of a joint, often in an abnormal position, usually resulting from destruction of articular cartilage, as in rheumatoid arthritis.

annulus Dense fibrous ring surrounding the tympanic membrane.

anosmia Absence or impairment of the sense of smell.

anterior Referring to the front.

anterior triangle (of the neck) Landmark area for palpating the submaxillary, submental, and anterior cervical lymph modes; sectioned by the anterior surface of the sternocleidomastoid muscle, the mandible, and an imagined line running from the chin to the sternal notch.

anthropometrics Measurement of body composition and growth; includes measurement of height, weight, body mass index, head circumference, and skinfold thickness.

anular Type of lesion that forms a ring around a center of normal skin.

anuria Complete absence of urine production; may also be used to describe situations in which urine output is less than 100 cc per day.

apathy Lack of emotional expression; indifference to stimuli or surroundings.

aphakia Absence of the crystalline lens of the eye.

aphasia Absence or severe impairment of the ability to communicate through speech.

aphthous ulcer (canker sore) Painful ulcer on the mucous membrane of the mouth.

apical Refers to the top portion (apex) of an organ or part.

apnea Absence of breathing.

apocrine sweat glands Secretory dermal structures located in the axillae, nipples, areolae, scalp, face, and genital area; they develop at puberty and respond to emotional stimulation.

arcus senilis Gray ring composed of lipids deposited in the peripheral cornea; commonly seen in older adults. Also called *arcus cornealis.*

areola Circular, darkly pigmented area around the nipple of the breast.

arteriosclerosis General term denoting hardening and thickening of the arterial walls.

ascites Accumulation of serous fluid in the peritoneal cavity.

assessment Process of gathering and analyzing subjective and objective client data to summarize a client's status.

asterixis Flapping movement or tremor best seen with outstretched hands; associated with metabolic disorders, especially hepatic failure.

asthenopia General eye discomfort or fatigue resulting from use of the eyes.

asthma Paroxysmal dyspnea that is accompanied by wheezing and caused by spasm of the bronchial tubes or by swelling of their mucous membranes.

astigmatism Visual distortion resulting from an irregular corneal curvature that prevents light rays from being focused clearly on the retina.

ataxia Inability to coordinate muscular movement.
atelectasis Shrunken, airless alveoli or collapse of lung tissue.
atherosclerosis Formation of plaques within arterial walls resulting in thickening of the walls and narrowing of the lumen; end organs supplied by these vessels receive diminished circulation.
athetosis Condition in which there are slow, irregular, involuntary movements in the upper extremities, especially the hands and fingers.
atrophy Diminution of size or wasting; can also refer to loss of elastic tissue resulting in a slightly sunken epidermis that wrinkles easily when pulled to the side.
attrition of teeth Wearing away of the occlusal surfaces of the teeth from many years of chewing or excessive grinding.
auricle Flap of the external ear; also called the *pinna.*
auscultatory gap Phenomenon sometimes noted by an examiner listening for blood pressure sounds; temporary silent interval between systolic and diastolic sounds that may cover a range of 40 mm Hg; commonly occurs with hypertensive clients with a wide pulse pressure.

B

balano- Prefix that denotes the glans penis. *Example: Balanitis* means inflammation of the glans penis.
ballottement Technique of palpating a floating structure by bouncing it gently and feeling it rebound.
Bartholin's glands Two mucous-secreting glands located within the posterolateral vaginal vestibule.
bigeminal pulse Abnormal pulse characterized by a strong beat and a weaker one in close succession, followed by a pause when no beat is felt; pulse is irregular in rhythm.
bilateral Relating to or referring to two sides.
Biot breathing Breathing characterized by several short breaths followed by long, irregular periods of apnea.
bisferious pulse Abnormal pulse characterized by two main peaks; occurs with aortic stenosis and/or regurgitation.
blepharitis Inflammation of the eyelid.
blocking Interruption in a train of thought, a loss of an idea, or a repression of a feeling or idea from conscious awareness; can be a normal behavior or, in extreme form, indicative of abnormality.
body mass index (BMI) Method to evaluate height-weight ratio; calculated by dividing the weight (kilograms) by the height (meters).
borborygmi Abdominal sounds produced by hyperactive intestinal peristalsis that are audible at a distance.
boutonnière deformity Common deformity of the hands seen in patients with rheumatoid arthritis; involves flexion of the proximal interphalangeal joint and hyperextension of the distal interphalangeal joint.
bradycardia Abnormally slowed heart rate, usually under 60 beats per minute.
bradykinesia Abnormal slowness of movement.
bradypnea Breathing that is abnormally slow.
bronchial breath sounds High-pitched breath sounds normally heard over the trachea and the area around the manubrium; considered abnormal if heard anywhere over the posterior or lateral chest.
bronchitis Inflammation of the bronchi.
bronchophony Increased vocal resonance detected over a bronchus that is surrounded by consolidated lung tissue.
bronchovesicular breath sounds Refers to breath sounds at a pitch intermediate between bronchial or tracheal sounds and alveolar sounds.
Brudzinski's sign Examination technique used to detect meningeal irritation by flexing the neck of a supine patient forward.
bruit Audible murmur (a blowing sound) heard when auscultating over a peripheral vessel or an organ.
bruxism Grinding of the teeth; usually an unconscious act occurring during sleep.
buccal Pertaining to the inside of the cheek.
bulbar conjunctiva Thin, transparent mucous membrane that covers the sclera and adjoins the palpebral conjunctiva, which lines the inner eyelid.
bulla Elevated, circumscribed, fluid-filled lesion greater than 1 cm in diameter.
bunion Abnormal prominence on the inner aspect of the first metatarsal head, with bursal formation; results in lateral or valgus displacement of the great toe.
bursa Fibrous, fluid-filled sac found between certain tendons and the bones beneath them.
bursitis Inflammation of a bursa.

C

cachexia Severe malnutrition and wasting of muscles associated with a chronic illness such as cancer.
callus Hyperkeratotic area caused by pressure or friction; usually not painful.
canthus Outer or inner angle between the upper and lower eyelids.
carpal tunnel syndrome Painful disorder of the wrist and hand induced by compression of the median nerve between the inelastic carpal ligament and other structures within the carpal tunnel.
cataract Opacity of the crystalline lens of the eyes.
cauliflower ear Thickened, disfigured ear caused by repeated trauma such as blows to the ear.
cellulitis Diffuse spreading infection of the skin or subcutaneous or connective tissue.
cerumen Waxy secretion of the glands of the external acoustic meatus; earwax.
chalazion Small, localized swelling of the eyelid caused by obstruction and dilation of the meibomian gland.
circinate Circular.
circumduction Circular movement of a limb.
circumscribed Well-defined, limited, and encircled.
clonus Abnormal pattern of neuromuscular functioning characterized by rapidly alternating involuntary contraction and relaxation of skeletal muscles.

clubbing Broadening and thickening of the fingernails or toe nails associated with an increased angle of the nail greater than 160 degrees; associated with chronic hypoxia.
coarctation Stricture or narrowing of the wall of a vessel.
cochlea Conical bony structure of the inner ear; perforated by numerous appertures for passage of the cochlear division of the acoustic nerve.
cognitive functioning Appraisal of an individual's perception of his intellectual awareness, his potential for growth, and his recognition by others for his mental skills and contributions.
cogwheel rigidity Abnormal motion in the muscle tissues characterized by jerky movements when the muscle is passively stretched.
coherency Conversation and behavior that conveys thoughts, feelings, ideas, and perceptions in a logical and relevant manner.
compulsive behavior Repetitive act that usually originates from an obsession; extreme anxiety emerges if the act is not completed.
condyloma acuminatum (wart) Soft, warty, papillomatous projection that appears on the labia and within the vaginal vestibule; viral in origin and sexually transmitted.
condyloma latum Slightly raised, moist, flattened papules that appear on the labia or within the vaginal vestibule; a sign of secondary syphilis; sexually transmitted.
confabulation Fabrication of events or sequential experiences often recounted to cover up memory gaps.
confluent Describes lesions that run together.
consolidation Increasing density of lung tissue caused by pathologic engorgement.
contusion (bruise) Swelling, discoloration, and pain without a break in the skin.
Cooper ligaments Suspensory ligaments of the breast.
corn Hyperkeratotic, slightly raised, circumscribed lesion caused by pressure over a bony prominence, usually on the fourth or fifth toe; painful if pressure or friction is persistent.
costal angle Costal margin angle formed on the anterior chest wall at the base of the xiphoid process, where the ribs separate.
crackles Abnormal respiratory sound heard during auscultation characterized by discontinuous bubbling sounds; heard over distal bronchioles and alveoli that contain serous secretions; formerly called *rales.*
crepitus Dry, crackling sound or sensation heard or felt as a joint is moved through its range of motion.
cricoid cartilage Lowermost cartilage of the larynx.
crust Dried serum, blood, or purulent exudate on the skin surface.
cryptorchism (undescended testis) Failure of one or both of the testicles to descend into the scrotum.
cyanosis Bluish-gray discoloration of the skin resulting from the presence of or abnormal amounts of reduced hemoglobin in the blood.
cycloplegia Paralysis of the ciliary muscle resulting in a loss of accommodation and a dilated pupil; usually induced with medication to allow for examination or surgery of the eye.
cystocele Bulging of the anterior vaginal wall caused by protrusion of the urinary bladder through relaxed or weakened musculature.

D

darwinian tubercle Blunt point projecting up from the upper part of the helix of the ear.
database Collection or store of information.
Subjective: Portion of the client data that is supplied by the client; the client's perceptions of himself.
Objective: Portion of the client data that is perceived by the examiner through physical examination or obtained from other external sources (such as laboratory studies).
deciduous teeth Twenty teeth that appear normally during infancy: four incisors, two canines, and four molars in the upper and lower jaw.
delusion Persistent belief or perception that is illogical or improbable.
dementia Broad term that indicates impairment of intellectual functioning, memory, and judgment.
depersonalization Sense of being out of touch with one's environment; loss of a sense of reality and association with personal events.
desquamation Sloughing process of the cornified layer of the epidermis; when accelerated, the process can cause peeling, scaling, and loss of the deeper layers of the skin.
diaphragmatic excursion Extent of movement of the diaphragm.
diarthrotic joint Joint that permits relatively free movement; types of diarthortic joints include hinge joints, pivot joints, condyloid joints, ball and socket joints, and gliding joints.
diastole Period of time within the cardiac cycle in which ventricles are relaxed and filling with blood.
diffuse Spread out, widely dispersed, copious.
diplopia Double vision; usually caused by an extraocular muscle malfunction or a muscle innervation disorder.
distal Refers to the area furthest away from a point of reference.
dizziness Sensation of faintness.
dorsal Referring to the back or posterior part of an anatomic structure. *Example:* Dorsal aspect of the hand.
dorsiflexion Backward bending or flexion of a joint.
dysarthria Speech disorder involving difficulty with articulation and pronunciation of specific sounds; results from loss of control over the muscles of speech.
dysesthesia Sensation of something crawling on the skin or of pricks of pins and needles.
dyskinesia Refers to a reduced ability to perform voluntary movements.
dyslexia Impairment of the ability to read (with no impairment of mental or intellectual function); letters or words may appear reversed or the reader may have difficulty distinguishing right from left.

dysmenorrhea Abnormal pain associated with the menstrual cycle. Mild, self-limiting premenstrual pain is considered normal. Pain becomes abnormal when it is severe, disabling, or accompanied by other severe symptoms, such as nausea, vomiting, fainting, or intestinal cramping.
dysmetria Inability to fix the range of movement in a muscular activity.
dyspareunia Pain associated with sexual intercourse; most often use to describe female conditions including vaginal spasms, lack of lubrication, or genital lesions.
dysphagia Difficulty swallowing.
dysphasia Speech disorder involving difficulty in the use of language to convey meaning to others; not as severe as aphasia.
dysphonia Difficulty in controlling laryngeal speech sounds; can be a normal event, such as male vocal changes occurring at puberty.
dyspnea Breathing that is labored or difficult.
dyssynergia Failure of muscular coordination; also known as *ataxia.*
dysuria Difficulty, pain, or burning sensation associated with urination.

E

ecchymosis Discoloration of skin or a mucous membrane caused by leakage of blood into the subcutaneous tissue; can also be a bruise.
eccrine sweat glands Secretory dermal structures distributed over the body that secrete water and electrolytes and regulate body temperature; heat, emotional reactions, and physical exercise are the primary stimulants for secretion from these glands.
ectopic Term used to describe an event that occurs away from its usual location; in reference to the heart, it could pertain to an extra beat or contraction.
ectropion Abnormal outward turning of the margin of the eyelid.
eczematous Superficial inflammation characterized by scaling, thickening, crusting, weeping, and redness.
edema Excessive accumulation of fluid within the interstitial space.
egophony Abnormality in vocal resonance; when lungs are auscultated, the client says "e-e-e," but the nurse hears "a-a-a"; suggests pleural effusion.
embolus Foreign object (composed of air, fat, or clustered cellular elements) that circulates through the blood and usually lodges in a vessel, causing some degree of occlusion.
emotional functioning Appraisal of an individual's access to his own feelings, his satisfaction with those feelings, his ability to express those feeling effectively, and his capacity to resolve or deal with stressors.
emphysema Chronic pulmonary disease characterized by overdistended lung tissue.
enophthalmos Abnormal backward placement of the eyeball.
entropion Abnormal inward turning of the margin of the eyelid.
enuresis Any involuntary urination, especially during sleep.
epicondyle Round protuberance above the condyle (at the end of a bone).
epididymitis Inflammation of the epididymis (tightly coiled, comma-shaped structure overlying the posterolateral surface of the testis).
epiphysis End of a long bone that is cartilaginous during early childhood and becomes ossified during late childhood.
epispadias Congenital defect in which the urinary meatus opens on the dorsum of the penis.
epistaxis Bleeding from the nose.
epulis Any growth on the gum.
erosion Wearing away or destruction of the mucosal or epidermal surface; often develops into an ulcer.
erythematous Redness (of the skin).
euphoria Sense of elation or well-being; can be a normal feeling or exaggerated to the extent of distorting reality.
eustachian tube Tube lined with mucous membrane that joins the nasopharynx and the tympanic cavity, and allows for the equalization of air pressure with atmospheric pressure.
eversion Outward turning, as with a foot, or an inside out position, as with an eyelid.
exacerbation Increase in intensity of signs or symptoms.
excoriation Scratch or abrasion on the skin surface.
exophthalmos Abnormal forward placement of the eyeball.
extension Movement that brings a joint into a straight position.
external rotation Outward turning of a limb.
extrapyramidal system Motor pathways lying outside the pyramidal tract that help to maintain muscle tone and to control body movements such as walking; includes nerve pathways between the cerebral cortex, the basal ganglia, the brainstem, and the spinal cord.

F

fasciculation Localized, uncoordinated, uncontrollable twitching of a single muscle group innervated by a single motor nerve fiber.
fissure Linear crack in the skin.
flaccid Referring to muscles that lack tone.
flail chest Unstable, flapping chest wall caused by fractures of the sternum and ribs.
flank Part of the body between the bottom of the ribs and the upper border of the ilium.
flatulence Presence of excessive amounts of gas in the stomach or intestines.
flexion Movement that brings a joint into a bent position.
fontanel Unossified space or soft spot lying between the cranial bones of an infant.
Fordyce spots Small yellow spots on the buccal membrane that are visible sebaceous glands; a normal phenomenon seen in many adults that is sometimes mistaken for abnormal lesions. Also called *Fordyce granules.*

fornix (plural: fornices) General term designating a fold or an archlike structure. The vaginal fornix is the ringed recess (pocket) that forms around the cervix as it projects into the vaginal vault; although continuous, this fornix is anatomically divided into the anterior, posterior, and lateral fornices.
fourchette Small fold of membrane connecting the labia minora in the posterior part of the vulva.
frenulum (lingual) Band of tissue that attaches the ventral surface of the tongue to the floor of the mouth.
friction rub Sound produced by the rubbing of the pleura around the lung or the pericardium around the heart.
functional assessment Appraisal of an individual's perception of his capacity to maneuver within a defined environment.

G

gallop rhythm Audible extra heart sound produced by an abnormal third or fourth heart sound.
gingiva Pertaining to the gum.
glaucoma Eye disease characterized by abnormally increased intraocular pressure caused by obstruction of the outflow of aqueous humor.
glossitis Inflammation of the tongue.
goiter Hypertrophy of the thyroid gland, usually evident as a pronounced increase in its size.
gout Metabolic disease associated with abnormal uric acid metabolism that is a form of acute arthritis; marked by inflammation of the joints.
graphesthesia Ability to recognize symbols, numbers, or letters traced on the skin.
gravida Denotes number of pregnancies. *Example: Multigravida* indicates more than one pregnancy.
guarding Protective withdrawal or positioning of a body part during an injury.
gynecomastia Abnormally large mammary glands in the male.

H

hallucination Sensory perception that does not arise from an external stimulus; can be auditory, visual, tactile, gustatory, or olfactory.
health history Collection of subjective data by interview from a patient as a component of health assessment.
heave Palpable, diffuse, sustained lift of the chest wall or a portion of the wall.
helix Margin of the external ear.
hemangioma Benign tumor found predominately in subcutaneous tissue or skin; caused by newly formed blood vessels.
hematuria Presence of blood in the urine.
hemoptysis Coughing up blood or referring to bloody sputum.
hepatojugular reflux Phenomenon indicating right heart failure in which venous pressure rises when the upper abdomen is compressed for 30 to 45 seconds; upon upper right quadrant compression, increased prominence of the jugular vein is noted.
hernia Abnormal opening in a muscle wall or cavity that permits protrusion of its contents.
herpetiform Describes a cluster of vesicles resembling herpes lesions.
hirsutism Excessive body hair, usually in a masculine distribution, owing to heredity, hormonal dysfunction, porphyria, or medication.
Homan's sign Calf pain associated with rapid dorsiflexion of the foot, often indicative of thrombophlebitis.
hordeolum (stye) Infection of a sebaceous gland at the margin of the eyelid.
hydramnios Excess formation of amniotic fluid during pregnancy.
hydrocele Nontender, serous fluid mass located within the tunica vaginalis (layered, hollow membrane adjacent to the testis).
hymenal remnants Small, irregular, fleshy projections that are remnants of a ruptured hymen; a normal phenomenon that may or may not be present at the vaginal introitus in varied sizes and shapes.
hyoid U-shaped bone suspended from the styloid process of the temporal bone.
hyperesthesia Abnormally increased sensitivity to sensory stimuli such as touch or pain.
hyperextension Refers to the extension of a body part beyond normal limits of extension.
hyperkinesis Hyperactivity or excessive muscular activity.
hyperkinetic Hyperactive.
hyperopia (farsightedness) Refractive error in which light rays focus behind the retina.
hyperresonance Sound elicited by percussion; its pitch lies between that of resonance and tympany.
hypertension Refers to abnormally high blood pressure.
hypoesthesia Decreased or dulled sensitivity to stimulation.
hyposmia Decreased sense of smell.
hypospadias Congenital defect in which the urinary meatus opens on the ventral aspect of the penis; opening may be located in the glans, penile shaft, scrotum, or perineum.
hypotension Refers to abnormally low blood pressure.
hypoxemia Abnormal reduction of oxygen content in the arterial blood.
hypoxia Abnormal reduction of oxygen delivery to body tissue; oxygen deficiency.
hypovolemic Pertaining to decreased blood volume; usually refers to a state of shock resulting from massive blood loss and inadequate tissue perfusion.

I

illusion Perceptual distortion of an external stimulus. *Example:* A mirage in a desert.
"inching" Recommended method for moving the stethoscope over the precordium while listening for heart sounds; small, sliding movements (rather than lifting and lowering the stethoscope from side to side) may enable the listener to hear more sounds.

incidence Number of times an event occurs.
incus One of three ossicles in the middle ear; resembling an anvil, it communicates sound vibrations from the maleus to the stapes.
induration Hardening of the skin, usually caused by edema or infiltration by a neoplasm.
infancy First year of life.
infarct Localized area of tissue necrosis caused by prolonged anoxia.
inferior Lower surface of an organ; refers to a position that is lower in relation to another.
infection Redness or congestion of a part of the body caused by dilation of blood vessels secondary to an inflammatory or infectious process.
intermittent claudication Condition characterized by symptoms of pain, aching, cramping, and localized fatigue of the legs that occur while walking but that can be quickly relived by rest (2 to 5 minutes); discomfort occurs most often in the calf but may arise in the foot, thigh, hip, or buttock; caused by prolonged ischemia.
internal rotation Inward turning of a limb.
introitus General term denoting an opening or the orifice of a cavity or hollow structure.
inversion Turning inside out or upside down.
inverted nipple Nipple that is turned inward.
ischemia Diminished supply of blood to a body organ or surface; characterized by pallor, coolness, and pain.
isthmus glandulae thyroideae Narrow portion of the thyroid gland connecting the left and right lobes.

K

keloid Hypertrophic scar tissue; prevalent in nonwhite races.
keratosis Overgrowth and thickening of the cornified epithelium.
Kernig's sign Diagnostic sign of meningeal irritation characterized by inability of a supine client to completely extend the leg when the knee and hip are flexed on the abdomen.
kinesthetic sensation Ability to detect the position of a body part when it is moved through space.
Koplik spots Lesions that appear in the prodromal stage of measles; they appear as small blueish-white lesions with irregular borders on the buccal mucosa opposite the molar teeth.
Korotkoff sounds Sounds heard during the taking of blood pressure.
Kussmaul respiration Rapid deep respiration, often associated with ketoacidosis.
kyphosis Abnormal convexity of the posterior curve of the spine.

L

labile emotions Unpredictable, rapid shifting of expression of feelings.
labyrinth Complex structure of the inner ear that communicates directly with the acoustic nerve by transmitting sound vibrations from the middle ear through the fluid-filled network of three semicircular canals that join at a vestibule connected to the cochlea.
lateral Referring to the side; position away from the middle.
Leopold's maneuvers Series of palpation techniques used to determine fetal presentation, position, and lie.
leukoplakia Thickened, white, well-circumscribed patch that can appear on any mucous membrane; sometimes precancerous; often a response to chronic irritation, such as pipe smoking.
leukorrhea White vaginal discharge; can be a normal phenomenon that occurs (or increases) with pregnancy, the use of birth control medication, or as a postmenstrual phase; can also be an abnormal sign indicating malignancy or infection.
lichenification Thickening of the skin characterized by accentuated skin markings; often the result of chronic scratching.
light reflex Triangular landmark area on the tympanic membrane that most brightly reflects the examiner's light source.
lordosis Abnormal anterior concavity of the spine.
lower motor neurons Nerve cells that originate in the anterior horn cells of the spinal column and travel to innervate the skeletal muscle fibers; injury or disease of this area will result in decreased muscle tone, reflexes, or strength.
lymphadenitis Inflammation of the lymph nodes.
lymphoma General term for the growth of new tissue in the lymphatic area; generally refers to malignant growth.

M

macule Flat, circumscribed lesion of the skin or mucous membrane that is 1 cm or less in diameter.
malleus Innermost ossicle of the middle ear; resembling a hammer, it is connected to the tympanic membrane and transmits sound vibrations to the incus, which communicates with the stapes.
mastitis Inflammation of the breast.
mastoid process Conical projection of the temporal bone extending downward and forward behind the external auditory meatus.
McBurney point Point of specialized tenderness in acute appendicitis that is situated on a line between the umbilicus and the right anterosuperior iliac spine about 1 or 2 inches above the latter.
medial Referring to the middle; the median plane of the body.
mediastinum Space within the thoracic cavity positioned behind the sternum, in front of the vertebral column, and between the lungs.
menarche Onset of menstruation in adolescence or young adulthood.
menorrhagia Abnormally heavy or extended menstrual periods.
metrorrhagia Any uterine bleeding that is not related to menstruation.
midaxillary line Vertical line extending downward from the midaxillary fold; used in assessment as an anatomical reference point.

midclavicular line Vertical line extending downward from the middle of the clavicle; used in assessment as an anatomical reference point.
miosis Condition in which the pupil is constricted, usually drug-induced; agent that induces this reaction is called a *miotic.*
Montgomery tubercles Small sebaceous glands located on the areola of the breast.
Murphy's sign Sign of gallbladder disease consisting of pain when taking a large breath when the examiner's fingers are pressing on the approximate location of the gallbladder.
myalgia Tenderness or pain in the muscle.
mydriasis Dilation of the pupil, usually drug-induced; agent that induces this reaction is called a *mydriatic.*
myoclonus Twitching or clonic spasm of a muscle group.
myopia (nearsightedness) Refractive error in which light rays focus in front of the retina.

N

nabothian cyst (retention cyst) Small white or purple firm nodule that commonly appears on the cervix; forms within the mucus-secreting nathobian glands, which are present in large numbers on the uterine cervix.
nares (singular: naris) Nostrils; anterior openings of the nose.
necrosis Localized death of tissue.
neonate Newborn infant during the first 28 days of life; referring to the time from birth to 4 weeks of age.
neurosis Ineffective or troubled coping mechanism stemming from anxiety or emotional conflict.
nevus Congenital pigmented area on the skin. *Example:* Mole, birthmark.
nicking Abnormal condition showing compression of a vein at an arteriovenous crossing; visible through an ophthalmoscope during a retinal examination.
nodule Solid skin elevation that extends into the dermal layer and that is 1 to 2 cm in diameter.
nystagmus Involuntary rhythmical movement of the eyes; oscillations may be horizontal, vertical, rotary, or mixed.

O

objective data Data obtained from examination, measurements, or diagnostic tests; observable by the examiner.
obsession Persistent thought or idea that preoccupies the mind; not always realistic and may result in compulsive behavior.
oligomenorrhea Abnormally light or infrequent menstruation.
oliguria Inadequate production or secretion of urine (usually less than 400 ml in a 24-hour period).
orchi- Combining form that denotes the testes. *Example: Orchitis* means inflammation of one or both of the testes.
orthopnea Difficulty breathing in any position other than an upright one.
osteoarthritis Form of arthritis in which one or many of the joints undergo degenerative changes.
otalgia Pain in the ear.
otitis externa Infection of the external canal or auricle of the ear.
otitis media Infection of the inner ear.

P

Paget's disease of the nipple Condition characterized by an excoriating or scaling lesion of the nipple extending from an intraductal carcinoma of the breast.
palmar Relating to the palm of the hand.
palpebral conjunctiva Thin, transparent mucous membrane that lines the inner eyelid and adjoins the bulbar conjunctiva, which covers the sclera.
palpebral fissure Opening between the upper and lower eyelids.
palpitation Sensation of pounding, fluttering, or racing of the heart; can be a normal phenomenon or caused by a disorder of the heart.
papilla General term for a small projection; dorsal surface of the tongue is composed of a variety of forms of papillae that contain openings to the taste buds.
papule Solid, elevated, circumscribed, superficial lesion 1 cm or less in diameter.
paradoxical pulse Diminished pulse amplitude on inspiration with an increased amplitude on expiration; an exaggeration of a normal response to respiration; often associated with obstructive lung disease.
paranoia Sense of being persecuted or victimized; suspicion of others.
paraphimosis Condition characterized by the inability to pull the foreskin forward from a retracted position; glans is usually swollen and inflamed.
paresthesia Abnormal sensation such as numbness or tingling.
parity Denotes the number of viable births.
paronychia Inflammation of the skinfold that adjoins the nail bed; characterized by redness, swelling, and pain; may be pustular.
paroxysmal nocturnal dyspnea (PND) Periodic acute attacks of shortness of breath while recumbent; relieved by sitting or standing.
pars flaccida Small portion of the tympanic membrane between the mallear folds.
pars tensa Larger portion of the tympanic membrane.
patch Flat, circumscribed lesion of the skin or mucous membrane that is more than 1 cm in diameter.
peau d'orange Dimpling of the skin that resembles the skin of an orange.
pectoralis major muscle One of the four muscles of the anterior upper portion of the chest.
pectus carinatum Abnormal prominence of the sternum.
pectus exacvatum Abnormal depression of the sternum.

periodontis (pyorrhea) Inflammation and deterioration of the gums and supporting alveolar bone; occurs in varying degrees of severity; if neglected, this condition will result in loss of teeth.

peristalsis Alternating contraction and relaxation of the smooth muscles of the intestinal tract to propel contents forward.

perlèche (cheilosis, cheilitis) Fissures at the corners of the mouth that become inflamed; caused by overclosure of the mouth in an edentulous client, marked loss of the alveolar ridge, or riboflavin deficiency; saliva irritates the area, and moniliasis is a common complication.

petechiae Tiny, flat, purple or red spots on the surface of the skin resulting from minute hemorrhages within the dermal or submucosal layers.

phimosis Tightness of the foreskin that results in an inability to retract it; usually caused by adhesions of the prepuce to the underlying glands.

phobia Uncontrollable and often unreasonable intense fear of a specific object or event.

photophobia Ocular discomfort caused by exposure of the eyes to bright light.

physical functioning Appraisal of an individual's perception of his ability to control and manipulate his physical environment, as well as his judgement of the ability of his inner resources to control and use his body effectively.

pilonidal fistula (or sinus) Abnormal channel containing a tuft of hair that is situated most frequently over or close to the tip of the coccyx; may also occur in other regions of the body.

pinna Auricle or projected part of the external ear.

plantar flexion Extension of the foot so that the forepart is depressed with respect to the position of the ankle.

plantar Referring to the bottom surface of the foot.

plaque Solid, elevated, circumscribed, superficial lesion more than 1 cm in diameter.

plaque (dental) Film that accumulates on the surface of the teeth; made up of mucin and colloidal material from saliva; subject to bacterial invasion.

pleximeter Finger placed on the skin surface to receive the taps from the percussion hammer or plexor; used in percussion.

point of maximum impulse (PMI) Specific area of the chest where the heartbeat is palpated most clearly; usually the apical impulse, a brief systolic beat in the fourth or fifth intercostal space along the midclavicular line.

posterior Referring to the back.

posterior triangle (of neck) Landmark area for palpating the posterior cervical chain, the supraclavicular chain, and the occipital lymph chain; sectioned along the anterior border by the sternocleidomastoid muscle, the posterior border by the trapezius muscle, and the bottom by the clavicle.

precipitating factor Event or entity that hastens the onset of another event.

precordium Area of the chest that overlies the heart and adjacent great vessels.

predisposing factor (risk factor) Event or entity that contributes to the cause of another event. *Example:* A family history of obesity increases a client's risk for obesity.

presbycusis Impairment of hearing in old age.

presbyopia Loss of accommodation (ability to focus on near objects) associated with aging.

pre-school age Refers to children between the ages of 3 and 5 years.

problem list Compilation of findings that appear at the end of a database; may be diagnoses (medical or nursing), clusters of interrelated findings, or isolated findings that the examiner wishes to pursue but cannot label or attach to other findings.

pronate To turn the forearm so that the palm faces downward or to rotate the leg or foot inward.

proprioception Awareness of body posture, movement, and changes in equilibrium originating from sensory nerve endings (proprioceptors) within muscles and tendons.

pruritus Itching.

psychosis Any major mental disorder characterized by greatly distorted perceptions and severe disorganization of the personality.

psychosocial functioning Appraisal of an individual's capacity to attain and maintain satisfactory intimate and social relationships with others.

ptosis Drooping of the upper eyelid; can be unilateral or bilateral; usually results from innervation or lid muscle disorder.

ptyalism Excessive salivation.

pudendum Collective term denoting the external genitalia; for the female it includes the mons pubis, labia majora, labia minora, vaginal vestibule, and vestibular glands; for the male it includes the penis, scrotum, and testes.

pulse deficit Discrepancy between the ventricular rate auscultated over the heart and the arterial rate palpated over the radial artery.

pulse pressure Difference between systolic and diastolic pressures, usually within the range of 30 to 40 mm Hg; tends to increase as systolic pressure rises with arteriosclerosis of the large vessels (specifically the aorta).

pulsus alternans Alternating pulse; abnormal pulse characterized by a regular rhythm in which a strong beat alternates with a weaker one.

purpura Hemorrhage into the tissue, usually circumscribed; lesions may be described as petechiae, ecchymoses, or hematomas, according to size.

pustule Vesicle or bulla that contains pus.

pyramidal tract Bundle of upper motor neurons that coordinate voluntary movements originating in the motor cortex of the brain; nerve fibers travel through the brainstem and the spinal cord, where they synapse with anterior horn cells; responsible for the coordinated response of voluntary movements.

pyrosis Burning sensation in the epigastric and sternal region with the raising of acid liquid from the stomach; also called *heartburn*.

pyuria Presence of white cells (pus) in the urine.

R

rebound tenderness Sign of inflammation in the peritoneum in which pain is elicited by a sudden withdrawal of a hand pressing on the abdomen; often found in clients with appendicitis.

rectocele Bulging of the rectum and posterior vaginal wall through relaxed or weakened musculature of the vagina.

red reflex Red glow over the pupil created by light illuminating the retina.

refraction Deviation of light rays as they pass from one transparent medium into another of different density.

remission Disappearance or diminishment of signs or symptoms.

reticular Describes a netlike pattern or structure of veins on a tissue surface.

retraction Shortening or drawing backward of the skin.

rheumatoid arthritis Chronic, destructive collagen disease characterized by inflammation, thickening, and swelling of the joints.

rhino- Combining form that denotes the nose.

rhonchus Loud, low-pitched, coarse sound like a snore heard on auscultation of an airway obstructed by thick secretions, muscular spasm, neoplasm, or external pressure; also called a *sonorous wheeze.*

Romberg's test Test that evaluates an individual's ability to maintain a given position when standing erect with feet together and eyes closed.

S

scale Small, thin flake of epithelial cells.

schizoid Exhibiting behaviors or having characteristics that resemble schizophrenia.

school age Refers to children between the ages of 6 and 12 years.

scoliosis Lateral curvature of the spine.

scotoma Defined area of blindness within the visual field; can involve one or both eyes.

sebaceous glands Secretory dermal structures that produce sebum, an oily substance; puberty stimulates production of sebum; the primary areas for secretion are in the face, chest, and upper part of the back.

seborrhea Group of skin conditions characterized by noninflammatory, excessively dry scales or by excessive oiliness.

sensorium Status of level of consciousness and orientation to surroundings.

shifting dullness Change in the dull sounds heard with palpation; at first the dull sound is heard in one location, then in a different location.

shotty node Small lymph node that feels hard and nodular; generally moveable and nontender; may show evidence of having been infected many times in the past.

sign Objective finding perceived by the examiner.

significant negative Absence of a finding that is often significant in clarifying the client's condition.

Skene's glands (periurethral) Mucus-secreting glands that lie just inside the urethral orifice of women; not visible during examination.

smegma Secretion of sebaceous glands, especially the cheesy, foul-smelling secretion sometimes found under the foreskin of the penis and at the base of the labia minora near the glans clitoris.

spasticity Increased tone or contractions of muscles causing stiff and awkward movements; seen with upper motor neuron lesions.

spermatocele (epididymal cyst) Painless, fluid-filled epididymal mass that contains spermatozoa.

spiritual state Individual's version of his effectiveness in developing and sustaining a belief and value system that assists him in self-acceptance and in his relationship to others and to a higher being.

spondylitis Inflammation of one or more of the spinal vertebrae; usually characterized by stiffness and pain.

sprain Traumatic injury to the tendon; characteristics are pain, swelling, and discoloration of the skin over the joint.

stapes One of the ossicles in the middle ear; resembles a tiny stirrup and transmits sound vibrations from the incus to the internal ear.

stereognosis Ability to recognize objects by the sense of touch.

sternocleidomastoid muscle Major muscle that rotates and flexes the head; originates by two heads from the sternum and clavicle and inserts on the mastoid process and the occipital bone.

stoma General term that means opening or mouth. *Example: Stomatitis* refers to a general inflammation of the oral cavity.

strabismus Condition in which the eyes are not directed at the same object or point.

strain Temporary damage to the muscles usually caused by excessive physical effort.

striae Streaks of linear scars that often result from rapidly developing tension in the skin; also called *stretch marks.*

stridor Shrill, harsh sound heard during inspiration and caused by laryngeal obstruction.

subjective data Data obtained from a health history; data the client provides to the examiner.

subluxation Partial or incomplete dislocation of a joint.

superior Upper surface of an organ; refers to a position that is higher in relation to another.

supernumerary nipple Extra nipple.

supinate To turn the forearm so that the palm faces upward or to rotate the foot and leg outward.

symptom Subjective indicator or sensation perceived by the client.

systole Period of time within the cardiac cycle in which the ventricles are contracted and ejecting blood into the aorta and pulmonary arteries.

T

tachycardia Rapid heart rate (more than 100 beats per minute).

tachypnea Rapid breathing; respiratory rate that is faster than normal.

tactile fremitus Vibratory sensations of the spoken voice felt through the chest wall on palpation.

tail of Spence Upper outer tail of the breast that extends into the axillary region.
telangiectasia Dilation of a superficial capillary or network of small capillaries that produces fine, irregular, red lines on the skin surface.
tendinitis Inflammation of a tendon.
thrill Palpable murmur; feels like the throat of a purring cat.
thrombophlebitis Inflammation of a vein; often associated with clot formation.
thrombus Blood clot attached to the inner wall of a vessel; usually causes some degree of occlusion.
tic Spasmodic muscular contraction most commonly involving the face, head, neck, or shoulder muscles.
tinnitus Tinkling or ringing sound heard in one or both ears.
toddlerhood Refers to the ages of 12 to 36 months.
tophus Calculus that contains sodium urate deposits that develops in periauricular fibrous tissue; associated with gout.
torsion (of spermatic cord) Twisting of the spermatic cord that results in an infarction of the testis.
torus palatinus Exostosis or benign outgrowth of bone located on the midline of the hard palate.
tragus Cartilaginous projection in front of the exterior meatus of the ear.
trapezius muscle Major muscle that rotates and extends the head; originates along the superior curved line of the occiput and the spinous processes of the seventh cervical and all thoracic vertebrae and inserts at the clavicle, acromion, and base of the scapula.
tremor Continuous involuntary trembling movement of a part or parts of the body.
trimester Refers to a period of time during pregnancy. There are three trimesters during pregnancy; each trimester lasts a period of 3 months.
tumor Solid skin elevation that extends into the dermal layer and that is more than 1 cm in diameter.
turbinates Extensions of the ethmoid bone located along the lateral wall of the nose; these fingerlike projections are covered with erectile mucosal membranes that become swollen or inflamed in response to allergy or viral invasion.
turgor Normal resiliency of the skin.
two-point discrimination Ability to identify being touched by two sharp objects simultaneously.
tympany Low-pitched note heard on percussion of a hollow organ such as the stomach.

U

ulcer Circumscribed crater on the surface of the skin or mucous membrane that leaves an uncovered wound.
umbo Central depressed portion of the concavity of the lateral surface of the tympanic membrane; marks the spot where the malleus is attached to the inner surface.
unilateral Relating to or referring to one side.
upper motor neurons Nerve cells that originate in the cerebral cortex and project downward; make up the corticobulbar and pyramidal tracts and end in the anterior horn of the spinal cord; responsible for the fine and discrete conscious movements.
urticaria (hives) Pruritic wheals; often transient and allergic in origin.

V

vaginitis Inflammation of the vaginal vault; has various causes.
valgus Bending outward.
varicocele Abnormal tortuosity and dilation of spermatic veins; spermatic cord is described as feeling like a bag of worms; condition is not painful but involves a pulling or dragging sensation.
varus Turning inward.
vellus hair Soft nonpigmented hair that covers the body.
verge (anal) External ring at the opening of the anus.
vermilion border Demarcation point between the mucosal membrane of the lips and the skin of the face; common site for recurrent infections such as herpes infections and carcinoma; blurring of this border may be an early sign of lesion development.
vertigo Sensation of moving around in space (whirling motion; subjective vertigo) or of objects moving about oneself (objective vertigo); results in disturbance of the individual's equilibrium.
vesicle Fluid-filled, elevated, superficial lesion 1 cm or less in diameter.
vesicular breath sounds Normal breath sounds heard over most of the lungs.
vestibule Middle part of the inner ear located behind the cochlea and in front of the semicircular canals.
vocal fremitus Vibratory sensations of the spoken voice felt through the chest wall on palpation; also known as tactile fremitus.
volar Referring to or denoting the palmar aspect of the hand or the plantar aspect of the foot.
vulva External female genitalia; also referred to as the *pudendum.*

W

wheal Elevated, solid, transient lesion; often irregularly shaped but well demarcated; an edematous response.
wheeze High-pitched, musical noise that sounds like a squeak; heard during auscultation of a narrowed airway.
whispered pectoriloquy Transmission of whispered words through the chest wall, heard during auscultation; indicates solidification of the lungs.

X

xerostomia Dryness of the mouth.

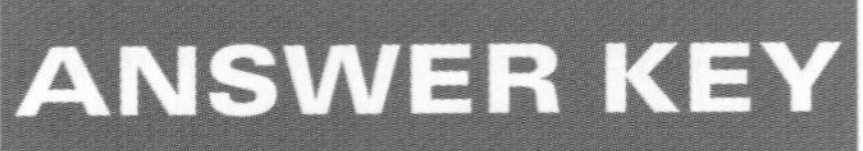

ANSWER KEY

Answers to **CRITICAL THINKING QUESTIONS** *and* **CASE STUDIES** *at the End of Each Chapter*

CHAPTER 1

CRITICAL THINKING QUESTIONS

1. This would be a focused assessment because of the urgency and priority of the child's (and the mother's) needs at this time. The assessment would focus on the injury to the forearm, as well as assessing for complications associated with that injury. The assessment would also focus on the immediate response of the mother and child to the injury (e.g., pain and anxiety). The assessment is focused on these two areas in order to provide immediate and appropriate care to the child.
2. This would be a comprehensive assessment because the nurse will need to collect baseline data to plan care for this child on an ongoing basis. The baseline data will be valuable to the nurse and other health care providers in order to monitor the child's progress (note changes), identify variables that may affect his progress, and develop an appropriate and realistic teaching plan for the child and the mother. Additionally, because the child is in no acute distress at this time, he can actively participate with his mother in a comprehensive assessment.

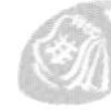

CASE STUDY

CASE 1

1. Subjective data:
   Abdominal pain in right abdomen.
   Pain feels like a knife and goes to shoulder.
   Client is nauseated.
   Client feels exhausted.
   Client has not slept for three nights; pain keeps her awake.
   Client hurts too much to get up and move.
2. Objective data:
   Dark circles under eyes.
   Vital signs: Blood pressure (BP), 132/90 mm Hg; Pulse, 104 beats/min; Respirations 22 per minute; Temperature, 101.8° F (38.8° C).
   Elevated white blood cell (WBC) count.
   Client lying in fetal position.
3. Functional health patterns:
   Nutrition–metabolic
   Activity–exercise
   Cognitive–perceptual
   Sleep–rest
4. Applicable NANDA-approved nursing diagnoses include the following:
   Risk for altered body temperature: hyperthermia.
   Pain.
   Sleep pattern disturbance.
   Risk for fluid volume deficit.

CASE 2

1. Functional health pattern: cognitive–perceptual.
   Nursing diagnosis: *pain* related to right leg injury.
   a. Subjective data:
      Complains of pain in right leg.
      Pain medication helps only a little bit and "butt hurts" because she can't move.
   b. Objective data:
      Client has fractured femur.
      Right leg in skeletal traction.
      Taking Percocet orally for pain every 6 hours.
2. Functional health pattern: elimination.
   Nursing diagnosis: *colonic constipation* related to inactivity and analgesics.
   a. Subjective data:
      No bowel movement for 3 days.
      Stool looked like "hard, dry rabbit turds."
      Normal bowel elimination daily.
   b. Objective data
      Client is on bed rest in skeletal traction.
      Fluid intake average = 1000 ml/day.
      Eating 30% of meals.
      Abdomen slightly distended.
      Active bowel sounds.
      Taking Percocet for pain.
3. Functional health pattern: nutrition–metabolic.
   Nursing diagnosis: *risk for impaired skin integrity* related to immobility.
   a. Subjective data:
      "My butt hurts because I can't move around."
      "The food is horrible."
   b. Objective data:
      Client is on bed rest in skeletal traction.
      Fluid intake average = 1000 ml/day.
      Eating 30% of meals.
      2-inch diameter redness over sacrum (skin intact).
4. Functional health pattern: activity–exercise.
   Nursing diagnosis: *diversional activity deficit* related to complete bed rest.
   a. Subjective data:
      Client complains she is so bored she can't stand it.
      "I am used to being active so being stuck in bed is driving me crazy."
      "TV shows are not worth watching."
   b. Objective data:
      Client is on complete bed rest with right leg in skeletal traction.
      Client is alert, agitated, and restless.

CHAPTER 2

CRITICAL THINKING QUESTIONS

1. Blended families usually involve stepparents and stepchildren. A biologic parent lives elsewhere, and children are commonly transferred between homes of two families, forcing the parents and stepparents to deal with a part-time relationship with one child. Duvall's tasks of the family may apply; however, the first few stages may not occur.
2. In single-parent families, children live with one biologic parent. Both sustain a loss from the absence of the other biologic parent. There may be great variation in involvement of the absent parent from active involvement to no involvement. Financial difficulties are a common stressor. Duvall's tasks of the family may apply until children leave the home; however, later stages (middle-age parents and aging family members) do not apply.
3. Intergenerational families include those in which multiple generations of a family live together under one roof, or those where grandparents and/or great-grandparents raise and care for the children. Duvall's tasks apply only to middle tasks. Couples may be married, but may not have time to themselves. After children leave home, there may be no sense of an "empty nest."
4. Foster families occur when a child has sustained a loss of his or her biologic parents. Typically, the child is placed in a household where an adult couple serves as head of the household. Siblings may be part of more than one household, and adults in the family may have minimal to no legal relationship with the children. Duvall's tasks may be very difficult to apply because of significant changes and variability associated with foster child care.

CASE STUDY

1. Subjective data:
   Client recently lost spouse (5 months ago).
   Son says his mother has "gone downhill."
   Son indicates client is no longer keeping her house clean, nor cooking appropriate meals.
   Son reports significant change in client's personal hygiene habits (she no longer has an interest in getting her hair done or getting dressed for the day).
   Son reports that client becomes angry when he talks about other living options; client states, ". . . . you think I am helpless and want to lock me away."
2. Objective data: Client is a 78-year-old female who sits quietly during conversation.
   Overall hygiene—client appears clean.
   Her hair is matted, and her clothes do not match and are badly wrinkled.
   Client's speech is clear.
   Her overall affect is very dull; she makes no eye contact with her son or the nurse.
   Age-consistent findings with physical examination; no overt physical problems identified.
3. Mrs. Cobb is in Erikson's stage of ego integrity versus despair.
4. Mrs. Cobb may be struggling with the following developmental tasks: dealing with the death of her spouse; adapting to living arrangements; adjusting to relationships with adult children and grandchildren; adjusting to slower physical and intellectual responses; managing leisure time and remaining active; maintaining physical and mental health; finding the meaning of life.
5. Additional assessment needs to be done in the area of skills of daily living verses mental health/depression. Some of the changes noted by the son may be indicative of physical/cognitive decline, or they may be a result of depression and apathy from the loss of a husband. There are several developmental tests that may enlighten the nurse as to what kind of help may be necessary.
6. Any of the tools that focus on stress—Social Readjustment Rating Scale, Stokes/Gorden Stress Scale, Geriatric Scale of Recent Life Events—should be considered. Also, any of the tools that assess behavioral functioning may help to determine Mrs. Cobb's ability to perform activities of daily living and to assess her behavior. These include the Chrichton Geriatric Rating Scale and the Sandor Clinical Assessment—Geriatric.

CHAPTER 3

CRITICAL THINKING QUESTIONS

1. Ask the mother/grandmother about the cloth. This may be a home remedy or the treatment of a medicine healer. You should ask permission to remove the cloth long enough to examine the abdomen with the understanding that it may be placed back on when you are finished. To remove it without asking, or to insist that it stay off sends a message that you do not value the clients' beliefs. In addition, it may be helpful to ask the purpose of the cloth. Asking about the purpose helps the nurse to understand and acknowledge the family's perceived value of the treatment.
2. First, it is important to understand that it is a common Hispanic practice for an entire family (including extended family) to visit a hospitalized loved one, particularly an elder. The visitation "rules" may create conflict for the family and client. The nurse must determine to what extent the visitors are affecting the client and the staff's

ability to provide care and look for solutions to meet the needs of the family and the health care provider.

3. *Health belief and practices*: What does illness mean to you? How do you perceive your health? What do you currently do to treat your illness and to help you stay healthy? *Religious and ritual influences*: Are there any special religious practices or beliefs that are practiced? Are there any special practices or beliefs that may affect health care when patient is ill or dying? *Dietary practices*: What does the family eat? Who prepares the food? How is food prepared? *Family relationships*: Describe the roles of family members. Who is responsible for child rearing?

CHAPTER 4

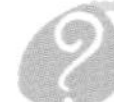

CRITICAL THINKING QUESTIONS

1. The past health history for a 6-week-old infant includes the mother's health status during the pregnancy, information regarding the labor and delivery process, and the infant's health status immediately after birth.
2. With newborns and infants, the focus of psychosocial status is the infant's impact on the family. This includes questions to the parents about parenting skills, stressors the infant is placing on the family, child care arrangements, and sibling rivalry. With children, the focus of psychosocial status is still on the family but also includes developmental milestones reached by the child behavioral patterns of the child, and the child's friends and school. With adolescents, the focus of psychosocial status is on friends and family and influences affecting the adolescent.
3. A health history organized by functional health patterns collects and organizes data in 11 areas of functioning as opposed to the traditional body system. Both formats collect similar data; it is the organization of the data that differs. Although proponents of both the systems approach and functional health patterns will argue that one approach is better than the other, both are readily used and both have value. For this reason, it is important to have familiarity with both.

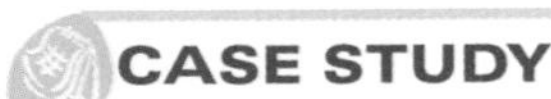

CASE STUDY

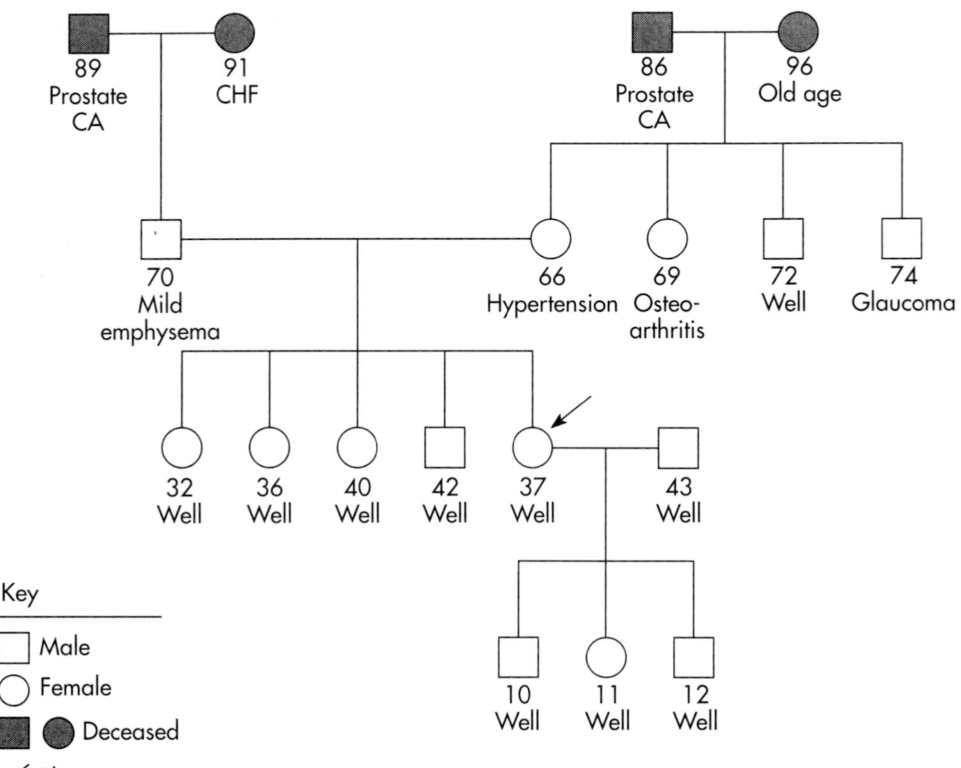

CHAPTER 5

CRITICAL THINKING QUESTIONS

1. Many institutions prefer the use of the tympanic thermometer, even for infants. Unless the child has a fever, the axillary route using either an electronic or a mercury-in-glass thermometer is also appropriate. The rectal route for temperature measurement should be avoided in the infant. There is risk of rectal perforation while taking a rectal temperature on a newborn.
2. The nurse must wash hands before and after the examination and after an examination procedure that could result in transmission of organisms (even when gloves are worn). During certain parts of a physical examination, personal protective equipment should be used by the examiner for protection against contamination and infection. For any part of the examination in which the examiner anticipates the possibility of contact with body fluids or mucous membranes, personal protective equipment should be used. Gloves should be worn to touch the inside of the mouth, open lesions, and the perineal area. Masks and gowns are not routinely indicated.
3. The two types of equipment used to assess fetal heart sounds for routine assessment are the fetoscope and the Doppler. The fetoscope is a special stethoscope which uses bone conduction to enhance the heart sounds of the fetus. The fetal heart tones cannot usually be auscultated with a fetoscope until 17 to 19 weeks' gestation. The Doppler makes use of a continuous ultrasound to assess fetal heart tones. The Doppler requires a conduction gel applied to the skin, and the sounds are amplified. The Doppler is more sensitive than a fetoscope, thus fetal heart tones are usually audible with a Doppler by 10 to 12 weeks' gestation.
4. The goal is to provide a latex safe environment by avoiding use of any latex produce for his care. A latex allergy alert should be posted in the patient record and/or in the computer to inform all healthcare workers of this allergy. A "latex precautions" sign should be posted outside the patient's room—and a special supply cart with latex-free equipment could be set up outside the door of the patient's room. Additionally, it would be a good idea to post a list of products containing latex in an area for easy reference.

CHAPTER 6

CRITICAL THINKING QUESTIONS

1. First, use the stethoscope correctly. Check to be sure that the diaphragm side of the head is engaged; also be sure to point the ear pieces of the stethoscope forward as you place them in your ears. Second, be sure to always place the stethoscope directly against the client's skin. Unfortunately, some examiners do not take the time to do this, and attempt to auscultate through the clothing. This is not appropriate because it reduces transmission of sound and can cause interference. Third, be sure to hold the stethoscope firmly on the skin, between the index and second finger. If you lightly lay the stethoscope on the skin, or if you hold the head of the stethoscope incorrectly, if will affect your ability to hear sounds.
2. Routine measurement for growth and development includes weight, recumbent length, and head circumference. Chest circumference is measured at birth, but routine measurement following birth is not done unless an abnormal head or chest size is suspected. Weight, recumbent length, and head circumference measurments are plotted by age on growth charts.
3. 5′5″ = 65 inches; 140 lb = 63.64 kg. This client falls around the 50th percentile for weight and over the 50th percentile in skinfold thickness.

CHAPTER 7

CRITICAL THINKING QUESTIONS

1. Anxiety can occur with stress. Assessment of a person who is stressed includes such questions as "Have there been recent changes in your life? Were these changes stressors for you? How do you deal with stress?" The person who is stressed would describe recent changes in his or her life or a number of stresses for which his or her usual coping strategies did not work. The individual usually can name one or several events that have contributed to the stress. Assessment of a person who is anxious includes questions such as "Have you had difficulty concentrating or making decisions? Have you been preoccupied or forgetful?" Since anxiety varies from mild anxiety to panic, there is a wide range of behavior. Also it is not as common as stress, so a person usually cannot name coping strategies he or she use when anxious. The anxious person usually cannot name a particular event that caused the anxiety. As the anxiety gets worse, they develop a narrow field of perception and have difficulty making decisions.
2. Appropriate dress; body posture; facial expression; tone of voice.
3. *Fetal alcohol syndrome:* Physical features are noted during infancy such as low birth weight, growth deficiency, and malformed facial features. Cognitive manifestations include learning disabilities and sometimes mental retardation.

   Narcotic abstinence syndrome: These features are manifested within 48 to 72 hours after birth as a result of withdrawal from the substance abused by the mother. Manifestations include tremors, restlessness, increased muscle tone, and high-pitched shrill cry.

Fetal cocaine exposure: Infants tend to have low birth weight, smaller than average head circumference, and are at risk for cerebral, renal, and cardiac anomolies. These problems are associated with decreased placental perfusion due to cocaine use.

4. *Similarities:* Both are associated with disorganized thought and confusion, so the clinical findings may initially be similar.

   Differences: Delirium is an acute problem of short duration—it responds to treatment. Dementia, however, is a chronic, progressive disease that does not respond to treatment.

CASE STUDY

1. Unkempt general appearance; crying behavior; excessive sleeping; self-deprecating, slow speech with flat affect.
2. Ask about the onset of symptoms and current stressors. Ask about recent changes in her life, and identify coping mechanisms. Ask about interpersonal relationships with friends and with boyfriend. May consider doing a Holmes stressor scale. Ask her if she takes any medications.
3. Coping–stress management.
   Self-perception–self-concept.
   Sleep–rest.
   Nutrition–metabolic.
4. *Risk for ineffective coping.*
   Risk for self-esteem disturbance.
   Risk for sleep pattern disturbance.
   Risk for altered nutrition: more than body requirements.

CHAPTER 8

CRITICAL THINKING QUESTIONS

1. Similarities will be in the use of the ABCDs of subjective pain assessment. Under **D**escription of pain, use the symptom analysis approach to ask client to describe the location (where does it hurt?), quality (how bad?), chronology (when?), setting (in what environment?), alleviating factors (what make the pain better?) and aggravating factors (what makes the pain worse?). Determine the **A**ffective response (what is his or her attitude toward the pain?), the **B**ehavioral response (how does he or she react to the pain?) and the **C**ognitive response (what has been his or her experience with this type of pain?).

   The cognitive assessment will help to determine differences as clients reveal their past experiences with pain, expectation for pain relief, and the meaning of pain for them. The cultural reaction to pain that each client has learned also affects the pain response. Ms. Baker is African American and may be verbal about her pain. She may willingly describe it and request pain medication. Because she is experiencing acute pain, she can know that the pain will subside as her operative site heals.

   Mr. Sanford is experiencing chronic cancer pain but also may be having acute pain from his surgical site. He may have some physiologic signs of pain. As his cancer progresses, he may need higher doses of analgesics for the same level of pain relief. He may willingly request pain medication. Since he is an older adult, he may not want to bother anyone for pain medication. The assessment helps to individualize his care.

   Ms. Martinez may be experiencing chronic, nonmalignant pain from her rheumatoid arthritis in addition to acute pain from her recent surgery. Thus she may have some physiologic signs of pain from her surgical site. Hispanic people often do not report their pain because they think it is a sign of weakness. The assessment determines if this is the way this client believes.
2. Table 8-1 provides data about the "typical" pain responses of people from these ethnic groups. Your responsibility is to individualize your care by assessing these individual clients to compare their responses to what you know to be typical.

   Those clients who probably will not initiate their own request for pain relief are the woman from Cambodia, the man from China, and the woman from the Philippines. The woman from Cambodia will not ask for pain relief until the pain is severe. If the pain is acute, the physiologic signs of pain may help with this assessment. The man from China learned to be stoic about his pain, and when pain medication is offered, it may be refused the first time. Remember to offer pain-relief medication more than once. The woman from the Philippines may believe that God will give her the strength to endure the pain. Pain medication can be offered as an adjunct to her religious beliefs.

   The clients who probably will initiate their own request pain relief are the man from Israel and the man from Iraq. The man from Israel may provide great detail of the pain and expect pain relief. The man from Iraq will expect immediate pain relief, but the expression of the need for the pain relief may come from a family member or close friend.

CASE STUDY

1. Mr. Moore's description of pain indicates some sort of acute problem—this indicates a need to search for the source of the problem. Also, Mr. Moore has observable symptoms consistent with acute pain.
2. Ask if the pain radiates to any other site. Ask if there are any symptoms associated with urination,

such as blood in the urine or pain with urination? Ask Mr. Moore if he has ever had pain like this before. If so, describe. Ask Mr. Moore if he has noticed anything that reduces the intensity. Has he taken any medications or tried any self-treatment. Ask Mr. Moore what his past experiences with pain have been. Assess the heart and lungs. Perform fist percussion over the costovertebral angle to assess kidney tenderness.

3. Cognitive–perceptual.
4. *Pain* related to inflammatory process.
   Nausea related to inflammatory process and acute pain.
   PC: Renal calculi.

CHAPTER 9

CRITICAL THINKING QUESTIONS

1. Sleep is necessary for health and affects how the client feels. Sleep provides relief from anything distressing, disturbing, or tiring and creates mental calm. During sleep the body restores itself (e.g., repair of epithelial and specialized cells occur during sleep). During sleep the workload of the heart is decreased. The heart rate slows from the usual 70 to 80 beats/min to 60 to 70 beats/min accompanied by a 5% to 10% reduction in systemic blood pressure.
2. When clients are deprived of sleep, they have difficulty coping with stress, their immune system becomes impaired, and they feel fatigued, with decreased ability to concentration. They may demonstrate perceptual difficulties such as confusion, paranoia, and hallucinations with increased anxiety and short-term memory loss.
3. **a.** A nap for a 2-year old is an expected behavior. The sleep obtained during the night is not sufficient. A nap for an 85-year old client is an expected behavior. Old-old adults tend to sleep 6 hours during the night and awaken frequently. A nap for a 3-year old is not as common but occasionally these will occur. By this age naps are not needed. A nap for a 16-year old is not an expected behavior.
   b. 2-year old needs the sleep. 3-year old may be tired or may suggest psychosocial issues. The 16-year old may nap occasionally, but regular napping may point to sleep deprivation. The 85-year old may nap due to changes in nighttime sleeping.
   c. What do you think is the cause for needing naps? How often are naps taken? How long are the naps? Has there been a change in your usual activities? Have you had difficulty sleeping during the night? Has the time of sleep changed (e.g., are you staying up later than usual and/or getting up earlier than usual)? What factors prevent you from sleeping? Discomfort? Environmental disturbances? Work or school–related issues? Personal relationships? Stress? Anxiety? Do you drink alcohol or caffeine prior to sleep at night? What do you usually do to help you sleep? Have these methods been unsuccessful for you at this time?

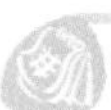

CASE STUDY

1. Complains of not sleeping well and never feels rested; descriptions of ineffective sleep; stress in life; divorce and possible bankruptcy; alcohol intake in evening.
2. How long has this been going on? How often does this occur (how many nights a week)? What medications is he currently taking? Questions about coping mechanisms—how does he best handle stress; who does he have in his life to talk about problems, etc.
3. Coping–stress tolerence.
   Sleep–rest.
4. *Sleep pattern disturbance* related to change in sleep routine as manifested by statement that he never feels rested.
   Risk for ineffective coping related to multiple stressors.

CHAPTER 10

CRITICAL THINKING QUESTIONS

1. Determine the BMI and the DBW. Ask what his usual body weight was prior to the CVA, and calculate the percentage of body weight lost in last 3 months. Complete a dietary assessment, evaluating the client's food habits—perhaps a 24-hour recall and food-frequency questionnaire. A serum albumin level should be determined along with the serum cholesterol level. Assess for muscle wasting and oral mucosa; assess the oral cavity as well. Also observe the client while eating and drinking to assess for chewing and swallowing difficulties. Assess/review the client's activities of daily living. Also assess social factors such as income, living arrangements, and social activities.
2. Measure length, weight, and head circumference. Ask the mother about feedings, including the type of feeding (breast milk or formula), frequency, and length of time or amount of feeding. Evaluate skin color, turgor and texture, edema and rashes; assess physical activity, noting muscle tone, lethargy. Note rooting reflex and suck effort.
3. The BMI is an indicator of total body fat—this number is based on a calculation of height and weight; therefore it is a relative number. Normal BMI range is 20 to 25 for people of all heights. In this example, even though they are very different in size, they are almost identical in the percentage of body fat they carry.
4. BMI = 20.8; DBW = 165 lb. Currently he is 12% below DBW; in the last 6 months he has had a 15% decrease in body weight from his usual body weight. A 15% loss in body weight over 6 months is a serious finding. He is in need of referral.

CASE STUDY

1. Subjective data:
   Fatigue.
   Shortness of breath.
   Change in diet.
   Weight loss.
   Perception of health.
   Objective data:
   Height for weight.
   Scaling of skin.
   Hair findings.
   Cracks in corner of mouth.
   Pale conjunctiva.
2. Ask about other symptoms she may be experiencing; ask if her appetite has been affected; ask if weight loss has been intentional; ask what her usual body weight is; ask her if she has a history of weight loss; assess her knowledge regarding vegetarian diet. Calculate the BMI (18.9), the DBW (120), her current percentage of DBW (9% below), and her percentage body weight change in 4 months from her UBW. She might be a good candidite for MAMC and MAMA calculations.
3. Health perception–health management.
   Nutrition–metabolic.
   Activity–exercise.
   Cognitive–perceptual.
4. *Altered health maintenance* related to lack of knowledge regarding change in diet.
   Altered comfort related to cracks in mouth.
   Activity intolerance related to decrease in energy.
   PC: Malnutrition.

CHAPTER 11

CRITICAL THINKING QUESTIONS

1. Teach him the **ABCD Early Signs. A** = Asymmetry: Melanoma lesions are asymmetrical in shape and appearance. **B** = Border: Melanoma lesions have irregular, indistinct, and sometimes notched borders. **C** = Color: Melanoma lesions tend to have uneven and variegated color. Lesions may vary from brown to pink to purple or have a mixed pigmentation. **D** = Diameter: Melanoma lesions are usually over 6 cm (2 inches) in diameter.
2. The examiner should note the following: location (where the lesion is found); distribution (isolated lesions or confluent); color; size; pattern (clustered, linear, etc.); shape; elevation (flat, raised); characteristics (hard, soft, crusty, fluid-filled, solid, draining).
3. Typically, injuries consistent with a fall are on bony prominences, as the normal reaction during a fall is to stretch out arms for protection. A large soft-tissue injury to the upper arm could occur if the child struck an object during the fall. Multiple bruises, particularly if they are of different ages, are concerning because most 9-month-old children are not yet walking and do not typically bruise themselves.

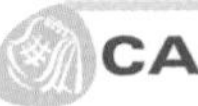

CASE STUDY

1. Foul-smelling odor; loss of appetite; flat affect; 6′2″, 153 pounds; skin breakdown; minimal activity.
2. Ask the client if he is aware of the skin breakdown. Ask about recent weight loss with loss of activity. Assess ulcers to determine stage and presence of infection. Assess other pressure areas for evidence of skin breakdown. Perform a nutritional assessment.
3. Nutrition–metabolic.
   Activity–exercise.
   Health perception–health management.
4. *Impaired skin integrity* related to reduced mobility and nutritional status.
   Risk for infection related to nutritional status.
   Risk for self-care deficit related to weakness.
   Risk for impaired home maintenance management related to weakness and depression.
   Altered nutrition: less than body requirments related to decreased appetite, depression.

CHAPTER 12

CRITICAL THINKING QUESTIONS

1. **a.** At the angle of the mandible is the retropharyngeal or tonsillar lymph node. This node is enlarged due to an inflammatory process.
   b. Determine what additional data to collect by remembering that the retropharyngeal node drains the tonsils, posterior palate, thyroid, and floor of the mouth. Ask the client is she has had a sore throat or pain in her mouth. Inspect the posterior pharynx for enlarged tonsils, redness, pustules. Inspect the posterior palate and floor of the mouth. Inspect and palpate the thyroid for enlargement.
2. **a.** The node behind the mastoid process is the postauricular node, and the node in the groin is the inguinal node. They could be enlarged due to an inflammatory process; however, considering the client's age and locations of the nodes, they may be "shotty" nodes, which are normal variations at this age.
   b. If the nodes are "shotty" nodes, they will be small (1 cm), firm, and mobile, but nontender. Also remember where the lymph that drains to these nodes flows from (refer to Table 12-1). The postauricular nodes receive drainage from the scalp and external auditory canal. Thus, ask the caregiver about any signs of inflammation from these areas and inspect and palpate these areas

to determine if inflammation is present. The inguinal nodes receive drainage from the legs and in males from the penis and scrotum. Again, ask about a history of inflammation here and inspect and palpate these areas for signs of inflammation. If no signs of inflammation are found and there is no history of inflammation from these areas, then you can determine that these node are probably "shotty," a normal variation that requires no action except documentation

3. A lymph node that is tender and less discrete usually is caused from inflammation, whereas a lymph node to which a malignancy has spread is harder and tends to be more discrete.

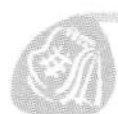

CASE STUDY

1. Fatigue/weakness; maculopapular rash; enlarged lymph nodes.
2. Ask if there is tenderness to lymph nodes. Ask if client has been ill recently. Ask if he has had recent weight loss. Ask if he has been eating properly and getting adequate sleep. Assess lymph nodes in axilla; note size, consistency, mobility, borders, and tenderness of lymph nodes.
3. Activity–exercise.
   Self-perception–self-concept.
4. *Activity intolerance* related to excessive energy demands as manifested by fatigue and statements of "running out of breath easily."
   Fatigue related to hypermetabolic state as manifested by complaint that fatigue and weakness are interfering with school and basketball performance
   Self-esteem disturbance related to altered role performance as manifested by statements that he feels he is "letting everyone down" based on his poor performance.

CHAPTER 13

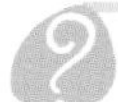

CRITICAL THINKING QUESTIONS

1. Migraines affect women more than men; they have an aura before the headache, pain is typically unilateral and throbbing, lasting typically 4 to 6 hours. Accompanying symptoms include depression, irritability, photophobia, nausea, and vomiting. Cluster headaches affect men more than women; they frequently have slight nausea at the onset of the headache. Pain is usually unilateral and described as burning, stabbing pain behind an eye typically lasting 30 to 60 minutes but recurring over days to weeks. Accompanying symptoms include ipsilateral lacrimation, nasal stuffiness, nasal drainage, and ptosis. Tension headaches affect both genders. The headache starts off slowly. The pain is usually bilateral and described as a tight band around the head lasting several days. Accompanying symptoms include contraction of skeletal muscles of face, jaw, and neck.
2. The position for palpating the fontanel is the sitting position to allow cranial contents to move away from the fontanel by gravity. Ask if the infant has been crying, which can cause a bulging fontanel. Finally compare the head circumference measurement at this visit with the last visit of the infant and/or with physical growth charts to see if it is too large. If the fontanel is bulging with the infant in a sitting position, infant has not been crying, and the head circumference is abnormally large for the age, weight, and height of the infant, then you have reason for a referral.

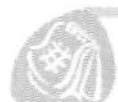

CASE STUDY

1. Patient complaints of severe, reoccuring headache; nasal stuffiness occurs with headache; nothing seems to help headache.
2. Get more information about the headaches including the following:
   Pattern of headaches—frequency, time of day they occur; onset of headache.
   Characteristics of headache—Where is pain? What is pain like? How long does pain last? How severe is the pain?
   Precipitating factors—What brings the headache on?
   Treatment—What has Rob done to try to treat the headaches?
   History—any past or recent trauma to the head? Assess the range of motion in the neck, if possible, and attempt to palpate the neck for lymph nodes.
3. Sleep–rest.
   Coping–stress tolerance.
   Cognitive–perceptual.
   Self-perception–self-concept.
4. *Pain* related to discomfort caused by headache.
   Risk for ineffective individual coping related by repeated headaches.
   Sleep pattern disturbance related to disruption of sleep from pain.
   Anxiety related to lack of knowledge of etiology and treatment and uncertainty of recurrence of headache.
   Hopelessness related to ineffective treatment modalities.

CHAPTER 14

CRITICAL THINKING QUESTIONS

1. The nurse should discuss with the client problems associated with routine use of a nasal spray—

specifically a "rebound" effect that will actually make the problem worse.

2. Hoarseness may be associated with a known irritation such as overuse of the voice of laryngeal irritation from smoking, inhaling irritating fumes, allergies, or even a change in the weather. Hoarseness that cannot be traced to an irritation—in other words, having an unknown cause—should definitely be evaluated for possible malignancy.
3. The nurse should tell the mother that babies who suck on a bottle while they sleep are at higher risk for cavities, especially if the bottle has milk or juice in it. If the mother wants to give her baby a bottle, the nurse should encourage her to fill it with water. Furthermore, the nurse should tell the mother that tooth care needs to begin when the teeth erupt. A gentle brushing of the baby's teeth with a small soft toothbrush will not hurt the baby. Furthermore, the mother should be encouraged to take the baby to a dentist between the ages of 2 and 3.

CASE STUDY

1. Client claims to have had a painful sore in his mouth for about a year or more; he has self-treated the lesion, with no improvement; client has been a smoker for 40 years (at risk for oral cancer); examination reveals palpable, tender lymph nodes of jaw and neck (may indicate chronic infection or malignancy); possible leukoplakia lesions are linked with smoking (thought to be precancerous); large lesions with irregular borders are present under tongue (need to rule out malignancy).
2. Ask him when he first noticed the lesion. Ask him about the pain with the lesion. Ask him if he has done anything else to self-treat this problem other than using the cream recommended by the dentist. Ask him about any odors from his mouth. Ask him if the painful sore has affected his ability to eat. Ask him if he has had any weight loss. Attempt to scrape off white lesions to determine whether lesions are leukoplakia, thrush, or leukoedema. Palpate the tongue for irregularities. Inspect and palpate for the presence of lesions. Inspect the condition of the gums.
3. Health perception–health management.
   Nutrition–metabolic.
   Cognitive–perceptual.
   Self-perception–self-concept.
4. *Altered health maintenance* related to unhealthy lifestyle as manifested by history of smoking and lesions in mouth.
   Altered comfort related to lesions in mouth as manifested by complaints of pain.
   Fear related to perceived outcome as evidenced by statements fearing cancer and mutilation.
   Risk for altered nutrition: less than body requirements related to painful lesions in mouth.
   PC: Cancerous lesions in mouth.

CHAPTER 15

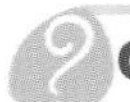

CRITICAL THINKING QUESTIONS

1. Discuss the three preferred methods: cleaning wax from the ear canal with a cotton swab, cleaning the ear canal by irrigating with water, and cleaning by use of ear drops that soften the wax to aid removal. The most effective method is a combination of ear drops to soften the wax followed by irrigation of the ear canal to remove the wax. These techniques should not be performed in the presence of myringotomy tubes, otitis media, or ruptured membranes.
2. Appropriate screening tests: whispered voice test; finger-rubbing test; Rinne test; Weber's test; Romberg's test
3. Evaluating the fluctuation of the tympanic membrane (TM) assists the examiner in determining retraction or bulging. This is done by gently squeezing the bulb attachment of an otoscope so that puffs of air are transmitted to the tympanic membrane. Slight fluctuation of the membrane is a normal response.
4. Differentiating redness associated with crying versus otitis media is done by looking for other clinical signs, primarily bulging and mobility of the tympanic membrane.

CASE STUDY

1. Fever; complaints of ear pain; presence of drainage in ear canal; TM perforation; reduction of hearing in left ear; quiet affect; limited talking.
2. Ask what treatment the child has received for the ear pain from the medicine man in the past. Ask if she has ever seen drainage from ear with past problems. Ask if the child has been treated at a hospital or clinic for ear pain in the past. Ask mother if child acts withdrawn or demonstrates disruptive behavior. Complete a Rinne test and also assess developmental level.
3. Health perception–health management.
   Role-relationship.
   Cognitive-perceptual.
4. *Impaired verbal communication* related to hearing loss in left ear.
   Risk for injury related to decreased hearing acuity.
   Pain related to inflammation of the middle ear.
   Risk for parental role conflict related to illness of the child.
   Risk for altered growth and development related to impaired hearing.

CHAPTER 16

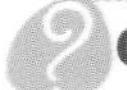

CRITICAL THINKING QUESTIONS

1. The first clue is the size; retinal arteries are about one-fourth narrower than retinal veins. The second

difference is the color. Arteries appear as a very light red color and may have a narrow band of light reflex in the center. Veins, on the other hand, are darker in color and do not have a band of light reflex.
2. Observe the sclera for redness. Note blank stare, excessive tearing of eyes, and swelling of eyelids. Note whether pupil is constricted or dilated. Note whether pupil reaction to light is slow or absent. Note presence of nystagmus or inability to maintain convergence. Note presence of a decreased corneal reflex.
3. General inspection of external structures of the eye should be done. Visual acuity should be checked with a Snellen E chart. A red reflex should be checked; corneal light and reflex/cover-uncover should also be done. Finally, examination of extraocular movements and cranial nerves III, IV, and VI should be done, including asking the child to follow through the six cardinal fields of gaze.

CASE STUDY

1. Data deviating from normal: history of poorly controlled diabetes; sudden change in vision; significant visual acuity findings; ophthalmoscope findings; new vessels and presence of hemorrhage vessels.
2. Ask the client whether he has pain. Ask whether the change in vision has been gradual and progressive or intermittent. Ask whether he has any other symptoms associated with the change in vision, such as intolerance to light. Ask him whether he currently wears contact lenses or glasses. Ask how long he has had diabetes. It is important to determine the last visual acuity results to compare with the current one.
3. Health-perception–health management.
   Activity–exercise.
   Self-perception–self concept.
4. *Anxiety* related to possible loss of eye sight as manifested by concern over losing job or ability to manage disease.
   Risk for injury related to visual impairment.
   Risk for self-care deficit related to visual impairment.
   Risk for ineffective management of therapeutic regimen related to visual impairment.

CHAPTER 17

CRITICAL THINKING QUESTIONS

1. Attempt to comfort the child. Ideally, you should allow the parent or primary caregiver to hold the child. If this does not work, you or the parent may also attempt to offer the child a pacifier or try a bottle.
2. Ask what has changed. The mother said the family moved recently, so ask about the new home and environment and possible irritants within the new home. Also ask about ventilation and air conditioning and exposure to smoke and pets in or around the home.
3. Mr. Stein should start with healthy habits, including hand washing, drinking plenty of fluids, eating nutritious meals, and getting adequate rest each night (7 to 8 hours). He should be encouraged to avoid individuals with colds and the flu or to wear a mask if interaction is unavoidable. If possible he should avoid exposure to air pollutants as well. An annual flu vaccine may also be helpful.
4. These symptoms are consistent with tuberculosis. High risk groups include American Indians, and immigrants from Mexico. He should be placed in droplet isolation until diagnosis is made.
5. He has 9-year history at ⅓ pack a day (3 pack years); a 15-year history at ½ pack a day (7 ½ pack years); and a 32-year history of 1 pack a day (32 pack years). Total = 42 ½ pack year history.

CASE STUDY

1. History of shortness of breath; limitation in activity; interrupted sleep (requires pillows); smoking history; labored breathing with tachypnea; presence of cyanosis; underweight/protruding ribs; increased AP diameter; reduced chest wall movement; diminished tactile fremitus; adventitious breath sounds and diminished breath sounds.
2. Ask about chest pain with shortness of breath. Ask about the presence of cough. Ask how old client was when she started smoking. Ask how long she has been smoking as much as she currently is. Assess oxygen saturation, body weight, and rhythm of breathing pattern. Assess for presence of retratction. Percuss chest for tone and diaghragmatic excursion. Count how many words she can say without taking a breath to assess dyspnea.
3. Activity–exercise.
   Sleep–rest.
   Nutrition–metabolic.
   Self-perception–self-concept.
4. *Impaired gas exchange* related to alveolar hypoventiliation.
   Ineffective airway clearance related to expiratory airflow obstruction.
   Activity intolerance related to dyspnea.
   Sleep pattern disturbance related to dyspnea.
   Risk for altered nutrition: less than body requirements related to poor appetite and labored breathing.
   Risk for anxiety related to dyspnea.
   Risk for self-care deficit related to dyspnea and fatigue.
   PC: Hypoxia.

CHAPTER 18

CRITICAL THINKING QUESTIONS

1. Look for polyarthritis, chorea, erythema marginatum, subcutaneous nodules, arthralgia, an increase in the sedimentation rate or leukocytosis.
2. The posterior tibial and dorsalis pedis pulse cannot be palpated. Try a Doppler to determine if you can hear the pulsation. Check the capillary refill in the toes of his right foot and the color and temperature to verify whether there is any perfusion to his right foot. If the foot has a dorsalis pedis pulse with a Doppler, with capillary refill is about 2 seconds and is warm and tan colored (appropriate for race), then you know there is some perfusion of the right foot. If, however, you cannot get a dorsalis pulse by Doppler, the capillary refill is greater than 2 seconds, and the right foot is cool to cold and pale, you know the perfusion is altered. Also compare the right leg pulses with the left leg pulses.
3. Nocturia occurs with heart failure in individuals who are ambulatory during the day. Lying down at night promotes reabsorption of the fluid and its excretion. Additional questions include the following: Does he get short of breath? When? When he lies down? How many pillows does it take to ease his breathing? Do his feet swell during the day? Does the swelling go away after a night's sleep? Does he have a cough? Is he coughing up anything? What does the sputum look like?
4. Infants with cardiovascular disease do not eat well and tend to have poor weight gain. An infant with congestive heart failure takes only a few ounces during each feeding. There are other problems associated with poor weight gain as well; therefore, additional clinical findings should be considered.

CASE STUDY

1. Complaint of shortness of breath; complaint of fatigue that interferes with routine activities; complaint of sleeping difficulty; labored breathing with elevated respiratory rate, pulse rate, and blood pressure; pitting edema in lower extremities; frothy-looking phlegm.
2. Complete a symptom analysis on the shortness of breath and fatigue. Ask the client if he has symptoms associated with chest pain, cough, or nocturia. Ask the client about cardiovascular history. Perform a precordial assessment, including inspection, percussion, palpation, and auscultation.
3. Activity–exercise.
   Sleep–rest.
   Coping–stress tolerance.
   Self-perception–self-concept.
4. *Activity intolerance* related to fatigue.
   Anxiety related to breathlessness.
   Sleep pattern disturbance related to nocturnal dyspnea.
   Impaired gas exchange related to dyspnea.
   Risk for ineffective individual coping related to altered lifestyle.
   Risk for self-care deficit related to dyspnea and fatigue.
   PC: Hypoxemia.

CHAPTER 19

CRITICAL THINKING QUESTIONS

1. Risk factors for breast cancer include that the client is female, she is over the age of 40, she had an early onset of menarche, she had her first and only child at the age of 36, and she has a strong family history of breast cancer. Although one cannot predict who will and will not develop breast cancer, this woman certainly has very strong risk factors.
2. Do a symptom analysis. Determine onset, which breast, whether discharge is spontaneous or expressed, and ask client to describe the character of discharge in addition to its color. Also ask her if she has noticed other symptoms, such as lumps or pain. (Since the client is 78, it is unnecessary to ask if the discharge is associated with menstrual cycle.) During the examination, be sure to wear gloves. Note if the discharge is spontaneous or expressed, and note color and consistency of the discharge. Finally, prepare a slide with discharge for cytologic evaluation.
3. Offer the following information:
   Perform a breast self-examination every month at the same time every month. Undress and stand in front of a mirror. Look at your breasts in the following three positions: (1) standing with hands on hips, (2) standing with arms extended above your head, and (3) leaning forward with your hands outstretched. Watch for any changes in the way your breast appears, such as a dimpling, puckering or change in size. Palpate your breasts. Raise your left arm over your head. Starting at the nipple of the left breast, firmly press the fingers from your right hand in a circular motion, working outward and feeling every part of your breast. You are feeling for any lump or mass. After you palpate your breast, squeeze the nipple and look for any discharge. Repeat this procedure with other breast. You may do this procedure standing and/or lying down. If you feel any lumps or see any discharge from your nipple, you should contact your primary health provider.

CASE STUDY

1. Client has a history of nontender breast lump, noticeable for about 9 months; mass has increased

in size over 9 months; risk factors include early onset of menarche and the fact that the client is childless; palpable lump is present in the left upper outer quadrant; dimpling noted on left breast; left nipple is retracted; bloody discharge is noted from nipple when squeezed.

2. Ask about personal or family history of breast disease. Ask client whether she does regular breast self-examinations. Ask whether she has ever had a mammogram. Ask about the location of the lump. Ask whether the lump is tender now. Ask whether she has noticed nipple discharge. Ask about changes in the lump size in relation to menstrual cycle. Inspect the areolae. Besides location, the following characteristics must be assessed with a breast mass: size, shape, consistency, tenderness, mobility, and borders. Palpate the axilla. It is especially important to note any lumps or masses in the left axilla.
3. Cognitive–perceptual.
   Self-perception–self-concept.
   Coping–stress tolerance.
4. *Ineffective denial* realted to delay in seeking health care for known problem.
   Knowledge deficit related to inaccurate perception of health status.
   Risk for body image disturbance related to probable breast surgery.
   Risk for ineffective individual coping related to possible disfigurment from breast surgery.

CHAPTER 20

CRITICAL THINKING QUESTIONS

1. Listen to the abdomen for bruits in the aortic, renal, iliac, and femoral arteries. A bruit in these arteries may indicate stenosis or an aneurysm. Listen in the umbilical area for a venous hum (soft, low pitched, and continuous). A venous hum suggests increased collateral circulation between portal and systemic venous systems and may indicate portal hypertension. A friction rub is high pitched and may be heard in association with respiration. It may indicate inflammation of the peritoneal surface from tumor or infection.
2. Hepatitis B immunization is now recommended for infants. Mrs. Quintana should be told this is a series of three shots given over a period of months; stress the importance of getting all three injections to gain adequate immunization.
3. *Questions for subjective data:* Ask them about the location of pain. Mr. Nguyen reports his pain is diffuse, whereas Mrs. Martinez states her pain is in the left lower quadrant. Ask them about associated symptoms. Mr. Nguyen reports he has had nausea, vomiting, and diarrhea; Ms. Martinez says she had has diarrhea. Ask them what makes the symptoms better. Mr. Nguyen says there is some relief with vomiting and diarrhea; Ms. Martinez reports feeling better after she has a bowel movement or flatus.

   Assessment findings for objective data: Mr. Nguyen has hyperactive bowel sounds in all quadrants and a nontender abdomen to palpation. Ms. Martinez has normal bowel sounds in all quadrants and tender descending colon to deep palpation.

   Conclusion: Mr. Nguyen's findings may indicate gastroenteritis, whereas Ms. Martinez's findings may indicate irritable bowel disease.

CASE STUDY

1. Abdominal pain (progressively worse); loss of appetite and nausea; guarded position; hot skin, possibly indicating fever; absence of bowel sounds; pain to palpation and guarding RLQ; positive rebound tenderness in RLQ.
2. Ask client about vomiting with her nausea. Ask about her menstrual cycle (LMP) and about the possibility of pregnancy. Ask her about bowel elimination (last BM) and appearance of stool. Check vital signs (of particular interest is temperature). Auscultate for arterial bruits and venous hums. Percuss kidney for CVA tenderness. Perform iliopsoas muscle test and obturator muscle test.
3. Cognitive–perceptual.
   Self-perception–self-concept.
   Nutrition–metabolic.
4. *Pain* related to abdominal inflammation.
   Altered comfort: nausea related to abdomen inflammation.
   Anxiety related to uncertainty of diagnosis and pain.
   PC: Hyperthermia.

CHAPTER 21

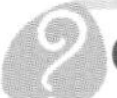

CRITICAL THINKING QUESTIONS

1. Discuss Kegel exercises. These are exercises that help to decrease stress incontinence by strengthening the muscles of the perineum. Kegel exercises should be done at least 4 times a day while urinating. Stop the urine flow by tightening the muscles, then start the stream again, repeating this 12 to 24 times.
2. An imperforate hymen becomes a problem at the onset of menses because the vaginal opening is blocked, preventing menstrual flow from exiting the vagina. As the volume of fluid increases, pressure is applied to surrounding structures, including the bladder. Symptoms most commonly include urinary frequency, bladder fullness, and abdominal discomfort.
3. The history is vital to obtain. At this age, it will be necessary to talk with her while her parents are out of the room. Questions should be simple, gentle,

and nonjudgmental. These will greatly improve the accuracy of the information she is willing to share. There is no one set rule to determine the age when a full examination of the genitalia is necessary. However, a good rule of thumb is that if the person is sexually active, an examination should be done. The examination should be similar to that of an adult.

4. The Pap smear should always be taken first. Since the specimen needed for chlamydia and gonorrhea needs to be from the os or endocervix (depending on the type of culture done), this should be done second. Finally, the slide for wet mount and KOH preparation is usually done last, as the specimen is vaginal secretions.

CASE STUDY

1. History suggests some type of acute inflammation. It is also suggestive of multiple sex contacts, and primary partner has multiple sex contacts. Mass with inflammation, discharge, and extreme pain to palpation needs further evaluation.
2. Discussion is needed regarding past sexual history and associated medical problems, if any. Identification of protection (or lack of it) is also important to discuss. Obtain a culture of the discharge for evaluation. If client is too uncomfortable for internal examination, this may need to be delayed until the inflammation has resolved.
3. Health perception–health management.
   Nutrition–metabolic.
   Cognitive–perceptual.
4. *Altered comfort: pain* related to verbalization of discomfort in perineal area.
   Altered health maintenance related to sexual activity.
   Risk for infection transmission related to sexual activity.

CHAPTER 22

CRITICAL THINKING QUESTIONS

1. Discuss why genital self-examination is done—to screen for testicular cancer and to identify sexually transmitted diseases. Discuss how to perform genital self-examination. This should include the following: inspection of the tip for evidence of swelling, sores, or discharge; palpation of the entire shaft of the penis, from base to glans to feel for lumps or tenderness; and examination of the scrotum for color, texture, and presence of lesions. Client should also palpate his scrotum for presence of lumps, swelling, or tenderness.
2. Be sure one of the child's parents is present. Explain to the child what you must do and why (to be sure all his body parts are healthy). It may be necessary for the parent(s) to reassure the child that it is OK for this person to see their "privates."
3. He should be encouraged to use condoms for barrier protection during sexual intercourse. Discussion should also include the risk of sexually transmitted infection (STI) with oral-genital and rectal sex as well.
4. Advantages and disadvantages of circumcision should be discussed; advantages include decreased incidence of glans penis inflammation, cancer of the penis, urinary tract infections in infants, and sexually transmitted infection (particularly syphilis, gonorrhea, and warts). Disadvantages include potential for infection and pain from the procedure. Since circumcision is largely based on cultural practice, this should be explored.

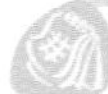

CASE STUDY

1. Protrusion or mass noted in left groin area. History suggests possibly a hernia.
2. Discuss level of discomfort and other related symptoms by completing a symptom analysis. Determine if there is past history of this problem. Need to determine if this hernia is reducible. If it is nonreducible, it may require prompt surgical intervention. Also full examination of genitalia is in order.
3. Cognitive–perceptual.
   Health perception–health management.
4. *Altered comfort: pain* related to swelling and inflammation.
   Risk for injury related to lifting activities.
   PC: Inguinal hernia.

CHAPTER 23

CRITICAL THINKING QUESTIONS

1. With acute prostatitis, the patient will have an inflamed prostate; therefore the prostate will be tender, and the patient will likely have a fever. Symptoms of obstruction develop more quickly than with the other two problems. With palpation, the prostate will be tender and possibly asymmetric. Additionally, the seminal vesicles may be dilated and tender to palpation. With benign prostate hypertrophy, symptoms will develop gradually, with complaints of hesitancy, decreased force of stream, dribbling, and incomplete emptying of the bladder. With palpation, the prostate will feel rubbery, symmetric, and enlarged. With prostatic carcinoma, the symptoms of obstruction gradually occur. With palpation, the prostate is hard, irregular, and feels asymmetric; the median sulcus is obliterated.
2. When did bleeding start? How much bleeding have you noticed? When/where do you see the bleeding? What does the blood look like? Do you have any

other symptoms associated with the bleeding such as pain, gas, cramping, weight loss, fatigue, etc.? What do you think is causing the bleeding?

3. Sexually transmitted infection (associated with multiple partners and "occasional condom use"); rectal trauma (related to recipient of anal intercourse); loss of anal sphincter tone (associated with frequent recipient of anal intercourse).
4. Reduce fate intake to 30% of total caloric intake; limit alcohol use to two drinks a day; limit intake of smoke or charbroiled meats; choose foods that are high in vitamin A, vitamin C, vitamin E; and eat generous portions of food high in fiber.

CASE STUDY

1. Sensation of rectal fullness, rectal bleeding, blood in stool, palpable mass in the rectum, enlargement of prostate, fatigue, and weight loss.
2. This client needs an extensive interview. Among several things that must be explored, try to find out how much blood he has been seeing. Also, ask him about changes in bowel elimination pattern or the change in the appearance of the stools (besides the presence of blood). Ask about abdominal discomfort or distention. Ask about problems with urination—problems with starting or the force of the stream. Ask about sexual history. Find out his past medical history and family history. The examination should include a guaiac test and inguinal lymph node assessment; as part of abdominal assessment specifically consider the possibility of pelvic or abdominal masses.
3. Activity–exercise.
   Coping–stress tolerance.
   Cognitive–perceptual.
   Nutrition–metabolic.
4. *Activity intolerance* related to generalized weakness.
   Fear related to physical condition.
   Pain related to rectal fullness.
   Risk for altered nutrition: less than body requirements.
   PC: Anemia.

CHAPTER 24

CRITICAL THINKING QUESTIONS

1. Muscle strain results if a muscle is stretched or torn beyond its functional capacity. A sprain is a stretching or tearing of a supporting ligament of a joint. A fracture is a partial or complete break in the continuity of the bone. Since the injury involves the joint, muscle strain is not likely. Both fractures and sprains are associated with pain and swelling and can have a bluish discoloration, so it is not always easy to differentiate these. If Mark had walked in bearing weight on the affected ankle, it would be doubtful that a fracture resulted; if he was unable to bear weight at all, it could be a fracture or a severe sprain—thus an x-ray examination is usually the final diagnostic indicator.
2. Inspect the knees for symmetry and erythema; palpate the knee for edema and tenderness. The client has two risk factors for osteoarthritis: over 50 years of age and obese. If you find the left knee to be asymmetric due to edema in addition to being red and tender, you may conclude he has osteoarthritis.
3. The left arm would have tricepts and biceps strength of 5/5, elbow ROM 160°, nontender to palpation. The right arm would have triceps and biceps strength of less than 5/5, perhaps 3/5 or 4/5; elbow ROM less than 160°, perhaps 110°, due to slight contracture since the elbow has been in the same position for the time the cast was on; and would be nontender to palpation. Comparing the size of the left and right arms, you find the size of the right arm to be smaller than the left due to muscle atrophy from nonuse.

CASE STUDY

1. Diagnosis of RA; significant joint pain; limitations in self-care activities; limitations in socialization; difficulty with posture and gait; deformities to joints; tender inflamed joints with palpation; subcutaneous nodules at the ulnar surface of the elbows.
2. Ask the client what medications she is taking for the RA; find out whether she is involved with any other nonpharmaceutical therapies; ask her whether these things help or make a difference; ask if she has any assistive devices that she uses and/or if she receives any assistance with self-care activities. Document ROM in various joints. Use of a goniometer would be particularly helpful.
3. Cognitive–perceptual.
   Activity–exercise.
   Self-perception–self-concept.
   Role–relationship.
4. *Pain* related to joint inflammation.
   Risk for impaired physical mobility related to joint pain and stiffness.
   Risk for self care deficit related to loss of dexterity.
   Body image disturbance related to statements made by client.
   Risk for social isolation related to consequences of chronic illness and body image.

CHAPTER 25

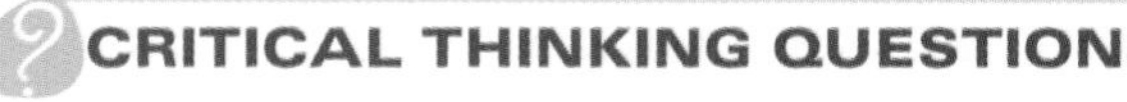

CRITICAL THINKING QUESTIONS

1. Kevin's findings are invalid because he did not adjust his tool to determine two-point discrimination. Different body surfaces have varying

sensitivity; depending on what body surface is being tested, the distance between two points on tool must be adjusted. For instance, on the fingertips, the minimal distance for the two points is 2/32 to 5/16 inch (2 to 8 mm). The only body surfaces able to detect more than 1 inch are the chest and forearm (1.5 inch or 3.75 cm), back (1.5 to 2.75 inches or 3.75 to 7.0 cm), and upper arms and thighs (3 inches or 7.5 cm). The abdomen is not a body part that is able to detect two-point discrimination.

2. These findings represent abnormal findings of the cranial nerves. Deficit of the tongue indicates glossopharyngeal cranial nerve (IX), deficit of uvula indicates the glossopharyngeal and vagus cranial nerves (IX and X), the abnormality of the tongue indicates the hypoglossal cranial nerve (XII), and the shoulder weakness indicates the spinal accessory cranial nerve (XI). All of these cranial nerves originate in the medulla oblongata (see Fig. 25-7). The tumor is probably in the medulla oblongata. The purpose of this question is to reinforce the fact that health assessment is a method to check the function (physiology) of the body (e.g., since these cranial nerves were not functioning, they revealed abnormal findings to you).
3. Conductive hearing loss of left ear may be indicated since the whispered voice is decreased to 25%, the bone conduction is greater than air conduction (BC > AC) and vibration lateralizes to the left ear.
4. Referring to the dermatome map, you see that L2 (second lumbar spinal nerve) innervates the upper, outer thigh, L3 innervates the medial aspect of the inner lower thigh, and L4 innervates the medial aspect of the lower leg. These data indicate that this client has a spinal lesion at L3 on the right and L4 on the left.

CASE STUDY

1. The client has been diagnosed with right CVA; he had headache preceding incident; the client is unable to talk; he has absence of sensation and a trace to no muscle strength on the left arm and leg; he requires assistance for mobility; and the client avoids eye contact and cries.
2. Ask Mr. Thomas if he feels he can swallow normally. Ask him whether he has any pain or discomfort. Ask Mrs. Thomas about medical and family history; ask about medications he may be currently taking. Ask Mrs. Thomas if her husband lost consciousness or had a seizure with this incident. Assess gag reflex. Test reflexes (deep tendon). Assess for drooling.
3. Cognitive–perceptual.
   Activity–exercise.
   Nutrition–metabolic.
   Self-perception–self-concept.
4. *Impaired physical mobility* related to altered neuromuscular function.
   Impaired verbal communication related to expressive aphasia.
   Self-care deficit syndrome (total) related to left hemiplegia.
   Self-esteem disturbance related to loss of function.
   Risk for impaired skin integrity related to immobility.
   Risk for altered nutrition: less than body requirements related to inability to feed self.

CHAPTER 26

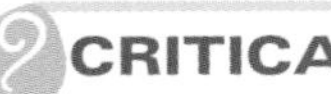

CRITICAL THINKING QUESTIONS

1. The blood pressure (BP) is high; it would be helpful to know what the prepregnancy blood pressure is to determine how much change has occurred with pregnancy. Any systolic BP over 160 mm Hg or a diastolic pressure over 90 mm Hg should be evaluated further.
2. First, a 40-year-old woman has less than optimal ova for pregnancy. Second, there is a tremendous change in the cardiovascular, respiratory, and musculoskeletal systems associated with pregnancy. This is typically better tolerated by younger individuals, although if in good heath, women of this age can tolerate pregnancy without difficulty.
3. The presumptive signs of pregnancy are a woman's first clue that she may be pregnant. These, in themselves, do not indicate pregnancy, but they are significant enough to make most women suspicious. A commonly used probable sign most women rely on is the home pregnancy testing. This is considered probable because it is possible to have a false positive result. The most accurate way to determine pregnancy is with the positive signs—presence of fetal heart tones and visualization of fetus by ultrasound.

CASE STUDY

1. Subjective:
   Symptoms of puffiness to hands and feet.
   Backache.
   Fear of excessive labor pain.
   Objective:
   Increase in BP.
   Sudden, excessive increase in weight.
   3+ protein in urine.
2. Assess FHT; palpate fetal movement. Assess the extent of the edema, including how far up on the legs and the degree of edema; if pitting. Check her visual acuity. Conduct a neuroassessment—particularly check reflexes. Ask her about her diet, specifically sodium intake, as this may be

contributing to the edema. Get more information about the back discomfort; do a symptom analysis. Determine her knowledge level of labor and delivery process; assess pain experiences.

3. Nutrition–metabolic.
   Cognitive–perceptual.
   Self-perception–self-concept.
4. *Fluid volume excess.*
   Altered comfort related to edema and changes in spinal position.
   Anxiety related to perceived threat to comfort secondary to labor and delivery.
   PC: Preeclampsia.

ILLUSTRATION CREDITS

American Academy of Dermatology and Institute of Dermatologic Communication and Education, Schaumburg, Ill.

American College of Rheumatology: *Clinical slide collection of the rheumatic diseases,* 1991, 1995, 1997, Atlanta, American College of Rheumatology.

American Nurses Association: *Standards of clinical nursing practice,* Kansas City, 1991, The Association.

Baden HP: *Diseases of the hair and nails,* Chicago, 1987, Year Book.

Baran R, Dawber RR, Levene GM: *Color atlas of the hair, scalp, and nails,* St. Louis, 1991, Mosby.

Barkauskas VH et al: *Health and physical assessment,* ed 2, St. Louis, 1998, Mosby.

Beaven DW, Brooks SE: *Color atlas of the nail in clinical diagnosis,* ed 2, London, 1994, Times Mirror International Publishers.

Beck AT, Beck RW: Screening depressed patients in family practice: a rapid technique, *Postgrad Med* 52:81, 1972.

Bedford MA: *Color atlas of ophthalmological diagnosis,* ed 2, London, 1986, Wolfe.

Belcher AE: *Cancer nursing,* St. Louis, 1992, Mosby.

Bingham BJG, Hawke M, Kwok P: *Atlas of clinical otolaryngology,* St. Louis, 1992, Mosby.

Black JM, Mattassarin-Jacobs E: *Medical-surgical nursing: clinical management for continuity of care,* ed 5, Philadelphia, 1997, WB Saunders.

Bowers AC, Thompson JM: *Clinical manual of health assessment,* ed 4, St. Louis, 1992, Mosby.

Cannobio MM: *Cardiovascular disorders,* St. Louis, 1990, Mosby.

Chipps EM, Clanin NJ, Campbell VG: *Neurologic disorders,* St. Louis, 1992, Mosby.

Cohen BA: *Atlas of pediatric dermatology,* London, 1993, Wolfe.

Crichlow RW, Kaplan EL, Kearney WH: *Ann Surg* 175:490, 1972.

DeWeese DD et al: *Otolaryngology head and neck surgery,* ed 7, St. Louis, 1988, Mosby.

Diagnostic picture tests in clinical medicine, St. Louis, 1984, Mosby.

Dickason EJ, Silverman BL, Schult MO: *Maternal-infant nursing care,* ed 2, St. Louis, 1994, Mosby.

Doughty DB, Jackson DB: *Gastrointestinal disorders,* St. Louis, 1993, Mosby.

Dunlap C, Barker BF: *Oral lesions,* ed 3, 1991, New York, Colgate-Hoyt.

Edge V, Miller M: *Women's health care,* St. Louis, 1994, Mosby.

Farrar WE et al: *Infectious diseases: text and color atlas,* ed 2, London, 1992, Gower.

Folstein M et al: The meaning of cognitive impairment in the elderly, *J Am Geriatr Soc* 33(4):228, 1985.

Fortunato N, McCullough SM: *Plastic and reconstructive surgery,* St. Louis, 1998, Mosby.

400 self-assessment picture tests in clinical medicine, London, 1984, Wolfe.

Francis CC, Martin AH: *Introduction to human anatomy,* ed 7, St. Louis, 1975, Mosby.

Frankenburg WK et al: *Denver II: technical manual,* Denver, 1990, Denver Developmental Materials, Inc.

Gallager HS et al: *The breast,* St. Louis, 1978, Mosby.

GI series, 1981, AH Robbins Co.

Goldman MP, Fitzpatrick RE: *Cutaneous laser surgery: the art and science of selective photo thermolysis,* St. Louis, 1994, Mosby.

Goldstein BG, Goldstein AO: *Practical dermatology,* ed 2, St. Louis, 1997, Mosby.

Greenberger NJ, Hinthorn DR: *History taking and physical examination,* St. Louis, 1993, Mosby.

Grimes DE: *Infectious diseases,* St. Louis, 1991, Mosby.

Habif TP: *Clinical dermatology: a color guide to diagnosis and therapy,* ed 2, St. Louis, 1990, Mosby.

Habif TP: *Clinical dermatology: a color guide to diagnosis and therapy,* ed 3, St. Louis, 1996, Mosby.

Helveston EM: *Surgical management of strabismus: an atlas of strabismus surgery,* ed 4, St. Louis, 1993, Mosby.

Hill MJ: *Skin disorders,* St. Louis, 1994, Mosby.

Hilt NE, Schmitt EW: *Pediatric orthopedic nursing,* St. Louis, 1975, Mosby.

Isaacs JH: *Textbook of breast disease,* St. Louis, 1992, Mosby.

Kamal A, Brockelhurst JC: *Color atlas of geriatric medicine,* 1991, Wolfe.

Kaufman RH et al: *Benign diseases of the vulva and vagina,* ed 4, St. Louis, 1994, Mosby.

Lawrence CM, Cox NH: *Physical signs in dermatology: color atlas and text,* St. Louis, 1993, Wolfe.

Lewis SM, Collier IC, Heitkemper MM: *Medical-surgical nursing: assessment and management of clinical problems,* ed 4, St. Louis, 1996, Mosby.

Lewis SM, Heitkemper MM, Dirksen SR: *Medical-surgical nursing: assessment and management of clinical problems,* ed 5, St. Louis, 2000, Mosby.

Lloyd-Davies RW et al: *Color atlas of urology,* ed 2, London, 1994, Wolfe.

Lowdermilk DL, Perry SE, Bobak IM: *Maternity and women's health care,* ed 6, St. Louis, 1997, Mosby.

Lowdermilk DL, Perry SE, Bobak IM: *Maternity nursing,* ed 5, St. Louis, 1999, Mosby.

Mansel R, Bundred N: *Color atlas of breast disease,* St. Louis, 1995, Mosby-Wolfe.

Marks JG, DeLeo VA: *Contact and occupational dermatology,* St. Louis, 1992, Mosby.

Marshall WA, Tanner JM: *Arch Dis Child* 44:291, 1969.

McCaffery M, Pasero C: *Pain: clinical manual,* ed 2, St. Louis, 1999, Mosby.

McCance KL, Huether SE: *Pathophysiology: the biologic basis for disease in adults and children,* ed 3, St. Louis, 1998, Mosby.

McCullough DC: *Pediatric neurosurgery,* Philadelphia, 1989, WB Saunders.

McKenry LM, Salerno E: *Mosby's pharmacology in nursing,* ed 20, St. Louis, 1998, Mosby.

McLaren DS: *A colour atlas and text of diet-related disorders,* ed 2, St. Louis, 1992, Wolfe.

Melzack R, Katz J: Pain measurement in persons with pain. In Wall PD, Melzack R, editors: *Textbook of pain,* ed 3, New York, 1994, Churchill-Livingstone.

Monteleone JA: *Recognition of child abuse for the mandated reporter,* ed 2, London, 1996, GW Medical Publishing.

Mourad LA: *Orthopedic disorders,* St. Louis, 1991, Mosby.

Nesi FA et al: *Smith's ophthalmic plastic and reconstructive surgery,* ed 2, St. Louis, 1998, Mosby.

Newell FW: *Ophthalmology: principles and concepts,* ed 7, St. Louis, 1992, Mosby.

Phipps WJ, Sand JK, Marek JF: *Medical-surgical nursing: concepts and clinical practice,* ed 6, St. Louis, 1999, Mosby.

Potter PA, Perry AG: *Basic nursing: theory and practice,* ed 2, St. Louis, 1991, Mosby.

Potter PA, Perry AG: *Basic nursing: a critical thinking approach,* ed 4, St. Louis, 1999, Mosby.

Prior JA, Silberstein JS, Stang JM: *Physical diagnosis: the history and examination of the patient,* ed 6, St. Louis, 1981, Mosby.

Raj PP: *Practical management of pain,* ed 2, St. Louis, 1992, Mosby.

Rudy EB: *Advanced neurological and neurosurgical nursing,* St. Louis, 1984, Mosby.

Scully C, Welbury R: *Color atlas of oral diseases in children and adolescents,* London, 1994, Wolfe.

Seeley RR, Stephens TD, Tate P: *Anatomy and physiology,* ed 3, St. Louis, 1995, Mosby.

Seidel HM et al: *Mosby's guide to physical examination,* ed 3, St. Louis, 1995, Mosby.

Seidel HM et al: *Mosby's guide to physical examination,* ed 4, St. Louis, 1999, Mosby.

Shipley M: *A colour atlas of rheumatology,* ed 3, London, 1993, Mosby-Year Book Europe.

Sigler BA, Schuring LT: *Ear, nose, and throat disorders,* St. Louis, 1993, Mosby.

Stein HA, Slatt BJ, Stein RM: *The ophthalmic assistant: fundamentals and clinical practice,* ed 5, St. Louis, 1988, Mosby.

Swartz MH: *Textbook of physical diagnosis: history and examination,* ed 2, Philadelphia, 1994, WB Saunders.

Symonds EM, MacPhearson MBA: *Color atlas of obstetrics and gynaecology,* London, 1994, Mosby-Wolfe.

Tanner JM: *Growth at adolescence,* ed 2, Oxford, England, 1962, Blackwell Scientific Publications.

Thibodeau GA, Patton KT: *Anatomy and physiology,* ed 2, St. Louis, 1993, Mosby.

Thibodeau GA, Patton KT: *Anatomy and physiology,* ed 4, St. Louis, 1999, Mosby.

Thompson JM et al: *Mosby's clinical nursing,* St. Louis, 1986, Mosby.

Thompson JM et al: *Mosby's clinical nursing,* ed 3, St. Louis, 1993, Mosby.

Thompson JM et al: *Mosby's clinical nursing,* ed 4, St. Louis, 1997, Mosby.

Van Wieringen JC et al: *Growth diagrams 1965 Netherlands. Second national survey on 0-24-year-olds,* Groningen, Netherlands, 1971, Wolters-Noordhoff.

Varcarolis EM: *Foundations of psychiatric mental health nursing,* ed 3, Philadelphia, 1998, WB Saunders.

Von Noorden GK: *Binocular vision and ocular motility: theory and management of strabismus,* ed 4, 1990.

Weston WL, Lane AT: *Color textbook of pediatric dermatology,* St. Louis, 1991, Mosby.

Weston WL, Lane AT, Morelli JG: *Color textbook of pediatric dermatology,* ed 2, St. Louis, 1996, Mosby.

White GM: *Color atlas of regional dermatology,* St. Louis, 1994, Mosby-Wolfe.

Wilson HS, Kneisl CR: *Psychiatric nursing,* ed 3, Menlo Park, Calif, 1988, Addison-Wesley.

Wilson SF, Thompson JM: *Respiratory disorders,* St. Louis, 1990, Mosby.

Wong DL et al: *Whaley and Wong's essentials of pediatric nursing,* ed 5, St. Louis, 1997, Mosby.

Wong DL et al: *Whaley and Wong's nursing care of infants and children,* ed 5, St. Louis, 1995, Mosby.

Wong DL et al: *Whaley and Wong's nursing care of infants and children,* ed 6, St. Louis, 1999, Mosby.

Yesavage JA, Brink TL: Development and validation of a geriatric depression screening scale: a preliminary report, *J Psychiatr Res* 17:37, 1983.

Zitelli BJ, Davis HW: *Atlas of pediatric physical diagnosis,* ed 2, 1992, Mosby .

Zitelli BJ, Davis HW: *Atlas of pediatric physical diagnosis,* ed 3, 1997, Mosby.

REFERENCES

Acute Pain Management Guideline Panel: *Acute pain management: operative or medical procedures and trauma,* AHCPR Publication No. 92-0032, Rockville, MD, 1992, Agency for Health Care Policy and Research, Public Health Service, U.S. Department of Health and Human Services.

Advisory Committee in Immunization Practices, American Academy of Pediatrics and the American Academy of Family Physicians: Childhood Immunization Schedule, *Pediatrics* 191(1):154-157, 1998.

Agency for Health Care Policy and Research: *Colorectal Cancer Screening,* AHCPR Publication No. 98-0033, Rockville, MD, Agency for Health Care Policy and Research, 1998.

Alagaratnam TT, Wong J: Limitations of mammography in Chinese females, *Clin Radiology* 36:175, 1985.

Albertson PC: Prostate disease in older men: benign hyperplasia, *Hospital Practice,* vol. 32 #5, pp. 61-81, 1997.

Alliance to End Childhood Lead Poisoning, July 15, 1999, *http://www.aeclp.org/.*

American Academy of Nursing (AANN) Expert Panel Report: Culturally competent health care, *Nursing Outlook* 40(6):277-283, 1992.

American Cancer Society: *Cancer facts and figures,* Atlanta, 1998, American Cancer Society.

American College of Obstetrics and Gynecology: Hypertension in pregnancy, *ACOG Tech Bull,* pp. 219, 1996.

American Nurses Association: *Standards of clinical nursing practice,* Kansas City, 1991, The Association.

American Psychiatric Association: *Diagnostic and statistical manual of mental disorders (DSM-IV),* ed 4, Washington DC, 1994, The Association.

Arnault DS: Framework for culturally relevant psychiatric nursing. In Varcarolis EM: *Foundations of psychiatric mental health nursing,* ed 3, Philadelphia, 1998, Saunders.

Astle B, Allen M: Management of persons with problems of the eye. In Phipps WJ, Sands JK, Marek JF: *Medical-surgical nursing: concepts and clinical practice,* ed 6, St. Louis, 1999, Mosby.

Ault D, Schmidt D: Diagnosis and management of gastroesophageal reflux in infants and children, *The Nurse Practitioner* 23(8):78, 81-82, 88-89, 94, 99-100, 1998.

Baden A, Karkeck J, Chernoff R: Geriatrics. In Gottschlich MM, Matarese LE, Shront EP, eds: *Nutrition support dietetics core curriculum,* ed 2, Gathersburg, MD, 1993 Aspen Press.

Baren R, Tosti A: Nails. In Freedberg et al, eds: *Dermatology in general medicine,* ed 5, New York, 1999, McGraw-Hill.

Barrett J: Nursing management of adults with ear disorders. In Beare PG, Myers JL: *Adult health nursing,* ed 3, St. Louis, 1998, Mosby.

Barry MJ et al: The American Urological Association symptom index for benign prostatic hyperplasia, *The Journal of Urology* 148(11):1549-1557, 1992.

Bayley N: *Bayley scales of infant development,* New York, 1993, Psychological Corporation.

Beare PG, Myers JL: *Adult health nursing,* ed 3, St. Louis, 1998, Mosby.

Beck AT, Beck RW: Screening depressed patients in family practice: a rapid technique, *Postgrad Med* 52:81-85, 1972.

Berarducci A, Lengacher CA: Osteoporosis in perimenopausal women: current perspectives, *The American Journal for Nurse Practitioners* 2(9):914, 1998.

Bingham BJ, Hawke M, Kwok P: *Atlas of clinical otolaryngology,* St. Louis, 1992, Mosby.

Bjorgen S: Herpes zoster, *American Journal of Nursing* 98(2):46-47, 1998.

Black JM, Matassarin-Jacobs E: *Medical-surgical nursing: clinical management for continuity of care,* ed 5, Philadelphia, 1997, Saunders.

Blackman M: You asked about adolescent depression, *Canadian Journal of Continuing Medical Education,* May 1995, *www.mentalhealth.com.*

Borum ML: Does age influence screening for colorectal cancer? *Age & Aging* 27:509-511, 1998.

Branch DW, Porter TF: Hypertensive disorders of pregnancy. In Scott JR, DiSaia PJ, Hammond CB, Spellacy WN, eds: *Danforth's obstetrics and gynecology,* ed 8, Philadelphia, 1999, Lippincott Williams & Wilkins.

Braunstein GD: Gynecomastia. In Harris JR, Lipman ME, Morrow M, Hellman S, eds: *Diseases of the breast,* Philadelphia, 1996, Lippincott-Raven.

Brazelton TB: Neonatal behavioral scale, ed 2, *Clinics in Developmental Medicine,* No. 88, London, 1983, Spastics International Medical Publications; Philadelphia, Lippincott.

Broome M et al: Children's medical fears, coping behaviors, and pain perception during a lumbar puncture, *Oncology Nursing Forum* 17:361, 1990.

Brown M: *Readings in gerontology,* St. Louis, 1978, Mosby.

Brown S, Parker N, Stegbauer C: Managing allergic rhinitis, *The Nurse Practitioner* 24(5):107-108, 110-111, 115-117, 120, 1999.

Burton BT, Foster WR: Health implications of obesity: an NIH consensus development conference, *J Am Diet Assoc* 85(9):1117-1121, 1985.

Buti RL: Herniated lumbar discs: diagnosis and management, *Journal of the American Academy of Nurse Practitioners* 10(12):547-550, 1998.

Butler JM: Playing detective assessing skin lesions in primary care, *Advance for Nurse Practitioners,* pp. 41-43, August 1997.

Camargo C et al: Prospective study of moderate alcohol consumption and mortality in U.S. male physicians, *Archives of Internal Medicine,* 157:79-85, January 13, 1997.

Campinha J, Yahle T, Lanenkamp M: The challenge of cultural diversity for nurse educators, *J Continuing Ed Nsg* 27:2, 1996.

Center for Disease Control and Prevention: Guidelines for treatment of sexually transmitted diseases, *MMWR* 47 (No. RR-1), pp. 1-118 1998.

Cerrato P: Improving the odds of a healthy birth, *RN* 9(55):71-73, 1992.

Chandrasoma P, Taylor C: *Concise pathology,* ed 3, Stamford, CT, 1998, Appleton & Lange.

Chari RS, Frangieh AY, Sibai BM: Chronic hypertension in pregnancy, *Comprehensive Therapy* 21(5):227-234, 1995.

Chew AL: *The lollipop test: a diagnostic screening test of school readiness,* Atlanta, 1992, Humanics Limited.

Christianson RE et al: Incidence of congenital anomalies among white and black live births with long-term follow-up, *Am J Public Health* 71:1333, 1981.

Cleary BL: Age-related changes in the special senses. In Matteson MA, McConnell ES, Linton AD: *Gerontological nursing,* ed 2, Philadelphia, 1997, Saunders.

Coddington RD: The significance of life events as etiologic factors in diseases of children. Part II: a study of a normal population, *J Psychosomatic Res* 16:205-213, 1972.

Cole FL: Temporal variation in the effects of iced water on oral temperature, *Res Nurse Health* 16(2):107-111, 1993.

Crigger N, Forbes W: Assessing neurologic function in older patients, *AJN* 97(3):37-40, 1997.

Cronin SN: Nursing care of clients with disorders of the lower airways and pulmonary vessels. In Black JM, Mattassarin-Jacobs E: *Medical-surgical nursing: clinical management for continuity of care,* ed 5, Philadelphia, 1997, Saunders.

Cropley C, Lester P, Pennington S: Assessment tool for measuring maternal attachment behavior. In McNall LK, Galeener JT, eds: *Current practice in obstetrics and gynecologic nursing,* Vol. 1, St. Louis, 1976, Mosby.

Cruikshank DP: *Malpresentations and umbilical cord complications.* In Scott JR, DiSaia PJ, Hammond CB, Spellacy WN, eds: *Danforth's obstetrics and gynecology,* ed 8, Philadelphia, 1999, Lippincott Williams & Wilkins.

Cunningham F et al: *Williams obstetrics,* ed 20, Stamford, 1997, Appleton & Lange.

Cutter J: Recording patient temperature: are we getting it right? *Professional Nurse* 9(9):608-616, 1994.

DeJong M: Infective endocarditis, *AJN* 98(5):34-35.

Deters GE: Cancer. In Phipps WJ, Sands JK, Marek JF: *Medical-surgical nursing: Concepts and clinical practice,* ed 6, St. Louis, 1999, Mosby.

Deters GE: Management of persons with problems of the breast. In Phipps WJ, Sands JK, Marek JF: *Medical-surgical nursing: concepts and clinical practice,* ed 6, St. Louis, 1999, Mosby.

Denver Developmental Materials Catalog of Screening and Training Materials, Denver, 1994, DDM, Inc.

Donovan DA, Nicholas PK: Prostatitis: diagnosis and treatment in primary care, *The Nurse Practitioner* 22(4):144-156, 1997.

Dugan K: Caring for patients with pericarditis, *Nursing 98* 28(3):50-51.

Duvall EM, Miller BC: *Marriage and family development,* ed 6, New York, 1985, Harper & Row.

Eekhof JA, de Bock GH, Laat J, Dap R, Springer MP: The whispered voice: the best test for screening for hearing impairment in general practice? *British Journal of General Practice,* 1996.

Erikson EH: *Childhood and society,* ed 2, New York, 1963, Norton.

Espeland K: Identifying the manifestations of inhalant abuse, *Nurse Practitioner* 20(5):49-53, 1995.

Ferreira N: Sexually transmitted *chlamydia trachomatis, Nurse Practitioner Forum* 8(2):70-76, 1997.

Finlay LD: Cardiovascular system. In Lewis SM, Collier IC, Heitkemper MM: *Medical-surgical nursing: assessment and management of clinical problems,* ed 4, St. Louis, 1996, Mosby.

Fitzpatrick TB, Bernhad JD, Cropley TG: The structure of skin lesions and fundamentals of diagnosis. In Freedberg et al, eds: *Dermatology in general medicine,* ed 5, New York, 1999, McGraw-Hill.

Fogel CI, Woods NF, eds: *Women's health care: a comprehensive handbook,* Thousand Oaks, 1995, Sage Publishers.

Folstein M et al: The meaning of cognitive impairment in the elderly, *J Am Geriatr Soc* 33(4):228, 1985.

Frankenburg WK et al: The Denver II: a major revision and restandardization of the Denver Developmental Screening Test, *Pediatrics* 89:91-97, 1992.

Frisancho AR: New norms of upper limb fat and muscle areas for assessment of nutritional status, *American Journal of Clinical Nutrition* 34:2540-2545, 1981.

Frongilli EA, Rauschenbach BS, Roe DA, Williamson DR: Characteristics related to elderly persons not eating for 1 or more days: implications for meal programs, *Am J Public Health* 82:600-602, 1992.

Gambert SR: The crucial prostate exam, *Emergency Medicine* 29(1):45-52, 1997.

Garner JS: Guideline for isolation precaution in hospital practice, *Infection Control Hospital Epidemiology* 17:53-80, 1996.

Gaziano J et al: Moderate alcohol intake, increased levels of high-density lipoproteins and its subfractions, and decreased risk of myocardial infarction, *New England Journal of Medicine* 329:1829-1834, 1993.

Geissler EM: *Cultural assessment,* ed 2, St. Louis, 1998, Mosby.

Giardino AP, Christian CW, Giardino ER: *A practical guide to the evaluation of physical abuse and neglect,* Thousands Oaks, 1997, Sage Publications.

Giger JN, Davidhizar RE: *Transcultural nursing: assessment and intervention,* ed 2, St. Louis, 1995, Mosby.

Goldblum K, Collier IC: Vision and hearing problems. In Lewis SM, Collier IC, Heitkemper MM: *Medical-surgical nursing: assessment and management of clinical problems,* ed 4, St. Louis, 1996, Mosby.

Goldenring JM, Cohen E: Getting into adolescent heads, *Contemporary Pediatrics* 75-90, July 1998.

Goldstein BG, Goldstein AO: *Practical dermatology,* ed 2, St. Louis, 1997, Mosby.

Goldstein G, Hersen M: *Handbook of psychological assessment,* New York, 1984, Pergamon Press.

Goodenough FL: *Measurement of intelligence by drawings,* New York, 1926, World Book.

Goolsby MJ: Screening, diagnosis, and management of prostate cancer: improving primary care outcomes, *The Nurse Practitioner* 23(3):11-35, 1998.

Gordon MJ: *Nursing diagnosis: process and application,* ed 3, St Louis, 1994, Mosby.

Gorin SS, Arnold J: *Health promotion handbook,* St. Louis, 1998, Mosby.

Grap MJ: Protocols for practice: applying research at the bedside—pulse oximetry, *Critical Care Nurse* 18(1):94-98, 1998.

Green JM: Expectations and experiences of pain in labor: findings from a large prospective study, *Birth* 20(2):56-72, 1993.

Gritter M: The latex threat, *AJN* 98(9):26-32, 1998.

Grundy SM, Bilheimer D, Chait A et al: Summary of the Second Report of the National Cholesterol Education Program Expert Panel on Detection, Evaluation, and Treatment of High Blood Cholesterol in Adults, *JAMA* 269:3015-3023, 1993.

Habif TP: *Clinical dermatology: a color guide to diagnosis and therapy,* ed 3, St. Louis, 1996, Mosby.

Haddock BJ, Merrow DL, Swanson MS: The falling grace of axillary temperatures, *Pediatric Nursing* 22(2):121-125, 1996.

Hairston L: Physical examination of the prepubertal girl, *Clinical Obstetrics and Gynecology* 40(1):127-134, 1997.

Hardcastle JM: Colorectal cancer, *CA—A Cancer Journal for Clinicians* 47(2):66-68, 1997.

Harlan WR, Harlan EA, Grillo GP: Secondary sex characteristics of girls 12-17 year of age: the U.S. health examination survey, *Journal of Pediatrics* 96(6):1074-1078, 1980.

Harris DB: *Children's drawings as measures of intellectual maturity,* San Diego, CA, 1983, Harcourt Brace Jovanovich.

Harris JR, Lipman ME, Morrow M, Hellman S, eds: *Diseases of the breast,* Philadelphia, 1996, Lippincott-Raven.

Himes JH, Dietz WH: Guidelines for overweight in adolescent preventive services: recommendations from an expert committee, *Am J Clin Nutr* 54:307-316, 1994.

Holmes TH, Rahe RH: The social readjustment rating scale, *Journal of Psychosomatic Research* 11:213-218, 1967.

Houlihan MJ: Fibroadenoma and hamartoma. In Harris JR, Lipman ME, Morrow M, Hellman S, eds: *Diseases of the breast,* Philadelphia, 1996, Lippincott-Raven.

House-Fancher MA, Griego L: Congestive heart failure and cardiac surgery. In Lewis SM, Collier IC, Heitkemper MM: *Medical-surgical nursing: assessment and management of clinical problems,* ed 4, St. Louis, 1996, Mosby.

Hwang MY: Benefits and Dangers of Alcohol, *www.ama-assn.org,* 1/5/99.

Jacobs LK, Lin YJ, Orkin BA: The best operation for rectal prolapse, *Surgical Clinics of North America* 77(1):49-70, 1997.

Jacox AK: Assessing pain, *AJN* 79:895, 1979.

Jessup JM, Menck HR, Fremgen,A, Winchester DP: Diagnosing colorectal carcinoma: clinical and molecular approaches, *CA—A Cancer Journal for Clinicians* 47(2):70-92, 1997.

Johansson CB, Johansson JC: *Manual supplement for the career assessment inventory,* Minneapolis, 1978, National Computer Systems.

Johnston L, O'Malley P, Bachman J: National survey results on drug abuse. In *Monitoring the Future* study, Rockville, MD, 1993, National Institute on Drug Abuse.

Kane R, Kane RL: *Assessing the elderly,* Lexington, MA, 1984, Lexington Books.

Kaufman M, McMurrian TT: *Humanics national child assessment form,* 1992, Humanics Limited, P.O. Box 7447, Atlanta, GA 30309.

Kemper DW, Giuffre J, Drabinski G: *Pathways,* Boise, Idaho, 1986, Healthwise, Inc.

Kicklighter RH, Richmond BO: *Children's adaptive behavior scale revised and expanded manual,* Atlanta, 1983, Humanics Limited.

Kirton C: Assessing edema, *Nursing 96* 26(7):54.

Knobf MT: *Breast cancers.* In McCorkle R, Grant M, Frank-Stromborg M, Baird SB, eds: *Cancer nursing,* ed 2, Philadelphia, 1996, Saunders.

Kolcaba KY: Comfort as process and product, merged in holistic nursing art, *Journal of Holistic Nursing* 13:117, 1995.

Krumholz H, Seeman T, Merrill SS et al: Lack of association between cholesterol and coronary heart disease mortality and morbidity and all-cause mortality in persons older than 70 years, *JAMA* 272:1335-1340, 1994.

Kuczamarski RJ, Flegal K, Campbell S, Johnson C: Increasing prevalence of overweight among U.S. adults: The national health and nutrition examination surveys 1960-1991, *JAMA* 272:205-211, 1994.

Landis SH, Murray T, Bolden S, Wingo PA: Cancer statistics, 1999, *CA—A Cancer Journal for Clinicians* 49(1):8-11, 1999.

Landis SH, Murry T, Bolden S, Wingo PA: Cancer statistics 1999, *CA—A Cancer Journal for Clinicians* 49(1):8-31, 1999.

Lawson EJ: A narrative analysis: a black woman's perceptions of breast cancer risks and early breast cancer detection, *Cancer Nursing* 21(6):421-429, 1998.

Leffel DJ, Fitzgerald DA: Basal cell carcinoma. In Freedberg et al, eds: *Dermatologoy in general medicine,* ed 5, New York, 1999, McGraw-Hill.

Lester N: Cultural competence: a nursing dialogue, *AJN* 98(8):26-33, 1998.

Lewis SM, Heitkemper MM, Dirksen SR: *Medical-surgical nursing: assessment and management of clinical problems,* ed 5, St. Louis, 2000, Mosby.

Lewis SM, Collier IC, Heitkemper MM: *Medical-surgical nursing: assessment and management of clinical problems,* ed 4, St. Louis, 1996, Mosby.

Libertino JA: *International perspectives in urology,* Vol. 5, Baltimore, 1982, Williams and Wilkins.

Lindblade DD, McDonald M: Removing communication barriers for the hearing-impaired elderly, *Medsurg Nursing* 4(5):370-385, 1995.

Lowdermilk DL, Perry SE, Bobak IM: *Maternity and women's health care,* ed 6, St. Louis, 1997, Mosby.

Ludwig-Beymer PA: Transcultural aspects of pain. In Andrews MM, Boyle JS, eds: *Transcultural aspects of nursing care,* Philadelphia, 1995, JB Lippincott.

Lueckenotte AG: *Gerontologic nursing,* St. Louis, 1996, Mosby.

Lueckenotte AG: *Pocket guide to gerontologic assessment,* ed 2, St. Louis, 1994, Mosby.

Lunneborg PW: *Vocational interest inventory manual,* Los Angeles, 1981, Western Psychological Services.

Lusk SL: Noise exposures: effects on hearing and prevention of noise induced hearing loss, *AAOHN Journal* 45(8):397-405, 1997.

Mannia J: Finding an effective hearing testing protocol to identify hearing loss and middle ear disease in school-aged children, *Journal of School Nursing* 13(5):23-28, 1997.

Marantides D, Lottman M: Management of persons with hematological problems. In Phipps, WJ, Sands JK, Marek JF: *Medical-surgical nursing: concepts and clinical practice,* ed 6, St. Louis, 1999, Mosby.

Marantides D, Marek J, Morgan J: Management of persons with problems of the kidney and urinary tract. In Phipps WJ, Sands JK, Marek JF: *Medical-surgical nursing: concepts and clinical practice,* ed 6, St. Louis, 1999, Mosby.

Marek J: Management of persons with inflammatory and degenerative disorders of the musculoskeletal system. In Phipps WJ, Sands JK, Marek JF: *Medical-surgical nursing: concepts and clinical practice,* ed 6, St. Louis, 1999, Mosby.

Matteson MA: Age-related changes in the integument. In Matteson MA, McConnell ES, Linton AD: *Gerontological nursing,* ed 2, Philadelphia, 1997, Saunders.

Matteson MA, McConnell EC, Linton AD: *Gerontological nursing: concepts and practice,* ed 2, Philadelphia, 1997, Saunders.

Matsunaga E: The dimorphism in human and normal cerumen, *Ann Hum Genet* 25:273, 1962.

Maxwell-Thompson C, Yuan A: Management of persons with vascular problems. In Phipps WJ, Sands JK, Marek JF: *Medical-surgical nursing: concepts and clinical practice,* ed 6, St. Louis, 1999, Mosby.

McCaffery M, Pasero C: *Pain: clinical manual,* ed 2, St Louis, 1999, Mosby.

McCance KL, Huether SE: *Pathophysiology: the biologic basis for disease in adults and children,* ed 3, St. Louis, 1998, Mosby.

McCubbin HI, Thompson AI, eds: *Family assessment inventories for research and practice,* Madison, WI, 1987, The University of Wisconsin-Madison.

McKenry LM, Salerno E: *Mosby's pharmacology in nursing,* ed 20, St. Louis, 1998, Mosby.

Mebust WK, Bostwick D, Grayhack J, Jolgrewe L, Wasson J, Kirby R, Mostofi K: Scope of the problem: indications for treatment and assessment of benign prostate hyperplasia and its relationship to cancer, *Cancer* 70 (1, suppl):369-70, July 1, 1992.

Metcoff J: Clinical assessment of nutritional status at birth, *Pediatr Clin North Am* 41:875, 1994.

Miola ES: The otoscope: an update on assessment skills, *Journal of Pediatric Nursing* 9(4):283-286, 1994.

Minuchin S: *Families and family therapy,* Cambridge, Mass, 1974, Harvard University Press.

Mitchell JT: Nursing role in management: lower respiratory problems. In Lewis SM, Collier IC, Heitkemper MM: *Medical-surgical nursing: assessment and management of clinical problems,* ed 4, St. Louis, 1996, Mosby.

Monteleone JA: *Recognition of child abuse for the mandated reporter,* ed 2, London, 1996, G.W. Medical Publishing.

Moos RH, Moos BS: A typology of family social environments, *Fam Process* 15:357-371, 1976.

Morrison C: The significance of nipple discharge: diagnosis and treatment regimes, *Primary Care Practice* 2(2):129-140, 1998.

Murphy C: Assessment of fathering behaviors. In Johnson SH: *High-risk parenting: nursing assessment and strategies for the family at risk,* Philadelphia, 1979, Lippincott.

Myers I, Briggs-Myers PB: *Gifts differing,* Palo Alto, CA, 1980, Consulting Psychologists Press.

NANDA: *Nursing diagnoses: definitions and classification 1999-2000,* Philadelphia: North American Nursing Diagnosis Association, 1999.

National Cancer Institute: *Racial/ethnic patterns of cancer in the United States 1998-1992,* Bethesda, Maryland: NIH Publication No. 96-4104, 1996.

National High Blood Pressure Education Program, *Heart Memo,* National Institutes of Health, National Heart, Lung, and Blood Institute, Winter 1999, pp. 4-6.

National Institute for Occupational Safety and Health (NIOSH): *National occupational research agenda,* U.S. Department of Health and Human Services, Public Health Service, Centers for Disease Control and Prevention, Publication No. 96-115, Cincinnati, OH, 1996, National Institute for Occupational Safety and Health Publications Dissemination.

National Institute for Occupational Safety and Health: *NIOSH alert: preventing allergic reactions to natural rubber latex in the workplace,* June 1997.

National Institutes of Medicine: *Nutrition during pregnancy, part I: weight gain; part II: nutrient supplements,* Washington, DC, 1991, National Academy Press.

Neinstein LS: *Adolescent health care: a practical guide,* ed 2, Baltimore, 1991, Williams & Wilkins.

Neubauer D, Smith P, Earley C: Sleep disorders. In Barker LR, Burton J, Zieve P, eds: *Principles of ambulatory medicine,* ed 5, Baltimore, 1998, Williams & Wilkins.

Nicol NH: Assessment of clients with integumentary disorders. In Black JM, Matassarin-Jacobs E: *Medical-surgical nursing: clinical management for continuity of care,* ed 5, Philadelphia, 1997, Saunders.

Nichols BS, Misra R, Alexy B: Cancer detection: how effective is public education? *Cancer Nursing* 19:98-103, 1996.

Northourse PG, Northouse LL: *Health communication: strategies for health professionals,* Norwalk, 1992, Appleton & Lange.

O'Connor DL: Preventing sports injuries in kids, *Patient Care for the Nurse Practitioner* 1(4):24-32, June 1998.

O'Day MP: Cardio-respiratory physiological adaptation of pregnancy, *Seminars in Perinatology* 21(4):286-275, 1997.

O'Hanlon-Nichols T: The adult cardiovascular system, *AJN* (12):34-40, 1997.

O'Hanlon-Nichols T: Neurologic assessment, *AJN* 99(6):44-50, 1999.

O'Hanlon-Nichols T: Gastrointestinal assessment, *AJN* 98(4):48-53.

O'Toole S: Alternatives to mercury thermometers, *Professional Nurse* 12(11):783-786, 1997.

Olson DH: Circumplex model VII: validation studies and FACES III, *Family Process* 25:337-351, 1986.

Overfield T: *Biologic variation in health and illness: race, age and sex differences,* Melano Park, CA, 1985, Addison Wesley.

Pagana KD, Pagana TJ: *Mosby's manual of diagnostic and laboratory tests,* St. Louis, 1998, Mosby.

Parker SL, Johnston D, Wingo PA, Ries L, Heath CW: Cancer statistics by race and ethnicity, *CA—A Cancer Journal for Clinicians* 48(1):31-48, 1998.

Parker SL, Tong T, Bolden S, Wingo PA: Cancer statistics 1997, *CA—A Cancer Journal for Clinicians* 47(1):5-27, 1997.

Parsons, MT, Spellacy WN: Premature rupture of membranes. In Scott JR, DiSaia PJ, Hammond CB, Spellacy WN, eds: *Danforth's obstetrics and gynecology,* ed 8, Philadelphia, 1999, Lippincott Williams & Wilkins.

Petrakis NL: Cerumen genetics and human breast cancer, *Science* 173:347, 1971.

Phipps, WJ, Sands JK, Marek JF: *Medical-surgical nursing: concepts and clinical practice,* ed 6, St. Louis, 1999, Mosby.

Piaget J, Inhelder B (translated by Helen Weaver): *The psychology of the child,* New York, 1969, Basic Books.

Portage Project, Portage, WI, 1994, Cooperative Educational Service Agency 5 (CESA 5).

Porter LW: A study of perceived need satisfactions in bottom and middle management jobs, *Personnel Journal* 59:907-912, 1961.

Potter PA, Perry AG: *Basic nursing: a critical thinking approach,* ed 4, St. Louis, 1999, Mosby.

Potter PA, Perry AG: *Fundamentals of nursing: process and practice,* ed 4, St. Louis, 1997, Mosby.

Powell ML: *Assessment and management of developmental changes and problems in children,* ed 2, St. Louis, 1981, Mosby.

Psychological Corporation: *Tests and other products for psychological assessment,* San Antonio, TX, 1995, Harcourt Brace.

Purnell LD, Paulanka BJ: *Transcultural health care: a culturally competent approach.* Philadelphia, 1998, F.A. Davis.

Puskar M: Smoking cessation in women, *Nurse Practitioner* 20(11):80-89, 1995.

Reeder SJ, Martin LL, Koniak-Griffin D: *Maternity nursing,* ed 18, Philadelphia, 1997, Lippincott.

Reidy M, Thibaudeau MF: Evaluation of family functioning: development and validation of a scale which measures family competence in measures of health, *Nursing Papers* 16:42-56, 1984.

Report of the Expert Committee on the Diagnosis and Classification of Diabetes Mellitus, *Diabetes Care* 20(7):1183, 1997.

Report of the Second Task Force on Blood Pressure Control in Children: *Pediatrics* 79(1):1-25, 1987.

Report of the U.S. Preventive Services Task Force: *Guide to clinical preventive services,* ed 2, Baltimore, MD, 1996, Williams & Wilkins.

Ridker et al: Association of moderate alcohol consumption and plasma concentration of endogenous tissue-type plasminogen activator, *Journal of the American Medical Association* 272:929-933, 1994.

Robinson RA: The diagnosis and prognosis of dementia. In Anders WF, ed: *Current achievements in geriatrics,* London, 1964, Cassell.

Rofles SR, DeBruyne LK: *Life span nutrition: conception through life,* New York, 1990, West Publishing Company.

Rosenthal SI, Burklow KA, Biro FM, Pace LC, Devellis RF: The reliability of high-risk adolescent girls' report of their sexual history, *Journal of Pediatric Health Care* 10(5):217-220, 1996.

Ross C: A comparison of osteoarthritis and rheumatoid arthritis: diagnosis and treatment, *The Nurse Practitioner* 22(9):20-39, 1997.

Ruggles DJ: Depression in the elderly: a review, *Journal of the American Academy of Nurse Practitioners* 10(11):503-507, November 1998.

Scariati PD, Grummer-Strawn LM, Fein SB: Water supplementation of infants in the first month of life, *Arch Pediatr Adolesc Med* 151(8):830-832, 1997.

Schaefer MT, Olson DH: Assessing intimacy: the pair inventory, *J Marital Family Therapy* 7:47-60, 1981.

Schmitt M: Evaluating the shoulder, *Patient Care for the Nurse Practitioner* 2(3):42-50, 1999.

Schmitz T, Bair N, Falk M, Levine C: A comparison of five methods of temperature measurement in febrile intensive care patients, *American Journal of Critical Care* 4(4):286-292, 1995.

Schneider J: Management of chronic non-cancer pain: a guide to appropriate use of opioids, *Journal of Care Management* 4(4):10-20, August 1998.

Schonberg SK, ed: *Substance abuse: a guide for health professionals,* Elk Grove, Illinois, 1988, American Academy of Pediatrics.

Schuster C, Ashburn S: *The process of human development: a holistic life-span approach,* Boston, 1992, Lippincott.

Schwartz RA, Stoll HL: Squamous cell carcinoma. In Freedberg et al, eds: *Dermatology in general medicine,* ed 5, New York, 1999, McGraw-Hill.

Scripture D: Hyperthyroidism: an unusual case presentation, *The Nurse Practitioner* 23(2):50-55, 1998.

Scott JR: Placenta previa and abruption. In Scott JR, DiSaia PJ, Hammond CB, Spellacy WN, eds: *Danforth's obstetrics and gynecology,* ed 8, Philadelphia, 1999, Lippincott Williams & Wilkins.

Secor MC: Skills workshop part I: the challenging pelvic examination, *Patient Care for the Nurse Practitioner* 2(7):36-45, 1999.

Seidel HM et al: *Mosby's guide to physical examination,* ed 4, St. Louis, 1999, Mosby.

Seller R: *Differential diagnosis of common complaints,* ed 3, Philadelphia, 1996, Saunders.

Sepe S: *Life saving vaccines under-used by minority adults: closing the gap,* Office of Minority Health, Bethesda, Maryland: U.S. Department of Health and Human Services, November, 1998, p. 4.

Shader RI, Harmatz JS, Salzman C: A new scale for clinical assessment in geriatric populations: Sandoz Clinical Assessment Geriatric (SCAG), *J Am Geriatr Soc* 22:107-113, 1974.

Shugars D, Patton L: Detecting, diagnosing, and preventing oral cancer, *The Nurse Practitioner* 22(6):105, 109-110, 113-115, 119-120, 129, 1997.

Sieh A, Brentin LK: *The nurse communicates,* Philadelphia, 1997, Saunders.

Sinatra FR, Sinatra GM: Food fads and special diets: facts and fallacies, *Contemporary Pediatrics* 13(2):56-68, 1996.

Sixth Report of the Joint National Committee on Prevention, Detection, Evaluation, and Treatment of High Blood Pressure, National Institutes of Health, National Heart, Lung, and Blood Institute, NIH Publication No. 98-4080, November 1997.

Smith CM, Schmann L: Differential diagnosis of headache, *Journal of American Academy of Nurse Practitioners* 10(11):519-524, 1998.

Smith AD: Causes and classifications of impotence, *Urology Clinics of North America* 8:79, 1981.

Smith-Dijulio K: People who depend upon substances of abuse. In Varcarolis EM: *Foundation of psychiatric mental health nursing,* ed 3, Philadelphia, 1998, Saunders.

Smith L, Schumann L: Differential diagnosis of headache, *Journal of the American Academy of Nurse Practitioners* 10(11):519-524, 1998.

Smith PC, Kendall LM, Hulin CL: *The measurement of satisfaction in work and retirement,* Chicago, 1969, Rand-McNally.

Snyder M, Lindquist R: *Complementary/alternative therapies in nursing,* ed 3, New York, 1998. Springer Publishing Co.

Spencer-Cisek PA: Overview of cancer prevention, screening, and detection, *Nurse Practitioner Forum* 9(3):134-146, 1998.

Steinberg S: Childbearing research: a transcultural review, *Soc Sci Med* 43(12):1765-1784, 1996. *Danforth's obstetrics and gynecology,* ed 8, Philadelphia, Lippincott Williams & Wilkins.

Stokes S, Gordon S: *Development of a tool to measure stress in the older individual,* New York, 1986, Stewart Research Conference, Nursing in the 21st Century, Perspectives and Possibilities.

Swartz MH: *Textbook of physical diagnosis: History and examination,* ed 2, Philadelphia, 1994, WB Saunders.

Tanner JM: *Growth at adolescence,* ed 2, Oxford, England, 1962, Blackwell Scientific Publications.

Thomas CR, Gale M, Evans N: *Racial differences in the incidence of colon and rectal cancer in patients under the age of forty,* Abstract 345, Proceedings of the Third International Conference on Anticancer Research, 1990.

Thompson SD: Ovarian cancer screening: a primary care guide, *Primary Care Practice* 2(3):244-250, 1997.

Tierney LM, Whooley MA, Saint S: Oxygen saturation: a fifth vital sign? *West J Med* 166(4):285-6, 1997.

Tobin L: Evaluating mild to moderate hypertension, *The Nurse Practitioner* 24(5):22, 25-26, 29-30, 32, 38, 40-41, 1999.

Tolson D: Age-related hearing loss: a cause for nursing intervention, *Journal of Advanced Nursing* 26(6):1150-1157, 1997.

Turk DC, Melzack R: The measurement of pain and assessment of people experiencing pain. In Turk DC, Melzack R, eds: *Handbook of pain assessment,* New York, 1992, Guilford Press.

Turk DC, Okifji A: Chronic pain and pain associated with cancer: do men and women respond differently? National Institute of Health, April 1998, from *wwwl.od.nih.gov/painresearch/genderand pain/abstract/dturk.htm.*

Uphold C, Graham M: *Clinical guidelines in family practice,* ed 2, Gainesville, FL, 1997, Baramarrae Books.

U.S. Department of Health and Human Services: Tobacco use among high school students—United States, *MMWR* 47:229-233, 1998.

U.S. Department of Health and Human Services, Public Health Service: *Health United States,* 1995, Bethesda, Maryland Publication No. (PHS) 96-1232.

U.S. Preventive Services Task Force: *Guide to clinical preventive services,* ed 2, Baltimore, 1996, Williams & Wilkins.

Vader L: Eye disorders. In Black JM, Matassatin-Jacobs E: *Medical-surgical nursing: clinical management for continuity of care,* ed 5, Philadelphia, 1997, Saunders.

Valassi K, Clark HM: Nutrition and digestive function. In Burke MM, Walsh MD, eds: *Gerontologic nursing,* St. Louis, 1992, Mosby.

Varcarolis EM: Reducing stress and anxiety. In Varcarolis EM: *Foundations of psychiatric mental health nursing,* ed 3, Philadelphia, 1998, Saunders.

Verdon ME: Issues in the management of human papillomavirus genital disease, *American Family Physician* 55(5):1813-1819, 1997.

Visher ED, Visher JS: *Step-families: a guide to working with stepparents and stepchildren,* Secaucus, NJ, 1979, The Citadel Press.

Von Eschenbach A, Ho R, Murphy GP, Cunningham M, Lins N: American Cancer Society guideline for the early detection of prostate cancer: update for 1997, *CA—A Cancer Journal for Clinicians* 47(5):261-264, 1997.

Warmkessel J: Caring for a patient with colon cancer, *Nursing 97* 27(4):34-39.

Waxweiler RJ et al: Monitoring the impact of traumatic brain injury: a review and update, *Journal of Neurotrauma* 12(4), 1995.

Weaver P, Harrison B, Eskander G et al Colon cancer in blacks: a disease with worsening prognosis, *Journal National Medical Association* 83:133-136, 1991.

Wechsler H, Rigotti NA, Giedhill-Hoyt J, Lee H: Increased levels of cigarette use among college students, *JAMA* 280(19):1673-1678, 1998.

Weilitz PB, Sciver TV: Nursing role in management: obstructive pulmonary disease. In Lewis SM, Collier IC, Heitkemper MM, eds: *Medical-surgical nursing: assessment and management of clinical problems,* ed 4, St. Louis, 1996, Mosby.

Weinstock H, Dean D, Bolan G: Chlamydia trachomatis infections, *Sex Transm Dis* 8:797-819, 1994.

Wheeler L: Well woman assessment. In Fogel CI, Woods NF, eds: *Women's health care: a comprehensive handbook,* Thousand Oaks, 1995, Sage Publishers.

Whitney E, Cataldo C, and Rolfes S: *Understanding normal and clinical nutrition,* ed 5, Belmont, CA, 1998, West/Wadsworth.

Wilke D, Boss B: Nursing assessment and role in management: pain. In Lewis SM, Collier IC, Heitkemper MM: *Medical-surgical nursing: assessment and management of clinical problems,* ed 4, St. Louis, 1996, Mosby.

Wilkins RL, Krider SJ, Sheldon RL: *Clinical assessment in respiratory care,* ed 3, St. Louis, 1995, Mosby.

Williams SR: *Essentials of nutritional and diet therapy,* ed 7, St. Louis, 1999, Mosby.

Wong DL et al: *Whaley and Wong's nursing care of infants and children,* ed 5, St. Louis, 1995, Mosby.

Wong DL et al: *Whaley and Wong's nursing care of infants and children,* ed 6, St. Louis, 1999, Mosby.

Wong DL, Perry SE: *Maternal-child nursing care,* St. Louis, 1998, Mosby.

Woodhead GA, Moss MM: Osteoporosis: diagnosis and management, *The Nurse Practitioner* 23(11):18, 23-27, 31-35, 1998.

Wright LM, Leahey M: *Nurses and families: a guide to family assessment and interventions,* Philadelphia, 1984, F.A. Davis.

Wynsberghe D et al: *Human anatomy and physiology,* ed 3, New York, 1995, McGraw-Hill.

Yamada T, ed: *Handbook of gastroenterology.* Philadelphia, 1998, Lippincott-Raven.

Yanovski SZ: A practical approach to the treatment of the obese patient, *Arch Fam Med* 2:309-316, 1993.

Yantis MA: Sleep apnea: what you need to know, *AJN* 99(9), 1999.

Zanca J: Adult vaccines: who should get what, and when? *Closing the Gap,* newsletter of the Office of Minority Health, U.S. Department of Health and Human Services, pp. 13-14, November 1998.

Zeman FJ, Ney DM: *Applications of clinical nutrition,* Englewood, CA, 1988, Prentice Hall.

Ziegfeld CR: Differential diagnosis of a breast mass, *Primary Care Practice* 2(2):121-128, 1998.

INDEX

A

D

E

F

F

M

O

Q

R

W

X

Y

Z

Special Features

AGE-RELATED VARIATIONS

CASE STUDIES

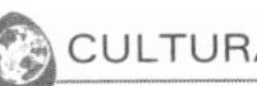

CULTURAL NOTES

ETHNIC & CULTURAL VARIATIONS BOXES